Concepts in
Medical Physiology

Concepts in Medical Physiology

Julian Seifter, MD
Associate Professor of Medicine
Associate Master, Walter Bradford Cannon Society
Harvard Medical School
Cambridge, Massachusetts

Austin Ratner, MD
Adjunct Assistant Professor of Bioethics
Case Western Reserve School of Medicine
Cleveland, Ohio

David Sloane, MD
Attending Physician, Division of Rheumatology, Allergy and Immunology
Brigham and Women's Hospital
Boston, Massachusetts

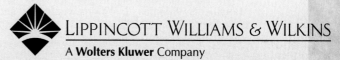
LIPPINCOTT WILLIAMS & WILKINS
A **Wolters Kluwer** Company
Philadelphia • Baltimore • New York • London
Buenos Aires • Hong Kong • Sydney • Tokyo

Executive Editor: Betty Sun
Senior Developmental Editor: Kathleen H. Scogna
Marketing Manager: Joe Schott
Production Editor: Kevin Johnson
Designer: Risa Clow
Compositor: Maryland Composition
Printer: Quebeccor Dubuque

Library of Congress Cataloging-in-Publication Data

Seifter, Julian.
    Concepts in medical physiology / Julian Seifter, David Sloane, Austin Ratner.
        p. ; cm.
    Includes bibliographical references and index.
    ISBN 0-7817-4489-X
  1. Human physiology.   I. Sloane, David, 1968-   II. Ratner, Austin.   III. Title.
    [DNLM: 1.   Physiological Processes.   QT 4 S459c 2006]
  QP34.5.S52 2006
  612–dc22

                                                                                    2005016358

To Betsy, Andrew, and Charlie
JULIAN SEIFTER

To Kristin and Virgil
AUSTIN RATNER

In honor of seven: Marcia, Fay, Richard, Susan, Tsila, Nesya, and Avi
And in memory of three: Joseph, Irv, and Joan
"How about that?"
DAVID SLOANE

Preface

Authors of textbooks frequently cite students as their source of inspiration. Our students have undoubtedly been an inspiration, but they've also been more than that. They were actually involved in the composition of this book.

We sought to combine two principal strategies in order to create a text uniquely suited to the needs of medical students, who are faced with the daunting task of simultaneously learning critical concepts about the function of the body, preparing for clinical responsibilities on the wards, and preparing for the U.S. Medical Licensing Examination (USMLE). First, we sought out successful students and formally involved them. Medical students with recent USMLE and course experience at the Harvard and Johns Hopkins Schools of Medicine submitted their ideas about the content and style of explanation. They gave their views of which physiology topics were most important and which most difficult to understand, they submitted questions, and they submitted their own written attempts at explaining the material to their peers. We used these contributions as starting points for the construction of a physiology text that medical students *wished* they had had when they were studying.

Second, we assembled an authorial team with special expertise not only in basic science, but also in education, clinical medicine, and the written word. Armed with insight into the perspective of the medical student, we tried to achieve a new standard of clear communication with our readers. We sought to avoid common pitfalls of medical writing, such as long lists of unprioritized or disorganized information and undefined jargon. We worked to create fresh concept diagrams, tables, and figures alongside verbal explanations of quantitative concepts, including helpful new analogies and metaphors. In order to simplify material that medical students found particularly difficult, we gave it extra attention and attempted to connect the complex physiology to simpler underlying concepts in physics, biochemistry, and cell biology. In so doing, we provided explanations not seen in other texts, and our students found this conceptual approach to aid them not only in comprehension, but also in *retention*. Once difficult topics are understood clearly on the basis of previously mastered first principles, it seems there is suddenly less to remember. We've so far won great approval from students with our new ways of handling difficult topics like the alveolar gas equation, acid-base homeostasis, countercurrent multiplication in the kidney, the lung/chest wall counterbalance, the Frank-Starling relationship in the heart, the menstrual cycle, and many others.

Several other features reinforce the conceptual approach to physiology. "Integrated Physiology" inserts are provided to help establish the themes found across different organ systems, maintaining a focus on underlying concepts. Concept-focused summaries are included at the end of each chapter to facilitate study and to underscore the main ideas, while keeping an eye on the "big picture."

In addition, we loaded our text with clinical material, including the following in every chapter:

- Pathophysiology sections that show how the major pathologic conditions can be predicted (and therefore easily remembered!) by a knowledge of the *physiologic functions* and what can go wrong with them.

- "Clinical Application" inserts with minicases that discuss the diagnosis, course, and treatment of common conditions and illnesses.

- "Clinical Application" inserts that discuss common tests, treatments, and procedures and how they work.

- Suggested reading with referrals to reviews on common illnesses from core clinical journals.

- USMLE-type questions with answers, composed with the help of students and recent medical school graduates who have taken the USMLE.

We also included longer clinical cases with discussions of differential diagnosis for each major organ system. In general, we tried our utmost to connect physiology to the practical issues students will face on the wards and in residency and to help students prepare for the USMLE.

With the unusual skill set of our author team and the involvement of actual medical students, we hope we have created a text that uniquely addresses the needs of medical students and is uniquely integrated with clinical medicine.

INTENDED READERSHIP AND PREREQUISITES

This book was written with first-year medical students especially in mind, but it should be a useful reference for medical students in years two, three, and four, and for practitioners (residents and beyond) who want a review of basic concepts or of the physiological basis of clinical practice. Because of the book's focus on the foundations of physiological knowledge and its attention to the difficulties encountered by students new to the material, it should also be a useful introduction for other students in the health sciences or biological sciences. Advanced undergraduates, graduate students of biology, students of dentistry and nursing, and others may not need all of the clinical material but should find the basic physiological concepts accessible and useful. In most cases, students will require an introductory background in cell biology and biochemistry before using our book, though we have tried to review the relevant cell biology and biochemistry.

THE ORGANIZATION OF *CONCEPTS IN MEDICAL PHYSIOLOGY*

Our text begins with a series of chapters that review basic cell biology and some of the basic themes across organ systems, such as the principles of homeostasis or of solute transport. We then proceed through each organ system in the traditional manner, including some chapters and sections not found in many physiology texts—for example, a more extensive section on blood and the immune system than is usually present in physiology texts, a chapter on the gastrointestinal immune system, and a chapter on hepatic physiology and pathophysiology, focusing on the liver's role in detoxification, its role in the production of blood proteins, and the differential diagnosis of jaundice. In each chapter, we first review the system structure, taking an inventory of the gross anatomy, histology, and molecules involved. We then proceed to the main discussion of system function and conclude with a pathophysiology discussion that shows how the functions just learned can go awry, leading to system dysfunction.

AUTHOR BIOGRAPHIES

Julian L. Seifter, MD, Associate Professor of Medicine and Associate Master of the Walter Bradford Cannon Society at Harvard Medical School

Dr. Seifter has codirected the human physiology course and directed the human pathophysiology course at Harvard Medical School. He has widely published original reports in the fields of nephrology and internal medicine, as well as papers on the subject of medical education, and contributed many chapters to well-known texts such as *Harrison's Principles of Internal Medicine* and *Cecil's Textbook of Internal Medicine*. Dr. Seifter has received 12 teaching awards from the students and house staff at Harvard Medical School, where he has been teaching for over 20 years, and directed the training programs in nephrology at Brigham and Women's Hospital, where he is an attending on the general medical service and the nephrology consult service. He was recently recognized in *Boston Magazine*'s list of top doctors as best of Boston in nephrology.

Austin Ratner, MD, Adjunct Assistant Professor of Medical Humanities, Case School of Medicine

Dr. Ratner is a full-time freelance writer. He is a graduate of the Johns Hopkins School of Medicine and former writer and content director for an educational healthcare web site. He studied English literature at Yale and the University of Michigan. Dr. Ratner is author of the novel *Killing Goliath*, and winner of the 2000 *Missouri Review* Fiction Prize.

David Sloane, MD, Attending Physician, Division of Rheumatology, Allergy and Immunology, Brigham and Women's Hospital

After graduating from Washington University in St. Louis with a major in English literature and minors in mathematics and philosophy, David Sloane received his MD from Harvard Medical School where, like so many of his classmates, he fell in love with physiology, thanks in large part to the lectures and informal discussions of Dr. Seifter. He has taught and tutored students of science and medicine for over 10 years. In addition to caring for patients, he is engaged in basic science research into the cellular and molecular basis of allergic inflammation. He likes to think he can write about and explain biology well and with some humor, but his mother, wife, children, and bosses know better.

CONTRIBUTORS AND REVIEWERS

Concepts in Medical Physiology benefited from the efforts of many students and faculty over a period of many years. They contributed to varying degrees—some enormously, some in smaller ways—but all were important to the success of the final product. They are listed alphabetically below along with the chapter or chapters to which they contributed.

Student Contributors

Our student contributors have graduated and moved on since their work on the book, but they are identified according to their level of training at the time of their contribution. HMS, Harvard Medical School; JHSM, Johns Hopkins School of Medicine.

Student	Contribution
Rich Abramson, HMS	Ch 28 Control of Gastrointestinal Motility and Secretion
Chris Alessi, HMS	Ch 16 The Mechanics of Breathing
Jen Ang, HMS	Ch 27 Nutrition, Digestion, and Absorption
Dan Barouch, HMS	Part III Blood and Lymph
James Beckerman, HMS	Ch 24 The Regulation of Potassium Balance
Steve Boorjian, HMS	Chs 3 and 31 Cell-to-Cell Communication and The Endocrine Pancreas
Marisa Brett, HMS	Ch 32 The Pituitary Gland
Fina Canas, HMS	Ch 19 The Regulation of Breathing
Aaron Cheng, HMS	Ch 28 Control of Gastrointestinal Motility and Secretion
Jim Cheung, HMS	Ch 28 Control of Gastrointestinal Motility and Secretion
Christine Chung, HMS	Ch 20 Renal Functions, Renal Circulation and Glomerular Filtration
Renn Crichlow, HMS	Ch 8 Bone Physiology
Carl Deirmengian, HMS	Chs 3 and 31 Cell-to-Cell Communication and The Endocrine Pancreas
Akshay Desai, HMS	Chs 12 and 13 The Vasculature and The Heart as a Pump
Sanjay Desai, HMS	Chs 13 and 14 The Heart as a Pump and The Electrical Activity of the Heart
Jennifer Furin, HMS	Ch 30 The Gastrointestinal Immune System
Patricio Gargullo, HMS	Chs 3 and 31 Cell-to-Cell Communication and The Endocrine Pancreas
Daniel Garibaldi, JHSM	Ch 19 The Regulation of Breathing
Naomi Hamburg, HMS	Ch 25 Acid-Base Homeostasis
Joan Han, HMS	Ch 20 Renal Functions, Renal Circulation, and Glomerular Filtration
Michael House, HMS	Chs 2 and 22 Membrane Transport and The Regulation of Blood Pressure and Extracellular Fluid Volume
Sara Ann Hughes, HMS	Ch 28 Control of Gastrointestinal Motility and Secretion
Sean Ianchulev, HMS	Ch 23 Osmoregulation
Doug Johnston, HMS	Ch 27 Nutrition, Digestion, and Absorption
David Kaczorowski JHSM	Ch 21 Tubular Transport

Ken Katz, HMS	Chs 1 and 15 Homeostasis and Exercise Physiology
Pamela Kirschner, HMS	Ch 35 Hormonal Regulation of Calcium and Phosphate Metabolism
Susan Lee, JHSM	Ch 22 The Regulation of Blood Pressure and Extracellular Fluid Volume
Carlos Lerner, HMS	Ch 20 Renal Functions, Renal Circulation, and Glomerular Filtration
Moe Lim, HMS	Ch 18 Gas Transport
Alex Lin, JHSM	Ch 21 Tubular Transport
Jennifer Lin, HMS	Ch 21 Tubular Transport
Annie Luetkemeyer, HMS	Ch 34 The Adrenal Gland
Anjli Maroo, HMS	Ch 15 Exercise Physiology
Eric Morrow, HMS	Ch 5 An Overview of Nerve Cell Physiology and the Autonomic Nervous System
Geoff Nguyen, JHSM	Ch 33 The Thyroid Gland
Jean Ou, HMS	Chs 26 and 37 Micturition and The Male Reproductive System
Ryan Putzer, HMS	Ch 4 Signal Transduction
Lecia Sequist, HMS	Ch 36 The Female Reproductive System
Andrew Yee, HMS	Ch 35 Hormonal Regulation of Calcium and Phosphate Metabolism

Faculty Contributors

Faculty Member	Contribution
Carlo Brugnara, MD, Harvard Medical School	Part III Blood and Lymph
Alan Cormier, PhD, Medica Corporation	Ch 17 Gas Exchange in the Lungs
Lisa Hark, PhD, RD, University of Pennsylvania	Ch 27 Nutrition, Digestion, and Absorption
Stephen C. Hauser, MD, Mayo Clinic College of Medicine	Chs 27 and 28 Nutrition, Digestion, and Absorption and Control of Gastrointestinal Motility and Secretion
Landon King, MD, Johns Hopkins School of Medicine	Part V Pulmonary Physiology Case Study
L. Christine Turtzo, MD, Johns Hopkins School of Medicine	Parts V and VI Pulmonary Physiology and Renal Physiology
Charles Wiener, MD, Johns Hopkins School of Medicine	Part V Pulmonary Physiology

Faculty Reviewers

Faculty Member	Contribution
Bill Bowerfind, MD, Johns Hopkins School of Medicine	Part V Pulmonary Physiology
Cindy Brown, MD, Johns Hopkins School of Medicine	Part V Pulmonary Physiology
Anna Hemnes, MD, Johns Hopkins School of Medicine	Part V Pulmonary Physiology
Laura Herpel, MD, Johns Hopkins School of Medicine	Part V Pulmonary Physiology
Courtney Schreiber, MD, University of Pittsburgh School of Medicine	Part VIII Endocrine Physiology
David Wolk, MD, Harvard Medical School	Part III Blood and Lymph Case Study

Acknowledgments

In addition to our many contributors and reviewers, we owe special thanks to several other people who have had a shaping influence on our book. Leonard Lilly helped to pave our way with his fine collaboration between medical students and faculty, *Pathophysiology of Heart Disease*, now in its 3rd edition from Lippincott Williams & Wilkins. Betty Sun, Executive Editor at Lippincott, stayed with us through a long and challenging developmental process of several years, never flagging in her belief in or attentiveness to the project. Kathleen Scogna, Senior Developmental Editor, maintained complete command of our ambitious and unwieldy endeavor, while simultaneously shouldering the burden of many other projects. Betty and Kathleen contributed numerous suggestions for improvements and for the book's design, and the book would not have been possible without their expertise or their patience. Betsy Dilernia took on the huge task of thoroughly line-editing a draft of the book, and her diligent editorial oversight and detailed suggestions were critical. Rob Duckwall at the Dragonfly Media Group, veteran of such projects as *Grant's Anatomy*, gave his fine artistic and technical skills to our illustrations and always answered the call, even while on vacation!

Table of Contents

Part VIII

ENDOCRINE PHYSIOLOGY 495

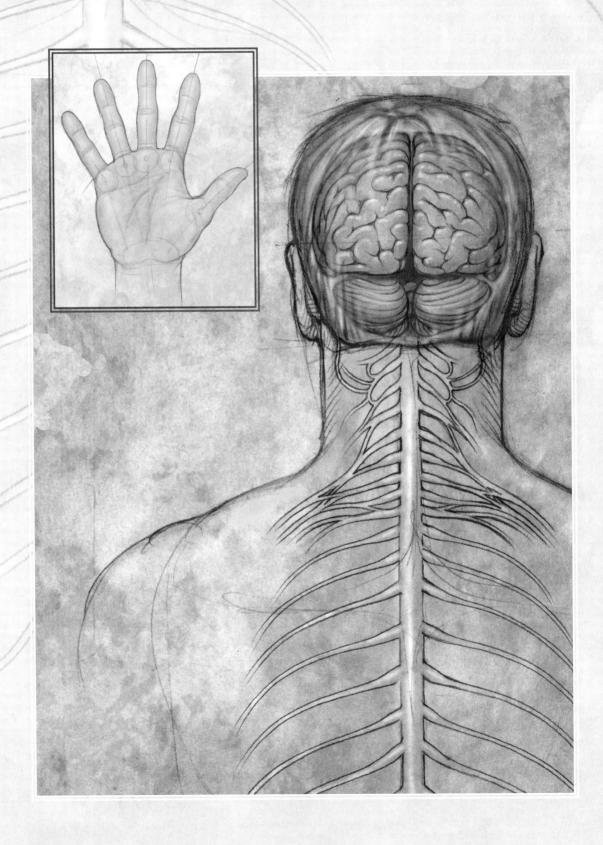

GENERAL PRINCIPLES

1

Homeostasis

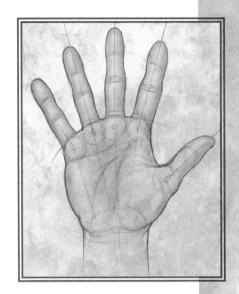

INTRODUCTION

"A fairly constant or steady state, maintained in many aspects of the bodily economy even when they are beset by conditions tending to disturb them, is a most remarkable characteristic of the living organism. . . . Since. . .circumstances are often present, which, if not controlled, would profoundly modify the constancy of the state, we must assume that controlling factors are at hand ready to act whenever the constancy is imperiled" (Cannon, 1926).

So wrote Walter B. Cannon, the eminent American physiologist. While previous investigators had appreciated this same characteristic of living systems, Cannon first proposed a term for it. He called it **homeostasis** (from the Greek *homeo-* meaning "same" and the Latin *-stasis* meaning "standing"). Homeostatic processes defend the body against the perturbing forces of the environment. If water is scarce, homeostasis conserves water to keep the amount of fluid in our bodies constant. If the environment is hot, homeostasis purges heat to maintain a constant body temperature.

When homeostatic processes are working properly, the body achieves a steady state. A **steady state** is a condition in which the inputs of matter and energy to a system equal the outputs. Homeostasis maintains such a state over the long term, but not necessarily from instant to instant. For example, ingestion of a large amount of fluid will temporarily expand the extracellular fluid volume in the body. Over the long term, however, homeostatic mechanisms will purge excess fluid through urination, restoring the steady state level of fluid volume.

While inputs of matter and energy equal outputs in a steady state, this doesn't mean the internal system is similar in content to the external environment. On the contrary, a steady state means the system maintains its differences from the environment—for example, by staying carbon-rich in a carbon-poor environment. Similarly, the system is not internally uniform in a steady state. For example, most of the body's potassium is concentrated inside cells, while most of the body's sodium is concentrated outside cells. In a steady state, there are concentration gradients and there is flow through the system. Homeostasis not only controls matter and energy exchange with the outside environment, but also preserves the concentration gradients and other polarities of the internal environment. In contrast to a steady state, an **equilibrium** exists when conditions are uniform, there are no concentration gradients, and there is hence no net flow through the system.

Explaining how the body's homeostatic mechanisms maintain a steady state is the aim of physiology. Pathophysiology is the study of how and why the body's homeostatic mechanisms fail, and what happens when they do. An understanding of both physiology and pathophysiology depends on a firm conceptual grasp of homeostasis.

AN ELECTROMECHANICAL EXAMPLE OF HOMEOSTASIS

Let's consider a nonbiological example of a homeostatic system—cruise control. You're driving across the country. To relieve an incipient ache in your plantar-flexed right foot, you engage the cruise control system at 65 mph. While you lean back and tune in your favorite radio station, the cruise control maintains a constant speed.

The Structure of a Homeostatic System

Your car's cruise control is maintaining a steady state—in this case, a speed that is generally constant over time. How does this system work? A simple model consists of four components (FIGURE 1.1).

- *Sensor.* This is the speedometer, which determines the speed of the car and relays the information to a computer elsewhere in the car.
- *Control center.* This is the car's onboard computer, which compares the input from the speedometer with the speed you've programmed for cruise control (65 mph in this case). The computer then determines whether the car should speed up, slow down, or continue at its present speed.
- *Effector.* This is the engine, which translates the commands of the computer into action to alter the car's speed.
- *Transmission pathways*: This is the wiring in your car's electrical system. The speedometer sends information to the computer along an incoming or **afferent pathway**, and the

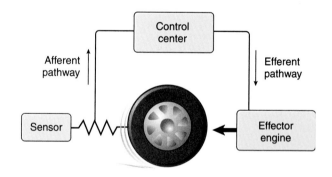

Figure 1.1 The basic components of a homeostatic system. This simple model of a cruise control system has a sensor that detects the current speed of the car. The sensor sends this information via the afferent transmission pathway to the computer control center, where a comparison of the current speed is made with the set point. The control center makes a decision to increase, decrease, or maintain the speed. It sends a signal via the efferent transmission pathway to the effector engine to adjust the work it does in order to affect the speed appropriately.

computer sends information to the engine along an outgoing or **efferent pathway**.

These four basic components are found in biological as well as nonbiological control systems.

The Function of a Homeostatic System

Despite varying topography, your car's cruise control system constantly maintains the 65 mph speed. However, you notice that your speed is not always precisely 65 mph; the cruise control system is always reacting to, rather than anticipating, outside conditions. Only a perceived decrease in speed by the speedometer can trigger the computer to rev up the engine. Therefore, your car must already be chugging up a hill, for example, and slowing down to a speed less than 65 mph, before the car's computer realizes it should signal the engine to work harder. The more sensitive the system is to deviations from the set point, the higher the system's "gain." The higher your cruise control's gain, the less will be the variation from the set point speed of 65 mph.

Likewise, if you start down a hill and surpass the set point speed, this information is relayed to the computer, which causes the engine to slow down back toward the set point of 65 mph. The result is that the speed of the car fluctuates around the 65 mph mark. The amplitude and frequency of the fluctuations depend on both changing outside conditions and the system's gain (FIGURE 1.2).

FEEDBACK SYSTEMS

Fluctuations around a preset value are characteristic of homeostatic systems like the cruise control system. A **feedback system** is one in which the system adjusts its activity by monitoring its own output. Feedback can be either negative or positive. Three types of systems—negative-feedback, positive-feedback, and feed-forward—contribute to maintaining homeostasis in the body.

Negative-Feedback Systems

A **negative-feedback system** responds to an altered output by restoring itself toward a predetermined set point (FIGURE 1.3). In the case of cruise control, an increase in speed slows down your engine, which could be achieved either by decreasing the flow of gas to the engine or by applying the brakes (or both). A decrease in speed prompts the computer to increase speed back toward the set point (65 mph) by augmenting effective engine activity, either by increasing the flow of gas to the engine or by decreasing the braking force (or both).

Because negative-feedback systems check themselves, they are very stable and are crucial to the

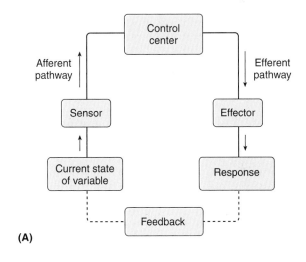

(A)

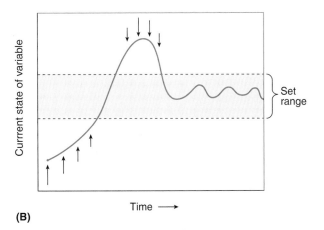

(B)

Figure 1.3 A negative-feedback system. **A.** A model of the system. **B.** The system's function and the changes in the variable. The *curve* represents the value of the variable, and the *arrows* represent the work done by the homeostatic system to return the variable to the set range. The length of the arrow is proportional to the effort exerted by the system.

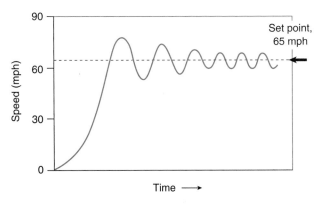

Figure 1.2 Fluctuations of a variable around a set point. A homeostatic system, such as the cruise control system, increases the variable when it is under the set point and decreases it when it is above the set point. Depending on the gain of the system, the variable "floats" around the set point. Other stimuli may perturb the variable, necessitating further work by the homeostatic system to correct the perturbation.

maintenance of homeostasis in the body. Negative-feedback systems contribute to the control of various physiologic variables, such as blood pressure and the concentration of blood glucose. Some processes of feedback regulation are considered **compensations**. Examples of compensatory mechanisms include changes in respiratory or renal functions in response to a challenge in acid-base balance and thickening of the muscle of the left ventricle in response to hypertension to enable a greater force of contraction. Long-term **adaptations** in structure and function of cells and organs are used to maintain the normal steady state. In adaptation to the low inspired oxygen of high altitude, there is an increase in the number of oxygen-carrying red blood cells in the circulation.

Positive-Feedback Systems

A positive-feedback system responds to a disturbance in steady-state conditions by moving variables farther away from the initial set point (FIGURE 1.4). Consider another nonbiological example, a population "explosion." As the birth rate increases, there

will be a larger population and subsequently a greater birth rate—exactly the opposite behavior a negative-feedback system would exhibit. In economics, an example of positive-feedback would be increased prices leading to an increased cost of living, which would in turn promote increased wages, increased cost of production, and ultimately even higher prices. The explosive behavior of positive-feedback systems makes them inherently unstable.

While they are less common than negative-feedback systems in maintaining the steady state in the body, positive-feedback systems do play a role in maintaining homeostasis. For example, the opening of some voltage-gated cell membrane ion channels, leading to the initiation of an action potential in neurons, depends on a positive-feedback system. As the membrane potential increases from the resting potential, the channels open, allowing more positively charged ions to enter the cell. This further increases the membrane potential, thereby triggering more channels to open. Such systems either possess an intrinsic mechanism or depend on a companion antagonistic system that shuts down the activity of the system and resets the physiologic variable to its original set point.

Feed-Forward Systems

Unlike feedback systems, a **feed-forward system** is proactive; it has a sensor that can anticipate environmental changes and prompt the system to act before the alterations begin to affect it (FIGURE 1.5). Consider a cruise control equipped with both a comprehensive topographic road map and a sensor to detect your exact position and direction on any road. Anticipating an uphill climb, for example, the computer would know to tell the engine to work harder before the topography changes. Thus, the system could maintain its set point speed even before changing conditions perturbed it.

As an example of how your body uses a feed-forward system, imagine yourself about to run with (or, you hope, ahead of) the bulls in the traditional Running of the Bulls event in Pamplona, Spain. The prospect that large-horned fauna will soon be stampeding behind you gets your heart racing. In physiologic terms, your autonomic nervous system provides an increased cardiac output even before your leg muscles demand more oxygen-laden blood to fuel your dash to safety (see Chapter 5). The production of saliva in anticipation of a good meal is another example of a feed-forward system.

FUELING HOMEOSTASIS

It's fine to kick back in your car and cruise along at 65 mph (more or less), as long as you keep one eye on the fuel gauge. Your car might be in perfect running

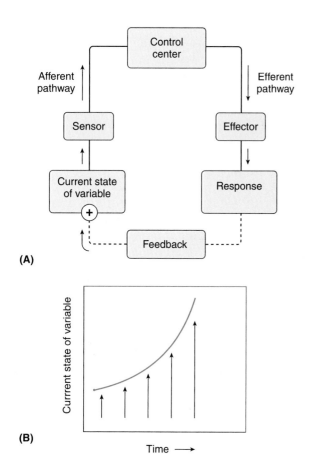

Figure 1.4 Positive-feedback system. **A.** A model of the system. **B.** The system's function and the changes in the variable. In a positive feedback system, the response moves the variable farther away from the starting point.

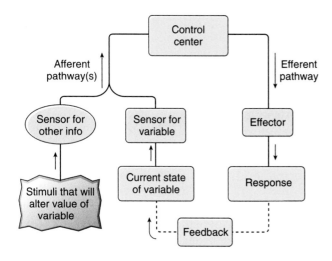

(A)

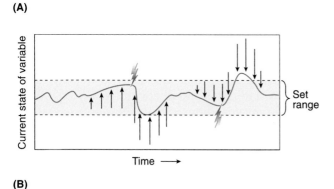

(B)

Figure 1.5 A feed-forward system. **A.** The control center uses information beyond the current state of the variable and anticipates that the variable is going to be "pushed" from the set range by some stimulus. It therefore activates the compensatory mechanism(s) preemptively, so that the time and degree of perturbation of the variable may be limited. **B.** The curve shows that the system begins to adjust the variable *before* the stimuli (*lightning bolts*) affect the variable.

diture is devoted to keeping potassium inside cells and sodium outside cells.

COMPONENTS OF A HOMEOSTATIC SYSTEM IN THE BODY

Powered by fuel in the gas tank, your car's cruise control system uses hardware (speedometer, wires, computers, and engine) to maintain your speed at 65 mph. These four hardware components are the elements common to all homeostatic mechanisms: a sensor, transmission pathways, a control center, and an effector. In the body, receptors are the body's sensors, which can detect chemical, electrical, or mechanical changes. The body's transmission pathways include neural and vascular "highways," as well as the chemical transmitters or signaling molecules that carry information along the pathways. The body's control centers are the nervous system and endocrine system, which determine the body's responses to changes in its environments. Its effectors are muscles, secretory tissues, and other end organs that ultimately produce the body's response to a given stimulus.

A major difference between many physiologic homeostatic systems and the electromechanical homeostatic systems exemplified by cruise control is that physiologic homeostatic systems often have a set range instead of a set point. This means that many physiologic variables do not have a single normal value but a normal range of values. For example, the normal range of serum potassium is 3.5 to 5.0 mmol/L, as opposed to the cruise control set point speed of 65 mph.

Understanding each homeostatic mechanism in the body requires knowing the specific components of the particular system. What is the receptor, and to what is it responding? How is information transmitted from the receptor to the control center and from there to the effector? What is the effector, and how does it modulate one or more physiologic variable(s)? What is the body's response to its own modified function? Analyzing homeostatic mechanisms in a systematic way provides insight into the normal function of cells, tissues, organs, and organ systems in the body and into the causes and results of diseases.

PATHOPHYSIOLOGY

Physiologic homeostatic systems can fail in one or more of three ways: intrinsic defects, extrinsic defects, and deleterious long-term effects of acute compensatory changes.

With intrinsic defects, the system itself malfunctions. An *intrinsic defect* is an inherited or acquired defect in any component of the system—sensor, trans-

order, but without gas in the tank, the cruise control system (and the entire car, for that matter) is useless.

The body's equivalent of gas is food. Usually in the presence of oxygen, the body converts chemical energy in ingested food into other forms of chemical energy, most importantly adenosine triphosphate (ATP). As long as it has an adequate stock of ATP, the body can convert this chemical energy into whatever form it needs to maintain homeostasis. When body temperature drops, ATP in your muscles fuels their contractions, causing shivering; the thermal energy released in the process increases body temperature. When faced with charging bulls, your heart muscle converts ATP to kinetic energy, increasing blood flow to muscles you use to escape. The chemical energy of the body can be converted to mechanical, thermal, and electrical energies that support all biological processes. Almost a quarter of the body's energy expen-

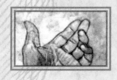

AUTONOMIC CONTROL OF ARTERIAL BLOOD PRESSURE

Many neurohormonal systems act in concert to maintain blood pressure (see Chapters 12 and 22). Arterial blood pressure is a function of cardiac output (how frequently and how intensely the heart muscle contracts) and blood vessel resistance. These relationships are quantified in analogy to Ohm's law (see Chapter 12), but the homeostatic mechanism underlying autonomic control of blood pressure can be appreciated qualitatively without this equation.

Suppose there is a drop in blood pressure. How does the body respond? First, pressure-sensitive receptors (baroceptors) in the carotid sinuses and aortic arch detect the pressure drop. The receptors actually are stretch receptors that detect a pressure change across the vessel wall. In response to this blood pressure drop, the carotid-sinus receptors decrease their rate of stimulation of cranial nerves IX and X. These cranial nerves ultimately synapse on neurons in the medulla of the brain stem, which respond to the decreased rate of stimulation by increasing sympathetic nervous outflow and decreasing parasympathetic nervous outflow (see Chapter 5). This alteration in autonomic outflow mediates three peripheral changes: increased heart rate, increased contractility of the cardiac ventricles, and vasoconstriction of systemic arteries and veins (increasing blood vessel resistance).

These changes result in an increase in blood pressure. This increase is sensed by the baroceptors, which subsequently increase their rate of firing, causing a compensatory readjustment of sympathetic and parasympathetic outflow (FIGURE B1.1). Conversely, an increase in blood pressure sensed by the baroceptors triggers a decrease in heart rate, ventricular contractility, and blood vessel resistance, leading to a fall in blood pressure. In either case, blood pressure is restored toward the previous level.

The components of this homeostatic mechanism are:

- Sensors: Baroceptors in the carotid sinus.
- Afferent transmission pathway: Cranial nerves IX and X.
- Control center: Neurons in the medulla.
- Efferent transmission pathway: Sympathetic and parasympathetic nerves.
- Effectors: Cardiac myocytes and vascular smooth muscle.

This system is a negative-feedback system. (Note: the kidney is also critical to blood pressure control. For simplicity, the kidney's contribution is not included in this brief discussion.)

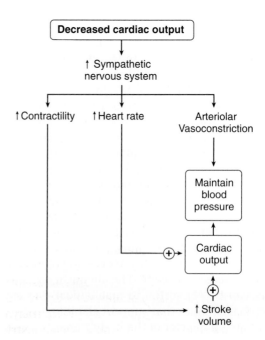

Figure B1.1 Blood pressure regulation by the autonomic nervous system (ANS). A decrease in blood pressure below the set range is detected by the system and leads to changes in heart contraction and blood vessel resistance that increase the pressure. An increase in blood pressure above the set range is detected by the system and results in the opposite changes in the heart and blood vessels that lower the pressure.

mission pathway, control center, or effector. Such is the case in type I diabetes mellitus, in which the immune system destroys insulin-producing beta islet cells in the pancreas, leading to hyperglycemia (i.e., high blood glucose levels). This beta cell deficiency constitutes sensor, control center, and transmission pathways defects because pancreatic beta cells sense the plasma glucose concentration and respond by secreting insulin when the concentration is above the normal set range (see Chapter 31). Type I diabetics no longer have enough beta cells to produce an adequate supply of insulin to maintain glucose homeostasis. In Type II diabetes mellitus, there is a peripheral tissue resistance to insulin action. Insulin may be secreted in increased amounts owing to hyperglycemia, but the end-organ effector sites cannot respond normally to the insulin.

With *extrinsic defects*, a homeostatic system responds normally but is responding to an abnormal stimulus, and in trying to "do its job," propagates a disease state. For example, a patient in congestive heart failure may have a cardiac left ventricle that can no longer pump blood effectively. This pump failure leads to a backup of blood in the lungs and a deficiency in perfusion (i.e., supply of blood) to peripheral tissues, including the kidneys. In response, the kidneys react as they do whenever they are inadequately perfused—they secrete the hormone renin, setting off a hormonal cascade (the renin-angiotensin-aldosterone axis) that ultimately causes increased salt (and water) re-absorption by the nephrons. The body thus holds on to more fluid. This response is expected from a normal, though underperfused, kidney. However, the lungs are liable to "drown" from retention of even more fluid that cannot be pumped forward fast enough by the failing heart (see Chapter 22). Here the kidney homeostatic mechanisms are working properly, but their function exacerbates the situation for the damaged heart. There is an intrinsic defect of the heart and an extrinsic abnormality involving the kidney.

Deleterious long-term effects of acute compensatory changes result when the body's attempts to maintain homeostasis are initially helpful but ultimately counterproductive. This is the cost of running for a long time (chronically) a homeostatic mechanism intended for short-term (acute) use. Consider again a case of congestive heart failure due to left ventricular dysfunction. There is inadequate blood pressure to sufficiently perfuse peripheral tissues. The decrease in systemic blood pressure is sensed by the arterial baroceptors (See Clinical Application Box *Autonomic Control of Arterial Blood Pressure* and Chapter 5). These baroceptors, sensing decreased perfusion pressure, trigger more sympathetic and less parasympathetic outflow, leading to peripheral vasoconstric-

tion. While leading to a higher blood pressure through an increased vascular resistance in the short term, this response forces the failing heart to pump against even higher resistance, which further compounds the heart failure over the long term.

Using medication, surgery, radiation, and other modalities, therapeutic interventions aim to reverse, or correct, pathophysiologic functioning of homeostatic mechanisms. Managing congestive heart failure may include augmenting the heart's ability to pump blood, changing the hemodynamics of blood flow through the arteries, or interfering with the kidney's efforts to rev up the renin-angiotensin-aldosterone axis. The physician's job is to know how control systems like the ones at work in congestive heart failure ought to function, how and why they sometimes do not, and what to do in such cases.

Summary

- Homeostasis is the maintenance of a steady state.
- Homeostatic systems must have one or more sensors, transmission pathways, a control center, and one or more effectors.
- Negative-feedback systems work to decrease a variable when it is too high and increase it when it is too low.
- Positive-feedback systems work to increase a variable when stimulated.
- Feed-forward systems use predictive information to anticipate how a variable is going to change and preemptively compensate for that change.
- Physiologic homeostatic systems often have a set range for a variable, rather than a single set point value. They require energy in the form of organic molecules such as ATP.
- Pathophysiology may result from an intrinsic defect in a homeostatic system, from a normal response to an abnormal stimulus (an extrinsic defect), or from the chronic (i.e., long-term) effects of a homeostatic compensatory mechanism.

Suggested Reading

Cannon WB. Some general features of endocrine influence on metabolism. Trans Cong Am Phys Surg. 1926; 13:31–53.

Shannon CE. A mathematical theory of communication. Bell System Tech J. 1948;27:379–423, 623–656.

REVIEW QUESTIONS

Directions: Each of the numbered items or incomplete statements in this section is followed by answers or by completions of the statement. Select the ONE lettered answer or completion that is BEST in each case.

1. Pancreatic beta cells monitor the blood glucose concentration. When the glucose concentration is above the normal set range, they secrete insulin to lower the concentration. When the concentration is below the normal set range, they decrease or stop insulin secretion. In this homeostatic system, insulin is

   (A) the sensor.
   (B) the afferent transmission pathway.
   (C) the control center.
   (D) the effector.
   (E) the efferent transmission pathway.

2. An 84-year-old man suffers a heart attack. His left ventricular function is impaired and his blood pressure goes down. Which of the following best describes the autonomic nervous system (ANS) response?

   (A) The ANS is a negative-feedback system and will work to decrease blood pressure.
   (B) The ANS is a negative-feedback system and will work to increase blood pressure.
   (C) The ANS is a positive-feedback system and will work to decrease blood pressure.

(D) The ANS is a positive-feedback system and will work to increase blood pressure.

3. A 78-year-old woman has heart failure and relatively normal kidney function. Sensing poor perfusion from the failing heart, her kidneys activate the renin-angiotensin-aldosterone axis. Although her blood pressure rises slightly, she becomes short of breath and has swelling in her legs as fluid accumulates in her lungs and extremities. This is an example of

(A) a failure of proper sensing by the kidney's homeostatic system.
(B) a failure of the kidney control center.
(C) a failure of the kidney's effector mechanisms.
(D) a proper kidney homeostatic response that worsens the disease.

ANSWERS TO REVIEW QUESTIONS

1. **The answer is** E. Insulin is the efferent transmission pathway. In the pancreatic islet cell, an elevated blood sugar is recognized by a cell surface receptor (sensor) that transmits an intracellular signal (afferent transmission pathway) through the metabolism of glucose, to the control center in the same cell, which stores insulin. Insulin is then released into the circulation (the efferent transmission pathway), where it binds to specific receptors in muscle and fat cells that then remove glucose from the circulation (effector sites), lowering the blood sugar. The pancreatic receptors, noting a fall in sugar levels, then decrease insulin output by a process of negative feedback.

2. **The answer is** B. When blood pressure is low, the ANS works to increase it back toward the normal set range. Once the blood pressure reaches the normal set range, the ANS should stop trying to further increase it. This is a negative-feedback system. If the ANS were a positive-feedback system, it would continue to raise blood pressure beyond the set range. Lowering blood pressure further would be an inappropriate response to a variable already perturbed below the set range.

3. **The answer is** D. The kidney is underperfused, so it activates the renin-angiotensin-aldosterone axis in an attempt to increase blood volume and pressure to augment perfusion. This is an appropriate response by the kidney, which sensed low blood pressure and responded accordingly. However, because the root cause is not low blood volume but heart pump failure, the kidney's response exacerbates the disease.

2

Membrane Transport

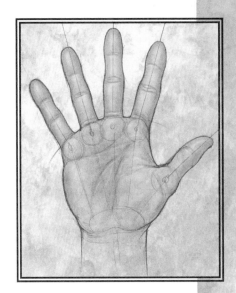

INTRODUCTION

The contents of cells are sealed off from the extracellular environment by a lipid barrier called the **plasma membrane**. The plasma membrane serves homeostasis by protecting the cell's interior from the changing conditions of the extracellular fluid. This helps maintain the specific chemical milieu that supports the intracellular metabolic processes of life. Proteins embedded in the membrane help to control molecular traffic across the lipid barrier—functioning like immigration officers to retain desired constituents and deny entry to undesired ones. In addition, such controlled membrane transport enables cells to react to or act on the extracellular environment, thereby serving particular specialized functions on behalf of the whole organism. For example, intestinal absorptive cells have membrane proteins that allow them to take up nutrients from the gut, while renal tubular cells possess different membrane proteins that enable them to excrete metabolic waste products from the blood into the urine.

A special type of cellular reaction involves the passage of ions (and hence electrical charge) across the membrane. The cell membrane, in fact, oversees membrane transport to create a constant ion gradient where the concentration of positive ions outside the cell exceeds that of the cell interior. This affords each cell a resting membrane electrical potential, which is critical to cell excitability. Cell excitability is the change in the membrane potential that is necessary for cellular responses in various tissues, including nerve, muscle, and cardiac tissue.

COMPONENTS OF THE CELL MEMBRANE

The plasma membrane is composed predominantly of phospholipids, cholesterol, and proteins. The established model for the structure of the plasma membrane is known as the **fluid mosaic model**.

Phospholipids

Phospholipids have a polar head group and two hydrophobic fatty acyl chains that give them a unique conformation, favoring the formation of a lipid bilayer (FIGURE 2.1). The most abundant phospholipids are phosphatidylcholine and sphingomyelin, which are found primarily in the outer layer of the plasma membrane. Phosphatidylserine and phosphatidylethanolamine are located preferentially with the inner layer. Phosphatidylglycerol and phosphatidylinositol are other examples of common membrane phospholipids.

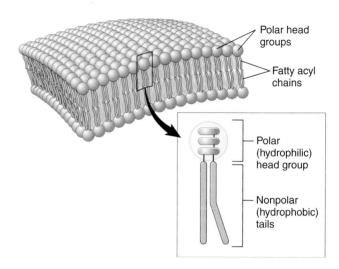

Figure 2.1 Plasma membrane phospholipids. Membrane phospholipids contain a hydrophilic polar head group and two hydrophobic nonpolar tails. Phospholipids are arranged in the membrane with the head groups "out" and the tails "in," thus forming a bilayer.

Cholesterol

Cholesterol (FIGURE 2.2), integrated within the lipid bilayer, enables the lipid membrane to remain fluid even at reduced temperatures. It is unique to animal cell membranes, as plants lack cholesterol. Although cholesterol has become infamous for its role in the development of atherosclerosis, which may lead to heart disease and stroke, this molecule is essential for plasma membrane function—so much so, that even if our diet contains no cholesterol whatsoever, the liver synthesizes it.

Glycolipids

Another class of lipids found within the plasma membrane is the glycolipids. Glycolipids contain carbohydrate side groups extending into the extracellular space.

Proteins

Membrane proteins include channel proteins, carrier proteins, transporters, hormone receptors, cell adhesion molecules, and enzymes. Membrane proteins are classified as either integral (intrinsic) or peripheral (extrinsic), depending on whether they are embedded within the plasma membrane or simply associated with the membrane surface, respectively (FIGURE 2.3). An example of an integral membrane protein is an ion channel, which may have multiple membrane-spanning hydrophobic α helices traversing the lipid bilayer (FIGURE 2.4).

According to the fluid mosaic model of the structure of the plasma membrane, integral membrane

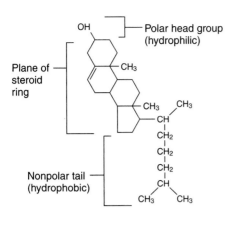

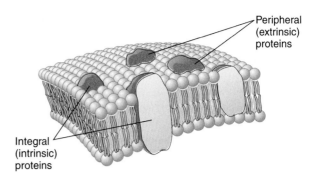

Figure 2.3 Integral and peripheral membrane proteins. Integral membrane proteins are embedded in the lipid bilayer, while peripheral proteins are associated with either the inner or outer face of the membrane.

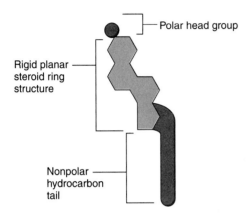

Figure 2.2 Cholesterol. Like the phospholipids, cholesterol has a hydrophilic polar head and a hydrophobic nonpolar tail.

proteins are free to move within the plane of the plasma membrane and to "flip-flop," or reverse their orientation (the extracellular end becomes the intracellular end and vice-versa). However, such proteins may generally localize to certain areas of the

membrane called *lipid rafts,* and they typically assume a specific polarity (i.e., they do not flip-flop much) owing to selective anchoring of the intracellular end to the cytoskeleton. As a result, the plasma membrane is a heterogeneous structure. Its outer and inner faces are asymmetric, and different regions may have very different contents. Examples of integral membrane proteins are shown in Figure 2.4A-D.

Peripheral membrane proteins are located both extracellularly and intracellularly (Figure 2.4E-F). They may associate with the plasma membrane's integral proteins via charge–charge interactions, noncovalent bonds between a positively charged area on one protein and a negatively charged area on another. Some membrane proteins are covalently attached to fatty acid chains, prenyl groups, or phospholipids intercalated within the plasma membrane.

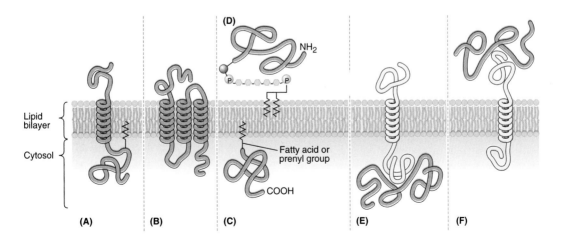

Figure 2.4 The association of proteins with the plasma membrane. **A-B.** Integral membrane proteins may have one or more alpha helices that cross the lipid bilayer. They may also be covalently bound to phospholipids (A.). **C.** Other integral membrane proteins may be bound only by phospholipids, prenyl groups, or fatty acids. **D.** Still other integral membrane proteins are bound through oligosaccharides to glycolipids or phospholipids. **E-F.** Peripheral proteins are noncovalently bound to either the intracytoplasmic or the extracellular domains of transmembrane proteins.

TYPES OF TRANSPORT

Because the plasma membrane is made up predominantly of hydrophobic (or lipophilic) molecules, other hydrophobic molecules are able to enter or exit cells through dissolution—by dissolving into or through the membrane. Hydrophilic molecules, however, must cross the plasma membrane through water-filled channels or via specific carrier proteins.

Transport Across the Plasma Membrane

Transport across the plasma membrane occurs by several mechanisms, including diffusion, osmosis, endocytosis, exocytosis, and protein-mediated transport (FIGURE 2.5).

Diffusion and Osmosis   The **diffusion** of molecules across the plasma membrane is not carrier-mediated and does not require energy expenditure. Diffusion is the net flow of a solute from an area of high solute concentration to an area of low solute concentration. When these areas are separated by a membrane, diffusion takes place across the membrane. The molecules of solute always cross the membrane in both directions, with more crossover from the high concentration area to the low. The magnitude and direction of diffusion are described quantitatively by Fick's law of diffusion:

$$J = -P \times A \times (C1 - C2)$$

where J represents the net rate of diffusion from compartment 1 into compartment 2; P is the permeability coefficient, which is proportional to molecular size and to the solubility of the molecule in the medium (diffusivity), and inversely related to the thickness of the membrane and the viscosity of the medium; A denotes the area for diffusion; and C1 and C2 represent the respective concentrations of the molecule across the permeability barrier. According to this equation, small, uncharged molecules diffuse easily, whereas large or highly charged molecules will not, and they will require protein-mediated transport to cross the membrane.

Osmosis is the diffusion of water across a semipermeable membrane from a solution of low solute concentration to one of higher solute concentration. The concentration of "free" water molecules is greater in a solution with a lower solute concentration because less water is occupied in charge interactions with the solute. The increased amount of free water molecules on one side of a membrane is what drives the diffusion of water from low solute concentration to high. Like diffusion, osmosis does not require energy.

Endocytosis and Exocytosis   **Endocytosis** is a mechanism for transporting substances too large for diffusion or passage through protein channels from the outside of the cell to the cell interior. In this process, extracellular material is brought into the cell without actually passing through the lipid bilayer (FIGURE 2.6). Rather than crossing the membrane, the material is surrounded by the plasma membrane and enclosed within a small sphere of bilayer that pinches off. This envelope derived from the membrane is called a vesicle, and it moves within the cytoplasm. Although the

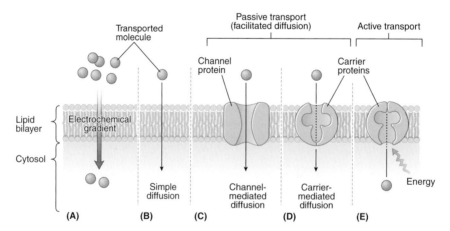

Figure 2.5   The transport of solutes across the plasma membrane. **A.** An electrochemical gradient favors the movement of a solute from the extracellular to the intracellular space. **B.** If the solute is small and lipid-soluble, it may pass through the membrane via simple diffusion. **C.** The solute may require a protein channel to facilitate passive diffusion across the membrane. **D.** The facilitated diffusion may require a protein carrier to passively carry the solute down its gradient. **E.** In active transport, the carrier protein requires metabolic energy to fulfill its transport function because transport of the solute against its electrochemical gradient costs energy.

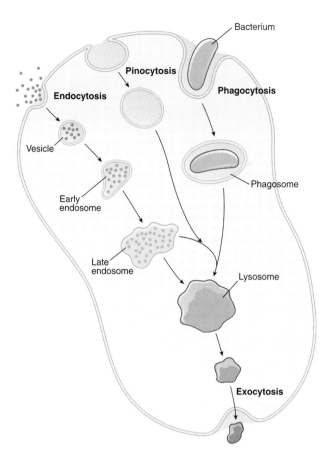

Figure 2.6 Endocytosis and exocytosis. A cell can take up material by enclosing it in an envelope of lipid bilayer that then pinches off of the plasma membrane. When the engulfed material is solid, the process is called phagocytosis. When the enveloped material is mostly liquid, the process is called pinocytosis. Because the substances remain inside membrane-enclosed spheres called vesicles, they are topologically still "outside" the cell. After being metabolized, the cell can extrude waste materials by fusing the vesicle back to the plasma membrane. This process of exocytosis is the reverse of endocytosis. It is used by the cell to export important products made intracellularly into the extracellular environment.

the plasma membrane than the other, a concentration gradient is present. A **concentration gradient** promotes diffusion of the substance from the space of higher concentration to the space of lower concentration ("down the gradient") and opposes movement of the substance in the opposite direction ("up the gradient"). Similarly, if electrical charges are unequally distributed on the two sides of the cell membrane, an **electrical gradient** is present (FIGURE 2.7). Often, an unequal distribution of a charged substance on the two sides of the cell membrane will cause a chemical gradient and an electrical gradient to coexist. In such a situation, the net force acting on a given particle of this substance is called an **electrochemical gradient**, a name that accounts for both the concentration and the charge components.

In some instances, cells need to take up ions or molecules from the extracellular space into the cytoplasm or move intracellular substances out of the cell against forces that oppose such transport. This requirement occurs, for example, when a molecule cannot freely diffuse through the plasma membrane because it is too large and/or too hydrophilic, even if a concentration gradient favors the necessary movement. Alternatively, the cell may need to transport a substance up a chemical or electrical gradient. Both these mechanisms are facilitated by specific protein transporters embedded in the cell membrane.

Protein-mediated membrane transport involves integral proteins that are specific carriers or channels. These proteins are carriers for facilitated diffusion or active transporters, depending on whether they move molecules down or up an electrochemical gradient, respectively.

vesicle is inside the cell, the vesicle contents are still extracellular, topologically speaking. Later, the vesicle can fuse with the plasma membrane again. Endocytosis, an energy-dependent process, has other names depending on the material taken up. It is called **phagocytosis** when particulate matter enters the cell, **pinocytosis** when soluble small molecules in a volume of fluid enter, and **receptor-mediated endocytosis** when specific extracellular molecules are bound to integral proteins prior to being endocytosed.

Exocytosis is the opposite process, whereby intracellular material in a vesicle is expelled from the cell when the vesicle fuses with the plasma membrane. Like endocytosis, exocytosis requires energy.

Facilitated Diffusion and Active Transport When the concentration of a substance is greater on one side of

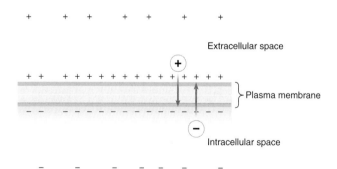

Figure 2.7 An electrical gradient across the plasma membrane. The intracellular space is negatively charged. This is because the Na$^+$/K$^+$ pump creates a high intracellular K$^+$ concentration, and K$^+$ flows out of the cell, leaving behind an excess of anions. The stoichiometry of the pump also makes a contribution, pumping out more positive charges (3 Na$^+$s) than it pumps in (2 K$^+$s). The negative charge inside cells creates an electrical gradient that draws cations into the cell and repels anions.

Facilitated diffusion is the movement of a substance that cannot freely cross the membrane down an electrochemical gradient. Such a process does not require metabolic energy because it works "downhill" much like simple diffusion, except that the net flux of molecules is much greater because of facilitation by the protein carrier or channel (FIGURE 2.8). An example of facilitated diffusion is provided by the insulin-dependent glucose transporter (GLUT), which allows plasma glucose to enter cells.

The various ion-specific channels for Na^+, K^+, Cl^-, and others participate in facilitated diffusion because they allow ion entry into cells only in the presence of a favorable "downhill" electrochemical gradient. Many ion channels are gated, meaning that they alternate between an open and a closed conformation, depending on the presence of an "opening" stimulus (FIGURE 2.9). Ion channels that open in response to an extracellular hormone are termed *ligand-gated ion channels*. For example, the nicotinic acetylcholine receptor, nAChR, is a ligand-gated Na^+ channel triggered by acetylcholine at the synaptic cleft. Some ion channels open when the resting membrane electrical potential of the plasma membrane reverses, a process known as *depolarization*. Such channels are called *voltage-gated ion channels*. A *mechanical-gated channel* opens under the influence of hydrostatic or osmotic pressure (Figure 2.9).

Active transport is either primary or secondary, depending on the source of energy used. Primary active transporters use ATP directly to carry specific ions against an electrochemical gradient. The best example of a primary active trans-

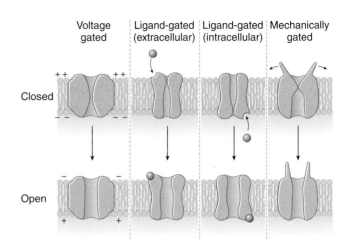

Figure 2.9 Gated membrane protein channels. A gated channel is one that alternates between a closed state, which does not allow solutes to go down their electrochemical gradient, and an open state, which does. Such channels may be opened in response to changes in the membrane electrical potential (voltage-gated), the presence of an extracellular or intracellular ligand (ligand-gated), or the application of a mechanical force such as stretch or pressure (mechanically gated).

porter is the ubiquitous Na^+/K^+-ATPase, a protein pump that transports both Na^+ and K^+ against their respective electrochemical gradients (FIGURE 2.10). By simultaneously transporting three Na^+ ions out of the cell and two K^+ ions in, the Na^+/K^+-ATPase (also called the Na^+/K^+ pump) maintains a high extracellular and low intracellular Na^+ concentration and a high intracellular and low extracellular K^+

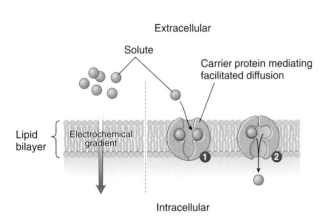

Figure 2.8 Facilitated diffusion. Solute S has an electrochemical gradient favoring movement into the cell, but it is unable to cross the plasma membrane via simple diffusion because it is either too large or too hydrophilic (or both). Solute S enters by facilitated diffusion with the help of a carrier protein without energy expenditure. In the model shown, the carrier can exist in two conformational states: state 1, in which solute S binds to the protein on the outside, and state 2, in which the solute diffuses into the cell. This arrangement is known as a "ping-pong" mechanism.

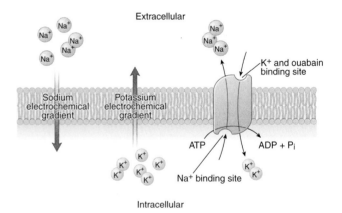

Figure 2.10 The Na^+/K^+-ATPase active transporter. Na^+ has an electrochemical gradient favoring movement into the cell, while K^+ has a gradient favoring movement out of the cell. The Na^+/K^+-ATPase creates and maintains these gradients by moving Na^+ out of the cell and K^+ into the cell, against their respective gradients. Each iteration of the transporters moves three Na^+ out and two K^+ in and uses one molecule of ATP as the energy source. Each iteration contributes to the resting membrane potential because more positive charges move out than in, so the cell interior is relatively negative compared to the extracellular space. Such a transporter is electrogenic.

concentration. The establishment and maintenance of such ion gradients are responsible for the resting membrane electrical potential, discussed below. Other examples of active transporters are the Ca^{2+}-ATPase found in the sarcoplasmic reticulum, renal tubules, intestine, and cardiac muscle. The Ca^{2+}-ATPase sequesters cytosolic Ca^{2+} within the sarcoplasmic reticulum or transports Ca^{2+} out of the cell. The H^+/K^+-ATPase, located on the lumenal surface of gastric parietal cells, is another primary active transporter. This transporter pumps H^+ against an unfavorable electrochemical gradient into the lumen of the stomach, acidifying gastric contents.

Secondary active transport involves a pump like the Na^+/K^+ ATPase and a **cotransporter**. First, the pump establishes a Na^+ gradient. Then, the Na^+ diffuses down its concentration gradient across the cotransporter. The cotransporter couples this movement of Na^+ to the movement of another solute. ATP is used indirectly, in that transmembrane gradients created by primary active transporters (e.g., the Na^+/K^+-ATPase) are used to drive the transport of other solutes against unfavorable concentration or electrical gradients.

When a cotransporter moves two solutes in the same direction, it is called a *symporter* (FIGURE 2.11). Examples of symporters are the Na-K-2Cl cotransporter found in the ascending limb of the renal tubule, the Na^+-glucose cotransporter in the intestinal mucosa, and the Na^+-amino acid cotransporter in the proximal renal tubule.

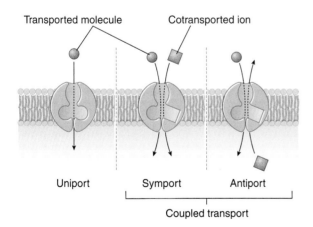

Figure 2.11 Plasma membrane transporters. Uniporters carry one solute across the membrane. If this movement is down the electrochemical gradient, it requires no added energy, but if it is against the gradient, energy must be spent. Cotransporters move more than one solute. Symporters carry two solutes in the same direction, while antiporters transfer them in opposite directions. If both solutes are moving down their respective gradients, no energy is needed. If one of the solutes is going down its gradient, it may supply enough energy to move the other against its gradient. If both solutes are transported against their gradients, energy is required.

An *antiporter* transports two solutes in opposite directions across the cell membrane (see Figure 2.11). The Ca^{2+}/Na^+ antiporter found in cardiac muscle uses the Na^+ gradient created by the Na^+/K^+-ATPase to drive intracellular Ca^{2+} out of cells against its electrochemical gradient. The Cl^-/HCO_3^- antiporter prevents the cytosol from becoming too basic during intracellular accumulations of HCO_3^- by extruding intracellular HCO_3^- and taking up Cl^- in exchange.

RESTING MEMBRANE POTENTIALS

The Na^+/K^+-ATPase establishes chemical gradients of both Na^+ and K^+ across the plasma membrane, which favor the inward movement of Na^+ and the outward movement of K^+ through ion-specific channels. Because the Na^+-K^+ pump moves three Na^+ ions out of the cell but only two K^+ ions into the cell with each iteration, it generates a net negative charge within the cytoplasm, relative to the extracellular environment. The separation of negative charges on the intracytoplasmic side of the membrane from positive charges on the extracellular side gives the cell a *resting membrane potential*, which is the voltage drop across the membrane. If this were the Na^+/K^+ pump's only contribution to resting membrane potential, the potential would be very small (around -5 mV). However, the pump makes a second, much larger, contribution to resting membrane potential. By creating concentration gradients across the cell membrane, the pump sets up a flow of ions down their concentration gradients, across the membrane, and this ion flow creates a much larger separation of charge. Net Na^+ flows into the cell through Na^+ channels, making the inside of the membrane more electropositive. Net K^+ flows down its gradient out of the cell, rendering the inside of the membrane more electronegative. The chemical gradient thus creates an electrical gradient.

Furthermore, the chemical and electrical gradients oppose one another. A high intracellular K^+ concentration drives K^+ efflux, K^+ efflux renders the cytoplasm more negative, and this negative electrical potential holds onto the positive ion, opposing K^+ efflux and driving its influx. As more net K^+ flows out of the cell, the chemical gradient declines, lessening the force for efflux, while the electrical gradient increases, increasing the force for K^+ influx. As the chemical force falls and the electrical rises, the two forces eventually become equal and the rates of K^+ efflux and influx equilibrate with no net flux of K^+. The membrane potential at this equilibrium point is called the **equilibrium potential** or the Nernst potential.

The Nernst equation expresses the direct relationship between an ion's equilibrium concentration

Table 2.1 **NORMAL RANGES FOR INTRACELLULAR AND EXTRACELLULAR CONCENTRATIONS AND CALCULATED NERNST POTENTIALS FOR SELECTED IONS**

Component	Intracellular Concentration (mmol)	Extracellular Concentration (mmol)	Nernst Potential (mV)
Cations[a]			
Na^+	5–15	135–145	69.7
K^+	140	3.5–5	−91.0
Mg^{2+}	0.5	1–2	14.3
Ca^{2+}	10^{-4}	1–2	125.3
H^+	7×10^{-5} ($10^{-7.2}$ M or pH 7.2)	4×10^{-5} ($10^{-7.4}$ M or pH 7.4)	45.4
Anions[b]			
Cl^-	5–15	100–110	−65.6

[a]The concentrations of Ca^{2+} and Mg^{2+} given are for the free ions. There is a total of about 20 mmol Mg^{2+} and 1–2 mmol Ca^{2+} in cells, but this is mostly bound to proteins and other substances and, in the case of Ca^{2+}, stored within various organelles.
[b]In addition to Cl^-, the cell contains many other anions not listed in this table; in fact, most cellular constituents are negatively charged (HCO_3^-, PO_4^{3-}, proteins, nucleic acids, metabolites carrying phosphate and carboxyl groups, etc.).

gradient and its equilibrium electical potential. The larger the equilibrium concentration difference, the larger must be the electrical potential that opposes it. The Nernst equation is:

$$V = RT/zF \times \ln(C_o/C_i)$$

where V equals the equilibrium potential, R is the gas constant, T is the absolute temperature, F is Faraday's number, z is the charge number of the ion, and C_o and C_i represent extracellular and intracellular ion concentrations, respectively. Using the known values for R, T, and F, and simplifying, the equation can be

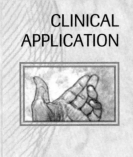

CLINICAL APPLICATION

DRUGS AFFECTING MEMBRANE TRANSPORTERS

The cardiac glycosides are a group of drugs derived from the leaves of the foxglove plant. They have been in clinical use for centuries as therapy for heart diseases, such as congestive heart failure. Of the cardiac glycosides, digoxin is the most therapeutically important. Its effects on cardiac contractility are related to its action on the Na^+/K^+-ATPase of the cardiac myocyte cell membrane. By binding to the K^+-binding site of the transporter, digoxin inhibits the Na^+/K^+ pump. This causes an increase in intracellular Na^+. The elevated intracellular Na^+ diminishes the electrochemical gradient favoring Na^+ entry into the cell. The Na^+ gradient is critical to the Na^+/Ca^{2+} antiporter. The Na^+/Ca^{2+} antiporter is responsible for extruding intracellular Ca^{2+} following cardiac depolarization and contraction. With decreased function of the Na^+/Ca^{2+} antiporter, there is an increase in the intracellular concentration of Ca^{2+}. This in turn leads to an increased store of Ca^{2+} in the intracellular sarcoplasmic reticulum. This augmented Ca^{2+} supply is released with future cardiac myocyte depolarizations. The added Ca^{2+} release from the sarcoplasmic reticulum enhances the force of contraction because Ca^{2+} has an integral role in the actin-myosin interaction that underlies muscle contraction. The net result is an increase in the contractile force of the heart, which ameliorates heart failure due to poor cardiac muscle contraction.

Local anesthetics (e.g., lidocaine, bupivacaine, procaine, etc.) also function by inhibiting a membrane transporter. Local anesthetics block nerve cell activation (action potential generation) by blocking voltage-gated Na^+ ion channels. Without the influx of Na^+ that occurs with nerve stimulation, axons are not depolarized. Thus, nociceptive (pain) signal transmission is inhibited, resulting in anesthesia.

reduced to:

$$V = 60 \text{ mV}/z \times \log_{10}(C_o/C_i)$$

The Nernst equation calculates the potential created by an ion given its equilibrium concentration difference. TABLE 2.1 lists the normal ranges for the intracellular and extracellular concentrations of Na^+, K^+, Mg^{2+}, Ca^{2+}, and Cl^-, as well as their calculated Nernst potentials. When many different ions are distributed across the plasma membrane, each ion creates a transmembrane potential according to its Nernst equation. The cell's overall resting potential will reflect the cumulative effects of each ion's Nernst potential contribution. Because facilitated diffusion of ions is responsible for establishing the resting potential, the ion with the greatest membrane permeability, and hence the greatest net flux across the plasma membrane, will have the largest weight and will push the overall resting membrane potential toward its own Nernst equilibrium. In general, for a cell at rest, facilitated diffusion of K^+ out of the cell exceeds the transmembrane flux of other ions; therefore, the cell's resting membrane potential approaches the Nernst potential for K^+, with minor contributions from the other ion gradients.

For an average cell, the resting membrane potential is approximately -70 to -90 mV, reflecting the importance of K^+. Of course, different cell types may have different resting potentials, depending on varying densities of ion channels and carriers that will affect the net flux of a particular ion and change its contribution to the resting membrane potential.

As the Nernst equation makes clear, small changes in the concentration of some ions may have larger effects on the resting membrane potential. The most important examples are changes in the extracellular concentration of K^+. Lowering $[K^+]_o$ from 5 to 2 mmol will decrease the equilibrium potential from -87 to -111 mV, while raising the concentration to 8 mmol will increase the potential to -75 mV. Although such alterations may seem small, they affect the activity of nerve, muscle, and heart cells profoundly, causing potentially life-threatening diseases. (See Clinical Application Box *Drugs Affecting Membrane Transporters*.)

Summary

- The plasma membrane is made up of phospholipids, cholesterol, glycolipids, and proteins.
- Diffusion and osmosis are passive processes that require no energy. Fick's law of diffusion is $J = -P \times A \times (C1 - C2)$.
- Integral membrane proteins are necessary for facilitated diffusion and active transport. Endocytosis, exocytosis, and active transport require energy.
- Differences in the extracellular and intracellular concentrations of charged ions produce electrical gradients. These gradients contribute to the cell resting membrane potential according to the Nernst equation: $V = 60 \text{ mV}/z \times \log_{10}(C_o/C_i)$.
- The extracellular concentration of K^+ is critical to maintenance of the normal resting potential. Deviation above or below the normal range of $[K^+]_o$ (3.5–5 mmol) may cause life-threatening disturbances in the membrane potential.

Suggested Reading

Chieregatti E, Meldolesi J. Regulated exocytosis: new organelles for non-secretory purposes. Nat Rev Mol Cell Biol. 2005;6(2):181–187.

Jacobson K, Sheets ED, Simson R. Revisiting the fluid mosaic model of membranes. Science. 1995;268(5216):1441–1442.

REVIEW QUESTIONS

Directions: Each of the numbered items or incomplete statements in this section is followed by answers or by completions of the statement. Select the ONE lettered answer or completion that is BEST in each case.

1. Which of the following processes requires energy?

    (A) Diffusion
    (B) Facilitated diffusion
    (C) Osmosis
    (D) Active transport

2. A patient with kidney failure has a serious heart rhythm disturbance because the resting membrane potential of his cardiac cells has increased. This condition is most likely due to which of the following disturbances?

    (A) Decreased $[K^+]_i$
    (B) Decreased $[K^+]_o$
    (C) Increased $[K^+]_i$
    (D) Increased $[K^+]_o$
    (E) Increased K^+ flux

3. The membrane transporter directly responsible for acidification of the gastric lumen is the

    (A) Na^+/K^+-ATPase
    (B) Na^+-amino acid symporter
    (C) Ca^{2+}/Na^+ antiporter
    (D) Cl^-/HCO_3^- antiporter
    (E) H^+/K^+-ATPase

ANSWERS TO REVIEW QUESTIONS

1. **The answer is D.** The first three processes all involve the movement of solutes down an electrochemical gradient and thus require no input of energy. Active transport, however, is the movement of solute against such a gradient and therefore does require energy expenditure.

2. **The answer is D.** Kidney failure almost invariably causes an increase in the extracellular concentration of K^+, and it is this alteration in the equilibrium potential (as predicted by the Nernst equation) that increases the resting membrane potential. Decreasing $[K^+]_o$ or increasing $[K^+]_i$ would have the opposite effect (i.e., the membrane potential would decrease further). While a decrease in $[K^+]_i$ would also raise the membrane potential, this is less likely to occur because the Na^+/K^+-ATPase maintains a high intracellular K^+ concentration.

3. **The answer is E.** The lumenal surface of gastric parietal cells possesses a membrane transporter that extrudes protons (H^+) into the stomach lumen. It is this transporter that is inhibited by some drugs used to treat or prevent stomach ulcers, because disabling the H^+/K^+-ATPase decreases gastric acidity.

Cell-to-Cell Communication

3

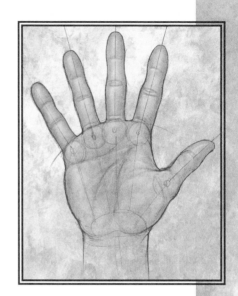

INTRODUCTION

It is no surprise that cells communicate with each other. Signaling is essential for coordinating the function and differentiation of nearby cells. Cells located close to one another communicate in three main ways:

1. If the cells are connected by a gap junction, one cell can send a signal through the gap junction directly into the adjoining cell's cytoplasm.

2. If the cells are close enough to make contact with each other, a signal can be communicated by direct interaction of membrane receptors.

3. A cell can secrete a molecule into the extracellular space, signaling those cells that are close enough to make contact with the molecule.

In addition to signaling between nearby cells, the functioning of the human body depends on the ability of organs and tissues to communicate with each other at a distance. For example, if a stimulus contacts your toe, the message needs to travel the full length of your body to reach the sensory regions of your brain. Sometimes it is important for the whole body to receive a message. For example, if your eyes and ears notice a growling lion racing at you, this message must be sent from your eyes and ears to every part of your body so you can react in a coordinated and efficient manner. Tissues and organs use two main mechanisms to communicate with each other throughout the body:

1. An organ can secrete a substance into the bloodstream, thereby delivering the signal to almost every cell of the body.

2. An organ can use the nervous system to communicate with another region of the body.

MECHANISMS OF CELL-TO-CELL COMMUNICATION

If we attach names to the five modes of communication introduced above and add one more, we get six major mechanisms of cell-to-cell communication: gap junction communication, juxtacrine communication, autocrine communication, paracrine communication, endocrine communication, and neuronal communication (FIGURE 3.1).

Gap Junction Communication

In **gap junction communication**, a signal travels from one cell's cytoplasm directly into an adjoining cell's cytoplasm through a gap junction. A **gap junc-**

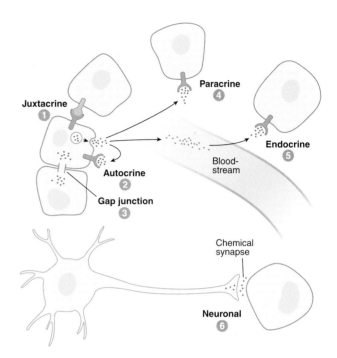

Figure 3.1   Six mechanisms of cell-to-cell signaling.

tion is a channel made of the protein connexin, which allows communication between the cytoplasm of adjacent cells. The signal may be an ion, a small molecule, or a metabolite, as long as it is small enough to travel through the gap junction. One function of gap junction communication is to enable adjacent cells in a tissue to share the same cytosolic environment, providing for equal growth and differentiation. Electrical signals are often propagated through gap junctions.

Juxtacrine Communication

Juxtacrine communication is cell-to-cell communication through the direct contact of plasma membranes. Transmembrane proteins (e.g., pro-TGF-α) and phospholipids (e.g., platelet activating factor) are two types of cell membrane molecules that can convey a signal to another cell by direct contact. Juxtacrine communication allows a cell to restrict a signal only to cells with which it is in direct contact, thereby providing spatial regulation.

Another advantage is that the signal cannot diffuse away. For example, endothelial cells on blood vessels at a very specific part of the body may need to recruit and activate inflammatory cells in response to infection. A membrane-bound signal not only tethers the inflammatory cells to the correct location, but also avoids being washed away by the blood. It has long been known that adhesion molecules on cell surfaces are responsible for binding cells together. In recent years, it has become increasingly clear that these contacts often result in intracellular changes in one or both of the cells making contact.

Paracrine and Autocrine Communication

Other modes of communication work through secreted molecules. **Paracrine communication** occurs when the secreted molecule acts on other cells by traveling through the extracellular matrix. Paracrine communication provides the means of sending a message to cells within a certain diffusion space, without affecting cells that are beyond this space. The signaling molecules are destroyed in local tissues before they have a chance to enter the bloodstream. It is this rapid, local, enzymatic inactivation that restricts the signaling molecule action to a certain space. Local growth, differentiation, and metabolism are coordinated through paracrine communication.

Autocrine communication is a subset of paracrine communication. **Autocrine communication** occurs when the secreted molecule acts on the same cell that secreted it. Growth factors often work through this mechanism. Of course, in order for this mechanism to work, the cell generating the signal must also possess the proper receptor. This makes the signaling cell the target as well.

Endocrine Communication

In addition to secretion into the extracellular matrix, signals can be secreted into the blood stream and travel relatively great distances to reach target cells. This is called **endocrine communication**. The endocrine signaling molecules are called **hormones**. The most important aspect of endocrine signaling is the ability of hormones to affect cells that are far from the signal source.

Gap junction, juxtacrine, autocrine, and paracrine communication all operate to coordinate growth, differentiation, and metabolism in a local setting. The endocrine system, along with the nervous system, facilitates the integration of organ system function.

Neuronal Communication

In **neuronal communication**, a signal is released from a presynaptic neuron and travels through the synaptic cleft to reach the postsynaptic cell. The postsynaptic cell may be another neuron, a muscle fiber, a gland, a cardiac cell, and so on. The signaling neuron uses the synaptic cleft structure to direct its signal toward targets. Molecules secreted into the synaptic cleft that transmit a neural signal are called **neurotransmitters**. Although the signaling event is quite local, the length of axons allows for signaling that affects the whole body.

Neurons with cell bodies at great distances from target cells can communicate by this method because neurotransmitters only need to travel across the relatively small synaptic cleft. The synapse, where the neuron terminal is close to the target cell, is thus a specialized version of paracrine communication. The nervous system is responsible for not only local signaling, but also signaling between the various organ systems.

RECEPTORS AND LIGANDS

Cell-to-cell communication requires a signaling cell, a molecular signal, and a target cell that receives the molecular signal. The target cell is equipped with a **receptor** that recognizes the molecular signal and causes intracellular changes. Receptors can be intracellular or plasma membrane associated, and they are usually proteins. The signal molecules that interact with receptors are called **ligands**. Ligands come from all classes of biomolecules and may act on intracellular or cell membrane associated receptors. Some receptors accommodate more than one ligand, and some ligands bind to more than one receptor.

The main classes of ligands are peptides or proteins, catecholamines, steroids, thyroid hormones, and eicosanoids (FIGURE 3.2). Each class of ligands has a core structure that gives the molecule certain properties. These properties are often useful in predicting a specific molecule's characteristics and mechanisms of action. A signaling molecule may be either hydrophilic or hydrophobic. **Hydrophilic** molecules dissolve well in water but not in lipids. These molecules are often polar, charged, and can interact favorably with water, sometimes using hydrogen bonding. Hydrophilic molecules are soluble in blood and can be stored in membrane vesicles because they cannot diffuse freely through lipids.

Hydrophobic molecules do not dissolve well in water but dissolve well in lipids. They are not very polar, are often uncharged, and cannot form stabilizing interactions with water molecules. Most often, hydrophobic molecules have hydrocarbon structures. They do not dissolve well in blood and must bind to carrier proteins in the blood in order to participate in endocrine signaling. They cannot be stored in membrane vesicles because they are soluble in lipids and would escape the vesicle by diffusion.

Amphipathic molecules are part hydrophilic and part hydrophobic. They are often found in membranes, partly exposed to and partly hidden from water.

Hydrophilic Ligands

Hydrophilic ligands do not cross the lipid bilayer and typically bind to membrane-bound protein receptors. Most peptide and protein hormones are hydrophilic. Catecholamines are hormones based on a single amino acid.

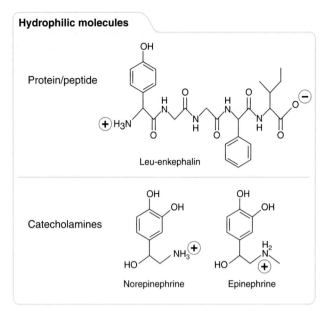

Hydrophilic molecules

Protein/peptide

Leu-enkephalin

Catecholamines

Norepinephrine   Epinephrine

Hydrophobic molecules

Steroids

Cortisol   Testosterone

Estradiol

Thyroid hormone

Thyroxine

Eicosanoid

Prostaglandin E2

Figure 3.2 Examples of some hydrophilic and hydrophobic signal molecules.

examples of the many **peptide or protein hormones**. These protein ligands are hydrophilic. Synthesized like other cellular proteins, they possess a signal sequence called a **signal peptide** that directs them for secretion. After translation has begun in the cytoplasm, a signal recognition complex binds the signal peptide and halts translation. The complex then binds a docking protein on the endoplasmic reticulum. Translation continues and the resulting protein is transported into the endoplasmic reticulum. A signal peptidase enzyme cleaves the signal peptide away, and the protein is transported to the Golgi apparatus. In the Golgi, the protein may be further cleaved or otherwise modified, such as by glycosylation and phosphorylation. Finally, the protein is packaged into a secretory vesicle located in the cytoplasm.

The original translated protein is called a *preprohormone.* After the signal peptide is removed, the protein is called a *prohormone.* The prohormone is then further cleaved either in the Golgi or in the secretory vesicle to form the final hormone product. Because the peptide/protein hormones are hydrophilic and cannot easily cross membranes, they remain stored in secretory vesicles until they are rapidly released for signaling.

Catecholamines   The amine signaling molecules include the catecholamines and the thyroid hormones. Although both are derived from the amino acid tyrosine, **catecholamines** have a second hydroxyl group on the aromatic tyrosine ring, whereas thyroid hormones have an iodinated aromatic ring. The catecholamines are hydrophilic, but thyroid hormones are hydrophobic.

The catecholamines are synthesized by enzymes such as tyrosine hydroxylase, dopamine decarboxylase, and dopamine hydroxylase, which modify the basic tyrosine structure. Because the amines are hydrophilic, they are stored in secretory vesicles like the protein hormones.

Hydrophobic Ligands

Hydrophobic hormones dissolve in the lipid bilayer and typically bind to intracellular receptors. Steroids, thyroid hormone, and eicosanoids are hydrophobic hormones.

Steroids   **Steroids** are hydrophobic, uncharged molecules that are poorly soluble in water. They diffuse freely through lipid membranes. There are five major classes of steroids: glucocorticoids, mineralocorticoids, androgens, estrogens, and progestins (FIGURE 3.3). The adrenal glands, testes, ovaries, and placenta are the main steroid producers

Peptides and Proteins   Follicle-stimulating hormone (FSH), thyroid-stimulating hormone (TSH), adrenocorticotropic hormone (ACTH), cholecystokinin (CCK), insulin-like growth factor (IGF), endothelial growth factor (EGF), angiotensin, and insulin are all

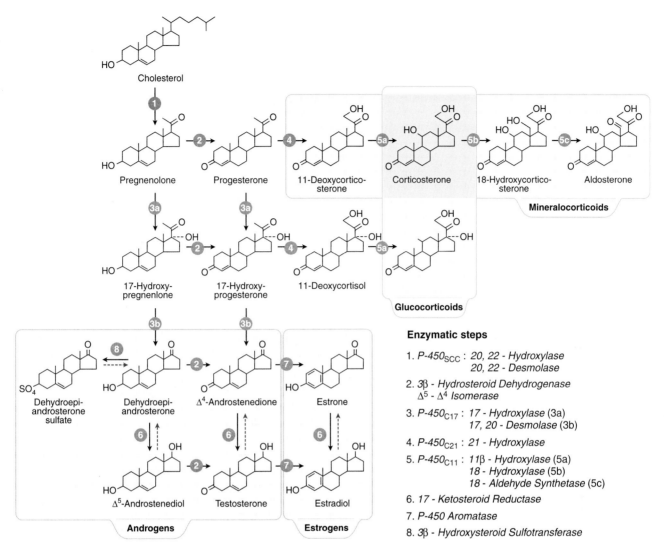

Figure 3.3 Structures and synthetic pathways of steroid hormones. Note that the rate-limiting step in steroid synthesis is the conversion of cholesterol to pregnenolone by the P450 hydroxylase or desmolase enzymes.

in the human body. All steroids are synthesized from cholesterol. The rate-limiting step in steroid synthesis is the conversion of cholesterol to pregnenolone by the desmolase complex. Pregnenolone is then converted to progesterone, and progesterone can be modified in various ways to form different steroid molecules. Much of steroid synthesis is ultimately regulated by the hypothalamus through the anterior pituitary gland. Steroids cannot be stored in any significant quantity because they are hydrophobic hydrocarbons and will pass freely through lipid membranes. Cells need no special mechanism to secrete the steroids because they can diffuse out of the cell after synthesis.

Thyroid Hormones   The **thyroid hormones** thyroxine (also called T_4) and triiodothyronine (also called T_3) are, like the catecholamines, derivatives of the amino acid tyrosine and are produced by the thyroid

gland. They are charged but possess a large hydrophobic hydrocarbon region that makes them poorly soluble in water (see Figure 3.2). Because of their hydrophobicity, they diffuse through lipid membranes. However, they are also carried across membranes by transport systems.

Because the thyroid hormones are hydrophobic and pass through membranes, a special storage mechanism tightly regulates their release. Thyroglobulin is a protein produced in thyroid follicular cells and stored in secretory vesicles. Iodide ions are taken up by these cells and chemically added to some tyrosine residues on the protein (a process called *iodination* or *organification*). An intramolecular reaction between two iodinated tyrosine residues on thyroglobulin occurs, forming T_3 and T_4, depending on whether there are three or four iodide ions, respectively (FIGURE 3.4). At this point, T_3 and T_4 are still covalently bonded to the protein, so that the thyroid

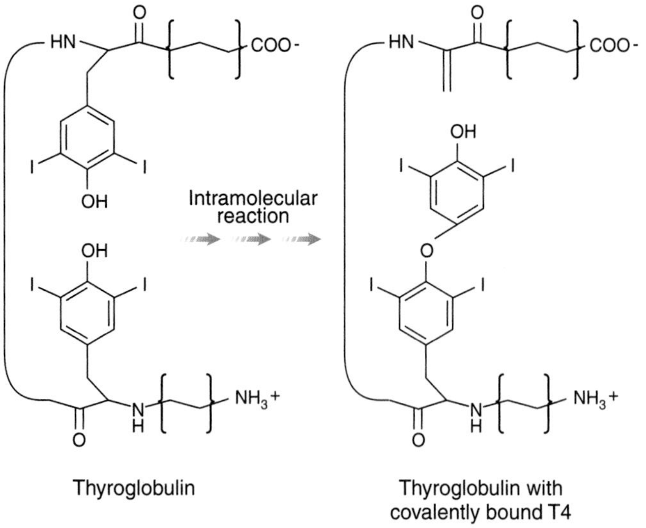

Figure 3.4 The synthesis of thyroxine (T₄) on thyroglobulin. Iodinated tyrosine residues on thyroglobilin combine to form T₄. The hormone cannot reach the circulation and act on its target tissues until it is cleaved from its protein framework by proteolysis.

hormones are unable to diffuse out of the cell in an unregulated manner.

The modified protein is then secreted into the follicular lumen and stored there, where it is termed *colloid*. Upon stimulation by TSH from the anterior pituitary, the follicular cell endocytoses the modified thyroglobulin protein. The endosome then fuses with a lysosome, and acid proteases and peptidases cleave thyroglobulin in multiple places, releasing T_3 and T_4. The hydrophobic T_3 and T_4 are then free to diffuse out of the cell.

Eicosanoids Synthesized by cells in almost every part of the body, **eicosanoids** are hydrophobic hydrocarbons that resemble fatty acids. They are poorly soluble in water and diffuse freely through membranes. The class of eicosanoids includes the prostaglandins (see Figure 3.2), the leukotrienes, and the thromboxanes.

To synthesize eicosanoids, cell membrane lipids (e.g., linoleic acid) are converted to arachidonic acid by enzymes called phospholipases. The enzyme cyclooxygenase converts arachidonic acid into the prostaglandin series of molecules, while the enzyme 5-lipoxygenase converts arachidonic acid into the leukotriene series of molecules. The eicosanoids are not stored because they diffuse freely through membranes.

THE CHRONOLOGY OF CELL-TO-CELL COMMUNICATION

Just as the molecular structure of a signaling molecule dictates its storage and secretion, structure determines a ligand's mode of transport, action on target cells, and eventual inactivation (TABLE 3.1).

Storage and Secretion

The stored signaling molecules are hydrophilic (except for the thyroid hormones) and cannot diffuse through lipid membranes to escape secretory vesicles. Thus, after synthesis, proteins, peptides, and catecholamines are stored in lipid membrane-enclosed vesicles (FIGURE 3.5). The thyroid hormones are also stored; however, as described above, they are bound to thyroglobulin in the follicular space

Table 3.1   THE MAIN CLASSES OF CELL-TO-CELL COMMUNICATION MODULES

	Protein/Peptide	Catecholamine	Steroid	Thyroid Hormone	Eicosanoid
Structure	Hydrophilic	Hydrophilic	Hydrophobic	Hydrophobic	Hydrophobic
Synthesis	Translation machinery	Modification of tyrosine	From cholesterol	Modification of tyrosine	From arachidonic acid
Storage	Membrane vesicles	Membrane vesicles	No	Covalently bonded to thyroglobulin	No
Blood Carriers	Usually not	Usually not	Albumin and specific proteins	Albumin and specific proteins	Usually not
Receptor Site	Cell membrane receptor	Cell membrane receptor	Intracellular receptor	Intracellular receptor	Cell membrane receptor
Inactivation	Uptake + Proteases	Uptake and COMT and MAO	Conjugated by liver and excreted by kidney	Sequential deiodination by microsomal deiodinases	Degraded by widely distributed enzymes

COMT, catechol-O-methyltransferase; MAO, monoamine oxidase.

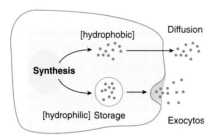

Figure 3.5 Synthesis and secretion of signaling molecules. Hydrophobic molecules are not stored; they leave the cell that produces them via diffusion through the plasma membrane. Hydrophilic ligands, however, are often stored in membrane-enclosed vesicles until they are released via exocytosis.

until released by proteolysis. Signaling molecules that are stored in secretory vesicles can be secreted from a cell faster than molecules that are not stored, because the former do not need to be newly synthesized but accumulate in their vesicles. In general, the stored signaling molecules react to rapid changes in the body that require an immediate response. For example, norepinephrine is a catecholamine neurotransmitter stored in the secretory vesicles of a neuron. It can be secreted from the neuron in the short time it takes for exocytosis of the secretory vesicles. For this reason, norepinephrine is well suited for rapidly responsive neural communication.

The secretion of signaling molecules stored in a vesicle occurs by fusion of the vesicle with the cell membrane. The mechanism involves the cytoskeleton, calcium receptors, and other proteins involved in vesicular exocytosis. This complex process of vesicle movement within the cytosol and its subsequent fusion with the plasma membrane has not been fully elucidated. A number of signals can initiate a rise in intracellular calcium that eventually leads to movement of the vesicle toward the cell membrane, vesicular exocytosis, and secretion of the signaling molecule. Impairment of this process leads to abnormal cell-to-cell communication.

The steroids and eicosanoids cannot be stored and are secreted as they are synthesized (see Figure 3.5). These molecules diffuse out of the cell through the plasma membrane to reach the extracellular space. Because synthesis may take hours, the steroids may be secreted hours after the signal for their secretion was initiated.

The regulation of signaling molecule secretion is quite complex. However, certain general concepts are important to understand. Often, the secretion of a hormone is regulated by **negative feedback.** In order to prevent progressive increases in concentration, some hormones can inhibit their own secretion. Negative feedback may be accomplished by the signaling molecule inhibiting one or more of the mecha-

nisms that lead to its own synthesis and secretion. Conversely, a drop in signal molecule concentration can stimulate increased synthesis and release of the ligand as negative feedback is relieved. These mechanisms are important in stabilizing and preventing sudden changes in signaling molecule levels. Maximum-dose responsiveness is another mechanism that prevents excess hormone action. **Positive feedback** is an opposite mechanism of regulation. Instead of inhibiting, a signal molecule may actually stimulate its own synthesis and secretion. This action enables rapid elevations in hormone levels in response to small stimuli.

Transport

When a given signaling molecule is secreted into the extracellular space, it exists in equilibrium between two "pools." A certain amount is found free in solution while the remainder is bound to one or more proteins. In general, the free molecules in solution are active in cell-to-cell communication because they can leave the capillaries. The hydrophobic signaling molecules, such as the steroids and thyroid hormones, are mainly bound to proteins synthesized by the liver. Albumin may nonspecifically bind these molecules. There are also ligand-specific transport proteins, such as thyroid hormone-binding globulin and sex hormone-binding globulin. Up to 99% of thyroxine (T_4) may be bound to serum proteins during transport in the blood. The protein-bound pool acts as a reservoir that replenishes the free molecules in solution as they are removed from solution by degradation, uptake, or immobilization. It also provides homogeneous delivery of the signaling molecules to all parts of the circulation. The bound pool is usually not subject to degradation or renal excretion, which extends the serum half-life of a hormone. As a result, these hormones often have longer half-lives and long-lasting effects.

In contrast, the water-soluble hydrophilic signaling molecules, such as proteins, peptides, and catecholamines, are generally not bound to proteins (though there are exceptions). Generally, they travel freely in the blood and tissues to their sites of action. Because little or none of these hormones are bound to protein, these molecules are readily subjected to inactivating mechanisms, so they often have short half-lives and short-lasting effects.

Action

As stated previously, signaling molecules either act on cell-surface receptors, or they enter the cell and act on intracellular receptors. Because the hydrophilic signaling molecules do not diffuse well through lipid membranes, they generally act on cell-surface receptors. Some hydrophobic molecules, such as the eicosanoids, also act on cell-surface receptors.

Cell-surface receptors can be divided into three main types (FIGURE 3.6). **Channel-linked receptors** change ion conductance through the plasma membrane after a ligand binds. **Enzyme-linked (catalytic) receptors** have an intracellular portion that acts enzymatically when the extracellular portion is bound by ligand. **G-protein–linked receptors** affect other membrane channels or enzymes when bound by ligand (see Chapter 4). The peptide or protein signal molecules, catacholamines, and eicosanoids act through cell membrane receptors.

Hydrophobic signaling molecules, such as steroids and thyroid hormones, can diffuse through lipid cell membranes and generally act on intracellular receptors. The intracellular receptors may be in the cytoplasm or in the nucleus. Once the signaling molecule binds to a receptor, the complex moves into the nucleus (if binding occurred in the cytoplasm), where it regulates gene transcription by binding to DNA regions called *hormone response elements (HRE)*. Ligand and receptor binding to an HRE may augment or inhibit transcription of the particular target gene (FIGURE 3.7). Transcriptional activation may take an hour to significantly affect mRNA concentrations; however, the hormone effects may last hours to days.

Although altering transcription is the classically accepted mechanism of steroid action, steroids may also act by binding cell membrane receptors. Certain steroid actions, such as neuronal effects and changes in sperm head calcium concentration, occur too rapidly to be mediated through transcription. Recent experiments have identified steroid action at $GABA_A$ and NMDA cell membrane receptors. This implies that steroids may be clinically useful in managing stress, seizure disorders, memory, and postpartum depression.

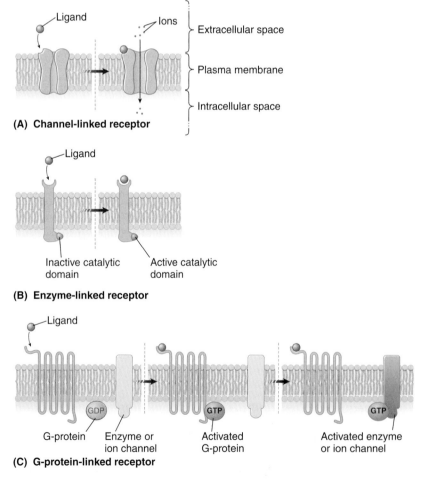

(A) Channel-linked receptor

(B) Enzyme-linked receptor

(C) G-protein-linked receptor

Figure 3.6 Three types of cell surface receptors.

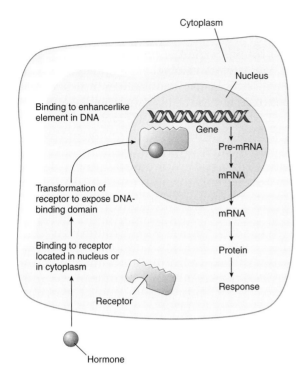

Figure 3.7 The action of steroid hormones on target cells. Hydrophobic steroid hormones cross the plasma membrane to enter the cytoplasm. There, they bind to their receptors and are translocated to the nucleus where the ligand-receptor complex regulates gene transcription. The DNA segments to which ligand-receptor complexes bind are called hormone response elements.

Inactivation and Uptake

After a signaling molecule is secreted, one or more mechanisms may remove it from the extracellular space. Enzymes in the circulation and tissues may enzymatically inactivate signaling molecules. The liver, the site of degradation for many signaling molecules, performs phase I and phase II reactions that chemically modify signaling molecules, making them more water-soluble, so that they may be excreted by the kidney. In general, these enzymatic processes are not active on the protein-bound pool of a signaling molecule. Thus, ligands with large protein-bound pools tend to have longer half-lives.

Signaling molecules may also be removed from the extracellular space by reuptake into the intracellular space. In the synapse, signals from many neurotransmitters are terminated by reuptake of the molecules into nerve terminals. In the case of some ligands, reuptake is a form of recycling, as the same molecules are repackaged into secretory vesicles and can be reused when a subsequent depolarization activates the nerve cell. Other neurotransmitters, such as acetylcholine (ACh), are first metabolized by synaptic enzymes, after which the catabolic products can be taken up by nerve terminals and used to build new signaling molecules.

One way to quantify the removal of a signaling molecule is by defining its *metabolic clearance rate (MCR)*, the volume of plasma cleared of the molecule per unit time (e.g., mL/min). The MCR is a clinically useful index that describes the removal of a molecule from the blood and is inversely proportional to the serum half-life.

PATHOPHYSIOLOGY

When cell-to-cell communication malfunctions, a variety of disorders ensue, depending on the nature of the signal and the direction of displacement from the homeostatic range of the signal (i.e., too much or too little signal; FIGURE 3.8). Hypofunction of a signaling pathway can result from reduced synthesis, reduced secretion, reduced action, and/or excessive inactivation or uptake of the signal molecule. Common examples are enzyme deficiencies, secretion abnormalities, and inactivating receptor mutations. Hyperfunction results from excessive synthesis, excessive secretion, excessive action, or reduced inactivation or uptake of the ligand. Abnormalities of signal receptors may also contribute to disease. Mutations or antagonism of a receptor that block the effect of ligands attenuate signal pathway activity, while other receptor mutations may cause inappropriate hyperfunction, with activation of the receptor in the absence of ligand or oversensitivity of the receptor for ligand.

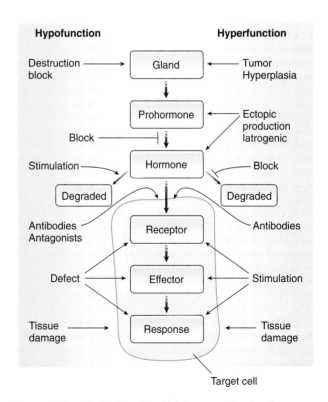

Figure 3.8 Mechanisms by which hormone signal pathways may hyperfunction or hypofunction.

One example of impaired ligand synthesis is ***congenital adrenal hyperplasia* (CAH)**, a group of diseases caused by deficiency in cortisol synthesis. The most common form of CAH is a deficiency in the cytochrome P450 enzyme 21–hydroxylase, which is important for the synthesis of both cortisol and aldosterone in the adrenal gland. Patients with CAH have two major manifestations. They exhibit salt wasting, a disturbance in sodium and potassium homeostasis, because the synthesis of aldosterone is decreased. Without aldosterone, these patients fail to conserve sodium properly and present neonatally with hyponatremia (low serum sodium), hyperkalemia (high serum potassium), and hypovolemic (low blood volume) shock.

Patients also exhibit androgen excess. As cortisol synthesis is deficient, it cannot provide negative feedback to inhibit ACTH secretion by the anterior pituitary. ACTH levels therefore rise and steroid synthesis is increased, especially at the step where cholesterol is converted to pregnenolone. The precursors to cortisol and aldosterone build up in the cell. However, because there is a deficiency in cortisol and aldosterone synthesis, the precursors are used to synthesize androgens. The excess androgens have a variety of physiologic effects. For example, females are born with ambiguous external genitalia as a result of elevated androgens. In summary, the deficiency of 21-hydroxylase leads to symptoms from the lack of products (salt wasting) and also leads to symptoms from the failure of feedback inhibition (androgen excess).

An example of pharmacologic or toxic antagonism of signal molecule synthesis is sometimes seen in patients treated with aspirin. Such patients may develop gastrointestinal symptoms, including ulcer formation. Although factors that damage the stomach and duodenum are normally balanced by protective mechanisms, a change in balance may lead to ulcer formation. Aspirin inhibits the action of cyclooxygenase, an important enzyme in the synthesis of prostaglandins. The positive effects of aspirin, such as pain relief and fever control, are related to this inhibition of prostaglandin synthesis. Unfortunately, prostaglandins also have a protective effect on the GI wall. The decreased synthesis of prostaglandins after exposure to aspirin impairs GI wall protection and increases the probability of ulcer formation.

An example of abnormal signal molecule secretion is the **Lambert-Eaton syndrome**, which is characterized by muscle weakness, especially in the proximal muscles and trunk. Other symptoms include blurred vision, decreased sweating, and a dry mouth. Most patients (70% to 80%) have a malignancy, such as oat cell carcinoma of the lung. Others have autoimmune diseases, such as rheumatoid arthritis and thyroiditis. Patients with Lambert-Eaton syndrome make proteins called antibodies that bind to and block the calcium channel at the presynaptic nerve terminal of the motor endplate. As a result, calcium cannot rush into the cell fast enough to cause the appropriate exocytosis of vesicles and secretion of neurotransmitter. Communication of a neural signal is impeded, and muscle weakness results. Thus, it is an inability to properly exocytose storage vesicles at the neuromuscular junction that leads to the symptoms of Lambert-Eaton syndrome.

Type II diabetes, the most prevalent endocrine disorder, is an example of decreased effect of a signal molecule—in this case, insulin. Patients exhibit hyperglycemia (high blood glucose), glucosuria (glucose in the urine), polyuria (high volume of urine), and polydypsia (excessive thirst). Although various theories exist to explain the disease, it appears that insulin resistance plays a large role in the pathogenesis of this form of diabetes. *Insulin resistance* is a state in which the body does not react properly to circulating levels of insulin. Although there is production, secretion, and receptor binding of insulin, the insulin receptors fail to activate sufficiently. A variety of factors can cause this signaling failure, including insulin receptor mutations and the existence of autoantibodies to the insulin receptor.

Summary

- The major types of cell-to-cell signaling are gap junction, juxtacrine, autocrine, paracrine, endocrine, and neuronal communication.
- Molecular structure determines the properties of a signaling molecule.
- The major classes of molecules used for signaling are peptides or proteins, catecholamines, steroids, thyroid hormones, and eicosanoids.
- The steps in cell-to-cell communication are synthesis, storage, secretion, transport, action, and inactivation or reuptake.
- Malfunctioning in cell-to-cell signaling leads to pathophysiology due to shortage or excess of the signal.

Suggested Reading

Snyder SH. The molecular basis of communication between cells. Sci Am. 1985 Oct;253(4):132–141.

REVIEW QUESTIONS

Directions: Each of the numbered items or incomplete statements in this section is followed by answers or by completions of the statement. Select the ONE lettered answer or completion that is BEST in each case.

1. Which of the following signal molecules is not a protein?
   (A) Follicle-stimulating hormone (FSH)
   (B) Thyroid-stimulating hormone (TSH)
   (C) Thyroxine (T_4)
   (D) Insulin
   (E) Insulin-like growth factor (IGF)

2. Hydrophobic signaling molecules that bind to intracellular receptors generally affect cell function by
   (A) binding to DNA and regulating transcription
   (B) binding to DNA and regulating translation
   (C) binding to RNA and regulating transcription
   (D) binding to RNA and regulating translation
   (E) binding to RNA and regulating conductance

3. The action of a signal molecule can be decreased by each of the following, except
   (A) negative feedback
   (B) positive feedback
   (C) ligand inactivation
   (D) ligand reuptake
   (E) receptor removal

ANSWERS TO REVIEW QUESTIONS

1. **The answer is** C. Unlike the other signal molecules listed, thyroxine (T_4) is not a protein; it is derived from organification or iodination of tyrosine residues of thyroglobulin. In keeping with its hydrophobic molecule structure, T_4 passes through the plasma membrane and binds to an intracellular receptor. This is in contrast to the majority of hydrophilic protein signal molecules that must act on cell-surface receptors.

2. **The answer is** A. While signal molecules that bind intracellular receptors may influence cell function via numerous mechanisms, the majority do so mainly by complexing with their receptor, translocating to the nucleus (if binding occurs in the cytoplasm), and then binding to stretches of DNA called hormone response elements (HRE). This binding often changes the rate and/or efficiency at which nearby genes are expressed by either increasing or decreasing transcription of DNA into RNA.

3. **The answer is** B. Negative feedback occurs when a signal molecule acts to inhibit its own production and/or secretion. Ligand inactivation is the metabolism of a signal molecule to one that has less or no signal activity. Ligand reuptake removes the signal molecule from its receptor. Receptor removal accomplishes the same end. However, positive feedback will increase the synthesis and/or secretion of a ligand, thereby (all else being equal) augmenting its effects.

4

Signal Transduction

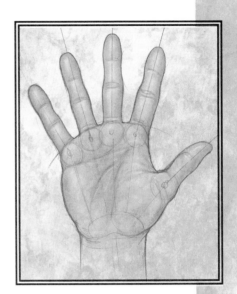

INTRODUCTION

As described in the previous chapter, cell-to-cell signaling occurs via direct contact between cells or across a distance. In the former case, information is passed by means of cell-surface proteins that link cells together biophysically and biochemically. In the latter case, cells communicate by means of molecules secreted from a "talking" cell (the one sending a signal) and picked up by one or more target or "listening" cells. Once a signaling molecule reaches a target cell, it effects changes in that cell that constitute the biological response to the message. While the last chapter focused on extracellular transmission, this chapter focuses on the intracellular changes that occur after a signal has been received from outside the cell.

The changes in the target cell that a signaling molecule brings about may occur in fractions of a second, minutes, hours, days, or even years. However, only some of these changes are the "final goals" the signaling molecule is designed to elicit, and these final goals are often the last in a long chain of intracellular biochemical reactions. The intermediate changes leading up to the final effects are the steps of **signal transduction**, the passage of the message from the initial signaling molecule to the final target cell changes. The word *transduction* (from the Latin meaning "to lead across") refers to various solutions to a simple but important problem: How can information outside the cell get into the cell when the prime function of the plasma membrane (and the nuclear membrane) is to separate the intracellular environment from the extracellular (and the cytoplasmic environment from the nuclear)? Signal transduction systems transport information across the cell membrane and/or nuclear membrane. This chapter focuses on the mechanisms by which information carried by hydrophilic messenger molecules crosses the cell membrane and alters intracellular activity, often culminating in intranuclear changes as well.

RECEPTORS AND LIGANDS IN SIGNAL TRANSDUCTION

Signaling molecules that carry information from a transmitting cell to target cells may be amino acids, peptides, proteins, lipids, nucleotides, even gas molecules. As indicated in Chapter 3, a signaling molecule may be either hydrophilic ("water-loving"), dissolving well in water but not in lipids, or hydrophobic ("water-fearing"), dissolving well in lipids. In addition to heterogeneous chemistry, signaling molecules are characterized by variability in size (e.g., from single amino acids to many thousands in a large protein). Unlike hydrophobic (lipophilic) messengers, which cross the receiving cell's plasma membrane and interact directly with intracellular targets, hydrophilic signaling molecules generally cannot pass through the plasma membrane. Instead, they interact with receptors on the cell surface and relay information by inducing changes on the intracellular face of such receptors.

The physical interaction whereby a hydrophilic signaling molecule fits into the extracellular portion of a cell membrane receptor is known as binding. The Latin word *ligare* means "to bind, connect, join, tie." Signaling molecules (hydrophilic and hydrophobic) are called **ligands** (as described in the previous chapter), and the binding of a messenger molecule to its receptor(s) is called **ligation**.

A signaling molecule may be a ligand for more than one receptor. A single ligand may bind to one, two, or more receptors simultaneously (FIGURE 4.1A). In such a situation, the ligand brings the receptors close together to bring about biochemical changes. If a single ligand molecule connects two receptors, the process is called *receptor dimerization*; if three receptors are ligated, it is called *receptor trimerization*. The receptors so joined may be identical or different.

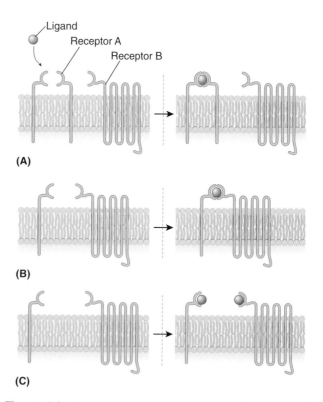

(A)

(B)

(C)

Figure 4.1 Ligands and receptors. **A.** A single ligand molecule may bind to two or more of the same type of receptor. **B.** It may simultaneously bind two or more different types of receptors. **C.** If there are multiple ligand molecules in the environment of the cell, they may bind to different receptors with different binding affinities.

Even if a single ligand molecule only binds one receptor at a time, it may be accommodated by two or more types of receptor (Figure 4.1B), and the different receptors may have different affinities for the ligand as they compete for it (Figure 4.1C).

SIGNALING PATHWAYS, CASCADES, AND NETWORKS

Once a ligand binds to its receptor, it induces a number of biochemical changes in the target cell (FIGURE 4.2). Information is encoded in structural changes, and structural changes can cause functional changes in molecules. A single ligand, even if it binds to a single receptor, may activate an enzyme that metabolizes a substrate 10, 100, or 1,000 times before being "shut off." In other reactions, a single enzyme may lead to the generation of two or more different products (e.g., by cleaving a single molecule into multiple pieces), both or all of which carry important information. Frequently, two or more molecules that were separate when the system was "at rest" combine transiently when the system is activated. Thus, signal transduction systems are characterized by *amplification*, *signal splitting* (e.g., bifurcation, trifurcation), and *signal merging* (the opposite of signal splitting).

Analogies can help clarify signal transduction systems. Portions of a signal transduction system that are linear—that is, where one reaction follows another in series and without amplification, signal splitting, or signal merging—are like a chain reaction or bucket brigade. The components of a signal transduction system are like dominoes set up in a row, such that tipping over the first sets off a cascade that tumbles the others, or like the people in a bucket brigade, each with a different bucket and position in line, at first receiving and then transmitting information (the water or sand in the bucket).

However, the steps of signal transduction systems occur in parallel in some places, especially after a signal is split, so that linear models (signal transduction pathways and cascades in series) may be misleading. More accurate analogies depict the nonlinearity of these systems. Signaling networks are like webs, with a particular molecule "node" receiving inputs and generating outputs that affect multiple components of the system. Often, the output signal affects the "node" itself. Such signaling webs or networks are characterized by feedback loops (positive and negative) and counter-regulatory or antagonistic components. Perhaps the best analogy compares signal transduction systems to language. Ligands are like words, phrases, or clauses, while receptors are like the ears and brains that receive and interpret messages. Just as a single word may have more than one meaning in a given context or to different

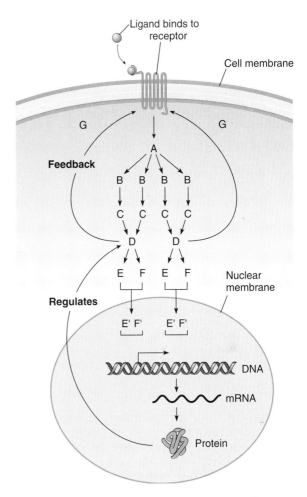

Figure 4.2 A generalized signal transduction system. When a signaling molecule binds to a receptor, an electrochemical or physical change occurs in the receptor and/or proteins associated with the receptor. This change is propagated and transformed, carrying the information away from the ligand-receptor complex. The signal may be amplified, where one A generates many Bs. The signal may integrate, where more than one C is required to induce a single D. Alternatively, the signal may split, where one D gives rise to multiple different changes (E, F, and G, a trifurcation). Often, one or more downstream effects (E and F) converge on the nucleus to alter gene transcription (E′ and F′). Signals are frequently involved in feedback mechanisms, where a downstream change may impact the molecular machinery that helped bring it about (G). Each step is a biochemical or biophysical change in the target cell. Such steps are often (rapidly) reversible and may be points where the target cell regulates its response to signaling molecules (as a protein regulates the function of step D).

audiences, one ligand may have different effects on different cells at different times and under different circumstances. A given ligand often acts on a target cell, while many other ligands are doing the same, thereby creating a context in which many signals are received in series and in parallel.

The human body consists of diverse populations of differentiated cells. Cell populations differ widely in the expression of cell-surface receptors, as well as in downstream signaling machinery. (The term "downstream" is used to indicate events occurring after an initiating event.) These differences in cells account for the variability and specificity of signaling effects (particularly in the case of hormones, which are diffusely distributed). Receptor expression, for example, may vary from cell to cell; the same signaling molecule produces different effects in different cells, depending on the abundance and the subtype of receptor expressed. The same is true for the intracellular components of signaling networks. Because every element of a signaling network is potentially a regulatory site, the differential expression of regulatory molecules is another potential source of diversity. Moreover, cellular "decisions" (e.g., whether or not to grow, divide, secrete factors, or express certain genes) are made by integrating signals from multiple pathways, which often have overlapping and interacting regulatory species.

THREE TYPES OF PLASMA MEMBRANE RECEPTORS

The receptors for hydrophilic ligands are proteins embedded in the cell's plasma membrane. They may be composed of one or many polypeptide chains. The extracellular portion contains the ligand binding site(s). One or more *transmembrane domains* cross the plasma membrane and anchor the receptor, although receptors may "float" within the plane of the membrane. The intracellular portion of the receptor is the part that alters the cell interior in response to ligand binding. Thus, in the strictest sense, it is the receptor that transduces extracellular signals, carrying information across the plasma membrane from the extracellular space to the intracellular cytoplasm. There are three main types of cell-surface receptors: ion channel-linked, G-protein–linked, and enzyme-linked.

Ion Channel-Linked Receptors

Ion channel-linked receptors are either associated with or are themselves pores in the plasma membrane that, when open, allow specific ions to pass from one compartment to another (e.g., from the extracellular to the intracellular space). When an ion channel-linked receptor binds its ligand(s), an alteration in cell membrane permeability to one or more ions occurs because the pore in the membrane changes its state; if it was closed, it opens, or vice-versa. This type of receptor is critical for the function of such cells as neurons and muscles, where the transmembrane electrical potential is tightly regulated and changes in that potential are critical to cell activity (see Chapter 5). An important example of an ion channel-linked receptor is the *acetylcholine receptor*. When a ligand such as acetylcholine (ACh) binds to AChR, the receptor undergoes a steriochemical change. A pore, or water-filled channel, opens in its center, allowing ion(s), such as Na^+ and Ca^{2+}, normally relatively restricted to the extracellular space, to cross the plasma membrane. The change in the concentrations of such ions across the cell membrane causes the transmembrane electrical potential to change as well. The direction and magnitude of the change in membrane potential depend on the types of ions involved, and how much and in what way their extracellular and intracellular concentrations are altered. The Goldman equation quantifies the alteration in the membrane electrical potential on the basis of different extracellular and intracellular ion concentrations (see Chapter 5).

G-Protein–Linked Receptors

G-protein–linked receptors are single proteins that have seven transmembrane domains (i.e., they cross the cell membrane seven times). Their extracellular portions contain the ligand binding domain(s), determining the specificity of the receptor. These receptors are named for the ability of their intracellular domain to associate with a three-component complex called a *trimeric GTP binding protein*, or more simply, *G-protein*. There are many different types of G-proteins, with distinct downstream effects. As the first part of their name implies, however, all *trimeric* G-proteins are made up of three distinct subunits: α, β, and γ. G-proteins adhere to the inner leaflet of the plasma membrane via the α and γ subunits. Important examples of G-protein–linked receptors are those for epinephrine.

FIGURE 4.3 shows signal transduction by a G-protein–linked receptor. Before a ligand binds to the G-protein–linked receptor, the α subunit of the G-protein binds to a molecule of guanosine diphosphate (GDP) and associates with the β and γ subunits. When a signal molecule binds to the receptor's extracellular ligand binding domain, an allosteric (or conformational) change in the receptor allows the G protein's α subunit to bind, linking the activated receptor to the inactive G protein. Once the receptor's intracellular segment associates with a G protein, the α subunit releases its molecule of GDP and binds a molecule of guanosine triphosphate (GTP). This exchange of GDP for GTP results in dissociating the α subunit from the β + γ dimer and activating both these components of the G-protein. The GTP binding, activated α subunit goes on to activate its target protein(s), depending on the specific type of G-protein. For example, the α subunit of the G-protein G_s binds to and activates the membrane-bound enzyme adenylyl cyclase. In contrast, the α

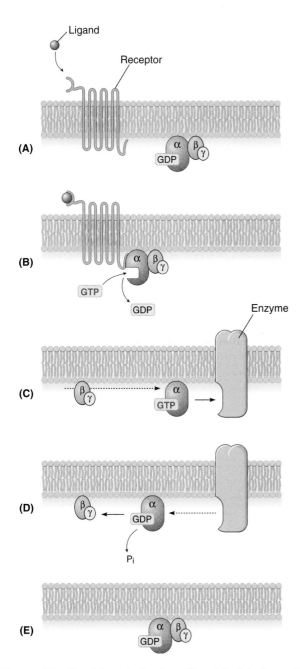

Figure 4.3 Signal transduction by a G-protein–linked receptor. **A.** At rest, the receptor's extracellular domain is unoccupied and the trimeric GTP binding protein is unactivated, with a molecule of GDP bound to the α subunit. **B.** When a ligand binds, the receptor is activated, allowing the binding of the G-protein and exchange of GDP for GTP by the α subunit. **C.** The activated α subunit dissociates from the β + γ dimer and alters its target(s). The β + γ dimer also transmits signals to other targets (not shown). **D.** Eventually, the α subunit cleaves the terminal phosphate (P_i) from its bound GTP, forming GDP, and thereby inactivating itself. **E.** The inactive α subunit then re-associates with the β and γ subunits to restore the G protein to its resting state.

subunit of G_i inhibits adenylyl cyclase, among other actions. The α subunit of G_q activates a different membrane-bound enzyme, phospholipase C-β (PLC-β). Meanwhile, the activated β + γ dimer may alter the function of its target protein(s) as well. The

activated β + γ subunit of some G-proteins may interact with transmembrane ion channels to alter their state. A crucial feature of signal transduction systems is the ability to "reset" the molecular machinery back to the resting state. Activating signals have to be shut off, and inhibitory signals that may be tonically active, once shut off to stimulate a cell, have to be restarted. In the case of G-protein–linked receptors, this is accomplished by the intrinsic GTP-ase enzymatic activity of the α subunit. The activated α subunit not only transmits signals by altering targets such as adenylyl cyclase, but also cleaves the third (terminal) phosphate off of GTP, producing a molecule of GDP and an inorganic phosphate. In so doing, the activated α subunit shuts itself off. Once the GTP has been cleaved to GDP, the inactive α subunit re-associates with the β + γ dimer, and the trimeric G-protein reassumes its resting state.

Second Messenger: Cyclic AMP   Signaling molecules are sometimes called *first messengers* because they are the first in the chain to carry information from the "talking" cell that releases them to target "listening" cells. Hydrophilic first messengers cannot cross the plasma membrane to enter the cell. Their binding to cell-surface receptors initiates signal transduction, but the signal has to be transmitted from the plasma membrane to the target cell's interior.

Some intracellular molecules are generated in response to the binding of first messenger to cell-surface receptors; as the internal counterparts to first messengers, they are called *second messengers*. Just as first messengers are released by one or more cells and travel through the extracellular space until they reach receptors on target cells, second messengers are generated by enzymes closely associated with ligand-bound, activated cell-surface receptors and travel through the intracellular space until they reach their target(s). Second messengers are often small molecules or even ions. The production of second messengers is often a point of amplification in a signal transduction pathway, and because second messengers may have great effects on cell function, their concentrations are carefully monitored and their generation tightly regulated. Two important examples of second messengers are cyclic adenosine monophosphate and ionic calcium (Ca^{2+}).

First, we turn to **cyclic AMP (cAMP)**. The activated α subunit of G_s increases the enzymatic activity of adenylyl cyclase. This enzyme converts ATP by the removal of the two terminal phosphate groups and cyclization, the creation of a new bond between the remaining phosphate group and the 3′ carbon of the sugar component of adenosine (hence, *cyclic* AMP). The intracellular concentration of cAMP in the absence of stimulatory signals is approximately 50 to

100 nM (0.5–1 × 10^{-7} M). Activation of adenylyl cyl-case can lead to a rapid increase in this concentration to more than 1 μM (1 × 10^{-6} M).

Prominent among the effects of cAMP is the activation of the enzyme *protein kinase A (PKA)*. A **kinase** is an enzyme that adds one or more phosphate groups to a substrate, often a very important mechanism for altering the structure and/or function of the substrate. The substrates for kinases are frequently proteins and enzymes. Kinases typically add phosphate groups to specific amino acids on target proteins; some kinases are specific for serine and threonine residues, while others phosphorylate only tyrosines. PKA is a serine/threonine kinase. The effects of kinases are balanced or antagonized by **phosphatases**, enzymes that remove the phosphate group(s) added to substrates by kinases. Many kinases and phosphatases differ in structure, substrate specificity, the mechanisms by which their activities are regulated, and the cells and subcellular compartments where they are expressed and function.

The process of PKA activation by cAMP is shown in FIGURE 4.4. In a resting state, dimers of PKA are bound by dimers of regulatory proteins that keep the kinases inactive. These inhibitory regulatory proteins can bind cAMP. In the resting state, the low intracellular concentration of cAMP makes this uncommon. However, activation of adenylyl cyclase leads to increased intracellular cAMP concentrations. The greater availability of cAMP results in the binding of this second messenger to the regulatory proteins, which undergo a conformational change and release PKA. The kinase is then free to phosphorylate its substrates.

An important example of such a PKA target is the skeletal muscle enzyme phosphorylase kinase. When PKA phosphorylates phosphorylase kinase, it activates it, resulting in the breakdown of glycogen stores into glucose, which is used by the muscle cell to fuel contraction. By this mechanism, the hormone epinephrine enhances muscle performance: Epinephrine binds to the β adrenergic receptor on the surface of skeletal muscle cells, activating the G_s α subunit, which increases adenylyl cyclase synthesis of cAMP. The increased intracellular concentration of cAMP liberates PKA, which leads to the activation of phosphorylase kinase and the breakdown of glycogen into glucose. The increased availability of glucose allows muscle to contract more than it otherwise could (see Chapter 6).

A number of important genes have *cAMP response elements (CRE)*, DNA sequences that regulate transcription of these genes. When a *CRE binding (CREB) protein* binds to the CRE sequence, transcription of the genes is increased. However, in order to bind to the CRE, CREB must be phosphorylated and

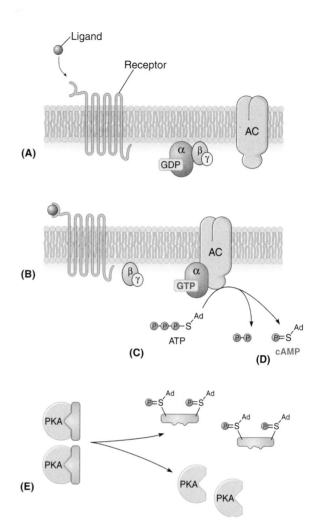

Figure 4.4 The activation of PKA by cAMP. A G_s α subunit activates adenylyl cyclase (AC), leading to increased cAMP production and activation of PKA. **A.** The G_s α subunit is activated by exchanging GDP for GTP. **B.** Adenylyl cyclase is activated. **C.** AC cleaves off the two terminal phosphates of ATP and cyclizes the molecule. **D.** cAMP is created. **E.** cAMP binds to the regulatory proteins that inhibit PKA, causing them to release the kinase.

bound by yet another protein, called *CREB binding protein (CBP)*. PKA phosphorylates CREB, allowing CBP to bind to it, and for this heterodimer (CBP + phosphorylated CREB) to bind to the CRE DNA sequence (FIGURE 4.5). Thus, when intracellular cAMP concentrations rise and PKA is activated, the kinase, liberated from its regulatory proteins, moves to the nucleus where it phosphorylates CREB. Phosphorylated CREB binds to CBP, and together they bind to the CRE and augment transcription (see Figure 4.5).

How does such a subsystem, once activated, get shut off? The enzymatic GTP-ase activity of the G_s α subunit ensures that, in time, the stimulation of adenylyl cyclase ceases. In addition, the activated α subunit of G_i inhibits adenylyl cyclase, so that a ligand binding to a G_i-linked receptor may antagonize

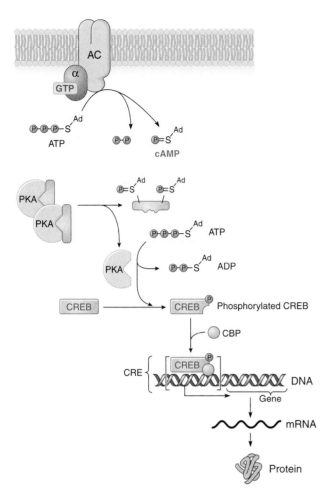

Figure 4.5 PKA activation and CREB phosphorylation. The activation of PKA leads to the phosphorylation of CREB, which can then bind to CREB binding protein (CBP). This heterodimer binds to the cAMP response elements (CRE) on specific genes and augments their transcription, leading to more mRNA production and greater protein synthesis.

the effects of a ligand binding to a G_s-linked receptor. A single ligand that binds to both types of receptor but with different affinities and/or time courses may thereby regulate its own effects on target cells. (See Clinical Application Box *Abnormalities of Signal Transduction in Human Diseases.*)

FIGURE 4.6 illustrates what happens to the increased intracellular concentration of cAMP. Counteracting adenylyl cyclase is the enzyme cAMP phosphodiesterase (cAMP PDE), which breaks the bond between the phosphate group and the 3′ carbon of adenosine's sugar, thus converting cAMP into AMP. When adenylyl cyclase activity decreases to the resting level, cAMP PDE works to restore the intracellular cAMP concentration to the prestimulation value. As the cAMP concentration decreases, molecules of the second messenger dissociate from the PKA regulatory proteins, which then reassume their original conformation, re-associate with PKA,

and again inhibit their kinase activity. Likewise, protein targets of PKA that have been phosphorylated may return to their unphosphorylated state by the action of one or more phosphatases that counteract PKA activity.

Second Messenger: Calcium Some signaling molecules, including acetylcholine and vasopressin, mediate some of their effects by means of seven transmembrane receptors associated with the G_q protein. Unlike G_s and G_i, which mediate their effects through adenylyl cyclase, G_q works through the enzyme phospholipase C-β (PLC-β). PLC-β cleaves the phosphoinositide 4,5-bisphosphate (PI(4,5)P$_2$), a component of the inner leaflet of the plasma membrane. PI(4,5)P$_2$ has two fatty acid chains connected to a three-carbon glycerol backbone. Attached to the third carbon is a phosphate group. This phosphate group is linked to an inositol molecule at carbon 1, while two other phosphates are at carbons 4 and 5. When a ligand binds to a G_q-coupled receptor, the α subunit exchanges GDP for GTP and activates PLC-β. PLC-β then enzymatically breaks the chemical bond between the phosphate group at carbon 1 and the glycerol backbone. This cleavage produces two products: (1) the glycerol backbone and the two fatty acid chains, called *diacylglycerol (DAG)*, which remains embedded in the cell membrane; and (2) the inositol molecule with three phosphate groups—inositol 1,4,5-triphosphate (IP$_3$), which is free to diffuse into the cytosol. Both DAG and IP$_3$ participate in the G_q induced signaling cascade.

IP$_3$ introduces the second messenger of this signaling pathway by binding to and opening an ion channel in the cell's endoplasmic reticulum (ER). In the cytosol, ion pumps maintain a low intracellular Ca^{2+} concentration, typically about 1×10^{-7} M. Within the ER and outside the cell, however, the Ca^{2+} concentration is 10,000-fold greater. When IP$_3$ opens the ion channel in the ER, there is a rapid release of Ca^{2+} into the cytosol, increasing the intracellular Ca^{2+} concentration 10 to 20 times.

Meanwhile, the DAG that remained embedded in the plasma membrane allows another enzyme, *protein kinase C (PKC)*, to bind or "dock," but PKC bound to DAG is not fully active until it also binds Ca^{2+} ions. Thus, the two arms of the G_q pathway that arose when PLC-β cleaved PI(4,5)P$_2$ into IP$_3$ and DAG reunite: DAG localizes PKC to the inner leaflet of the plasma membrane, while IP$_3$ effects the increase in intracellular Ca^{2+} necessary for full PKC activation (see FIGURE 4.7). Activated PKC, a serine/threonine kinase, phosphorylates a number of cell-specific targets, including the signal transduction enzyme mitogen-activated protein kinase (MAPK) and the inhibitor (IκB) of the transcription factor nuclear factor κB (NFκB).

CLINICAL APPLICATION

ABNORMALITIES OF SIGNAL TRANSDUCTION IN HUMAN DISEASES

A number of diseases bring about changes in cell, tissue, organ, and organ system physiology because, at the molecular level, they alter signal transduction network activity. The bacterium *Vibrio cholera*, for example, produces a protein toxin. When this cholera toxin enters epithelial cells lining the gastrointestinal tract, it enzymatically removes an ADP ribose from intracellular NAD^+ and adds it to the α subunit of G_s. This modification inhibits the intrinsic GTP-ase activity of the α subunit, making it impossible for this molecule to shut itself off. The chronically activated α subunit continues to stimulate adenylyl cyclase, with subsequent overproduction of cAMP. The pathologically elevated intracellular cAMP concentration induces epithelial cells to secrete tremendous amounts of Cl^- and water into the lumen of the GI tract. This massive Cl^- and water efflux is the basis of the voluminous diarrhea that characterizes **cholera**.

Similarly, the bacterium *Bordetella pertussis* produces a toxin that ADP ribosylates the α subunit of G_i, inhibiting it from binding to seven transmembrane receptors. This kills or impairs immune cells that would eradicate the bacteria. *Bordetella pertussis* is the lung pathogen responsible for **whooping cough**.

A fascinating example of signal transduction dysregulation occurs in the blood cancer called **chronic myelogenous leukemia (CML)**. Cells in patients with CML often have a chromosomal abnormality in which there is a fusion between the long arms of chromosomes 9 and 22. This leads to the formation of a new gene that encodes an unregulated tyrosine kinase called BCR-ABL. The hyperfunction of BCR-ABL is critical to the proliferation of the cancerous white blood cells. Recently, a small molecule that can fit into the ATP binding site of BCR-ABL and blocks its function has been shown to be effective in the treatment of this serious malignancy.

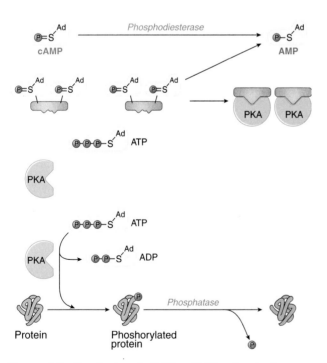

Figure 4.6 The cleaving of cAMP into AMP by phosphodiesterase. Phosphodiesterase breaks the cyclic structure of cAMP, forming AMP. As the intracellular concentration of cAMP declines, the PKA inhibitory proteins reassume their native shape, and with it their ability to bind and inhibit PKA. The protein substrates that have been phosphorylated by active PKA may be dephosphorylated by specific phosphatases.

Ca^{2+} is a powerful second messenger used by other signal transduction systems in addition to G-protein–linked receptors. Among the other mechanisms by which Ca^{2+} effects changes in cells is the binding of four Ca^{2+} to the protein calmodulin. When the intracellular concentration of Ca^{2+} increases, more ions are available to bind to calmodulin, which alters the protein's conformation. The Ca^{2+}-calmodulin complex then binds to and activates a number of protein kinases, known collectively as *Ca^{2+}-calmodulin-dependent protein kinases (CaM-kinases)*. Activation of such kinases leads to the phosphorylation of their respective substrates. As with other systems, the activity of various phosphatases antagonizes that of the kinases, so that activation signals are shut off and the cascade is reset (FIGURE 4.8). ATP-fueled ion pumps return the intracellular Ca^{2+} concentration to its resting value by either extruding Ca^{2+} from the cytosol into the extracellular space or sequestering it in the ER.

Enzyme-Linked Receptors

Enzyme-linked receptors are transmembrane proteins that are enzymes themselves or are closely associated with enzymes. Enzyme-linked receptors are important in processes such as cell growth, adherence,

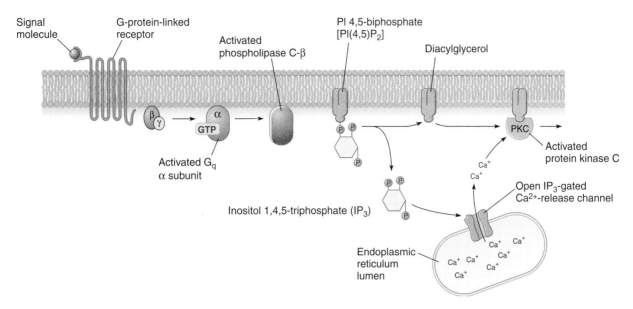

Figure 4.7 Activation of phospholipase C-β (PLC-β) by activation of the G_q α subunit. PLC-β cleaves PI(4,5)P_2 into IP_3 and DAG. IP_3 induces the efflux of Ca^{2+} from intracellular stores such as the ER, while DAG binds to and activates (in conjunction with Ca^{2+}) PKC.

and movement. Unlike G-protein–linked receptors, most enzyme-linked receptors have only one transmembrane domain. This type of receptor can be subdivided into those with kinase activity and those with phosphatase activity.

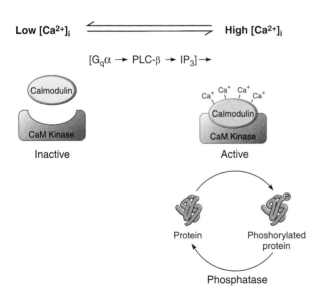

Figure 4.8 Increased intracellular Ca^{2+} concentrations ([Ca^{2+}]$_i$) and the activation of CaM kinases. CaM kinases require calcium-bound calmodulin. Once activated, CaM kinases phosphorylate target substrates. As ion pumps resequester Ca^{2+} ions into the ER or extrude them from the cell, the [Ca^{2+}]$_i$ decreases, Ca^{2+} dissociates from calmodulin, and the CaM kinases are inactivated. Target proteins that have been phosphorylated may resume their previous state by being dephosphorylated by specific phosphatases.

Kinases Among the best characterized enzyme-linked receptors are those with an intracytoplasmic segment that has one or more domains with tyrosine kinase activity. Importantly, the intracytoplasmic tails of such receptors also have tyrosine residues, often both inside and outside the kinase domain(s). Whereas with G-protein–linked receptors, a single molecule of ligand may bind to and activate a receptor, this is generally not true of receptor tyrosine kinases. Instead, ligand (monomer, dimer, trimer, or higher-order oligomer or polymer) binds to and thereby connects (or "cross-links") two (dimerization), three (trimerization), or more (oligomerization) receptors. As a result, the intracytoplasmic domains of the receptors are aggregated. Activation of these aggregated receptors occurs when a kinase domain of one receptor phosphorylates one or more tyrosine residues on a neighboring receptor's intracytoplasmic tail. This reciprocal process (i.e., each receptor tail both phosphorylates and is phosphorylated by another) is called *autophosphorylation* (FIGURE 4.9). If the tyrosines that are phosphorylated are inside a kinase domain, this tends to increase kinase activity; phosphorylation of tyrosines outside a kinase domain often generates a docking site for other proteins in the signal transduction network.

Proteins and other molecules do not simply stick to each other at random; they have domains that mediate specific binding to one or more amino acid sequences called motifs. The Src-homology 2 (SH2) domain, one of the most important types of domains, specifies the binding of the protein having such a domain with another having a sequence containing a phosphorylated tyrosine (or phosphotyro-

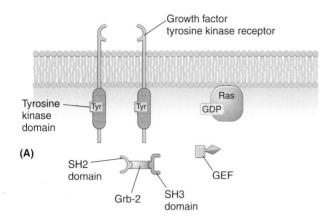

(A)

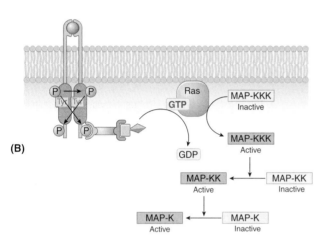

(B)

Figure 4.9 The oligomerization and activation of enzyme-linked receptors by ligands. Ligand binds to the extracellular domains of two or more tyrosine kinase receptors, causing them to autophosphory-late. This allows SH2-containing proteins such as GRB-2 to bind to the phospho-tyrosine residues on the receptors. In this example, GRB-2 binds to Ras GEF by the GRB-2 SH3 domain. GEF expedites the exchange by Ras of GDP for GTP, and the subsequent activation of this critical signaling molecule. Activated (i.e., GTP-bound) Ras activates mitogen-activated protein kinase kinase kinase (MAP KKK), which activates MAP KK, which activates MAP K, which phosphorylates and activates a number of targets, eventually altering gene expression.

sine). When tyrosine kinase receptors autophosphorylate in response to ligand-mediated oligomerization and activation, they allow SH2-containing proteins to dock. These proteins may have enzymatic activity of their own, or they may be linkers, allowing additional proteins to dock near the activated receptors.

An important example of this mechanism is the activation of the Ras signaling molecule (see Figure 4.9). Like the α subunit of trimeric G-proteins, Ras is active when it binds to GTP and inactive when it binds to GDP. Cross-linking of some growth factor receptors leads to tyrosine autophosphorylation. A

linker molecule called GRB-2 binds to a phosphotyrosine on the receptor by means of the GRB-2 SH2 domain. GRB-2 also has an SH3 domain that mediates binding to motifs containing proline residues. Like GRB-2, many important signaling proteins have more than one SH2 and/or SH3 domains, allowing them to aggregate two, three, or more network components.

Other important enzyme-linked receptors do not have kinase activity themselves. Instead, they have intracytoplasmic domains that associate with nonreceptor tyrosine kinases. These kinases are activated when the receptors are cross-linked and often phosphorylate their receptors. Examples of this subtype of enzyme-linked receptor are the growth hormone receptor and antigen receptors on T cells.

Phosphatases It was once generally accepted that a cell remained "at rest" until it received one or more activating signals. Once such a signal was received and the cell responded by changing shape, dividing, secreting substances, and so on, researchers thought that termination of activation would occur when ligands drifted off of activating receptors and were removed or metabolized, the activating receptor was internalized (sequestered) or chemically modified so that it could no longer respond to ligand (desensitized), and/or the cell would "slow down on its own" from a type of metabolic inertia. Cells that did not slow down, such as cancer cells, were thought to suffer from chronic activation. Increasingly, however, an appreciation for the importance of antagonistic signaling systems has arisen. Some cell-surface receptors are inhibitory and actively stop or prevent the cell from responding to activation signals. In other words, cells are like cars that have both gas pedals (activating receptors) and breaks (inhibitory receptors); they don't just slow down by letting up on the gas. Cells that are chronically activated may have one or more defects in such inhibitory receptors.

Many inhibitory receptors are enzyme-linked and have phosphatase activity (FIGURE 4.10). Often, the intracytoplasmic domain of such a receptor does not have phosphatase activity itself, but has tyrosine residues that, when phosphorylated by the kinase activity of an activating receptor, allow a nonreceptor phosphatase to dock. Once it docks, such a nonreceptor phosphatase may also be tyrosine phosphorylated by a kinase (e.g., from an activating receptor), and thereby activated. The activated phosphatase then enzymatically clips off the phosphate groups the kinase has added to its substrates, thus undoing the activation work of the kinase.

An important example is the family of killer inhibitory receptors (KIR) on the surface of immune

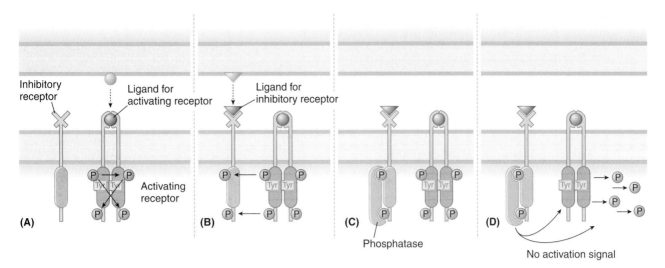

Figure 4.10 Enzyme-linked receptors with associated phosphatases as inhibitory receptors. **A.** The ligand for an activating receptor is presented to the lower cell by the upper cell, causing receptor protein tyrosine kinase aggregation (cross-linking) and autophosphorylation, with the generation of an activation signal. However, if the presenting upper cell also displays the ligand for an inhibitory receptor, the two types of receptor are coligated. **B.** The tyrosine kinases of the activating receptors phosphorylate the intracellular domain of the inhibitory receptor. **C.** This creates a docking site for a nonreceptor tyrosine phosphatase. **D.** This phosphatase then dephosphorylates the activating receptor (and perhaps its own receptor, and even itself) to inhibit or terminate an activation signal.

cells called natural killers. *Natural killer (NK) cells* patrol the body and destroy invaders or body cells that have been damaged or compromised by infection or mutation. But normal, healthy body cells have to have a way of escaping destruction by NK cells, so natural killers display KIR on their surface. The ligands for the KIR are MHC I proteins expressed on the surface of healthy cells, but not on the surface of bacteria or some cancer cells. When an NK cell meets an invader or cancer cell, it latches on by means of an activating receptor that initiates a signal transduction system in the NK cell, causing activation and destruction of the target. When an NK cell encounters a normal cell, it likewise binds with an activating receptor. However, the NK cell also engages the target cell's MHC I by means of one or more KIR. A ligand-bound KIR can recruit a phosphatase that inhibits activation signals, effectively preventing the NK cell from destroying the target cell.

Summary

- Signaling molecules may be hydrophobic or hydrophilic. Hydrophobic signaling molecules can pass through the plasma membrane to transmit signals directly, but hydrophilic molecules need to transmit information across the plasma membrane via one or more receptors.

- Extracellular hydrophilic messenger molecules that bind to cell membrane receptors are called ligands.

- The three main types of cell-surface receptors are ion channel-linked, G-protein–linked, and enzyme-linked.

- When a ligand binds to an ion channel-linked receptor, the channel changes its state (i.e., the probability that it is opened or closed, depending on the cell, the receptor, and the ligand). Changes in ion channel state alter the ion permeability of the plasma membrane and, with it, the membrane potential.

- G-protein–linked receptors have seven transmembrane domains and associate with trimeric GTP-binding proteins.

- Among the G-proteins, the α subunit of G_s activates adenylyl cyclase, which leads to increased production of cAMP and activation of protein kinase A (PKA). The α subunit of G_q activates PLC-β, which leads to intracellular Ca^{2+} release and activation of PKC.

- Ligand binding to cell-surface receptors often leads to changes in the intracellular concentrations of second messengers such as cAMP and Ca^{2+}.

- Receptor protein kinases often must be cross-linked by ligands to autophosphorylate each other.

- Specific protein domains, such as SH2 and SH3 domains, mediate specific binding of one protein to another.

- Many important receptors are inhibitory. Some recruit protein phosphatases that enzymatically remove phosphate groups from proteins that have been activated by one or more kinases.

Suggested Reading

Attisiano S, Wrana JL. Signal transduction by the TGF-β superfamily. Science. 2002;296:1646–1647.

Morris AJ, Malbon CC. Physiological regulation of G protein-linked signaling. Physiol Rev. 1999 Oct;79(4): 1373–1430.

Neves SR, Ram PT, Iyengar R. G protein pathways. Science. 2002;296:1636–1639.

REVIEW QUESTIONS

Directions: Each of the numbered items or incomplete statements in this section is followed by answers or by completions of the statement. Select the ONE lettered answer or completion that is BEST in each case.

1. Cholera toxin works by
   (A) ADP ribosylating the G_s α subunit
   (B) ADP ribosylating the G_i α subunit
   (C) ADP ribosylating the G_q α subunit
   (D) ADP ribosylating the G_s β subunit
   (E) ADP ribosylating the G_i γ subunit

2. Pertussis toxin works by

(A) ADP ribosylating the G_s α subunit
(B) ADP ribosylating the G_i α subunit
(C) ADP ribosylating the G_q α subunit
(D) ADP ribosylating the G_s β subunit
(E) ADP ribosylating the G_i γ subunit

3. In chronic myelogenous leukemia, the 9;22 translocation produces

(A) a dysregulated ion channel-linked receptor
(B) an abnormally expressed G-protein–linked receptor
(C) an overactive G_s α subunit
(D) an abnormal tyrosine kinase
(E) an underactive tyrosine phosphatase

4. A 58-year-old woman develops breast cancer. Histopathology demonstrates a mutant Ras protein that is constitutively (i.e., always) activated. Such a protein may have a defect in

(A) ATP binding
(B) GTP binding
(C) cleaving ATP into ADP
(D) cleaving GTP into GDP
(E) exchanging ADP and GDP for ATP and GTP

ANSWERS TO REVIEW QUESTIONS

1. **The answer is A.** Cholera toxin works by adding an ADP ribose to the $G_s \alpha$ subunit, impairing its intrinsic GTP-ase activity. Thus, this subunit, when activated by exchanging GDP for GTP, is unable to shut itself off by cleaving the terminal phosphate on GTP to form GDP. It therefore continues to activate adenylyl cyclase, which increases the intracellular concentration of cAMP. This leads to an abnormally high efflux of Cl^- and water out of cells that line the GI tract, causing the profuse watery diarrhea of cholera.

2. **The answer is B.** Pertussis toxin adds an ADP ribose to the $G_i \alpha$ subunit, preventing it from interacting with seven transmembrane receptors. This leads to dysfunction and the death of immune cells that would combat the *Bordetella pertussis* bacterium that causes whooping cough.

3. **The answer is D.** In CML, the translocation (9;22) creates a new gene that encodes an unregulated tyrosine kinase that chronically stimulates affected white blood cells. The proliferation of these cells constitutes the malignancy.

4. **The answer is D.** Like G_α, Ras is inactive when it is bound to GDP and active when bound to GTP. The protein GEF catalyzes the exchange of GDP for GTP, leading to Ras activation. In order to shut off, Ras, with the help of a molecule called GTP-ase activating protein (GAP), enzymatically cleaves off the terminal phosphate of its GTP molecule, transforming it into GDP. A mutant Ras molecule unable to perform such an enzymatic step would be unable to turn off and would continue sending stimulatory signals to the affected cell. This is a common mutation in many human cancers.

5

An Overview of Nerve Cell Physiology and the Autonomic Nervous System

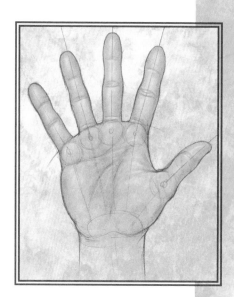

INTRODUCTION

The nervous system is arguably the most complex and least understood body system. Intriguing subjects such as the gathering and processing of sensory information, balance and muscle coordination, language, thought, emotion, and consciousness are outside the scope of this text. However, the nervous system actively participates in, regulates, and integrates all the other body systems. This chapter focuses first on the cellular physiology of **neurons** (nerve cells) and then on the **autonomic nervous system (ANS)**, a subsystem that seems to work autonomously; that is, it generally influences physiology independent of and undetected by conscious awareness. Individual neurons gather, process, and transmit information by means of electrochemical signals. The ANS receives information from the other body systems (the internal environment) and from the surroundings (the external environment) and automatically adjusts the activity of different systems to match the overall needs of the body. The function of the ANS is critical to maintaining healthy homeostasis, and its dysfunction may have a profoundly negative influence, contributing significantly to disease.

NERVE CELL PHYSIOLOGY

The neuron is the basic cellular unit of the nervous system. A single nerve cell is capable of carrying out many of the quintessential features of the system, such as the gathering, integration, and transmission of information. The more complex, "emergent" properties of the nervous system arise from neural networks, in which hundreds, thousands, or millions of highly interconnected nerve cells communicate with one another.

Nerve Cell Structure

Neurons generally resemble other cells in having a nucleus, cytoplasm, cell membrane, and an internal environment kept distinct from the extracellular milieu. However, they also possess specialized structures that support their functions of information processing.

Nerve Cell Morphology FIGURE 5.1 illustrates some of the morphologic features of nerve cells. Although there is great variability among neurons, these cells are often thin and elongated. Relatively short, branching projections called **dendrites** are found at one end of the neuron (Figure 5.1). The dendrites are cytoplasmic extensions near the neuron's **cell body**, which contains the nerve cell's nucleus and much of the molecular machinery necessary for gene expression, protein production, and cell

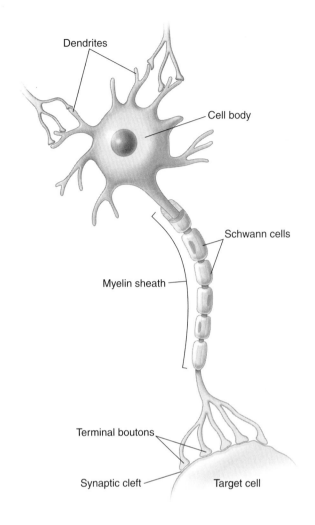

Figure 5.1   Structure of a neuron. Dendrites are the thin, branching cytoplasmic extensions of the neurons cell membrane. The axon terminals of other neurons synapse on the dendrites. The cell body contains the nucleus and other organelles. The elongated axon is covered by a myelin sheath. The myelin sheath is the cell membrane of support cells such as oligodendrocytes or Schwann cells that wraps around the axon. Terminal boutons are specialized endings of the axon. The synapse or synaptic cleft separates the axon terminals from the membrane of target cells.

metabolism. The relatively long projection of the neuron from the cell body is called the **axon**. Many nerve cell axons are normally covered by a layer of specialized membrane called **myelin**. This myelin sheath is not truly part of the neuron; rather, it is the plasma membrane of cells that support neurons wrapped around their axons. In the central nervous system (CNS), such support cells are called *oligodendrocytes*, while in the peripheral nervous system they care called *Schwann cells*. The axon ends in branches with specialized endings. Figure 5.1 illustrates axon endings called **terminal boutons** found in neurons such as those of the motor system (see Chapter 6). In other nerve cells, such as those of the

ANS, the axon terminals have a different shape and are called **varicosities** (see Chapter 7 and Figure 7.5).

Generally, a nerve cell that communicates with another cell (receiving or sending information from or to another neuron or a target tissue cell) does not touch that other cell. Instead, the terminal boutons or varicosities of a neuron are closely apposed to the cell membrane of a target tissue cell or the dendrites of another neuron. The **synapse** is the gap between a nerve cell and a target cell or other neuron. The synapse is not a simple "empty space" but has a complex molecular structure with cytoskeletal elements that maintain the association of the nerve terminals of the *presynaptic* neuron with their *postsynaptic* targets. In addition, important enzymes may reside in the synaptic cleft (FIGURE 5.2).

Nerve Cell Organelles   Like most other cells, neurons have organelles like mitochondria, the Golgi apparatus, and endoplasmic reticulum that support basic metabolic functions. Cytoplasmic vesicles are especially important small, membrane-bound compartments that contain specialized signaling molecules called **neurotransmitters** (Figure 5.2).

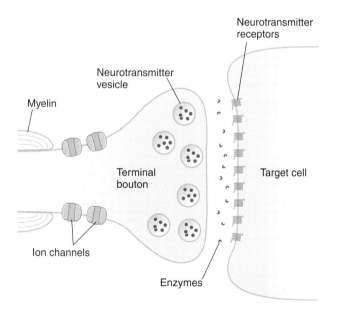

Figure 5.2 A close-up view of a nerve terminal and the synapse. The terminal bouton on the left contains a number of membrane bound vesicles, small subcellular compartments holding chemical neurotransmitters. The synapse between the terminal bouton and the target cell has enzymes that can cleave neurotransmitter molecules once they are released from the nerve terminal. The cell membrane of the presynaptic neuron has embedded ion channels and the N^+-K^+-ATPase transporter, while the plasma membrane of the postsynaptic target cell has embedded neurotransmitter receptors. Note how the neurotransmitter-containing vesicles and the neurotransmitter receptors cluster at the synapse, where a nerve terminus is juxtaposed with the target cell membrane.

Such vesicles may be found throughout the cell but are especially prominent and functionally important at the nerve terminals.

Nerve Cell Membrane   The neuron plasma membrane is critical not only in maintaining the integrity of the intracellular environment but in receiving signals and allowing the electrochemical state of the nerve cell to change in a regulated way. As in other cells, the cell membrane is a lipid bilayer with embedded proteins. One such membrane protein is the Na^+-K^+-ATPase ion transporter that uses the energy liberated by cleavage of the terminal high-energy phosphate of ATP to extrude three Na^+ from the cell and transport two K^+ into the cell. Two classes of membrane proteins essential to nerve cell function are *ion channels* and *neurotransmitter receptors*.

Ion channels are found in specialized regions of the axon cell membrane and regulate the passage of ions such as Na^+, K^+, Cl^-, and Ca^{2+} into or out of the cell. Some ion-specific channels, called *ungated*, are almost always open, making the plasma membrane somewhat permeable to K^+ or Na^+, for example. However, other ion-selective channels oscillate among three states: closed, open, and locked. When they are closed, such channels do not allow their specific ion to cross the cell membrane, but when they are open, they permit the specific ion to traverse the plasma membrane. When such a channel is locked, it is closed and unable to open. Such channels are called *gated ion channels*. A gated channel spontaneously shifts among the closed, open, and locked states, but the probability that it will be in one or another state is related to the presence of a specific stimulus. Two subclasses of gated ion channels critical for neuron function are **voltage-gated ion channels** and **ligand-gated ion channels**. A voltage-gated ion channel is more likely to be open when there is a change in the electrical potential of the nerve cell membrane, while a ligand-gated ion channel is more likely to be open when a specific neurotransmitter binds to it.

Neurotransmitter receptors are present on the dendrites of postsynaptic neurons and the plasma membrane of nonneuronal target cells and bind their respective neurotransmitter ligands that have been released into the synaptic cleft (Figure 5.2).

Nerve Cell Ions, Resting Membrane Potential, and Electrochemical Gradients   As described in Chapter 2, the plasma membrane is semipermeable, allowing some substances to pass between the intracellular and the extracellular spaces but restricting the movement of others. When the concentration of a solute differs on one side of the membrane from the other, a chemical gradient exists. Such a gradient favors the movement (by diffusion) of the solute from the area of higher concentration to that of lower concentration until equilibrium is established and the concentrations on both sides of the membrane are equal. Movement of a substance down a chemical gradient disperses the potential energy that is present in the system before equilibrium is reached.

When a solute and the cell membrane each have an electrical charge, electrostatic force also affects the movement of that solute. Ions such as Na^+, K^+, Ca^{2+}, Cl^-, and HCO_3^- are electrically charged solutes whose intracellular and extracellular concentrations are tightly controlled and whose transmembrane movements are the basis of electrochemical signaling in neurons and muscle cells.

Why is there an electrical potential difference across the plasma membrane? Three factors contribute to the establishment and maintenance of a separation of electrical charges between the intracellular and extracellular spaces. First, the interior of a cell contains negatively charged solutes, such as amino acids and nucleic acids that are unable to traverse the cell membrane. Second, because the Na^+-K^+-ATPase enzyme in the plasma membrane transports three Na^+ out of the cell and two K^+ into the cell, there is a net loss of one positive charge from the cytoplasm. The Na^+-K^+-ATPase is therefore called an *electrogenic ion pump*. Third, leakage of K^+ out of the cell down its chemical gradient through membrane channels removes more positive charges from the cell. These factors collude to make the intracellular space electrically negative compared to the extracellular space, and this baseline electrical polarization of the cell membrane is called the **resting membrane potential (E_m)**. Mathematically, E_m is simply the difference in electrical potential between the inside and the outside of the cell: $E_m = E_{in} - E_{out}$. A typical human neuron has an E_m of -60 to -70 mV, with the negative sign indicating the relative excess of negative charges (or dearth of positive charges) intracellularly.

The resting membrane potential influences the movement of charged solutes. Consider a typical neuron, in which the intracellular concentration of K^+ is approximately 120 mmol/L and the extracellular concentration is approximately 4.0 mmol/L. If there were no difference in the voltage across the cell membrane and the solute were uncharged, the only force driving the movement of K^+ would be the concentration favoring diffusion from the intracellular space into the extracellular space. However, because E_m is negative, an electrostatic force attracts the K^+ cation, opposing the concentration gradient (FIGURE 5.3A). Both electrical and chemical forces act on Na^+ and Cl^- as well (Figures 5.3B and C). Thus, there is a combined **electrochemical gradient** acting on each

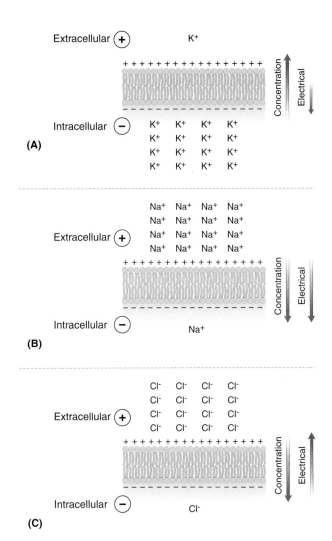

Figure 5.3 Electrochemical gradients of K^+, Na^+, and Cl^-. **A.** A large concentration gradient favors the movement of K^+ out of the cell, but the negative resting membrane potential, $E_m = -60$ to -70 mV, partially opposes this. **B.** Both a concentration gradient and an electrical gradient favor the movement of Na^+ into the cell. Only the relative impermeability of the cell membrane and the action of the Na^+-K^+-ATPase maintain this high Na^+ electrochemical gradient. **C.** Cl^- has a concentration gradient similar to Na^+, but because its charge is -1 the negative resting membrane potential opposes the movement of Cl^- into the cell.

of the ions. The sum of the chemical potential (from the concentration gradient) and the electrical potential (from the ion's charge and E_m) of a mol of ion X is called the *electrochemical potential* and is defined by the equation

$$\mu = \mu_0 + RT\ln[X] + zFE \tag{5.1}$$

where μ_0 is the reference state electrochemical potential; $R = 8.3145$ J/(K)(mol) is the universal gas constant; T is the absolute temperature in degrees Kelvin, approximately $310°K$ at body temperature; ln [X] is the natural logarithm of the concentration of the ion X; z is the electrical charge on X ($+1$ for K^+ and Na^+, $+2$ for Ca^{2+} and Mg^{2+}, and -1 for Cl^- and

HCO_3^-); $F = 9.6485 \times 10^4$ Coulombs/mol is the Faraday constant; and E is the the electrical potential. The difference in electrochemical potential across a cell membrane is defined as $\Delta\mu = \mu_{in} - \mu_{out}$. Since μ_0 is constant, substituting equation (5.1) yields

$$\Delta\mu = RT\ln([X]_{in}/[X]_{out}) + zF(E_{in} - E_{out}) \quad (5.2)$$
$$= RT\ln([X]_{in}/[X]_{out}) + zFE_m$$

$\Delta\mu$ is called the *electrochemical potential difference*. It quantifies the electrochemical gradient, the combined chemical ($RT\ln([X]_{in}/[X]_{out})$) and electrical ($zF(E_{in} - E_{out})$) forces acting on an ion X. As equation (5.2) depicts, the electrochemical gradient acting on a particular ion depends on the ratio of the intracellular and extracellular concentrations of the ion, the ion's charge, and E_m (Figure 5.3)

Ionic Electrochemical Equilibrium and the Nernst Equation

Equation (5.2) quantifies the chemical and electrical potentials of an ion. What if the two forces (chemical and electrical) are of equal magnitude but oriented in opposite directions? Under such a condition, the ion would be in equilibrium across the cell membrane, with the movement of ions from the intracellular space to the extracellular space balanced by a movement of ions in the opposite direction, resulting in no net change. Then $\Delta\mu$ must equal 0, and by definition, $RT\ln([X]_{in}/[X]_{out}) = -zFE_m$. Given the charge (z) of the particular ion and the membrane potential E_m, this relationship can be solved for $[X]_{in}/[X]_{out}$, the ratio of the intracellular and extracellular concentrations of the ion that will result in electrochemical equilibrium. Conversely, measuring the intracellular and extracellular concentrations of the ion *in equilibrium* allows one to solve for E_m, the membrane potential that maintains the balance.

$$E_m = \frac{RT\ln([X]_{in}/[X]_{out})}{-zF} \quad (5.3)$$

Converting from natural logarithm (ln, $\log_e$) to $\log_{10}$ by the equation $\ln = (2.303)\log_{10}$ and substituting in the known values of R, T, and F results in the **Nernst equation**.

$$E_m = (-61.5 \text{ mV/z})\log_{10}([X]_{in}/[X]_{out}) \quad (5.4)$$

The Nernst equation provides the value of E_m (the *Nernst potential* or *equilibrium potential*) that results from an ion being in equilibrium at the measured intracellular and extracellular concentrations. Alternatively, the Nernst potential can be thought of as that membrane potential needed for the given ion to be in equilibrium at the given concentrations.

The Nernst potential depends on the particular ion's charge and its distribution across the cell membrane. For example, the Nernst potential for K^+, E_K^+,

is $(-61.5 \text{ mV/}+1)\log_{10}(120/4.0) = -91$ mV. Given the measured intracellular and extracellular concentrations of K^+, the value of approximately -65 mV for E_m is not sufficiently negative to equal E_K^+. Thus, although the negative membrane potential opposes the concentration gradient for K^+, it is of insufficient magnitude to bring K^+ into equilibrium, and the net electrochemical gradient still favors the efflux of K^+ from the cell into the extracellular space.

For Na^+, the Nernst potential, E_{Na}^+ is approximately $(-61.5 \text{ mV/}+1)\log(10/140) = +70$ mV. Because E_m is far from the Na^+ equilibrium potential, both the concentration and electrical components of the electrochemical gradient favor the influx of Na^+ into the cell. For Cl^-, the Nernst potential, E_{Cl}^- is approximately $(-61.5 \text{ ml/}-1)\log(9/105) = -65.6$ mV. Because E_{Cl}^- is very close to E_m, it is near equilibrium, with the chemical gradient favoring the influx of Cl^- into the cell balanced by the electrical gradient favoring the efflux of Cl^- out of the cell.

Membrane Permeability, the Chord Conductance Equation, and the Goldman Equation

If the measured resting membrane potential E_m is not equal to the Nernst potential for a given ion, there will be a nonzero electrochemical gradient favoring the movement of that ion. If it is able to cross the membrane through open, nongated ion channels, the ion will do so down this gradient and subsequently alter both its intracellular and extracellular concentrations and the distribution of electrical charges across the membrane. The passage of ions across the membrane produces a *transmembrane current* that may have large effects on membrane electrical potential while effecting negligible changes in the ion concentrations inside and outside the cell.

If the resting membrane potential E_m is stable and yet unequal to the Nernst potential for any single ion, there must be a steady state of transmembrane ionic currents. For example, if E_m is -65 mV and nongated K^+ channels allow K^+ to exit the cell, there will be a small transmembrane current I_K^+. If I_K^+ is unopposed, it will result in the loss of positive charges from the cell and the shift of E_m toward the equilibrium potential for K^+ until E_m eventually reaches E_K^+ and the system achieves equilibrium. However, nongated Na^+ channels in the membrane allow this ion to cross the membrane according to its electrochemical gradient—i.e., Na^+ leaks into the cell, with the resulting current I_{Na}^+ adding positive charge to the cell interior and driving E_m toward E_{Na}^+. A similar argument holds for I_{Cl}^-, though this current is very small because the resting membrane potential E_m is so close to the Nernst potential for Cl^- E_{Cl}^-.

At rest, E_m is stable because there is no *net* transmembrane current. That is, $I_K^+ + I_{Na}^+ + I_{Cl}^- = 0$.

According to Ohm's law, each ionic current I is the result of dividing that ion's electrical potential (driving force) by the resistance of the membrane to the passage of that ion: $I_X = (E_m - E_X)/R_X$. The *conductance* g_X of the membrane to a particular ion is defined as the inverse of the membrane's resistance to the passage of that ion—i.e., the conductance is directly proportional to how leaky the membrane is to that ion while the resistance is inversely proportional to this leakiness. Thus, $I_X = (E_m - E_X)(g_X)$, and (by substitution) at equilibrium $(E_m - E_K^+)(g_K^+) + (E_m - E_{Na}^+)(g_{Na}^+) + (E_m - E_{Cl}^-)(g_{Cl}^-) = 0$. Solving for E_m yields the **chord conductance equation**:

$$E_m = \frac{(E_K+)(g_K+) + (E_{Na}+) \times (g_{Na}+) + (E_{Cl}-)(g_{Cl}-)}{g_m} \quad (5.5)$$

where $g_m = g_K^+ = g_{Na}^+ = g_{Cl}^-$, the total conductance of the membrane to the three ions. The chord conductance equation states that E_m is the weighted average of the membrane conductances for the relevant ions. In the resting, steady state, the relatively small leakage of Na^+ and K^+ down their electrochemical gradients is opposed by the electrogenic Na^+-K^+-ATPase pump so that the gradients are maintained. The current I_{Cl}^- is very small in the resting state because E_m is very close to E_{Cl}^-. If the conductance of the membrane to a given ion were to change, E_m would change in accordance. For example, if a toxin (such as tetrodotoxin from the puffer fish) were used to completely block the Na^+ ion channels, making the membrane impermeable to Na^+, g_{Na}^+ would equal 0, there would be no I_{Na}^+, and E_m would be the weighted average of K^+ and Cl^- currents only. However, if the membrane conductance to Na^+ were to dramatically increase while the conductances to K^+ and Cl^- remained stable, the larger value of g_{Na}^+ in the chord conductance equation predicts that E_m would shift toward E_{Na}^+. Thus, the greater the conductance of the plasma membrane to an ion, the more E_m will be driven toward the equilibrium potential of that ion.

A third expression combining the information from the Nernst and chord conductance equations is the **Goldman equation**:

$$E_m = (RT/F) \ln \times \left(\frac{P_K^+[K^+]_{out} + P_{Na}^+[Na^+]_{out} + P_{Cl}^-[Cl^-]_{in}}{P_K^+[K^+]_{in} + P_{Na}^+[Na^+]_{in} + P_{Cl}^-[Cl^-]_{out}} \right) \quad (5.6)$$

where P_X is the permeability of the cell membrane to that ion, a measure similar (but not identical) to the conductance of the membrane for that ion. Like the Nernst equation, the Goldman equation calculates a membrane potential on the basis of the intracellular and extracellular concentrations of ions. Like the chord conductance equation, the Goldman equation states that the resting membrane potential is the weighted average of membrane permeability to the ions K^+, Na^+, and Cl^-. Just as the chord conductance equation predicts that a dramatic increase in the conductance of an ion would drive E_m toward the Nernst potential for that ion, the Goldman equation states that an increase in the membrane permeability to an ion will shift E_m toward that ion's Nernst potential. In fact, if the permeability of one ion greatly exceeds those of the other ions, the Goldman equation essentially reduces down to the Nernst equation. For example, if P_{Na}^+ were to suddenly increase to be much greater than P_K^+ and P_{Cl}^-, the K^+ and Cl^- terms would drop out, the P_{Na}^+ factors would cancel, and the Goldman equation would equal the Nernst equation for Na^+.

Nerve Cell Function

Neurons receive and transmit information in the form of electrochemical impulses. More precisely, a signaling neuron can be thought of as a binary element in a signaling network—it can be in either one of two states, "on" or "off" (but not both) at any given time. The "on" and the "off" states of the nerve cell are different electrochemical conditions of the cell. At rest, a neuron is in the "off" state. When it receives a sufficient activating signal, the cell undergoes an electrochemical shift into the "on" state for a brief period and then returns to the "off" state. The change in the electrochemical state of the neuron is a patterned alteration of the cell membrane potential, E_m.

Thresholds and Electrotonic Conduction   The activation of a nerve cell requires the following five components: a stimulus, one or more receptors for that stimulus, an intact plasma membrane, ion channels, and ion gradients. Different neurons are sensitive to different stimuli. Some, for example, are triggered by energy, such as pressure (mechanical energy) or temperature (thermal energy), while others are activated by matter, such as the presence of a particular chemical. When an appropriate stimulus reaches a neuron, it causes a change in the neuron's resting membrane potential. An activating stimulus *depolarizes* the membrane, making it less negative with respect to the extracellular space. Conversely, an inhibitory stimulus *hyperpolarizes* the membrane, making it more negative. For example, an activating stimulus might shift E_m from its resting value of -65 to -55 mV, depolarizing the membrane, while an inhibitory stimulus might drive E_m to -90 mV, hyperpolarizing it.

Not every exposure to an activating stimulus guarantees a response by the neuron. Whether the stimulus is sufficient to activate the nerve cell depends on whether that stimulus depolarizes the membrane to the neuron's **threshold membrane potential**. The threshold varies among different neurons but is typically −55 to −50 mV. A subthreshold stimulus depolarizes the membrane slightly (e.g., from the resting value of −65 to −58 mV) but not to the threshold potential. Such a subthreshold stimulus causes a few gated Na^+ channels in the specific area of the membrane where the stimulus was received to open, increasing the local membrane conductance (g_{Na}^+) and membrane permeability (P_{Na}^+) to Na^+ and allowing positive charges to flow into the neuron. As predicted by the chord conductance and Goldman equations, this shifts E_m away from its resting value, depolarizing the membrane toward the Nernst potential for Na^+ of +70 mV. The Na^+ ions that enter the cell rapidly diffuse from their site of entry, and an intracellular current carries the depolarization to adjacent membrane segments. Because of the resistance of the cytoplasm, the change in E_m decreases exponentially with distance from the site of membrane stimulation. The passive spread of local ionic currents is called **electrotonic conduction**, but the magnitude of membrane depolarization is insufficient to reach the threshold, and E_m decays back down to its resting value as the positive charges leak across the membrane. Some Na^+ ions that entered the cell are returned to the extracellular space by the Na^+-K^+-ATPase as well.

Action Potential Generation and Voltage-Gated Ion Channels A dramatically different response occurs when a stimulus of sufficient magnitude reaches a neuron. Such a stimulus depolarizes the membrane to the threshold value and triggers a self-propagating membrane depolarization cascade called an **action potential**, the patterned alteration in E_m that is the "on" state of the nerve cell. In this case, a greater inward flow of Na^+ causes the local membrane potential to reach −50 mV (FIGURE 5.4A). The local ionic current depolarizes an adjacent segment of membrane, but instead of decaying, the permeability (and thus the conductance) of this second membrane segment to Na^+ rapidly increases, producing a new depolarizing transmembrane current. The process repeats as the new depolarization moves down the membrane, depolarizing a third segment of membrane. In the mean time, the first area of depolarization returns to the resting E_m, a process called membrane *repolarization* (Figure 5.4B)

The basis of the action potential is the sequential opening and subsequent locking of voltage-gated ion channels (FIGURE 5.5). Unlike ungated channels, voltage-gated channels are sensitive to changes in E_m. When a stimulus depolarizes the membrane to

threshold, the increase in E_m causes a conformational shift in the tertiary and quaternary structure of the voltage-gated Na^+ channel, increasing the probability that it will go from the closed state to the open state. Voltage-gated channels only allow their specific ion to pass through their central pore and traverse the cell membrane when they are in the open state. As some Na^+ channels open, P_{Na}^+ and g_{Na}^+ increase, and the influx of Na^+ further depolarizes the membrane. As E_m rises, more and more voltage-gated Na^+ channels open, driving E_m toward E_{Na}^+. This positive feedback loop is responsible for the explosive depolarization phase of the action potential.

Like most positive feedback loops, the depolarization phase of the action potential eventually has to be limited and reversed for the neuron to return to its resting state. The limitation of the action potential depolarization of a given segment of membrane occurs because after membrane depolarization initially shifts voltage-gated Na^+ channels from the closed to the open state, it subsequently causes them to go from the open to the locked state. The locking of the

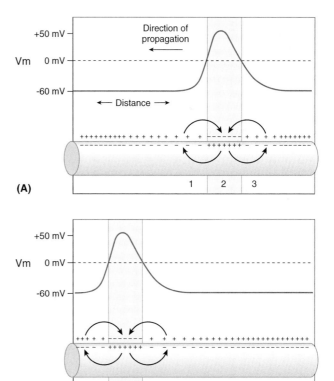

Figure 5.4 Triggering and propagation of an action potential. **A.** An action potential occurs when a region of the neuron membrane is depolarized to the threshold value. The positive charges that flow into the cell quickly diffuse, creating local currents. This passive electrotonic conduction depolarizes adjacent segments of the membrane. **B.** The action potential moves unidirectionally because local currents can initiate an action potential in an area of the membrane that has not been stimulated in some time but cannot do so in an area of the membrane that is recovering from an action potential and is in the refractory state.

Closed

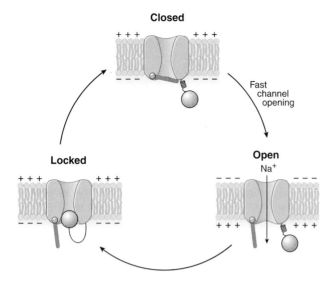

Figure 5.5 Voltage-gated ion channels shift sequentially among three states. At rest, the voltage-gated Na$^+$ channel is closed. When membrane depolarization occurs, it increases the probability that the channel will open, allowing Na$^+$ to enter the cell. After some time in the open state, membrane depolarization causes the channel to enter the locked state. Only membrane repolarization can reset the channel to the closed state. During the time that most of the Na$^+$ channels are locked, the neuron is unable to respond to additional stimuli and is in the refractory state.

Na$^+$ channels curtails the influx of Na$^+$, and Na$^+$ starts to leave the cell through ungated ion channels and the Na$^+$-K$^+$-ATPase. While locked, voltage-gated Na$^+$ ion channels are unable to open in response to a depolarizing stimulus. Early in the course of an action potential and shortly after, the neuron membrane is therefore in a *refractory state*. The refractory state is made up of two periods. When the majority of channels are locked, the neuron is in the *absolute refractory period* and cannot produce an action potential to any stimulus, no matter how much greater than threshold it is. Thereafter, as some Na$^+$ channels convert from the locked to the closed state, the neuron is in the *relative refractory state* and can produce another action potential only in response to a stimulus that exceeds the threshold. Finally, when all of the voltage-gated Na$^+$ channels reenter the closed state, that area of the membrane is reset and can respond to any threshold stimulus with a full action potential.

The reversal of the action potential, membrane repolarization, occurs because depolarization causes voltage-gated K$^+$ channels to shift from the closed state to the open state. This increases P_K^+ and g_K^+, allowing K$^+$ to exit the cell down its electrochemical gradient (made all the steeper by E_m being driven so far from E_K^+ by the action potential), which removes positive charge from the interior of the cell and restores the charge distribution of the resting state. The K$^+$ voltage-gated ion channel differs in two important ways from the Na$^+$ voltage-gated ion channel.

First, the K$^+$ channels open more slowly in response to membrane depolarization than the Na$^+$ channels, so that the repolarizing efflux of K$^+$ starts as the Na$^+$ channels lock. Thus, first P_{Na}^+ and g_{Na}^+ rise, driving E_m toward E_{Na}^+, then P_{Na}^+ and g_{Na}^+ decrease as the Na$^+$ channels lock. Simultaneously, P_K^+ and g_K^+ increase as the K$^+$ channels open, and E_m is driven down toward E_K^+. A second difference between the voltage-gated K$^+$ and Na$^+$ channels is that some K$^+$ channels do not lock in response to prolonged depolarization. At the end of the action potential, when the Na$^+$ channels are locked or closed and the K$^+$ channels have not yet reverted to the closed state, the continued flow of K$^+$ out of the cell causes a transient hyperpolarization—i.e., E_m becomes more negative than the resting value, approaching E_K^+ more closely (FIGURE 5.6). Thereafter, the K$^+$ voltage-gated channels close, and E_m returns to its resting value.

Myelin, Nodes of Ranvier, and Saltatory Conduction
Action potentials do not dissipate as they propagate down the neuron membrane. Although the local currents that carry depolarization from one region of the membrane to an adjacent region decay exponentially with increasing distance from the site of membrane depolarization, the electrotonic conduction in this case (unlike the situation with a subthreshold depolarization) is sufficient to bring the next segment of membrane to threshold, thus regenerating the action

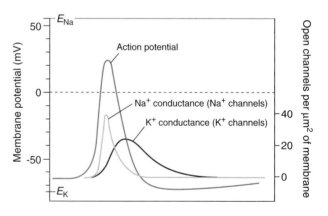

Figure 5.6 Changes in membrane permeability and ion conductances with an action potential. When a stimulus causes membrane depolarization sufficient to drive E_m to the threshold potential, there is an explosive increase in the membrane's permeability to Na$^+$ (P_{Na}^+) and therefore in Na$^+$ conductance (g_{Na}^+) as voltage-gated Na$^+$ channels open and allow Na$^+$ to enter the cell. This depolarizes the membrane, explaining why the rapid depolarization phase of the action potential is concurrent with the increase in P_{Na}^+ and g_{Na}^+. At the peak of the action potential, P_{Na}^+ and g_{Na}^+ decrease rapidly as the voltage-gated Na$^+$ channel lock. The voltage-gated K$^+$ channels open more slowly than the Na$^+$ channels, and the peak in P_K^+ and g_K^+ coincides with membrane repolarization. Because the K$^+$ channels close slowly, unlike the Na$^+$ channels that quickly lock, the efflux of K$^+$ drives E_m beyond the resting value toward E_K^+, briefly hyperpolarizing the membrane.

potential there. As the action potential progresses, the voltage-gated Na$^+$ channels in the region behind the action potential are in their locked refractory state, preventing the local currents from causing another action potential to arise there. Thus, the action potential propagates unidirectionally (Figure 5.4).

The resistance of the neuron's cytoplasm limits the rate at which an action potential can be conducted down the axon. This can be partly overcome by increasing the cross-sectional area of the axon, which reduces the resistance to current flow. However, this solution is limited by the competing interest of resource and spatial economy. An alternative solution that satisfies both the need for rapid action potential propagation and the limitation on neuron size is the myelin sheath wrapped around the axon. This insulting layer greatly reduces the leakiness of the cell membrane to ions, and thus increases the distance and efficiency of action potential propagation by electrotonic conduction. Despite the improved integrity of local currents, the neuron cannot rely on them alone for the propagation of the action potential, which decays if it is not periodically regenerated. Therefore, there are gaps called the **nodes of Ranvier** in the myelin sheath at roughly regular intervals. The nodes of Ranvier are locations where the action potential is regenerated as it travels down the axon. There are higher densities of voltage-gated Na$^+$ and K$^+$ channels at the nodes than at those portions of the cell membrane covered by myelin. This solution is metabolically economical for at least two reasons. First, by strategically locating the ion channels at the nodes rather than expressing them homogeneously on the axon membrane, it decreases the total number of proteins the neuron has to synthesize. Second, by increasing the efficiency, the rate, and the range of electrotonic conduction, fewer Na$^+$ ions are needed to enter the cell, which saves work for the Na$^+$-K$^+$-ATPase.

The axon membrane is thus divided into two qualitatively distinct regions. The regions covered by myelin allow the action potential to be rapidly propagated but does not regenerate it. The nodes of Ranvier regenerate the action potential, but this occurs more slowly than local transmission by electrotonic conductance. Thus, the action potential appears to start, move rapidly down the axon, slow down at a node of Ranvier to regenerate, and then continue down the axon quickly until it reaches the next node. Such a pattern is called **saltatory conduction** from the Latin word *saltare* meaning "to jump" (FIGURE 5.7A). Loss of the myelin sheath, as occurs in diseases such as multiple sclerosis, can cause profound neurological dysfunction, as saltatory conduction fails and action potentials are propagated slowly or even decay completely (Figure 5.7B).

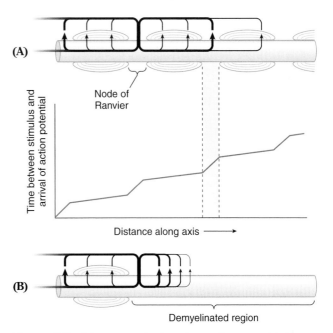

Figure 5.7 Saltatory conduction of an action potential down a myelinated axon. **A.** An action potential is generated when the membrane at a node of Ranvier is depolarized to threshold. Local currents carry the depolarization down the axon and an intact myelin sheath prevents leakage of current across the membrane, increasing the rate and the distance electrotonic conduction can occur. When the depolarization reaches the next node of Ranvier, it slows down and regenerates the action potential. The alternating velocity at which the action potential propagates is called saltatory conduction. **B.** If the myelin sheath is damaged or lost, as occurs in diseases such as multiple sclerosis, charge leaks out the membrane. The action potential propagates more slowly and may even dissipate completely before it reaches the next node of Ranvier.

Transmission Across the Synapse   An action potential propagates down the axon and reaches the axon terminals, but it is unable to cross the synaptic cleft to reach the next neuron or target cell. To overcome this problem, the information encoded in the action potential must be transformed from a membrane voltage change into a medium that can cross the synapse and affect the target cell. If the target cell is another neuron, the information must be translated back into an action potential so that it can propagate down the next axon. The language that allows the action potential to cross the synaptic cleft is that of the neurotransmitters.

At rest, these chemical substances are stored in membrane-bound vesicles clustered at the axon terminals. When an action potential depolarizes the terminal membrane, it causes specialized *voltage-gated Ca^{2+} channels* to open. Like Na$^+$, Ca^{2+} has a large electrochemical gradient favoring its influx into the cell, where ion pumps maintain relatively low cytoplasmic concentrations of this ion ([Ca^{2+}]$_{in}$). Because the intracellular Ca^{2+} concentration is kept so low, the increase in membrane permeability

$(P_{Ca^{2+}})$ and conductance $(g_{Ca}{}^{2+})$ to Ca^{2+} bring about a nonnegligible increase in $[Ca^{2+}]_{in}$ (FIGURE 5.8A). This is in contrast to ions such as Na^+ and K^+, whose brief flow across the membrane in response to an action potential causes significant alterations in the membrane potential but not in their intracellular concentrations. The increase in $[Ca^{2+}]_{in}$ induces programmed changes in the cytoskeleton that cause neurotransmitter vesicles to fuse with the cell membrane of the axon terminals and release neurotransmitters into the synaptic space (Figure 5.8B).

Once released, neurotransmitters diffuse across the synaptic cleft and bind to receptors on the surface of a target cell. These neurotransmitter receptors are *ligand-gated ion channels* that open in response to the binding of their ligands (Figure 5.8C). If the neurotransmitter receptor is a ligand-gated Na^+ channel and sufficient numbers of such receptors are induced to open, the membrane of the postsynaptic cell is depolarized, and a new action potential is generated (Figure 5.8D). If the neurotransmitter receptor is a ligand-gated K^+ channel, the membrane of the postsynaptic cells is hyperpolarized, decreasing the likelihood that the target cell will be activated. In order to limit the effect of neurotransmitters, these molecules are either broken down by specialized enzymes resident in the synaptic cleft or taken up and recycled by the axon terminals of the presynaptic neuron.

Complexity in Neurons and Neural Networks Neuron action potentials are binary events—all or nothing depolarizations. Neural networks, however, oversee complex functions, integrate various types of information, and respond in finely graded ways. How do relatively simple action potentials encode such complexity? On the level of a single neuron, complexity may arise from a number of places. Different neurons respond to different stimuli according to their receptors. Different parts of a neuron may have different sensitivities to stimulation. For example, a neuron's dendrites may be more sensitive to stimuli than the axon but not as sensitive as the cell body where signals are integrated. There are many different types and subtypes of voltage-gated ion channels, and they differ in their responsiveness to membrane depolarization. The function of the various voltage-gated ion channels can be modified by extracellular and intracellular stimuli. For example, phosphorylation of a channel may profoundly alter its response to depolarization. Likewise, there are many different neurotransmitters and neurotransmitter receptors, and the receptors (like the voltage-gated ion channels) can be modified by intracellular and extracellular stimuli. Finally, although an isolated action potential is a binary phenomenon, information may be encoded by trains of action potentials of various frequencies.

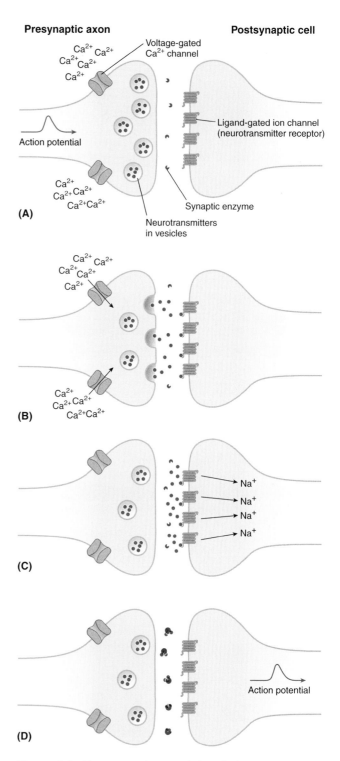

Figure 5.8 Trans-synaptic transmission. **A.** An action potential reaches the axon terminals and the depolarization of the terminal membrane opens voltage-gated Ca^{2+} channels. **B.** The influx of Ca^{2+} causes neurotransmitter vesicles to fuse with the plasma membrane and release neurotransmitter molecules into the synaptic cleft. **C.** The neurotransmitter diffuses across the synapse and binds to ligand-gated ion channels on the dendrites of the postsynaptic neuron, depolarizing the membrane. **D.** If sufficient activating stimuli reach the postsynaptic neuron, an action potential will be generated and conducted. Meanwhile, enzymes in the synaptic cleft metabolize the neurotransmitter so that signaling is limited.

On the multicellular level, a single neuron may receive input from tens, hundreds, or thousands of other neurons, some of which stimulate and others of which inhibit it according to which neurotransmitters they release and which receptors it possesses. The neuron has to integrate these signals continuously to decide whether or not to fire an action potential. Feedback loops and highly branched networks may have complex outputs that vary according to a few simple rules and many interactions.

AUTONOMIC NERVOUS SYSTEM STRUCTURE

The ANS has a bodywide range, collecting information from and distributing instructions to the skin and organs, such as the eyes, and the visceral organs, such as the heart and blood vessels, lungs, gastrointestinal (GI) tract, bladder, and reproductive organs. The structural basis for a system that can gather information from disparate organs and the environment, integrate the data, and transmit impulses throughout the body reflects its function: The ANS is literally a network of highly branching and interconnected nerve cells.

The ANS is composed of two divisions, the **sympathetic nervous system (SNS)** and the **parasympathetic nervous system (PNS)**. Their distinct structures support different but complementary functions, which are described below. Many consider the complex neuronal network of the GI enteric nervous system (ENS) to be a third division of the ANS because it, too, generally works unconsciously (see Chapter 28 for a description of the ENS).

The ANS shares many basic structural and functional characteristics with the neurologic system involved in the control of skeletal muscle, the *motor system* (see Chapter 6). For example, the general structure of a nerve cell and the initiation and propagation of action potentials in the ANS resemble those of the motor system. However, there are critical differences between the two systems. The primary distinction is that the motor system is under conscious control, while the ANS works largely unconsciously. In what follows, it is useful to compare and contrast the structure and function of the ANS with those of the motor system.

Autonomic Nervous System Tissues

As with all homeostatic systems, the ANS monitors the function of target tissues, transmits the information on target tissue function via afferent pathways, integrates the information in central control centers, and sends instructions back to the target tissues via efferent pathways. This section describes these basic components starting from periphery and moving centrally.

Target Tissues While the effector tissues of the motor system are skeletal muscles, the major tissues influenced by the ANS are smooth muscles (such as those of blood vessel walls, the alimentary canal, and the urinary bladder); glands (such as the sweat glands and those of the respiratory and GI tract); and cardiac muscle and cardiac electrical conduction system.

Peripheral Nerves Information enters the ANS through nerves supplying the skin, internal organs, and their associated blood vessels. Just as afferent nerves of the motor system transmit specialized information on the stretch status of skeletal muscles, the specialized endings of **afferent ANS nerves** gather and communicate organ-specific information relevant to homeostasis. Chemoreceptors send signals about variables such as the pH and partial pressure of oxygen in their tissues. Nerve endings in blood vessels and viscera, such as the GI and urinary tracts, measuring wall tension (and, as a derivative, estimate the pressure in the organ) are called *mechanoreceptors* or *baroreceptors*. An exception to the general rule of the unconscious workings of the ANS are the *nociceptors*, afferent nerves that relay signals interpreted as pain when viscera are damaged and/or overdistended.

ANS afferent neurons have long processes that go from their specialized endings in peripheral tissues to their cell bodies in the dorsal root ganglia of the spinal cord. Information is transmitted to the spinal cord by short axons where it can be processed, integrated with other signals, and acted on via autonomic reflexes of varying complexity.

Once signals are processed and appropriate responses are "decided," they are transmitted via efferent ANS nerves. Among the most prominent ANS nerves is the vagus nerve, also called cranial nerve X, of the PNS.

Peripheral Ganglia A collection of interconnected ANS neurons is known as a *ganglion*, and ganglia are found only in the ANS. The sympathetic **paravertebral ganglia** are arranged in two longitudinal (rostrocaudal) chains, one on either side of the spinal column. In addition, three sympathetic **prevertebral ganglia** are nerve tissue nodes anterior to the spinal column in the midline. They are situated around and take their names from three major branches of the descending aorta: the celiac ganglion, also called the solar plexus, (the celiac trunk), the superior mesenteric ganglion (the superior mesenteric artery), and the inferior mesenteric ganglion (the inferior mesenteric artery) (FIGURE 5.9)

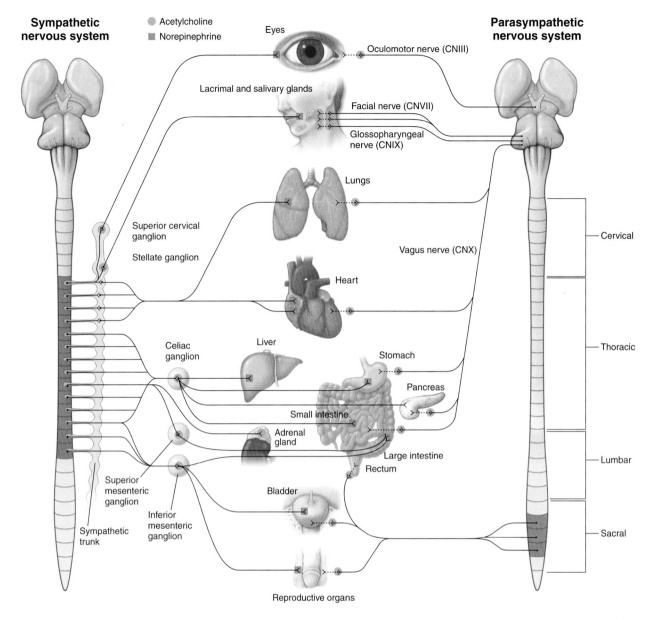

Figure 5.9 Components of the autonomic nervous system. Sympathetic preganglionic neurons from the thoracic and lumbar levels of the spinal cord send out relatively short axons and synapse either in the paravertebral or prevertebral ganglia. An exception is the neurons that go all the way to the adrenal medulla. The parasympathetic preganglionic neurons have relatively long axons and synapse on ganglia very near or actually embedded in the target organs or tissues. CN, cranial nerve.

The PNS is neuroanatomically distinct from the SNS by having its ganglia located very near or actually embedded in the walls of its target organs (Figure 5.9)

Spinal Cord Levels Another major neuroanatomic distinction between the SNS and the PNS is in the location of the cell bodies of their respective preganglionic neurons. Those of the SNS are in the thoracic and lumbar levels of the spinal cord, explaining why the SNS has also been called the *thoracolumbar* division of the ANS. Parasympathetic preganglionic neurons may originate from one of four cranial nerve nuclei in the brain stem or from sacral spinal cord seg-

ments. The four cranial nerve nuclei are the oculomotor (cranial nerve III), the facial (cranial nerve VII), the glossopharyngeal (cranial nerve IX), and the vagus (cranial nerve X) (Figure 5.9). The PNS has therefore also been called the *craniosacral* division of the ANS.

Central Integration Centers The powerful homeostatic control exerted by the ANS requires the integration of signals indicating the state of individual organs and the external environment. In addition to the peripheral ganglia and the spinal cord, a number of structures within the central nervous system (CNS) are important in this respect. Within the brain stem are a number of vital centers that coordinate autonomic reflexes involved in the maintenance of homeostasis by influencing variables such as blood pressure and respiration. Information, for example, from the carotid body baroreceptors and other vascular and cardiac structures is interpreted in the medulla oblongata so that low blood pressure causes reflex increases in heart rate and contractility. Similarly, a decrease in blood pH detected by the carotid body chemoreceptors will stimulate an increase in respiratory rate so that the lungs "blow off" CO_2, thus raising blood pH.

The hypothalamus is a complex collection of neurons called nuclei, located in the diencephalon, just superior to the midbrain and below the thalamus and cerebral hemispheres. A stalk with a portal system connects it to the pituitary gland. The central location of the hypothalamus reflects its primary position in the CNS—receiving information from and sending instructions to other systems. The hypothalamus not only receives input from unconscious subsystems like the ANS, but processes sensory data from the forebrain along with information from the limbic system on the emotional responses to experiences (such as anger or fear), some or all of which may register in consciousness. Among the many homeostatic variables it can modify are body temperature, thirst, hunger, and sleep.

Autonomic Nervous System Efferent Neurons

ANS efferent neurons differ importantly from lower motor neurons of the motor system. As mentioned above, the axon terminals of lower motor neurons are terminal boutons, while the axon terminals of ANS efferent neurons are varicosities (see Chapter 7 and Figure 7.5). In the motor system, an upper motor neuron (with its cell body in the motor cortex) sends its axon down the spinal cord, where it synapses on a lower motor neuron (that has its cell body in the ventral horn of the spinal cord), which in turn sends its axon out to the periphery, where it synapses directly on skeletal muscle. The ANS, however, generally has two neurons in series, forming a path from the spinal cord to the effector organs. The first of these, like the lower motor neuron, has its cell body in the spinal cord, but its axon terminates in one or more (due to branching) ANS ganglia. The second ANS neuron has its cell body in the ganglion, and its axon projects to the periphery, ending near target tissues. The two neurons are therefore called the **preganglionic neuron** and the **postganglionic neuron**, respectively (Figures 5.9 and 5.10). The axons of sympathetic preganglionic neurons that exit the spinal cord via the ventral root and enter a paravertebral ganglion often branch, sending collaterals up and down the chain to superior and inferior ganglia. A single sympathetic preganglionic neuron may thus synapse on up to 20 sympathetic postganglionic neurons. This divergence allows coordinated (i.e., simultaneous) sympathetic stimulation of multiple target tissues. Such divergence is absent in the parasympathetic division.

Autonomic Nervous System Neurotransmitters and Their Receptors

Among the myriad molecules, intracellular and extracellular, involved in the metabolism, signal transduction, information transmission, interpretation, and response functions of the ANS are the neurotransmitters and their receptors. Again paralleling the motor system, ANS neurotransmitters are the chemical signaling molecules released from axon terminals to bridge information-bearing neurochemical signals in the form of an action potential across the synaptic cleft separating a neuron from target cells.

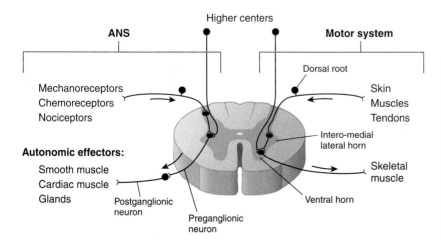

Figure 5.10 The ANS versus the motor system. The ANS has a two-neuron pathway from the spinal cord to the target tissue, a preganglionic and a postganglionic neuron in series. The relatively high diversification (branching) of the sympathetic neurons is not shown, but it allows one preganglionic cell to synapse on up to 20 postganglionic cells in different ganglia. In the motor system, upper motor neurons from the cerebral cortex send axons down the spinal cord that synapse on lower motor neurons whose axons exit to the periphery and synapse directly on skeletal muscle cells. Arrows indicate the flow of information.

Acetylcholine Acetylcholine (ACh) is a critical neurotransmitter for both the motor system and the ANS. In the motor system, it mediates stimulation at the neuromuscular junction by binding to **nicotinic ACh receptors** on the sarcolemma, thereby inducing membrane-depolarizing ion fluxes. (These receptors are so-named because the tobacco plant poison nicotine binds to and activates them.) In the ANS, ACh is found in both the SNS and PNS, where it mediates the connections between preganglionic and postganglionic neurons. ACh is also found in the axon terminals of sympathetic postganglionic neurons that end on sweat glands, and at the ends of all parasympathetic postganglionic neurons. The ACh receptors at ANS ganglia (i.e., on the postganglionic neurons) are nicotinic (though a different subtype than those of the motor system), while those on the peripheral target tissues at parasympathetic postganglionic synapses are **muscarinic ACh receptors**. (They are so-named because the mushroom alkaloid muscarine binds to and activates them.) Collectively, the receptors that bind ACh (acetylcholine) are described as *cholinergic*.

Norepinephrine Norepinephrine (NE) is an important neurotransmitter found in the vesicles of postganglionic sympathetic neurons (except the ones that terminate on sweat glands). (NE is also known as *noradrenaline*.)

Epinephrine Epinephrine (Epi) (also called *adrenaline*) is a powerful neurotransmitter, but its release into the circulation by the medulla of the adrenal glands and its subsequent far-reaching effects justify calling this chemical a hormone as well. Epinephrine binds to the same receptors as NE. Because the alternate names of both NE and Epi are derived from the root *adren-*, their receptors are called *adrenergic*. As with the cholinergic (ACh) receptors, there are a number of different subtypes of adrenergic receptors, which differ in their anatomic distribution, the affinities with which they bind ligands such as NE and Epi, and the signal transduction systems through which ligand binding effects changes in target cell function. Among the most important and best characterized adrenergic receptors are α_1, α_2, β_1, β_2, and β_3 (TABLE 5.1).

Because parasympathetic postganglionic neurons release Ach, the PNS has also been called the cholinergic division of the ANS. Likewise, since most sympathetic postganglionic neurons release NE and/or Epi, the SNS has also been called the adrenergic division of the ANS.

Neuropeptides A number of larger signaling molecules are also found in the axon terminals of ANS neurons. Among them are *substance P*, released by afferent fibers synapsing in the spinal cord in response to nociceptive signals from the periphery; *neuropeptide Y*, found along with NE in the varicosities of sympathetic postganglionic neurons innervating blood vessels; and *vasoactive intestinal peptide* (VIP), present in terminal vesicles of parasympathetic postganglionic neurons in saliva glands.

AUTONOMIC NERVOUS SYSTEM FUNCTION

The effects of the ANS on specific organs, organ systems, and the whole body can be divided into three basic categories: coping with a threat of harm (e.g., escaping or combating an attacker), consuming and digesting food, and reproducing. Most effector tissues, such as the heart, the GI tract, and the genitourinary system are innervated by both the SNS and the PNS. In some cases, their effects are antagonistic, in that parasympathetic stimulation will drive a physiologic variable one way (e.g., decrease heart rate) while sympathetic activation will do the opposite (e.g., increase heart rate). Under relatively normal circumstances, there is a baseline activity of the sympathetic system called **sympathetic tone**. Stressful situations (real or perceived) that demand emergency responses precipitate increased (and coordinated) sympathetic activity and concomitant decreased parasympathetic stimulation. Thus, the SNS is dominant in the catabolic preparation for fight-or-flight responses. The PNS promotes digestion and absorption of food and other more anabolic functions when the individual enjoys a respite from danger. However, it would be a mistake to conclude that the SNS and PNS are always at odds with one another. In fact, they often work additively or synergistically, as in the control of male reproductive organ function. It is the balance between the activity of the two subsystems at any one time that determines the target value, direction, and magnitude of the shift in a given variable. Table 5.1 lists the organ specific effects of SNS and PSN stimulation, some of which are detailed below.

Effects on the Cardiovascular System

Sympathetic stimulation, mediated largely by the binding of NE and/or Epi to β_1-adrenergic receptors, increases heart rate and the force of contractility. Both of these changes work to increase blood pressure and cardiac output, providing organs such as the brain and skeletal muscle (where sympathetic stimulation causes vasodilation) with increased oxygen and glucose for defense (fight) or for escape (flight). Parasympathetic stimulation slows the heart rate, thereby decreasing cardiac output and blood pressure. Interestingly, the vagus nerve, which carries

Table 5.1   EFFECTS OF ANS STIMULATION ON TARGET ORGANS

Organ	Function	SNS Effect [adrenergic receptor]	PNS Effect
Heart	Rate	Increase [β_1]	Decrease
	Contraction	Increase velocity and force [β_1]	Decrease
Blood vessels			
–Skin and internal organs	Contraction	Increase [α_1]	None
–Skeletal muscle	Contraction	Decrease [β_2]	None
Eye			
–Pupil sphincter	Constriction	None	Increase
–Radial pupil muscle	Dilation	Increase [α_1]	None
–Lacrimal glands	Tearing	Increase	Increase
Lungs	Broncho-constriction	Increase [β_2]	Decrease
Kidney	Renin secretion	Increase [α_1, β_1]	None
GI tract			
–Tract walls	Contraction	Decrease [β_2]	Increase
–Sphincters	Contraction	Increase [α_1]	Decrease
–Glands	Secretion of enzymes	Increase mucus [α_1, α_2] and ions	Increase
–Liver	Glycogenolysis	Increase [β_2]	None
GU Tract			
–Bladder	Contraction	Decrease [β_2]	Increase
–Trigone + Sphincter	Contraction	Increase [α_1]	Decrease
–Penile	Erection	Promotes	
	Ejaculation	Promotes [α_1]	
Adrenal Medulla	Epi and NE secretion	Increase [nicotinic AchR]	None
Posterior Pituitary	ADH secretion	Increase [β_1]	None

PNS signals, tonically slows the heart rate, so that the heart normally beats at a lower rate than its intrinsic pacemaker would direct. Disrupting the vagus nerve (as occurs in patients who receive a heart transplant) allows the heart to beat at its higher intrinsic rate.

Effects on the Gastrointestinal System

If danger threatens, resources should not be used for the processes that build up body structures over the course of hours, days, and years. The individual needs to employ emergency procedures to survive what is hopefully a short-term (acute) stress, and worry about long-term issues later. Thus, sympathetic stimulation decreases peristaltic contractions that propel food in the GI tract, relaxes the gallbladder, and constricts sphincter muscles such as the sphincter of Oddi. Parasympathetic stimulation opposes these actions, increasing smooth muscle contraction to produce peristalsis, inducing contraction of the gallbladder, and relaxing sphincter muscles.

Effects on the Renal System

Sympathetic innervation of the kidney is a critical control center for the regulation of blood pressure. Adrenergic stimulation augments the secretion of renin, leading to the generation of angiotensin II, a powerful vasoconstrictor that elevates blood pressure. When pressure is high enough or the demand for increased pressure resolves, sympathetic stimulation decreases, inducing a decrement in renin release. This is another example of control by one division of the ANS by regulation of tone rather than antagonization by the other division, as the contribution of the PNS to this renal function seems to be minimal.

Effects on the Genitourinary System

The process of urination (micturition) is complex, in that at least four systems participate in its control. Sympathetic signals from SNS (adrenergic) neurons in the lumbar spinal cord cause relaxation of the detrussor muscles of the urinary bladder wall and contraction of the trigone and internal urethral sphincter, thus inhibiting the outflow of urine. Parasympathetic preganglionic neurons in the sacral spinal cord synapse on parasympathetic postganglionic (cholinergic) neurons in the bladder wall, and these promote detrussor contraction and trigone and internal urethral sphincter relaxation.

A third control system is the micturition reflex center in the brainstem, which receives information on bladder wall tension (and thus bladder pressure) from afferent nerves and, when pressure rises, inhibits sympathetic neurons that prevent voiding. A fourth level of control is the contraction or relaxation of the external urethral sphincter, which is skeletal muscle under voluntary control with lower motor neurons in the sacral spinal cord. Thus, lower spinal cord injury can cause profound problems with urinary incontinence and incomplete voiding.

The regulation of male sexual function is another example of cooperation rather than antagonization between the two divisions of the ANS. The parasympathetic system mediates erection, while the sympathetic system controls ejaculation.

Effects on the Dermatologic System

Unlike other systems, the components of the skin, especially its blood vessels and sweat glands, are exclusively under sympathetic influence, without parasympathetic input. Activation of the SNS results in the constriction of dermal vessels, secretion by the sweat glands, and contraction of the pilomotor muscles that raise body hair. These responses are important in thermoregulation. Adrenergically mediated vasoconstriction shunts blood away from the skin where heat is lost to the environment, thus helping maintain body temperature in cold conditions. Decreased SNS signaling allows for vasodilation (partly mediated by local metabolites) when conditions are hot, allowing more heat to dissipate to the surroundings. Sympathetic stimulation of sweat glands helps cool the body. In animals, pilo-

erection helps conserve heat and give a threatened creature a fierce appearance, but in humans it mostly causes goose bumps. In order to effect consistent responses that would not antagonize each other when temperature control is the goal, the invocation of vasoconstriction, sweating, and piloerection has to be selective. In large-scale adrenergic activation (see below), all of these effects occur simultaneously.

A separate ANS reaction in the skin is the vasodilator response to injury. Afferent ANS neurons near skin areas that suffer traumatic damage release substance P both at the site of injury and in the spinal cord. Branches of their axons that innervate blood vessels cause the relaxation of smooth muscle and vasodilation. This increases the volume and decreases the speed of blood flow, allowing inflammatory and repair cells from the blood to access the site of damage.

Effects on the Pulmonary System

Sympathetic stimulation, working through β_2-adrenergic receptors, causes relaxation of the smooth muscle investing the bronchioles, resulting in bronchodilation. This provides greater ventilation during exertion for fight or flight. Parasympathetic activity opposes this action, causing bronchoconstriction and increased secretion by bronchial glands.

Effects on the Endocrine System

Receiving information about a threat or the need to respond to stress, the hypothalamus releases corticotropin-releasing hormone (CRH), which reaches the anterior pituitary and causes the release of adrenocorticotropic hormone (ACTH). ACTH reaches the adrenal cortex and induces the production and release of glucocorticoids that have profound and diverse effects on salt and water balance, immune function, and glucose supply and metabolism (see Chapter 32).

The most rapid and dramatic autonomic endocrine response is sympathetic stimulation of the adrenal medulla. Structurally and functionally, this subsystem is distinct from the rest of the ANS in that the adrenal gland is supplied by *pre*ganglionic, not postganglionic, sympathetic neurons. The chromaffin cells of the adrenal medulla resemble postganglionic sympathetic neurons, warranting their designation as neuroendocrine cells. Sympathetic preganglionic neurons whose axons exit the spinal cord synapse directly on these medullary cells, and activation causes the secretion of potent adrenergic mediators. Whereas most sympathetic postganglionic neurons release NE into the limited extracellular space of a target tissue, adrenal neuroendocrine cells release a combination of Epi (80%) and NE (20%) into the bloodstream, in amounts large enough to transiently maintain relatively high serum concentrations. These powerful mediators circulate widely, acting like sympathetic hormones.

Integrated Responses

Most of the time, the SNS and PNS mediate the physiologic adjustment of one organ or target tissue independent of the others; that is, the demands of a given circumstance may require, for example, a decrease in heart rate but an increase in sweating. An increase in PNS activity and a decrease in SNS activity in the cardiac conduction system will achieve the first change, while and increase in sympathetic signals in the skin will effect the second.

Two aspects of the SNS, however, suggest the ability for large scale, coordinated activity that organizes many or all of the body systems in response to stress (actual or imagined). The first is the high degree of divergence in the SNS. Because a single preganglionic neuron may send axon branches to numerous ganglia, multiple end organs or tissues may be activated at the same time. The second is the adrenal medullary response described above. Since Epi is released and circulates widely, it agonizes adrenergic receptors throughout the body simultaneously. Such widespread sympathetic activity stimulates the heart to increase its rate and contraction and dilates lung bronchioles to provide the oxygen to sustain exertion. Vasodilation in the skeletal muscle brings the increased blood flow from the heart to the tissues needed for fight or flight. The catabolism of glycogen in the liver and lipids in adipose tissues liberates glucose and fatty acids, the easily used fuels of brain and muscle. Such conditions recruit all the skin responses: vasoconstriction of dermal vessels causes the skin to turn pale, increased sweating cools the skin, and piloerection causes goose bumps—the very picture of a frightened patient suffering a heart attack, or of a patron of an effective horror movie. While such reactions can be life-saving under some conditions (e.g., when chased by a predator), they can be deleterious under others. (See Clinical Application Box *Drugs That Modify the Sympathetic Nervous System*.)

AUTONOMIC NERVOUS SYSTEM PATHOPHYSIOLOGY

When the ANS operates properly, it regulates and integrates organs and organ systems to promote healthy homeostasis. When the ANS does not function normally, it causes organ-specific or organ system–specific disease.

Horner's Syndrome

Autonomic innervation of the eye includes both sympathetic and parasympathetic contributions. The sympathetic preganglionic neurons send axons up the paravertebral chains where they synapse on cells in the superior cervical ganglion. Postganglionic neurons from here innervate the iris radial muscle that dilates the pupil, the lacrimal glands that produce tears, and the muscles that help raise the eyelids. The parasympathetic preganglionic neurons of cranial nerve III synapse on cells of the ciliary ganglion, which in turn stimulate the iris pupillary sphincter muscle that constricts the pupil. When the SNS is damaged or inhibited, the affected side has a loss of sympathetic tone, producing an imbalance between the SNS and PNS. The decreased pupil dilation, eyelid raising, and tear production leaves the parasympathetic forces inducing constriction unopposed, and a triad of miosis (small, contracted pupils), ptosis (eyelid drooping), and anhydrosis (decreased tear production) results, a condition called **Horner's syndrome**.

Lesions to the Hypothalamus

Complex functions such as appetite and weight control, thirst and osmolality control, and thermoregulation under the influence of the hypothalamus can be disturbed by lesions—often ischemic (i.e., impaired blood flow, as in a stroke); neoplastic (i.e., cancer); or traumatic—to this compact brain center. However, the exact manifestations of hypothalamic dysfunction depend on the particular hypothalamic nuclei and/or tracts affected. Some experimental lesions in animals produce dramatic increases in appetite and body weight (hyperphagia), while others induce a loss of appetite (anorexia) that can be fatal. Thermoregulation in patients who have suffered hypothalamic lesions can be difficult, as they become hypothermic when their heat-conserving mechanisms fail and body temperature falls toward room temperature.

Vasovagal Episode

The initial response to painful stimuli is often an increase in sympathetic activity that elevates the heart rate, cardiac contractility, and therefore, the blood pressure. Shortly thereafter, the increased blood pressure can trigger baroreceptors in the heart and arteries and lead to a reflex increase in parasympathetic activity that decreases the heart rate and dilates blood vessels to reduce the blood pressure. When such a compensatory reflex over-

DRUGS THAT MODIFY THE SYMPATHETIC NERVOUS SYSTEM

The subtypes of adrenergic receptors that mediate the effects of the sympathetic neurotransmitters norepinephrine (NE) and epinephrine (Epi) were originally differentiated by their ligand binding and their activating or inhibiting sympathetic signals. Such receptors differ in their structure and the signal transduction machinery they employ. While sympathetic responses may be life-saving in some circumstances, they contribute adversely to diseases such as high blood pressure (hypertension). The ability to modulate adrenergic receptor subtypes by pharmacological agents is a mainstay of modern medicine. In the case of hypertension, medications such as metoprolol, which antagonize the β_1-adrenergic receptors in the heart, are useful in decreasing heart rate and contractility, reducing cardiac output and blood pressure.

Consider an example of a situation where sympathetic discharge is harmful: a patient suffers an acute heart attack, with damage to the ventricular muscle that pumps blood (see Chapter 13). The patient may be frightened and in pain, leading to activation of his sympathetic system and the subsequent release of NE and Epi. These neurotransmitters stimulate the heart, increasing its firing rate and contraction. However, making the heart work harder induces a greater demand for oxygen and other nutrients supplied by the blood at the very moment when blood flow to the heart is dangerously restricted. This may actually further damage the weakened heart. Thus, such patients are routinely given drugs like metoprolol to limit the oxygen demand of their hearts.

An opposite situation occurs in patients suffering from an exacerbation of asthma, where one or more stimuli induce constriction of the bronchi, limiting the flow of air into and out of the lungs. Such patients can be treated with rapidly acting drugs that agonize β-adrenergic receptors. An example is the inhaled drug albuterol. As one might expect, albuterol, which can relieve the airflow obstruction of asthma by binding to the β_2 receptors on bronchioles, can also induce (as a side effect) an increase in heart rate (tachycardia) when it is absorbed systemically and agonizes cardiac β_1 receptors.

---

compensates and parasympathetic activity is too high, the blood pressure can drop precipitously. The low blood pressure during such an excessive PNS reflex is often accompanied by a mixture of PNS and SNS effects, including profuse sweating, clammy and pale skin, nausea, and lightheadedness and possibly fainting (syncope). Because excessive activity of the vagus nerve (cranial nerve X) is responsible for the vasodilation and other cardiovascular manifestations, this group of symptoms is called a **vasovagal episode**.

Summary

- Neurons are the basic cellular elements of the nervous system.

- A neuron's **dendrites** receive input from other cells, the **axon** conducts information, and the release of **neurotransmitters** at the axon terminals allows information to cross the **synapse** between a neuron and a target cell.

- Like most cells, neurons possess a **resting membrane potential (E_m)** owing to the unequal distribution of ions (Na^+, K^+, and Cl^-) between the intracellular and extracellular spaces. The average resting membrane potential of a typical neuron is -60 to -70 mV. The *electrogenic* Na^+-K^+-ATPase pump helps maintain the concentration gradients for Na^+ and K^+.

- The combination of electrical and chemical forces influencing an ion's movement across the cell membrane is called the **electrochemical gradient**.

- The **Nernst equation** defines the equilibrium potential of each ion. This Nernst potential is the membrane voltage needed to just balance the concentration gradient of the particular ion.

- The **chord conductance** and **Goldman equations** express the membrane potential as the weighted average of the membrane conductances (g_X) and membrane permeabilities (P_X), respectively, for each of the relevant ions. If the membrane permeability to one ion, such as Na^+, greatly exceeds that of the others, the Goldman equation reduces down to the Nernst equation and the membrane potential will shift toward the Nernst potential for that ion.

- Stimuli that depolarize the neuron membrane to or above the **threshold** value trigger an **action potential**, a limited positive feedback loop of membrane depolarization caused by the sudden increase in P_{Na}^+ (and therefore g_{Na}^+). The repolarization portion of the action potential is caused by the increase in P_K^+ and therefore g_K^+).

- The basis of the action potential is the sequential opening, locking, and resetting of **voltage-gated Na^+ and K^+ channels**.

- The action potential propagates down the axon like a regenerating wave of depolarization. In many neurons, the **myelin** sheath increases the efficiency and the rate of action potential conduction. An action potential in such a neuron propagates rapidly by **electrotonic conduction** in myelinated areas and slows down to regenerate at **nodes of Ranvier**. This mode of transmission is called **saltatory conduction**.

- At axon terminals, an action potential induces an increase in the membrane conductance to Ca^{2+}, which causes neurotransmitter vesicles of the presynaptic cell to fuse with the membrane and release neurotransmitter molecules into the synaptic cleft. The neurotransmitters bind to their receptors on the postsynaptic cell and depolarize it, establishing a new action potential.

- The ANS works largely unconsciously and integrates information from the internal and external environments to maintain total body homeostasis.

- The ANS has two divisions, the **sympathetic nervous system (SNS)** (also called the *thoracolumbar* or *adrenergic* division) and the **parasympathetic nervous system (PNS)** (also called the *craniosacral* or *cholinergic* division).

- Because the SNS preganglionic neuron cell bodies are in the thoracic and lumbar levels of the spinal cord, the SNS is also called the *thoracolumbar* division of the ANS. Because the PNS preganglionic neuron cell bodies are in some cranial nerve nuclei located in the brainstem while other cell bodies are in the sacral segments of the spinal cord, the PNS is also called the *craniosacral* division of the ANS.

- The major neurotransmitters of the ANS are **acetylcholine (Ach)**, **norepinephrine (NE)**, and **epinephrine (Epi)**, though a number of neuropeptides and other signaling molecules are important as well.

- Both SNS and PNS preganglionic neurons release Ach.

- Because most SNS postganglionic neurons release NE and/or Epi, the SNS is also called the **adrenergic** division of the ANS. Because all PNS postganglionic neurons release Ach, the PNS is also called the **cholinergic** division of the ANS.

- Many target tissues are influenced by both the SNS and PNS, which may work antagonistically or cooperatively.

- Widespread, simultaneous activation of the SNS induces the preparation for the fight-or-flight response.

- Dysfunction of the ANS causes organ-specific or organ system-specific disease. In **Horner's syndrome**, lack of sympathetic tone causes miosis, ptosis, and anhydrosis on the affected side. Excessive PNS activity carried by the vagal nerve (cranial nerve X) can cause a **vasovagal episode**, with hypotension and possible syncope.

Suggested Reading

Beers WH, Reich E. Structure and activity of acetylcholine. Nature. 1970;228(5275):917–922.

Exton JH. Mechanisms involved in alpha-adrenergic phenomena. Am J Physiol. 1985;248(6 Pt 1):E633–667.

Hirst GD, Edwards FR. Sympathetic neuroeffector transmission in arteries and arterioles. Physiol Rev. 1989;69(2):546–604.

REVIEW QUESTIONS

Directions: Each of the numbered items or incomplete statements in this section is followed by answers or by completions of the statement. Select the ONE lettered answer or completion that is BEST in each case.

1. A 36-year-old man is exposed to diisopropyl phosphofluoridate (DFP), a biological toxic agent that blocks the acetylcholinesterase enzyme, which catabolizes ACh at synapses. Which of the following would you expect among his symptoms?

    (A) High heart rate (tachycardia) and high blood pressure (hypertension)

(B) Hypersalivation and hyperlacrimation (increased tearing and salivation)
(C) Constipation
(D) Urinary retention
(E) Ejaculation

2. A 28-year-old woman injects cocaine into her bloodstream. This drug causes the accumulation of norepinephrine and would be expected to manifest as

(A) urinary incontinence
(B) bowel incontinence
(C) elevated heart rate and blood pressure

(D) depressed heart rate and blood pressure
(E) miosis

3. Which of the following drugs might help a patient with low blood pressure and a slow heart rate?

(A) Metoprolol, a drug that blocks cardiac β-adrenergic receptors
(B) Atropine, a drug that block the cardiac effects of ACh
(C) Acetylcholine
(D) Diisopropyl phosphofluoridate (DFP), a drug that blocks the breakdown of ACh

4. Which of the following is the predominant neuro-transmitter at both sympathetic and parasympathetic ganglia?

   (A) Epinephrine (Epi)
   (B) Norepinephrine (NE)
   (C) Substance P
   (D) Acetylcholine (Ach)
   (E) Vasoactive intestinal peptide (VIP)

5. A 64-year-old man presents to an emergency department with a broken toe. He is accidentally given an injection of atropine, a drug that antagonizes the effects of Ach at muscarinic receptors, instead of an analgesic. Which of the following symptoms do you expect him to have?

   (A) Tachycardia (a high heart rate)
   (B) Hypertension (high blood pressure)
   (C) Cool, clammy, pale skin
   (D) Diarrhea
   (E) Increased tearing and salivation

ANSWERS TO REVIEW QUESTIONS

1. **The answer is B.** Exposure to DFP causes the accumulation of ACh, which mimics hyperactivity of the parasympathetic division of the ANS. Thus, increased salivation and tearing are expected, along with a decrease in the heart rate (bradycardia) and blood pressure (hypotension), increased contraction of the peristaltic and bladder wall muscles (causing defecation and urination), and penile erection.

2. **The answer is C.** Because NE is a major neurotransmitter for the SNS, its overabundance would mimic the fight-or-flight response. Cocaine thus causes tachycardia (increased heart rate) and hypertension (increased blood pressure). All the other symptoms are manifestations of excessive or unopposed parasympathetic activity.

3. **The answer is B.** By inhibiting the parasympathetic neurotransmitter ACh, atropine essentially produces a pharmacologic vagotomy, blocking the parasympathetic break on heart rate and causing the pulse to increase. This, in turn, can elevate blood pressure. All the other substances would either inhibit sympathetic tone (metoprolol) or increase parasympathetic signals, which would further decrease the heart rate and blood pressure.

4. **The answer is D.** Both SNS and PNS preganglionic neurons release ACh at synapses with their postganglionic counterparts.

5. **The answer is A.** By inhibiting the actions of Ach on muscarinic receptors, atropine produces a constellation of symptoms that in some organ systems resembles an increase in sympathetic tone. Thus, its effects on the heart include an increase in the pulse and blood pressure, which makes this drug useful in patients suffering from hypotension due to a low heart rate. In the GI tract, it decreases motility and impairs salivation. It likewise inhibits lacrimation. In the skin, where sympathetic postganglionic neurons release Ach to induce secretion by sweat glands, atropine does not mimic a hyperadrenergic state. Instead, sweating is decreased and the skin becomes dry, hot, and red. In addition, the antagonization of muscarinic receptors can produce mydriasis (dilation of the pupil) with subsequent difficulty seeing, and toxic doses of the drug can cause profound behavioral changes including delirium, characterized by restlessness and confusion. The clinic picture of atropinism has been encapsulated in the mnemonic: "Fast as a hare, red as a beet, hot as an iron, blind as a bat, and mad as a hatter."

Part II

MUSCULOSKELETAL PHYSIOLOGY

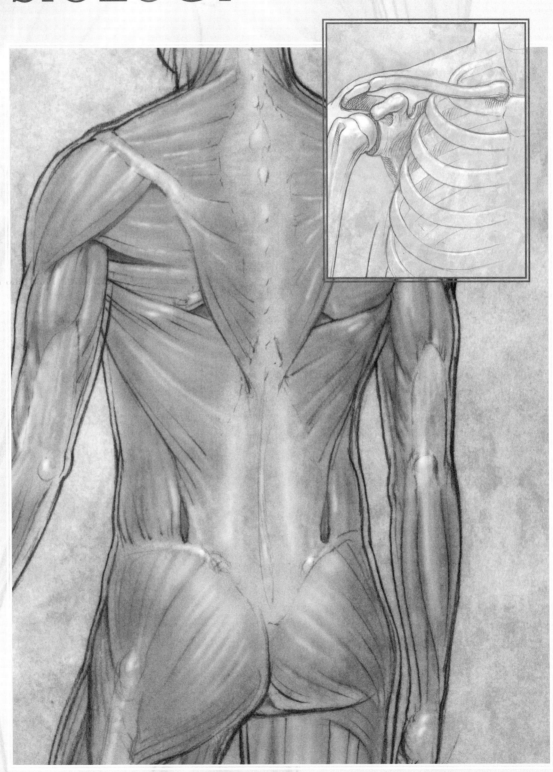

6

The Neuromuscular Junction and Skeletal Muscle

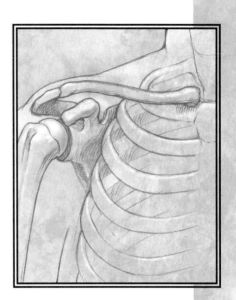

INTRODUCTION

There are three different types of muscle: skeletal, cardiac, and smooth. These three types are differentiated based on their distinct control systems (neuronal, neurohormonal); their anatomic locations; and their specialized cellular structure, function, and biochemistry. Because skeletal muscle is under voluntary control, it allows activities as fundamental as walking and as advanced as accurately wielding a scalpel. It is the type of muscle adherent to bones that moves joints. Although this chapter focuses on skeletal muscle and its neuronal control, much of the discussion of the molecular basis of the contractile machinery of skeletal muscle applies to cardiac and smooth muscle as well.

The major function of **skeletal muscle** is its role as the effector organ in voluntary movement. It mediates the transformation of central nervous system electrical activity into purposeful mechanical actions such as maintaining posture, moving limbs and digits, and speaking. Skeletal muscle also has a number of secondary roles. It is a potential source of metabolic energy. In cases of stress, such as starvation, skeletal muscle tissue can be catabolized (broken down) to provide energy. In addition, skeletal muscle contributes to body heat generation. The precise control of muscle activity by the nervous system is necessary for effective reflexive and conscious movement.

SYSTEM STRUCTURE

Three organ systems are involved in movement: nerves, muscles, and bones. This chapter will discuss nerves and muscles. While bones have their own physiological functions and regulatory systems (see Chapter 8), for our present purposes, we will regard them as the scaffolding of the body.

Neuromuscular Organs

Three organs are essential for conscious movement: the brain, the spinal cord, and skeletal muscles. Many reflexive movements, however, require only the spinal cord and the skeletal muscles.

Central Nervous System   The central nervous system is composed of the brain and spinal cord. Higher areas of the brain generate instructions for purposeful, conscious movements and modify lower systems that carry out unconscious movements and reflexive muscle contractions. The spinal cord performs two critical functions. First, it carries information in two directions: sensory input important in planning movements is transmitted from the periphery to the brain while instructions that originate in the brain are conveyed to the skeletal muscles in the periphery. Second, the simplest reflex movements are organized in the spinal cord and may occur without input from the brain.

Skeletal Muscles   Skeletal muscles are found throughout the body. They are connected to bones via tendons. Collectively, skeletal muscles make up 45% to 50% of total body mass and receive variable percentages of cardiac output depending on the activity level. Their various sizes and shapes correlate with their skeletal attachments and motor functions.

Neuromuscular Tissues

Tissues important in the generation, modification, and execution of instructions for movements include specific areas of the brain and spinal cord as well as the skeletal muscles.

Motor Nerve Tissues   FIGURE 6.1A illustrates some of the brain tissues involved in the generation and transmission of motor instructions. The *premotor cortex* and *supplementary motor area* are located in the frontal lobe. The premotor cortex receives input from the *cerebellum*, which provides important signals regulating balance and coordination. The supplementary motor area receives input from the *basal ganglia*, a complex subcortical tissue involved in the prioritization of movement programs and their components. In addition, both the premotor cortex and the supplementary motor area are connected to networks of sensory and association neurons that provide information important for planning and executing movements. The *primary motor cortex* is a strip of frontal lobe cerebral cortex that receives input from the premotor cortex, the supplementary motor area, the cerebellum, and higher sensory and association areas of the brain. The primary motor cortex is arranged as a modified body map called a *homunculus.*

The axons of the neurons in the motor areas travel through the *internal capsule* to reach the brain stem and spinal cord (Figure 6.1B). A number of spinal cord tracts are involved in the transmission of movement instructions to and from higher centers. Among these, the *lateral corticospinal tract* is critical in voluntary limb movement. The cell bodies of neurons of the lateral corticospinal tract are in the primary motor cortex and their axons comprise part of the internal capsule and then constitute part of the lateral column of the spinal cord. The axons of many, but not all, motor tract neurons cross the midpoint somewhere between their origin and termination, which explains why neurons with cell bodes on the left side of the brain control muscles on the right side of the body and vice versa. Such a crossing of an axon from one side to the other is called a *decussation.*

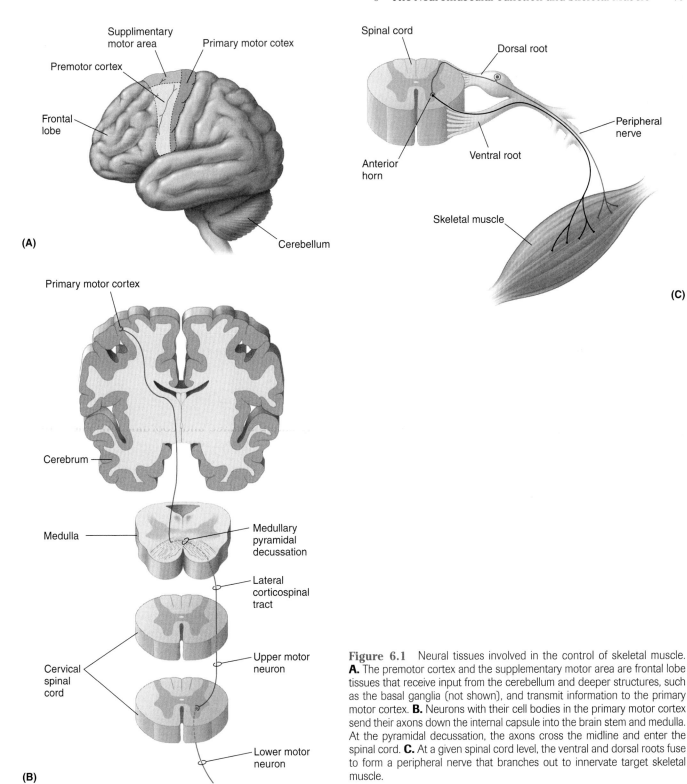

(A)

(B)

(C)

Figure 6.1 Neural tissues involved in the control of skeletal muscle. **A.** The premotor cortex and the supplementary motor area are frontal lobe tissues that receive input from the cerebellum and deeper structures, such as the basal ganglia (not shown), and transmit information to the primary motor cortex. **B.** Neurons with their cell bodies in the primary motor cortex send their axons down the internal capsule into the brain stem and medulla. At the pyramidal decussation, the axons cross the midline and enter the spinal cord. **C.** At a given spinal cord level, the ventral and dorsal roots fuse to form a peripheral nerve that branches out to innervate target skeletal muscle.

The peripheral nerves that control voluntary muscles have their cell bodies in the *anterior horn* of the spinal cord gray matter (Figure 6.1C). Their axons exit the spinal cord via ventral roots, and fuse with dorsal roots to form spinal nerves. Spinal nerves branch out into peripheral nerves, a large collection of which is called a *plexus* (e.g., the brachial plexus). Peripheral nerves continue to branch out until they reach their target muscles.

Skeletal Muscle Tissue Skeletal muscle tissue is surrounded by a collagen-containing layer called the

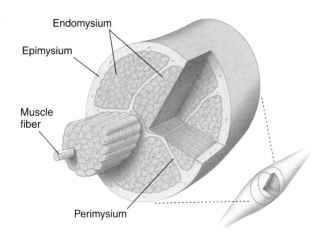

Figure 6.2 Skeletal muscle subdivisions. The epimysium is the external covering layer of the entire skeletal muscle. The perimysium separates groups of muscle fibers. The endomysium divides individual muscle fibers from one another.

epimysium. A block of skeletal muscle tissue is subdivided into bundles of muscle cells by *perimysium*. A single bundle is subdivided by the *endomysium*, which insulates individual muscle cells (FIGURE 6.2).

Neuromuscular Cells

Three cell types are critical to basic movements: efferent neurons that carry instructions to skeletal muscles, afferent neurons that relay information from skeletal muscles to the central nervous system, and the cells of skeletal muscle.

Nerve Cells   Neurons in higher brain centers such as the lateral corticospinal tract are called **upper motor neurons** (FIGURE 6.3). The nervous system cells involved in transmitting instructions for voluntary movements from the spinal cord to skeletal muscles are specialized efferent neurons called **lower motor neurons**. Their cell bodies are in the anterior horns of the gray matter of the spinal cord, while their axons project out sequentially via ventral roots, spinal nerves, and peripheral nerves to the skeletal muscles they innervate. Schwann cells myelinate the axon and terminal branches of the motor neurons. The lower motor neuron axons end in specialized terminal branch structures called terminal boutons. Peripheral nerves also contain afferent sensory neurons that relay information from peripheral tissues, including skeletal muscles, back to the spinal cord.

Skeletal Muscle Cells   Skeletal muscles cells, or *muscle fibers*, are long and cylindrical (FIGURE 6.4). They result from the fusion of numerous precursor cells during development. In histologic terms, skeletal muscle is described as *striated* because cells appear striped under the light microscope.

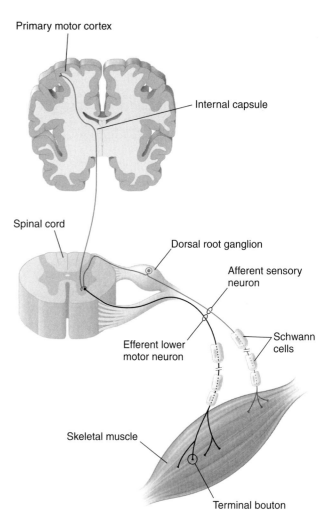

Figure 6.3   Innervation of skeletal muscle. The neurons with their cell bodies in the primary motor cortex are called upper motor neurons. After their axons travel through the internal capsule and decussate, they synapse on efferent lower motor neurons, which have their cell bodies in the anterior horn of the gray matter of the spinal cord and transmit information from the spinal cord to skeletal muscles. The axons of lower motor neurons exit the spinal cord through the ventral roots. Schwann cells wrap their cell membranes round lower motor neuron axons to myelinate them. Peripheral nerves branch and finally synapse on skeletal muscle cells. The lower motor neuron axon terminals are called terminal boutons. Peripheral nerves also contain afferent sensory neurons, which transmit information from skeletal muscles to the spinal cord. Such afferent sensory neurons have their cell bodies in the dorsal root ganglia.

Neuromuscular Organelles

Like most other cells, motor neurons and skeletal muscle cells have a number of organelles, including one or more nuclei, endoplasmic reticulum, ribosomes, and the Golgi complex. Although each of these is essential for proper cell function, the following discussion focuses on those organelles critically involved in movement.

The Neuromuscular Junction   The **neuromuscular junction** is the meeting point between the peripheral

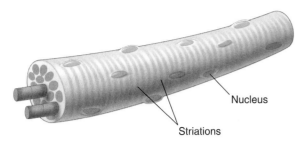

Figure 6.4 A skeletal muscle fiber. Skeletal muscle fibers are long, cylindrical cells. Because they result developmentally from the fusion of many precursor cells, they have numerous nuclei. The prominent stripes are called striations.

nervous system and skeletal muscle. The neuromuscular junction is a chemical synapse between a lower motor neuron and a skeletal muscle cell (FIGURE 6.5). On the *presynaptic* side of the neuromuscular junction is the terminal bouton of the lower motor neuron axon. Synaptic vesicles in the presynaptic lower motor neuron contain the neurotransmitter **acetylcholine (ACh)**. These synaptic vesicles aggregate at specific sites called *active zones*.

The nerve and muscle cells do not touch; they are separated by a narrow gap called the *synaptic cleft*. The synaptic cleft is a complex, amorphously structured extracellular space containing carbohydrates and enzymes. On the *postsynaptic* side of the neuromuscular junction is the muscle cell.

The Sarcolemma and T Tubules As Figure 6.5 shows, the muscle cell membrane is called the **sarcolemma**. At the points where lower motor neurons synapse with muscle fibers, the sarcolemma forms a shallow depression, or synaptic trough, into which the terminal bouton fits. At the trough, the sarcolemma invaginates into synaptic folds, forming pits. The "mouths" of synaptic fold pits are located directly under the active zones and are studded with numerous ACh receptors. This area of the sarcolemma is also referred to as the *motor end plate*.

The sarcolemma has a system of deep invaginations that topologically extend the extracellular space into the muscle fiber. By means of this system of *T tubules*, subcellular structures even in the center of the muscle fiber are not far from the extracellular space (FIGURE 6.6). (T stands for transverse.)

The Sarcoplasmic Reticulum Along with the T tubules, the skeletal muscle fiber contains a structurally and functionally specialized endoplasmic reticulum called **sarcoplasmic reticulum (SR)**, a

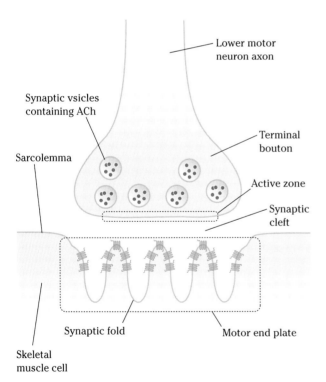

Figure 6.5 The neuromuscular junction. The terminal bouton has numerous neurotransmitter vesicles that contain acetylcholine (ACh). The vesicles aggregate at active zones. The terminal bouton does not touch its target muscle cell—it is separated from the muscle fiber by the synaptic cleft. The muscle cell membrane, or sarcolemma, apposed to the terminal bouton has numerous synaptic folds where ACh receptors are present in high density. The segment of the sarcolemma with such synaptic folds is known as the motor end plate.

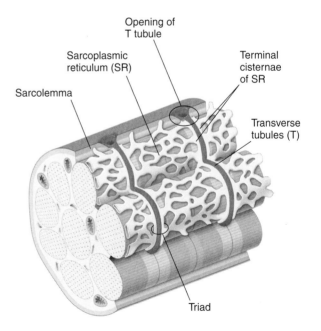

Figure 6.6 The T tubule system and sarcoplasmic reticulum of a skeletal muscle fiber. The T tubules are complex invaginations of the sarcolemma. The sarcoplasmic reticulum is a set of interconnected membrane-bound spaces. This drawing from an electron micrograph shows a T tubule flanked by the terminal cysternae of the SR on both sides, forming a triad.

system of closed membrane pouches (i.e., they do not open to the extracellular space). These membrane-enclosed spaces are longitudinal in the middle and have lobulated ends called *terminal cisternae* (Figure 6.6). The SR has a high internal concentration of calcium.

When a muscle fiber is viewed under an electron microscope, each T tubule invagination is seen to be flanked on either side by a terminal cisterna. Together, a T tubule and the two terminal cisternae are called a *triad*. Triads occur at regular intervals along the long axis of the muscle fiber (Figure 6.6).

Myofibrils and Sarcomeres   Striated muscle appears striped when viewed under the microscope because of the regular arrangement of its contractile components, specialized protein aggregates. A longitudinal section through a muscle fiber reveals many closely packed parallel **myofibrils** with alternating light and dark bands or cross-striations. Myofibrils are long, tubular structures with longitudinal axes parallel to the longitudinal axis of the whole muscle cell (Figure 6.7A). The alternating light and dark cross striations of a single myofibril are in register with the striations of neighboring myofibrils.

A myofibril has five main components (Figure 6.7B). An *I band* is the light cross striation, and a *Z line* is a dark line in the center of an I band. Although these structures have two-dimensional names, they are three-dimensional. An I band appears as a circle in

transverse section through the same myofibril. Thus, an I band is really a squat cylindrical substructure of the larger cylindrical myofibril, which is in turn a cylindrical component of the even larger muscle fiber. Likewise, a Z line is a round plate when viewed in transverse section, like a thin slice out of a cucumber. For this reason, a Z line is sometimes referred to as a Z disk.

An *A band* is the dark cross-striation. Like an I band, it is a three-dimensional cylindrical structure. An A band has a relatively lighter *H band* in its center. In the center of the H band is a dark structure called an *M line*. Like a Z line, an M line is actually a disk.

A **sarcomere**, a portion of a myofibril between two consecutive Z lines, is the basic functional contractile unit of skeletal muscle. As mentioned above, triads occur at regular intervals along the length of the muscle fiber. Each sarcomere has two associated triads, one at each of the I band and A band borders.

Neuromuscular Molecules

The molecules of motor neurons are responsible for the electrochemical events that transmit information such as instructions for movement down a nerve cell axon and across the synaptic clefts that separate upper motor neurons from lower motor neurons and lower motor neurons from skeletal muscle cells. The molecules of skeletal muscle cells constitute the contractile machinery ultimately responsible for movement.

Motor Neuron Molecules   Motor neurons have many proteins embedded in their cell membranes. Among the most important membrane proteins for neuronal control of skeletal muscle contraction are the channels and ion pumps.

Each synaptic vesicle of a motor neuron terminal contains approximately 10,000 molecules of ACh, the fundamental neuromuscular neurotransmitter that activates skeletal muscle. **ACh receptors (AChRs)** are found in high concentrations on the sarcolemma, clustered around the mouths of the synaptic folds (Figure 6.5). The AchR is a complex protein pentamer embedded in the lipid bilayer of the sarcolemma. Although each receptor has five subunits, two of the five are identical (the α subunits); therefore, there are really only four different proteins (and four corresponding genes): α, β, γ, and δ. Because the α subunit has the ACh binding site, each ACh receptor can accommodate two neurotransmitter molecules. The five subunits combine to form a central ion channel.

The enzyme **acetylcholinesterase (AChE)** is associated with the extracellular surface of the sarcolemma via hydrophobic interactions. It is therefore an inhabitant of the synaptic cleft.

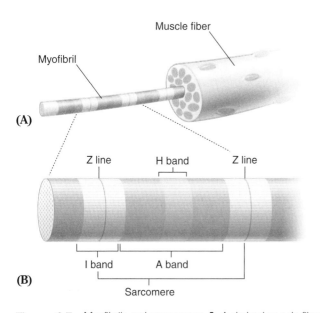

Figure 6.7   Myofibrils and sarcomeres. **A.** A skeletal muscle fiber is composed of numerous myofibrils—closely packed, parallel cylindrical structures. **B.** A single myofibril is a series of alternating dark and light bands. The sarcomere is the basic unit of the myofibril and extends from one Z line to the next. The sarcomeres of a given myofibril are in register with those of adjacent myofibrils, accounting for the striations of a skeletal muscle cell.

Skeletal Muscle Proteins   Like motor neurons, skeletal muscle cells have a number of molecules essential for motor function. The most important of these are the proteins that combine to form the contractile machinery and are responsible for the striated appearance of skeletal muscle fibers. The two large divisions of the contractile proteins are the thin filaments and thick filaments.

Thin Filaments   The light I bands of the sarcomere are composed of protein polymers called **thin filaments**. Thin filaments have three subcomponents: actin polymers, tropomyosin polymers, and troponin complexes (FIGURE 6.8A). Minor proteins bind thin filaments to a Z line.

G-actin is the monomeric (globular) form of the protein *actin*. G-actin monomers are polarized, having a plus end and a minus end. G-actin monomers polymerize into double helical strands of F (filamentous)-actin. Seven consecutive G-actin monomers constitute a single turn of the F-actin double helix. Because the constituent G-actin monomers are polarized, F-actin polymers are also polarized, and "point" out from the Z line to which they are attached. Each Z line has thin filaments anchored upon it, projecting out in both directions, that is, from both its sides (left and right in a longitudinal view, front and back in a transverse view).

The F-actin double helix has a groove on either side. This groove is occupied by a thin supercoiled double helix protein called *tropomyosin*. Each tropomyosin molecule extends the length of seven G-actin monomers on an F-actin polymer.

Each tropomyosin molecule has associated with it a three-part regulatory protein complex called *troponin*. These three constituents of the troponin complex are called troponin T (TnT), troponin I (TnI), and troponin C (TnC) on the basis of their respective regulatory functions (see below).

Thick Filaments   The dark A bands contain another protein polymer essential to the molecular basis of muscle contraction. This second polymer is called the **thick filament**, and it is composed primarily of the protein *myosin*.

A single myosin molecule has a long, straight double-helical "tail" and a double "head" portion at one end (Figure 6.8B). Between the long tail and the head is a flexion or hinge ("neck") point. The result can be likened to two golf clubs wrapped around each other and then bent near the two heads. Myosin molecules aggregate with their tails together to form thick filaments. The head of the individual myosin molecules projects out from the cylindrical mass of tails at regular intervals and angles.

Like the F-actin polymers of thin filaments, thick filaments are polarized. The center of each thick filament is a *bare zone*, with only myosin tails and no

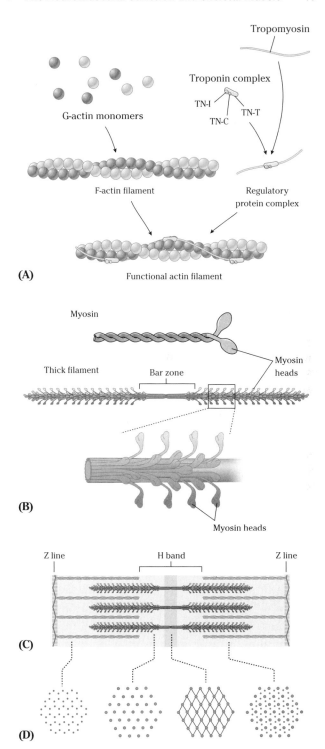

Figure 6.8   Component proteins of the sarcomere. **A.** Thin filaments are composed of G-actin polymerized into a double helix of F-actin, tropomyosin, and the three-part regulatory trponin complex. The three proteins of the troponin complex are TnT, TnI, and TnC. **B.** Thick filaments are composed of myosin. Each mysosin monomer has a long tail, a neck, and a head. The tails of two myosin monomers form a double helix. Multiple myosin helices comprise a thick filament. The bare zone in the center of the thick filament lacks myosin heads. **C.** Thin filaments protrude from Z lines and interdigitate with thick filaments. Minor proteins keep adjacent filaments in register. The bare zones of thick filaments make up the sarcomere's H band. **D.** Sections through different parts of the sarcomere may show only thin filaments, only thick filaments, or the crystalline array where they overlap.

heads jutting out. This bare zone constitutes part of the central, lighter H band of the A band. Just as polarized thin filaments protrude out from a Z line to either side, polarized half thick filaments protrude out from either side of the bare zone. Minor proteins in the bare zone help keep parallel thick myosin filaments aligned, and these minor proteins constitute the central M line of the A band.

A fundamental property of skeletal muscle structure and function is that thin filaments of the I band overlap with thick filaments of the A band (Figure 6.8C). The sarcomere thus has the following molecular structure as one "reads along" its length: A Z line at one end has thin filaments projecting from it, forming the I band. At some point, thin and thick filaments meet, interdigitating as the I band ends and the A band starts. Moving farther along the sarcomere, the thin filaments at one end terminate and there are only thick filaments, with a central bare (H band) zone at the center of the sarcomere (M line). After the bare zone, thick filaments oriented in the opposite direction from those before the bare zone protrude (the other half of the H band). Still farther, thick and thin filaments again interdigitate, making a new A band. As with the thick filaments, this second set of thin filaments is oriented in the opposite direction from the first set. Proceeding along the sarcomere, the A band ends and the second I band starts. Finally, the thin filaments of the second I band end by anchoring in the other Z line that defines the single sarcomere. The sarcomere is therefore an envelope structure: Z line 1-thin filaments 1 (I band 1)-thick filaments 1 (A band 1)-bare zone (H band and M line)-thick filaments 2 (A band 2)-thin filaments 2 (I band 2)-Z line 2.

Viewed in transverse section, thin and thick filaments form lattices with crystalline regularity (Figure 6.8D). If the section is made through the I band, only thin filaments are seen. If the section is made through the H zone, only thick filaments are seen. If the section is made through the overlap portion of the A band, both thick and thin filaments are seen.

Other important proteins include the many calcium ion pumps and channels embedded in the sarcoplasmic reticulum membrane, and dystrophin. Dystrophin is a large structural protein bound to the cytoplasmic side of the sarcolemma.

Neuromuscular Cations

If skeletal muscle proteins constitute the contractile machinery, cations are the battery power of the electrochemical events of motor neuron and skeletal muscle cell function. Although anions such as chloride (Cl^-) are important in nerve cell and muscle cell physiology, three cations deserve particular attention: sodium (Na^+), potassium (K^+), and calcium (Ca^{2+}).

Sodium and Potassium As described in Chapter 5, the concentration of Na^+ ions is approximately 10 times greater in the extracellular fluid than in the cytoplasm of motor neurons. However, the K^+ concentration is approximately 27 times greater in the neuron cytoplasm than in the extracellular fluid. Thus, there is a large concentration gradient favoring the influx of Na^+ ions into the nerve and a second concentration gradient favoring the efflux of K^+ out of the neuron. The Nernst and Goldman equations allow the calculation of the equilibrium potentials for Na^+ and K^+ as well as Cl^- and of the neuronal cell membrane potential. The differential distribution of the charged ions across the nerve cell membrane produces a neuron membrane potential of approximately -60 to -70 mV. Because of this relative negative charge of the inside of the neuron with respect to the outside, there is an electrical gradient (in addition to the chemical gradient) that greatly favors Na^+ influx. Although this same membrane potential opposes the efflux of K^+, it is not powerful enough to overcome the great concentration gradient promoting K^+ efflux.

The situation is similar with the muscle fiber, which has a resting membrane potential of -90 mV.

Calcium Both lower motor neurons and muscle fibers depend on the presence of a Ca^{2+} ion gradient. The Ca^{2+} concentration outside lower motor neurons is much greater than that in the nerve cell cytoplasm. In conjunction with the negative resting membrane potential of the lower motor neuron, there is a large electrochemical gradient favoring the influx of Ca^{2+} into the nerve cell.

The situation is more complex with the muscle fiber. While there is still a large electrochemical gradient promoting the influx of Ca^{2+} from the extracellular fluid into the cytoplasm, the more important gradient is the one favoring the efflux of Ca^{2+} from the lumen of the SR (which has a high relative Ca^{2+} concentration) into the cytoplasm.

SYSTEM FUNCTION

Skeletal muscle is arguably the organ system with the tightest relationship between structure and function. The activity of motor neurons and skeletal muscle cells is the direct result of the orderly movement of their components, starting from the scale of cations and proceeding through the scale of molecules to that of whole cells. The integration of cellular activities constitutes the function of the entire organ system.

Neuromuscular Cations and the Action Potential

As detailed in Chapter 5, an **action potential** is a wave of membrane depolarization, a change in the electrical charge of a cell membrane from a negative resting membrane potential to a brief positive membrane potential. Changes in membrane permeability and conductance of ions are responsible for the generation and spread of action potentials in both nerves and muscle cells.

In the case of the lower motor neuron, an action potential, caused by increased membrane permeability and conductance to Na^+, propagates down the axon to the many nerve terminals. At the terminal, depolarization increases membrane permeability and conductance of Ca^{2+}, which subsequently enters the nerve terminal down its electrochemical concentration gradient. This Ca^{2+} influx results in the release of ACh from the nerve terminal.

On the other side of the synapse, muscle fiber depolarization triggered by ACh is mediated by increased sarcolemma permeability and conductance of Na^+ into the cell. The depolarization propagates across the entire sarcolemma and spreads via the T tubule system into the muscle fiber. The action potential triggers Ca^{2+} efflux from the terminal cisternae into the cytoplasm.

After an action potential has passed, membrane cation permeabilities and conductances return to their previous levels and the membrane potential repolarizes, going back to its resting negative value. Neurons and muscle fibers restore electrochemical gradients by extruding Na^+ and taking in K^+ by means of ion pumps such as the Na^+-K^+-ATPase.

Neuromuscular Molecules

The cations and molecules of excitable cells such as motor neurons and skeletal muscle have a reciprocal relationship. On the one hand, an action potential is the result of the function of molecules such as the ion pumps and channels in the membrane of motor neurons and skeletal muscle cells. On the other hand, the release of neurotransmitters and the activation of the contractile proteins are the result of changes in the intracellular cation concentrations brought about by the action potential.

Excitation Contraction Coupling **Excitation contraction coupling** is the process by which electrical events (action potentials) are transformed into mechanical events (muscle contractions). Excitation contraction coupling starts in the motor neuron when information in the form of an action potential travels from the central nervous system to the periphery via lower motor neurons. Membrane permeabilities and conductances to Na^+ and K^+ increase from the opening of neuronal membrane ion channels, which allow ions to flow down their electrochemical gradients. As these ion channels open in response to an increase in membrane potential (depolarization), they are called voltage-gated. Because they contribute to additional increases in membrane potential, the process is self-promoting; the opening of a voltage-gated channel causes additional membrane depolarization, which promotes the opening of still more channels.

Calcium is the ion essential to the function of sarcomere contractile molecular machinery, and is the means by which electrochemical events (the action potentials of the motor neuron and the muscle fibers) are converted into mechanical events (muscle contraction). Thus, the essential step in excitation contraction coupling is the opening of voltage-gated Ca^{2+} channels.

Acetylcholine Acetylcholine (ACh) is the neurotransmitter molecule responsible for "ferrying" the neuronal action potential across the synapse and initiating a new action potential on the muscle fiber sarcolemma. Neurons produce ACh by transferring an acetyl group from acetyl CoA to a molecule of choline. ACh is stored in the synaptic vesicles of motor neurons.

When an action potential arrives at a motor neuron terminal, the transient increase in the membrane conductance of Na^+ and Ca^{2+} leads to an influx of Na^+ and Ca^{2+} down their respective electrochemical gradients that causes vesicle fusion with the nerve terminal membrane and the release of ACh into the synaptic cleft. Approximately 60 vesicles release their contents for each action potential.

Once released from the presynaptic neuron, ACh diffuses across the synapse and two molecules of ACh bind to each ACh receptor, resulting in transformation of the neuronal action potential into a muscle fiber action potential by way of a chemical signal. ACh soon diffuses from the receptor binding sites and is cleaved by synaptic acetylcholinesterase (AchE) into acetate and choline, thus inactivating the neurotransmitter signal. Approximately 50% of the choline thus produced is taken up by the nerve terminal and recycled into new ACh.

How does ACh engender a new action potential in the sarcolemma? The binding of two molecules of Ach to an Ach receptor leads to a conformational shift in the AchR, with the opening of the ion channel and an increase in the sarcolemma permeabilities and conductances for Na^+ and K^+. Thus, the AChR is a *ligand-gated* ion channel (ACh is called the AChR's *ligand*; that which binds to the AChR.) With opening of the AChR cation channel, Na^+ enters the muscle fiber down its electrochemical gradient, and the sarcolemma is depolarized. The action potential propagates along the sarcolemma and via T tubules into the muscle fiber. Depolarization is transmitted from the T tubules to the membrane of sarcoplasmic reticulum, which has numerous voltage-gated Ca^{2+} channel proteins on its surface. These include the L-type calcium channel, involved in slowly activated sustained conductance; and the dihydropyridine (DHP) receptor, which acts as a voltage sensor that relays the stimulus to release calcium from the SR. With depolarization, the SR channels open, releasing Ca^{2+} from the SR. Calcium ions thus diffuse into the cytoplasm.

Calcium release from the sarcoplasmic reticulum stores is mediated by membrane protein receptors known as ryanodine-sensitive calcium release channels (RyR). These channels trigger the calcium-activated physiologic pathways, not only in skeletal and smooth muscle, but also in the heart and brain. The RyR is one of two types of calcium-release channels important in excitation-contraction coupling. The other channel, more abundant in smooth muscle, is the inositol 1,4,5-triphosphate-stimulated channel (IP3).

Crossbridge Cycling The diffusion of Ca^{2+} into the cytoplasm is the linchpin of the molecular events responsible for the transformation of action potential into muscle contraction. Contraction depends upon the binding of thick filament myosin heads to thin filament F-actin at specific binding sites. When myosin heads do bind to actin, they give the appearance of small *crossbridges* connecting the thick and thin filaments. In the resting (uncontracted) state of the sarcomere, myosin heads are blocked from binding to actin because tropomyosin occupies the F-actin double-helical groove and sterically inhibits such binding. Troponin T functions as a connector between the regulatory troponin complex and the tropomyosin molecule. Tropomyosin maintains its blocking position in the F-actin groove owing to the function of troponin I (I is for inhibition of crossbridge binding).

The key event that allows contraction is the depolarization-induced increase in available Ca^{2+} in the cytoplasm. Four Ca^{2+} ions bind to the troponin C (C is for calcium binding) subunit and trigger a conformational shift in TnC. This change in TnC conformation shuts off TnI, and the entire troponin-tropomyosin complex shifts out of the F-actin groove, unmasking the previously blocked myosin crossbridge binding site on actin. With the removal of binding inhibition, myosin crossbridges bind to actin and contraction ensues by means of crossbridge cycling.

Crossbridge cycling is the sequence of molecular events underlying muscle contraction (FIGURE 6.9A). The myosin head is both an enzyme and a motor. It contains an enzymatic active site that binds the energy molecule ATP and cleaves it into ADP + P_i (P_i is inorganic phosphate). In the relaxed state, the myosin head binds a molecule of ATP and has a low affinity for actin. The myosin head then cleaves the ATP into ADP + P_i, which remain in the myosin head active site. This mechanism temporarily stores in the myosin head the chemical energy of the cleaved high-energy phosphate bond and gives the myosin head a high affinity for actin.

When (and only when) the skeletal muscle cytoplasmic Ca^{2+} concentration is high enough to unmask the crossbridge binding site on actin, the myosin head binds to the thin filament. The ADP and P_i are then released from the active site and the myosin head undergoes a conformational change called the *power stroke*. The power stroke reduces the angle the myosin head makes with the thick filament from 90 to 45 degrees, and the thin actin filament is essentially dragged a short distance by the myosin crossbridge power stroke. With the completion of the power stroke, the crossbridge is stuck to the thin filament. A new molecule of ATP then binds to the empty active site on the myosin head, which again has a low affinity for actin and separates from the thin filament binding site. The process of binding and cleavage of the new ATP "resets" the myosin head to its 90-degree angle and restores its high affinity for actin, preparing the system for another round of this crossbridge cycling.

Sliding Filaments The sliding filament model explains the molecular basis of muscle contraction (Figure 6.9B). How does crossbridge cycling translate into muscle contraction? Recall that thick and thin filament overlap is indispensable to contraction—myosin heads can not bind to actin unless there is such overlap—and that crossbridge cycling involves the dragging of thin filaments by the myosin head power stroke. The direction of the power stroke is always the same and the thin filament is pulled into the center of the sarcomere toward the M line.

Crossbridge cycling causes thin filaments to slide over thick filaments. As this occurs, the overlap between thick and thin filaments increases and the Z lines at either end of the sarcomere are pulled toward each other. The I band (where thin filaments do not overlap with thick filaments) and the H band (where thick filaments do not overlap with thin filaments) progressively narrow as many sequential rounds of crossbridge cycling take place. The width of the A band is unchanged. The length of the filaments remains the same, but since their overlap increases, the entire sarcomere shortens. In fact, the degree of

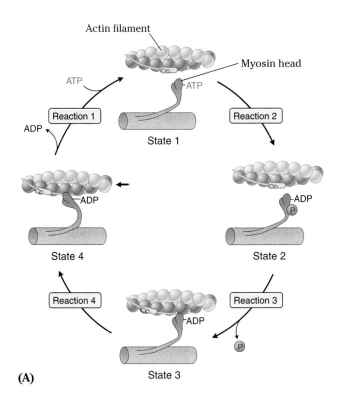

(A)

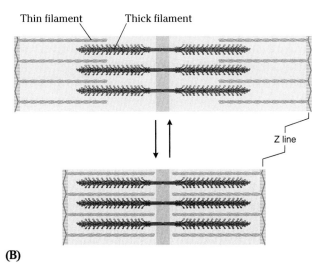

(B)

Figure 6.9 Crossbridge cycling and the sliding filament model. **A.** The myosin heads of thick filaments progress through four chemical reactions. In reaction 1, the myosin head binds a molecule of ATP. In reaction 2, the ATP is cleaved into ATP + P_i. In reaction 3, the P_i is released and the myosin head binds to the thin actin filament. The binding to the thin filament can only occur if an increase in intracellular calcium ions causes the inhibitory troponin complex to shift tropomyosin away from the myosin head's actin binding site. In reaction 4, the myosin head bends at the neck region, creating the power stroke that drags the thin filament a short distance. When reaction 1 is repeated, the myosin head releases the ADP and binds another molecule of ATP, resetting the head for another power stroke. **B.** Consecutive crossbridge cycles by many myosin heads cause the thin and thick filaments to slide over one another, shortening the sarcomere.

filament overlap is directly proportional to (and one of the major determinants of) the force a muscle can generate.

Contraction Cessation   The cessation of contraction is as critical for muscle function as contraction itself. How do the motor neuron and muscle shut off? A neuronal action potential is a self-limiting phenomenon because the voltage-gated Na^+ channels lock on their own. Likewise, when ACh diffuses from the AChR, the muscle fiber's ligand-gated channels close, thus ending the muscle cell action potential. The electrogenic Na^+-K^+-ATPase ion pump in the neuronal membrane and the sarcolemma restores the electrochemical gradients that were dissipated slightly by the action potential by transporting three Na^+ cations out of the cell in exchange for two K^+ cations that are imported. In addition, the increase in cell membrane permeability and conductance to K^+ that occurs as Na^+ voltage-gated ion channels are locking helps repolarize the membrane. Both of these processes help reset the neuron and the muscle cell for another action potential.

Crossbridge cycling is therefore self-limiting as well. Once an action potential in the muscle cell ends, the Ca^{2+} channels in the SR close, and the powerful Ca^{2+} pumps in its membrane rapidly move Ca^{2+} from the cytoplasm into the lumen. The decrease in available Ca^{2+} leads to the diffusion of Ca^{2+} from TnC, which resumes its previous conformation. This allows TnI to move tropomyosin back into the F-actin groove where the interaction of myosin crossbridge heads with their actin binding sites is inhibited. With the cessation of myosin head binding and crossbridge cycling, contraction ends and passive relaxation occurs.

A clinical condition associated with over-activity of calcium release in relation to re-uptake is known as malignant hyperthermia, in which the muscles are rigid and produce muscle damage and excessive lactic acid production. A drug called dantrolene can inactivate that abnormal calcium release.

ATP, Creatine Phosphate, and Creatine Kinase   If skeletal muscle proteins are the contractile machinery and cations are the battery power of the electrochemical events of motor neuron and skeletal muscle cell function, **adenosine triphosphate (ATP)** is the energy "fuel" or "currency" of the muscle fiber, and crossbridge cycling depends on the maintenance of a readily available pool of it. When crossbridge cycling takes place, ATP is rapidly hydrolyzed. Without a reserve of high-energy phosphate bonds, rapid depletion of the available ATP pool with subsequent inhibition of muscle contraction would result. The molecule **creatine** is found in muscle fibers and is phosphorylated to **creatine phosphate**.

CREATININE, CREATINE PHOSPHOKINASE, AND THE TROPONINS T AND I

Apart from the importance of the creatine system for maintaining ATP supplies and muscle function, this system has two extremely important clinical roles. The first involves creatinine (Cr), a metabolite of creatine and creatine phosphate. Creatinine is produced by and secreted into the bloodstream from skeletal muscle at a roughly regular rate. Because it is freely filtered from the blood by the kidney and is excreted in the urine, the Cr serum level is a marker of renal function. When a patient's renal function is impaired, the kidney's glomerular filtration rate falls and the serum Cr concentration typically rises. The higher the serum Cr concentration, the worse the glomerular filtration rate. Kidney function is routinely assessed in the clinical setting by reporting a patient's baseline and current serum Cr concentration (see Chapter 20).

The second clinical role is the measurement of serum levels of the enzyme creatine phosphokinase (CPK). Distinct isoforms of CPK are found in different tissues. Skeletal muscle has a CPK isoform called MM, while cardiac (heart) muscle has an isoform called MB. When one of these tissues is damaged and cells are lysed (broken apart), there is a release of the tissue-specific CPK isoform from the cells into the blood-stream. Measurement of the specific CPK isoform serum concentration allows for the assessment of specific tissue damage. An elevated CPK-MM concentration may indicate skeletal muscle trauma or necrosis (cell death and lysis) from disorders such as *polymyositis* and *rhabdomyolysis*. Elevated CPK-MB is diagnostic of *myocardial infarction* (or heart attack, the death or infarction and subsequent necrosis of cardiac muscle cells).

Just as muscle cell necrosis leads to the release of CPK enzymes, specific cardiac isoforms of the regulatory molecules troponin T and troponin I can be measured in blood. In the setting of suspected heart attack, cardiac troponin assays are very sensitive and specific, and are routinely performed in the diagnosis of acute coronary syndromes such as myocardial infarction.

When crossbridge cycling starts to hydrolyze the available ATP to ADP + P_i, creatine phosphate can donate a high-energy phosphate to ADP, restoring it to ATP. This reacting is catalyzed by the enzyme **creatine phosphokinase (CPK)**. A clinically important metabolite of creatine is called **creatinine**. (See Clinical Application Box *Creatinine, Creatine Phosphokinase, and the Troponins T and I.*)

How does the skeletal muscle cell generate ATP? Anaerobic glycolysis and oxidative phosphorylation are the two main metabolic pathways for ATP production. They both use glucose as their main fuel, but the former process does not require oxygen and generates only two new ATP for each molecule of glucose, whereas the latter requires oxygen and produces 38 ATP molecules per glucose molecule.

Dystrophin   **Dystrophin** is a large structural protein found on the cytoplasmic side of the sarcolemma. It binds the muscle fiber cytoskeleton to the sarcolemma, so that myofibrin shortening with contraction is transmitted to the sarcolemma. Mutation of the gene that codes for the dystrophin protein causes

a dysfunctional protein and the disease *muscular dystrophy*, which is characterized by muscle weakness.

Neuromuscular Organelles

The movements of two organelles are essential for skeletal muscle function. First, motor neuron synaptic vesicles must move to release ACh into the synaptic cleft. Second, muscle fiber sarcomeres maintain relatively fixed positions within the cell but must shorten.

Motor Neuron Vesicle Fusion   As discussed above, a single nerve terminal depolarization leads to an increased neuron cytoplasmic Ca^{2+} concentration that causes the fusion of approximately 60 ACh-containing vesicles with the nerve terminal cytoplasmic membrane and exocytosis of the neurotransmitter. The subsequent depolarization of the muscle cell membrane is called an **end-plate potential (EPP)**. A "safety" mechanism is built into this system, as the neuronal action potential results in the opening of approximately ten times the minimum number of ACh receptors needed for a muscle fiber depolarization and contraction. This overabundance is called a *physiologic reserve*.

The large end-plate potential is actually the sum of discrete small depolarizations called **miniature end-plate potentials (MEPPs)** (FIGURE 6.10A). Each MEPP has an amplitude of 0.4 mV and corresponds to the fusion of one synaptic vesicle and the release of a single quantum or packet of ACh. At rest, there is a random release of one or a few vesicles, with generation of MEPPs of different integer multiples of 0.4 mV (Figure 6.10B).

Sarcomere Shortening   The molecular events of crossbridge cycling and the sliding filament model discussed above explain the shortening of a single sarcomere. When the effect of a small shortening of one sarcomere is multiplied by the many sarcomeres in series in a single myofibril, the shortening of a single myofibril is considerable. When the shortenings of many myofibrils are summed, the whole muscle fiber likewise shortens. The shortening of many muscle fibers manifests as contraction of the entire muscle, with change in muscle length and the generation of force.

Neuromuscular Cells

Although the previous discussion detailing the structure and function of the skeletal muscle system on the subcellular level has treated the constituent cells generically, there is significant variability among motor neurons and among skeletal muscle cells. The differences among these cells are anatomical, structural, and functional.

Functional Heterogeneity of Lower Motor Neurons   Lower motor neurons are heterogeneous. Type I lower motor neurons are small diameter nerves that typically conduct an action potential at a high speed and are easily triggered. Such small nerves synapse on only a few muscle fibers. Type II lower motor neurons are large-diameter nerves that have even higher action potential conductance rates, but require greater stimulation to be triggered. These large nerves synapse on many muscle fibers.

Functional Heterogeneity of Skeletal Muscle Fibers   Like motor neurons, skeletal muscle fibers vary, and their names reflect differences in their structure, biochemistry, function, and (gross or microscopic) appearance. Type I cells are also referred to as "slow," "oxidative," and "red." They produce slow, sustained, powerful contractions for functions such as weight bearing and posture, do not fatigue easily, and depend upon oxidative phosphorylation for energy production. Type II fibers produce faster, shorter contractions and use glycolysis for ATP generation. Because they have fewer mitochondria, these "fast," "glycolytic" cells appear "white" under the microscope. Muscle fibers with intermediate numbers of mitochondria have a microscopic appearance between those of red and white fibers.

Neuromuscular Tissues

In order to produce physiologically useful contractions, the functions of skeletal muscle cells need to be coordinated in both space and time. There are two types of coordination: one that operates among cells during a single contraction and one that operates within cells during a series of contractions.

Motor Units   A single lower motor neuron branches out and synapses on numerous muscle fibers (FIGURE 6.11A). This provides the first type of coordination, which operates among cells. In large muscles that are

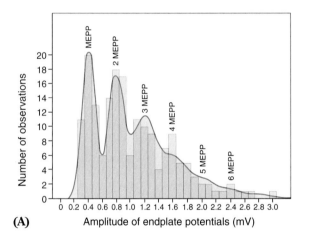

(A)

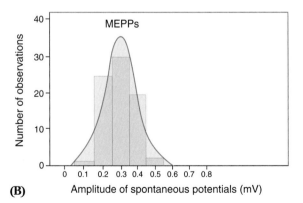

(B)

Figure 6.10   End-plate potentials (EPP) and miniature end-plate potentials (MEPP). **A.** Stimulating a lower motor neuron with low level electrical shocks induces a depolarization known as an end-plate potential of the associated skeletal muscle. The histogram shows the frequency of EPP of different magnitude and demonstrates that the most common EPP are multiple of 0.4 mV. Each 0.4 mV depolarization is defined as a miniature end-plate potential and corresponds to the fusion of a single lower motor neuron synaptic vesicle and release of its ACh. A physiologic EPP corresponds to 60 MEPPs. **B.** Even at rest, spontaneous MEPPs occur as single neurotransmitter vesicles release their contents into the synapse.

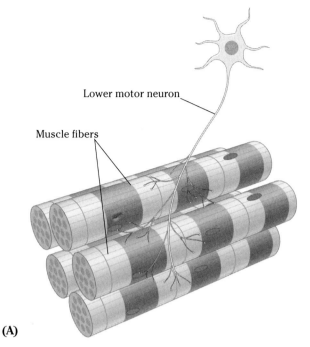

Lower motor neuron

Muscle fibers

(A)

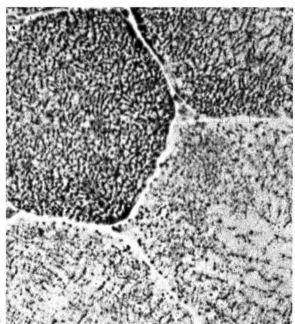

(B)

Figure 6.11 The motor unit. **A.** A lower motor neuron generally synapses on more than one muscle fiber. A single lower motor neuron and all the muscle fibers on which it synapses constitute a motor unit, the basic physiologic unit of skeletal muscle contraction. **B.** A single muscle is comprised of numerous motor units. Since the type of lower motor neuron determines some of the biochemical features of its associated muscle fibers, a sample of skeletal muscle has a checkerboard appearance, with type I (*lightly stained white*) and type II (*darkly stained*) muscle fibers mixed together.

responsible for powerful, gross contractions, a single lower motor neuron may synapse on over a thousand muscle fibers. In small muscles that mediate very precise movements, a single neuron may synapse on as few as two or three muscle fibers. Lower motor neu-

rons are only stimulatory; there are no inhibitory lower motor neurons. Any given muscle fiber is innervated by only one motor neuron. A single lower motor neuron and all of the muscle fibers it innervates is termed a **motor unit**. A motor unit is the functional contractile unit of skeletal muscle.

Like their component nerve and muscle cells, motor units are heterogeneous. Type I motor units are composed of a small nerve synapsing on a few muscle fibers and generating a small force in muscles used for precision movement, such as the muscles of the eye. Type II motor units have large nerves that synapse on numerous muscle cells and produce large, gross forces in strength muscles, such as the quadriceps (TABLE 6.1). Since the type and function of the lower motor neuron determine the type of muscle cell, all the muscle fibers in a single motor unit are the same type. Since different motor unit types are present in a single muscle, a random sample of a tissue demonstrates a checkerboard appearance of differently staining muscle fibers (Figure 6.11B).

Twitch and Tetanus   A single action potential causes the release of sufficient SR calcium ions to produce a transient muscle contraction. Because the Ca^{2+} is rapidly pumped back into the SR, however, the contraction from a single action potential is a small **twitch,** which generates a force and a lengthening less than the maximum the muscle can achieve (FIGURE 6.12). If a series of action potentials stimulates contraction, but the time interval between action potentials is long enough to allow complete relax-

Table 6.1   TYPES OF SKELETAL MUSCLE MOTOR UNITS

	Type I	Type II
Lower motor neurons		
Cell diameter	Small	Large
Rate of action potential Conduction	Fast	Very fast
Excitability	High	Low
Skeletal muscle cells		
Alternate names	Slow, oxidative, red	Fast, glycolytic, white
Rate of myosin ATPase	Slow	Fast
Oxidative capacity	High	Low
Glycolytic capacity	Low	High
Examples of function	Posture	Limb movement

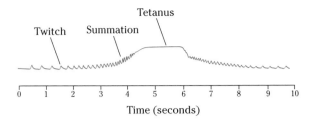

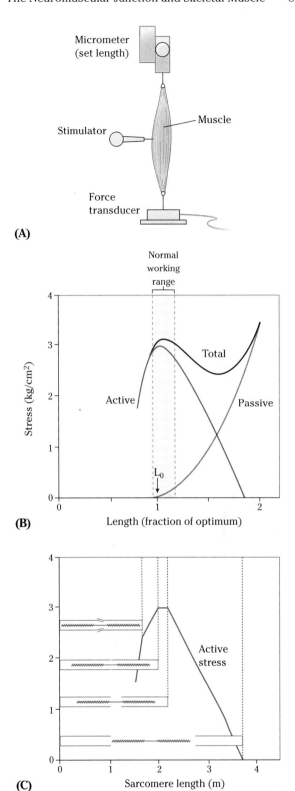

Figure 6.12 Twitch and tetanus. If a skeletal muscle is stimulated with a brief electrical shock, a single twitch occurs. If a series of electrical shocks is used but the frequency of stimulation is low enough, each twitch resolves as the muscle relaxes completely between stimulations. However, if the frequency is increased, summation occurs and individual twitches stack onto one another, leading to the sustained maximal muscle contraction known as tetanus.

ation of the muscle tissue, the result will be a series of twitches.

However, if the time interval between action potentials is shortened so that the SR can not recollect all of the Ca^{2+} that it released into the cytoplasm before the next action potential arises, complete relaxation does not take place before the next contraction occurs. In this case, the new contraction starts with a partially contracted muscle, and contractile forces "stack" onto each other. If the frequency of action potentials is high enough, twitches fuse together in a process called *summation* and the muscle achieves **tetanus**, a state of maximum contractile force and shortening. Tetanus provides the second type of coordination, which operates within cells during a series of contractions.

Skeletal Muscle Organs

The integrated function of many neuromuscular tissues gives rise to the gross behavior of skeletal muscles. Although skeletal muscles play important roles in the metabolism of protein, fat, and glucose, and the generation of body heat, the present discussion focuses on the physiology of muscle contraction.

Length-Stress Relationships As shown in FIGURE 6.13A, a muscle can be attached by its two ends to a device that keeps its length fixed and measures the stress it generates before and during stimulation by an electric shock. Such a system allows for the measurement of both the *passive stress,* the stress in the system before the muscle is stimulated, and the *total stress*, the stress measured when the stretched muscle is stimulated (Figure 6.13B). The total stress is the sum of the passive stress and the active stress caused by contraction.

As the muscle is stretched increasingly farther from its relaxed state, the elastic components of the contractile machinery and cytoskeleton generate the passive stress of the muscle. Passive stress is directly

Figure 6.13 Skeletal muscle length-stress relationships. **A.** A skeletal muscle can be isolated and suspended in a device that can control the muscle length, measure the stress it generates, and stimulate the muscle electrically. **B.** The total stress in a muscle preparation is the sum of passive stress from stretch and active stress from contraction. **C.** When thick and thin filament overlap is optimal, the force generated by contraction is maximal, and so is the active stress. When overlap is too great or too little, less active and total tension are achieved.

proportional to stretch. The total stress, however, starts to increase with stretching; it then achieves a maximum, after which more stretching of the muscle results in less than maximum total stress. Why does this occur? Since increased stretching always increases the passive stress, the decrease in total tension must result from a decrease in active stress with stretching of the muscle beyond an optimal point.

The sliding filament model of muscle contraction explains this phenomenon (Figure 6.13C). When the muscle is unstretched and is at a length less than the optimum, the thick and thin filaments overlap so much that they may interfere with each other when crossbridge cycling takes place. As the muscle is stretched and reaches the optimum length (L_o in Figure 6.13B), the overlap between thick and thin filaments is optimized, and the resulting active stress generated is at its maximum. When stretched even farther, however, the filaments overlap less as the thin filaments are too far away for some myosin heads to reach and bind to thin actin filaments. This less-than-optimal overlap results in less-than-maximal force generation, and the total stress therefore decreases.

Isometric and Isotonic Contractions   Experimentally and in living physiology, muscles are capable of two types of contraction: isometric and isotonic. An **isometric contraction** generates a force while the length of the muscle is unchanged. An **isotonic contraction** generates a constant force while the length of the muscle changes.

In common physiologic movements, both types of contraction occur in stages. As an example, consider picking up a glass of water on a table and bringing it to your lips to drink. The first phase is when your hand grasps the glass and your biceps and brachioradialis muscles start to contract. This initial contraction generates an isometric force, and the muscles do not shorten yet. In the second phase, an isotonic contraction starts, as the force generated by your muscles overcomes the gravitational and inertial forces keeping the glass on the table. The glass starts to rise as your muscles shorten and your elbow bends, and the force generated by your muscles as the glass is moving is constant. As the initial isometric contraction takes place, more and more motor units are recruited, staring with the smaller ones and progressively adding larger ones, until such time as the object starts to move and the contraction becomes isotonic.

The shape and connections of a muscle are related to its gross function, so that the forces transmitted to the skeleton are not wasted. Most muscles are anatomically arranged so that their resting length is at or near the optimum length, where filament overlap and active force generation are maximized. In addition, many muscles cross over joints so that a small change in muscle length at the proximal end of a limb produces a small change in joint angle that translates into a large movement in the distal limb. Growth and exercise may alter the maximum force and/or velocity with which a skeletal muscle contracts. (See Clinical Application Box *Growth and Exercise.*)

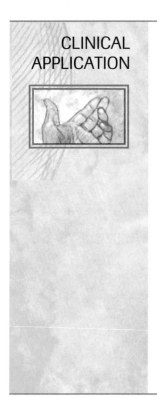

CLINICAL APPLICATION

GROWTH AND EXERCISE

Lengthening of muscle fibers occurs with normal growth, so that skeletal muscle can keep pace with skeletal growth. Lengthening results from the addition of new sarcomeres *in series* with old sarcomeres, so that myofibrils, muscle fibers, and the entire muscle are longer. The muscle can increase its shortening velocity, though it does not increase force generation. With exercise (training and repeated use), a muscle fiber increases in diameter because of the production of new myofibrils *in parallel* to old ones. This enlargement of the muscle is called **hypertrophy**, and a hypertrophic muscle cell is able to generate greater forces. In contrast to hypertrophy, **hyperplasia** is the appearance of new muscle cells from cell division. Mature muscle cells have a limited ability to divide, but some increase in muscle cell number can occur and result in increased force-generating capacity.

With prolonged exertion, actively contracting muscles deplete ATP supplies. The creatine phosphate pool provides only a few seconds of reserve, and oxidative phosphorylation is too slow a process to provide sufficient ATP to keep pace. Thus, contracting muscles depend on glycolysis, and each molecule of glucose that is catabolized produces two molecules of lactic acid. The buildup of lactic acid and resultant decrease in pH, along with the depletion of available ATP, results in muscle fatigue. When exercise ends, the muscle metabolizes the lactic acid by means of oxidative phosphorylation. This continued oxygen consumption during rest after exertion is referred to as *repayment of the oxygen debt.*

PATHOPHYSIOLOGY

Because the primary function of skeletal muscle is effecting voluntary movement, diseases involving skeletal muscle are characterized by movement or strength problems or both. **Paralysis,** the inability to make a voluntary movement, may occur because of dysfunction anywhere along the path from impulse generation in the motor cortex of the brain, down the axons of upper motor neurons in the spinal cord to the lower motor neurons, along the lower motor neuron axon, across the synapse, or in the muscle fibers themselves. **Paresis** is weakness of voluntary muscle contraction.

Denervation, Hypersensitivity, and Renervation

If a lower motor nerve is cut or destroyed, the muscle cells of the motor unit no longer receive stimulation in the form of ACh. The result is flacid paralysis, in which the muscle lacks normal tone and is flabby. Reflex arcs are disrupted, and a patient may have decreased or absent reflexes in the involved muscle. The muscle fibers, starved for stimulation, adapt by increasing their production of ACh receptors; the denervated muscle is thus hypersensitive to ACh.

If a lower motor neuron axon regrows and synapses again on the muscle fibers, there can be a return of function. In some instances, when multiple axons are damaged and regrowing, the new axon and synaptic terminals are of a different type than the original. The result is a change of muscle fiber type, and microscopic examination of a sample of such muscle reveals an abnormal homogeneity of muscle fiber types and a loss of the normal checkerboard intermingling of cell types. This condition is called *fiber type grouping*. The change in a muscle fiber's type with renervation was once thought to be due to different trophic factors from nerve terminals, but evidence now indicates that different stimulation patterns between small and large lower motor neurons determine fiber type.

Fasciculations and Fibrillations

Fasciculations are visible twitches of single motor units. They commonly appear in lower motor neuron diseases, such as damage to the anterior horn cell bodies, characteristic of *amyotrophic lateral sclerosis (ALS)* and *polio*. Clinically, they look like brief ripples under the skin. **Fibrillations** are spontaneous contractions of single muscle fibers. Unlike visible fasciculations, fibrillations are invisible to the eye but can be identified by electromyography, a technique that measures electrical activity in muscle cells.

Botulism

Clostridium botulinum is a gram-positive rod-shaped bacterium that produces a potent protein toxin. If a person contracts a *C. botulinum* infection through a contaminated skin wound or ingests the bacterium's preformed toxin in spoiled foods, the botulinum toxin enters motor nerve terminals and inhibits the release of ACh, leading to paralysis. It is one of the most potent toxins known, and as little as 1 µg can be deadly to a person.

Contractures and Atrophy

If a limb is immobilized for long periods by paralysis or physical restraint, the process of growth is reversed. Sarcomeres are removed in series from the myofibrils, resulting in a shortening of muscle called a **contracture**. Patients with paralyzed limbs must therefore have physical therapy so that contractures do not occur. With denervation, muscle cells shrink in size, the process of **atrophy**. Over months, atrophic cells can degenerate completely and be replaced by fat or connective tissue.

Muscular Dystrophy

The dystrophin protein mentioned earlier is one of many cytoskeletal proteins that link the contractile machinery of the muscle cell to the sarcolemma and to other cells. Dystrophin is encoded by a very large gene on the X chromosome. If this gene is mutated so that no dystrophin is produced, **Duchenne's muscular dystrophy (DMD)**, a congenital X-linked hereditary disorder, results. DMD manifests as progressive muscle weakness. It is present in 1 out of every 3,500 male newborns and is fatal by age 20 to 30 from events such as respiratory muscle failure and/or aspiration pneumonia. A less severe form of the disease, called *Becker's muscular dystrophy*, is caused by a different mutation in the gene that results in a decreased amount or abnormal size of the dystrophin molecule.

Rigor Mortis

With death, there is eventual depletion of the muscle fiber's pool of ATP. Without new ATP to fill the active site of the myosin head, the crossbridge can not release from its actin binding site (Figure 6.9A, reaction 1). This causes a stiffening of the muscle, a freezing in midcontraction known as **rigor mortis** ("the stiffness of death").

Myasthenia Gravis

Myasthenia gravis is an autoimmune disorder of the neuromuscular junction that manifests as progressive skeletal muscle weakness and fatigability. The prevalence is approximately 1 in 10,000. Like many autoimmune disorders, women are affected more frequently than men. Myasthenia gravis may affect a person at any age, but peak incidences occur in women in their twenties and thirties and in men in their fifties and sixties.

The defect in myasthenia gravis is a depletion of ACh receptors and a distortion of the synaptic folds. This aberration arises because the immune system inappropriately produces antibodies against the AChR. Antibodies are proteins that normally bind to foreign molecules and tag them for destruction in order to protect the individual from invaders such as parasites, bacteria, and viruses (see Chapter 11). In myasthenia gravis, as in other autoimmune disorders, the body's immune system misidentifies a normal protein (in this case, the AChR) as a foreign or dangerous one and attempts to eradicate it by producing anti-AChR antibodies. These antibodies bind to the AChR and interfere with neuromuscular function in three ways: by augmenting the rate of AChR endocytosis and destruction, by steric hindrance of the ACh binding sites, and by precipitating the formation of the immune system's complement membrane attack complex, which then damages the muscle cell membrane.

The paucity of AChRs on the surface of the muscle fibers means that there are fewer ACh binding sites when an action potential arrives at the lower motor neuron terminal and subsequently releases ACh. With fewer open ACh receptors, there is less depolarization of muscle fibers, and many fibers that would normally reach threshold and contract do not have an action potential. Repeated stimulation leads to progressive neuromuscular fatigue and manifestly poorer performance as the nerve terminal is depleted of ACh with each subsequent stimulation.

Symptoms include generalized proximal limb weakness and fatigability with repeated activity; these symptoms subside with rest. Drooping of the eyelids (*ptosis*) and double vision (*diplopia*) occur with weakness of the lid and extraocular muscles, respectively. If facial muscles suffer, a flattened smile or a snarl when attempting to smile may occur. Patients may have difficulty chewing and swallowing. "Mushy" or nasal speech may develop, and there may be weakness with neck extension. Difficulty breathing, sometimes severe enough to require hospitalization and mechanical ventilation—referred to as a *crisis*—can result if the diaphragm is affected.

There are two general categories of treatment. One is the use of inhibitors of AChE, so that the ACh released from nerve terminals into the synapse is not rapidly catabolized, but can bind to the remaining ACh receptors for a longer time. A short-acting AChE inhibitor (edrophonium) is used to diagnose myasthenia gravis by demonstrating an improvement in muscle weakness with the inhibitor.

Because myasthenia gravis is an autoimmune disorder, the other category of treatment is directed at the immune system. These modalities include surgical resection (removal) of the thymus, where much immune function occurs; the use of immunosuppressive agents (such as corticosteroids); removal of the anti-AChR antibodies from the blood by a process called *plasmapheresis*; and the use of intravenous immune globulin, an injection of other antibodies that block the anti-AChR antibodies by a mechanism that is not well understood. Treatments have significantly reduced the mortality of the disease, but in most cases, patients require lifelong medical therapy.

Summary

- There are three types of muscle: skeletal muscle (under voluntary control), smooth muscle (involuntary), and cardiac or heart muscle.

- The organs essential for voluntary movements are the brain, the spinal cord, and the skeletal muscles.

- **Upper motor neurons** start in the *primary motor cortex* of the brain and send their axons down the spinal cord. **Lower motor neurons** start in the anterior horn of the spinal cord, synapse on muscle fibers, and propagate action potentials by means of the neurotransmitter **acetylcholine (ACh)**.

- When ACh is released from the terminals of a lower motor neurons, it diffuses across the synapse and binds to **ACh receptors** embedded in the muscle cell membrane. This binding leads to the opening of the ACh receptor *ligand-gated ion channel* and triggering of an action potential in the muscle cell.

- An **end-plate potential (EPP)** is the muscle cell depolarization induced by an action potential in a lower motor neuron and corresponds to the fusion of approximately 60 neurotransmitter vesicles with release of their ACh. A **miniature end-plate potential (MEPP)** is the 0.4 mV depolarization of the muscle cell membrane that corresponds to the fusion of a single neurotransmitter vesicle.

- Muscle cell **myofibrils** are the microscopic cross-striations of skeletal muscle. A **sarcomere**, the distance between two Z lines, is the basic contractile unit of a skeletal muscle cell.

- Each sarcomere is an arrangement of overlapping thin and thick filaments. The **thin filaments** are composed of *F-actin*, *tropomyosin*, and the three-part *troponin* complex. The **thick filaments** are composed of *myosin*.

- The **sarcoplasmic reticulum (SR)** is a skeletal muscle organelle comprised of membrane-bound spaces that store relatively large amounts of calcium ions.
- **Excitation contraction coupling** is characterized by an action potential that causes the release of calcium ions from the SR, which allows myosin heads to bind to actin.
- The myosin head *power stroke* drags the thin filament a short distance. The splitting of the terminal phosphate group of a molecule of ATP allows the myosin head to detach from a binding site on actin and "reset" in preparation for another power stroke. The complete sequence of myosin binding, power stroke, releasing, and resetting is known as **cross-bridge cycling**.
- Repeated crossbridge cycling causes the thin and thick filaments to slide over one another, leading to shortening of the sarcomere.
- Type I lower motor neurons are small, easily triggered, conduct action potentials rapidly, and synapse on only a few muscle fibers. Type II lower motor neurons are large, are not easily triggered, conduct action potentials very rapidly, and synapse on many muscle fibers.
- Type I skeletal muscle cells contract relatively slowly, use oxidative metabolism, and appear red under the microscope. Type II skeletal muscle cells contract relatively quickly, use glycolytic metabolism, and appear white under the microscope.
- A single lower motor neuron and all associated muscle fibers constitute a **motor unit**.
- A **twitch** is the contraction of skeletal muscle in response to a single lower motor neuron action potential. **Tetanus** is the "stacking" of sequential muscle cell contractions from depolarizations temporally close enough together so that complete relaxation cannot occur between them.
- An **isometric contraction** of a muscle is one in which stress increases while the length of the muscle is constant. An **isotonic contraction** is one in which the length of the muscle decreases while the stress is constant.
- Diseases affecting the skeletal muscle system may interfere with any step from action potential generation through sarcomere shortening. **Paralysis** is the inability to move. **Paresis** is weakness of movement.

Suggested Reading

Ebashi S. Excitation-contraction coupling and the mechanism of muscle contraction. Annu Rev Physiol. 1991;53:1–16.

Gordon AM, Homsher E, Regnier M. Regulation of contraction in striated muscle. Physiol Rev. 2000;80(2):853–924.

Rios E, Pizarro G, Stefani E. Charge movement and the nature of signal transduction in skeletal muscle excitation-contraction coupling. Annu Rev Physiol. 1992;54:109–33.

REVIEW QUESTIONS

Directions: Each of the numbered items or incomplete statements in this section is followed by answers or by completions of the statement. Select the ONE lettered answer or completion that is BEST in each case.

1. Which of the following ions is stored in the sarcoplasmic reticulum?
   - (A) Na^+
   - (B) K^+
   - (C) Ca^{2+}
   - (D) Cl^-
   - (E) HCO_3^-

2. A 27-year-old woman presents to the emergency department with progressive weakness, drooping eyelids (ptosis), double vision (diplopia), and appears to snarl when asked to smile. She most likely has antibodies directed against which of the following?
   - (A) Acetylcholine
   - (B) AChE
   - (C) Presynaptic voltage-gated Ca^{2+} channels
   - (D) Postsynaptic ACh receptors
   - (E) Dystrophin

3. A 54-year-old man with amyotrophic lateral sclerosis has spontaneous movements of his tongue that are visible to the naked eye. Such movements are called
   - (A) fibrillations
   - (B) fasciculations
   - (C) tetanus
   - (D) palsies
   - (E) twitches

4. A 64-year-old man comes to the emergency department with chest pain. His electrocardiogram (ECG) indicates he has had a myocardial infarction (heart attack). Which of the following would you *not* expect to be greatly elevated in his blood?
   - (A) Actin
   - (B) Troponin I
   - (C) Troponin T
   - (D) CPK-MB isoform

ANSWERS TO REVIEW QUESTIONS

1. **The answer is C.** The sarcoplasmic reticulum is a major storage site for Ca^{2+}. When an action potential travels along the sarcolemma to the T tubules, it triggers voltage-gated Ca^{2+} channels on the SR to open and release the stored Ca^{2+}. Although other ions may be contained in the SR, Ca^{2+} is the most prominent and important for skeletal muscle contraction.

2. **The answer is D.** This patient has symptoms consistent with myasthenia gravis, an autoimmune disease characterized by the production of antibodies directed against the receptor for ACh. A disease with a distinct but somewhat similar presentation is Eaton Lambert syndrome, in which antibodies directed against the presynaptic Ca^{2+} channel interfere with ACh release from the terminals of lower motor neurons. Unlike myasthenia gravis, Eaton Lambert syndrome often occurs in patients with lung cancer. Dystrophin is the protein whose gene is mutated in muscular dystrophy.

3. **The answer is B.** Fasciculations are contractions of the muscle fibers in a single motor unit and are visible to the naked eye. Fibrillations are deporarizations resulting from one or a few vesicles of ACh being release by a presynaptic neuron. They may be detected by electromyography but are not visible to the naked eye. Tetanus is the achievement of maximal muscle contraction by means of "stacking" muscle fiber depolarizations on one another without full recovery in between successive stimulations. A palsy is dramatic, uncontrolled movements of the body. Twitch is a term generally reserved for electrical stimulation of muscle fibers and corresponds to the skeletal muscle contraction induced by a single action potential.

4. **The answer is A.** Muscle fiber necrosis results in the release of a number of muscle specific proteins. The CPK, troponin I, and troponin T proteins are routinely used to diagnose cardiac muscle cell death, the definition of a myocardial infarction or heart attack. All of these would be expected to be elevated in this patient. Actin is not routinely measured in such situations.

Smooth Muscle

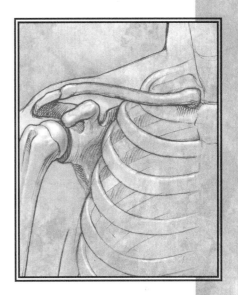

7

INTRODUCTION

Smooth muscle and skeletal muscle have similarities as well as significant differences. Although they share some basic structures that allow them to contract, each type of muscle has individual properties (anatomic distribution, histologic appearance, biochemistry, etc.) that suit its function. This chapter describes smooth muscle physiology by comparing and contrasting it with that of skeletal muscle (see Chapter 6).

Like skeletal muscle, the primary function of **smooth muscle** is contraction. However, while skeletal muscles often attach to bones and cross joints so that contraction produces limb movement, smooth muscle typically forms tissues within organ systems (vascular, respiratory, gastrointestinal, etc.) to regulate the movement of liquids (blood), gases (air), and/or solids (food) within hollow tubular structures (blood vessels, bronchi, alimentary tract). Smooth muscle also has synthetic functions that are important physiologically and in pathophysiologic conditions.

SYSTEM STRUCTURE

Just as skeletal muscle function requires the integration of three organ systems (nervous system, skeletal muscle system, and skeletal system), smooth muscle function also requires neural input, smooth muscle itself, and a framework organ system to which the smooth muscle is physically associated and on which contraction occurs. However, while skeletal muscles use bones as their framework, smooth muscles use various other organs and tissues.

Smooth Muscle in Organs

With the possible exceptions of the urinary bladder and the uterus, there are no true smooth muscle organs. Instead, smooth muscle is a component of many organ systems. Often, these organ systems are hollow, and smooth muscle is a component of the walls of the constituent organs. In this respect, smooth muscle can be thought of as a contractile tissue which, like connective tissue, serves a roughly consistent function in many anatomic locations.

Smooth Muscle Tissues

Smooth muscle is present in the following tissues:

- The walls of arteries, veins, and lymphatic ducts of the cardiovascular system (FIGURE 7.1)
- The walls of bronchi of the respiratory tract (FIGURE 7.2)

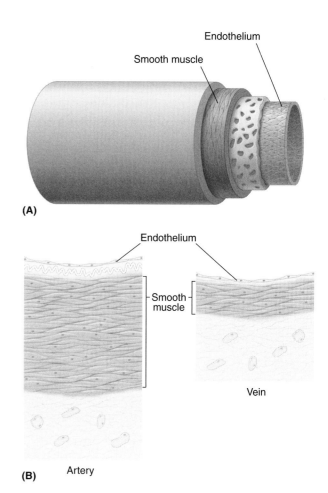

Figure 7.1 Smooth muscle layers in the wall of peripheral blood vessels. **A.** A longitudinal section of an artery reveals the smooth muscle tissue layer beneath the endothelium. Note that smooth muscle cells are oriented circularly around the vessel lumen, so that even slight contraction will cause important changes in the radius of the lumen. **B.** The thickness of the smooth muscle layer is greater in arteries than in veins.

- The walls of the esophagus, stomach, small intestine, and colon of the gastrointestinal (GI) tract (FIGURE 7.3). Different layers are oriented in various directions. Some smooth muscle bands spiral around the GI tract, while others are more circular. Other hollow organs (e.g., the gall bladder) associated with the GI tract also contain smooth muscle within their walls
- The ureters and urinary bladder of the genitourinary tract
- The myometrium of the uterus consists of four strata of smooth muscle, each oriented in a different direction

Smooth muscle cells form sheets and layers (FIGURE 7.4A). In longitudinal section, the individual cells

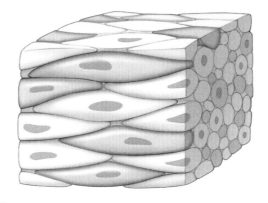

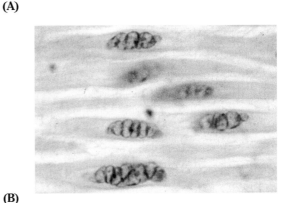

(A)

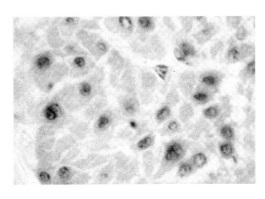

(B)

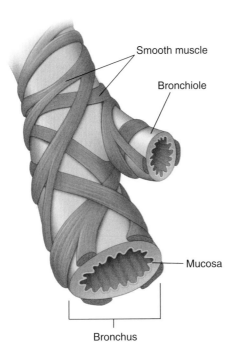

Figure 7.2 Smooth muscle in the walls of bronchi and bronchioles. Strips of smooth muscle beneath the respiratory mucosa wind obliquely down the airways of the lung.

appear tightly packed in a staggered array (Figure 7.4B). This staggering means that in transverse section, the single plane of section "catches" different cells at different points along the longitudinal axis—some at one end, others in the middle (Figure 7.4C).

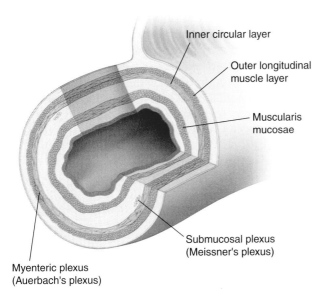

Figure 7.3 Smooth muscle in the walls of the GI tract. Note that there are both circular layers, which alter the lumen radius, and longitudinal layers which facilitate the movement of gastrointestinal contents (peristalsis). In addition, the muscularis mucosae allows the mocosal layer of the GI tract to move. The submucosal Meissner's) and myenteric (Auerbach's) plexuses are collections of autonomic neurons that modulate smooth muscle contraction.

(C)

Figure 7.4 Sheets and layers of smooth muscle cells. **A.** Smooth muscle cells are packed tightly together and are staggered in a block of tissue. **B.** A longitudinal plane of section displays the fusiform shape of the cells and how the thicker central part of a given smooth muscle cell is often apposed to the thinner ends of adjacent cells. **C.** A transverse plane of section catches different cells in different places along their long axis.

Smooth Muscle Cells

Both the muscle cells themselves and the nerve cells with which they are physically associated differ between the skeletal muscle system and the smooth muscle system. Their histologic differences are the basis of functional differences among these cells.

Innervation Skeletal muscle cells and lower motor neurons make up the neuromuscular junction, or synapse, discussed in Chapter 6. Smooth muscle cells

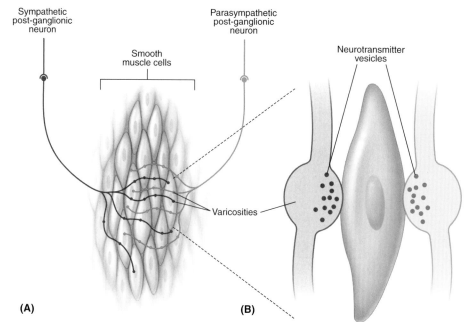

Figure 7.5 Autonomic neuron endings in near smooth muscle. **A.** Unlike the arrangement between skeletal muscle cells and lower motor neurons, there is no synapse between smooth muscle cells and autonomic neurons. **B.** Instead, terminal varicosities, which contain neurotransmitter-laden vesicles, are closely apposed to the smooth muscle cell membrane.

are often associated with neurons as well, but these nerve cells are part of the autonomic nervous system (see Chapter 5). Many smooth muscle tissues have dual innervation, with neurons from both the sympathetic and parasympathetic branches of the autonomic nervous system. Instead of terminal boutons, the axons of these autonomic nerves end in dilated structures called *varicosities*. Although these varicosities are closely approximated to the cell membrane of smooth muscle cells, they do not form neuromuscular junctions as lower motor neurons do with skeletal muscle cells (FIGURE 7.5).

Histology When relaxed, a single smooth muscle cell is fusiform, or long and tapered at both ends. The staggered arrangement of cells allows for close packing: the thickest middle portion of one cell typically is

surrounded by the smaller ends of adjacent cells, and vice versa (Figure 7.4A). These cells are called smooth because, unlike skeletal muscle cells, they have no striations. They have a homogeneous appearance under the light microscope.

Smooth Muscle Organelles

When examined by electron microscopy, a number of organelles are visible in smooth muscle cells. There is a single, centrally located nucleus. Like skeletal muscle, smooth muscle contains myofilaments, both thick and thin. Skeletal (striated) muscle is characterized by the almost crystalline regularity of its thick and thin filaments, and it is this structural regimentation into sarcomeres that produces the striations (FIGURE 7.6A,B). The absence of such striations in

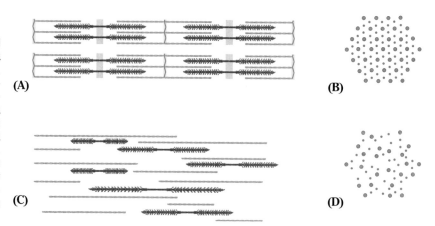

Figure 7.6 Thick and thin filaments in skeletal and smooth muscle. **A.** In skeletal muscle, thick and thin filaments are arranged into sarcomeres. **B.** A transverse section of a sarcomere is characterized by an almost crystalline regularity of filaments and demonstrates the 1-to-2 ratio of thick to thin filaments in this type of muscle. **C.** Smooth muscle cells have thick and thin filaments but lack this highly organized pattern of sarcomeres. **D.** A transverse section of smooth muscle reveals a ratio of thick to thin filaments of approximately one-to-ten. Nevertheless, the contractile machinery and sliding filament model are largely the same in both types of muscle cells.

smooth muscle cells is a direct consequence of the different arrangement of thick and thin filaments. Smooth muscle cells have no sarcomeres and no regularly ordered association or ratio between the different contractile protein polymers (Figure 7.6C,D). Instead of the skeletal muscle ratio of two thin filaments for every thick filament, there is a looser, approximately 10-to-1 thin-to-thick filament ratio.

While sarcomeres in skeletal muscle are connected in series to form myofibrils parallel to the long axis of the muscle fiber, the contractile machinery of smooth muscle cells, lacking sarcomeres, is not limited to this one alignment but is often oriented obliquely. Smooth muscle cells also have intermediate filaments that interconnect various components of the cytoskeleton (FIGURE 7.7A). *Dense bodies* are protein anchoring structures to which thin filaments attach. They are thus the smooth muscle analogue of skeletal muscle Z lines. Dense bodies may be entirely within the cytoplasm, or they may be bound to the inner aspect of the cell membrane.

As in other metabolically active cells, smooth muscle cells contain mitochondria where ATP is generated. Because some smooth muscle cells have synthetic functions (e.g., they may produce cytokines, growth factors, and components of the extracellular matrix such as collagen), they have ribosomes, rough ER, and Golgi apparatuses. Skeletal and smooth muscle cells both have sarcoplasmic reticulum (SR), a collection of closed membranes that store Ca^{2+}. Smooth muscle cell SR is not as well developed as that of skeletal muscle. As in skeletal muscle cells, the smooth muscle cell membrane is called the *sarcolemma* and the cytoplasm is called the *sarcoplasm*.

While skeletal muscle fibers are the result of the fusion of numerous precursor cells, smooth muscle cells remain distinct, but in different anatomic and functional contexts these individual smooth muscle cells may be more or less interconnected. Gap junctions, desmosomes, and other structures can mechanically, electrically, and chemically couple adjacent smooth muscle cells (Figure 7.7A,B). While smooth muscle cells lack the T tubules of skeletal muscle, they do possess sarcolemma invaginations called *caveolae*, which perform a similar function.

Smooth Muscle Molecules

As in skeletal muscle, thick filaments in smooth muscle are composed of myosin. However, the smooth muscle isoform is different from that of skeletal muscle. Thin filaments contain actin and tropomyosin but lack the troponin regulatory complex. Among the many cytoskeletal molecules are desmin and vimentin. Extensive extracellular connective tissue networks contain elastin, collagen, and reti-

culin. Smooth muscle cells, like skeletal muscle cells, have ion channels and ion pumps in their sarcolemma.

Smooth Muscle Cations

As in skeletal muscle cells, there are three cations differentially distributed between the intracellular and extracellular spaces: sodium (Na^+), potassium (K^+), and calcium (Ca^{2+}). The electrochemical gradient for Na^+ greatly favors its influx into a smooth muscle cell. The opposite is true for K^+, which exits the cell when K^+-specific ion channels open. The cytoplasm of a smooth muscle cell normally has low concentration of Ca^{2+} relative to the extracellular space and the lumen of the SR, so that a large electrochemical gradient favors the entry of this cation into the sarcoplasm.

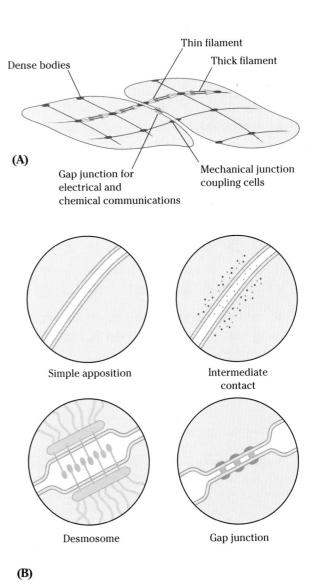

Figure 7.7 Organelles of smooth muscle. **A.** Dense bodies in the cytoplasm or inside the sarcolemma anchor the contractile filaments. **B.** Smooth muscle cells may be joined by desmosomes, gap junctions, simple apposition, or intermediate contact, depending on the tissue.

SYSTEM FUNCTION

Like skeletal muscle, the main function of smooth muscle is contraction. However, while skeletal muscle contraction is largely under conscious control by motor neurons and moves limbs, smooth muscle contraction is largely under unconscious control by the autonomic nervous system and often alters the shapes of organs and the flow of material through them. As with their structures, the contractile mechanisms of skeletal and smooth muscle are similar on many scales but differ importantly and reflect their distinct physiologic roles.

Smooth Muscle Cations

As in other excitable cells such as skeletal muscle cells and neurons, the movement of cations up or down their electrochemical gradients can cause and result from changes in the cell membrane electrical potential. The relationship between changes in the membrane potential and contraction in different smooth muscle cells, however, is not as rigid or as universal as that of excitation contraction coupling in skeletal muscle cells. Nevertheless, contractions in both smooth and skeletal muscle depend on an increase in the intracellular concentration of Ca^{2+}.

Smooth Muscle Membrane Electrical Potential
Skeletal and smooth muscle differ in their dependence on sarcolemma electrical potential changes to effect contraction. For skeletal muscle, an action potential is absolutely necessary for contraction. However, there is no consistent relationship between changes in smooth muscle membrane potential and contractility. There is great variability from one smooth muscle subtype to another. Some smooth muscle cells manifest regular, intrinsic, sinusoidal alterations in membrane potential that are unaccompanied by a change in contractile state (FIGURE 7.8A). Other smooth muscle cells are activated by an action potential. These cells often exhibit contractile summation and tetanus like skeletal muscles if action potentials "stack" in rapid succession (Figure 7.8B).

As with many cell types, the smooth muscle cell's resting membrane potential is the function of the variable permeability to and different intra- and extracellular concentrations of sodium, potassium, chloride, bicarbonate, and other ions. Ion pumps and membrane channels similar to those in skeletal muscle maintain electrochemical gradients.

Calcium   Skeletal and smooth muscle contraction and relaxation share dependence on changes in the intracellular calcium concentration. Influx and efflux of Ca^{2+} into the sarcoplasm determine the sarcoplasmic Ca^{2+} concentration, but the sources of Ca^{2+} vary

from one type of smooth muscle cell to another. Some Ca^{2+} enters from the extracellular pool by means of sarcolemmal ion channels. These sarcolemmal Ca^{2+} channels may be voltage-gated (i.e., they open with membrane depolarization) or ligand-gated (i.e., they open when the appropriate signaling molecule binds). Some such Ca^{2+} channels that are neither voltage-gated nor ligand-gated remain open for relatively long periods and are therefore called *leak channels*. Furthermore, there are mechanically-gated Ca^{2+} channels that respond to stretch by inducing the release of calcium. This mechanism may be important in blood vessels, relating volume-induced stretch to muscle contraction.

Some smooth muscle cells have significant Ca^{2+} caches in sarcoplasmic reticulum. When smooth muscle is stimulated, the entry of extracellular Ca^{2+} may trigger the release of sarcoplasmic stores through *calcium-gated calcium channels*. In other cells, stimulatory ligands may activate receptors and generate second messengers such as IP_3 and DAG (see Chapter 4) which may liberate sarcoplasmic Ca^{2+}. Whatever the mechanism, stimulation increases the intracellular Ca^{2+} concentration (FIGURE 7.9A).

Smooth Muscle Molecules

A number of molecules are important in smooth muscle contraction and relaxation. Among them are regulatory mediators, contractile proteins, kinases, and phosphatases that modulate the contractile proteins, channels and pumps that control the

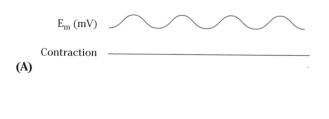

(A)

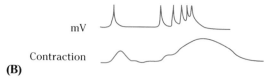

(B)

Figure 7.8   The relationship between electrical activity and contraction in smooth muscle. **A.** Unlike excitation-contraction coupling in skeletal muscle, spontaneous, periodic membrane depolarization may not cause contraction in some smooth muscle cells. **B.** In other smooth muscle tissues, a depolarization must reach or exceed a threshold value to cause contraction and rapid sequences may generate tetanus. Various stimuli may induce contraction or relaxation in smooth muscle from different anatomic locations. The critical factors determining a given smooth muscle cell's response to an agent are the type and number of cell surface receptors and their associated signal transduction mechanisms.

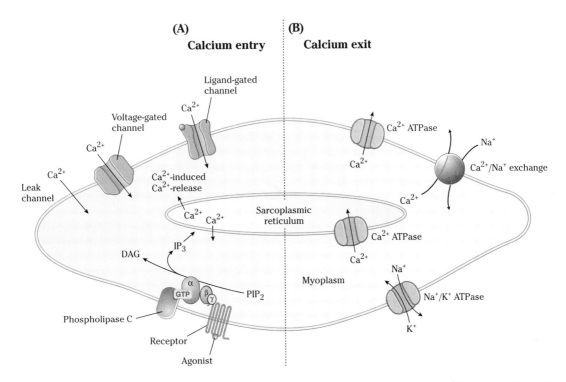

Figure 7.9 The movement of calcium into and out of smooth muscle. **A.** Extracellular Ca^{2+} may enter the cell through voltage-gated or ligand-gated channels in the sarcolemma. Leak Ca^{2+} channels open independent of membrane voltage changes or the binding of ligand and spend a relatively large amount of the time open, allowing Ca^{2+} to enter the cell. Ca^{2+} itself, or second messengers, such as IP_3, may induce the release of Ca^{2+} from the sarcoplasmic reticulum. **B.** Specialized ion pumps in the sarcolemma remove Ca^{2+}, extruding it into the extracellular space. Some of these use the energy liberated by the cleavage of ATP, while others use the energy of the steep electrochemical gradient favoring the influx of Na^+. Other ATP-requiring Ca^{2+} pumps sequester Ca^{2+} in the sarcoplasmic reticulum.

movement of cations, and the small molecules that fuel contraction.

Regulatory Mediators The regulation of smooth muscle contraction varies from one type of smooth muscle to another. A number of well-characterized mediators influence smooth muscle contractility; those that promote and those that inhibit contraction depend on the particular smooth muscle subtype. These mediators include epinephrine, norepinephrine, endothelial derived relaxing factor (EDRF; later identified as nitric oxide, NO), prostacyclin (PGI_2), acetylcholine (ACh), serotonin, histamine, bradykinin, adenosine diphosphate (ADP), estrogen, and progesterone.

Like neurons, smooth muscle cells receive both stimulatory and inhibitory signals. Stimulatory signals may be in the form of mediators that depolarize the smooth muscle cell and/or increase sarcolemmal permeability to Ca^{2+}. Inhibitory signals may hyperpolarize the cell and/or decrease sarcolemmal permeability to Ca^{2+}. Inhibitory signals may prevent contraction and may also promote relaxation in smooth muscle cells. A given smooth muscle cell will integrate numerous signals, some stimulatory and some inhibitory, at any given time. A mediator that stimulates a certain type of smooth muscle cell may

have an inhibitory effect on smooth muscle in another location.

Contraction What happens when smooth muscle is stimulated? Although skeletal and smooth muscle resemble each other in their dependence on Ca^{2+} for regulation of contraction and relaxation, the resemblance is somewhat superficial. While increases in skeletal muscle sarcoplasmic Ca^{2+} initiate contraction by binding to troponin and exposing the myosin binding site on actin filaments, smooth muscle cells lack troponin and possess a different Ca^{2+}-sensitive contraction and relaxation control mechanism.

When stimulation of smooth muscle leads to an increase in sarcoplasmic Ca^{2+}, four Ca^{2+} ions bind to a regulatory protein called *calmodulin*. The Ca^{2+}-calmodulin complex activates **myosin light-chain kinase (MLCK)**. As its name (kinase) implies, this enzyme phosphorylates (and thereby activates) the smooth muscle thick filament myosin light chain. Phosphorylation of myosin leads to crossbridge cycling with actin, and thereby contraction (FIGURE 7.10). Crossbridge cycling in smooth muscle is similar to that in skeletal muscle, with attachment of the myosin head to an actin binding site, a power stroke, the release of ADP and inorganic phosphate,

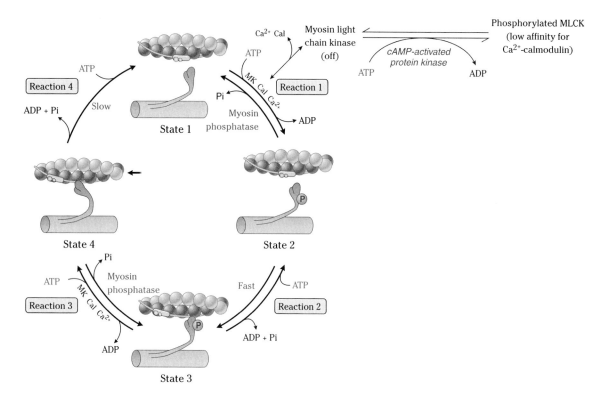

Figure 7.10 The role of Ca^{2+} in smooth muscle contraction. The mysoin heads of smooth muscle progress through four chemical reactions similar to those in skeletal muscle. Reaction 1, in which the myosin head is neither phosphorylated nor bound to actin, depends on Ca^{2+} binding to calmodulin. This complex then activates the enzyme myosin light-chain kinase (MLCK), which adds a phosphate group taken from ATP to myosin. This greatly increases the affinity of myosin for actin and the rate of reaction 2, crossbridge cycling, thus augmenting contraction. Myosin phosphatases can remove the phosphate group from myosin, whether the myosin is bound to actin (reaction 3) or not (the reverse of reaction 1), returning it to its lower cycling rate. Note that when the unphosphorylated myosin head is bound to actin and is associated with ADP + P_i, it produces the latch bridge state responsible for smooth muscle tone. In reaction 4, substitution of an ATP for ADP + P_i resets the myosin head by decreasing its affinity for actin. Any stimulus that increases intracellular concentrations of cAMP will activate protein kinases that phosphorylate MLCK, decreasing its affinity for the Ca^{2+}-calmodulin complex and thus inhibiting contraction.

binding of a new ATP molecule, the release of myosin from the actin binding site, and resetting of the myosin head for a new power stroke by splitting the terminal high-energy phosphate bond of the ATP molecule. The rate of smooth muscle crossbridge cycling is much lower than that of skeletal muscle.

As in skeletal muscle, contractile filaments have different states. There are four such states in smooth muscle. The myosin head may be phosphorylated or unphosphorylated, and it may be bound to actin or unbound (Figure 7.10). In the unphosphorylated state, the rate of myosin crossbridge cycling is very low. In the phosphorylated state, the rate is much higher, although it is still much lower than the skeletal muscle rate.

Crossbridge cycling in smooth muscle consumes ATP. Note, however, that ATP is used in some different reactions compared to skeletal muscle. Activated MLCK uses ATP to phosphorylate myosin and thus regulate the rate of crossbridge cycling. As in skeletal muscle, the myosin head consumes an ATP to reset itself for another power stroke, and the many ion pumps (Na^+-K^+-ATPase, sarcolemma Ca^{2+}, and sarcoplasmic reticulum Ca^{2+}) require ATP (Figure 7.10).

When smooth muscle stimulation decreases, sarcolemma and sarcoplasmic reticulum membrane transporters pump Ca^{2+} out of the cell and into the sarcoplasmic reticulum, respectively, thereby decreasing the sarcoplasmic Ca^{2+} concentration. Ca^{2+} dissociates from calmodulin, which inactivates MLCK. A separate enzyme called *myosin phosphatase* removes phosphate groups from the myosin light chain. However, while the dephosphorylated myosin has a lower rate of crossbridge cycling, it also has a lower rate of detachment from actin than does the skeletal muscle isoform. It thus enters a *latch bridge state,* where it stays attached to the thin filament, maintaining contraction for prolonged periods despite low sarcoplasmic Ca^{2+} concentrations and with minimal ATP consumption. This is what allows smooth muscle cells to maintain a state of prolonged partial contraction known as **tone.**

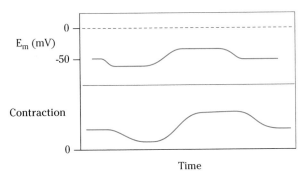

Figure 7.11 Relaxation of smooth muscle in response to membrane hyperpolarization. Among the many stimuli that can induce smooth muscle relaxation, hyperpolarization of the sarcolemma may close voltage-gated Ca^{2+} channels in some smooth muscle cells. The resulting decrease in cytoplasmic Ca^{2+} allows such cells that are tonically contracted to relax.

Relaxation How does smooth muscle relax? In time, in the setting of a low sarcoplasmic Ca^{2+} concentration, the dephosphorylated myosin heads do detach from actin, and the contractile filaments relax. Mediators that bind to sarcolemma receptors that activate the adenylate cyclase-cyclic AMP (cAMP) second messenger system (see Chapter 4) will activate protein kinases that phosphorylate MLCK, which decreases its affinity for the Ca^{2+}-calmodulin complex, so that it remains relatively inactive (Figure 7.10). An example of this is the binding of epinephrine to the β_2-adrenergic receptor, which relaxes vascular smooth muscle and causes vasodilation. In addition, mediators that increase intracellular concentrations of cyclic GMP (cGMP) will also activate protein kinases. These kinases increase the activity of myosin light chain phosphate (Figure 7.10) and modulate the activity of Ca^{2+} ion pumps, increasing the extrusion and/or sequestration of Ca^{2+}, decreasing the sarcoplasmic Ca^{2+} concentration and thereby promote relaxation (Figure 7.9B). Such mediators may be inhibitors of contraction and/or promotors of relaxation. Likewise, hyperpolarization of the sarcolemma may close voltage-gated Ca^{2+} channels, decreasing the influx of Ca^{2+} and allowing the tonically contracted smooth muscle to relax (FIGURE 7.11).

ATP Smooth muscle uses significantly less ATP than skeletal muscle. Although ATP is expended in the regulation of smooth muscle contraction, the latch bridge mechanism allows smooth muscle to generate and sustain significant forces with a net saving of ATP over skeletal muscle. This economy lets smooth muscle function at a low metabolic rate, and oxidative phosphorylation is sufficient for producing the necessary ATP.

Smooth Muscle Organelles

As in other cells, mitochondria produce ATP via oxidative phosphorylation. Ribosomes, rough ER,

and the Golgi apparatus are important in the production and secretion of collagen, elastin, proteoglycans, and other extracellular matrix components by smooth muscle cells. Thus, smooth muscle cells have synthetic and secretory abilities similar to those of fibroblasts.

Smooth Muscle Cells

When a smooth muscle cell contracts, the outer membrane wrinkles and the nucleus takes on a "corkscrew" appearance (FIGURE 7.12). Smooth muscle contractions are of two distinct patterns depending on the functional requirement. Vascular and sphincter smooth muscle cells maintain tone. Stimuli that promote contraction increase tone, while those that inhibit contraction and/or induce relaxation decrease tone. Contraction of smooth muscle in the GI and genitourinary tracts is intermittent, or *phasic*, in order to propel materials (food, feces, urine, etc.) forward.

Smooth Muscle Tissues

To induce changes of sufficient magnitude on the organ and whole body levels, a single smooth muscle cell must coordinate its contractile activity with hundreds, thousands, or millions of other smooth muscle cells. There are two mechanisms that allow such coordination of distinct smooth muscle cells into organized smooth muscle tissues. One is the chemical

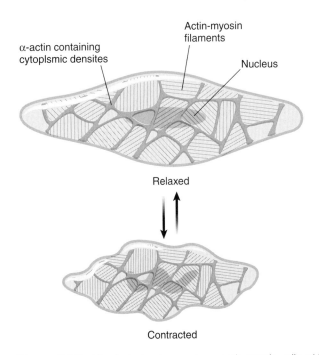

Figure 7.12 Morphologic changes in smooth muscle cells with contraction. Because the contractile proteins of smooth muscle cells are arranged obliquely instead of in parallel sarcomeres, contraction induces a dramatic shape change in the cell. The sarcolemma wrinkles, and the nucleus takes on a corkscrew-shaped appearance. These changes are reversible with relaxation.

and mechanical interconnection of cells. The other is the regulation of contraction by soluble mediators that harmonize the responses of an individual smooth muscle cell with others in a tissue.

Unitary versus Multiunit Tissues   Some smooth muscle tissues are characterized by a high degree of electrochemical coupling between adjacent cells, owing to the presence of numerous gap junctions. In such tissues, the stimulation of one cell will cause contraction in the group of connected cells, known as a *syncytium*. These are called **unitary tissues** and are found in the sphincters of the GI and genitourinary tracts (FIGURE 7.13A). Other smooth muscle tissues, such as those of the vas deferens and the iris, are called **multiunit tissues** because of the relative paucity of electrochemical cell-cell interconnections; each cell in such a tissue must be stimulated independently in order to contract (Figure 7.13B). Often, the cells of multiunit tissues are controlled by neural and endocrine factors.

The degree of cell-cell interconnection is a graded phenomenon; unitary and multiunit tissues are two ends of a spectrum. Generally, smooth muscle tissues that maintain tone (vascular, sphincters) are closer to the unitary end and do not exhibit

action potentials, whereas phasically contracting tissues are more likely to have action potentials and are closer to the multiunit end.

Cell–cell interconnection in a given tissue may change over time, as gap junctions are dynamic structures. Neurohormonal influences can increase or decrease their number. The uterus, which generally has a multiunit structure, demonstrates a great increase in gap junctions and movement toward the unitary end of the spectrum at the end of pregnancy in anticipation of labor.

The Control of Contraction   Smooth muscle contraction is involuntary, unlike skeletal muscle, which is under conscious control. Smooth muscle in vessels and sphincters must maintain tone, but they must be able to adjust how much tone is present. Tissues that contract phasically must be able to modify the frequency and the strength of such intermittent contractions.

The various stimuli that cause and/or influence smooth muscle contraction reflect the heterogeneity of different smooth muscle tissues. Skeletal muscle is neurally controlled, but smooth muscle contraction is often independent of neurons, and some smooth muscle has no neural input at all. Other smooth muscle tissues are neurally *modified*. Smooth muscle tissue is very heterogeneous with respect to the factors that regulate contraction. Smooth muscle tissue contraction is often modified by both sympathetic and parasympathetic influences, one increasing and the other decreasing the likelihood or frequency of contraction. However, there is great diversity in the types of innervating neurons, the neurotransmitters, and the response of the smooth muscle. In some tissues, sympathetic input promotes contraction and parasympathetic influences decrease it. In other tissues, the exact opposite is true.

For example, GI smooth muscle is innervated by sympathetic, parasympathetic, and enteric neurons. This smooth muscle increases contraction in response to ACh (which stimulates the PLC-IP$_3$-DAG second messenger system to increase the sarcoplasmic Ca^{2+} concentration; see Chapters 4 and 5) and decreases contraction in response to norepinephrine. However, vascular smooth muscle (which typically has only sympathetic innervation) increases contraction to norepinephrine.

The response of vascular smooth muscle is especially confusing because different smooth muscle receptors produce different (or opposite) changes in contraction, even though a single neurotransmitter is at work. An example is the effect of epinephrine on vascular tone. In low concentrations, stimulation of β$_2$-adrenergic receptors (via the adenylate cyclase-cAMP pathway) leads to relaxation of smooth muscle

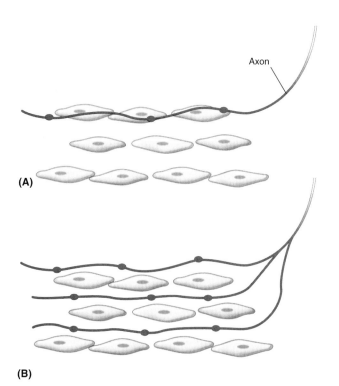

(A)

Axon

(B)

Figure 7.13   Unitary versus multiunit smooth muscle tissues. **A.** In unitary tissues, the smooth muscle cells are electrochemically linked into a single syncytium. **B.** Multiunit tissues are composed of cells that act separately and must be individually stimulated to contract or relax. Note the different arrangement of autonomic nerve cell neurotransmitter-containing vesicles between the two tissues.

and subsequent vasodilation. In higher concentrations, α_1-adrengeric receptors are activated, leading to smooth muscle contraction and vasoconstriction (by means of the PLC-IP$_3$-DAG system). The type of smooth muscle receptor and its associated second messenger system determine the response to a given mediator.

Endocrine factors can have an effect on smooth muscle. Estrogen and progesterone alter uterine phasic contraction. Estrogen induces phasic hyperpolarizations in the sarcolemma while progesterone hyperpolarizes it nonphasically. Angiotensin II is a potent mediator that increases vascular tone. Inhibiting angiotensin II generation or action with medications such as angiotensin converting enzyme inhibitors (ACEI) or angiotensin II receptor antagonists is an important means of correcting high blood pressure and treating kidney disease, respectively.

In addition, many smooth muscle tissues are influenced by the paracrine factors of nearby or adjacent cells other than neurons. The best example of this is the effect of endothelium on vascular smooth muscle. If an isolated vascular smooth muscle tissue is exposed to ACh, activation of the PLC-IP$_3$-DAG second messenger system results in contraction. However, a sample of vascular smooth muscle with an intact endothelium will relax when exposed to ACh, because the ACh binds to endothelial receptors and promotes the production of nitric oxide. The NO diffuses from endothelial cells and increases smooth muscle cell cGMP levels, resulting in relaxation. Other paracrine and autocrine factors are bradykinin and histamine.

Local metabolites, such as adenosine, carbon dioxide, and protons (H^+), can influence smooth muscle. Often, these markers of increased metabolic activity promote vascular smooth muscle relaxation in order to induce vasodilation and increase local tissue blood flow. This is an important example of a homeostatic mechanism (see Chapter 1). In tissues that increase their metabolic rate and/or suffer a decrease in their blood supply, the local concentrations of these metabolites increase. The increased concentrations induce vascular smooth muscle relaxation and therefore vasodilation. Vasodilation increases blood flow to the tissue to meet the metabolic demand. This action, in turn, corrects the demand-supply imbalance and "washes out" the metabolites, diluting the stimuli for smooth muscle relaxation and vasodilation. Thus, the contractile state of the vascular smooth muscle is constantly modified to match the metabolic needs of the tissues.

Mechanical forces such as stretch, also stimulate smooth muscle contraction. This is another important homeostatic mechanism. In tonically contracted smooth muscle tissues, as in the vascular system, this response is a critical component of blood pressure autoregulation. Increased blood pressure stretches the smooth muscle in the walls of blood vessels. If the smooth muscle relaxes and the vessels dilate, the resistance to blood flow decreases, thereby lowering the blood pressure (see Chapter 12). In phasically contracting tissues, such as in the GI and genitourinary systems, stretch is a stimulus to increase activity, facilitating the movement and digestion of food and the removal of waste products.

Neurohormonal and mechanical influences can promote an increase in smooth muscle cell size, called *hypertrophy*. This may be a physiologic adaptation to states such as pregnancy or a pathophysiologic condition such as chronic high blood pressure (hypertension).

Smooth Muscle and Organ Functions

Changes in the state of contraction of smooth muscle tissues have organ-specific effects that depend on both the physical arrangement of the smooth muscle tissues in the particular organ and on the material contained in that organ. For example, the smooth muscle in blood vessel walls is typically in a state of partial contraction. A limited relaxation of vessel wall smooth muscle tends to increase blood vessel diameter and increase blood flow, but excessive relaxation may cause stasis of blood. Likewise, excessive contraction of vascular smooth muscle can completely close the vessel lumen, obstructing blood flow entirely. In the GI tract, the rate of phasically contracting smooth muscle tissue regulates the movement of food and feces, with slowing of the rate leading to stasis and increasing of the rate leading to augmented motility. Smooth muscle tissues have length-stress relationships similar to but distinct from those of skeletal muscle.

Smooth Muscle Orientation The arrangement of smooth muscle tissues within different organs reflects the function of the tissue in that particular organ. In blood vessels, smooth muscle is circumferentially arranged so that contraction will decrease the radius of the vessel lumen (Figure 7.1). In the GI tract, different orientations of distinct smooth muscle layers within the walls allow mixing and peristalsis, the propulsion of the luminal contents (Figure 7.3 and Chapter 28).

Resistance in Tubular Structures Recall that Ohm's law describes the relationship among the flow of something (electrons, fluids); the gradient that drives this flow (potential difference, pressure differences); and the resistance to this flow (see Chapters 12 and 16). In many tissues, smooth muscle regulates the value of the last of these variables—the resistance. This is especially true in the vascular and respiratory systems, where changes in smooth muscle contractility alter tube caliber and therefore the resistance to the flow of materials.

In the cardiovascular system, Ohm's Law takes this form:

$$BP = CO \times TPR$$

where BP is blood pressure, CO is cardiac output, which is the product of heart rate and stroke volume, and TPR is total peripheral resistance. In conjunction with Poiseuille's law, we can rearrange this relationship and express it in this way:

$$TPR = 8\eta l/\pi r^4$$

where η is the viscosity of the fluid (blood), l is the length of the tube (vessel), and r is the radius of the tube (vessel). This equation quantifies the exquisite sensitivity of the resistance to the vessel radius. Smooth muscle contraction decreases this radius and dramatically increases TPR. Conversely, relaxation decreases TPR by allowing the vessel radius to increase.

Length-Stress Relationships Smooth muscle manifests length-stress relationships qualitatively akin to those of skeletal muscle. Total stress generation is the sum of passive and active stress. Active stress generation follows a parabolic curve with a central maximum, representing optimum overlap between thick and thin filaments. However, smooth muscle contraction occurs over a broader range of lengths than skeletal muscle (FIGURE 7.14A,B). The maximal shortening velocity of skeletal muscle is many times greater than that of smooth muscle, though smooth muscle can generate forces equal to or greater than skeletal muscle (Figure 7.14C).

Smooth muscle typically exhibits *viscoelastic* or (plastic) homeostatic properties. In hollow tubular structures such as blood vessels, smooth muscle tone determines the baseline pressure exerted on the luminal contents. When a stimulus stretches the muscle, it initially resists this stimulus and a counterstress is generated, thereby increasing the pressure inside the tube. In time, however, the muscle relaxes and takes on a new (greater) resting length in order to return to its previous level of baseline stress generation and bring the internal pressure back to its original value.

The faster the development of the stretching stimulus, the greater the transient counterstress generated, and the higher the brief increase in content pressure, but the faster the "decay" to a new resting length and return to the baseline stress and pressure. A stretching stimulus that evolves more slowly produces a smaller counterstress and in-

crease in pressure, but it decays to baseline more slowly (Figure 7.14D).

An opposite stimulus causes the reverse of these changes. A decrease in luminal contents brings about a decrease in luminal pressure and wall stress. The smooth muscle shortens and increases its degree of contraction in order to restore the baseline force and maintain luminal pressure (Figure 7.14E).

PATHOPHYSIOLOGY

Disease states resulting from problems with smooth muscle can affect any of the organ systems in which smooth muscle functions. Disorders in contractile function typically occur when smooth muscle contracts too much or too little, often producing a pathologic alteration in the resistance to flow in hollow tubular structures. Pathologic smooth muscle synthetic function may also contribute to disease.

Cardiovascular

Because of its prominent structural and functional roles in blood vessels, smooth muscle dysfunction has dramatic consequences for cardiovascular homeostasis. Alterations in blood pressure are often due to changes in the contractile state of smooth muscle. In some clinical situations, changing the amount of stress in the walls of blood vessels caused by smooth muscle can be used therapeutically to alter blood pressure. (See Clinical Application Box *Vasodilators and Vasopressors*.)

Septic Shock In serious infections, the release of endogenous and exogenous chemical mediators during the inflammatory response may cause the relaxation of smooth muscle in many vascular beds, lowering peripheral resistance to blood flow as many blood vessels dilate. As predicted by Ohm's law the blood pressure decreases, sometimes precipitously and to dangerously low levels, a condition known as *shock*. Because of the infectious basis, this type of reaction is known as **septic shock**.

Cardiogenic Shock Since cardiac output is the product of stroke volume of blood ejected per cardiac contraction and heart rate (contractions per minute), any serious impairment in cardiac contractility, such as a severe heart attack, will reduce the stroke volume and thus the cardiac output. A decrease in heart rate may do the same. In either situation (or when the two concur), a life-threatening decrease in blood pressure known as **cardiogenic shock** may ensue. In response to the low blood pressure (*hypotension*), the homeostatic systems of the body attempt to maintain the blood pressure by

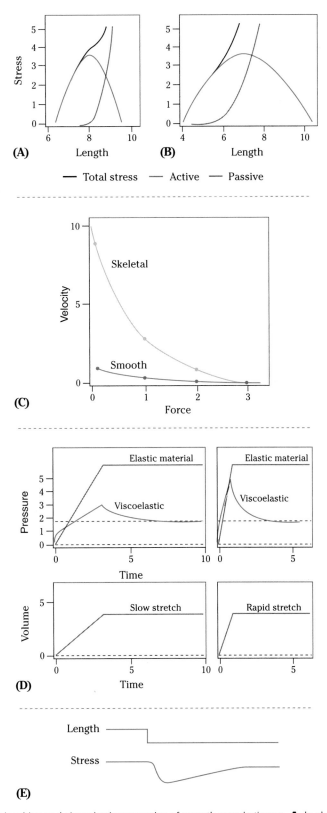

Figure 7.14 Length-stress relationships and viscoelastic properties of smooth muscle tissues. **A.** In skeletal muscle, total stress generation is the sum of passive stress and active stress. **B.** Smooth muscle behaves in a qualitatively similar manner but can generate active stress over a broader range than skeletal muscle can. As a smooth muscle cell is stretched, the overlap of thick and thin filaments is at first improved, then optimized, but then falls away from the optimum length. Active stress generation is maximal when the degree of filament overlap is optimal. **C.** Although smooth muscle can generate stress and force equal to those generated by skeletal muscle, the velocity of shortening of smooth muscle is significantly lower than that of skeletal muscle. **D.** Smooth muscle displays viscoelastic properties. In a three-dimensional model system, smooth muscle in the wall of a hollow tube exerts a tonic pressure on the contents of the tube. Stretching the smooth muscle slowly results in a small increase in the pressure that decays slowly to baseline, while stretching the smooth muscle rapidly produces greater pressure that decays more quickly. **E.** In a linear model of the reverse process, shortening a smooth muscle results in an early loss of stress followed by a gradual recovery toward baseline as the muscle adapts to the new length.

VASODILATORS AND VASOPRESSORS

A number of pharmacological agents are used to alter blood pressure. In hypertension, where blood pressure is pathologically elevated, a group of antihypertensive agents called nitrates can rapidly lower blood pressure by inducing smooth muscle relaxation and a lowering of TPR. Since the relaxation of vascular smooth muscle causes an increase in the diameter of the blood vessel, nitrates and related agents are known as *vasodilators*. Nitrates are metabolized to NO, which rapidly enters the cytosol of smooth muscle cells and activates the enzyme guanylate cylase. This enzyme converts guanosine triphosphate (GTP) into cyclic GMP (cGMP). Increased intracellular concentrations of cGMP activate a cGMP-dependent kinase which phosphorylates MLCK, thereby inactivating it and phosphorylate myosin light chain phosphatase, thereby hyperactivating it. This in turn shifts the balance between the activities of MLCK and myosin light chain phosphatase toward the dephosphorylation of myosin and thus the relaxation of smooth muscle.

In hypotension, where blood pressure is pathologically decreased, such as occurs in states like cardiogenic shock, agents known as *vasopressors* can raise blood pressure. Most of these drugs increase blood pressure by means of a number of mechanisms such as increasing the contractility of the heart (and thereby the stroke volume) and the heart rate. Only some of these agents increase the contraction of vascular smooth muscle and thus the TPR, one example being norepinephrine. Other agents, such as epinephrine, dopamine, and dobutamine, which all increase blood pressure, have diverse effects on TPR. Depending on the expression of different adrenergic receptors by the smooth muscle in a particular vascular bed, the affinity of the various agents for different adrenergic receptors, the compensatory reflexes of the autonomic nervous system, and other variables, different vasopressors may cause vasoconstriction in one area, vasodilation in another area, have no effect in a third area, and induce relaxation in the bronchial, GI, and genitourinary smooth muscle tissues.

increasing peripheral resistance. This is accomplished by a general increase in vascular smooth muscle tone. The result is a patient whose skin is cool and sometimes blue (cyanotic) from arterial constriction in the skin that slows down the flow of deoxygenated blood.

Raynaud's Phenomenon and Prinzmetal's Angina
Vascular smooth muscle occasionally spasms inappropriately. In peripheral tissues, this may lead to a deprivation of blood flow that brings oxygen and nutrients and washes out metabolic wastes. This situation is called **ischemia**. When ischemia occurs in a place in the extremities (fingers and toes) in response to minor cold exposure, it is known as **Raynaud's phenomenon**, and it can threaten the viability of the involved digits. If this smooth muscle spasm occurs in the coronary arteries of the heart, it will induce cardiac ischemia. A patient suffering from this disorder may have an abrupt onset of chest pain called **Prinzmetal's angina**. If prolonged, the spasm may lead to heart tissue death (*myocardial infarction,* or a heart attack).

Thermoregulation   Although thermoregulation is a physiologic homeostatic mechanism for maintaining core body temperature, numerous pathologic conditions can alter the balance between heat generation and heat dissipation. One of the major mechanisms by which the body rids itself of excess thermal energy is peripheral artery dilation. By bringing more blood to the skin, more body heat is "dumped" into the environment. Thus, in patients with fever or heat stroke, relaxation of the smooth muscle in dermal blood vessels occurs, and fair-skinned patients may appear flushed. Conversely, in exposure to excessive cold, peripheral artery vasoconstriction shunts blood away from the skin and minimizes heat loss. In such cases, light-skinned individuals may appear pale (decreased blood flow to the skin) or even blue (stasis of deoxygenated blood in the skin).

Diabetic Peripheral Autonomic Neuropathy and Orthostatic Hypotension   Diabetes mellitus of long duration often damages peripheral nerves; this condition is known as **diabetic neuropathy**. When sympathetic neurons that regulate arterial smooth muscle tone are lost, smooth muscle relaxation and loss of reflexive constriction can occur. In such patients, changes of position from lying to sitting and sitting to standing are no longer accompanied by reflexive vascular smooth muscle contraction, which increases peripheral resistance to blood flow and maintains blood pressure. Instead, there is a gravity-mediated pooling of blood and decreased venous return to the heart, with a subsequent decrease in cardiac stroke volume and loss of blood pressure. Known as **orthostatic hypotension**, this disorder can manifest as lightheadedness (presyncope) or even frank fainting/loss of consciousness (syncope).

Atherosclerosis Most heart attacks, many strokes, and much peripheral vascular disease are the result of progressive arterial wall damage and inflammation called **atherosclerosis**. Smooth muscle cells, along with endothelial cells, platelets, and monocyte-macrophages, as well as myriad inflammatory mediators, growth factors, and cholesterol, are believed to be the major effectors of this process. However, the role of smooth muscle cells may have less to do with their contractile functions than with their synthetic functions.

An atherosclerotic area of an artery is essentially a complex sore (or lesion) on the inner aspect of the vessel wall. Smooth muscle cells in such an area have been observed to alter their appearance and migrate from the vessel media through the fenestrations in the elastic lamella and into the intima (FIGURE 7.15A,B). As they do so, they activate or augment numerous synthetic and proinflammatory mechanisms. In fact, some researchers refer to the change in function in smooth muscle cells a shift from the "contractile" to the "synthetic phenotype."

The *response to injury* hypothesis postulates that recurrent or consistent mechanical and chemical insults cause the vessel wall to undergo changes, including intimal thickening, fatty streak formation, and finally development of an *atheromatous plaque* (Figure 7.15C). The slowly growing plaque gradually occludes the artery lumen and limits blood flow to tissues. In the heart, this arterial narrowing causes cardiac ischemia, which may manifest as angina and/or cardiomyopathy with heart failure. The rupture of a plaque results in blood clot formation (thrombosis), which occludes the vessel lumen. When this occurs in a coronary artery, a heart attack ensues. In the central nervous system, such an event results in damage to and/or death of part of the brain—a stroke.

Pulmonary

Just as the dysfunction of smooth muscle tissue profoundly affects blood pressure and blood flow sys-

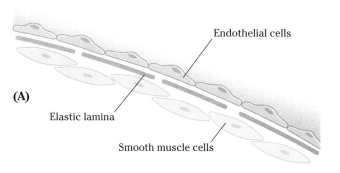

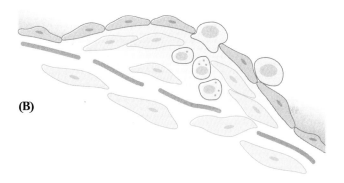

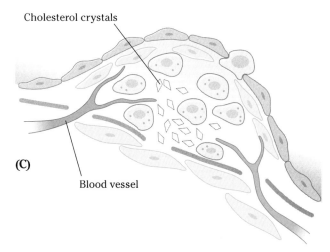

Figure 7.15 The role of smooth muscle cells in atherosclerosis. **A.** In the wall of a healthy artery, the smooth muscle cells have a contractile phenotype and occupy a place in the media, beneath the endothelium that rests on the elastic lamella. **B.** As vessel walls are damaged by such stimuli as high blood pressure and toxic cholesterol metabolites, the smooth muscle cells change from a contractile to a proliferative, synthetic phenotype, and move into the vessel intima through fenestrations in the elastic lamella. **C.** There, colluding with dysfunctional endothelial cells, macrophages, and platelets, they elaborate inflammatory mediators and contribute to the formation of a lesion called an atheromatous plaque.

temically, it can do so in the pulmonary vascular tree as well. **Pulmonary hypertension** results from the dysregulation of smooth muscle contraction in the blood vessels of the lungs. However, much more common is excessive contraction and hypertrophy of the smooth muscle tissues of the bronchi, which can cause impairment of airflow and therefore of gas exchange.

Asthma Smooth muscle contraction in respiratory passages increases resistance to airflow (again in accordance with Ohm's law). Excessive airway smooth muscle contraction in response to such trigger stimuli as allergens, cold air, and exercise may cause attacks of **asthma**, a disease characterized by intermittent airflow obstruction accompanied by reversible bronchoconstriction. The bronchi of people with asthma are termed "hyper-responsive" because smooth muscle constriction with profound resistance to airflow occurs on exposure to relatively low concentrations (compared to non-asthmatics) of stimuli. During an attack of airway bronchoconstriction, a patient may have shortness of breath (called dyspnea), coughing, chest tightness, and turbulent airflow in the contracted bronchi and bronchioles that often produces audible wheezing. An acute attack of asthma may be temporarily ameliorated by the patient inhaling a β_2-adrenergic receptor agonist medication that induces smooth muscle relaxation and bronchodilation. Inflammation of the airways is thought to contribute to smooth muscle hyper-responsiveness, and the most effective long-term treatment for asthma are anti-inflammatory drugs, such as inhaled steroids.

Gastrointestinal

Because smooth muscle tissues are components of the GI tract from the esophagus to the end of the colon, increased contraction or decreased contraction can affect almost any part of the tract. In addition, since the contraction of smooth muscle tissue in the walls of the GI tract is phasic and effective peristalsis depends on the orderly sequence of contractions in segments of the tract, any disorder in contraction can disrupt the movement of food and/or feces.

Achalasia The lower esophageal sphincter is composed of smooth muscle. In the condition known as **achalasia**, inappropriate tonic contraction of this muscle inhibits the normal passage of food and fluid beyond a sphincter that cannot relax. Patients may experience difficulty swallowing and may have chest pain as well.

Diabetic Peripheral Autonomic Neuropathy and Gastroparesis Diabetic peripheral autonomic neuropathy in the GI system can result in decreased esophageal and gastric motility and emptying. This impairment in stomach motility is known as **gastroparesis**. Patients may experience nausea, vomiting, and acid reflux when the alimentary tract contents do not move along normally because normal peristalsis does not occur.

Hirschsprung's Disease The failure of neural crest cells to migrate to the distal colon during development results in an absence of ganglion cells (Meissner's and Auerbach's plexuses, portions of the parasympathetic-enteric nervous system; Figure 7.3). Without these neurons, smooth muscle in the distal colon cannot relax, producing an obstruction to the movement of feces. The result is tremendous dilation of the normal colon that is proximal to the segment lacking autonomic ganglia, a syndrome called **Hirschsprung's disease** (also known as *congenital megacolon*).

Genitourinary

Like smooth muscle tissues in the GI tract, those in the genitourinary tract such as in the wall of the urinary bladder depend on autonomic neurons to regulate the passage of organ contents. Any irritation of the bladder wall, such as that inflammation which accompanies a **urinary tract infection** (also called *cystitis*), may induce spasms of bladder wall smooth muscle and thus urinary incontinence. Conversely, inhibition of or damage to the parasympathetic neurons that increase bladder contraction can impair bladder emptying.

Diabetic Peripheral Autonomic Neuropathy and Bladder Dysmotility Just as diabetic peripheral autonomic neuropathy may affect vascular and GI smooth muscle, it may also affect bladder contractility. Patients suffer from *urinary retention* when parasympathetic neurons are lost because smooth muscle in the bladder wall does not generate sufficient contractile force to empty the bladder. As more and more urine fills the bladder, the smooth muscle is increasingly stretched and moves to that portion of the length-stress curve where active force generation is impaired (poor contractile filament overlap). Eventually, the overstretched bladder, with its very thin wall, is almost unable to contract, establishing a vicious cycle in which urinary retention begets more urinary retention. The loss of sympathetic neurons, which normally cause bladder wall smooth muscle relaxation, can cause the opposite problem, with inappropriate contraction causing bladder spasms that result in urinary incontinence. These two problems of insufficient and excessive bladder contractility may coincide in a single patient, a condition known as **bladder dysmotility**.

Summary

- Smooth muscle is a component of the walls of many hollow or tubular organs, including blood vessels, bronchioles, the GI tract, and the genitourinary tract.

- While skeletal muscle contraction is controlled by motor neurons, smooth muscle contraction is modulated by autonomic neurons. Therefore, smooth muscle, unlike skeletal muscle, is generally not under voluntary control.

- Although smooth muscle, like skeletal muscle, has thin filaments made of actin and thick filaments made of myosin, smooth muscle does not have a regular arrangement of these contractile proteins into sarcomeres.

- Numerous mediators can alter the contractile state of smooth muscle tissue. Whether a given mediator causes contraction or relaxation depends on the receptor and associated signal transduction machinery in a given cell. Different smooth muscle tissues are very heterogeneous in their responses to different regulatory mediators.

- A stimulus inducing smooth muscle contraction increases the intracellular concentration of Ca^{2+}. The Ca^{2+} binds to *calmodulin*, and the Ca^{2+}-calmodulin complex binds to and activates the enzyme **myosin light-chain kinase (MLCK)**. MLCK phosphorylates the light chain of myosin thick filaments, increasing crossbridge cycling.

- *Myosin light chain phosphatase* dephosphorylates the light chain of myosin thick filaments, decreasing crossbridge cycling. Dephosphorylated myosin is still able to bind to thin actin filaments, inducing the *latch bridge state* that allows smooth muscle to maintain prolonged contraction known as **tone**.

- Like skeletal muscle contraction, smooth muscle contraction depends on ATP, but smooth muscle uses significantly less ATP than skeletal muscle. Smooth muscle cells use oxidative phosphorylation to generate ATP and depend less on glycolysis and repayment of an oxygen debt than skeletal muscle.

- The contractile activity of distinct smooth muscle cells are coordinated by intercellular chemical and mechanical connections and by regulatory mediators. **Unitary tissues** are highly interconnected and act as a *syncitium* while **multiunit tissues** are less tightly connected.

- In tubular structures such as blood vessels and the GI tract, the contraction of circumferentially oriented smooth muscle tissues leads to a decrease in the lumen of the tube and an increase in resistance to the flow of material in accordance with Ohm's law and Poiseuille's law. In the GI tract, longitudinally oriented smooth muscle tissues with *phasic* contraction generate peristalsis.

- Smooth muscle tissues display *viscoelastic* homeostatic properties in response to stretch.

- Pathophysiologic conditions arise when smooth muscle tissues contract too much, too little, or in a physically or temporally disordered manner.

- Excessive smooth muscle contraction may affect blood vessels (**Raynaud's phenomenon, Prinzmetal's angina**) causing **ischemia**, pulmonary bronchi (**asthma**), and the esophagus (**achalasia**).

- Insufficient smooth muscle contraction may affect blood vessels (**septic shock**).

- **Diabetic peripheral autonomic neuropathy** damages the nerve cells that regulate smooth muscle contraction in the cardiovascular system, the GI tract, and the genitourinary tract, producing **orthostatic hypotension, gastroparesis**, and **bladder dysmotility**, respectively. **Hirschsprung's disease** results from the failure of neural crest cells to migrate and form autonomic plexuses that control colonic smooth muscle relaxation.

- Smooth muscle cells have numerous synthetic functions as well as the ability to contract. Dysregulation of some of these synthetic functions contributes to the process of **atherosclerosis**.

Suggested Reading

Bolton TB, Prestwich SA, Zholos AV, Gordienko DV. Excitation-contraction coupling in gastrointestinal and other smooth muscles. Annu Rev Physiol. 1999;61:85–115.

Kuriyama H, Kitamura K, Itoh T, Inoue R. Physiological features of visceral smooth muscle cells, with special reference to receptors and ion channels. Physiol Rev. 1998;78(3):811–920.

Ross R. The pathogenesis of atherosclerosis: A perspective for the 1990s. Nature. 1993;362:801–809.

REVIEW QUESTIONS

Directions: Each of the numbered items or incomplete statements in this section is followed by answers or by completions of the statement. Select the ONE lettered answer or completion that is BEST in each case.

1. In smooth muscle, contraction depends on the binding of Ca^{2+} to

    (A) cacineurin

    (B) calmodulin

    (C) tropomyosin

    (D) troponin

    (E) myosin light-chain kinase

2. A 74-year-old man with poorly controlled type II diabetes for over 20 years, but no other medical problems might be expected to have each of the following EXCEPT

    (A) dizziness and near fainting when rising up out of bed too quickly

    (B) nausea and regurgitation or vomiting after large meals

(C) bronchial hyper-responsiveness and intermittent dyspnea and wheezing

(D) difficulty urinating

3. Which of the following is NOT caused by excessive smooth muscle contraction?

(A) Achalasia

(B) Prinzmetal's angina

(C) Raynaud's phenomenon

(D) Asthma

(E) Septic shock

4. An 88-year-old man has a severe heart attack and goes into cardiogenic shock. You would expect his peripheral vascular smooth muscle contraction to be _____ and his peripheral resistance to blood flow to be _____.

(A) decreased; decreased

(B) increased; decreased

(C) decreased; increased

(D) increased; increased

ANSWERS TO REVIEW QUESTIONS

1. **The answer is B.** In smooth muscle, Ca^{2+} from the extracellular space and/or the sarcoplasmic reticulum binds to calmodulin. The Ca^{2+}-calmodulin complex then activates myosin light-chain kinase, which phosphorylates the myosin head, increasing crossbridge cycling. Smooth muscle, unlike skeletal muscle, lacks troponin.

2. **The answer is C.** A patient with long-standing diabetes may have peripheral neuropathy. The nerve dysfunction results in loss of smooth muscle tone. When this occurs in the peripheral blood vessels, orthostatic hypotension ensues, with low blood pressure due to gravity-mediated blood pooling that is not compensated for. In the GI tract, loss of normal peristalsis results in gastroparesis with nausea and regurgitation after a large meal. When the bladder is affected, the ability to urinate completely may be impaired. Asthma, however, is characterized by excessive smooth muscle contraction in response to stimuli such as allergens, cold air, and exercise.

3. **The answer is E.** Septic shock occurs when a serious infection is accompanied by high concentrations of inflammatory mediators that cause widespread vascular smooth muscle relaxation and therefore vasodilation, decreased peripheral resistance, and low blood pressure. All the other conditions are characterized by inappropriate smooth muscle contraction causing blockage of the esophagus (achalasia), coronary vessels (Prinzmetal's angina), peripheral vessels (Raynaud's phenomenon), or airways in the lung (asthma).

4. **The answer is D.** In this situation where the heart is damaged and not pumping blood well (decreased stroke volume, therefore decreased cardiac output), the homeostatic mechanism (the baroreceptor reflex) invoked to maintain blood pressure is peripheral arterial smooth muscle contraction to increase peripheral resistance.

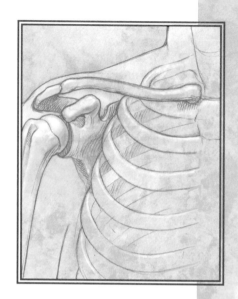

Bone Physiology

INTRODUCTION

The word skeleton comes from the Greek *skellein*, meaning to dry up; a dried-up body (*skeleton soma*) is one with only the bones remaining. Thus etymologically, but also in our cultural imagination, our bones refer to death. They are the only lasting remains of a human body. However, the skeleton is, like any other organ system, a system dedicated entirely to the functions of life. The human skeleton is made not only of minerals, but also of blood, proteins, and living cells. The skeletal system's diverse functions include mineral homeostasis, hematopoiesis, mechanical support for movement, protection, and the determination of body size and shape.

This chapter will outline the way in which bone as an organ interacts with the body to maintain homeostasis. We will cover the anatomy and composition of the various types of bone, how bone resorption and deposition are controlled and influenced, the types of fractures and how they heal, and diseases that affect the skeletal system.

SYSTEM STRUCTURE

Like many organs, bone is composed of living cells and an acellular matrix. There are at least three different cell types: **osteoblasts**, cells on the surfaces of bone that actively produce the protein component of the acellular matrix and regulate bone growth and degradation; **osteocytes**, quiescent osteoblasts suspended in the bone matrix; and **osteoclasts**, cells that promote bone degradation. The ends of many bones have a cartilage cap, produced by cells called **chondroblasts**.

Most extracellular matrices contain polysaccharide chains called **glycosaminoglycans**. These anionic chains bind water and repel one another, creating a viscous but fluid **ground substance**. Different body tissues supplement the ground substance with a particular amount of protein, depending on the character of the tissue matrix. Some tissues are mostly ground substance and therefore more fluid, while others are mostly protein and thus more solid. Bone is dominated by its extracellular matrix, with cells making up just a tiny percentage of the total weight. Bone is also a unique tissue in that its ground substance contains not only protein, but also a heavy proportion of inorganic minerals (FIGURE 8.1).

The Acellular Elements: Collagen and Hydroxyapatite

Bone is made up of collagen fibers and calcium phosphate crystals. It is sometimes compared to reinforced concrete: The collagen is analogous to the steel rods, and the calcium phosphate crystals are compared to the cement. The spindle- or plate-shaped crystals found on and within the collagen fibers are called **hydroxyapatite** and have the

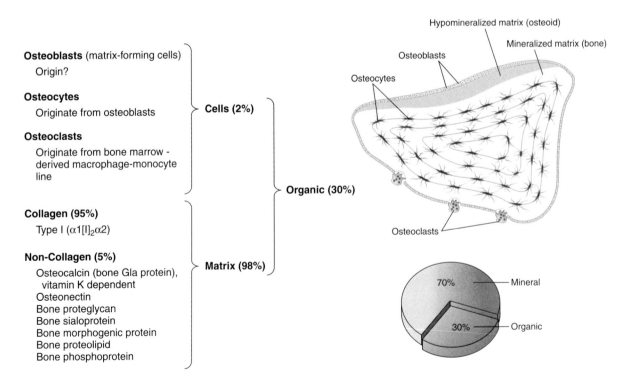

Figure 8.1 The composition of bone.

chemical formula $Ca_{10}(PO_4)_6(OH)_2$. These crystals are oriented preferentially along the long axis of the collagen fibers.

The collagen fibers in the bone matrix are composed of subunits called *tropocollagen*. Each tropocollagen is a triple-helical supercoil of three polypeptide chains. The tropocollagens are cross-linked to one another within the collagen fiber at hydroxylysine and lysine residues (FIGURE 8.2). These cross links stabilize the fiber, increase its resistance to deformation, and render it completely insoluble. About 85% to 90% of the total protein found in bone consists of collagen. Most of the collagen in bone is **type I collagen**. Other types of collagen are infrequent contributors to bone.

Noncollagen Proteins Noncollagen proteins (NCP) make up the majority of the remaining bone protein content. They can be classified into four groups that are somewhat overlapping: proteoglycans, cell attachment proteins, γ-carboxylated proteins, and growth factors. These proteins are largely serum-derived and bind to the mineral component of bone. Some of them may be incidentally trapped in the bone matrix during bone deposition.

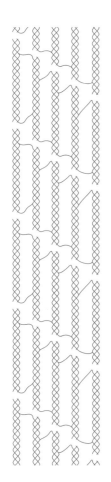

Figure 8.2 The structure of a collagen fiber.

The glycosaminoglycans of the ground substance are sometimes rooted to a protein backbone, in which case they are called **proteoglycans**. This is the case in the bone matrix. The proteoglycans in bone have an important role in fixing hydroxyapatite crystal to the collagen fibers and a poorly defined role in promoting and inhibiting mineralization. In general it seems that intact proteoglycans in high concentrations inhibit calcification, and partially degraded or sparse proteoglycans allow calcification to proceed.

Cell attachment proteins have the important job of anchoring osteoblasts and other bone cells to the bone matrix. Four proteins are recognized as having an integral role in cell attachment: fibronectin (FN), thrombospondin (TSP), osteopontin (OP), and bone sialoprotein (BSP). The exact physiologic role of the **γ-carboxylated proteins** is unclear, but measurements of one, called *osteocalcin*, have proven valuable as markers of bone turnover. Growth factors will be discussed below.

The protein **osteonectin** is an abundant NCP that comprises approximately 2% of the protein in bone. It binds Ca^{2+}, hydroxyapatite, collagen, and thrombospondin. Osteonectin also has a variety of functions in nonbone tissue and is expressed in wound repair. In bone, it may serve as a valuable osteoblast cell cycle regulator and may influence matrix mineralization.

Suspended in the bone matrix, the polypeptide **growth factors** influence the growth, development, and repair of bone. All of the following factors are produced by osteoblasts and elsewhere in the body and are found in the serum:

- Bone morphogenic proteins (BMP)
- Platelet-derived growth factor (PDGF)
- Insulin-like growth factor (IGF)
- Fibroblast growth factor (FGF)
- Transforming growth factor β (TGF-β)

These factors have various effects on bone and cartilage growth in the fetus and during postnatal life. They stimulate the proliferation of osteoblasts and chondroblasts and the proliferation and differentiation of progenitor cells in bone and cartilage cell lines. PDGF promotes chemotaxis in osteoblasts, and TGF-β, a major regulator of bone remodeling, enhances osteoblast activity. FGF may be particularly important in repairing injuries to bone, and IGF-1 is important in long bone growth. Defects in the IGF-1 receptor lead to dwarfism.

Cartilage versus Bone **Cartilage** is another form of extracellular matrix found in the body. Unlike the mineral composition of bone matrix, it is made out of proteoglycans and collagen or elastin. Cartilage composes the skeletal matrix of certain phylogenetically ancient fishes, such as sharks and skates. Cartilage covers the ends of bones inside joints; it is found in the trachea, in the tip of the nose, and in many other areas of the human body. In addition, it serves as a precursor to bone in the context of fetal development and bone growth prior to adulthood. When cartilage is mineralized (laden with hydroxyapatite) and converted to bone, it has undergone **ossification** (from the Latin *os*, meaning bone).

The Cellular Elements

While bone is mostly mineral, it is not a fixed and static entity. Even after an individual has reached maturity, bone is constantly being remodeled (destroyed and rebuilt) by cells within the matrix. The cellular constituents of bone are osteoblasts, osteocytes, and osteoclasts.

Osteoblasts are present at sites of bone formation called *remodeling sites*. Extensive rough endoplasmic reticulum and Golgi apparatus equip osteoblasts for abundant protein production. Embryologically, they are derived from condensing mesenchyme.

Osteocytes are osteoblasts encased in calcified bone. Approximately 15% of osteoblasts become osteocytes. When an osteoblast becomes totally encased in the calcified matrix, its metabolic activity decreases considerably. Gas and nutrients are in limited supply, arriving via very small channels called **canaliculi**. Canaliculi are formed around cytoplasmic processes that extend from the osteoblast during mineralization. The processes of many osteocytes are linked via gap junctions, allowing communication

and material transfer between cells. The osteocytes are eventually phagocytized by osteoclasts during bone resorption.

Osteoclasts are unique and highly specialized cells, present on all bone surfaces and especially at sites of actively remodeling bone. These large multinucleated cells (10–20 nuclei each) have many primary lysosomes and numerous mitochondria. Osteoclasts arise from the hematopoietic cell line in bone marrow. Their mononuclear precursors leave the marrow and circulate in the blood. At endosteal (i.e., inner bone) surfaces, they marginate, proliferate, and fuse, forming a ruffled border for bone resorption. This border is in fact an extracellular lysosome, sealed off by integrins that bind the osteoclast to the bone surface.

Patterns of Bone Composition

Osteoblasts deposit bone in two distinct patterns, lamellar and woven. **Woven bone** is formed when the osteoblasts deposit the collagen fibers randomly, "weaving" the collagen in a loosely organized pattern. Woven bone is normally present in the fetal skeleton and growth plates. It is produced quickly and has excellent strength in all directions. In an adult its presence always signifies pathology. It is formed at fracture sites, areas of infection, and is produced by tumors. Woven bone is typically replaced by **lamellar bone**, which is deposited more slowly and is stronger. Lamellar bone forms the characteristic **Haversian systems**, with concentric lamellae surrounding a central vascular bundle (FIGURE 8.3).

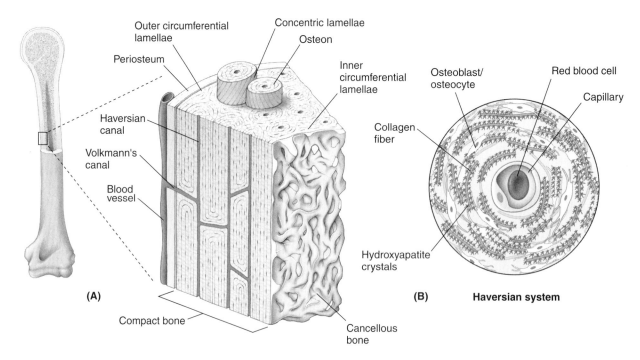

Figure 8.3 Lamellar bone. **A.** A macroscopic view. **B.** The Haversian system: a closer look.

There are two types of lamellar bone. **Cortical bone**, the tissue at the outer periphery of bones, is also called *compact bone*. **Trabecular bone,** the tissue inside of bones, is also called *spongy bone* or *cancellous bone*. Cortical bone is up to 20 times denser than trabecular bone, which is composed of a porous network of bony arches called **trabeculae** (the word is Latin for "little beams"). The bone marrow sits in these pores, which are large enough to be viewed with the naked eye. The fibrous **periosteum** is the outer covering of bone.

The Anatomy of Bones The skeleton is composed of two anatomically distinct types of bones—the **flat bones** of the skull, scapula, mandible, and pelvis; and the **long bones**, such as the tibia, femur, and humerus. These two bone types are formed by two different kinds of ossification. Flat bones are created in the fetus by **intramembranous ossification**, in which membranes of mesenchymal connective tissue are ossified. Long bones result from **endochondral ossification** during fetal life, the ossification of mesenchyme that has first differentiated into discrete cartilaginous forms.

Long bones are characteristically wider at the ends where the bone will articulate with another bone. The widened end of the bone is called the **epiphysis**, the long and thin shaft is called the **diaphysis**, and the end of the shaft just before the epiphysis is called the **metaphysis** (FIGURE 8.4). In growing children, a cartilaginous **growth plate** divides the epiphysis from the metaphysis. This is an active site of bone deposition. Arteries enter the bone through holes in the periosteum. The epiphyses contain a larger proportion of trabecular bone than is present in the diaphyses. The porosity of trabecular bone makes it more malleable and thus renders the bone better able to absorb the stress of bone-to-bone contact in the joint. The wideness of the epiphyses with respect to the diaphyses has a similar function. Increased surface area at the end of the bone distributes pressure and reduces the stress exerted per area of bone by the adjacent, articulating bone in the joint.

The epiphyses of bones are capped with cartilage. This cartilage may connect one epiphysis directly to another in a **cartilaginous joint,** such as the costochondral joints that connect ribs to the sternum, or may form a smooth surface for the articulation of two epiphyses in a **synovial joint,** such as the knee. In synovial joints, the space in which the two bones articulate is sealed in a fibrous capsule filled with lubricating synovial fluid. Muscles that attach to bones on either side of a joint can flex or extend the joint. Both muscles and ligaments stabilize joints.

SYSTEM FUNCTION

During adulthood, bone is always in a state of balance between simultaneous resorptive processes and depositional ones. Osteoclasts digest lacunae in bone and osteoblasts follow behind and fill them in with new bone. This process is called **remodeling**, or *bone turnover*. An increase in bone mass means that remodeling has been influenced in the direction of osteoblast function and bone deposition. Shrinkage of bone means remodeling has been influenced in the direction of osteoclast function and resorption.

Prior to adult life, bones undergo growth—a special form of bone deposition distinct from that in remodeling and driven in part by growth hormone. When osteoblasts conduct bone deposition as part of remodeling, they secrete the bone matrix directly onto preexisting bone. During growth, however, osteoblast activity is preceded by chondroblast activity. Cartilage is formed and then mineralized or ossified to become bone.

The Control of Remodeling

Two main factors govern the direction that remodeling takes: Ca²⁺ homeostasis and mechanical stress. We cover Ca^{2+} homeostasis in Chapter 33; for our present purpose, it suffices to say that parathyroid hormone (PTH) and vitamin D both promote osteoclastic bone resorption in order to liberate Ca^{2+}

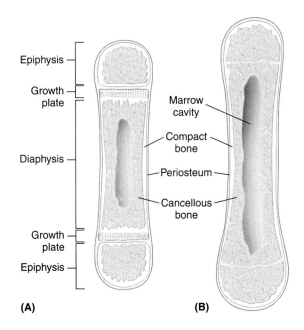

Figure 8.4 The structure of long bones. **A.** In childhood, the growth plate consists of a cartilaginous band between the diaphysis and the epiphysis. **B.** When long bone growth is complete, the growth plate becomes completely ossified. This is sometimes called closure of the epiphyses.

from hydroxyapatite and raise the serum Ca^{2+} concentration. Calcitonin from the parafollicular C cells of the thyroid inhibits bone resorption in order to suppress the serum Ca^{2+} concentration. (Several other endocrine axes have minor effects on bone remodeling as well. Glucocorticoids and thyroid hormone appear to promote resorption, while estrogen receptors in bone appear to mediate the inhibition of osteoclast activity.)

By mechanisms that remain unclear, mechanical stress also tips the balance in bone remodeling between resorption and deposition. More specifically, mechanical stress inhibits bone resorption and promotes bone deposition. Bone is in this sense extremely plastic (even while it is mostly mineral in composition), and the skeleton's outward appearance closely reflects the forces imposed upon it. When bones chronically bear weight or muscles chronically exert force upon them, the bones' trabeculae become dense and prominent (FIGURE 8.5). Bones protected from stress lose mass.

Julius Wolff first proposed this attribute of the bones in 1892 and the orthopedic notion that "form follows function" is sometimes called **Wolff's law.** Recently, investigators have suggested that bones possess a "mechanostat" that can detect strain, compare it with a set point, and influence osteoblasts and osteoclasts in accordance with this afferent information. The specific character and location of such a mechanostat remain to be discovered, but Harold Frost speculates that signals associated with stress could include electric potentials or "fluid shear over cell membranes."

Because of Wolff's law, chronic bed rest or lack of exercise with muscle weakness can put elderly people at risk of *osteopenia* (decreased bone mass) and fractures. Similarly, astronauts who spend extended

periods of time in space are threatened with osteopenia because the low gravity reduces the levels of mechanical stress on their bones and resorption becomes more active than deposition.

Finally, it should be noted that bone remodeling is to some extent a self-regulating phenomenon. As mentioned above, serum-derived growth factors are embedded in bone during deposition. When this bone is later resorbed, growth factors such as IGF-1, TGF-β, FGF, and PDGF are released. All these factors promote osteoblastic activity.

Bone Deposition in Remodeling

During remodeling, osteoblasts commence bone deposition by secreting a thick seam of type I collagen called the **osteoid.** Over the next 5 to 15 days, mineralization of the collagen fibers follows, also under the regulation of osteoblasts. The crystals formed are needle-like and lie alongside or penetrate the collagen fibers. The exact process whereby the osteoblasts control the precipitation of crystals is unclear. Under physiologic conditions, the extracellular fluid is supersaturated with hydroxyapatite, which should lead to uncontrolled crystal growth; yet, the process is somehow well controlled by the osteoblasts.

Bone Resorption

Osteoclasts are not activated directly, but rather by paracrine factors from osteoblasts. For example, the osteoblasts and not the osteoclasts bear the receptor for PTH, which causes the osteoblast to upregulate osteoclast proliferation, stimulating more bone resorption. The likely candidates for the paracrine factor are various *interleukins* (especially IL-6) and *granulocyte-monocyte-colony-stimulating factor (GMCSF)*. It appears that estrogen inhibits osteoclastogenesis by inhibiting osteoblast secretion of IL-6 and perhaps other interleukins. Recently, a receptor in the tumor necrosis factor receptor family, known as receptor activator of nuclear factor kappa B, or NF-κB (RANK), has been shown to be involved in the activation of osteoclasts and consequently bone resorption. In this model, preosteoclasts express RANK while RANK-ligand (RANKL) is expressed on the lining cells of the bone under stimulation by factors such as PTH, IL-1, and calcitriol (which is 1, 25 [OH]$_2$ vitamin D$_3$). The binding of RANKL to the osteoclast receptor RANK activates osteoclast differentiation and bone resorption. A free-floating decoy receptor known as osteoprotegerin (OPG) is produced by osteoblasts and competes for RANKL, thus modulating bone resorption. Estrogen increases OPG production and may prevent bone resorption by this mechanism.

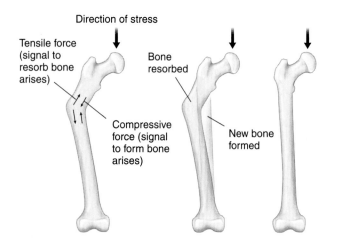

Figure 8.5 Wolff's law. Bone is remodeled in accordance with planes of stress.

Once encouraged by the osteoblasts, the osteoclasts resorb bone at the endosteal surfaces by forming extracellular lysosomes with integrin seals. The cells produce proteolytic enzymes and hydrogen ions in the sealed area under the ruffled border. Carbonic anhydrase generates protons, which are then extruded across the ruffled border via a variety of pumps, antiporters, and channels. Proteolytic enzymes are targeted to the area via mannose-6-phosphate receptors and are released via exocytosis. Osteoclastic resorption forms a small pit or lacuna in the bone, sometimes called *Howship's lacuna*. The osteoclast then moves on to a new area on the endosteal surface to start over. Meanwhile, bone resorption has released growth factors from the matrix that stimulate the osteoblasts. Once the osteoclasts vacate the lacuna, activated osteoblasts move in and begin to lay down osteoid to make new bone. Together, these events constantly renew the bone matrix and are referred to as the **activation-resorption-formation sequence** (FIGURE 8.6). (See Clinical Application Box *What Is Paget's Disease?*)

Bone Deposition in Growth

As mentioned above, flat bones are created in the fetus by intramembranous ossification, while long bones are the product of endochondral ossification. In endochondral ossification, the bone is modeled in cartilage before ossification occurs. This cartilaginous "bone template" is called an **anlagen**. The anlagen develops a bony sleeve under the periosteum. A marrow cavity forms, then centers of ossification grow in the marrow cavity, extending

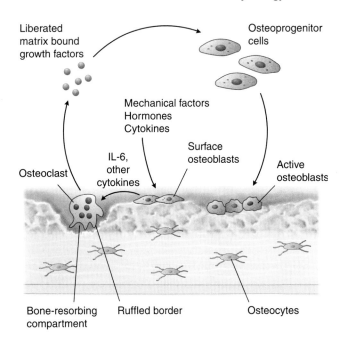

Figure 8.6 The activation-resorption-formation sequence. Osteoblasts are activated by mechanical or hormonal signals to trigger osteoclastogenesis. Osteoclastic resorption liberates growth factors from the matrix, which stimulate osteoblastic deposition.

trabeculae toward the bony sleeve, which serves as a scaffolding for the developing trabeculae, thereby determining the eventual shape of the mature bone. Muscular stress on bones may be important to the development of bones *in utero* as the fetus applies stress to immature bones by kicking and pushing against the uterine walls.

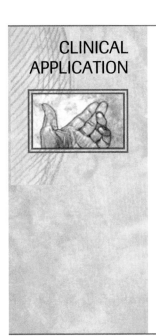

CLINICAL APPLICATION

WHAT IS PAGET'S DISEASE?

A newly acquired pitcher brought in to bolster the starting rotation of the Cleveland Indians leaves his first game at Jacobs Field with intense pain in his throwing arm. The x-ray shows a pathologic fracture of the right humerus, which is abnormally low in bone density. The pitcher is forced to miss the rest of the season and the Indians miss the playoffs. The diagnosis is Paget's disease, affecting the right humerus.

Paget's disease is a disorder of bone remodeling, characterized by an increase in osteoclast-mediated bone resorption and a compensatory increase in new bone formation. This increase in both osteoclast and osteoblast activity results in a disordered mosaic of woven and lamellar bone. This bone is larger, less dense, has increased vascularity, and is more malleable and susceptible to fracture.

Despite these abnormalities, most patients are asymptomatic, and it is estimated that up to 3% of the population over age 55 in North America and Europe is affected by this disorder. Those with symptoms may have bone pain, arthritis, bone deformity, and signs of peripheral nerve impingement. Although the precise etiology of Paget's disease remains unknown, it is possible that a virus may dysregulate the osteoclasts.

During childhood and adolescence, growth takes place in the long bones along the growth plate between the epiphysis and the metaphysis (Figure 8.4A). The growth plate contains functional zones distributed from the epiphysis to the metaphysis. The epiphysis contains quiescent chondrocytes, while the layers of the growth plate nearer the metaphysis contain active chondroblasts that are proliferating and laying down cartilage. Osteoblasts then mineralize this cartilage matrix, ossifying it and forming new trabeculae in the metaphysis. Orderly cartilage formation is necessary for orderly bone formation. If the cartilage matrix is too fluid, the chondrocytes move aberrantly, and anomalies such as dwarfism can result.

Growth hormone regulates the growth of bones indirectly by increasing the expression of IGF-1 by cells in the growth plate. IGF-1 then promotes chondroblast and osteoblast proliferation and enhances deposition of the bone matrix by osteoblasts. The exact mechanism of control over chondrocyte growth and differentiation is not completely clear. The *fibroblast growth factor receptor 3 (FGFR3)* appears to stop or slow the growth of chondrocytes in the proliferative zone of the plate. A second receptor active in the growth plate is the *parathyroid hormone-related peptide (PTHrP) receptor*. PTHrP receptors also appear to slow the rate of chondrocyte growth within the plate.

PATHOPHYSIOLOGY

Any defect in the regulation or mechanism of bone remodeling may lead to abnormalities in the quality and quantity of bone tissue. This, in turn, may lead to deformities and fractures. Among the causes of skeletal deformity and injury are abnormal Ca^{2+} homeostasis, fracture due to trauma, and osteoblast or osteoclast dysfunction.

Abnormal Calcium Homeostasis

Vitamin D deficiency results in poor intestinal Ca^{2+} absorption and hypocalcemia. The parathyroid glands secrete PTH in order to release Ca^{2+} from bone and raise the serum Ca^{2+} (which is critical for normal neuromuscular function). PTH activates osteoclasts, and bone resorption prevails over deposition. The increased osteoclastic activity results in demineralized and malleable bones. Histologically there is excess unmineralized matrix and wide osteoid seams. In growing children, the disease is called **rickets**, and the result is a weak skeleton and bones that deform under the strain of gravity or muscle tension. In adults, vitamin D deficiency with demineralization is called **osteomalacia**. Causes include malnourishment, inadequate sunlight exposure, and malabsorption.

Hyperparathyroidism is caused by the loss of normal negative-feedback control by high serum calcium. This leads to demineralization of bone as osteoclasts increase their activity. While resorption occurs in excess as it does in osteomalacia, in hyperparathyroidism, the serum Ca^{2+} is elevated rather than depressed, leading to a different pattern of bone destruction.

Fractures

Three forces cause **fractures** (bone breakage): tension, compression, and torsion. *Tension* stretches bone; *compression* compacts bone. Bending a bone causes the cortex on one side of the bone to experience tension, the other to be compressed, leading to breakage. *Torsion* causes part of a bone to rotate about its axis. Fractures are classified by the bone involved, the anatomic location, and the pattern of the fracture fragments. Fracture patterns are sometimes classified as follows:

- *Closed* versus *open*. In an open fracture, the bony fragment penetrates the skin.
- *Simple* versus *comminuted*. A simple fracture has a single fracture line. In a comminuted fracture, more than two fragments are created.
- *Extra-articular* versus *intra-articular*. In an intra-articular fracture, the fracture line enters the joint cavity.
- *Transverse*, *oblique*, or *spiral*. If the fracture line is perpendicular to the long axis of the bone, the fracture is transverse. A direct blow to a bone frequently causes a transverse fracture. If the fracture line is tilted up or down from the perpendicular line, it is called oblique. Twisting or wrenching (torsion) of bone causes a spiral fracture, in which the break occurs along more than one plane. This is commonly seen in skiing injuries.
- *Pathologic*. A fracture is called pathologic if it occurs in bone that is weakened from an underlying disease.

Bone is unique in its ability to completely reconstitute itself by reactivating processes that normally occur only in embryogenesis—the construction of an anlagen followed by woven bone. The four stages of bone healing are inflammation, soft callus, hard callus, and remodeling. The inflammatory phase begins immediately after injury and last for 7 days. During this time, a *hematoma* (blood clot) forms, filling gaps in the disrupted bone. The hematoma contains a fibrin meshwork that seals the site and forms a framework for incoming cells. Degranulating platelets at the

BONE SCANS AND BONE MINERAL DENSITY TESTS

Skeletal scintigraphy, otherwise known as a *bone scan*, can be used to evaluate metastatic bone disease, primary bone tumors, osteomyelitis (bone infection), aseptic necrosis (the death of bone tissue, often due to fracture and impaired blood supply), and other bone diseases. Bone scans are performed by administering a radionuclide that concentrates selectively in the bone matrix where bone turnover is most active.

The radionuclide administered is technetium-99m pertechnetate-labeled methylene diphosphonate, an analog of calcium phosphate. (The test is sometimes called a technetium scan.) About 2 to 3 hours after the technetium has been intravenously administered, a gamma camera takes a picture. The areas of increased bone turnover take up more technetium and appear darker or denser on the image produced. This imaging technique assists with localization of metastatic tumors, occult fractures, arthritis, or areas of infection—any portion of the bone where there is high osteoblastic and osteoclastic activity.

The bone scan is not to be confused with tests for osteoporosis that measure *bone mineral density (BMD)*. BMD tests use entirely different imaging techniques to assess bone density in the whole skeleton or in particular spots that are vulnerable to osteoporosis, such as the hip or wrist. A common test is *dual energy x-ray absorptiometry (DXA)*. BMD results obtained from an individual patient are compared with average values to assess whether osteopenia is present.

---

site release PDGF, TGF-β, and FGF. These signals activate bone growth. The hematoma anchors the bone for healing purposes but provides no significant structural stability. The proliferation of chondroblasts and the elaboration of cartilage marks the *soft callus* phase. Capillary buds invade, enabling more chondroblasts, osteoclasts, and osteoblasts to populate the callus. Next, the callus is gradually calcified and infiltrated by woven bone and is called a *hard callus*. Finally, the woven bone is remodeled to lamellar bone.

The callus can only bridge the fracture site under conditions of mechanical stability; that is, if the fractured bone is too mobile at the fracture site, a successful callus cannot form. This is the reason for splinting and casting fractures. In some cases, grafting of bone may be necessary to enable a callus to bridge the gap.

Osteoblast and Osteoclast Dysfunction

The most common disorder occurring at the level of osteoblast and osteoclast function is osteoporosis. **Osteoporosis** is a reduction in overall bone mass (osteopenia) that occurs in connection with aging. Since androgens and estrogens dampen osteoclastic activity, the postmenopausal drop in estrogen production puts postmenopausal women at particularly high risk for osteoporosis. In the absence of premenopausal estrogen levels, osteoblasts secrete more IL-6 and other cytokines that stimulate osteoclastogenesis, leading to increased bone resorption and more brittle bones. Although the entire skeleton is involved, disease in the femoral neck and vertebrae tends to pose the most clinical problems. Osteopenia in these locations predisposes sufferers of osteoporosis to hip fractures and spinal compression fractures even without significant trauma.

Exercise, bisphosphonate therapy, and calcium supplementation are treatments for osteoporosis. **Bisphosphonates** (such as alendronate or risedronate) bind to hydroxyapatite in bone and inhibit osteoclast activity or increase osteoclast cell death, helping restore the balance between resorption and deposition. Deposition occurs normally on top of the bisphosphonates, which become embedded and inactive in the matrix. (See Clinical Application Box *Bone Scans and Bone Mineral Density Tests.*)

Summary

- Bone is composed of cellular and acellular elements. The acellular element, or bone matrix, is made of collagen adorned with hydroxyapatite (calcium phosphate crystals).

- Woven bone is found in the fetus and in pathologic states. Lamellar bone, arrayed in a concentric circle around a blood vessel, is the usual pattern of bone deposition in postnatal life.

- Flat bones are the skull, pelvis, scapula, etc. Long bones are the humerus, femur, etc.

- Long bones have a diaphysis, metaphysis, and epiphysis. In growing children and adolescents, a growth plate divides the metaphysis and epiphysis.

- The inside of trabecular bone consists of porous network of bony arches called trabeculae. The pores are filled with bone marrow, where blood cells are made. More compact cortical bone surrounds and contains the trabecular bone.

- Osteoblasts deposit bone. Osteoclasts resorb bone. Osteoblasts control osteoclast proliferation with cytokines, such as IL-6.

- In adults, deposition and resorption go on all the time and remain in equilibrium. Thus, they preserve a relatively stable bone mass. Osteoclasts digest lacunae in the bone, and osteoblasts fill the lacunae with new bone. This process is called remodeling. Calcium homeostasis can shift bone turnover toward deposition or resorption in order to liberate Ca^{2+} from bone. Mechanical stress shifts remodeling toward deposition along planes of stress, and lack of stress shifts it toward resorption. This is Wolff's law: form follows function.

- During remodeling, osteoblasts deposit new bone (collagen and hydroxyapatite) directly on top of old.

- During fetal growth, bones are modeled in cartilage and then mineralized or ossified with woven bone.

- In childhood and adolescence, cartilage grows at the growth plate and is then ossified with lamellar bone.

- When bone is fractured, it grows a cartilaginous callus, which is then ossified with woven bone. The woven bone is later remodeled into lamellar bone.

- Growth hormone regulates long bone growth by inducing the expression of IGF-1.

Suggested Reading

Boyde A. The real response of bone to exercise. J Anat. 2003;203(2):173–189.

Delmas PD, Meunier PJ. The management of Paget's disease of bone. N Engl J Med. 1997;336(8):558–566.

Ettinger MP. Aging bone and osteoporosis: strategies for preventing fractures in the elderly. Arch Intern Med. 2003;163(18):2237–2246.

Frost HM. The biology of fracture healing. An overview for clinicians. Part I. Clin Orthop. 1989;(248):283–293.

Frost HM. From Wolff's law to the Utah paradigm: insights about bone physiology and its clinical applications. Anat Rec. 2001;262(4):398–419.

Wolff J. *The Law of Bone Remodeling*. Trans., Maquet PGJ, Furlong R. Berlin: Springer-Verlag; 1986.

REVIEW QUESTIONS

Directions: Each of the numbered items or incomplete statements in this section is followed by answers or by completions of the statement. Select the ONE lettered answer or completion that is BEST in each case.

1. Estrogen receptors are expressed on many different cells found in the bone matrix. Estrogen's inhibitory effect on osteoclastogenesis is probably mediated by estrogen receptors on which bone cell?

   (A) Osteoclasts
   (B) Osteocytes
   (C) Chondrocytes
   (D) Osteoblasts
   (E) Chondroblasts

2. A 96-year-old woman suffers a painful hip fracture with minimal trauma. If bone mineral density testing later shows that she has osteoporosis, her fracture could be described as

   (A) comminuted
   (B) pathologic
   (C) transverse
   (D) articular
   (E) open

3. An 81-year-old man complaining of back pain is diagnosed with prostate cancer after a transrectal biopsy. His bone scan shows dark areas at several lumbar and thoracic vertebrae, suggesting probable metastases. The dark areas reflect

   (A) increased bone resorption
   (B) increased bone deposition
   (C) increased bone resorption and deposition
   (D) cancellous bone
   (E) low radionuclide concentration

ANSWERS TO REVIEW QUESTIONS

1. **The answer is** D. Stimulation of the estrogen receptor on osteoblasts causes inhibition of osteoclastic activity. Osteoblasts control osteoclastogenesis through cytokines such as IL-6. Estrogen likely acts on the osteoblast, just as PTH acts on the osteoblast to up-regulate osteoclastic activity.

2. **The answer is** B. The patient has a pathologic fracture. A pathologic fracture is one that occurs in the context of underlying abnormalities in the bone. In this case, the abnormality is low bone mass owing to osteoporosis. She may also have a comminuted, transverse, articular, or (less likely) open fracture, but there is not enough information given to diagnose her with anything except a pathologic fracture.

3. **The answer is** C. The dark areas on the bone scan reflect increased bone remodeling, meaning increased resorption and deposition. The cancer promotes the resorption, and the osteoblasts respond to the increased resorption with increased deposition. The dark areas are highly concentrated with radionuclide, not the reverse.

BLOOD AND LYMPH

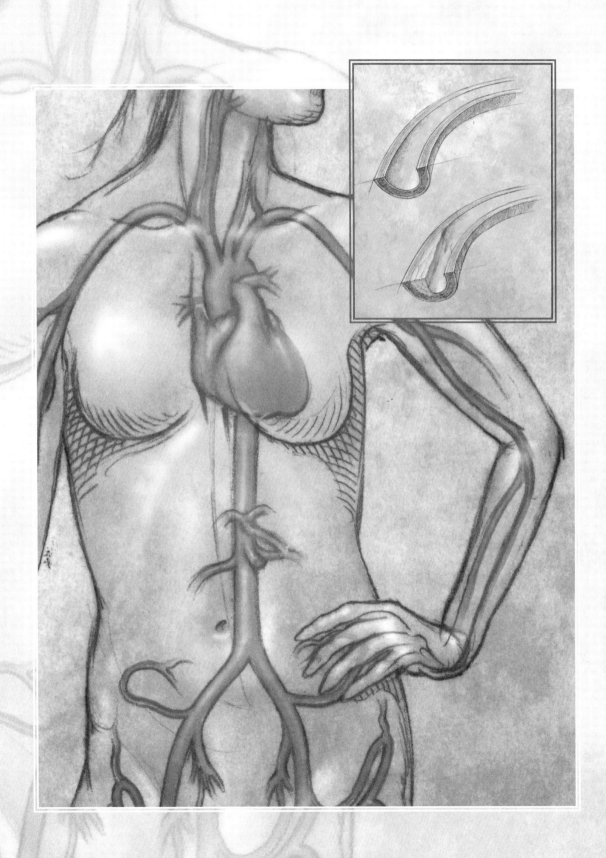

Blood

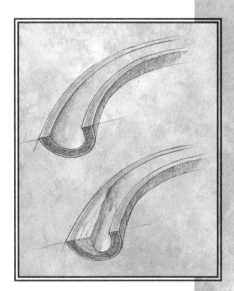

INTRODUCTION

The blood performs many key functions required for the viability of all other organs. Pumped by the heart through the circulatory system, blood is a major transportation route throughout the body. It brings oxygen and nutrients such as glucose to all living tissues of the body and removes carbon dioxide and other waste products. Blood also transports endocrine hormones and other substances throughout the body.

In the alveoli of the lungs, blood releases carbon dioxide and absorbs oxygen. It absorbs nutrients from the villi of the gastrointestinal tract. Wastes are removed by filtration of the blood by the nephrons of the kidney. Toxins are removed and proteins are added by the liver. New blood cells are produced by the bone marrow while old cells are removed in the spleen.

Blood maintains body temperature, provides protection against injury, and provides defense against infection and invasion. Thus, blood has the dual role of providing for the needs of individual tissues as well as integrating metabolism, respiration, communication, and homeostasis at the level of the whole organism.

SYSTEM STRUCTURE

The structure of blood differs in two related respects from that of other organ systems. First, blood is liquid under normal conditions rather than solid. Second, while most organs have relatively limited mobility if any, blood circulates throughout the body. These features are essential to the functions blood performs, and loss of either the liquidity of blood or its body-wide circulation can result in serious pathophysiology.

Blood Gross Anatomy

A normal, healthy adult has approximately 5 L of blood within the circulatory system. Blood cells are produced in bone marrow and circulate to body tissues in blood vessels, exerting most of their functions at the level of the tissue capillaries. The heart is the central pump of the system and the vessels are the conduits. Arteries bring blood from the heart to the capillary beds of peripheral tissues and organs, veins return blood to the heart, and lymphatic vessels return extracellular fluid to the vasculature. (See Part IV for a full description of the cardiovascular system.)

Blood Tissues

Blood is a specialized type of connective tissue that consists of two components: formed elements and plasma. **Formed elements** include red blood cells, white blood cells, and platelets. **Plasma** is the

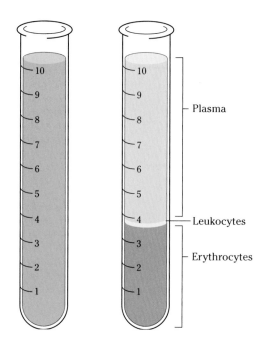

Figure 9.1   Hematocrit tubes before and after centrifugation. Blood from a patient is collected in a test tube. Before centrifugation (*left*), the blood appears to be homogeneously red from the abundance of erythrocytes. After centrifugation (*right*), the red cells fall to the bottom of the tube, the white cells form a small band called the buffy coat, and the plasma remains on top. By measuring the height of the packed red cells and dividing by the height of the total blood in the tube, the ratio is expressed as the hematocrit, or percentage of blood volume that is taken up by red cells.

aqueous medium that contains a variety of proteins, small molecules, and ions. These two components can be separated if a sample of blood is centrifuged. FIGURE 9.1 shows blood in tubes before and after centrifugation. After centrifugation, the lower layer is deep red in color; it is called the **hematocrit**. Consisting of red blood cells that have fallen to the bottom, the hematocrit constitutes 40% to 50% of the blood volume in a normal adult. The thin layer immediately above is whitish in color and is called the **buffy coat**. It consists of white blood cells and constitutes about 1% of the blood volume. The yellowish liquid that comprises the remainder of the blood volume is the plasma.

Blood Cells and Organelles

Blood cells are produced in bone marrow by **hematopoetic stem cells**. When the cells reach a sufficient degree of maturity (which may not necessarily be full maturity), they exit the bone marrow and circulate in the vasculature. The photomicrograph in FIGURE 9.2 shows a peripheral blood smear depicting numerous erythrocytes (red blood cells), leukocytes (white blood cells), and platelets. TABLE 9.1 lists the formed elements of human blood.

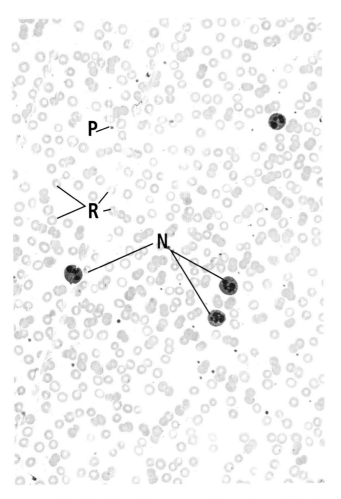

Figure 9.2 A peripheral blood smear. A drop of normal blood is smeared onto a glass slide, dried, stained, and examined under a light microscope. Note the shapes, relative numbers, and relative sizes of erythrocytes (*R*), neutrophils (*N*), and platelets (*P*).

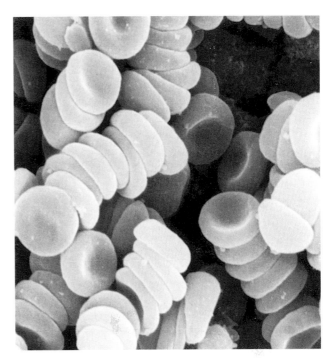

Figure 9.3 A scanning electron micrograph of typical erythrocytes (red blood cells). Note especially the biconcave-disk shape of the cells and their lack of a nucleus. During development, red cell precursors eject their nucleus, making them lighter and thus easier for the heart to pump throughout the circulatory system. The cytoplasm is filled largely with hemoglobin for carrying oxygen.

Erythrocytes are small cells with diameters of 6.5 to 8 μm, shaped like biconcave disks. There are about 4 to 6 million red blood cells per μL of blood; they are the most numerous of the formed elements. The center of the disk of an erythrocyte is characteristically

pale in color, as seen under a light microscope, reflecting the thinnest portion of the disk (FIGURE 9.3). Erythrocytes have no nucleus, no mitochondria, and no ribosomes; the lack of organelles reflects their specialized function. Using certain stains, erythrocytes typically appear intensely pink, indicative of their high protein content. Immature erythrocytes, known as *reticulocytes*, however, stain less intensely pink because they contain less protein and more RNA than mature erythrocytes, reflecting ongoing protein synthesis. Reticulocytes normally constitute approximately 1% of circulating red blood cells.

Leukocytes are somewhat larger than erythrocytes and far less numerous, about 4,000 to 10,000 per μL of peripheral blood. There are several different types of leukocytes, classified according to their nuclear shape and the presence and type of granules in their cytoplasm. FIGURE 9.4 shows photomicrographs of the five major types of human leukocytes as they would appear in a stained peripheral blood smear viewed under a light microscope.

Neutrophils, eosinophils, and basophils, known collectively as *granulocytes*, have diameters of 12 to 15 μm and are distinguished by the presence of numerous cytoplasmic granules. **Neutrophils**, also known as *polymorphonuclear leukocytes* (PMN or polys), have nuclei with 2 to 5 lobes linked by fine chromatin threads. Neutrophils have small primary

Table 9.1 THE FORMED ELEMENTS OF BLOOD

Cell	Size (μm)	Number[a]
Erythrocytes	6.5–8	Males: 4.1–6$\times$10^6/μL Females: 3.9–5.5$\times$10^6/μL 4,000–10,000/μL
Leukocytes		
Neutrophils	12–15	60%–70%
Eosinophils	12–15	2%–4%
Basophils	12–15	0%–1%
Lymphocytes	6–18	20%–30%
Monocytes	12–20	3%–8%
Platelets	2–4	1.5–4.5$\times$10^5/μL

[a]Some sources give these values per cubic millimeter (mm^3). Microliters and cubic millimeters are identical units.

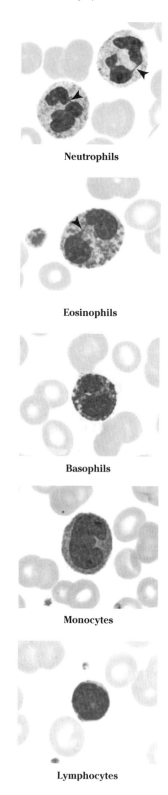

Neutrophils

Eosinophils

Basophils

Monocytes

Lymphocytes

Figure 9.4 Five types of leukocytes (white blood cells). Neutrophils, eosinophils, and basophils all have granules in their cytoplasm. These mediator-containing membrane-enclosed vesicles give these cells their collective name, granulocytes. In addition to the three types of granulocytes, the leukocyte population includes monocytes, which transform into macrophages at sites of inflammation, and lymphocytes, which circulate between the blood, peripheral tissues, and the lymphatic and lymph node system. There are tow subtypes of lymphocytes, T cells and B cells, but they cannot be differentiated from one another by light microscopy alone.

granules (also called azurophilic because they avidly take up an azure colored stain) and secondary granules (also called specific) granules that are near the limit of resolution of a light microscope. Neutrophils are the most numerous type of leukocyte, accounting for 60% to 70% of circulating white blood cells. Immature neutrophils, also known as *band forms*, have a nonsegmented C-shaped nucleus.

Far less numerous than neutrophils are eosinophils and basophils. **Eosinophils** account for 2% to 4% of leukocytes and are characterized by bilobed nuclei and numerous large granules that are bright red-orange (called eosinophilic because they bind the dye eosin) in stained smears. **Basophils** account for less than 1% of leukocytes and are characterized by irregular multilobulated nuclei that are obscured by numerous large blue granules (called basophilic because they stain with basic dyes).

The white blood cells without cytoplasmic granules are the monocytes and lymphocytes, also known as *mononuclear leukocytes* (because their nuclei are not lobed). **Monocytes** are large cells, 12 to 20 μm diameter, with a kidney-shaped nucleus; they are the precursors of **macrophages** in peripheral tissues. Some cells that appear similar to monocytes under light microscopy develop into **mast cells** when they enter tissues such as the skin and gastrointestinal (GI) tract. **Lymphocytes** are smaller cells approximately the size of an erythrocyte; they are characterized by a spherical nucleus that stains darkly and is surrounded by a very thin rim of cytoplasm. Lymphocytes can become significantly larger when they are activated. The different subclasses of lymphocytes, including **B cells** and **T cells,** are described in Chapter 11.

Platelets are small anucleate cell fragments with a diameter of 2 to 4 μm. There are 150,000 to 450,000 per μL in normal blood, making them more numerous than leukocytes but less numerous than erythrocytes. They are essentially membrane-enclosed sacs of cytoplasm that pinch off from large cells called **megakaryocytes**, which remain in the bone marrow. Platelets have numerous granules. Their role in controlling bleeding is described in Chapter 10.

Blood Molecules

Plasma contains over 100 different proteins, as well as numerous other molecules. TABLE 9.2 lists the major molecular constituents of plasma. The proteins in plasma can be separated using a technique known as **protein electrophoresis**, in which proteins exposed to an electrical field move through a solid gel based on their size and charge. Different proteins are distinguished by their respective mobility in the gel.

Electrophoresis separates plasma proteins into albumin and several groups of globulins termed α-, β-, and γ-globulin. **Albumin** is the principal plasma

Table 9.2 THE MOLECULAR CONSTITUENTS OF PLASMA

Proteins (gm/dL)	6.0–8.0
Albumin (g/dL)	3.4–5.0
Total globulin (g/dL)	2.2–4.0
Transferrin (mg/dL)	250
Haptoglobulin (mg/dL)	30–205
Hemopexin (mg/dL)	50–100
Ceruloplasmin (mg/dL)	25–45
Ferritin (μg/L)	15–300
Nonproteins	
Cholesterol (mg/dL)	140–250
Glucose (mg/dL)	70–110
Urea nitrogen (mg/dL)	6–23
Uric acid (mg/dL)	4.1–85
Creatinine (mg/dL)	0.7–1.4
Iron (μg/dL)	50–150

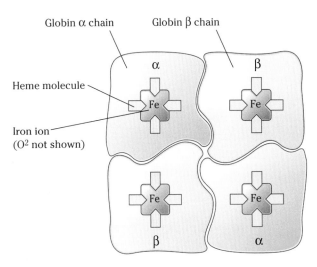

Figure 9.5 The structure of hemoglobin. Hemoglobin, the main oxygen-carrying molecule in erythrocytes, is composed of four protein chains: two α chains and two β chains. Each chain wraps around a heme molecule. Each heme molecule has a central coordinated iron atom (Fe), critical to binding molecular oxygen (not shown). Since each Fe atom can bind one O_2 molecule, a single molecule of hemoglobin can bind four molecules of O_2.

protein, and at a concentration of 3.4 to 5.0 g/dL, it accounts for nearly two thirds of total plasma protein mass. Total **globulin** accounts for 2.2 to 4.0 g/dL of plasma protein. The total plasma protein concentration normal range is approximately 6.0 to 8.0 g/dL. The functions of a number of these proteins as carriers, clotting factors, immunoproteins, hormones, or enzymes are detailed in subsequent chapters.

Blood proteins can be classified into those within cells (intracellular) and those in the plasma (extracellular). The principal intracellular protein of red blood cells is **hemoglobin**, which gives them their pink color in stained peripheral blood smears. Hemoglobin is a tetrameric protein with a molecular weight of 68,000 consisting of two α and two β polypeptide chains (the "-globin" part of hemoglobin). Within each subunit is a heme moiety (the "hemo-" part of hemoglobin), a planar molecule that contains a central iron ion capable of reversibly binding a molecule of oxygen (O_2) (FIGURE 9.5). The coordination of iron into the heme moiety is responsible for the brilliant colors of blood: red when well oxygenated and bluish-purple when poorly oxygenated. The catabolism of the heme moiety when red blood cells die produces the green, brown, and black colors of bile (biliverdin, bilirubin), stool (sterocobilin), and bruises (methemoglobin). (See Clinical Application Box *Sickle Cell Anemia, a Molecular Disease of Hemoglobin.*)

Besides proteins, other molecules in plasma include cholesterol, lipids, carbohydrates, and amino acids. Other constituents are degradation products of metabolism, such as urea, uric acid, and creatinine.

Blood Small Molecules and Ions

Plasma also contains dissolved electrolytes as well as molecular oxygen (O_2), nitrogen, and carbon dioxide. TABLE 9.3 lists the major ionic constituents of plasma. The major cations are sodium (134–146 mEq/L) and potassium (3.5–5.0 mEq/L), and the major anions are chloride (92–109 mEq/L) and bicarbonate

Table 9.3 IONIC CONSTITUENTS OF PLASMA

Cations	
Sodium (mEq/L)	134–146
Potassium (mEq/L)	3.5–5.0
Calcium (mg/dL)	8.0–10.4
Magnesium (mg/dL)	1.6–3.0
Hydrogen (pH)	7.36–7.44
Anions	
Chloride (mEq/L)	92–109
Bicarbonate (mEq/L)	24–31
Lactate (mEq/L)	1.0–1.8
Sulfate (mEq/L)	1.0
Phosphate (mg/dL)	2.6–4.6

SICKLE CELL ANEMIA, A MOLECULAR DISEASE OF HEMOGLOBIN

A number of important inherited diseases affect the genes that encode the protein chains of hemoglobin. Each person normally has two genes encoding the hemoglobin β chain (one inherited from the father and one from the mother) and four genes encoding the hemoglobin α chain (two from each parent). Perhaps the most famous of the genetic anomalies of hemoglobin is **sickle cell anemia**. In this disease, a mutation in the gene for the hemoglobin β chain produces a protein with a valine instead of the normal glutamate at the sixth amino acid position. Hemoglobin composed of this mutant β chain is called hemoglobin S (HbS) as opposed to normal adult hemoglobin (HbA).

Patients with one mutated β gene and one normal β gene (heterozygotes) have sickle cell *trait*, while those with two mutant β genes (homozygotes) have sickle cell *disease*. The small change in the β chain amino acid sequence allows deoxygenated HbS to polymerize and precipitate, deforming erythrocytes from their biconcave shape into curved (or sickle-shaped) cells. Such cells may break apart (hemolysis) or stick to capillary walls and each other, obstructing the flow of blood (vaso-occlusion).

The manifestations of sickle cell disease include attacks of anemia, heart and kidney damage, joint pains, and even death. Although sickle cell trait is not as dangerous, it puts the patient at increased risk of heart and kidney disease.

The mutant β chain gene is not uncommon, especially in people of African American descent: 8.6% of African Americans in the United States are heterozygotes for HbS, while 0.14% are homozygotes. Why would natural selection maintain such a potentially damaging gene? Interestingly, sickle cell trait protects the individual from the disease malaria, in which an invading parasite hides from the immune system by residing inside erythrocytes. A single mutant β chain produces enough HbS to make the red cell interior less hospitable to the malaria parasite, but generally not enough to produce full-blown sickle cell disease. Thus, natural selection favors the sickle cell trait in areas endemic for malaria, such as Africa, explaining the persistence of the gene in these populations.

(24–31 mEq/L). Determining the concentrations of these four plasma electrolytes ("chemistries") is among the most common laboratory tests ordered for patients.

SYSTEM FUNCTION

As detailed in the introduction, blood functions include the absorption and delivery of oxygen and nutrients, the removal of metabolic wastes, the movement of communication molecules between or among cells, body defense, and thermoregulation. Different functions are carried out by distinct blood structures of different scale. For example, as described below, hemoglobin absorbs oxygen in the lungs, while erythrocytes are the cellular containers that transport most of the body's hemoglobin molecules to tissues and prevent them from being lost by filtration at the kidney. The focus of this section is the physiology of erythrocytes. Other functions of blood are described in subsequent chapters.

Blood Ions

The ionic constituents of plasma are essential for providing a milieu compatible with cell function. They are important in determining plasma osmolality, which is approximately 280 to 290 mOsm/kg, and ionic electrochemical gradients across cell membranes (as described in Part I). The hydrogen ion concentration, reflected by the blood pH, is buffered to keep it in the narrow range of 7.36 to 7.44, which is critical for cellular physiology. The acid-base balance is maintained principally by the bicarbonate buffering system, although phosphates contribute as well.

Blood Molecules

The various proteins in blood perform many specialized functions. The function of hemoglobin is to carry oxygen from the alveoli of the lungs to the capillaries of tissues for aerobic respiration. Part V describes the details of gas exchange in the lungs and oxygen transport to the periphery. In pulmonary capillaries, the partial pressure of oxygen (or *oxygen ten-*

sion) is high, and each molecule of hemoglobin binds four oxygen molecules (one O_2 for each of the four heme units). In peripheral tissue capillaries, oxygen tension is low, and the oxygen is released from hemoglobin and diffuses into tissue cells.

The numerous intracellular proteins of white blood cells perform many functions, in contrast to the relative simplicity of red blood cells. TABLE 9.4 lists some of the proteins and enzymes within the granules of leukocytes. These include mediators of

Table 9.4 LEUKOCYTE GRANULE CONTENTS

Cells	Specific Granules	Azurophilic Granules
Neutrophils	Alkaline phosphatase	Acid phosphatase
	Collagenase	α-Mannosidase
	Lactoferrin	Arylsulfatase
	Lysozyme	β-Galactosidase
		β-Glucuronidase
		Cathepsin
		5′ Nucleotidase
		Elastase
		Collagenase
		Myeloperoxidase
		Lysozyme
		Acidic mucosubstances
		Cationic antibacterial proteins
Eosinophils	Acid phosphatase	
	Arylsulfatase	
	β-Glucuronidase	
	Cathepsin	
	Phospholipase	
	RNAse	
	Eosinophilic peroxidase	
	Major basic protein	
Basophils	Eosinophilic chemotactic factor	
	Heparin	
	Histamine	
	Peroxidase	

microbial killing and inflammation, which are described in more detail in Chapter 11. Briefly, the killing of invading microbes can be accomplished by several strategies, including enzymatic damage, oxidative damage, and the sequestration of essential nutrients. *Lysozyme* damages bacterial cell walls, *elastase* and *collagenase* degrade connective tissue (allowing antimicrobial cells and molecules to get access to invaders), *nucleotidase* degrades nucleic acids (destroying the DNA and RNA of microbial invaders), and *mannosidase* and *galactosidase* degrade carbohydrates critical to the function of some microbial glycoprotiens. Oxidative enzymes such as *myeloperoxidase* cause a "respiratory burst" that leads to the formation of chemically reactive and highly destructive compounds such as hydrogen peroxide, superoxide, hydroxyl radicals, and hypochlorite radicals. *Lactoferrin* is a protein that sequesters iron, a nutrient essential for bacterial metabolism.

Plasma proteins can be divided functionally into several groups by function: carrier proteins, clotting proteins, immunoproteins, hormones, and enzymes. Albumin is the major source of intravascular oncotic pressure since it cannot diffuse out of the vessels into the interstitial space (described further in Chapter 10). Albumin also binds and transports many compounds such as drugs, bilirubin, and fatty acids. Other binding and carrier proteins include **transferrin** for iron transport, **ferritin** for iron storage, *ceruloplasmin* for copper transport, *haptoglobin* for binding hemoglobin, *hemopexin* for binding free heme, *transcobalamin* for transporting cobalamin (vitamin B_{12}), specific hormone binding proteins, and **apolipoproteins** for cholesterol and lipid transport. Clotting proteins include **clotting factors** and control enzymes that lead to the formation of fibrin plugs to control bleeding (described further in Chapter 10). Immunoproteins include **complement proteins** and **antibodies** (also known as **immunoglobulins**) that constitute the large γ-globulin spike in protein electrophoresis (described further in Chapter 11). In addition, numerous specific hormones, enzymes, and enzyme inhibitors circulate in the plasma. In particularly high concentration are α_1-*antitrypsin* and α_2-*macroglobulin*, which are important in deactivating the potentially destructive proteases liberated by neutrophils and other leukocytes in response to microbial invaders. These protease inhibitors thus prevent excessive damage to the healthy cells and tissues of the body during the fight against infection.

Blood Cells and Organelles

The functions of the cells in blood are based on their major protein components. Erythrocytes, with limited organelles and packed with hemoglobin, are the oxygen-carrying cells of the blood. Under normal circumstances, they arise from precursor cells in bone marrow, live about 120 days, never leave the circulation, and are degraded by the reticuloendothelial systems of the spleen and liver. They pick up oxygen from the lung and deliver it to all tissues engaging in aerobic metabolism.

Leukocytes have a complex role and perform multiple functions in the inflammatory and immune responses (see Chapter 11). They travel in the blood but can exit the vasculature to enter tissues to fight invaders. Neutrophils live only about 6 to 8 hours in the blood and travel to sites of acute inflammation, constituting a principal defense against bacteria. They engulf (phagocytose) bacteria and kill them by fusing the phagosome (the intracellular, membrane-enclosed vesicle containing the engulfed invader) with lysosomes and specific granules, thus delivering destructive enzymes and toxic proteins directly to the phagocytosed material. This system restricts the pathogenic invader and the antimicrobial molecules to a small intracellular space, preventing damage to healthy cells and keeping the concentrations of enzymes and toxins high. Neutrophils also liberate the contents of azurophilic granules into their environments, thus damaging extracellular bacteria and host tissues by oxidative species and specific enzymes. Eosinophils have a high concentration of arginine-rich *major basic protein*, which gives them their characteristic staining pattern and, when released into the extracellular space, their effectiveness in defense against parasites. Basophils have numerous granules containing histamine and other mediators of inflammation and allergic immune responses. Monocytes exit the vasculature and develop into tissue macrophages that are particularly suited to phagocytosis of foreign bodies and invading pathogens. Mast cell precursors also exit the vasculature to complete their maturation in tissues, where these cells are packed with granules. Mast cells are important in allergic reactions and host defense. Lymphocytes generate and maintain specific (also called adaptive) immune responses against particular pathogens.

Platelets control bleeding when blood vessel integrity is breached. This process, termed hemostasis, is essential to preventing excessive bleeding (see Chapter 10). Platelets adhere to areas of denuded endothelium and release their granule contents, which causes platelet aggregation as well as activation of the coagulation system.

Blood Tissues

Bone marrow is the site of **hematopoiesis**, the production of new blood cells. *Pluripotent stem cells* are undifferentiated bone marrow cells that can divide and whose progeny can develop into all cell lineages. FIGURE 9.6 shows the basic steps of hematopoiesis. Erythroid precursors develop into erythrocytes, myeloid precursors develop into granulocytes and monocytes, lymphoid precursors develop into lymphocytes, and megakaryocytes produce platelets. These processes are tightly regulated by a large number of control proteins called *growth factors* and *cytokines* that are produced according to the body's need for these cells. For example, *thrombopoietin* is a hormone growth factor that increases the production of platelets by megakaryocytes. One of the best characterized of these maturation factors is **erythropoietin**, a hormone produced by the kidneys. Because the renal medulla operates at low oxygen tension and participates in the filtration of the blood, it is an excellent tissue for sensing and regulating the oxygen-carrying capacity of the blood. Since most of the oxygen carried by blood is bound to hemoglobin inside erythrocytes, the production of red blood cells is the logical variable for the kidneys to control in order to affect the oxygen concentration of the blood. Erythropoietin released by the kidneys travels via the blood to the bone marrow, where it stimulates erythroid precursor cells to enter and continue on the red cell developmental pathway. Thus, if the kidneys sense a drop in the partial pressure of oxygen, they release more erythropoietin, which augments bone marrow production of erythrocytes, and corrects the oxygen deficiency. The increased oxygen tension is sensed by the kidneys, which subsequently decrease their release of erythropoietin, completing the negative feedback loop.

The **capillary microcirculation** is the network of interconnecting capillaries that serves a small volume of tissue. A diagram of a typical tissue microcirculation is shown in FIGURE 9.7. An incoming arteriole gives rise to small capillaries whose diameters are only slightly larger than an erythrocyte (10 μm). Blood flow into the capillary bed can be greatly affected by contraction or dilitation of *precapillary sphincters*, which respond to the metabolic needs of the tissues as well as to neural and hormonal mediators. The exchange of nutrients, wastes, gases, and fluid occurs in the tiny tissue capillaries. **Metarterioles** are slightly larger vessels that arise from arterioles and then branch into capillaries. Capillaries then drain into a **venule** that returns the blood to the venous system. Occasionally, an *arteriovenous shunt* brings some arterial blood directly into the venous system, bypassing the capillary bed.

Variations on this general picture of microcirculation occur in each organ system. The alveolar capillaries of the lungs, the glomerular and peritubular capillary systems of the kidneys, the portal capillaries draining the GI tract, the myocardial capillaries of the heart, the vasa vasorum of arterial walls, the vasa

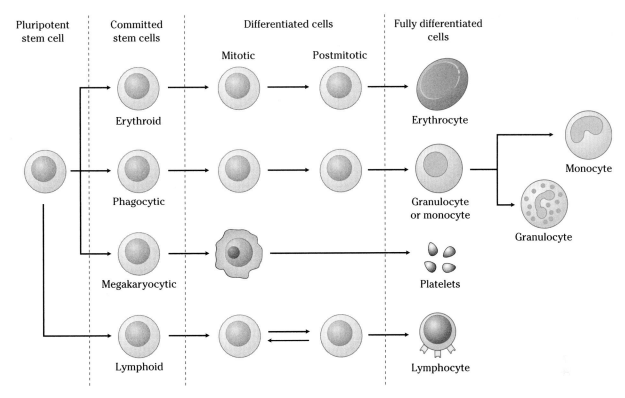

Figure 9.6 The process of hematopoiesis. Pluripotent stem cells in the bone marrow divide by mitosis and give rise to progeny that commit to one of four basic developmental pathways. The erythroid pathway results in red blood cells. The phagocytic pathway produces monocytes that mature further into macrophages, granulocytes (neutrophils, eosinophils, or basophils), or mast cells. Stem cells that enter the megakaryocytic pathway remain in the bone marrow, while fragments of their cytoplasm pinch off as platelets that leave the marrow to circulate with other blood cells. The lymphoid pathway leads to the production of T cells and B cells.

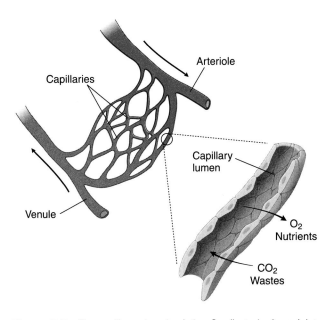

Figure 9.7 The capillary microcirculation. Small arteries branch into arterioles that have smooth muscle and sphincters that control the flow of blood. Capillaries, blood vessels with walls only one cell thick, constitute a three-dimensional net, carrying nutrients into and wastes out of tissues. Eventually, blood that travels through capillaries rejoin to bring the blood into the venous circulation, where it can travel back toward the heart and lungs to be reoxygenated and then recirculated.

nervosum of large nerves, and the tissue capillaries of muscle and skin all have their own distinguishing features, described in their respective chapters.

PATHOPHYSIOLOGY

The large number of constituents in the blood, each with their own distinctive functions, makes the pathophysiology of the blood very complex. Essentially, there can be quantitative or qualitative problems with any of the formed elements or plasma proteins, or distributive problems in circulating these cells and proteins to the appropriate tissues.

Quantitative problems can involve dysfunction in the production or destruction of any of the cells in the blood. Some common abnormalities are blood cell deficiencies. **Anemia** is a decrease in the concentration of erythrocytes, **leukopenia** is a decrease in the concentration of leukocytes, **thrombocytopenia** is a decrease in the concentration of platelets, and **pancytopenia** is a decrease in the concentrations of all cell lineages. Such decreases in the concentration of one or more cell lineages may be due to low cell numbers, as when cells are not produced rapidly enough to keep up with their loss or destruction. This may occur in three settings: a decreased rate of blood cell production by bone marrow when the life spans of blood cells are normal, an increased rate of blood cell loss and/or destruction when the rate of blood cell production is normal, and a combination of these. Pathologic decreases in the concentration of a cell lineage may also occur by means of *hemodilution*, as when a patient receives large volumes of cell-free intravenous fluid.

Other pathologic conditions are marked by abnormally high concentrations of formed elements. **Polycythemia** is an increase in the concentration of erythrocytes; **leukocytosis** is an increase in the concentration of leukocytes; and **thrombocytosis** is an increase in the concentration of platelets. Problems with excessive concentrations of formed elements are often the result of overproduction (in which case the total cell number is elevated), though they may be seen in conditions where a patient has lost a significant volume of vascular fluid without losing formed elements.

Qualitative problems involve the dysfunction of formed elements or plasma constituents. Distributive problems involve the scope of occlusive **vascular disease**, in which blood cells function adequately but are unable to reach the capillary microcirculation of a tissue or organ.

Pathology of the blood is manifested by an impairment of the essential functions described in this chapter, such as the delivery of oxygen and nutrients, the removal of waste products, adequate defense, and effective homeostasis. In quantitative or qualitative problems, consequences of this pathology often affect many organ systems. Because red blood cells are the major carriers of oxygen-carrying hemoglobin, anemia leads to pallor (a loss of color in the skin and mucous membranes resulting from decrease concentrations of the pigmented hemoglobin) and lethargy. Anemia may even precipitate damage to the heart and brain due to inadequate oxygen delivery (*ischemia*). Because white blood cells are essential to fighting invaders, leukopenia may lead to recurrent infections. Thrombocytopenia may lead to excessive bleeding secondary to inadequate blood clotting. Pathologically increased concentrations of formed elements may cause distributive problems as blood vessels are obstructed by clumps of red or white cells. Thrombocytosis commonly leads to vascular occlusion secondary to inappropriate blood clotting. In distributive problems, consequences of oxygen and nutrient deprivation, combined with the buildup of metabolic wastes, are localized to a particular organ and often lead to cell death known as *necrosis*. For example, coronary artery occlusion leads to myocardial infarction, and cerebral artery occlusion results in a stroke.

Iron Deficiency Anemia

Iron deficiency anemia is an extremely common pathological condition caused by a decrease in iron stores. Recall that iron is a component of the heme moiety in hemoglobin and directly binds oxygen. Iron deficiency can arise from insufficient dietary intake, impaired absorption, or an excessive loss of iron. Adult males require about 1 mg of iron per day to maintain iron stores in the face of obligate losses from the GI tract and skin. Rapidly growing children, menstruating women, and pregnant women require significantly more dietary iron. The impaired absorption of dietary iron, known as malabsorption, can occur with a variety of GI diseases. Excessive loss of iron can occur with any condition that causes bleeding, such as from the upper (esophagus, stomach, duodenum) or lower (colon) GI tract, the uterus (during menstruation), and trauma. Normally, senescent red blood cells are degraded by macrophages in the reticuloendothelial system of the liver and spleen, and their iron is recycled by complexing it with transferrin or ferritin. However, if blood cells exit the body, the lost iron must be replenished by the diet to avoid iron deficiency.

A deficiency of iron stores leads to an inability to incorporate sufficient iron into heme, and thus an inadequate production of functional hemoglobin. The hematocrit is low (anemia), and red blood cells are pale in appearance (hypochromic) and smaller in size (microcytic), resulting in a **hypochromic microcytic anemia**. The size of the red blood cells is measured in hospital laboratories and expressed at the *mean corpuscular volume (MCV)*, and the appearance and shapes are determined by examining a peripheral smear under the microscope. As shown in FIGURE 9.8, erythrocytes in iron deficiency anemia are small and irregularly shaped, with a narrow rim of cytoplasm and a large area of central pallor, indicating an insufficient quantity of hemoglobin. Compare the appearance of these erythrocytes with the normal ones in Figure 9.2.

The erythrocytes in iron deficiency anemia have a lower-than-normal oxygen carrying capacity. There is also laboratory evidence of decreased iron levels in the blood, decreased ferritin reflecting decreased iron stores, and increased transferrin. The transferrin concentration is also called the *total iron binding capacity (TIBC)* and its elevation in iron deficiency anemia reflects the body's attempt to mobilize as much iron as possible. An associated value is the percentage of transferrin saturation, calculated by dividing the concentration of serum iron by the concentration of transferrin. Normally the percentage saturation is 20% to 50%, but because the serum iron is low and the transferrin is high in iron defi-

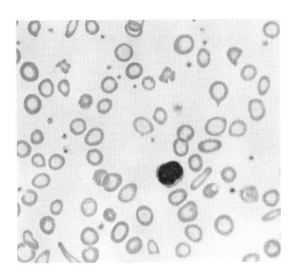

Figure 9.8 A peripheral blood smear of iron deficiency anemia. Note that the erythrocytes in this smear are small (microcytic) and have greater central pallor (hypochromic) because they contain less hemoglobin than normal red blood cells.

ciency anemia, the percentage saturation is typically well below 20% in this disease.

The clinical manifestations of iron deficiency anemia reflect the function of the defective red blood cells. Because their erythrocytes are unable to deliver adequate quantities of oxygen to tissues for cellular respiration, patients complain of weakness, fatigue, and lethargy. They appear pale and can even show signs of respiratory, cardiac, renal, or neurologic dysfunction if the anemia is severe. Other clinical signs that are more difficult to explain involve the effects of iron deficiency on the skin, nails, and mucosa, leading to dermal atrophy, brittle nails that have lost their normal convexity and have become "spooned" (*koilonychia*), and a smooth, sore tongue (*glossitis*). Another peculiar effect occasionally seen with iron deficiency anemia is known as *pica*, the desire to eat ice, dirt, and other nonnutritional substances.

Anemia of Chronic Renal Failure

Erythroid precursor cells in the bone marrow depend on erythropoietin for their growth and development into functional, mature red blood cells. But what if the kidneys are severely damaged, as in the **chronic renal failure** resulting from long-standing diabetes or hypertension (high blood pressure)? In such cases, the production of erythropoietin is greatly impaired, and anemia results from the subsequent deficiency. The mass production of recombinant human erythropoietin, which can be administered to patients with anemia due to low erythropoietin concentrations, has revolutionized the treatment of this type of anemia, correcting the hematocrit and often dramatically improving the symptoms of anemia in such patients.

Summary

- The overall function of the blood is to transport substances and cells from one organ to another, thus allowing the specialization of function of the different organ systems.

- Oxygen and nutrients are brought to cells while metabolic wastes are removed, maintaining tissue metabolism and respiration.

- **Hematopoetic stem cells** in **bone marrow** give rise to all blood cells.

- The blood transports the cells needed to provide defense from trauma and infection. **Erythrocytes** are the red blood cells that carry **hemoglobin** to transport oxygen. **Leukocytes** are the white blood cells that fight microbial invaders. **Platelets** are the anucleate cell fragments of **megakaryocytes** that are involved in blood clotting.

- Among the leukocytes are the granulocytes (neutrophils, eosinophils, and basophils), monocytes, and lymphocytes (T cells and B cells).

- Blood gases are exchanged at the lungs and the peripheral tissues, dietary nutrients are absorbed at the GI tract and delivered to tissues, and metabolic wastes are taken from peripheral tissues and removed by the lungs and kidneys.

- Blood transports hormones and other mediators throughout the body. Many such hormones are bound to carrier proteins such as **albumin**.

- The hormone **erythropoietin** is produced by kidney cells and stimulates the production of erythrocytes by the bone marrow. Other *cytokines* and *growth factors* expedite the maturation of megakaryocytes and the various white blood cells.

- The blood supply is essential for the viability of each individual organ as well as for the communication, homeostasis, and integration of the individual tissues and systems into a whole organism.

- Disorders of blood cells may be quantitative or qualitative. In quantitative disorders, the concentration of one or more cell lineages is too high or too low. In qualitative disorders, the concentration of a cell lineage is within the normal limits, but the cells are unable to perform one or more functions.

- **Anemia** is a pathologic decrease in the concentration of erythrocytes. **Leukopenia** is a pathologic decrease in the concentration of leukocytes. **Thrombocytopenia** is a pathologic decrease in the concentration of platelets.

- In **iron deficiency anemia**, a **hypochromic microcytic anemia** is observed. Symptoms relate primarily to impaired delivery of oxygen to tissues. In chronic renal failure, decreased production of erythropoietin leads to anemia that can be treated with injections of recombinant human erythropoietin.

Suggested Reading

Goodnight SH, Feinstein DI. Update in hematology. Ann Intern Med. 1998;128(7):545–551.

Weiss G, Goodnough LT. Anemia of chronic disease. N Engl J Med. 2005;352(10):1011–1023.

REVIEW QUESTIONS

Directions: Each of the numbered items or incomplete statements in this section is followed by answers or by completions of the statement. Select the ONE lettered answer or completion that is BEST in each case.

1. Which of the following type of blood cells does not normally leave the bone marrow?
   (A) Red blood cells (erythrocytes)
   (B) Neutrophils (polymorphonuclear cells or PMNs)
   (C) Lymphocytes (T cells and B cells)
   (D) Megakaryocytes
   (E) Basophils

2. Which of the following blood cells does NOT have granules?
   (A) Platelets
   (B) Erythrocytes
   (C) Neutrophils
   (D) Eosinophils
   (E) Basophils

3. An 84-year-old woman with a history of poorly controlled hypertension for the last 30 years and one heart attack has smoked one pack of cigarettes per day since she was 20 years old. She

has felt tired and "washed out" in the past year. Four months ago, she was told she might need to start dialysis soon. On physical exam, her skin and mucus membranes are pale. She has a hematocrit of 24%. Which of the following is a likely component for her anemia?

(A) Lung disease from smoking impairing the uptake of oxygen by her red blood cells

(B) Kidney disease from high blood pressure reducing the production of erythropoietin

(C) Heart disease from high blood pressure and the heart attack impairing her ability to pump blood through her arteries and veins

(D) Bone marrow disease from her age, reducing the production of erythrocytes

(E) Autoimmune disease, in which her own immune system mistakenly destroys her red blood cells

4. Which of the following patients would be expected to have a TIBC and percentage transferrin saturation in the normal range?

(A) An 80-year-old man with colon cancer that causes lower (colonic) gastrointestinal bleeding

(B) A 28-year-old woman, pregnant with twins, who hates taking prenatal vitamins

(C) A 29-year-old woman nursing the twins recently born via Caesarian section with significant blood loss during the procedure

(D) A 32-year-old woman with heavy periods that last 8 to 10 days for the last year

(E) A 64-year-old man with a hematocrit of 18 after being given large amounts of intravenous fluid in the emergency room because of low blood pressure and significant blood loss from trauma in a motor vehicle accident

ANSWERS TO REVIEW QUESTIONS

1. **The answer is D.** Megakaryocytes are large cells that normally remain in the bone marrow. Small volumes of their cytoplasm pinch off as membrane-enclosed, anucleate fragments called platelets, which do escape the marrow and circulate in the blood where they play critical roles in blood clotting (hemostasis). Erythrocytes, neutrophils, lymphocytes, and basophils all circulate in the blood after leaving the marrow.

2. **The answer is B.** Unlike platelets, neutrophils, eosinophils, and basophils, all of which have intracytoplasmic, membrane-enclosed vesicles containing important mediators such as enzymes and chemicals important in blood clotting (coagulation) or host defense (immunity), mature erythrocytes are mostly bags of hemoglobin and do not have granules.

3. **The answer is B.** This patient with long-standing hypertension has been told that she may soon need dialysis because she very likely has significant kidney disease. Severe damage to the kidneys reduces the production of erythropoietin, the hormone that stimulates the bone marrow to make red blood cells. If she had lung disease severe enough to impair the uptake of oxygen by her red blood cells, normal kidneys would detect this and increase their production of erythropoietin, resulting in an increase in the hematocrit, a condition known as polycythemia, which is essentially the opposite of anemia. Heart disease and age alone would not on their own produce anemia. Autoimmune destruction of red blood cells certainly occurs, but it is a separate disease from the kidney failure that she has. Replacing erythropoietin during dialysis may significantly improve the anemia.

4. **The answer is E.** The patient who suffered the traumatic accident likely has a low hematocrit because of acute blood loss and dilution of the remaining red cells by the intravenous fluids. Given the recent onset of his anemia and its mechanism, he probably has a low to normal transferrin and, because he has lost both transferrin and serum iron (and both have been diluted), he probably has a normal transferrin saturation. The more chronic blood loss of the patient with colon cancer, the woman with heavy menstruation, and the increased demands for serum iron owing to pregnancy and breast feeding are likely to result in iron deficiency anemia, characterized by increased transferrin (and therefore increased TIBC) and a low percentage iron saturation of transferrin.

10

Endothelial Function and Hemostasis

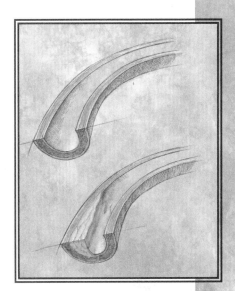

INTRODUCTION

This chapter describes the system that helps regulate the flow of blood and is essential in stopping the loss of blood from damaged vessels. Three components make up this system: the endothelium, platelets, and the proteins of the coagulation cascade. The **endothelium** is the single-cell-thick lining of the inner surface of all blood vessels. Endothelial cells, however, play far more than simply a structural role as a container for the cardiovascular system. They have a wide array of regulatory functions, including a primary role as the interface between blood and extravascular tissues. The physiologic response to endothelial disruption is known as hemostasis, and it involves the function of platelets and the coagulation system.

SYSTEM STRUCTURE

The regulation of blood flow through a vessel depends on cells in three interrelated structures: the walls of blood vessels, the lining of blood vessels, and some of the components of blood itself. Contraction of smooth muscle in the walls of blood vessels decreases blood flow, while smooth muscle relaxation increases blood flow (see Chapter 7). We describe two other cell types, the endothelium (which lines the walls of blood vessels) and platelets (which circulate in blood), below.

Endothelial Cells and Platelets

To understand the structure and function of endothelial cells in context, this section opens with a description of the vessel wall, including the endothelium. Unlike the relatively fixed endothelial cells, platelets circulate in blood under normal conditions. Both cell types have vesicles containing substances important in hemostasis.

The Vessel Wall and Endothelium   The walls of large blood vessels contain three layers, as shown in FIGURE 10.1. The inner layer, the **tunica intima**, consists of a single layer of endothelial cells and a small quantity of subendothelial connective tissue. An *internal elastic lamina* consisting of the connective tissue molecule elastin separates the tunica intima from the **tunica media**, which is composed of bundles of smooth muscle cells. The outer layer, the **tunica adventitia**, consists of collagenous and elastic connective tissue.

The walls of capillaries, in contrast, have a greatly simplified structure consisting of only a single endothelial cell. FIGURE 10.2 is an electron micrograph of the wall of a renal capillary. Note that only a thin rim of cytoplasm bordered by the endothelial cell

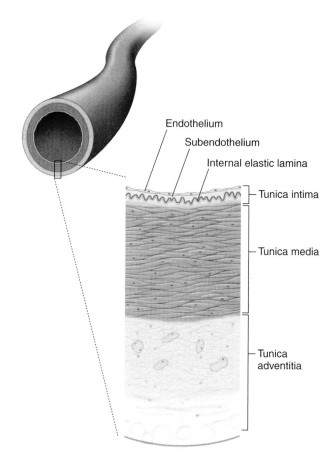

Figure 10.1   Layers of the wall of a large blood vessel. Note especially the endothelial lining, the subendothelial layer composed largely of collagen, and the smooth muscle layers of the tunica media.

membranes separates the intravascular space from the extravascular tissue interstitial space.

Endothelial cells generally are polygonal cells rolled into tubes, with the cell nucleus bulging into the capillary lumen. The total surface area of the

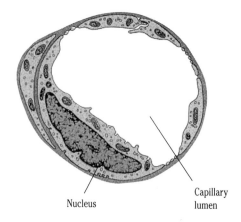

Figure 10.2   An electron micrograph of capillary endothelium. Capillaries are the smallest blood vessels, composed of a single-cell-thick layer of endothelium situated on a subendothelial basement membrane. Note the nucleus of the endothelial cell, bulging into the lumen of the capillary.

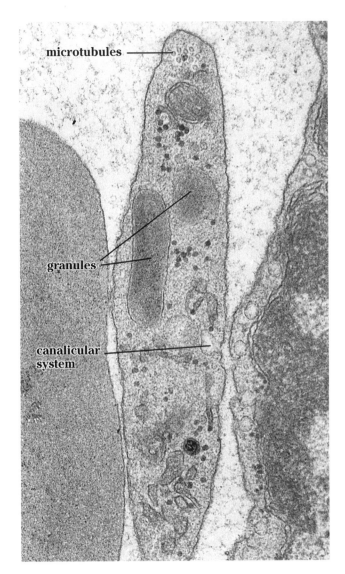

microtubules

granules

canalicular system

Figure 10.3 An electron micrograph of a platelet. Note the numerous granules of differing electron density, the microtubules, and the lack of a nucleus.

endothelium is massive, approximately 700 square meters. Endothelial cells have numerous vesicles known as **Weibel-Palade bodies** containing a protein called von Willebrand factor. Endothelial cells are held together by junctional complexes consisting of *zonulae occludentes* and some *gap junctions*.

Platelets Platelets are small anucleate cell fragments approximately one fourth the diameter of a red blood cell (FIGURE 10.3). They arise from megakaryocytes in the bone marrow. A rim of microtubules is present around the edges, maintaining the shape of the platelet. Numerous granules are present, including α granules, dense (δ) granules, and *lysosomes*. The α granules are slightly larger than the δ granules. Platelets also contain a canalicular system, a series of tubules thought to be important in platelet degranulation.

Endothelial and Hemostatic Molecules

A number of molecules are central to the control of blood flow. They may be part of the vessel wall (e.g., elastin and collagen), present on the surface of endothelial cells or platelets, or floating freely in the plasma. Others are stored in the granules of endothelial cells or platelets and are released in the process of hemostasis.

Endothelial Molecules Endothelial cells produce a large number of mediators that regulate several key biological processes (TABLE 10.1). Among these are substances that control the coagulation system. **Anticoagulant (antithrombotic) molecules** (molecules that inhibit blood clotting) include *prostacyclin (prostaglandin I₂)*, *thrombomodulin, ADPase, plasminogen activator*, and *heparin*. Endothelial derived **procoagulant (prothrombotic) molecules** (molecules that promote blood clotting) include *von Willebrand factor (vWF)* (stored in Weibel-Palade bodies), *platelet activating factor, tissue factor*, and *plasminogen activator inhibitor*.

Table 10.1 ENDOTHELIAL MOLECULES

Anticoagulant/ Antithrombotic Molecules	Procoagulant/ Prothrombotic Molecules
Prostacyclin	von Willebrand factor (vWF)
Thrombomodulin	Platelet activating factor
ADPase	Plasminogen activating inhibitor
Plasminogen activator	
Heparin and related molecules	
Vasoconstrictors	*Vasodilators*
Antiotensin II	Nitric oxide
Endothelin I	Prostacyclin
Selected prostaglandins	
Adhesion Molecules	
Selectins	
Integrins	
Immunoglobulin superfamily molecules	
Stimulatory Growth Factors	*Inhibitory Growth Factors*
Platelet-derived growth factor (PGDF)	Transforming growth factor (TGF)
Fibroblast growth factor (FGF)	

Endothelial cells also produce molecules that regulate vascular reactivity. **Vasoconstrictors** include *angiotensin II, endothelin-1,* and certain *prostaglandins.* **Vasodilators** include *nitric oxide (NO)* as well as prostacyclin. In response to inflammatory stimuli, endothelial cells express on their surface **adhesion molecules,** which bind to leukocytes traveling in the vessel lumen. They also produce mediators called *growth factors,* which can either promote or inhibit the growth and differentiation of other cells.

Thus, the endothelium can make multiple opposing mediators involved in the anticoagulant-procoagulant, vasoconstriction-vasodilation, adhesive-nonadhesive, and growth stimulation-inhibition systems. The physiologic antagonism achieved by these mediators enables the endothelium to achieve exquisite control of the balance set points and to manipulate these balances in adapting or responding to stimuli.

Platelet Molecules   Platelets have a number of cell-surface glycoprotein adhesion molecules called **integrins.** Platelet granule contents, listed in TABLE 10.2, contain numerous vasoactive and procoagulant agents.

Plasma Molecules   Plasma **clotting factors** are the central players in the coagulation cascade (TABLE 10.3). They are all synthesized in the liver, except for a portion of factor VIII, which is synthesized in endothelial cells and megakaryocytes. Many of the

Table 10.3 BLOOD CLOTTING FACTORS

Roman Numeral	Common Name(s)	Activated or Altered State
I	Fibrinogen	Fibrin
II	Prothrombin	Thrombin
III	Tissue thromboplastin; tissue factor	
IV	Calcium ions	
V	Proaccelerin	Altered proaccelerin (Va)
VII		VIIa
VIII		VIIIa
IX	Christmas factor	IXa
X	Stuart factor	Xa
XI	Plasma thromboplastin antecedent	XIa
XII	Hageman factor	XIIa
XIII	Fibrin-stabilizing factor	XIIIa
	Plasma prekallikrein	
	High-molecular-weight kininogen (HMWK)	

Table 10.2 CONTENTS OF PLATELET GRANULES

Dense Granules

Adenosine diphosphate (ADP)

Serotonin

Calcium

α-Granules

Clotting factors (fibrinogen, factor V, and factor VIII)

von Willebrand factor (vWF)

Thrombospondin

Platelet factor 4

β-*Thromboglobulin*

Platelet-derived growth factor (PDGF)

Lysosomes

Hydrolytic enzymes active at low pH

clotting factors are proenzymes that are activated by a proteolytic cleavage reaction. In addition to clotting factors, plasma also contains anticoagulant proteins that keep the coagulation process under control, such as antithrombin III, protein C, protein S, and tissue factor pathway inhibitor. Factors II, VII, IX, and X, as well as protein C and protein S, are synthesized in the liver and require a unique vitamin K-dependent carboxylation reaction that converts specific glutamate residues to γ-carboxyglutamate.

Calcium

Among the many atoms and ions important in general cell function, ionic calcium (Ca^{2+}) holds a place of particularly special import in the coagulation system for two reasons. First, as in other cells, a large electrochemical gradient favors the influx of Ca^{2+} into endothelial cells and platelets, and activation of these cells depends on Ca^{2+} entry. Second, many of the enzymes in the coagulation system require Ca^{2+} to cleave their substrates.

SYSTEM FUNCTION

The regulation of the flow of blood involves preventing hemostasis when there is no danger of bleeding, causing hemostasis when there is a danger of bleeding, and controlling the passage of some blood components from the vascular space into the tissues. Hemostasis, which prevents excessive blood loss when a vessel is damaged, is the result of four interrelated processes: vasoconstriction, endothelial cell activation, platelet activation, and coagulation. Both the prevention of hemostasis and the regulation of the passage of blood components such as proteins and cells into extravascular tissues are largely under the control of the endothelium. These cells and many of the cytokines, growth factors, and plasma proteins are also involved in the repair processes that ensue after blood vessel injury.

Endothelial Molecules, Hemostatic Molecules, and Calcium

Many of the steps in the process of hemostasis occur on the molecular scale. Although Ca^{2+} is essential for many of these reactions, most of the actual functions are carried out by glycoproteins. While many important molecules are soluble mediators or endothelial cell/platelet receptors, this section focuses on the plasma molecules, many of which have enzymatic activity.

Coagulation In multicellular organisms, blood must remain a fluid suspension of cells and molecules in order to circulate and perform its many integrative functions. However, because blood is a flowing liquid, the slightest disruption of the vasculature containment system threatens the organism with exsanguination, death due to the complete loss of blood. The physiologic solution to this problem is **hemostasis**, the process of stopping blood loss when a vessel is damaged. Hemostasis involves four interrelated processes: contraction of the smooth muscle in the blood vessel wall (vasoconstriction or *vasospasm*), endothelial cell activation, the binding and activation of platelets, and **coagulation**, the conversion of blood from a liquid to a solid. Hemostasis normally occurs only under just those conditions (the right places and the right times) where blood vessels have been compromised. Hemostasis is a complex reaction, a tightly regulated physiologic system that is usually inactive but can be triggered rapidly and effectively by stimuli such as endothelial disruption. Initial molecular signals are greatly amplified by a biochemical cascade—the **clotting cascade**—to produce a rapid and effective response.

The clotting cascade is a series of biochemical reactions involving the plasma clotting factors

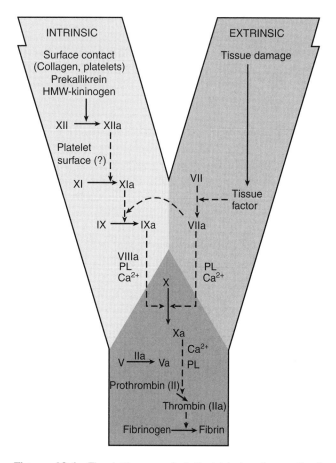

Figure 10.4   The clotting cascade. In the intrinsic pathway, stimuli such as foreign or activated platelet surfaces, high-molecular-weight kininogen, prekallikrein, or collagen, can activate factor XII. In the extrinsic pathway, thought to be the dominant one in vivo, the release of tissue factor from damaged cells initiates the cascade. Note that in either the extrinsic or the intrinsic pathway, Ca^{2+} and phospholipid surface (PL) are required cofactors for activating factor X, the first step of the common pathway, and that the same cofactors are required for the activation of factor II (prothrombin to thrombin).

(FIGURE 10.4). Many of the clotting factors have more than one name as well as a numeric designation (Roman numeral). To differentiate between the inactive proenzyme factors and those that have been proteolytically cleaved and are enzymatically active, a lowercase letter is appended to the Roman numeral. Thus, for example, prothrombin, also called factor II, is cleaved into the active enzyme thrombin, also called factor IIa.

The cascade is a series of proteolytic cleavage reactions triggered by endothelial disruption, and it culminates in the conversion of fibrinogen (factor I) into the cleavage product fibrin. Fibrin molecules polymerize, producing a fibrin plug that stops bleeding (**hemorrhage**) from a damaged blood vessel. All the coagulation factors involved circulate normally in the plasma but are inactive; they are activated by either conformational changes or limited proteolytic cleavage. Activation of the chain of events leading to coagulation can occur by two pathways, the extrinsic pathway and the intrinsic pathway, which ultimately converge to form a common pathway ending in the production of fibrin. The pathways can be likened to rows of standing dominoes. The tipping over (i.e., activating) of one piece (enzyme) initiates a chain reaction (Figure 10.4). The amplification component of the system is important. Unlike a linear system, in which one domino knocks over one domino, which knocks over one more domino, each activated coagulation cascade molecule may enzymatically cleave and activate tens, hundreds, or even thousands of substrate molecules.

Ironically, the **extrinsic pathway** is thought to be the predominant method of activating the clotting cascade *in vivo*. When tissue cells or endothelial cells are damaged, they expose the membrane-associated protein called **tissue factor (TF)**, also known as *thromboplastin*, to the circulating plasma clotting factors. It complexes with **factor VII**, and the TF/VII complex, in the presence of Ca^{2+} and a phospholipid membrane, slowly enzymatically cleaves **factor X** to its active form, Xa. Factor Xa, in turn, cleaves factor VII to VIIa, turning the TF/VIIa complex into an efficient enzyme that rapidly cleaves X to Xa, resulting in amplification of Xa production.

The **intrinsic pathway** is triggered when **factor XII**, also known as *Hageman factor* or *contact factor*, encounters a negatively charged surface, such as a site of endothelial injury with exposed subendothelial collagen, or a foreign surface such as the glass of a test tube. This surface causes factor XII to undergo a conformational change and become its active form, XIIa. Factor XIIa cleaves **factor XI** to form XIa, and XIa converts **factor IX** to IXa. In turn, IXa associates with the accessory **factor VIII**, Ca^{2+} ions, and a phospholipid surface, and converts factor X to Xa.

Both pathways converge by producing a "tenase" enzyme that converts factor X to Xa. Xa then associates with the accessory **factor V**, Ca^{2+} ions, and a phospholipid surface, and converts factor II (prothrombin) to factor IIa (thrombin), which is a highly reactive enzyme. Thrombin is the key enzyme of the clotting cascade and has a number of functions, including activating platelets, activating factors V and VIII to accelerate the cascade, converting **factor XIII** to **factor XIIIa**, and cleaving fibrinogen to fibrin. Fibrin polymerizes to form an initial clot, a meshwork of fibrin strands, which is then cross-linked and stabilized by factor XIIIa.

In summary, coagulation is initiated by the production and release of TF by damaged cells or by the activation of Hageman factor XII by a foreign surface. A cascade occurs in which factor X is activated, thereby converting prothrombin into the highly active enzyme thrombin. Thrombin cleaves soluble fibrinogen into fibrin, which aggregates and then is cross-linked to form a meshwork.

Clinically, the extrinsic pathway and the common pathway are evaluated by measuring the **prothrombin time (PT)** and the intrinsic pathway and common pathway are evaluated by measuring the **partial thromboplastin time (PTT)**. Each test measures the time it takes for clotting to occur, but in response to different triggers. If the PT is prolonged (i.e., it takes longer than normal for a clot to form) while the PTT is normal, there is a deficiency in the extrinsic pathway. If the reverse is true—the PTT is prolonged while the PT is normal—there is a defect in the intrinsic pathway. If both are prolonged, both pathways and/or the common pathway are affected.

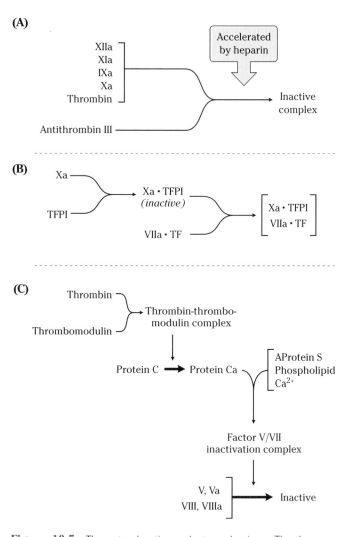

Figure 10.5 The natural anticoagulant mechanisms. The three mechanisms inhibit the clotting cascade by degrading or inactivating activated factors. **A,B.** The antithrombin III system and the TFPI system both inactivate factor Xa, the first member of the common final pathway. **C.** The powerful proteins C and S system, while largely restricted to factors V and VIII, can degrade both the active forms and the proenzymes.

Serum is the term used to describe the liquid phase of clotted blood, that is, plasma after the clotting factors have been consumed.

Anticoagulation and Fibrinolysis The coagulation system is potentially harmful if it leads to inappropriate or excessive clotting. Several **natural anticoagulant mechanisms**, depicted in FIGURE 10.5, inhibit the clotting cascade at a number of points. **Antithrombin III** is a protease inhibitor that binds and inactivates thrombin (factor IIa) as well as factors IXa, Xa, XIa, and XIIa. Its action is greatly potentiated by endothelial surface proteoglycans, as well as the commonly used anticoagulant drug **heparin** (see Clinical Application Box *Pharmacologic Anticoagulation*). Another important control point involves the proteins C and S system, which inactivates factors V and VIII. **Protein C** is activated by a complex of thrombin bound to *thrombomodulin* on endothelial cell surfaces. Thrombomodulin thus transforms (or "modulates," hence its name) thrombin from a procoagulant molecule that cleaves fibrinogen into an anticoagulant molecule by redirecting thrombin's enzymatic activity toward protein C. Activated protein C then combines with **protein S**, Ca^{2+} ions, and a phospholipid surface to form a complex that inactivates factors V and VIII, thus slowing the coagulation cascade. *Tissue factor pathway inhibitor (TFPI)* is another plasma protein that binds and inactivates factors Xa and VIIa.

Once a clot forms over an area of blood vessel damage, a complex process of repair and regeneration is initiated. Blood clots are meant to be transitory. Once the damage has been repaired, clots must be removed. The **fibrinolytic system** dissolves blood clots after they are formed and thus competes with procoagulant systems (FIGURE 10.6). A circulating protein called **plasminogen** is cleaved by plasminogen activators produced by endothelial cells to form the highly active enzyme **plasmin**. Plasmin cleaves fibrin into fragments called *fibrin split products (FSPs)*, thus degrading clots. Plasmin, like the activated proteins C and S system, also degrades factors V and VIII, giving it anticoagulant properties as well as fibrinolytic ones. Since plasmin is a highly destructive enzyme potentially capable of causing severe hemorrhage, it has its own series of inhibitors. The enzyme α_2-**antiplasmin** inhibits plasmin directly, and **type 1 plasmin activation inhibitor (PAI-1)** inhibits the conversion of plasminogen to plasmin. (See Clinical Application Box *Pharmacologic Thrombolysis*.)

Many of the enzymatic reactions of the clotting cascade require Ca^{2+} as a cofactor (e.g., activation of factors X and II). In fact, the dependence on the presence of Ca^{2+} is so great, that chemicals such as ethylene-diamine-tetraacetic acid (EDTA) which bind (or chelate) free Ca^{2+}, effectively prevent coagulation. EDTA is used in some test tubes into which blood is

---

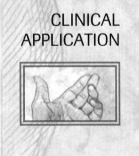

CLINICAL APPLICATION

PHARMACOLOGIC ANTICOAGULATION

A number of important drugs interfere with the coagulation cascade. Warfarin, frequently used in patients for long term anticoagulation, interferes with the vitamin K—dependent reaction necessary for the production of functional clotting factors II, VII, IX, and X, and reduces the levels of the activated proteins. The anticoagulant proteins C and S also require vitamin K, so they are decreased as well. Because proteins C and S have the shortest half life of the proteins requiring vitamin K-dependent γ-carboxylation of glutamate amino acids, plasma concentrations of these anticoagulant proteins are the first to diminish, leading to a paradoxical state of hypercoagulability early during the administration of this drug. Later, when the plasma concentrations of factors II, VII, IX, and X have decreased, the anticoagulant effects of warfarin exceed the procoagulant effects. Although factors II and X are in the common pathway of coagulation, factor VII is in the extrinsic pathway, and factor IX is in the intrinsic pathway. The laboratory test used most often to measure the effects of warfarin is the prothrombin time (PT), or its normalized derivative, the international normalized ratio (INR), which assesses the extrinsic and common pathways.

In contrast, heparins augment by a thousand-fold the activity of antithrombin III against factors XIIa, XIa, IXa, Xa, and IIa (thrombin) (Figure 10.5). Because the majority of these factors are part of the intrinsic pathway, the effect of heparins is measured by the following the partial thromboplastin time (PTT). In addition to high-molecular-weight heparin, the oldest member of the pharmacologic family of heparins, newer low-molecular-weight heparins are being used increasingly for anticoagulation, such as in the prevention of deep vein thrombosis.

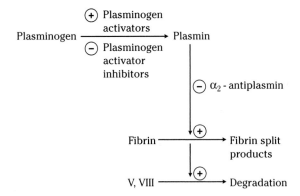

Figure 10.6 The fibrinolytic system. Once fibrinogen is converted to fibrin and fibrin is cross-linked to form the clot meshwork, it is sculpted and eventually degraded. This is achieved by the conversion of plasminogen, a proenzyme that binds to fibrin, to plasmin, which degrades fibrin into "split products" that can be measured clinically to qualitatively assess the activity of the coagulation system. Plasmin also cleaves factors V and VIII, giving it anticoagulative properties as well as fibrinolytic ones. Such a powerful enzyme must be tightly regulated by plasminogen activation inhibitors and α_2-antiplasmin.

collected, so that contact of the blood with the glass does not precipitate coagulation.

Endothelial Cells and Platelets

The endothelium has at least five major functions: (1) regulating hemostasis, (2) providing a permeability barrier between blood and tissues, (3) influencing vascular tone, (4) contributing to immunity and inflammation, and (5) modulating cell growth and differentiation. Because platelets play critical roles in hemostasis, their contributions are detailed along with those of the endothelium in controlling coagulation.

Regulating Hemostasis Intact endothelium has a number of natural anticoagulant and antiplatelet properties that maintain blood flow through undamaged vessels and prevent inappropriate clotting, which is the basis of a number of common and potentially deadly diseases. The endothelium normally covers the negatively charged subendothelial collagen layer of vessel walls and does not express tissue factor on its cell surface, preventing the activation of the clotting cascade. It also expresses thrombomodulin, which exerts anticoagulant effects through the proteins C and S system. Furthermore, it synthesizes the lipid mediator prostacyclin (PGI_2) and the enzyme ADPase, which specifically inhibit the activation of platelets.

Steps in the process of hemostasis are shown in FIGURE 10.7. When the endothelium is disrupted, exposed subendothelial collagen rapidly binds circulating **vWF**, a protein stored in and secreted by endothelial cells. Platelets, critical to hemostasis, express on their surface plasma membranes the glycoprotein receptor **gp 1b/IX** that specifically binds vWF. The vWF accumulates on connective tissue exposed by endothelial disruption and captures circulating platelets. By means of gp1b/IX and vWF, platelets bind to the surface denuded of endothelium and are activated. The entry of Ca^{2+} into platelets causes them to degranulate, releasing the contents of

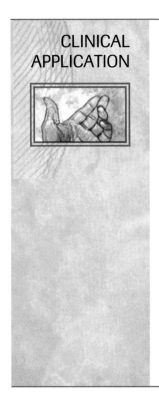

CLINICAL APPLICATION

PHARMACOLOGIC THROMBOLYSIS

"Clotbusters" are drugs that accelerate the breakdown of clots. They are especially useful in diseases in which a primary pathogenic component is the formation of a clot obstructing a major artery, such as a coronary artery (inducing cardiac ischemia and possibly a myocardial infarction) or a pulmonary artery (as in a pulmonary embolus). Such diseases are often characterized by the rapid onset of symptoms, and they require equally rapid treatment to avoid possibly lethal consequences. Once fibrinogen is cleaved to fibrin, the proenzyme plasminogen binds to the fibrin meshwork of the clot, poised to start dissolving it by degrading fibrin into "split products." However, to do so, plasminogen must itself be cleaved to the active enzyme plasmin. This is accomplished in vivo by tissue plasminogen activator that is released by endothelial cells (Figure 10.6).

Recombinant tissue plasminogen activator (rtPA) is the pharmacologic agent that achieves the same end. It rapidly initiates clot lysis and can restore blood flow through an obstructed artery, aborting a heart attack. In addition, because plasmin can degrade fibrinogen and factors V and VIII, rtPA has anticoagulant as well as fibrinolytic activities. A great advantage of rtPA is its high affinity for fibrin, ensuring that the activation of plasminogen is localized to the clot. Also, rtPA is specific for newly formed clots, so old clots (from ulcers, old injuries) are spared. Two drugs with similar plasminogen activating potential are streptokinase (produced by β-hemolytic streptococci) and urokinase (produced by kidney cells).

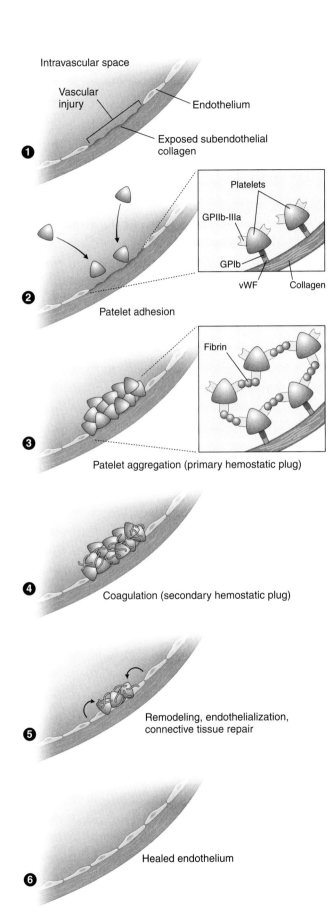

① Intravascular space

Vascular injury — Endothelium

Exposed subendothelial collagen

② Platelets

GPIIb-IIIa

GPIb

vWF   Collagen

Patelet adhesion

③ Fibrin

Patelet aggregation (primary hemostatic plug)

④ Coagulation (secondary hemostatic plug)

⑤ Remodeling, endothelialization, connective tissue repair

⑥ Healed endothelium

their α and δ granules. *Adenosine diphosphate (ADP)* and *serotonin* enhance platelet degranulation and aggregation. An extremely short-lived and active lipid mediator called *thromboxane A_2 (TXA$_2$)* is produced from arachidonic acid by platelets and greatly augments their activation and aggregation. The result is the **primary hemostatic plug**, an aggregate of platelets that achieves initial hemostasis. The primary hemostatic plug is like a pile of bricks with very little holding them together.

The next step is the activation of the coagulation system, which provides the fibrin "glue" that cements together the platelet bricks of the hemostatic plug. As described above, the negatively charged subendothelial connective tissue and tissue factor activate the clotting cascade. The activated platelets in the primary hemostatic plug greatly augment this process. Platelets express a glycoprotein receptor **gpIIb/IIIa** that binds fibrinogen, and the cell membrane of the platelets provides the phospholipid surface on which the coagulation reactions occur. Platelet degranulation also releases a number of procoagulant mediators, such as Ca^{2+}, factor V, *platelet factor 4* (which neutralizes antithrombin III), and *thrombospondin* (which also binds fibrinogen). The production and cross-linking of fibrin binds together the platelets and forms the **secondary (definitive) hemostatic plug**. The sticky strands of fibrin also trap some red blood cells, as shown in the scanning electron micrograph in FIGURE 10.8, giving the commonly appreciated red color of a blood clot.

The heparin-antithrombin III and proteins C and S mechanisms rapidly check the coagulation system. In addition, adjacent endothelial cells secrete prostacyclin, which limits coagulation to the site of endothelial injury. They also secrete plasminogen activators that activate the fibrinolytic system, which eventually degrades and remodels the clot as endothelial cells and fibroblasts proliferate and repair the injured area.

Figure 10.7 Hemostasis. Hemostasis becomes necessary when there is a break in the vascular endothelium (1), exposing subendothelial collagen. This subendothelial collagen soon binds circulating vWF and, by means of their gp1b/IX, platelets bind this vWF to adhere to the surface denuded of endothelium (2). This early primary hemostatic plug is fragile. It is reinforced by the end-product of the coagulation cascade, fibrin, which, binding to platelet gpIIb/IIIa receptors, cross-links the platelet aggregate (3). As the coagulation cascade progresses and the complex fibrin meshwork is woven, red and white cells, more platelets, and a number of regulatory proteins (such as plasminogen) are trapped in the matrix of cross-linked fibrin (4). The fibrinolytic system is activated as the endothelial cells bordering the damaged and denuded area initiate a complex system of repair and regeneration (5). As intact endothelium covers the previously "bare" spot, the clot dissolves, leaving the healed vessel interior (6).

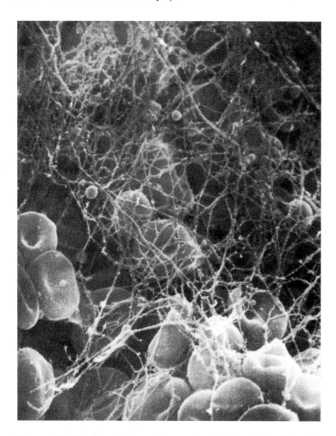

Figure 10.8 An electron micrograph of a blood clot. Note the complex three-dimensional web of cross-linked fibrin and the trapped red cells.

Providing the Permeability Barrier Between Blood and Tissues A second major function of the endothelium is to provide a selective permeability barrier at the interface between the intravascular space and the interstitial space, the extravascular space that bathes the tissue cells. The thin, single-cell barrier is ideally suited to the rapid diffusion of hydrophobic molecules, small hydrophilic metabolites, and gases such as oxygen and carbon dioxide (Figure 10.2). The tight junctions between endothelial cells limit the leakage (extravasation) of larger molecules such as proteins (particularly albumin) and prevent the inappropriate loss of blood cells into tissues. The fluid that passes out of the capillary vascular space enters the tissue interstitial space and is resorbed as lymph (see Chapter 11).

Three types of capillaries allow for different vascular permeabilities in different organs (FIGURE 10.9). **Continuous capillaries** have intact walls and basal lamina that largely limit the exchange of proteins and macromolecules. These are found in connective tissue, muscle, peripheral nerve, and the central nervous system (where they form the basis of the *blood–brain barrier*). **Fenestrated capillaries** have multiple fenestrae, or pores, but still have an intact

basal lamina. These are found where exchange of macromolecules occurs, including the gastrointestinal villi, the renal glomeruli, and endocrine glands. **Sinusoidal capillaries** (also called *discontinuous capillaries*) are large capillaries that have numerous fenestrae and a discontinuous basal lamina. Sinusoidal capillaries allow for the rapid exchange of large volumes of fluid and substances in the liver, spleen, and bone marrow.

Influencing Vascular Tone As described in Chapter 7, *vascular tone* is the degree of contraction of the smooth muscle cells in the tunica media. It can be quite dynamic, ranging between maximal relaxation and maximal contraction. In most vessels most of the

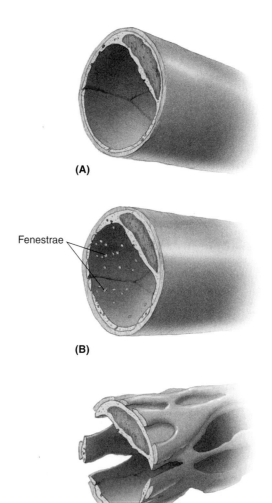

(A)

Fenestrae

(B)

(C)

Figure 10.9 Three types of capillaries. **A.** Continuous capillaries have numerous tight junctions fusing the membranes of adjacent endothelial cells. Only the smallest molecules (O_2, H_2O, CO_2, glucose, amino acids, etc.) can cross between tissue and blood space. **B.** Fenestrated capillaries have a number of larger openings. **C.** Sinusoidal capillaries, like those in the liver, have numerous large fenestrae (pores) that allow macromolecules to pass.

time, vascular tone is in an intermediate state. When the smooth muscle cells relax, the diameter (and therefore the cross-sectional area) of the vessel increases, and the resistance to blood flow drops. When the smooth muscle cells contract, the diameter of the vessel decreases, and the resistance to blood flow rises. Since the resistance of a tube to the laminar flow of a fluid is given by Poiseuille's law:

$$R = 8\eta l/\pi r^4$$

where R is the resistance, η is the viscosity of the fluid, l is the length of the tube, and r is the radius of the tube, small changes in the radius brought about by small changes in the contractile state of the vessel wall smooth muscle (tone) can have dramatic effects. Vessels dilate or constrict in order to alter the blood flow to tissues in response to neurotransmitters, tissue factors (including some metabolites), and exogenous drugs. The chemical mediators involved either have direct effects on vascular smooth muscle or work indirectly by stimulating the production of endothelial-derived vasoactive substances. Examples of the latter class are the conversion of angiotensin I to angiotensin II by angiotensin-converting enzyme (ACE) and the production of endothelin-1, which are both potent vasoconstrictors. Endothelial cells also produce nitric oxide (NO), previously known as endothelial-derived relaxing factor (EDRF), a powerful vasodilator.

Arachidonic acid (arachidonate) metabolites are lipid mediators that can act as either vasodilators or vasoconstrictors. Cleaved from membrane phospholipids by a phospholipase enzyme, arachidonic acid is cyclized by the enzyme **cyclooxygenase**. These intermediates can then form a number of different types of **prostaglandins**, depending on the cell type and the particular activation state of the cell. Two prostaglandins introduced earlier deserve mention again. The major prostaglandin produced by endothelial cells, prostacyclin (PGI_2), inhibits platelet function and is a vasodilator. In contrast, the major prostaglandin produced by platelets is thromboxane A_2 (TXA_2), which has the antagonistic functions of promoting platelet activation and aggregation and producing vasoconstriction to help control hemorrhage (FIGURE 10.10). Through the action of these molecules, platelet aggregation is catalyzed at sites of endothelial cell disruption but does not extend into adjacent segments of endothelial integrity (see Clinical Application Box *Pharmacologic Antiplatelet Agents*).

Contributing to Inflammation and Immunity
Endothelial cells perform a number of crucial functions in the inflammatory and immune responses. They normally prevent the extravasation of large amounts of fluid and retain white blood cells within the vascu-

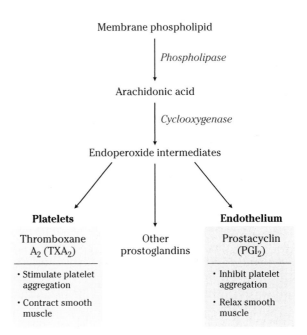

Figure 10.10 Arachidonate metabolism. Phospholipid molecules on the inner leaflet of the cell membrane are cleaved by the enzyme phosphopilase A₂, releasing the unsaturated fatty acid arachidonate. Arachidonate may be further modified by cyclooygenase to go down the prostaglandin or thromboxane pathway. In platelets, the major product is thromboxane A₂ (TXA₂), which activates platelets, while in endothelial cells the major product is prostacyclin (PGI₂).

lature. Inflammatory stimuli loosen the junctional complexes connecting endothelial cells. The result is increased permeability and a rapid flow of fluid and proteins, some of which are important in neutralizing foreign substances or microorganisms, into the affected area. The clinical appearance of the inflamed tissue is **edema**, or swelling. Concomitantly, vasodilation occurs, increasing the flow of blood to the area of inflammation. This not only augments the delivery of nutrients, immune cells, and proteins to the area, it explains why inflamed tissues get red and hot.

Inflammatory stimuli also up-regulate the surface expression of adhesion molecules on local endothelial cells, particularly those lining the postcapillary venules. These activated endothelial cells are "docking sites" for leukocytes. Although the vasodilation that is part of the inflammatory response increases the *volume* of blood per unit time delivered to the affected area, the *velocity* of blood flow decreases, allowing leukocytes to bind to the adhesion molecules and then exit the bloodstream by the process of diapedesis, thus entering the tissues and exerting their effects (see Chapter 11). In large part due to the contribution of endothelium, therefore, inflamed tissues clinically have the following characteristics (denoted by traditional Latin terms): swollen (*tumor*), red (*rubor*), hot (*calor*), painful (*dolor*), and dysfunctional (*functio laesa*).

PHARMACOLOGIC ANTIPLATELET AGENTS

Some very old and some very new drugs antagonize platelets. **Aspirin** acetylates and permanently inactivates the cyclooxygenase enzymes. In low doses, it affects platelets more than endothelial cells. Because platelets are anucleate cell fragments and do not reproduce, aspirin poisons platelets for their lifetime, and it is only by producing new platelets that the antiplatelet effects of aspirin are overcome. This property is exploited by using aspirin as a preventive and a treatment for conditions in which platelet aggregation, coagulation, and thrombosis are harmful, such as in coronary artery disease and stroke.

A newer approach to platelet inhibition is the use of humanized antibodies or small molecules that bind to and block the platelet receptor gpIIb/IIIa. These inhibitors have been successfully used in the prevention and treatment of acute coronary artery disease syndromes such as unstable angina and in patients who have undergone procedures such as the placement of a metal meshwork tube called a stent into an atherosclerotic coronary artery. Because they antagonize the binding of molecules like fibrin that cross-link platelets, they inhibit the aggregation and stabilization of hemostatic plugs. As expected, one of the major side effects of these antiplatelet drugs is bleeding.

Modulating Cell Growth and Differentiation Endothelial cells also produce a number of factors, such as **platelet-derived growth factor (PDGF)** and **fibroblast growth factor (FGF)**, that control the growth and differentiation of connective tissue elements, particularly smooth muscle cells and fibroblasts (see Table 10.1). They play an important role in healing and connective tissue repair and regeneration following injury. Other factors, such as **transforming growth factor (TGF)** suppress these processes. These factors also play a major in the physiologic and pathologic responses to chronic inflammatory stimuli.

PATHOPHYSIOLOGY

Any function of the endothelium or the hemostatic system can be disrupted and result in disease. Disruption of hemostasis leads to excessive bleeding or inappropriate clotting. Breakdown of the permeability barrier causes blood or some of its components to exit the vascular space and enter tissues. Endothelial dysfunction may also have profound effects on vascular tone, immune responses, and vessel wall cell growth. That many of the resulting pathological conditions—inherited or acquired—are life-threatening attests to the importance of the endothelium and the hemostatic system.

Disorders of Hemostasis

When the hemostatic response is inadequate or hypofunctional, the result of even limited damage to blood vessels is continued bleeding. Such is the case with major trauma, in which extensive damage to one

or more large blood vessels can lead to life-threatening low blood pressure and failure to perfuse vital organs if enough blood volume is lost—a syndrome called *hypovolemic shock*. Alternatively, significant bleeding can occur without major trauma if the components of the hemostatic response are absent or dysfunctional. Such bleeding diatheses include **hemophilia** (e.g., insufficient factor VIII), liver failure (insufficient production of multiple clotting factors), **von Willebrand's disease** (insufficient vWF), and thrombocytopenia (insufficient platelets).

When the hemostatic response is inappropriate or hyperfunctional, the result is excessive clotting, or **thrombosis**. Thrombosis often occurs in the iliac and femoral veins, leading to a dangerous condition known as *deep venous thrombosis (DVT)*. Hypercoaguable states include deficits of natural anticoagulants, such as **protein S deficiency, protein C deficiency,** or **antithrombin III deficiency**; a mutation of factor V known as **factor V Leiden**, which makes factor V resistant to enzymatic inactivation by activated protein C; and states such as malignancy and sepsis, which involve the production of mediators that inappropriately activate the clotting cascade. Blood also tends to clot more when it stops flowing and pools. The three general conditions that predispose to thrombosis are endothelial damage/dysfunction, hypercoaguable states, and blood stasis. These three constitute **Virchow's triad**, named after the legendary 19th century pathologist.

Disruption of the Permeability Barrier

When the permeability barrier function of the endothelium is insufficient, fluid leaks out of the vasculature into tissues with resultant edema. Many conditions, including congestive heart failure, liver failure, renal disease, and infection, can lead to edematous states (see Chapter 11). In patients who suffer from serious burns, the destruction of the endothelium may lead to significant fluid losses.

Abnormalities of Vascular Tone

When vascular tone is too low, the resultant low blood pressure (*hypotension*) can lead to insufficient perfusion of vital organs. Excessively high vascular tone can occur either systemically, as in the case of high blood pressure (*hypertension*), or focally, as in the case of vasospasm. Vasospastic disorders can occur in the digits, leading to **Raynaud's disease**; in the brain, contributing to **migraine headaches**; or in the heart, leading to a rare type of coronary artery disease known as **Prinzmetal's angina**.

Disorder of Immunity and Inflammation

Deficient inflammatory or immune responses result in immunodeficiency or immunosuppression that can lead to a wide array of infectious diseases. **Leukocyte adhesion deficiency** is an example of an imunodeficiency that results from an inability of phagocytic cells to bind to the endothelium and undergo diapedesis into the extravascular tissues. Dysfunction of the endothelium or hemostatic system is rarely a cause of the excessive or inappropriate immune reactions that cause chronic inflammatory diseases. However, the endothelium may play an important role in the development of allergic diseases by allowing benign foreign antigens to enter the body and elicit inappropriate immune responses (see Chapter 11).

Pathologic Cell Growth and Differentiation

Excessive and/or inappropriate growth signals from endothelium lead to hyperplasia of fibroblasts, smooth muscle cells, and connective tissue in the tunica intima of blood vessels, processes important in the development of plaques in **atherosclerosis**. These lesions result in vascular occlusion that manifest clinically as **coronary artery disease**, **cerebrovascular disease**, and **peripheral vascular disease**.

Hemophilia A

The structural defect in **hemophilia A** is an inherited deficiency of functional factor VIII. It can be caused by either a genetic lesion resulting in a reduced quantity of factor VIII, or one in which a normal amount of factor VIII is produced, but the protein has defective function. **Hemophilia B** is factor IX deficiency and involves an identical clinical picture. Hemophilia A and B are diseases that show X-linked recessive inheritance because the genes for these proteins are located on the X chromosome.

The functional consequence of factor VIII (or factor IX) deficiency is failure of coagulation and hemostasis with endothelial injury. Specifically, there is insufficient activation of the intrinsic pathway of the clotting cascade. Platelet function is notably normal, leading to normal production of the primary hemostatic plug. Without enough coagulation to produce the secondary (definitive) hemostatic plug, the initial "pile of bricks with very little holding them together" falls apart, leading to recurrent and intractable bleeding.

Minor injuries in people with hemophilia can lead to severe bleeding, sometimes massive enough to result in death by exsanguination. Occasionally the initial trauma is so minor that the bleeding appears spontaneous. The severity of the bleeding diathesis is dependent on the level of factor VIII present. Less than 1% of normal factor VIII activity leads to severe disease, 1% to 5% of normal activity leads to moderate disease, and 5% to 50% of normal activity leads to mild disease. Severe hemophilia is characterized by frequent nosebleeds, soft tissue hematomas, and intracranial hemorrhages. Blood is often found the urine and stool, reflecting urinary tract and gastrointestinal bleeds. A particularly difficult problem is bleeding into joints, or *hemarthroses*. This results in severe pain and swelling, and recurrent bleeds and the subsequent chronic inflammatory fibrosis produce crippling arthritis, deformities, and loss of function in the affected joints. The knees and ankles are most often afflicted.

Laboratory diagnosis of hemophilia A relies on measurement of deficient factor VIII activity. But suspicion that a patient has hemophilia is often sparked by the results of two common blood tests: the PT and the PTT. Individuals with hemophilia A show a normal PT and a prolonged PTT, indicating a deficiency in a clotting factor involved in the intrinsic pathway. Platelet levels are usually found to be normal, and the coagulation defect can be corrected in the laboratory by a "mixing study," in which deficient clotting factor is provided when the patient's blood is mixed with plasma from a normal donor.

Factor VIII replacement is the mainstay of clinical treatment for hemophilia. Sources of factor VIII include fresh frozen plasma, cryoprecipitate, affinity-purified factor VIII, and recombinant factor VIII. One of the tragedies of modern medicine is the contamination of pooled plasma stores with the human immunodeficiency virus (HIV) in the 1970s, which has led to HIV infection and AIDS in a large number of hemophiliacs receiving therapy during this time period.

Summary

- **Endothelium** lines blood vessels where it regulates hemostasis, provides a semipermeable barrier between the blood and extravascular tissues, influences vascular tone, contributes to immunity and inflammation, and modulates cell growth and differentiation.

- **Hemostasis** is the control of bleeding in response to blood vessel damage. It comprises four steps: *vasospasm*, endothelial activation, platelet adherence and activation, and **coagulation**.

- The **clotting cascade** is a series of proteolytic enzymatic reactions triggered either by the release of **tissue factor (extrinsic pathway)** or the activation of **factor XII (intrinsic pathway)**, ending in a common pathway producing a meshwork of **fibrin**.

- Platelets bind via **vWF receptors** to subendothelial collagen on vessel surfaces denuded of endothelium, forming a **primary hemostatic plug**. When the coagulation cascade is initiated, platelets bind to each other by means of **gpIIb/IIIa receptors** and fibrin, forming a **secondary hemostatic plug**.

- Defects in platelets or coagulation factors result in diseases with excessive bleeding (**hemorrhage**). Dysfunction of endothelial or circulating anticoagulant factors causes excessive or inappropriate **thrombosis** (clotting).

- **Virchow's triad** describes three conditions that predispose to thrombosis: endothelial damage/dysfunction, hypercoaguable states, and blood stasis.

- **Hemophilia A** is a genetic disease caused by mutations in the gene encoding factor VIII. **Hemophilia B** is caused by mutation in the gene encoding factor IX. Both diseases are characterized by bleeding because a defect in the coagulation cascade prevents primary hemostatic plugs from being converted to secondary hemostatic plugs.

REVIEW QUESTIONS

Directions: Each of the numbered items or incomplete statements in this section is followed by answers or by completions of the statement. Select the ONE lettered answer or completion that is BEST in each case.

1. Which of the following factors is an anticoagulant?
   - (A) Factor XII (Hageman factor)
   - (B) Factor VIII
   - (C) Prothrombin
   - (D) Thrombin
   - (E) Thrombomodulin

2. Which of the following would produce a predisposition to clotting?

   (A) Loss of factor VIII activity
   (B) Loss of factor IX activity
   (C) Loss of protein C activity
   (D) Decreased amounts of vWF
   (E) Antagonization of platelet receptor gpIIb/IIIa

3. A 98-year-old man with metastatic colon cancer has a perforation in his large bowel that leads to a bacterial infection in his blood. He is hospitalized with sepsis and treated with antibiotics and large volumes of intravenous fluids. Which of the following does NOT predispose this patient to suffering a deep venous thrombosis?

   (A) Lying in bed without getting up to walk
   (B) His malignancy
   (C) The presence of bacteria in his blood (bacteremia)
   (D) The IV fluids

4. A 12-year-old male has recurrent nosebleeds, large bruises from small or sometime no recalled trauma, and protracted bleeding when he brushes his teeth. Each the following might explain his bleeding EXCEPT

   (A) genetic mutation leading to insufficient prostacyclin (PGI$_2$) production by his endothelial cells
   (B) genetic mutation leading to decreased production of factor VIII by his liver
   (C) genetic mutation leading to normal amounts but enzymatically inactive factor VIII by his liver
   (D) an autoimmune disease that destroys his platelets
   (E) a genetic mutation leading to decreased production of von Willebrand factor (vWF) by his megakaryocytes and endothelium

ANSWERS TO REVIEW QUESTIONS

1. **The answer is E.** Activation of Hageman factor (factor XII) initiates the intrinsic pathway of clotting the cascade. Factor VIII, deficient or defective in hemophilia A, activates factor X. Prothrombin (factor II) is activated by factor Xa into thrombin (factor IIa), which cleaves fibrinogen into fibrin. These are all procoagulant factors, but thrombomodulin, expressed on the surface of endothelial cells, redirects the enzymatic activity of thrombin to activate protein C, which degrades factor V. Thus, thrombomodulin contributes to inhibiting coagulation and is therefore an anticoagulant.

2. **The answer is C.** Factors VIII and IX are part of the intrinsic coagulation pathway, and their loss produces hemophilia, a disease characterized by poor blood clotting and excessive bleeding. Since platelets adhere to subendothelial collagen exposed when endothelial cells are lost by means of vWF, and then stick to each other by means of gpIIb/IIa and fibrin, a loss of either vWH or gpIIb/IIa will favor bleeding. However, since protein C inactivates the procoagulant molecule factor V, a loss of protein C activity will predispose the blood to clot. A common related situation is the presence of a mutation in factor V (factor V Leiden), which makes factor V resistant to cleavage by activated protein C.

3. **The answer is D.** Deep venous thombosis is the formation of a blood clot in the veins, most commonly those of the lower extremity. The three general conditions that predispose to blood clotting are endothelial damage or dysfunction, hypercoagulable states, and blood stasis. The patient's lying in bed without getting up to walk allows the venous blood in his legs to pool (stasis), while the malignancy and the bacteremia make him hypercoagulable. The administration of large volumes of intravenous fluid, however, would not predispose him to thrombosis. Patients like these are treated prophylactically with pneumatic compression boots that fill with air to squeeze the calves periodically to increase venous return to the heart (to combat stasis) and with anticoagulants, such as low- or high-molecular-weight heparin (to combat hypercoagulability), to prevent deep vein thrombosis.

4. **The answer is A.** This patient has superficial bleeding that might be attributable to dysfunction of platelets or the coagulation system. Genetic lesions that decrease the amount or function of factor VIII produce hemophilia, a well-characterized bleeding disorder. Thrombocytopenia (abnormally low platelet counts) may occur with an autoimmune disease in which the body's own platelets are destroyed by the immune system. Since platelet adherence to subendothelial collagen exposed when endothelial cells are lost depends on vWF, genetic mutations in this protein produce the bleeding disorder identified by and named after von Willebrand. However, prostacyclin (PGI$_2$) is an endothelially derived antagonist of platelets and a vasodilator, so a loss of PGI$_2$ would, if anything, promote clotting, not inhibit it.

Suggested Reading

Moake JL. Thrombotic microangiopathies. N Engl J Med. 2002;347(8):589–600.

Simionescu M, Simionescu N. Functions of the endothelial cell surface. Annu Rev Physiol. 1986;48:279–293.

The Lymphatic System and the Immune System

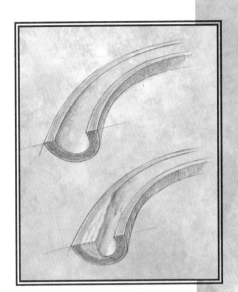

INTRODUCTION

This chapter describes the lymphatic system and the immune system. It departs from other discussions of these systems in two ways. First, the physiology of the lymphatic system has been put in the larger context of blood physiology, instead of being included in cardiovascular physiology, as has traditionally been done. Second, the discussion of lymphatic system physiology follows the description of endothelium in Chapter 10 and precedes that of immune system physiology (with which it has been paired) to emphasize how the lymphatic system functionally connects blood and endothelium with the immune system.

As discussed in Chapter 10, the capillary endothelium provides a semipermeable barrier that separates the intravascular space from the extravascular interstitial space. As arterial blood flows through capillaries, some fluid crosses this barrier, leaving the blood space and entering the interstitial space. Much of this fluid is resorbed by the venous end of the capillary, but an important fraction remains in the interstitial space. Somehow this volume of fluid has to be returned to the circulation so it does not continue to collect in the tissue space. This is the function of the lymphatic system. The fluid in the lymphatic vessels is called *lymph*. In addition to the acellular lymph fluid, the lymphatic system also transports and accommodates cells of the immune system, a complex set of interacting cells and their products that protect the body.

This chapter describes (a) the hydrostatic forces, oncotic forces, and filtration coefficients involved in fluid flow across capillary membranes, as well as the Starling equation, which quantitatively combines these forces into an expression generally applicable to all organ systems; (b) the interstitial space, the resorption of interstitial fluid, and fluid flow in the lymphatic vessels; (c) the connections between the lymphatic system and the vascular system; and (d) the basic features of the immune system.

LYMPHATIC SYSTEM STRUCTURE

The lymphatic system structures link the interstitial space and the intravascular space, returning fluids, solutes, and proteins filtered from the capillaries into the interstitial space back to the systemic circulation. In a 24-hour period, the lymphatic system transports 2 to 4 L of fluid, an amount equivalent to the body's total plasma blood volume. The lymphatic system includes vessels as well as lymph nodes, where the draining fluid is scanned by numerous leukocytes for the presence of bacteria and other foreign pathogens. Thus, the structures of the lymphatic system support two functions: fluid handling and immune surveillance. The first function is the topic of

the first half of this chapter, while the second function will be discussed in the second half.

The Extracellular Fluid

The extracellular fluid (ECF) occupies two compartments: about 25% of the ECF is within blood vessels as intravascular fluid, and 75% is within tissues as extravascular interstitial fluid. These two ECF compartments are dynamic, with component water molecules, ions, and macromolecules moving between them according to physical forces.

The Interstitial Space

The interstitial space is the space between tissue cells, the matrix containing the capillary microcirculation and tissue cells. Because the interstitial space is the immediate environment of tissue cells, it must be compatible with their function. The composition of the interstitial space is a collagenous framework filled with a gel-like solution containing negatively charged glycosaminoglycan polysaccharides (hyaluronan and proteoglycans), salts, water, and plasma-derived proteins (e.g., albumin). The particular composition varies greatly among different tissues, with anatomic locations. The skin, for example, has denser or "tighter" interstitial spaces with relatively high concentrations of collagen, hyaluronan, and albumin, whereas lung tissue has a "looser" matrix.

Lymphatic System Components

To return fluid from the interstitial space to the intravascular space, the lymphatic system has myriad small vessels in almost all tissues. This network of vessels is interrupted by lymph nodes where the immune surveillance is carried out. This section describes the structure of the lymphatic vessels, the lymph nodes, and the lymph fluid itself.

Lymphatic System Gross Anatomy The lymphatic system consists of **lymph nodes**, or encapsulated tissue masses, connected by a network of tubules called **lymphatic vessels**, or lymphatics. Lymph nodes are distributed unevenly throughout the body and are particularly numerous in the neck, axillae, and inguinal areas. Lymphatic vessels contain fluid known as **lymph**. Most of the body's lymphatic vessels lead into the *cisterna chyli*, a large lymph sac that connects to the largest lymph vessel, the *thoracic duct*. The thoracic duct feeds into the left subclavian vein, thus reconnecting lymph flow to the cardiovascular system. Lymph vessels from the right upper extremity, the right half of the thorax, and the right half of the head, lead to the *right lym-*

phatic duct, which feeds into the right subclavian vein (FIGURE 11.1). Other important organs of the lymphatic system, such as the spleen, thymus, tonsils, and Peyer's patches, are discussed in the context of the immune system.

Lymphatic System Tissues and Cells   **Lacteals** are lymphatic capillaries embedded within the interstitial space, along with blood vessels, capillaries, and tissue cells (FIGURE 11.2). These terminal lymphatic capillaries are thin, blind-ended channels lined by a single layer of endothelial cells. In contrast with vascular capillary endothelium (see Chapter 10), they have no fenestrations, no tight junctions, and virtually no basal lamina. FIGURE 11.3 is a photomicrograph of a lymphatic capillary showing a bileaflet valve, which ensures unidirectional flow of lymph (i.e., it prevents backflow). Anchoring filaments, consisting of elastic microfibrils, attach the initial portions of the lymphatic capillaries to the surrounding interstitial connective tissue framework and may keep the initial portion of the lymphatics open.

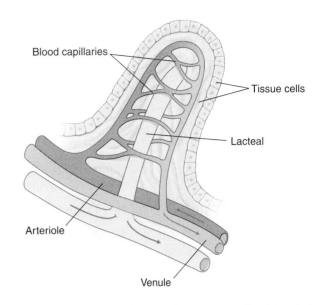

Figure 11.2   Lymphatics vessel components. Small lymphatic capillaries called lacteals are embedded in tissues. Lymph enters the sealed end and travels out of the tissue (*arrow*). Also shown is a nearby arteriole, blood capillary, and venule, with the flow of progressively deoxygenated blood indicated.

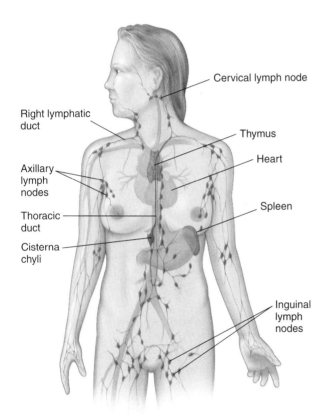

Figure 11.1   Gross anatomy of the lymphatic system. Although lymph nodes are found throughout the body, note their relatively high frequency in the neck, axillae, and inguinal regions. Lymphatic vessels often follow the general direction of large blood vessels. The majority of lymphatic vessels connect to the cisternae chyli and on into the thoracic duct, but lymphatics from the right side of the body lead to the right lymphatic duct. They all lead back to the venous circulation.

Lymph fluid itself typically contains very few cells, and generally only certain leukocytes (white blood cells). Because red cells do not ordinarily leave the vasculature, they are not found in normal lymph. White blood cells, on the other hand, can exit (or extravasate) from the postcapillary venules by the process of diapedesis (see Chapter 10) and enter tissues. The longer-lived cells of the immune system, lymphocytes and macrophages, often cycle repeatedly through the bloodstream, then the lymphatic system, and back again into the blood.

Lymph nodes are collections of tissue cells and leukocytes, such as macrophages and lymphocytes. A typical lymph node is shaped like a kidney bean. On the outer (convex) surface, one or more afferent lymphatic vessels "plug into" the node, penetrating the capsule. The deeper node is divided into an outer *cortex* and an inner *medulla*. Connective tissue *trabeculae* subdivide the outer cortex, where dynamic collections of immune cells called **follicles** are found. The arrangement of these resident immune cells into follicles and zones expedites their intercommunication functions (described later). The node's *hilum* is the area on the inner (concave) surface where efferent lymphatic vessels exit and where a feeding artery and a draining vein "plug into" the node (FIGURE 11.4).

Lymphatic System Molecules and Ions   Lymph is a clear aqueous fluid, occasionally slightly yellow or creamy. Because it is a filtrate of the blood, its ionic and molecular constituents are qualitatively similar to blood plasma, although they may occur in signifi-

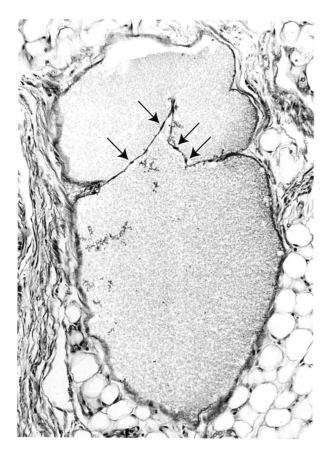

Figure 11.3 Microscopic view of a lymphatic vessel. Note the thin wall of endothelium and the bi-leaflet valve, which ensures that lymph flows unidirectionally (*arrows*).

LYMPHATIC SYSTEM FUNCTION

The many lymphatic vessels distributed in tissues absorb interstitial fluid and return it to the systemic circulation; but how is lymph formed, how does it enter the lymphatics, and how does it move from peripheral tissues into the bloodstream? This section described the forces driving the production and movement of lymph from the subcellular to the gross anatomic levels.

The Starling Forces

The three main determinants of filtration of fluid across a capillary membrane into the interstitial space are the net hydrostatic pressure, the net oncotic pressure, and capillary filtration. These three variables determine the direction and magnitude of fluid flux between the vascular space of a capillary and the interstitial space. The process of fluid moving from the vascular space of the capillary into the interstitial tissue is known as *transudation*. The hydrostatic and oncotic pressures are called **Starling forces** and are related to the capillary wall permeability and fluid flux by the Starling equation described below.

Hydrostatic Pressures There are two hydrostatic pressures, capillary hydrostatic pressure and interstitial hydrostatic pressure. **Capillary hydrostatic pressure (Pc)** is (quantitatively) the major force favoring

cantly different concentrations. Its composition is also dependent on the characteristics of the tissue it drains. For example, lymph from the gastrointestinal tract, known as *chyle*, is particularly opalescent owing to the high concentrations of absorbed fats, sugars, amino acids, and other nutrients.

The compositions of typical lymph and plasma are compared in TABLE 11.1. The ionic compositions of plasma, interstitial fluid, and lymph are nearly identical because of the rapid transport of these small ions across the endothelium and their diffusion. The major ions are sodium and chloride, with significant concentrations of potassium, calcium, and bicarbonate. In contrast, the tight junctions of most vascular endothelium prevent the free diffusion of proteins and large molecules into the interstitial space. Thus, the concentration of proteins (e.g., albumin and globulin) and other organic molecules (e.g., cholesterol) is significantly lower in lymph and interstitial fluid than in plasma. Finally, a number of important nutrient molecules found at high concentrations in the capillary circulation are present at lower concentrations in the lymph because tissue cells metabolize them.

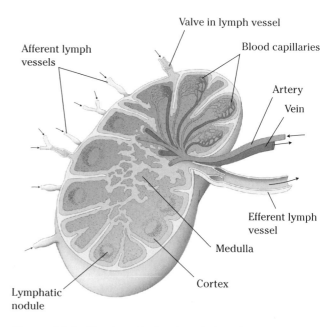

Figure 11.4 Structure of a lymph node. Lymph enters through afferent lymphatic vessels on the convex side of the node. Lymph then percolates through the node and exits via an efferent vessel at the node's hilum on the concave side. The hilum is also the point at which blood enters the node through an afferent arteriole and exits the node via an efferent venule.

Table 11.1   THE COMPOSITION AND CHARACTERISTICS OF LYMPH

	Lymph	Normal Serum	Lymph/Serum Ratio
Na^+ (mEq/L)	136.5 ± 3.0	135–145	1.02 ± 0.04
K^+ (mEq/L)	3.41 ± 0.1	3.5–5.0	0.98 ± 0.014
Cl^- (mEq/L)	107 ± 2.5	100–108	0.97 ± 0.02
Ca^{2+} (mEq/L)	6.2 ± 0.31	8.5–10.5	0.75 ± 0.03
Total protein (g/dL)	2.39 ± 0.04	6.0–8.0	0.39 ± 0.013
Albumin (g/dL)	1.68 ± 0.07	3.1–4.3	0.48 ± 0.02
IgG (mg/dL)	355 ± 9.3	614–1,295	0.28 ± 0.012
Urea (mg/dL)	39.3 ± 3.9	55–60	0.68 ± 0.08
Creatinine (mg/dL)	0.9 ± 0.1	0.6–1.5	1.0 ± 0.01
Glucose (mg/dL)	65.7 ± 4.5	70–110	0.84 ± 0.02
Cholesterol (total) (mg/dL)	21.7 ± 1.5	150–200	0.14 ± 0.024

the movement of fluid out of the capillary. Pc is determined by systemic blood pressure and the specific resistances of the local arterioles and venules. Systemic blood pressure is a function of total intravascular salt and water volume, pumping forces generated by the heart, and total vascular resistance (see Part IV). Pc is arbitrarily assigned a positive value, meaning that it is a force per unit area of capillary endothelium that pushes fluid out of the capillary circulation and into the interstitial space. Pc is approximately 32 mm Hg at the arteriolar end but decreases along the length of the capillary, reaching approximately 15 mm Hg at the venous end of a typical capillary.

Capillary hydrostatic pressure is opposed by **interstitial hydrostatic pressure (Pi)**, which is slightly negative, approximately −3 to 0 mm Hg. This slightly negative pressure, which actually (like Pc) favors the movement of fluid out of the capillary into the interstitial space, is thought to be due to the imbalance of opposing mechanical forces exerted by hyaluronan and collagen, as well as the affinity of hyaluronan for water. The difference between these pressures, Pc minus Pi, represents the net driving hydrostatic pressure for filtration, but because Pi is negative (i.e., the interstitial space "sucks" fluid out of the capillary while Pc pushes fluid out of the capillary), the total hydrostatic pressure (Pc minus Pi) exceeds Pc. For example, at the arteriolar end of the capillary where Pc = 32 mm Hg and Pi = −3 mm Hg, the net hydrostatic pressure (Pc minus Pi) = (32 mm Hg minus −3 mm Hg) = 35 mm Hg.

Oncotic Pressures   Just as there are two hydrostatic pressures, there are two oncotic pressures (one of the capillary and one of the interstitial space) that oppose their respective hydrostatic pressures,

preventing excessive fluid loss from their compartments. Since there are no large differences in salt concentrations between the interstitium and the plasma, the oncotic pressures are determined entirely by the differences in protein concentrations of the two compartments. **Capillary oncotic pressure (Πc)** is defined as the colloid osmotic pressure, the component of the total osmotic pressure that is contributed by plasma proteins. **Interstitial oncotic pressure (Πi)** is the colloid osmotic pressure exerted by the osmotically active proteins in the interstitium. Each pressure is a force per unit area of capillary endothelium that pulls fluid into the blood space, in the case of Πc, or into the interstitial space, in the case of Πi. The capillary endothelium allows essentially free diffusion of small solutes but severely restricts the filtration of protein so that most blood proteins (especially albumin) remain within the capillary lumen. Thus, the oncotic pressure of the capillary lumen is significantly higher (Πc of about 25 mm Hg) than the oncotic pressure of the interstitial space (Πi of about 0 to 5 mm Hg), leading to a difference of oncotic pressures, Πc minus Πi = 20 to 25 mm Hg, favoring fluid resorption. Oncotic pressure is dramatically affected by the relative permeability of a given solute to water, a factor quantified in the reflection coefficient σ. The reflection coefficient σ can range from 0 for a substance such as water that moves freely and exerts no oncotic pressure to 1 for a substance such as albumen that is restricted to one space (intravascular) and so exerts a large oncotic pressure. The equation for oncotic pressure is Π = σRT (ΛC), where R is the gas constant, T is the absolute temperature, and ΛC is the concentration difference between compartments.

FIGURE 11.5 shows the direction of the vectors for the two hydrostatic and two oncotic pressures. At the arteriolar end of the capillary, the hydrostatic forces for filtration exceed the oncotic forces for resorption, and the net effect is filtration. Owing to the drop in hydrostatic pressure across the capillary, the balance shifts at the venous side of the capillary, where oncotic forces exceed hydrostatic forces and the net effect is fluid resorption. In real capillary microcirculations, the local parameters are often more complex than in the idealized capillary show in the figure.

In most tissues, the volume of fluid that leaves the capillary and enters the interstitial space exceeds the volume of fluid that is resorbed from the interstitial space back into the capillary. Thus, there is a net loss of fluid from the circulation into the tissues. What happens to this fluid? If it continued to accumulate in the tissues, the result would be massive swelling of the tissues, or **edema**. To prevent edema, the excess filtered fluid enters the draining lymphatics and ultimately rejoins the vasculature. The lymphatics also remove the small quantity of plasma proteins that leak out of the capillaries, thus preventing their accumulation in the interstitial space. The lack of tight junctions and a very thin basal lamina in the lymphatic capillaries allow for their effective resorption of both fluid and proteins. These proteins are not effectively resorbed by capillaries, even at the venous side, owing to both the capillary membrane impermeability and the large albumin concentration gradient.

The Capillary Filtration Coefficient In addition to the net hydrostatic and net oncotic pressures, the third factor important in fluid flow across the capillary is **capillary filtration**. Capillary filtration is a function of two variables: the intrinsic hydraulic permeability of the endothelium and the other structural components of the capillary wall (known as *capillary wall permeability*) and the total surface area of the capillaries supplying a local area of tissue. Capillary filtration, the volume of fluid that can filter from the intravascular space of the capillary into the interstitium, is directly proportional to both capillary wall permeability and capillary wall surface area. The **capillary filtration coefficient (K_f)** is a quantitative measure of these two parameters. It is expressed in milliliters of fluid transported per minute per 1 mm Hg pressure per 100 g of tissue. The K_f is independent of hydrostatic and oncotic pressures and depends on the microscopic structure of the vessels and tight junctions between the endothelial cells. For example, if the capillary wall is damaged by toxins or inflammatory stimuli, then it becomes much more permeable, the K_f goes up, and much more plasma enters the interstitial space. Likewise, if the smooth muscle of small arterioles relaxes, opening (or recruiting) previously closed capillaries in a tissue bed, the total capillary surface area rises, the K_f increases, and transudation goes up.

The Starling Equation The relationship among hydrostatic pressures, oncotic pressures, and the K_f, as well as the flow of fluid across a capillary, can be expressed in a compact form known as the **Starling equation** (also known as the Starling-Landis equation, based on Landis's experimental confirmation of Starling's original 1896 hypothesis):

$$J = (K_f) \times [(Pc - Pi) - (\Pi c - \Pi i)]$$

The Starling equation states that the overall flow of fluid, J, expressed in units of volume per time in a given mass of tissue (mL of fluid transported per minute per 100 g tissue) is equal to the K_f times the differences between the hydrostatic and oncotic forces between the capillary lumen and interstitial space. A positive value for J indicates fluid filtration from the vasculature into the tissues (transudation), whereas a negative value for J indicates fluid resorption. The magnitude of J indicates the quantity of fluid flow.

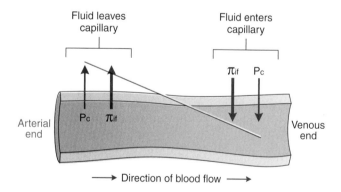

Figure 11.5 Forces determining fluid flux across a capillary endothelium. As blood flows from the arteriolar end of the capillary toward the venous end, the capillary hydrostatic pressure, Pc, decreases. The intersitial hydrostatic pressure (Pi), the capillary oncotic pressure (Πc), and the interstitial oncotic pressure (Πi) are also shown. At a critical point, the balance of forces shifts from favoring the efflux of fluid from the capillary lumen into the interstitium (transudation) to favoring the resorption of fluid from the interstitium back into the capillary (resorption). Filtration exceeds resorption, but the lymphatics maintain fluid homeostasis in the interstitium by absorbing the excess fluid.

The Flow of Lymph

The production of lymph takes place in all the major organs, with the exception of the brain, retina, bone marrow, cartilage, cornea, lens, intima of the large arteries, umbilical cord, and inner renal medulla. The lymphatics return fluids, proteins, and other substances that have been filtered but not resorbed by the tissue capillaries; but how does lymph flow in lymphatic vessels from peripheral tissues (e.g., in the legs) back to the central circulation (in the upper chest) without a heart to pump the fluid? The forces involved in transporting lymph through lymphatic vessels back to the subclavian veins include extrinsic forces and intrinsic forces. These forces are necessary because the return of lymph to the venous circulation is an uphill process, known as negative *vis a tergo*, or negative "force from behind." However, only small forces need to be generated owing to the presence of lymphatic valves, which impede backflow and assist the one-way flow of lymph toward the heart (see Figure 11.3).

Extrinsic forces that aid in the flow of lymph include any processes that lead to the generation of tissue compressive or suction forces. Most important are active striated muscle contractions, particularly limb movements during periods of standing and walking. Maximal lymph flow, therefore, occurs during periods of physical activity. This concept is shown in FIGURE 11.6, which depicts lymph flow during a typical 24-hour period. Other extrinsic forces include the rhythmic changes of intra-abdominal and intrathoracic pressure caused by respiration, intestinal peristalsis, and the pulsatility of arteries. It is easy to understand how long periods of lying in bed (e.g., during hospitalization) can lead to the stasis of lymph flow and can produce fluid accumulation in tissues.

Intrinsic forces that assist lymph flow are the intrinsic contractility of lymphatic vessels. Individual lymphatic segments between two valves can become distended and then contract, resulting in the propulsion of fluid upstream into the next segment in a peristaltic fashion. The contribution of intrinsic forces to overall lymph flow, however, is thought to be low. Sympathetic autonomic nervous system stimulation (see Chapter 5), through the action of catecholamines on α and β-adrenergic receptors, has also been shown to affect lymphatic contractility. In particular, large blood losses lead to an increase in thoracic duct flow, probably due to a catecholamine surge. Other mediators, including anesthetics such as pentobarbital and halothane, have been shown to cause a decrease in lymph flow. Both extrinsic and intrinsic forces are also thought to aid in generating a pressure gradient favoring the drainage of fluid from the interstitium into the terminal lymphatics (lacteals).

As mentioned earlier, lymph flowing from most of the body enters the cisterna chyli and thereafter the thoracic duct, eventually dumping into the left subclavian vein. Lymph from the right upper extremity, the right half of the thorax, and the right half of the head enters the right lymphatic duct and drains into the right subclavian vein.

LYMPHATIC SYSTEM PATHOPHYSIOLOGY

Any processes in lymph physiology, including filtration, resorption, or lymph flow, can become dysfunctional, resulting in disease. The aberrant accumulation of fluid in the interstitial space leads to edema. Edema occurs most commonly by one of four possible mechanisms: increased intravascular hydrostatic pressure, decreased intravascular oncotic pressure, increased capillary permeability, or lymphatic obstruction. The first three mechanisms are

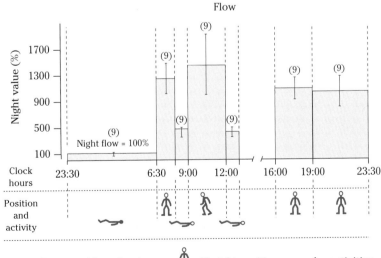

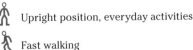

Figure 11.6 Variation in lymph flow over 24 hours. Because skeletal muscle contraction compresses lymphatics and helps propel lymph back toward the systemic circulation, physical activity greatly augments lymph flow. The x-axis shows the time of day and the symbol of the person shows the degree of activity. The y-axis shows the flow of lymph as a percentage of the average flow in a person asleep at night. The numbers in parentheses indicate the number of limbs in which lymph flow was measured. Mean ± SE refers to the mean and the standard error values for the flows indicated. The height of the boxes denotes the mean, and the lengths of the bars represent the standard error.

direct alterations in the parameters in the Starling equation and lead to a hyperfiltration state in the microcirculation. The fourth mechanism leads to reduced lymphatic flow due to obstruction in the lymphatic vessels or nodes.

Increased Intravascular Hydrostatic Pressure

Increased intravascular hydrostatic pressure (Pc) occurs in states of generalized increased intravascular plasma volume, such as total fluid overload. It can also result from a localized obstruction in which increased hydrostatic pressure occurs proximal to the obstruction. In congestive heart failure (CHF), impaired pumping function of the heart's left ventricle leads to increased pressure in the pulmonary venous circulation as blood backs up, leading to dangerous fluid accumulation in the lungs called **pulmonary edema**. This condition is extremely dangerous because the fluid interferes with the normal gas-exchange function of the lungs, thereby causing impaired uptake of oxygen by the blood (hypoxemia). In cirrhotic liver disease, obstruction to flow in the portal venous system owing to the destruction of liver parenchyma leads to portal hypertension (elevated Pc) and fluid accumulation in the abdominal cavity called **ascites**.

Decreased Intravascular Oncotic Pressure

Decreased intravascular oncotic pressure (Πc) occurs in states of hypoproteinemia, usually measured as **hypoalbuminemia**, a low concentration of albumin in the blood. This condition can result if protein intake is too low, as in cases of malnutrition, or if gastrointestinal malabsorption prevents ingested dietary protein from being efficiently taken up. Hypoalbuminemia may also occur if too little albumin is produced, as in liver failure, or if too much albumin is lost in the urine, as in the nephrotic syndrome.

Whatever the cause, decreased Πc impairs the ability of the venous end of the capillary to resorb fluid. Initially, the excess interstitial fluid is returned to the systemic circulation by the lymphatics, but once the volume of fluid exceeds the capacity of the lymphatics, edema results. This explains the appearance of severely malnourished children who paradoxically have protuberant abdomens: their peritoneal cavities are distended by ascites.

Increased Capillary Filtration Coefficient

Increased capillary permeability, expressed quantitatively as an increased CFC, occurs when the capillary endothelium is damaged. Examples are burns, in which connective tissue is destroyed; local inflammation, in which inflammatory stimuli loosen the tight junctions between endothelial cells; and toxic damage, in which endothelial cell dysfunction occurs, as in sepsis, pancreatitis, and inhalation injuries (e.g., damage from inhaling smoke). When such capillary damage affects the lungs, the acute respiratory distress syndrome (ARDS) results (see Chapter 17).

Lymphatic Obstruction

Lymphatic obstruction occurs in any disease in which lymphatic vessels or nodes are blocked. In lymphoma and some other metastatic cancers, neoplastic cells may invade and disrupt lymphatic channels. The same is true when lymph nodes are surgically removed, as is common with cancer surgery, and in certain parasitic infections such as filariasis, where small worms penetrate the system and obstruct lymph flow. In all cases, the resultant edema is localized to the area drained by the affected nodal group. A common example is lymphedema affecting a single upper extremity after extensive lymph node dissection for breast cancer.

IMMUNE SYSTEM TELEOLOGY

The immune system is arguably as complex as the nervous system. These two systems share a number of structural and functional features, and they, perhaps more than any other systems, contribute to individual identity by largely defining the difference between self and nonself. For example, identical twins, who have the same DNA and therefore have essentially interchangeable hearts, lungs, kidneys, and livers, differ most in their distinct immune systems and nervous systems.

The nervous system is largely a network for gathering, processing, and responding to energy, collecting environmental (internal as well as external) data, and turning energy (e.g., light, sound, touch) into information (electrochemical impulses such as action potentials). The immune system is a network for gathering, processing, and responding to matter. As mentioned in the introduction to this chapter, the many diverse structures and functions of the immune system can be thought of as thematically related using the metaphor of warfare carried out by the cells of the immune system in defense of the body. In this metaphorical war, immune system cells are the soldiers, immune system molecules are their tools and weapons, and the gathering, processing, and responding to matter are their defensive actions. In the most commonly accepted hypothesis about its purpose, the immune system protects the body from infection (the invasion of the body by pathogenic microbes). Immune system cells sample the matter contacting the body's borders, looking for evidence of pathogenic invaders. When such invaders are detected, the immune system is activated and responds with efforts to destroy or drive out the enemy. In addition to an increased susceptibility to infection, dysfunction of the immune system is often accompanied by certain diseases (e.g., malignancies) whose infectious basis is unproven. This has led some scientists to argue persuasively that the purpose of the immune system is really protection from danger (be it "foreign invaders" such as bacteria or "domestic terrorists" such as cancer cells).

Inflammation is the movement (by means of increased blood flow and increased vascular permeability) of active immune cells, fluid, and blood proteins into an area of the body. It is often observed when that anatomic area suffers trauma or infection (invasion by a pathogenic virus, bacteria, fungus, or parasite). Acutely inflamed tissue typically manifests some or all of the following: rubor (redness), dolor (pain), calor (heat), tumor (swelling), and functio laesa (loss of function). Inflammatory immune responses occur in nearly all tissues during infection or injury and are closely linked with the topics presented in prior chapters. The central players include leukocytes from the blood (see Chapter 9), which must interact with activated endothelial cells (see Chapter 10) to reach endangered tissues. The interactions among immune cells as they process and respond to foreign or dangerous materials occur largely in lymph nodes. These responses are usually protective and maintain homeostasis. When they are inadequate or excessively destructive, they contribute to disease. This section of the chapter introduces a conceptual framework of inflammation and immunity as physiologic responses to infection or irritation.

Innate and Adaptive Immunity

The body's defense against threats has three distinct but highly interrelated subsystems. The first line of defense against microbial invaders is preventing their entry by maintaining **physical barriers** such as intact skin and mucous membranes. This strategy is relatively (but not completely) nonspecific, meaning that it functions with little regard for the specific qualities of the invader.

The second line of defense is the **innate immune response**, in which certain white blood cells (e.g., macrophages, neutrophils, and eosinophils) and plasma protein systems, such as the complement cascade, recognize and respond to invaders. The innate immune cells detect microbes by means of cell-surface receptors, which are generally glycoproteins that bind to specific structures (called pathogen-associated molecular patterns [PAMPs])

that microbes have but human cells lack. When these *pattern recognition receptors* (PRRs) "grab hold" of an invader, the innate immune cell is activated and responds to the pathogen by creating inflammation.

Innate immune responses are somewhat specific, in that they depend on PAMPs, but PRRs are invariant, encoded by genes that do not change, and therefore cannot adapt. Innate immune responses are rapid, working within minutes to days to control and eradicate infection. They are involved in tissue repair following trauma and help contain injurious agents such as foreign bodies.

If the innate immune system cannot eradicate an invader, the third line of defense, the **adaptive immune response**, is invoked. It differs importantly from innate immunity in terms of time, specificity, plasticity, and memory. The major cells of adaptive immunity are lymphocytes: T cells and B cells. It takes days (as opposed to minutes or hours for the innate system) to mount the initial adaptive immune response to a new invader. In contrast, the adaptive immune response is not only highly specific for a given invader but it also changes to meet new demands. The cell-surface receptors of T and B cells recognize particular structures of microbes, and their derivation involves a dramatic reshuffling of genes. After a pathogen is eradicated, adaptive immune memory cells persist in the circulation, and if the same pathogen reinfects the host, they mount a more rapid and more exuberant secondary response. Often, the initial encounter between a particular microbe and a human host will produce disease as the host's adaptive immune system responds. On subsequent encounters, however, the adaptive immune response may be so rapid that the pathogen is eradicated before it can produce disease. This phenomenon is called **immunity**, the exquisitely specific response that differentiates "self" (the human host, in this case) from "nonself." Immunity protects the body by triggering a powerful response to neutralize and destroy pathogens, proteins, or cells that are nonself.

The three lines of defense are highly intertwined and interdependent. Innate immune cells detect invaders and signal adaptive immune cells about a threat. When in turn the adaptive immune system marshals its forces, it conscripts innate immune cells to do much of the fighting.

IMMUNE SYSTEM STRUCTURE

The immunologic organs include the barrier surfaces (skin, epithelial layers, and mucosae), the bone marrow, the thymus, the spleen, and the lymph nodes and other lymphoid tissues. Many important immune system cells move throughout the body but use fixed structures such as lymph nodes as headquarters for meeting and communicating with other cells. Among the hundreds of different immune system molecules, this section will focus on those important for the detection of pathogens, communication among immune cells, and eradication of invaders.

Immune System Organs and Tissues

The organs of the immune system constitute the physical barrier defenses of the body and are responsible for the production and "education" of immune cells. The spleen, lymph nodes, and lymphoid organs are analogous structures, each providing a headquarters or outpost for immune cells in a given anatomic location. The spleen screens the bloodstream, the lymph nodes screen the lymph, and lymphoid organs screen border regions such as the gastrointestinal tract and the upper airways.

Skin and Epithelia   Chief among the barriers representing the first line of defense is the skin. Keratinocytes in the epidermis adhere to one another, preventing microbes from freely entering the internal environs of the body, and breaches in this layer (burns, punctures, and other wounds) are important means by which pathogens enter the body. The epithelial linings of the alimentary canal and respiratory tract perform similar functions.

Bone Marrow   As discussed in Chapter 9, innate and adaptive immune cells, like other blood cells, all start life in the bone marrow, where they develop from stem cells. When stem cells undergo mitosis, some daughter cells remain stem cells, while others, under the influence of complex signal networks, differentiate (see Figure 9.6). Inherited or acquired deficiencies or dysfunction of the bone marrow thus leads to profound, possibly deadly, immune inadequacy. Such so-called immunodeficiency leaves the affected individual susceptible to infections.

The Thymus   The thymus, a lymphoid organ in the mediastinum, is critical to the "education" of the T cells of the adaptive immune system. It is divided by connective tissue septae into lobules, each of which has an outer cortex and an inner medulla. The thymus is most prominent in infants and children, and it involutes as we age.

The Spleen   Located in the left upper quadrant of the peritoneal cavity, the spleen is the circulation's largest lymphoid organ. Beneath its capsule, the splenic parenchyma is divided by incomplete connective tissue trabeculae. Histologically, the parenchyma is divided into red pulp and white pulp. Trabecular arteries penetrate the parenchyma, with central arterioles branching off, surrounded by white pulp. A periarteriolar lymphoid sheath (PALS) rich in T cells surrounds the central arteriole, and a corona rich in B cells is adjacent. Germinal centers are areas where stimulated immune cells reproduce. Blood eventually flows into trabecular veins (FIGURE 11.7). The spleen is important in immune surveillance of the bloodstream itself.

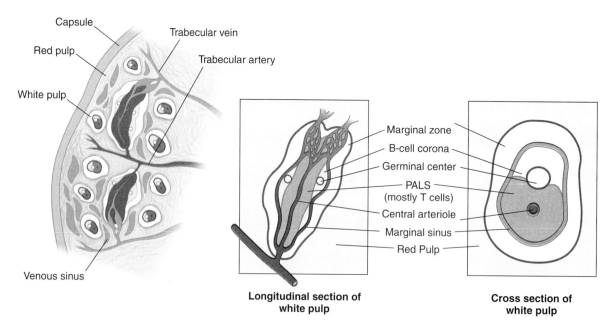

Longitudinal section of white pulp

Cross section of white pulp

Figure 11.7   The structure of the spleen. The parenchyma is divided into red pulp and white pulp. Central arteries are surrounded by periarteriolar lymphoid sheaths (PALS) populated largely by T cells. Germinal centers, where stimulated immune cells reproduce, and B cell coronae are also components of the white pulp.

Lymph Nodes and Other Lymphoid Tissues The numerous lymph nodes scattered throughout the body are important headquarters through which adaptive immune cells pass to receive and process information, communicate with one another, and reproduce. The gross structure is presented in Figure 11.4. As in the spleen, there are distinct but adjacent T cell-rich areas (paracortical) and B cell-rich areas (follicles). Lymph nodes harbor cells that monitor peripheral tissues for pathogenic invaders. Lymphoid tissues such as the tonsils of the pharynx and the Peyer's patches of the gastrointestinal tract are structurally and functionally similar to lymph nodes.

Immune System Cells

The cells of all three lines of defense of the immune system actively protect the body by varied means. Although the most superficial layers of the skin are dead and help prevent infection by adhering to one another, the living cells of the barrier surfaces (skin, endothelium, and epithelial and mucosal surfaces) reproduce; they secrete substances that frustrate, repel, or poison pathogens, and they communicate with and facilitate the function of innate and adaptive immune cells. The cells of the second and third lines of immune defense are more obviously dynamic.

Innate Immune Cells As mentioned above, innate immune cells are critical not only because they constitute the early defense systems of the body, but also because they alert, direct, and carry out orders from adaptive immune cells. Some innate immune cells circulate through the bloodstream, entering extravascular tissues only when needed to fight an invader. Others reside in tissue "outposts," monitoring the body's borders for invaders or other threats, leaving these tissues only to carry information to adaptive immune cells in lymph nodes. FIGURE 11.8A shows the major innate immune cells.

Granulocytes Among the innate immune cells, three (neutrophils, eosinophils, and basophils) are called *granulocytes* because they have numerous intracytoplasmic granules. Neutrophils are the most numerous granulocytes (normally constituting approximately 45% to 74% of leukocytes), followed by eosinophils (normally 0% to 7% of leukocytes), and then basophils (normally 0% to 2% of leukocytes). Until they are recruited to tissues, granulocytes circulate in the bloodstream.

Mast Cells Mast cells resemble basophils in having numerous intracytoplasmic granules and in containing certain chemicals and mediators associated with allergic reactions. However, basophils circulate in the blood as mature cells, while mast cells mature

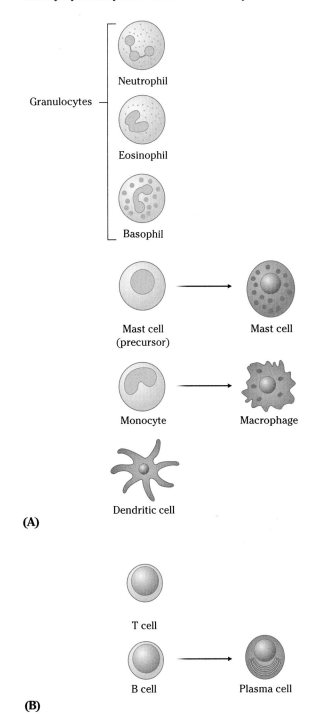

Figure 11.8 Innate and adaptive immune cells. **A.** Innate immune cells. Neutrophils, eosinophils, and basophils are called *granulocytes* because of their intracytoplasmic granules. Mast cells appear to be stuffed full of granules; they circulate as immature precursors, maturing in peripheral tissues. Monocytes differentiate into macrophages in tissues. Dendritic cells are named for their many branches. **B.** Adaptive immune cells. Lymphocytes (T cells and B cells) cannot be distinguished by light microscopy. B cells can differentiate into plasma cells.

only when they reach peripheral tissues such as the lung, the gastrointestinal tract, and the skin. Mast cells are powerful effector cells, and they are increasingly recognized as having important regulatory functions in immune responses.

Monocytes and Macrophages Monocytes are innate immune cells that have a single, bean-shaped nucleus. When circulating monocytes exit the bloodstream and enter tissues, they mature into macrophages. Macrophages, stimulated by the presence of an invader or activated by molecular signals of inflammation, may differentiate into epithelioid cells, and two or more may fuse, forming multinucleate giant cells.

Dendritic Cells Immature dendritic cells reside in peripheral tissues, where they have long projections and a central, oval nucleus. They are important innate immune system "border guards," sampling the tissue environment and staying vigilant for invaders. When they detect a pathogen, they migrate to a nearby lymph node and mature, then communicate with cells of the adaptive immune system.

Adaptive Immune Cells The adaptive immune cells are collectively called **lymphocytes** because they are the predominant cells found in lymph. However, they join other leukocytes in circulating in the blood as well. Viewed under the light microscope, all mature, resting lymphocytes appear essentially similar, having a central, round nucleus and a small volume of surrounding cytoplasm. Figure 11.8B shows the adaptive immune cells.

B Cells and Plasma Cells B cells are named for the bone marrow, where they are produced. Different B cells are designed to respond to different stimuli. Once a given B cell encounters its specific stimulus, it is activated and reproduces, creating a population (or clone) of identical daughter cells that all respond to the same specific stimulus. Some of these daughter cells undergo further maturation to become plasma cells, which are larger than resting B cells, have more cytoplasm with prominent Golgi apparatus and endoplasmic reticulum, and have a nucleus that resembles a clock face.

T Cells T cells originate in the bone marrow, and while still immature, they migrate to the thymus (for which they are named) to complete their early development. Like B cells, resting mature T cells have a central, round nucleus and little cytoplasm.

Immune System Molecules

Immune system cells gather, process, and respond to matter on the molecular level. The important molecules of the immune system fall into three broad categories: the nonself molecules detected by the immune system indicating the presence of an invader, the self proteins used to detect nonself molecules, and the molecules used by the immune system to fight invaders. This section describes some of the many molecules important in innate and adaptive immunity.

Antigens An **antigen** is any substance that provokes an immune response, or is *immunogenic*. An antigen may be a peptide or a protein, a lipid, a carbohydrate, or some combinations of these. An important example of a combination antigen is **lipopolysaccharide (LPS)**, a component of the cell wall of certain pathogenic bacteria. A molecule of LPS has a fatty acid-containing lipid A region bound to polysaccharide regions and is a powerful immunogen. An **epitope** is a region of an antigenic molecule that is specifically recognized by antibodies or T cell receptors (FIGURE 11.9A). Generally, small monomers, such as amino acids, nucleic acids, and single sugars, are too small to be effective antigens. Some small molecules that are, on their own, insufficient to be antigens become effective immunogens when bound to a normally inert host protein. Such small molecules are called **haptens** (see Figure 11.9B).

Major Histocompatibility Complexes The **major histocompatibility complex (MHC)** is a region of human chromosome 6 that contains a number of genes encoding proteins important in the function of the immune system. The name comes from the identification of the complex as a major determinant of

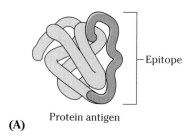

(A)   Protein antigen

Epitope

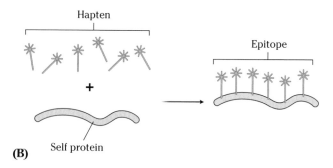

Hapten

Epitope

(B)   Self protein

+

Figure 11.9 Antigens, epitopes, and haptens. **A.** An antigen is a substance that elicits an immune response. The protein antigen shown here has a region on the right side, an epitope, that is specifically recognized by T cell or B cell receptors. **B.** Small molecules called haptens are not immunogenic on their own, but when bound to a host protein do constitute an effective antigen.

whether transplanted tissues are accepted (histocompatible) or rejected (histoincompatible), both in experiments with mice and in the care of humans. Mice are more likely to tolerate a transplant from another mouse having identical MHC genes than from a mouse with different MHC genes. The name is somewhat misleading, however, because transplantation is not a normal physiologic occurrence and the influence of MHC proteins on the fate of transplanted tissues is not their dominant physiologic function.

The MHC genes code for two sets of cell-surface receptors that hold protein fragments so that cells of the adaptive immune system can recognize them (the peptide antigens) as self or nonself. MHC molecules are therefore peptide-presenting proteins.

The two most important subtypes of MHC molecules are MHC I and MHC II. MHC I molecules are present on the surface of all nucleated body cells. MHC II molecules are generally restricted to the surface of immune cells; specifically, cells that can digest and "present" antigenic peptides to T cells (see below). The extracellular portion of the MHC molecules has a groove or cleft into which a peptide can fit (FIGURE 11.10). The human genome encodes a number of

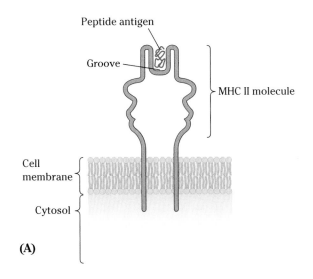

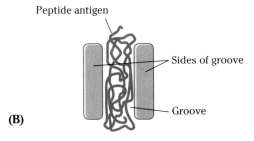

Figure 11.10 An MHC II molecule binding a peptide. **A.** Viewed from the side, the peptide is nestled in the groove of the MHC II molecule. **B.** Viewed from above, the walls of the MHC molecule and the fit between the peptide and the MHC II are appreciated from the perspective of cells such as T cells. Antigenic peptides fit into MHC clefts sort of like hot dogs fitting into buns.

MHC molecules, each able to accommodate a modest number of structurally related peptides. Thus, individuals with different MHC genes may differ in their ability to respond to a given antigen. If a person lacks all MHC genes encoding molecules that can accommodate a given peptide, he or she may not be able to mount an effective adaptive immune response against that peptide.

Antibodies **Antibodies** are proteins secreted by B cells that bind antigen. Because these proteins were recognized as products of the immune system, they were also called *immunoglobulins* (globulin is a term denoting a protein that can be coagulated by heat). There are five major **isotypes** of immunoglobulin (Ig), namely IgA, IgD, IgE, IgG, and IgM, and some subtypes (e.g., there are four subtypes of IgG).

Immunoglobulin monomers consist of two heavy chains and two light chains, arranged in a Y shape. Each branch of the Y is capable of binding a given epitope (FIGURE 11.11A). Because the two heavy chains and two light chains of a given antibody molecule are identical, the two branches of an Ig bind identical epitopes. The two branches of the antibody are thus called the *antigen binding fragment (F(ab′)$_2$)*, or the *F(ab′)$_2$ region*. The stem of an antibody molecule is called the *constant fragment Fc* or the *Fc region*. The Fc regions of antibodies of a given isotype are identical but differ from those antibodies of a different isotype. The F(ab′)$_2$ regions of antibodies that bind to different antigens are different. Thus, two different antibodies of the same isotype (e.g., an IgG$_1$ antibody that binds to an epitope of the bacterium *Streptococcus pneumoniae* and an IgG$_1$ antibody that recognizes a component of the Epstein-Barr virus) differ in their F(ab′)$_2$ regions but by definition have the same Fc portion. It is also possible (see below) for two antibodies of different isotypes to have the same antigen specificity; that is, they have different Fc portions but essentially identical F(ab′)$_2$ regions.

Once secreted by B cells or plasma cells, different antibody isotypes are directed to different locations in the body. IgG and IgM circulate in the blood; IgE circulates in the blood as well, but some binds to the surface of mast cells and basophils, waiting to activate these cells when antigen is encountered; and IgA is secreted at the mucosal surfaces, such as the gastrointestinal tract, to bind pathogens before they gain a foothold in the body. IgG, IgE, and IgD circulate as monomers, IgA as a dimer, and IgM as a pentamer (Figure 11.11B).

Antigen Receptors The exquisite specificity of the adaptive immune response resides in the precise binding of antigen receptors on B cells and T cells to specific epitopes. Because a given B cell or T cell pro-

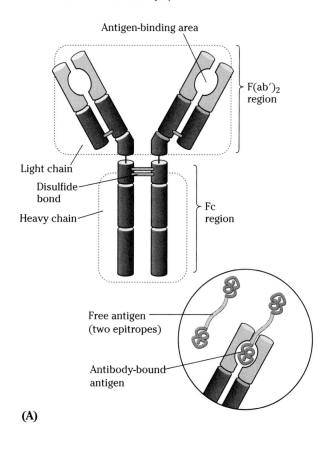

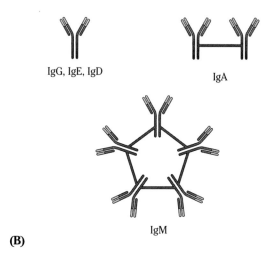

(A)

(B)

Figure 11.11 Antibodies. **A.** An antibody monomer, with identical antigen-binding areas formed by the ends of the heavy and light chains representing the F(ab')$_2$ region and the other ends of the heavy chains, bound together by disulfide bonds, making up the Fc region. **B.** Monomeric IgG, dimeric IgA, and pentameric IgM molecules.

duces antigen receptors of only one specificity, these receptors essentially determine the narrow range of substances to which the cell can respond. The cost of this precision is the need for great numbers of B cells and T cells, many of which produce nonfunctional receptors or receptors directed against antigens the host may never encounter.

B Cell Receptors   The antigen-specific receptors on B cells are essentially antibodies bound to the B cell surface (FIGURE 11.12A). A given B cell produces antibody of one specificity, but throughout its lifetime it may change the isotype of that antibody. Early in development, the antigen specificity of a particular B cell is determined. The immature B cell produces membrane-bound IgM of this specificity, and it is this cell-surface IgM that is the B cell receptor. If this specific B cell is activated by the presence of its antigen in the body, it may switch to the production of antibody (e.g., the secreted protein of its antigenic specificity). Thus, the B cell receptor is the cell-surface version of antibody or, seen from the other perspective, antibody is the secreted/soluble version of the B cell receptor. Furthermore, a given B cell that started producing antibody of a given isotype may switch to produce antibody of another isotype, say from IgM to IgG$_1$. Since each B cell is specific for one or a very few structurally related antigens, effective protection from the myriad pathogens in the world depends on the normal immune system having millions of B cells of different specificity.

T Cell Receptors   T cell receptors resemble B cell receptors in their ontogeny but differ from them in their structure and function (see Figure 11.12B). Like B cell receptors, they are made up of a number of proteins. However, T cell receptors remain bound to the cell surface and are not secreted. As with B cells, the receptors of a given T cell have the same antigenic specificity (i.e., they bind the same epitope or epitopes). Thus, a healthy immune system capable of dealing with a wide world full of different antigens must possess a large population of different T cells.

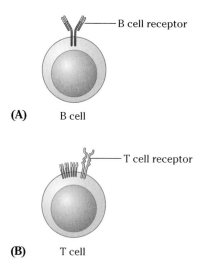

(A)   B cell

(B)   T cell

Figure 11.12 B cell and T cell receptors. **A.** The B cell receptor is a membrane-bound version of an antibody. It has the same antigen specificity as the antibody the B cell secretes. **B.** The T cell receptor does not have a secreted counterpart.

Cytokines, Chemokines, and Their Receptors   As in the nervous system, communication between and among cells is critical to the function of the immune system. While the electrochemical "language" of neurons is composed of ions and neurotransmitters, the language of the immune system is largely encoded by a large group of messenger molecules called **cytokines**. Cells secrete these molecular "words" in regulated ways and often in complex combinations simultaneously or in temporal sequence. However, just as spoken language requires a speaker and a listener (even if the latter and the former are the same person), so cytokines can have their effects only on cells equipped with appropriate receptors, many of which are expressed on the cell surface.

One particularly important subset of cytokines is a group of mediators that induce movement in target cells. Such chemotactic cytokines are called **chemokines**. Different chemokines draw different leukocytes (those having the appropriate receptors) to specific tissue sites. Other chemotactic molecules include bacterial products, complement components (such as C5a), and certain leukotrienes (such as LTB_4).

Adhesion Molecules   Since most innate and all adaptive immune system cells start off life in the bone marrow and then circulate in the blood, they must have a mechanism for exiting the circulation and reaching peripheral tissues. This process is called **diapedesis**, and it looks like a leukocyte in the bloodstream slowing down, rolling along and then sticking to the vessel wall, and finally squeezing its way through a gap between the endothelial cells of the vessel wall. The molecules involved in this critical and complex process include a group of cell surface proteins called **adhesion molecules**. There are three large families in this group: *selectins*, *integrins*, and some members of the *immunoglobulin superfamily*. As implied by their name, the members of the last family bear a structural resemblance to antibodies.

Effector Molecules   Once information about a threat has been transmitted to immune effector cells, and signaling molecules such as chemokines have attracted the cells to the front lines of the battle with a pathogen, the activated cells must fight the invader. Thus, in addition to molecules used for communication, many immune cells have an armamentarium of molecules they release to defend the body. **Vasoactive mediators** promote vasodilation and vascular permeability; they include histamine, serotonin, complement, certain cytokines (interleukin-1 and tumor necrosis factor), prostaglandins, leukotrienes, thromboxane, bradykinin, and nitric oxide. Such molecules have dramatic effects on blood vessels, causing smooth muscle relaxation and changes in epithelial cells that facilitate the passage of fluid, proteins, and cells from the circulation into tissues. Vasoactive mediators bring about many of the signs of inflammation: the redness, swelling, and heat of inflamed tissues all result in part from the increased blood flow. In addition, by increasing the diameter of the blood vessel and recruiting more capillaries, velocity of blood flow decreases, expediting diapedesis. If concentrations of vasoactive substances are high enough, these effects may extend from local to systemic. (See Clinical Application Box *Systemic Inflammatory Response Syndrome*.)

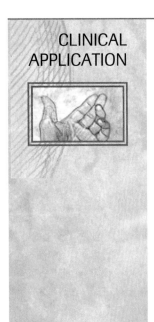

CLINICAL APPLICATION

SYSTEMIC INFLAMMATORY RESPONSE SYNDROME

If infection (especially with pathogenic bacteria) or traumatic tissue damage is widespread, the immune response may result in high concentrations of vasoactive mediators. Because these potent vasodilators dramatically increase the radius of a blood vessel lumen, the resistance to laminar flow of blood drops. In accordance with Ohm's law, the decrease in resistance correlates with lowered blood pressure (see Chapter 7). Thus, patients with severe bacterial infections in the blood (bacteremia) may also develop the **systemic inflammatory response syndrome (SIRS)**. In the case of bacterial infection, the term *sepsis* has also been used to describe the constellation of abnormal body temperature, low blood pressure (due in part to the vasodilation), high heart rate (compensatory tachycardia), and dysfunction of other organs such as the lungs, gastrointestinal system, and central nervous system. SIRS may also occur in situations where noninfectious inflammation runs out of control, such as severe pancreatitis or trauma.

It is difficult to treat SIRS or sepsis in part because the very immune response that eradicates the infection produces substances like the vasoactive mediators, which bring about the symptoms and signs of the syndrome. Too much of a good thing may be as harmful as a lack thereof.

Once activated leukocytes are in the heat of battle, they may release chemicals that damage pathogenic invaders, including degradative enzymes that catabolize proteins (proteases), lipids, or nucleic acids; oxygen free radicals; and proteins that puncture pathogen membranes. These effector molecules may also be destructive to host cells. Neutrophils are especially important inflammatory cells that, when activated, undergo an "oxidative burst" in which highly reactive oxidative species are produced by enzymes such as NADPH oxidase, which converts O_2 to O_2^- (superoxide) and H_2O_2 (hydrogen peroxide). Another neutrophil enzyme, myeloperoxidase, then converts H_2O_2 to HOCl (the hypochlorite radical), which is particularly toxic to bacteria.

The Complement System The **complement system** is a cascade of bloodborne innate immune system proteins analogous to the coagulation cascade (see Chapter 10). Most complement proteins (designated C1, C2, C3, etc.) are inactive plasma proenzymes under normal conditions. The complement proteins at the "top" of the cascade are activated by binding either to PAMPs on the surface of microbes or to the Fc regions of antigen-bound antibodies. When activated, these early complement proteins enzymatically cleave other components, activating them. Sequential activation of complement components results in two types of effector molecules. Small fragments of some complement proteins (e.g., C4a, C3a, and C5a, in the order of their production) attract and activate immune system cells to the area of inflammation. Larger "terminal" complement proteins (C5b to C9) combine to form a channel (or pore) called the *membrane attack complex*, which inserts into the cell membrane of an invader, causing potentially lethal damage to the microbe by cell lysis.

IMMUNE SYSTEM FUNCTION

To effectively defend the body against threats, the immune system must do more than fight invaders when they appear: it must produce and "train" cellular troops to detect pathogens, distinguishing between self and nonself. In addition, it prevents and limits invasion by maintaining fixed barriers, by stationing cells at tissue outposts, and by sending cells to patrol the body. Thus, even in the complete absence of active infection, the immune system is highly active.

Production of Immune Cells

With the exception of the cells involved in the barrier (first-line) defenses, cells of the innate and adaptive immune system originate in the bone marrow, derived from hematopoietic stem cells. Normally, granulocytes are released into the circulation as mature cells, capable of responding to pathogenic invaders. Mast cells, monocytes, and precursors of dendritic cells enter the blood incompletely differentiated and move into tissues to complete their maturation. Adaptive immune cells, however, have a more complex and protracted development.

Functional Classes of Immune Cells Some innate and some adaptive immune cells are either grouped together or differentiated based on similarities or differences in their activities (FIGURE 11.13). Among these functional classes of immune cells are (a) innate cells that are expert at engulfing pathogens, (b) cells that specialize in presenting antigen to T cells, (c) T cells that assist B cells and macrophages in fighting pathogens, and (d) T cells that are adept at destroying host cells co-opted by invaders.

Phagocytes **Phagocytes** are cells that take up material by phagocytosis (literally, "cell eating"); they include dendritic cells, macrophages, and neutrophils. All three of these innate immune cells posses cell-surface receptors that can bind to extracellular material and activate a complex program of cytoskeletal rearrangement, culminating in the engulfment of the material into the cell in a membrane-enclosed vesicle called an *endosome*. Endosomes are shuttled through the cytoplasm until they fuse with lysosomes, membrane-enclosed packets of digestive enzymes, leading to the demise and degradation of any invader unfortunate enough to be caught and intracellularly incarcerated. In the case of neutrophils, this is a major mechanism for combating infection and cleaning up the debris left when extracellular pathogens are killed. For dendritic cells and macrophages, this is also a critical step in the processing of antigens for presentation to T cells.

Antigen-Presenting Cells While many cells can process and present antigens to T cells under certain circumstances, the three types of antigen-presenting cells (APCs) specialized to do so (and therefore called professional APCs) are dendritic cells, macrophages, and B cells. Each one can take up materials in the immediate environment, digest them, and load fragments such as peptides into the groove of MHC II molecules. Once this is accomplished, they form close cell-to-cell connections called immunological synapses (another reminder of the parallel between the immune and nervous systems) with T cells, attempting to find a match between the peptide epitope in the MHC II cleft and the particular T cell's receptor. This attempted recognition of the MHC II-bound peptide by the T cell receptor is an essential

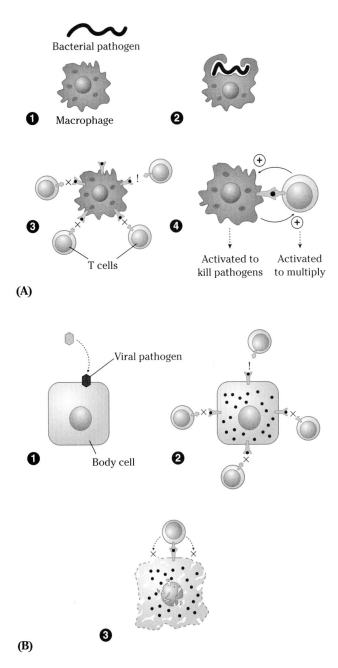

step in the activation of the adaptive immune system and the source of its specificity. Only those T cells whose receptor can bind to the peptide in the MHC II groove will be activated and stimulated to multiply (thus producing a population of daughter T cells, each with the same antigen specificity). Communication between an APC and a T cell is a true dialogue. Once the APC has communicated antigenic information to the T cell of the right specificity, the activated T cell responds by giving the APC (and, later, other cells) orders on how to proceed. To find the right match, an APC searches through myriad T cells of different specificities, often in an anatomic location such as a lymph node.

While the innate APCs (dendritic cells and macrophages) take up a broad range of materials in only a semispecific way, the B cell is highly restricted in what it can take up and process because its antigen uptake receptor is the specific B cell receptor. This also means that two dendritic cells or two macrophages are likely to resemble each other more in their ability to take up and present antigen than two different B cells, which may differ dramatically in their efficiency at taking up a given substance.

Helper T Cells   On the basis of the type of invader against which they respond and exactly how they respond, T cells are classified into two broad subsets. One subset consists of those that expedite the function of B cells and macrophages; they are therefore called **helper T cells**. A helper T cell is triggered by a match between its specific T cell receptor and the peptide in the groove of an MHC II molecule on the surface of an APC. If the APC is a B cell, the T cell releases cytokines that activate the B cell and direct it to make antibodies against the foreign antigen. If the APC is a macrophage, cytokine signals from the helper T cell activate the metabolism of the macrophage, encouraging it to intensify its chemical barrage against invaders trapped in endosomes (see Figure 11.13A).

Cytotoxic T Cells   The other subset of T cells consists of those that kill infected host cells and are therefore termed **cytotoxic T cells**. As with helper T cells, a cytotoxic T cell is activated by the binding of its specific T cell receptor to the peptide in the groove of an MHC molecule. However, unlike the situation with helper T cells, the MHC molecule in this case is an MHC I on the surface of a host cell that has been infected with an intracytoplasmic pathogen such as a virus (see Figure 11.13B). Since MHC I molecules are expressed by all nucleated body cells (as opposed to MHC II molecules, which are generally expressed on the surface of APCs), in a sense any nucleated host cell may act like an APC

Figure 11.13 Antigen-presenting cells, phagocytosis, helper T cells, and cytotoxic T cells. **A.** An extracellular pathogen such as a bacterium is bound (*1*) and phagocytosed (*2*) by a macrophage. The bacterium is digested, and peptides are loaded into the clefts of MHC II molecules and expressed on the cell surface. Helper T cells gather around the macrophage, seeking a good fit between their T cell receptors and the pathogen peptide (*3*). Most cells do not match (*x*), but eventually one or more does (*!*). Once the match is made (*4*), the macrophage stimulates the helper T cell, which divides, stimulating itself and the macrophage. **B.** An intracytoplasmic pathogen such as a virus (1) infects a nucleated body cell. The infected cell loads some MHC I molecules with peptides derived from the virus and expresses them on its surface. Cytotoxic T cells gather around the infected cell, seeking a good fit between their T cell receptors and the pathogen peptide (*2*). Most cells do not match (*x*), but eventually one or more does (*!*). Once the match is made (*3*), the cytotoxic T cell releases mediators that induce apoptosis (programmed cell death or cell "suicide") in the infected cell.

to cytotoxic T cells. Once stimulated, the cytotoxic T cell executes a highly regulated program in which it releases mediators such as perforin that puncture the infected cell's membrane, and enzymes such as granzymes that enter the infected cell through these membrane perforations and initiate a sequence of cell "suicide" called *apoptosis*. The virally infected cell thus gives up its life for the collective good of impeding the virus.

The Production of Adaptive Immune Cell Antigen Receptors

As already mentioned, a critical feature of the adaptive immune system is the specificity of T cell and B cell receptors for a given antigen. Such receptors are produced by a complex process of gene rearrangement particular to the immune system. Genes are instructions written in the language of DNA and collected into an instruction manual of the human genome. Most cells maintain an unedited and unabridged copy of the instruction manual but actually express only those genes they need. They "read" only the instructions germane to their function, while the other gene instructions go unread and unexpressed.

The genome "instruction manual" is not nearly large enough to have a fixed, separate set of instructions for encoding the billions or even trillions of possible B cell and T cell receptors, yet the adaptive immune system requires novel, distinct, and specific receptors to protect the body from the huge population of rapidly evolving pathogens. The solution to this problem is a set of genes encoding different portions of a B cell receptor or T cell receptor, and a given cell chooses (randomly) a particular gene for each of the segments and then strings them together into a cohesive and complete instruction code. For example, there are four segments to the heavy chain of a B cell receptor, called the V, D, J, and C segments. The genome encodes for not one but for 65 V genes, any one of which has to be juxtaposed with one D gene, one J gene, and one C gene to form a functional heavy chain gene. Because there are 27 D genes, six J genes, and nine C genes, the combinatorial possibilities are enormous. A similar gene structure and therefore potential for diversity exists for the light chain of the B cell receptor and both chains of the T cell receptor. Unlike other body cells, adaptive immune cells actually cut out of their copy of the genome "instruction manual" the unselected genes, leaving only the selected genes "stitched" or "pasted" together in a neat format. In a similar manner, B cells that have selected the structure of their F(ab′)$_2$ regions by this method can later in life switch this gene to another of the genes (called C genes for "con-

stant") encoding the Fc region of the antibody. This is how a B cell that started off producing IgM can change to another isotype (such as IgG or IgE) that recognizes the same epitope (FIGURE 11.14).

This system of genetic rearrangement introduces two new problems. First, there is the possibility that in the editing process, a given cell may make a mistake and fail to produce readable genetic instructions. Such cells generally undergo apoptosis. Second, because the selection process is random, there is the possibility that a cell may formulate a genetic instruction that encodes a receptor that will bind not (or not only) to a foreign epitope, but to a *self* epitope. Overcoming these problems is the function of adaptive immune cell education.

The Education of Adaptive Immune Cells

Once T cell precursors have rearranged their receptor genes, they are "educated" in the thymus, where they are "tested" for the ability of their T cell receptor to bind to the host's MHC molecules. If a given T cell has created a genetic instruction encoding a receptor completely unable to recognize the host MHC, that T cell is of no use to the host's immune system, no matter what peptide (self or nonself) it carries. Such cells are deleted or inactivated. On the other hand, T cells whose receptors bind too strongly to the host MHC and cause activation even when the peptide in the MHC groove is a benign self epitope will needlessly activate the immune system and cause unwanted damage. These, too, are deleted or inactivated. The middle path is the ideal: T cells selected to survive and circulate, looking for their antigens, are those that recognize the host's MHC molecules but will bind tightly only if there is a foreign peptide in the groove.

Encountering Pathogens

For T and B cells that survive their "education" but have not yet met up with their antigen, cellular life consists primarily of wandering through the blood and lymphatics, seeking to encounter their specific antigen. At this stage, they are known as *naïve* T or B cells. To understand the sequence of events, we shall follow a hypothetical patient through two infections.

Intracellular Pathogens Our patient's first infection is with a respiratory virus. Despite efficient first-line respiratory mucosa defenses such as intact epithelium, mucus production, and the beating of cilia, viral particles in respiratory droplets succeed in infecting cells in his respiratory tract. Some infected cells die,

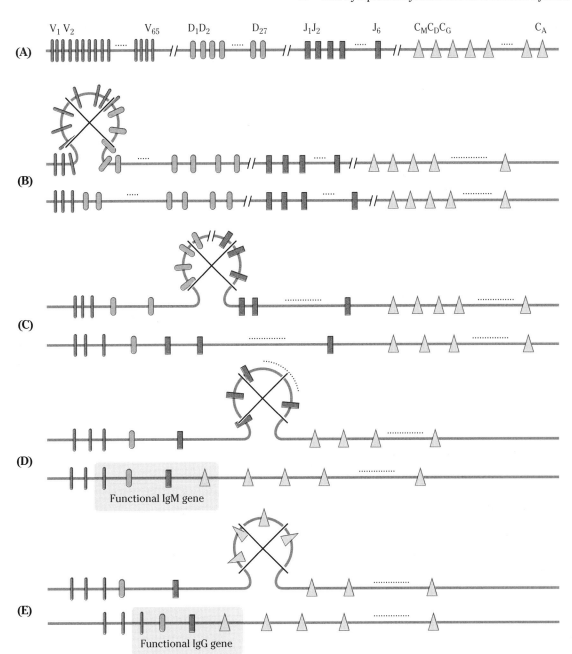

Figure 11.14 Genetic events in the production of the heavy chain of the B cell receptor and isotype switching. The various segments of the B cell receptor heavy chain that contributes to the F(ab')$_2$ region are called V, D, and J. The heavy chain C genes encode the different Fc regions of the antibodies that define isotypes (e.g., IgM, IgG, IgA). The human genome encodes 65 V genes, 27 D genes, and 6 J genes, and different B cells use different V, D, and J segments, stitching one of each of them together and deleting intervening DNA sequences to create a functional gene that encodes the F(ab') region of the antibody heavy chain. **A.** The intact genome with all the possible V, D, and J genes, as well as all nine C genes. **B.** In a highly regulated process, the DNA bends, breaks, and reseals, randomly bringing one V and one D gene together. **C.** The process repeats to join the previously juxtaposed V and D genes with a randomly selected J gene. **D.** Once this process is completed, the antibody specificity of the B cell is established and fixed, and the B cell produces membrane-bound IgM as its receptor by deleting unselected J genes and juxtaposing the selected VDJ genes with the gene encoding the constant region of IgM (C$_M$). **E.** After this B cell is stimulated, it can bend the DNA again and delete one or more constant region C genes to bring the VDJ gene into apposition with a different C gene; in this example, C$_G$, which leads to the production of a new isotype (here, IgG). Since the VDJ gene is unchanged, the new IgG has the same antigenic specificity as the IgM. This gene rearrangement process is a one-way street; deleted DNA cannot be pasted back in, so the alterations can only go forward, not backward. There is similar diversity in the B cell/immunoglobulin light chains and in the two chains of the T cell receptor.

releasing products normally sequestered intracellularly and alerting the cells of the innate immune system. Among these, macrophages are prominent, as they clean up the debris from dead cells.

The macrophages are activated, releasing inflammatory mediators such as *interleukin-1 (IL-1)*, which induces fever in the patient. However, the virus continues to spread. Infected cells load some viral peptides into MHC I molecules and display them on their surface, essentially sending out altruistic "red flags." In addition, the infected cells may secrete mediators called *interferons* that induce a relative state of viral resistance in the neighboring cells most at risk for infection by the spreading virus (thus interfering with the viral life cycle). Interferons and related signaling molecules have systemic effects like those of IL-1, causing fever, loss of appetite, weakness, and muscle aches. Eventually, cytotoxic T cells with receptors that recognize the viral antigens in the MHC I molecules displayed by infected cells arrive at the scene and kill off these compromised body cells. The infection is thus brought under control as the virus is eliminated.

Extracellular Pathogens Our patient's recovery from the viral illness involved the demise not only of the virus but also of infected cells of the respiratory epithelium. This resulted in a state of impaired first-line defense, and this "chink" in his living mucosal armor is exploited by a respiratory bacterial pathogen, *Streptococcus pneumoniae*. Unlike the intracellular viral pathogen, *S. pneumoniae* is extracellular. However, macrophages, neutrophils, and dendritic cells stationed in or patrolling the area bind onto the bacteria by means of PRRs that recognize PAMPs in the bacterial cell wall. These phagocytic cells engulf some of the bacteria and destroy them.

In addition, complement proteins, recognizing the foreign surface of the bacteria, initiate the complement cascade, which performs at least three important functions: (a) the chemotactic fragments C5a, C3a, and C4a (in order of decreasing potency) attract and activate more innate inflammatory cells; (b) complement proteins such as C3b deposited on the pathogen surface act like knobs onto which phagocytes can grab more efficiently, a process called **opsonization**; and (c) the formation of the "membrane attack complex" opens holes in the bacterial cell wall, damaging the pathogens.

Neutrophils release degradative enzymes and oxygen radicals that kill bacteria. The activated neutrophils are like kamikaze pilots, however, and many die along with the bacteria. The resultant mass of liquefied dead bacteria and cells is macroscopically recognized as **pus**, which, because of the metal content of some of the enzymes called metalloproteinases, is

yellow to green. The patient notes this as he starts to cough up purulent phlegm (sputum) and redevelops fever, malaise, and muscle and joint aches. However, he also starts feeling short of breath as the pus and the increasing number of bacteria and inflammatory cells pouring into the alveoli of his lungs impair gas exchange. He is now suffering from pneumonia. If he were to have his blood tested, there might well be an increase in the number of white blood cells, as they are recruited to fight the infection. A microscopic examination of a sputum sample would reveal bacteria, neutrophils, and debris.

Communication Among Immune Cells

The innate immune response was mobilized rapidly and effectively, but it could not keep up with the high rate of bacterial reproduction. However, it has successfully "bought time" for the adaptive immune response to be brought into play. APCs such as dendritic cells and macrophages, busy phagocytizing and degrading *S. pneumoniae*, load bacterial peptides into MHC II molecules and migrate to lymph nodes. Here, they encounter helper T cells and start the process of trying to find a match between the peptide epitopes of *S. pneumoniae* and helper T cell receptors.

At the same time, B cells are likewise trying to bind bacteria and/or the products of their degradation by means of their receptors. When B cells that can bind *S. pneumoniae* do so, they too process the antigenic proteins and present them to helper T cells. When appropriate matches are made, the helper T cells release mediators such as interleukin-2. They then proliferate and provide assistance to cells such as macrophages and B cells. In the latter case, helper T cells stimulate the B cells whose receptors bind *S. pneumoniae*, inducing them to mature into plasma cells that secrete large amounts of antibody against the pathogen.

Fighting Pathogens

The fight against the invading bacteria began with the phagocytic innate immune cells and proteins such as the complement cascade. When this defense was found to be insufficient, the adaptive immune system was invoked. These two halves of the immune system are functionally interrelated. Another way of dividing the immune response is by defining the effector mechanisms: cells or fluid molecules.

That part of the adaptive response that involves antigen-specific T cells is called the **cellular immune response** because the effectors are the cells themselves. The cellular immune response in our patient was the group of T cells whose antigen receptors bound *S. pneumoniae* epitopes in the context of MHC II molecules. Note, however, that a major portion of T cell–mediated immunity is the organization by T cells of the same cells that led the innate immune charge, namely macrophages and granulocytes. T cells alerted and directed by these innate cells now focus and enhance the effector functions of these same innate cells to intensify the fight against the pathogen.

That portion of the adaptive response that involves bloodborne molecules, especially antibodies, is called the **humoral immune response** because the molecules are serum factors, and blood or serum was considered one of the four "humors" in the medical literature of the 1600s. Thus, in our patient, the IgM and IgG antibodies directed against epitopes of the *S. pneumoniae* are key components of his humoral response. Antibodies are effective against pathogens because they can inhibit their entry into tissues or cells, bind to and neutralize toxic products of pathogens, and tag invaders for uptake and destruction.

Like the intertwining of innate and adaptive in the cellular immune response, there is cooperation between the innate and adaptive in humoral immunity. Antibodies produced by B cells, especially IgM, IgG_1, and IgG_3, are excellent activators of the complement cascade. When these antibodies bind to the surface of pathogens, the Fc regions precipitate complement, causing the deposition of complement fragments that, like the antibodies themselves, opsonize the bacteria. There are also strong links between humoral and cellular immunity. For example, macrophages have receptors for complement proteins and the Fc regions of antibodies, expediting phagocytosis.

Immunologic Memory

Another critical facet of the adaptive immune system (and another parallel with the nervous system) is its ability to retain information from an encounter with a given pathogen and recall that information to guide responses to subsequent encounters with that same pathogen. Our patient with pneumonia due to *S. pneumoniae*, either with or without the assistance of antibiotics (drugs that assist the immune system by poisoning bacteria), recovers from his infection. A year later, he breathes in respiratory droplets containing the same strain of bacteria, but this time he barely notices feeling sick. In fact, both cellular and humoral immune responses were invoked again, but much more rapidly and intensely than during the first infection, thus enabling him to defeat the bacteria without re-experiencing severe illness.

Immunologic memory occurs when, in the course of an adaptive response and the successful eradication of the invader, certain long-lived antigen-specific T and B cells called **memory cells** are produced. They spend the subsequent years or even decades patrolling the body, looking for evidence that their old nemesis (the same pathogenic invader) has reappeared. If they detect such a reinfection, they quickly marshal adaptive immune forces to stop the bacteria before disease occurs. Our patient is now immune to this strain of *S. pneumoniae*.

Immunologic memory and immunity, however, which do require previous exposure to the infectious agent, do not always and exclusively come at the price of illness. This disease-free route is **immunization**: the induction of immunity (i.e., protection from infection) by means of controlled exposure to either killed or disabled (attenuated) pathogen. By introducing, via **vaccination**, into a host, for example, defective viruses for hepatitis B, mumps, rubella, or smallpox, the adaptive immune system is given the chance to form antibodies and train memory B and T cells specific for the pathogens. If the vaccinated host later encounters the pathogen, the previously formed antibodies and memory cells prevent disease by quickly apprehending and neutralizing the invader.

IMMUNE SYSTEM PATHOPHYSIOLOGY

There are three basic types of immune system dysfunction. Underactivity of the immune system generally manifests as an increased risk of infection but is also associated with an increased risk of some types of cancer. Overactive immune system function may be directed at self antigens, in which case autoimmunity results. When the target of immune system activity is a harmless nonself antigen, the resulting disease is allergy.

Immunodeficiency

Immunodeficiency is a broad term indicating insufficient function of one or more components of the immune system. The many inherited and acquired causes of immunodeficiency share the general consequence of increased susceptibility to infection. However, the type and severity of the resulting illnesses vary widely with the mechanism and the immunologic subsystem affected.

Inherited immunodeficiencies can affect the production or proper function of any innate or adaptive cell or protein. Researchers have described deficiencies in the production or enzymatic activity of complement proteins and in cytokines, their receptors, or their signal transduction machinery. Loss of functional T cells and B cells is called *severe combined immunodeficiency (SCID)* and can be fatal without bone marrow transplantation or other interventions that restore adaptive immunity.

Equally complex and dangerous are **acquired immunodeficiencies**, which can result from insufficient nutrition, exposure to radiation or chemotherapeutic drugs that damage the production of functional immune cells, or even severe infection. Perhaps the best-known acquired immunodeficiency is the *acquired immunodeficiency syndrome (AIDS)*, which results from infection by the human immunodeficiency virus (HIV). By targeting a number of immune cells, especially helper T cells, HIV exploits the fact that, by infecting a host, the body will mobilize the immune system, making new targets for the virus, even as the T cells combat this rapidly reproducing and evolving pathogen.

Autoimmunity

As mentioned above, genetic rearrangement during B cell and T cell receptor production can result in receptors that recognize host proteins. Such adaptive immune cells are normally deleted (induced to undergo apoptosis) or silenced (a phenomenon called the induction of anergy). Sometimes, however, these protective measures fail to occur or, in the case of the unresponsive (anergic) state, are reversed or broken, resulting in autoimmunity. **Autoimmunity** is an immune response by the host directed against itself. In such cases, so-called autoreactive cytotoxic T cells may attack and kill healthy host cells, helper T cells may promote inflammation where none is needed, and B cells may produce autoantibodies that bind to self structures. Because these events lead to the initiation of the same immune responses that are normally directed at pathogenic invaders, inflammatory disease in the absence of infection results. Examples are rheumatoid arthritis and systemic lupus erythematosus, in which inflammation in the joints, skin, and other locations occurs. Therapies for such diseases currently rely on medications that suppress the immune system. While these treatments diminish inflammation, they carry the obvious danger of immunosuppression.

Allergy

Allergic diseases are the result of complex interactions among immune cells. Their exact pathogenesis is not completely understood, but epidemiologic data suggest they are increasing in wealthier nations

where, among other things, the burden of infectious diseases (especially parasitic infections) has decreased. In the simplest terms, **allergy** is a case of mistaken identity. The immune system somehow mistakes a common, benign component in the environment, such as cat dander, for something dangerous that has to be eradicated.

Allergy is closely related to **atopy**, a predisposition to produce IgE antibodies. These antibodies bind to mast cell and basophil receptors for the Fc region of the molecule, leaving their $F(ab')_2$ regions "waving in the wind," waiting to bind their antigen. When the antigen re-enters the body, it binds to the IgE on the surface of these cells and stimulates them to release chemical mediators such as histamine and leukotrienes, which cause itching, sneezing, and even symptoms of asthma, such as wheezing and shortness of breath.

Summary

- The lymphatic system of **lymphatic vessels** and **lymph nodes** resorbs the excess fluid filtering across capillaries, screens it for pathogenic invaders, and returns it to the systemic circulation.

- **Lacteals** are the blind-ended lymphatic capillaries in tissues. Bi-leaflet valves ensure the one-way flow of lymph from the tissue to eventually reach the venous circulation.

- The **Starling equation** quantifies the flux of fluid across the capillary wall by multiplying the **capillary filtration coefficient (CFC)** by the difference of the net **hydrostatic pressure** and the net **oncotic pressure**. The movement of fluid from the capillary lumen into the interstitial space is known as *transudation*.

- Intrinsic and extrinsic forces help lymph move from tissues toward the central systemic circulation.

- Dysfunction of the lymphatic system may result in the accumulation of fluid in peripheral tissues, known as **edema**. Edema generally results from one or more of four mechanisms: increased capillary hydrostatic pressure, decreased capillary oncotic pressure, increased capillary permeability, and lymphatic vessel obstruction.

- Increased capillary hydrostatic pressure is seen in **congestive heart failure (CHF)**, which may manifest as **pulmonary edema**. In **cirrhotic liver disease**, the accumulation of fluid in the peritoneal cavity is called **ascites**.

- Decreased capillary oncotic pressure is seen in **hypoalbuminemia** that may attend malnutrition, liver disease resulting in decreased albumin production, or conditions where albumin is lost at an increased rate.
- Increased capillary permeability is seen when the capillary endothelium is damaged, as occurs in burns, sepsis, and damage by toxins.
- Lymphatic obstruction is seen in a number of cancers, such as lymphoma, and after surgery where many lymph nodes are removed.
- The immune system protects the body from threats such as infection by pathogenic microbes (viruses, bacterial, fungi, and parasites).
- The immune system has three interdependent lines of defense for protecting the body: **physical barriers**, **innate immune responses**, and **adaptive immune responses**.
- The innate immune system acts rapidly but relatively nonspecifically to protect the host by using *pattern recognition receptors (PRRs)* that bind to the *pathogen-associated molecular patterns (PAMPs)* of microbes.
- The adaptive immune system of B cells and T cells is a highly antigen-specific response system that has **immunologic memory**. **Vaccination** can impart immunity by intentionally exposing the host to an attenuated pathogen unable to cause disease but able to stimulate the immune system and create immunologic memory.
- Innate immune cells include granulocytes (neutrophils, eosinophils, and basophils), mast cells, monocytes/macrophages, and dendritic cells. Adaptive immune cells include B cells and T cells.
- An **antigen** is any substance that elicits an immune response. A **hapten** is a nonself molecule too small to be immunogenic by itself, but which, when combined with a self protein, can be an antigen. An **epitope** is a region of an antigen specifically recognized by B cells and/or T cels.
- **Antigen-presenting cells (APCs)** present peptide antigens in the groove of **MHC II molecules** to **helper T cells**. All nucleated cells can present peptide antigens in the grooves of **MHC I molecules** to **cytotoxic T cells**.
- **Antibodies** are soluble versions of the B cell antigen receptor. The F(ab′)$_2$ region of the antibody binds to the antigen, while the Fc region determines the isotype (IgA, IgD, IgE, IgG, or IgM) of and the cellular response to the antibody. Antibodies bind to antigens to neutralize them and bind to pathogens to **opsonize** them, "tagging" them for destruction by innate immune systems such as the **complement cascade**.
- B cell and T cell antigen receptors are produced by a complex process of gene shuffling and DNA editing.
- Intracellular pathogens such as viruses are detected when their antigens are presented in MHC I molecules to cytotoxic T cells. Extracellular pathogens such as bacteria are detected when they are phagocytized and their antigens are presented in HMC II molecules to helper T cells.
- Insufficient immune system function results in **immunodeficiency**, which may be inherited or acquired (such as AIDS). Immune responses mistakenly directed against self antigens result in **autoimmunity** and manifest as inflammatory diseases such as rheumatoid arthritis. Immune responses mistakenly directed against benign nonself antigens result in **allergy**.

Suggested Reading

Aukland K, Reed RK. Interstitial-lymphatic mechanisms in the control of extracellular fluid volume. Physiol Rev. 1993;73(1):1–78.

Lankat-Buttgereit B, Tampe R. The transporter associated with antigen processing: function and implications in human diseases. Physiol Rev. 2002;82(1): 187–204.

Matzinger P. The danger model: a renewed sense of self. Science. 2002;296(5566):301–305.

Medzhitov R, Janeway CA Jr. Decoding the patterns of self and nonself by the innate immune system. Science. 2002;296(5566):298–300.

Olszewski WL, Engeset A. Immune proteins, enzymes and electrolytes in human peripheral lymph. Lymphology. 1978;11(4):156–164.

Walport MJ. Complement. First of two parts. N Engl J Med. 2001;344(14):1058–1066.

REVIEW QUESTIONS

Directions: Each of the numbered items or incomplete statements in this section is followed by answers or by completions of the statement. Select the

ONE lettered answer or completion that is BEST in each case.

1. A 68-year-old woman has a number of lymph nodes surgically removed from her right axilla because of breast cancer. Which of the following is a likely cause for her subsequent right arm swelling?

   (A) Decreased lymph removal
   (B) Decreased lymph production
   (C) Increased lymph protein content
   (D) Decreased lymph cell counts
   (E) Increased susceptibility to infection

2. A 36-year-old man is feeling well and has no evidence of illness. Which of the following cells would you expect to find in his lymph?

   (A) Neutrophils
   (B) Macrophages
   (C) Eosinophils
   (D) T cells
   (E) Liver cells

3. A 44-year-old man is infected with a virus. Which of the following molecules is the most likely to present antigenic epitopes from the virus on the surface of an infected cell?

   (A) A B cell receptor
   (B) An MHC I molecule
   (C) An integrin molecule
   (D) A T cell receptor
   (E) A cytokine molecule

4. Which of the following is *not* a function of antibodies?

   (A) Opsonization of invaders
   (B) Inhibiting the entry of pathogens into tissues or cells
   (C) Binding toxins
   (D) Presenting antigen to T cells
   (E) Activating the complement cascade

ANSWERS TO REVIEW QUESTIONS

1. **The answer is** A. The removal of a number of lymph nodes impairs the drainage of lymph from the affected limb, allowing the accumulation of edema fluid in the interstitial space. None of the other answers, except an increased susceptibility to infection, would result in fluid accumulation in the area. While areas swollen because of lymphatic dysfunction may indeed be more susceptible to infection, the cause-and-effect relationship in this case is less likely that immunodeficiency from the loss of a few lymph nodes leads to swelling than the reverse.

2. **The answer is** D. Lymphocytes, T and B cells, are the ones most commonly encountered in the lymphatics of healthy individuals. As these cells circulate from blood into tissues and lymph nodes, they enter the lymph and return to the central circulation. Although neutrophils, macrophages, and eosinophils are immune cells, they are not lymphocytes and would not be expected to be found in large numbers in the lymph of a healthy person. Liver cells (hepatocytes) do not normally leave the liver to circulate in the lymphatic vessels.

3. **The answer is** B. When intracellular, intracytoplasmic pathogens such as viruses infect cells, the infected cells load MHC I molecules with viral peptides and present them to cytotoxic T cells. B cell and T cell receptors "look" for antigen, and T cell receptors can detect antigen only when it is in the cleft of an MHC molecule. Integrins and cytokines do not bind antigenic epitopes for presentation to T cells. If an APC had phagocytosed some extracellular virus and digested it, peptide epitopes might have been loaded into MHC II molecules for presentation to helper T cells, but this was not a choice in this question.

4. **The answer is** D. Antibodies opsonize, inhibit movement, neutralize toxins, and precipitate complement. While the B cell receptor is essentially a membrane-bound antibody on the surface of B cells, its function there is to detect extracellular antigen and facilitate its uptake by the B cell. The MHC I and II molecules are important for antigen presentation to T cells.

CARDIOVASCULAR PHYSIOLOGY

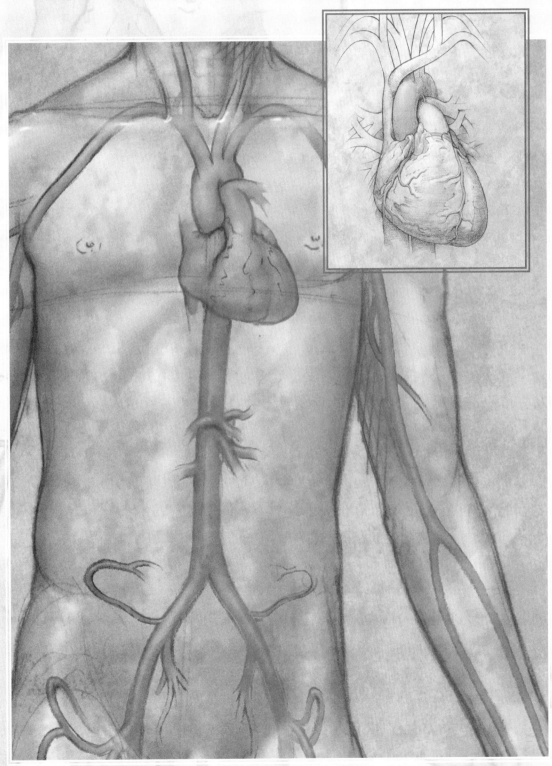

The Vasculature

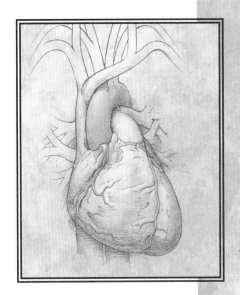

12

INTRODUCTION

The cardiovascular system is the principal transportation and distribution network of the body, delivering essential substances (e.g., glucose and oxygen) to the tissues and removing the by-products of metabolism (e.g., carbon dioxide, lactate, and heat). In its simplest formulation, the system is composed of three parts: a pump (the heart), a series of distributing and collecting tubes (the arterial and venous systems), and a transport medium (the blood). Part IV of this text focuses on the structure and function of the heart and the vasculature (blood vessels). The physiology of the blood and vascular endothelium was discussed in detail in Chapters 9 and 10.

This chapter focuses on blood flow through the vessels, on blood pressure in various parts of the vascular network, and on vascular resistance to flow. The relation between these three variables is expressed in analogy to Ohm's law, and the application of Ohm's law to the vasculature is the essence of this chapter. Further discussion of the regulation of systemic blood pressure appears in one of the renal physiology chapters (Chapter 22) because the renal and cardiovascular systems govern the blood pressure in concert. Chapters 13 and 14 discuss the mechanical action and electrophysiology of the heart. Chapter 15 discusses cardiovascular adaptations to exercise.

SYSTEM STRUCTURE

The **heart** comprises two hollow muscular pumps in series, dividing the circulation into pulmonary and systemic components (FIGURE 12.1). The **right ventricle** propels deoxygenated blood from the systemic veins into the pulmonary arteries and on to the lungs. After the exchange of oxygen and carbon dioxide in the pulmonary capillaries, the pulmonary veins return the oxygenated blood to the heart. This circuit from right ventricle to **left atrium** is the **pulmonary circulation**. Meanwhile, the **left ventricle** propels the oxygenated blood received from the pulmonary veins to the remaining tissues of the body through the aorta and its branches. The deoxygenated blood returns to the heart in the vena cava. This circuit from left ventricle to **right atrium** is the **systemic circulation**.

Within the systemic circulation, the various organ systems (e.g., the brain, the heart itself, the gastrointestinal tract, skeletal muscles, the kidneys) are connected in parallel, allowing for differential shunting of arterial blood flow between vascular beds based on moment-to-moment need (FIGURE 12.2). Regurgitant flow (backward flow) in the heart is

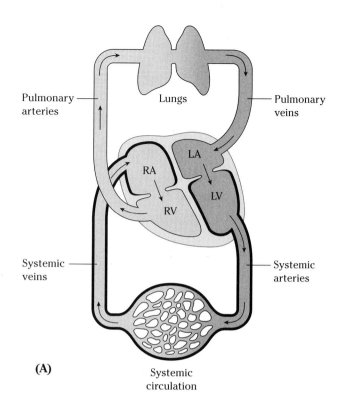

(A)

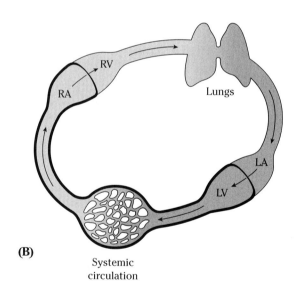

(B)

Figure 12.1 The pulmonary and systemic components of the vascular circuit. **A.** The anatomic arrangement of the circuit. **B.** A perspective of the circuit if the heart were cleaved right side from left and the right side were then "unkinked." Part B is an attempt to illustrate that while the pulmonary and systemic pumps are anatomically located side by side, they are in fact connected in one loop.

prevented by a series of unidirectional cardiac **valves** that guard the entrance and exit of each cardiac ventricle. The slamming shut of the cardiac valves create the "lub-dub" sound heard through the stethoscope over the *precordium* (the area of the chest over the heart).

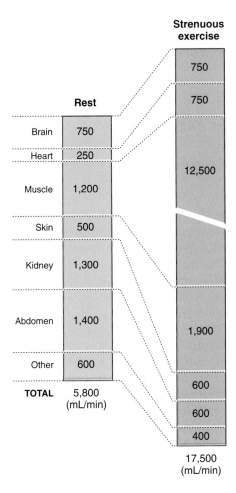

Figure 12.2 The distribution of blood to the body's organs and tissues at rest and during strenuous exercise.

Veins and Arteries

The concept of "blood pressure" will be explored below, but for now it suffices to say that there are high-pressure and low-pressure parts of the cardiovascular circuit. The arteries constitute the high-pressure part, the veins the low-pressure part. Arterial pressure is created not only by the heart but also by smooth muscle in the walls of the arteries, which squeezes the arterial blood. The vein walls are less muscular and highly distensible. Consequently, blood is squeezed from the high-pressure arteries into the high-capacity veins, leaving only around 20% of the total blood volume (1 out of 5 L) in the systemic arteries at any given time. If the normal blood volume is rapidly expanded (e.g., by blood transfusion) or contracted (e.g., through hemorrhage), most of the volume change is accommodated in the low-pressure portion of the circulation rather than in the arterial high-pressure circulation, whose volume remains relatively constant.

Another difference between arteries and veins is their elasticity. The high proportion of elastin in the walls of large arteries gives them **elastic recoil**, the tendency to shrink back down once stretched. This

property is particularly important in the aorta (described below). Elastic recoil is also critical in the parenchyma of the lung; this property drives the expiratory phase of breathing. Arteries and veins may also be distinguished by the property of vascular **compliance**, which is the distensibility of the vessel when exposed to a pressure gradient exerted across the vessel wall (the transmural pressure). Compliance is the change in volume in the vessel per change in pressure. Compliance is high when a large volume can be accommodated with small pressure changes, and low when small volume changes result in large pressure differences. Veins and venules have high compliance when pressure is low, while arterioles are of low compliance at low pressures. This property of veins allows for the accommodation of large volumes of blood in the circulation before development of high venous pressure. Thus the veins are sometimes described as "venous capacitance vessels." The high blood volume in the veins is available to return to the heart and lungs when needed, as in the case of exercise or other demand on cardiac output.

At high venous pressures, the compliance of a vein is close to that of arteries. This property allows for leg veins to be used in coronary artery bypass grafts. The venous pressure is also a driving force for movement of blood from veins back to heart, a flow known as **venous return**. (From the cardiac perspective, venous return is an important component of **preload**, a topic covered in Chapter 13). Normal gravitational forces oppose venous return and need to be overcome by developed venous pressures, particularly in the lower extremities. According to the relationship between compliance and pressure, it follows that the two ways to increase venous pressure are a fall in compliance and an increase in volume. Compliance may be decreased by compression of the peripheral veins by muscular contractions in the leg and by increased tone of the vessels (as by constriction mediated by the sympathetic nervous system).

From Large Arteries to Small

The contraction of the cardiac ventricles, an event called **systole**, drives blood into the pulmonary arteries and into the aorta. The ventricles then relax, an event called **diastole**. Systole expands the highly elastic aorta, and elastic recoil occurs during diastole, driving the blood out of the aorta and into the smaller arterial branches. Because both systole and diastole drive the blood forward, blood never stops moving. The continuous nature of blood flow despite its pulsatility is called the *Windkessel effect*. Flow is very pulsatile in the aorta and becomes less pulsatile as blood moves down the arterial system pulsatility is still measured, however, in small arteries. From the aorta, the blood travels through a branching network of vessels of progressively smaller caliber, terminating in the **capillaries**. Just before the level of the capillaries are the highly muscular **arterioles** (FIGURE 12.3). Arterioles are critical for the control of blood pressure and blood flow. By constricting some or all of the body's arterioles, the vasculature can direct the flow of blood to the organs that most need it, or it can elevate blood pressure throughout the cardiovascular circuit. The flow of blood into a given capillary bed may be controlled by muscular contraction in structures known as *precapillary sphincters*. When constricted, these sphincters result in a diversion through *thoroughfare channels* directly into the venous sinusoids, bypassing the capillary bed.

SYSTEM FUNCTION

To understand blood pressure, blood flow, and vessel resistance, it is useful to review some basic physics. In the following discussion, be careful to note the difference between the concepts of pressure and pressure difference. Ohm's law describes how voltage differences drive electrical flow (current). Similarly, blood pressure differences drive flow in blood vessels, and this relationship is described by an analogous equation (see below). Pressure *differences* rather than pressure at one site constitute the driving force. This concept was also covered in Chapter 2 in discussions of electrical and concentration gradients as driving forces that determine membrane transport events. These are all considered force-flow relationships:

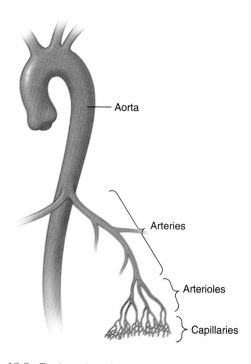

Figure 12.3 The branches of the vascular tree. The arterioles are noteworthy for their high smooth muscle content, which makes them the main sites of vasoconstriction and vasodilation in the body.

pressure differences drive volumes of fluid; voltage differences drive charge; electrochemical gradients drive moles of solute.

Pressure

Recall from basic gas laws that the pressure, P, of a gas in a container is proportional to the number of moles (n) in the container per volume (V) of the container:

$$P \sim n/V$$

(because $P = nRT/V$, where R is the gas constant and T is temperature in Kelvin). Reducing the container volume with a fixed amount (number of molecules) of substance in the container forces the molecules of that substance together. Because the molecules are more densely packed, they collide more often and hit the walls, exerting more force per area (i.e., pressure) on the container walls. Similarly, reducing the number of molecules of a substance in a container of fixed volume reduces the pressure in the container because there are fewer molecular collisions.

The situation for fluids in a tube (blood vessel) is analogous to that of a gas in a container. Shrinking the size of the vessels at a particular site in the cardiovascular circuit increases the pressure at that site. This is exactly what happens in the cardiac ventricles during systole, when the contraction of the cardiac muscles shrinks the vessel (ventricle) size. During diastole, aortic volume and pressure decline as the aorta empties its blood into the systemic circulation. (Similarly, loss of blood from the vessels due to hemorrhage decreases the number of molecules in the vessels and thus decreases the blood pressure.)

To shrink the ventricle or the aorta, work (W) must be done on the vessel walls (force, F, must be applied over a distance, d):

$$W = F \times d.$$

Thus, work or energy is necessary to drive the contraction of the vessels. In the heart, the energy of muscular contraction is derived from ATP. In the aorta, the kinetic energy of the blood entering from the heart pushes the aortic walls out, and that energy is stored as potential energy in the aortic elastin fibers. The potential energy is released and does the work of vessel contraction during diastole. Since the work is being done in three dimensions, the work equation can be rewritten for three dimensions:

$$W = P(\Delta V).$$

Work is the pressure exerted over a change in volume. Since pressure is force per area ($P = F/A$) and volume is equal to distance times area ($\Delta V = d \times A$), the equation $W = P(\Delta V)$ can be reduced to $W = (F/A)(d \times A)$, which is the same as the more familiar $W = F \times d$.

Pressure Difference

Two types of pressure need be considered in the cardiovascular system. First, a **transmural pressure** refers to a pressure gradient felt across the vascular wall, at one particular point in the vascular tree whether in the large cardiac chambers, the arteries, or the capillaries. Second is a **perfusion pressure or driving pressure,** which is the gradient of pressures between two places within the circulation. The transmural pressure at two points in the circulation creates the driving pressure forward through the circulation. Transmural pressure at one place in a vessel does not by itself make the vessel's contents move. If there is no opportunity for outflow, as in a closed container, an increase in transmural pressure is just that: an increase in pressure and nothing more. It is **pressure difference** that makes a gas or fluid flow from one location to another. When the pressure is 100 mm Hg at point A and 25 mm Hg at point B in a vessel, the fluid at point A will flow toward point B until the pressure difference is relieved. This is because the vessel wall at point A is pushing the fluid harder than the wall at point B (FIGURE 12.4). The **Ohm's law** analogy describes the flow of blood ($\dot{Q}$) in liters per minute from point A to point B:

$\dot{Q} = \Delta P/R$; or $\Delta P = \dot{Q}R$, where ΔP is the difference in pressure between point A and point B and R is the **resistance** to flow along the way from A to B.

Resistance is related to the amount of friction in the vessel between points A and B. The pressure difference is the net force pushing the fluid toward point B, while resistance is related to the net force opposing this movement (FIGURE 12.5). Resistance,

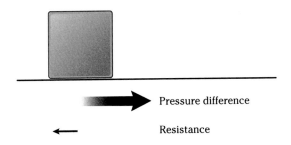

Figure 12.5 The forces at work on blood flow, depicted as a vector diagram.

like pressure, is a function of the size of the vessel or container. A narrow vessel creates more resistance than a wide vessel. Resistance is thus inversely proportional to vessel radius, as described in **Poiseuille's law**: $R = 8\eta l/\pi r^4$, where r is the vessel radius, l is the length of the tube, and η is the viscosity of the fluid. The length of the frictional surface and viscosity (which one might think of as the "internal friction" of a fluid, its own molecules rubbing against and interacting with its own molecules) also contribute to resistance, but they are three orders of magnitude less important than vessel radius (note the fourth-power function of the radius relationship).

Not only are pressure differences (also called "pressure drops") necessary to drive fluid across a length of vessel with resistance in it, but *resistance also creates pressure differences along vessels.* Consider two vessels, one with a high resistance and one with a low resistance (FIGURE 12.6). In the higher-resistance vessel, fewer molecules of fluid will be delivered to point B per unit time. Point B will hence have fewer molecules in it at the same container size;

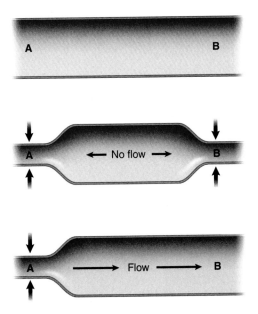

Figure 12.4 Pressure difference. Flow from point A to point B cannot occur in a vessel without a difference in the transmural pressure at point A versus point B.

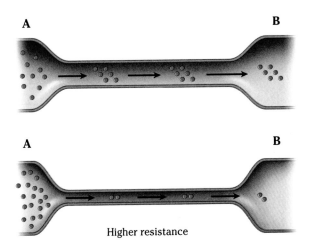

Figure 12.6 The genesis of a pressure difference. The dots represent molecules of fluid in the vessel. Higher resistance, and consequently decreased blood flow, leads to a buildup of fluid molecules upstream of the resistance and a dearth of molecules downstream of the resistance. Fewer molecules means less transmural pressure; more molecules means more transmural pressure.

as described above, this constitutes a lower transmural pressure at point B. Thus, as blood travels farther away from the heart, encountering resistance all the way, the pressure in the vessels gradually decreases. Likewise, in the higher-resistance vessel, point A will lose fewer molecules of fluid per unit time, will be more densely packed, and will have a higher transmural pressure. *Neural and humoral factors can increase muscle tone in arterioles to reduce flow and thus pressure to certain downstream areas or to boost upstream pressure.* This is the key to cardiovascular regulation of the blood pressure.

One of the more confusing aspects of vascular physiology is the fact that while compression in one place in the vascular tree increases pressure at that particular spot, it also affects the pressures upstream and downstream of the spot: it increases pressure upstream and decreases pressure downstream of the spot. This is because compression not only raises pressure in the compressed area, but also raises resistance in the area.

The flow of blood within the circulatory system is not only determined by favorable pressure gradients providing the energy for such flow. The relationship between vessel radius, velocity, and kinetic energy must also be considered. According to the Bernoulli principle, the total energy is a combination of potential energy observed in the gradients for pressure, and kinetic energy determined by the velocity of the moving fluid (blood). As blood moves from a larger vessel to a smaller vessel, velocity, and thus kinetic energy, increases, yet as a result of the increased velocity, transmural pressure falls. It is the kinetic energy that is maintaining the constancy of forward flow. The flow may actually proceed to an area of increased radius where transmural pressure is higher, giving the appearance of flow from an area of low to high pressure. Yet the total energy is what counts, and flow moves in the direction mandated by the total energy gradient. This principle is critical to understanding how flow continues past a vascular stenosis (narrowing by disease) and in understanding how the left ventricle can still eject blood into the aorta in late systole, when aortic pressure exceeds ventricular pressure.

Systemic Pressure, Resistance, and Flow

In the preceding discussion, flow, pressure, and resistance were discussed in relation to one container or vessel. However, these concepts may be applied to groups of vessels, or to the entire cardiovascular circuit. First, let's consider pressure.

MAP and SVR What is the pressure difference (ΔP) across the entire systemic arterial system? To answer this question, we must know the aortic pressure at the beginning of the systemic circulation and the pressure in the right atrium at the end of the systemic circulation. The aortic pressure is a weighted average of systolic and diastolic blood pressures. Since a large addition of blood enters the vasculature during systole (increasing the number of molecules with a limited increase in container size), the aortic pressure is higher during systole. Diastole involves pressure created by aortic elastic recoil, as described above, but this pressure is lower than that created during systole. The **mean arterial pressure (MAP)** is calculated from the systolic and diastolic pressure. Greater weight is given to diastolic because at low resting heart rates approximately two thirds of the cardiac cycle is diastole. At high rates, MAP is more closely approximated by the arithmetic mean of systolic and diastolic pressure. Thus, MAP = [(2 × diastolic pressure) + systolic pressure]/3. Usually the MAP is in a range of 70 to 110, but if it is <60 mm Hg, vital organs such as the brain and kidneys may be inadequately perfused.

Systolic and diastolic aortic pressures are usually estimated by measurements at the brachial artery (made with a blood pressure cuff and stethoscope) and referred to as *systemic blood pressure (SBP)*. The method of BP measurement gives a transmural pressure reading. Normal right atrial pressure is usually 5 mm Hg or less, so for a MAP of 100 mm Hg, the driving force for perfusion of the whole body, ΔP, is close to 100 mm Hg.

The resistance may also be estimated for the entire vascular circuit. This value is the **systemic vascular resistance (SVR)**, also called the *total peripheral resistance (TPR)*. The SVR is the sum of all the resistances in the circuit. The arterioles are muscular and of small diameter, and thus they contribute the most resistance to the SVR. The pressure drop across these resistance vessels is primarily related to the number of parallel vessels and their diameters (i.e., cross-sectional area). The blood downstream of the arterioles has a pressure of around 25 mm Hg.

Since the capillaries are the narrowest vessels in the body, one might wonder why they do not create a higher resistance than the arterioles (although they do contribute the next largest component to total resistance). They do not because so many capillaries arise from each arteriole that the total cross-sectional area of a capillary bed is very large, and the resistance is consequently less than at the arteriolar level. The blood downstream of the capillaries (i.e., in the veins) has a pressure of around 10 mm Hg and contributes <10% of the total resistance.

According to the Ohm's law analogy, the SVR can be calculated clinically as SVR = (Aortic − Right Atrial mean pressure)/Cardiac Output. (This is the same as saying $R = \Delta P/\dot{Q}$, since cardiac output equals blood flow.) Units are usually converted from mm Hg/liter/min to dynes/ sec/cm^{-5} by multiplying by 80. We'll return to the Ohm equation for the whole vascular tree after discussing blood flow.

Blood Flow and Cardiac Output   The blood flow through the circulation can be considered **laminar** or **turbulent**. Laminar flow is conceptualized streaming through an ideal tube with the characteristics described in Poiseuille's law; however, the circulation has numerous branchings and alterations within the surface of the wall that depart from the ideal conception. The *Reynolds number* is an index of the factors that determine whether flow will be laminar or turbulent. A high Reynolds number is associated with turbulent flow. The Reynolds number is proportional to the mean velocity of flow, the tube radius, and the density of the liquid, and inversely proportional to viscosity. Viscosity, in turn, is a direct function of forces acting horizontally on the flow of blood (shear stress) and inversely related to the varying velocities of layers of the liquid flowing downstream (shear rate). In laminar flow, the velocity of the stream is greatest at the center of the vessel and slowest at the outermost layer closest to the wall. In turbulent flow, with branching of vessels and eddying currents, the flow is more disorganized and the velocity more variable.

Turbulence is related to the separation of flow velocities. Factors such as narrowing of the vessel radius mean that vascular stenoses or even the constriction of the blood pressure cuff can lead to turbulent flow. Such flow is noisy and can be heard clinically over the narrowing as a murmur or bruit. Since viscosity is also a factor in turbulent flow, alterations in blood viscosity can increase or decrease turbulence. Anemia, or low hematocrit, leads to a decrease in viscosity and an increased Reynolds number. In fact, anemic patients may be found to have flow murmurs in the heart.

While blood flow may vary in different portions of the vascular circuit, net blood flow remains relatively constant given a steady state of physical and metabolic activity and environmental conditions. The *net blood flow* is defined as the volume of blood pumped out of the heart in 1 min. This value is called the **cardiac output (CO)**, and it is roughly 5 L/min in an adult. (Thus, the entire 5-L blood volume traverses the whole circuit each minute.) To standardize CO for individuals of varying size, the **cardiac index (CI)** is often used and is CO per body surface area in meter^2.

The CO is the product of the **heart rate (HR)** and the **stroke volume (SV)**: CO = (HR)(SV). HR is measured in beats per minute; SV, the volume of blood ejected into the aorta from the left ventricle with each systolic contraction, is measured in milliliters per beat. The SV is the end-diastolic volume of the left ventricle minus its end-systolic volume. The left ventricle does not completely empty during systole, so the SV is not equal to the entire volume of blood in the left ventricle at the end of diastolic filling (end-diastolic volume [EDV]); rather, it is a fraction, known as the **ejection fraction (EF)**. EF = (SV/EDV) × 100. The EF is normally greater than 60%. When the heart is working hard, the EF can increase to as much as 90% (during exercise); when heart contraction is impaired, EF can decrease to as low as 20% (in heart failure).

Capillary Hemodynamics   The capillaries serve as the interface between the circulation and the larger interstitial space. The movement of fluid and solutes from the plasma water is the basis of both the supply of necessary nutrients to the cells and the elimination process for cellular waste products. The high permeability to fluid and the large surface area of capillary networks in the tissues enable this critical transport function. The driving forces favoring fluid filtration across the capillary barrier are the capillary hydrostatic pressure (Pcap) and the oncotic pressure in the interstitial fluid (Πint). Forces opposing filtration are the hydrostatic pressure in the interstitium (Pint) and the capillary oncotic pressure (Πcap). Therefore, the net driving forces (NDF) from the plasma into the interstitial fluid can be described as NDF = (Pcap − Pint) − (Πcap − Πint).

The hydrostatic pressure in the capillary is close to venous pressure because of the precapillary arteriolar resistance, described above. The oncotic pressure in plasma is primarily due to the macromolecule albumin, which has low permeability across most capillary barriers. This permeability does vary from tissue to tissue, ranging from 0 (i.e., complete permeability) to 1 (i.e., zero permeability). A reflection coefficient, σ, is used to qualify ΔΠ. The new expression for driving forces then becomes NDF = (Pcap − Pint) − σ(Πcap − Πint).

In accordance with the Ohm's law analogy for driving forces and resistance as determinants of flow ($\dot{Q}$), both the driving forces in the above equation and a constant related to the resistance or conductance of the barrier determine the flow across that barrier. The constant, known as the ultrafiltration coefficient, K$_{uf}$, is in itself determined by the surface area, thickness, length, and intrinsic permeability properties of the capillary wall. The relationship, known as the **Starling law of the capillary**, is $\dot{Q} = K_{uf}[(\Delta P) - \sigma(\Delta \Pi)]$.

As fluid accumulates in the interstitium, it is removed by lymphatic drainage.

If L indicates the lymphatic flow rate, then the Starling relationship for net flow from the capillary becomes $\dot{Q} = K_{uf}[(\Delta P) - \sigma(\Delta \Pi)] - L$.

The interstitial space can increase its volume with minimal changes in pressure (high compliance), but when a large volume of fluid moves into the interstitial space, the high pressure that develops will further slow capillary ultrafiltration. The accumulation of interstitial fluid, clinically known as **edema**, can be detected by exerting pressure with a finger into the soft tissues, usually of the lower extremities, displacing the edema fluid. After releasing the external pressure, it takes time for the fluid to move back to its original location, so the indentation of the finger remains; this is known as *pitting edema*. Edema in the feet is usually greatest at the end of a period of standing because gravitational forces cause the greatest pressures to be exerted in the feet.

The Starling forces of the capillary will be addressed in the discussion of heart failure in Chapter 13; gas exchange in the lungs in Chapter 17; renal glomerular filtration in Chapter 20; renal tubular reabsorption in Chapter 21; gastrointestinal fluid absorption in Chapter 27; and cirrhosis of the liver in Chapter 29.

The Regulation of Blood Pressure

By substituting into Ohm's law ($\Delta P = \dot{Q}R$) MAP for ΔP, CO for $\dot{Q}$, and SVR for R, we get an equation descriptive of the whole vascular tree: MAP = (CO)(SVR). Of these three variables, blood pressure is monitored and regulated by the brain. Chapter 22 describes the homeostatic system for maintaining a constant blood pressure. The **baroreceptors** are the sensors by which the brain detects changes in blood pressure. There are low-pressure baroreceptors in the pulmonary vessels and in the cardiac atria. There are high-pressure baroreceptors in the aortic arch, carotid sinus, and in the renal arterioles. Baroreceptors in the carotid sinus communicate with the medulla predominantly through a branch of the glossopharyngeal nerve, whereas the aortic arch baroreceptors are innervated by the vagus nerve. The medulla in turn sends efferent signals to the systemic arterioles and heart in sympathetic and parasympathetic nerves. The medulla also neurally stimulates a hormonal response (adrenal secretion of circulating epinephrine), which acts at the heart and arterioles. The overall response is called the **baroreceptor reflex**.

The efferent signals influence the MAP through two different cardiovascular effector mechanisms. One is the modulation of CO; the other is the modulation of SVR. When the baroreceptors detect low blood pressure, they stimulate the heart to pump harder (increasing SV) and faster (increasing HR), thereby increasing CO. Increased CO forces more blood from the venous reservoir into the arteries, increasing the number of molecules inside a container of fixed size, thereby increasing the systemic arterial pressure. The stimulus of low blood pressure also causes arteriolar vasoconstriction in certain vascular beds. As described above, this increases SVR and increases the pressure upstream of the arterioles. Now there is adequate blood pressure for the perfusion of other vascular beds, such as in the brain and the heart itself (whose arterioles are not as much constricted by the baroreceptor reflex). *The baroreceptor reflex can work effectively only if it shuts down certain vascular beds (e.g., skin and intestine), thereby preserving blood pressure for the perfusion of other vascular beds (heart and brain) that remain unconstricted.* (See Clinical Application Box *Carotid Massage*.)

As Chapter 22 describes, these cardiovascular effector mechanisms are accompanied by renal ones. The most important renal response to low blood pressure is an increase in salt and water reabsorption in the renal tubules. This increases the extracellular fluid volume, which packs the arteries more densely with fluid, just as increased CO does.

The cardiovascular mechanisms of control are divided into central and local mechanisms. The central control mechanism was introduced above and will be discussed in more detail below. Local factors act in paracrine fashion (i.e., near their site of secretion) to influence arteriolar constriction. The degree of constriction in the arterioles, called **vasomotor tone**, is present all the time even in the absence of baroreceptor stimulation. (Without this basal level of arteriolar tone, the SVR and MAP would

---

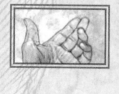

CLINICAL APPPLICATION

CAROTID MASSAGE

The baroreceptor reflex is occasionally used clinically to treat or diagnose *tachycardia* (rapid heart rate). Massaging the carotid arteries stimulates the baroreceptors there and sends a "high blood pressure" signal to the medulla. Increased parasympathetic output to the heart (intended to decrease HR, which would decrease CO and in turn decrease MAP) can then slow a dangerously rapid sinus tachycardia. Carotid massage can also elucidate the source of a supraventricular tachycardia, since only sinoatrial tachycardias will respond.

drop precipitously.) The central and local control systems act in concert to determine vasomotor tone, which may reflect a mixture of constrictive and dilatory influences.

Local control mechanisms are more important in some tissues, while central control mechanisms predominate in others. For example, in the skin and splanchnic regions, central regulation of vascular resistance predominates, whereas in the heart and brain, local control is more important. This makes sense, because the central homeostatic response to low blood pressure must spare the heart and brain from reflex vasoconstriction to achieve its intended result, as described above.

Local Control   The various local control mechanisms over vasoconstriction are sometimes called **autoregulatory mechanisms** because they act independently of the brain. Autoregulatory mechanisms have two primary functions: (a) maintaining constant blood flow to an organ with a steady metabolic rate in the face of changing blood pressure and (b) adjusting blood flow to an organ according to local changes in its metabolic activity.

There must first be a safeguard in place to maintain a relatively constant blood flow to the tissues in response to rapid changes in blood pressure. One safeguard is the **myogenic response**, in which vascular smooth muscle contracts in response to stretch and relaxes with a reduction in tension. When a person who has been lying down suddenly stands up, blood pools in the lower extremities, stretching the arterioles of the lower extremities. This stretch leads to arteriolar (precapillary) vasoconstriction, which prevents excess blood flow to the extremities, thereby avoiding accumulation of fluid and pressure that would otherwise lead to edema. A similar myogenic vasoconstrictor response protects the brain and kidney from the potentially damaging effects of a rapid rise in blood pressure. Cerebral blood flow is essentially constant over systolic blood pressures ranging from 60 to 160 mm Hg, and renal blood flow and glomerular filtration rate (see Chapter 20) are likewise constant from systolic pressures ranging from 80 to 200 mm Hg. The precise mechanism by which myogenic autoregulation occurs is poorly understood, but it is presumed that stretch of vascular smooth muscle activates transmembrane calcium channels, leading to muscular contraction.

A second autoregulatory mechanism depends on the release of factors from the vascular endothelium. Increases in the velocity of blood flow through a vessel lead to reflex secretion of nitric oxide (formerly called endothelial-derived relaxing factor [EDRF]) and other factors from the endothelium. Here again the mechanism is not clearly understood, but it is thought that the increased shear stress on the endothelium created by high flow stimulates the endothelium to synthesize or release paracrine substances.

The final autoregulatory component is a **metabolic mechanism**, which adjusts blood flow to a given tissue based on its oxygen needs. In this way, blood flow is directed toward the tissues that are metabolically active and away from those tissues that are resting. If blood flow falls in other organs when some organs increase flow, it is only because either perfusion pressure falls or resistance in the other organs increases. In most tissues, any shortfall in the oxygen supply relative to the metabolic demand is accompanied by an accumulation of metabolites (including CO_2, H^+ ions, ADP, AMP, adenosine, lactic acid, K^+ ions, and inorganic phosphates). These particular metabolites also serve as vasodilators. Decreased pO2, except in the lungs, can produce vasodilation that is independent of metabolite accumulation. This occurs through the direct action of hypoxia on smooth muscle mitochondrial energy production. However, vasoactive metabolites usually are the major contributors to hypoxic vasodilation.

Active or **functional hyperemia** describes the relationship between tissue metabolism and blood flow. The phenomenon of autoregulation of blood flow in response to changes in perfusion pressure is very important in the regulation of cerebral, coronary, and renal blood flow.

Reactive hyperemia refers to the situation in which metabolites accumulate, resulting in vasodilation. Such a situation prevails when an occlusive tourniquet is removed from the arm of a patient. On placing the tourniquet, blood flow (and the flow of oxygen and other nutrients) to and from the distal tissues is blocked, causing a local accumulation of metabolic by-products (such as those listed above), leading to vasodilation in an attempt to increase flow to the ischemic arm. Once the tourniquet is released, blood flow resumes in the now-dilated vascular bed, giving a transient deep-red color (hyperemia) to the forearm. As the vasoactive metabolites are flushed out of the arm with circulating blood, vasomotor tone returns to normal, restoring normal blood flow and arm color. The duration of this hyperemia can be increased either by prolonging the occlusion or by increasing the activity of the occluded extremity; both maneuvers enhance the cumulative hypoxia of the tissues, allowing the accumulation of vasoactive substances that promote blood flow to the region after the occlusion is removed.

The pulmonary circulation exhibits the opposite behavior in the context of tissue hypoxia. To maximize oxygenation of the blood, the lungs direct blood flow to the regions of greatest availability of O_2 and away from the regions with a low partial pressure of oxygen. Consequently, in the lungs, a low PO_2 results in vasoconstriction rather than vasodilatation, as seen in most parts of the systemic circulation.

Prostaglandins, leukotrienes, serotonin, and bradykinin all exert variable influences on arteriolar resistance in different vascular territories. Another important mediator of resistance in various vascular beds is the vasoconstrictor endothelin.

Adrenergic Receptors in Central Control We already described some of the central control of the blood pressure above. Now we will explore the effector mechanisms by which the nervous system influences blood pressure. Nervous control of blood vessels is modulated primarily by the sympathetic nervous system. (The parasympathetic nervous system's primary role in blood pressure control is decreasing the heart rate in response to high blood pressure.) The main transmitter released from postganglionic sympathetic nerve terminals is **norepinephrine (NE)**, which exerts different effects on vascular smooth muscle depending on the type of receptor expressed in the tissue. Adrenergic receptors are of two classes, α and β, each of which has two major subtypes. The arterioles supplying tissues other than the heart and brain carry α_1 receptors and β_2 receptors. Stimulation of α_1 **receptors** leads to vasoconstriction, and stimulation of β_2 **receptors** leads to vasodilatation. TABLE 12.1 summarizes the actions of the sympathetic (adrenergic) receptors on the vasculature. The α_2 adrenoreceptors are also found in blood vessels, particularly in smaller-resistance vessels.

The effects of sympathetic stimulation are complex, because in any given tissue both receptor types are expressed, and the net effect is thus a summative one. Whether the net result is vasodilatation or vasoconstriction depends on the number and affinity of each type of receptor in a given vascular bed. The situation is further complicated by the fact that both epinephrine and NE are also produced in the adrenal medulla, and catecholamines of adrenal origin seem to have less effect on blood pressure than those of neural origin (perhaps because neurotransmitters released into the circulation reach the receptors on vascular smooth muscle in lower concentrations). In skeletal muscle, for instance, epinephrine in low concentrations dilates resistance vessels (owing to the predominance of the β-adrenergic effect), while at high concentrations it produces vasoconstriction (predominant α-adrenergic effect). *Low blood pressure sympathetically stimulates vasoconstriction in all vascular beds besides the heart and brain and stimulates faster and harder cardiac contraction.* This boosts systemic blood pressure by increasing SVR and CO, providing an increased driving force for perfusion of the heart and brain. High blood pressure leads to decreased sympathetic output and increased parasympathetic output, thus relaxing the nonbrain, nonheart arterioles (which reduces SVR) and decreasing the heart rate (which decreases the CO).

The nervous control of the circulation described in the previous paragraphs is primarily a short-term regulatory mechanism, allowing rapid response to short-term variations in blood pressure. More long-term regulation of blood pressure is afforded by the release of vasoactive agents into the bloodstream, which not only increase vascular resistance but also promote the restoration of blood volume, which is ultimately key to resuscitating the hypotensive patient. Included among these agents that act from *within* the vessel lumen rather than at a nerve terminus are angiotensin, aldosterone, and vasopressin (antidiuretic hormone [ADH]).

Humoral Control The **renin-angiotensin-aldosterone axis (RAA)** is a key cardiovascular regulatory system that is important not only to normal compensatory responses but also to the pathophysiology of disease states such as congestive heart failure and hypertension. (The RAA axis will be discussed again in Chapters 20 and 22.) Renin is a proteolytic enzyme released from the juxtaglomerular apparatus (JGA) of the kidney into the afferent arteriole of the glomerulus in response to conditions signaling low-pressure or low-volume states. Circulating renin cleaves the pro-peptide angiotensinogen (produced in the liver) to a 10-amino acid peptide, angiotensin I, which has little biological activity. Angiotensin I is then rapidly converted to an eight-amino acid peptide angiotensin II (AII) by angiotensin-converting enzyme (ACE), located in large quantities in the vascular endothelium of the pulmonary vessels. AII is a direct, fast-

Table 12.1   ADRENERGIC RECEPTORS

Receptor	Primary Location	Effect of Stimulation
α_1	Blood vessels	Vasoconstriction
α_2	Central nervous system (CNS)	Vasodilation
β_1	Heart	Increase in heart rate (chronotropy) / cardiac contractility (inotropy)
β_2	Blood vessels	Vasodilation

acting, potent vasoconstrictor that works primarily by activating the angiotensin II, type 1 (ATI) receptor. In states of low blood pressure or arterial volume, the signal sensed at the level of the JGA leads to a cascade of events that generate a compensatory AII-mediated increase in peripheral vascular resistance. This serves to complement the baroreceptor reflexes noted above to help maintain blood pressure. Both ACE and ATI receptors are important antihypertensive, pharmacologic targets.

The role of AII in moment-to-moment regulation of blood pressure in the normal state, however, is limited. The RAA axis is most active in patients who are salt or volume depleted owing to a low-salt diet, sweating, or other fluid loss (e.g., hemorrhage). The vasoconstrictor effect of AII is limited to sensitive vascular beds such as the renal, cutaneous, and splanchnic circulations; the coronary, cerebral, and pulmonary circulations, as well as the entire venous system, are protected from its effects.

As will be discussed in long-term regulation of blood pressure (Chapter 22), AII is also an important regulator of blood volume. It exerts this effect as a potent stimulator of the hypothalamic thirst center, promoting oral intake of fluids and by direct actions on the renal proximal tubule to enhance the reabsorption of sodium and on the adrenal cortex to produce the mineralocorticoid aldosterone, which stimulates reabsorption of sodium from the collecting duct of the nephron.

Renin release is stimulated not only by renal arterial baroreceptors but also by sympathetic outflow from the medullary pressor centers to sympathetic nerve terminals that synapse on the JGA.

As noted previously, catecholamines such as NE and epinephrine (primarily the latter) may also be released into the circulation by sympathetic stimulation of the adrenal cortex (due to physical exertion, cold, heat, hypoglycemia, pain, hypoxia, fear, etc.). These hormones exhibit effects on different vascular beds depending on the distribution of receptor types expressed in a given tissue. Because of its greater affinity for β-adrenergic receptors, for example, low systemic concentrations of epinephrine caused by low-intensity stimulation of the adrenal medulla lead to relaxation of vascular smooth muscle and vasodilatation.

ADH, or vasopressin, is a 9-amino acid peptide hormone synthesized in the hypothalamus and released from the posterior pituitary primarily in response to a decrease in blood volume (as sensed at the level of arterial baroreceptors) or to an increase in plasma osmolality (as sensed by sensitive osmoreceptors in the hypothalamus). Other factors, including physiologic stress (from pain or extreme temperature), may also promote ADH release, while alcohol and a variety of medications may inhibit it. ADH has two primary effects. The first, mediated by the vasopressin type 2 (V2) receptor and the primary effect under normal conditions, is to promote the reabsorption of water from the distal collecting duct of the nephron The second, mediated by the type 1 receptor (V1), is to cause constriction of vascular smooth muscle. The pressor effect occurs only at higher serum concentrations of vasopressin. The role of ADH in the regulation of extracellular fluid volume is discussed in detail in Chapter 23.

Atrial natriuretic peptide (ANP), like ADH, is an important regulator of fluid volume whose release is triggered by the cardiac stretch receptors. It acts to antagonize the ADH effect, reduce plasma volume, and lower blood pressure through a mechanism of systemic vasodilation, mediated by cyclic GMP. In volume-expanded states, increases in ANP lead to a loss of salt and water in the urine, decreasing the extracellular volume. Levels of the related B-type polypeptide (BNP) are used clinically to help characterize states of volume expansion and heart failure. Both conditions are associated with elevated levels due to increased transmural pressures causing atrial and ventricular stretch that results in release of the natriuretic peptide.

PATHOPHYSIOLOGY

A step-by-step account of the body's response to hemorrhage (bleeding) serves as a review of blood pressure regulation. Consider a gastrointestinal hemorrhage of moderate to severe volume from a bleeding gastric ulcer. The initial loss of blood leads to an immediate decrease in the mass of blood contained in the vessels and hence a drop in blood pressure. This is sensed at the level of the baroreceptors in the carotid sinus and aortic arch. The decreased stretch in these receptors leads to a reduction in the rate of firing of the afferent impulses to the cardiovascular control center in the brain. The brain, in turn, responds with a compensatory increase in sympathetic outflow and a decrease in vagal (parasympathetic) tone to the periphery, leading to massive peripheral vasoconstriction and increased heart rate.

Meanwhile, poor blood flow to the periphery results in poor oxygen delivery and the release of vasodilatory metabolites. The reflex nervous adjustments compete with the local metabolic and autoregulatory adjustments to try to return cardiac output and blood pressure to a level sufficient to maintain perfusion to vital organs, such as the brain and heart.

Increased sympathetic outflow to the arterioles causes constriction of the resistance vessels and an

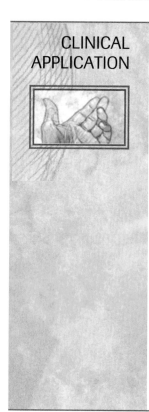

WHAT IS HYPERTENSION?

A 55-year-old man is observed on a routine physical to have a blood pressure of 150/100. He has no symptoms, and his ophthalmic examination is normal. The above-normal blood pressure is observed again on two subsequent visits. Attempts to take the blood pressure under relaxed circumstances at the end of the visit yield no different results.

Hypertension is defined as a systolic blood pressure (the first number) above 140 mm Hg and a diastolic blood pressure (the second number) above 90 mm Hg. Most cases of hypertension are of unknown cause and are called *essential hypertension*. Hypertension caused by other disease processes, such as atherosclerosis of the renal arteries (renal artery stenosis), is called *secondary hypertension*. The table below lists the classifications of hypertension, as delineated in the *Seventh Report of the Joint National Committee on Prevention, Evaluation, and Treatment of High Blood Pressure* (JNC 7).

Category	Systolic BP (mm Hg)		Diastolic BP (mm Hg)
Normal	<120	and	<80
Prehypertension	120–139	or	80–89
Hypertension, stage 1	140–159	or	90–99
Hypertension, stage 2	≥160	or	≥100

increase in peripheral vascular resistance, which increases blood pressure. The decrease in vagal tone and increase in sympathetic discharge to the heart increase heart rate and thus support cardiac output and blood pressure. Sympathetic outflow to the juxtaglomerular apparatus, as well as direct activation of the renal baroreceptors in the afferent arterioles of the nephron, leads to salt and water retention and the expansion of extracellular fluid volume. Meanwhile, sympathetic activation of the adrenal gland leads to the generation of circulating catecholamines, which increase vascular resistance and CO.

Local vasodilatory effects prevail in the heart and brain, sustaining blood flow to these areas, while central vasoconstrictive effects predominate in the muscles, gastrointestinal tract, and skin (and later in the kidneys), diverting blood flow to locations of high priority at the expense of lower-priority places. Clinically, this phenomenon manifests as cold, clammy extremities and decreased urine output in the patient who has had a moderate hemorrhage. (See Clinical Application Box *What Is Hypertension?*)

Summary

- The vascular circuit from right ventricle to left atrium is the pulmonary circulation. The circuit from left ventricle to right atrium is the systemic circulation.

- The blood volume is around 5 L, 4 L of which are contained in the low-pressure veins.

- The contraction of the cardiac ventricles is called systole; their relaxation is called diastole. Elastic recoil in the aorta propels blood onward during diastole, ensuring continuous flow (the Windkessel effect).

- The arterial system starts with the aorta and branches into smaller vessels. From large to small, these vessels are called arteries, arterioles, and capillaries. The arterioles are muscular and can be dilated or constricted by neural and hormonal influences.

- Changes in vessel volume with the mass of fluid remaining constant influence pressure at a point in the vascular circuit: $P \sim n/V$.

- The heart shrinks the vessel volume when it contracts, raising the pressure in its chambers. It must do work to compress the chamber walls: $W = P(\Delta V)$.

- Pressure difference (ΔP) makes a gas or fluid flow from one location to another. When the heart contracts, it creates a high pressure in the vascular circuit relative to spots downstream, causing blood to move forward through the vascular system

- Blood flow ($\dot{Q}$) is measured in liters per minute.

- Friction opposes the flow of blood. Resistance (R) is a measure of friction in the vessel. It is proportional to the vessel radius (r), a relationship described by Poiseuille's law: $R = 8\eta l/\pi r^4$.
- Ohm's law describes the relation between ΔP, $\dot{Q}$, and R: $\Delta P = \dot{Q}R$. The pressure difference between two points can be represented by Ohm's law.
- A greater pressure difference drives more blood flow, and for a given pressure difference, more resistance shrinks the blood flow.
- Resistance also creates pressure differences in vessels, though this is not the relationship between R and ΔP described by Ohm's law. Resistance creates pressure differences by increasing the mass of fluid upstream of the resistance and decreasing the mass of fluid downstream of the resistance.
- Ohm's law applied to the entire cardiovascular circuit is MAP = (CO)(SVR), where MAP is mean arterial pressure, CO is cardiac output, and SVR is systemic vascular resistance.
- MAP is controlled locally (by factors intrinsic to the vessels themselves) and centrally (by reflexes involving the brain) and by the kidneys.
- Local control includes the myogenic response (in which wall stretch leads to vasoconstriction and vice versa), the endothelial secretion of factors such as nitric oxide, and the release of metabolic vasodilators.
- Central control is through the baroreceptor reflex. Baroreceptors sense low pressure and stimulate the medulla, and the medulla increases sympathetic output. Increased sympathetic output increases CO (by increasing heart rate and contractility) and arteriolar constriction in vascular beds other than in the heart and brain.
- Humoral control involves important vasoconstrictors such as AII and ADH and vasodilators like ANP. These hormones, working in the short term on vascular resistance to control blood pressure, also have more long-term effects to regulate blood pressure by effects on renal control of the circulating volume.
- Arteriolar constriction raises systemic vascular resistance (SVR), which raises systemic blood pressure. The increased blood pressure drives perfusion (blood flow) into the heart and brain, whose arterioles are not constricted.

Suggested Reading

Andresen MC, Kunze DL. Nucleus tractus solitarius—gateway to neural circulatory control. Annu Rev Physiol. 1994;56:93–116.

Cowley AW Jr. Long-term control of arterial blood pressure. Physiol Rev. 1992;72(1):231–300.

Lanfranchi PA, Somers VK. Arterial baroreflex function and cardiovascular variability: interactions and implications. Am J Physiol Regul Integr Comp Physiol. 2002;283(4):R815–826.

Stauss HM. Baroreceptor reflex function. Am J Physiol Regul Integr Comp Physiol. 2002;283(2):R284–286.

REVIEW QUESTIONS

Directions: Each of the numbered items or incomplete statements in this section is followed by answers or by completions of the statement. Select the ONE lettered answer or completion that is BEST in each case.

1. A 22-year-old woman is brought to the emergency room with severe hemorrhaging from open wounds on her lower extremities and a blood pressure of 80/40. The following would best describe her blood vessels:
   - (A) Vasoconstriction in all vascular beds
   - (B) Vasoconstriction in CNS and coronary arteries only
   - (C) Vasodilation in all vascular beds
   - (D) Vasoconstriction in all vascular beds except CNS and coronary
   - (E) Vasodilation in all vascular beds except CNS and coronary

2. During pregnancy, vascular circuits are added in parallel to the systemic circulation as maternal blood vessels grow into the decidua basalis and fill the intervillous spaces with blood. The addition of parallel blood vessels or vascular spaces to the vascular circuit will:
   - (A) Increase SVR
   - (B) Decrease SVR
   - (C) Increase CO
   - (D) Decrease CO
   - (E) Not affect SVR or CO

3. Anxiety is known to raise the mean arterial pressure. It may do so by which of the following mechanisms?
   - (A) Increased stroke volume
   - (B) Increased parasympathetic output to the sinoatrial node of the heart
   - (C) Decreased sympathetic output to the arterioles
   - (D) Increased sympathetic output to the capillaries
   - (E) Sweat

ANSWERS TO REVIEW QUESTIONS

1. **The answer is D.** She has low blood pressure due to hemorrhage. This would trigger her baroreceptor reflex, causing widespread vasoconstriction of her arterioles with sparing of the coronary arteries in the heart and the arterioles of the brain. The widespread vasoconstriction boosts the SVR and the MAP, and the increased MAP helps sustain perfusion of the heart and brain.

2. **The answer is B.** An additional parallel vascular circuit decreases SVR. This is because adding circuits in parallel is effectively the same as increasing the cross-sectional area (hence radius) of the vascular tree. A larger radius means a lower resistance.

3. **The answer is A.** Anxiety increases sympathetic outflow from the CNS, which boosts the contractility of the heart, leading to larger stroke volumes. CO = heart rate times stroke volume, so increased stroke volume increases CO, elevating the blood pressure. Parasympathetic output slows the heart rate, decreasing CO and MAP. Anxiety can sometimes lead to increases in MAP, followed by parasympathetic reflexes that lower the MAP. This is called the vasovagal reflex (see Chapter 22).

13

The Heart as a Pump

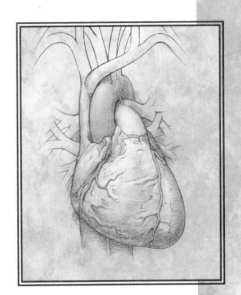

INTRODUCTION

In Chapter 12, we introduced the vascular analogy to Ohm's law. We saw that muscular contraction of the cardiac ventricles is necessary to create the pressure difference that drives blood flow through the cardiovascular system. In this chapter, we will examine more closely the mechanics of the pump that generates this pressure difference and the physiologic and pathophysiologic consequences of alterations in the function of the pump. Cardiac tissue has a heavy burden: it must contract in a responsive, controlled, and reliable manner more than 1 billion times in an average lifetime.

SYSTEM STRUCTURE

The human heart is a four-chambered pump surrounded by a fibrous sac (FIGURE 13.1). The most superficial tissue of the heart is the *pericardium*, a three-layered structure that encases the heart and the roots of the great vessels. The outer fibrous layer of the pericardium functions as a protective shell for the organ, while the inner serous layers secrete pericardial fluid into the potential space created between them. This potential space, the *pericardial sac*, provides a low-friction pocket in which the cardiac muscle can move as it contracts. Cardiac geography, as is so often the case, is described in precisely the opposite of common sense. The superior-most region of the heart (the top of the atria) is called its *base*, while the inferior-most region of the heart (the tip of the ventricles) is called its *apex*.

As suggested in Chapter 12, the heart can be thought of as two pumps. The right heart pumps deoxygenated blood into the pulmonary circulation, and the left heart provides oxygenated blood to the systemic circulation. Each pump contains two chambers: an atrium and a ventricle. The **atria** are thin-walled, low-pressure reservoirs that collect venous blood upon its return to the heart. The atria contract before the ventricles, forcing blood into the ventricle for pulmonary or systemic circulation. The **ventricles**, the major functional compartments of the heart, are thick-walled, muscular, high-pressure chambers. Each ventricle leads to an outflow tract into its respective arterial root. The **right ventricle (RV)** leads to the pulmonary root, and the **left ventricle (LV)** leads to the aortic root. The RV expels its contents into the relatively low-pressure pulmonary arterial tree, and as such its walls are considerably thinner than that of the LV. The RV generates approximately one seventh of the maximal LV pressure.

An extensive **conduction system** courses through both the atria and the ventricles, terminating in the conductive **Purkinje fibers**, which stimulate the muscle cells. This tissue, specialized for the

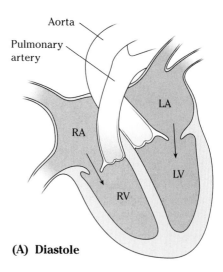

(A) Diastole

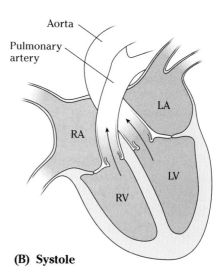

(B) Systole

Figure 13.1 Gross anatomy of the heart. The heart is shown during diastole (ventricular relaxation and filling) and systole (ventricular contraction and ejection). RA, right atrium; LA, left atrium; RV, right ventricle; LV, left ventricle.

transmission of action potentials, is arranged to ensure a pattern of three-dimensional contraction optimal for the successful pumping of blood. Thus, the atria contract essentially from the top of the heart toward the valves between the atria and ventricles, propelling blood down into the ventricular chambers. The ventricles contract from the bottom of the heart upward, propelling blood into the up-directed pulmonary and aortic arteries.

The final structural components of the heart pump are its valves. The valves are endothelialized fibrous structures secured to a dense, fibrous cardiac skeleton. As their name implies, the **atrioventricular (AV) valves** separate the atria from the ventricles. The right heart contains the three-leaflet **tricuspid valve**, while the bicuspid **mitral valve** resides in the left heart. The AV valves remain passively open while blood flows from the atria to the ventricles. As the ventricles contract, the increasing chamber pressure eventually forces the tricuspid and mitral valves to close. The endocardial surface of each ventricle contains muscular projections, known as *papillary muscles*, connected to the free edges of the AV valves through fibrous threads, known as *chordae tendineae*, and serve to anchor the valve leaflets during ventricular contraction. As the contraction signal spreads through the ventricles, it initiates papillary muscle contraction first, allowing the chordae tendineae to tense prior to the expulsion of blood. This anchoring inhibits the excursion of AV valve leaflets into the atrial cavities during contraction, thereby preventing *atrial regurgitation*, which could jeopardize the systemic circulation of blood.

The three-cusped **semilunar valves** separate the ventricles from their arterial roots. The semilunar valves remain closed until ventricular contraction when the intraventricular pressure builds, forcing the valves open. Their semilunate shape enables them to endure the tremendous force of blood flow encountered over their surfaces during ventricular contraction. The right heart contains the **pulmonic valve**, while the left heart contains the **aortic valve.** The cavities produced by the semilunar shape of the valve leaflets are the sinuses of Valsalva, and it is in the right and left aortic sinuses of Valsalva that the right and left coronary arteries originate.

Histology

The **myocardium**, or cardiac muscle tissue, is a special type of striated muscle. While the myocardium shares many of the properties of other vertebrate striated muscle, it also has certain unique features that distinguish it anatomically, histologically, electrophysiologically, and functionally. The basis of this specialization is the **cardiac myocyte**, or muscle cell, which is specialized for rhythmic conduction and contraction. The histology of the cells is similar to skeletal muscle in that the basic contractile unit remains the **sarcomere**, a group of *actin* and *myosin filaments* (myofibrils). The cell membrane of the myocytes is called the *sarcolemma* as in skeletal muscle, and the sarcolemma invaginates into a system of *T tubules* to excite the muscle cells, as in any other muscle cells.

There are, however, several important differences between cardiac muscle tissue and skeletal muscle tissue. A unique feature of myocardial tissue is the intercalated disc, seen histologically as a dark-staining band between myocytes. **Intercalated discs** are collections of gap junctions that provide low-resistance points of cytoplasmic communication between adjacent myocytes. They thereby enable efficient cell-to-cell transmission of charge and fulfill an important requirement of functional myocardium: the rapid conduction of action potentials. Rapid action potential conduction in turn allows the synchronous, ordered, and rapid contraction throughout the myocardium that is critical to the pumping of the heart.

Cardiac myocytes also have a high density of mitochondria. These organelles account for around 35% of the cell volume and provide the large supply of ATP necessary to fulfill its constant work requirement. The genesis of adequate amounts of ATP depends on the presence of oxygen, so cardiac tissue is also very well perfused. A nearly 1:1 ratio of capillary to myocyte ensures that the cardiac tissue has access to abundant oxygen and can also purge itself of its copious waste products.

SYSTEM FUNCTION

Cardiac function is in one sense extremely simple: the physics of its contraction recapitulate the physics of contraction of just one muscle cell. Consequently, we will examine the contraction of the individual cardiac myocyte as we discuss the contractile function of the organ as a whole. The essential concepts of this chapter are preload, afterload, and contractility, which apply to cardiac physiology on the cellular level and the organic level.

Excitation-Contraction Coupling

The contraction of an individual myocyte begins with stimulation by the Purkinje fibers or by an adjacent muscle cell. Stimulation means depolarization of the myocyte cell membrane, creating an action potential. To translate this electrical stimulation into action, the cell must couple this chemical excitation with a mechanical force, a process called **excitation-contraction coupling.** It does so via ionic calcium, whose intracellular release ultimately converts high-energy chemical bonds into mechanical cross-bridging of actin and myosin filaments (FIGURE 13.2).

The events occur as follows. During phase 2 of depolarization, the sarcolemma and network of T tubules become increasingly permeable to calcium. The channels open by means of a voltage-dependent mechanism that is modulated by cAMP-dependent phosphorylation of Ca^{2+} channels. This extracellular-sourced Ca^{2+} influx triggers the larger intracellular release of Ca^{2+} from the sarcoplasmic reticulum. The intracellular concentration of Ca^{2+} rises one to two orders of magnitude during this excitation to about 10^{-5} M. Unlike in skeletal muscle, the Ca^{2+} release

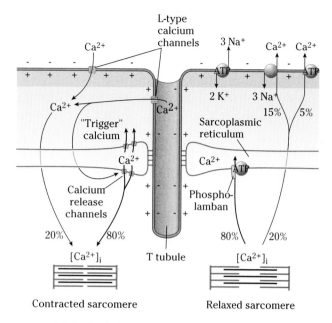

Figure 13.2 Excitation-contraction coupling. The left side of the diagram shows contraction; the right represents recovery.

from the sarcolemma and T tubule network plays a crucial role in achieving appropriate contraction in the myocyte.

At rest, the contractile proteins *troponin* and *tropomyosin* are arranged to interfere with the cross-bridging of actin filaments and myosin heads. However, once Ca^{2+} enters the cell, it allosterically binds to *troponin-C*, inducing a conformational change in the thin filament that subsequently promotes cross-bridge formation. Once phase 2 of the action potential ceases, Ca^{2+} release halts, and the intracellular Ca^{2+} is rapidly extruded from the cell and resequestered into the sarcoplasmic reticulum.

The resequestration of Ca^{2+} is accomplished by an ATP-driven Ca^{2+} pump stimulated by phosphorylated phospholamban. This last step illustrates the dual, conflicting role that phosphorylation plays in myocardial contraction. Cyclic-AMP-dependent protein kinase has two actions: (1) to accelerate contraction, via the phosphorylation of sarcolemmal Ca^{2+} pumps responsible for the initial Ca^{2+} influx during phase 2, and (2) to accelerate relaxation, via the phosphorylation of phospholamban, stimulating resequestration of Ca^{2+} during diastole.

For a more complete description of the various phases of cardiac electrical activity, see Chapter 14.

Three Determinants of Stroke Volume

Three variables affect myocardial function: preload, afterload, and contractility. Although these properties apply to the discussion of all myocardial tissue, they are best understood in the context of the

primary functional chamber of the heart, the left ventricle. The function ultimately affected by these variables is the amount of blood the LV ejects during a single contraction, known as the **stroke volume (SV)**.

Preload The **preload** is the degree of stretching of the myocardium and its myofibrils prior to contraction. It is closely related to the extent of chamber filling (with blood). The more blood that has entered a chamber prior to its contraction, the longer its myofibrils will be prior to contraction. *Stretched myofibrils generate more force.* This is because stretching results in more actin-myosin cross-bridging (FIGURE 13.3). Therefore, more venous return of blood to the heart, which fills the cardiac chambers to a greater extent, will result in more forceful cardiac contraction.

Experiments show that the tension developed during contraction increases with increasing initial length of the myofibril up to a plateau of maximal tension, beyond which the generated force is inversely related to initial length (FIGURE 13.4). This maximal tension, for myocytes, occurs at a length of 2.0 to 2.4 μm. At shorter lengths, <2.0 μm, the actin filaments actually begin to overlap and interfere with myosin-actin interactions. At lengths greater than 2.4 μm, there is limited actin-myosin interaction at best, producing little active tension.

Chamber filling of the LV just before contraction is called the **LV end-diastolic volume** (or, less commonly, the LV end-diastolic pressure). Filling occurs during diastole and contraction begins when diastole ends and systole begins. LV end-diastolic volume is an effective measurement of preload. Therefore,

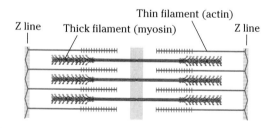

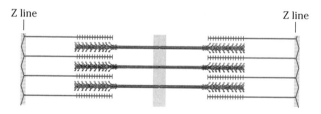

Figure 13.3 A sarcomere at varying lengths. At greater lengths, there is more actin-myosin cross-bridging, implying a greater force of muscular contraction. This is the basis of the Frank-Starling relationship.

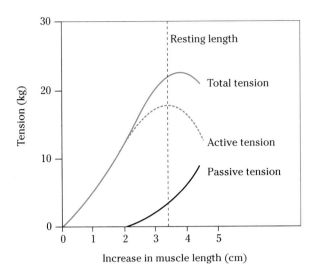

Figure 13.4 Muscle force versus muscle length.

within a certain physiological range, as the LV end-diastolic volume increases, the force generated by the LV will also increase, leading to a proportional increase in the volume expelled from the LV, or SV. This is known as the **Frank-Starling relationship.**

Afterload The **afterload** is the force opposing my-ocardial contraction. If a muscle fiber were attached to a weight on one end, the weight would be the af-terload (FIGURE 13.5). Whereas the preload is reflected in the initial length of the myofibrils (the initial degree of chamber filling), the afterload is reflected in the final length of the myofibrils. Afterload delimits how far the muscle can contract. The final length of muscle tissue contracting against a fixed afterload will be the same regardless of differences in preload; tissues with increased preload and the same after-load will simply contract a greater distance to rest at the same endpoint (by the Frank-Starling mecha-nism). Having started bigger (more full of blood) and contracting down to a fixed endpoint still involves more ejection of blood (a larger SV), so high preload with fixed afterload still increases SV.

Whereas LV preload was determined by the LV end-diastolic volume, the LV afterload is determined by the pressure in the aorta. The aortic pressure (afterload) hence determines how far the LV can contract during systole and sets the **LV end-systolic volume.** An LV end-systolic volume exists because the heart never completely empties itself of blood. The percentage of blood purged from the left ven-tricle during systole is called the **ejection fraction.** A normal ejection fraction is around 60%. For a fixed preload, an increase in afterload will result in a decreased SV and hence a decreased ejection fraction.

Contractility **Contractility** is the force generated by the myocardium under conditions of fixed preload and afterload. It is directly related to the availability of Ca^{2+} in the cell. It can be measured as the maximal force generated in isometric contraction (contrac-tion that increases tension but does not produce movement) at a fixed preload. Changes in contractil-ity are achieved hormonally, with inotropic agents such as norepinephrine. (Inotropy = contractility.) Norepinephrine and epinephrine increase the level of intracellular cAMP, which is critical to initiating contraction. With increased contractility comes increased contractile force and thus increased SV at any given preload and afterload. Afterload can there-fore limit contraction of the ventricle over a range of preloads, but only if the contractility is held constant. Increased contractility allows the ventricle to con-tract farther (to a smaller LV end-systolic volume) against a fixed afterload. This represents an increase in the ejection fraction. The ejection fraction, which can be measured by echocardiogram, is a critical indicator of the health of the myocardium. My-ocardium that is injured and scarred—for example, due to ischemia (poor perfusion from the coronary arteries)—generates a lesser force of contraction than a healthy heart at the same preload and after-load; in other words, injured myocardium possesses less contractility.

The Cardiac Cycle

One **cardiac cycle** is the period of time from the beginning of one ventricular contraction to the beginning of the next. There are several important physical, electrical, and audible phenomena that repeat during the cardiac cycle (FIGURE 13.6). The discussion below details the events of the cardiac cycle and will continually refer to the various trac-ings in the figure. While the cardiac cycle applies to both the left and right hearts, the discussion below focuses on the left heart. FIGURE 13.7 shows another way to look at the cardiac cycle: the pressure-volume loop.

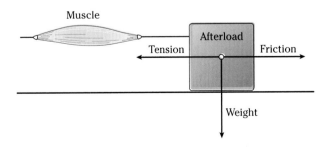

Figure 13.5 An analogy for afterload. In the analogy, friction is the afterload, which opposes the force of muscle tension.

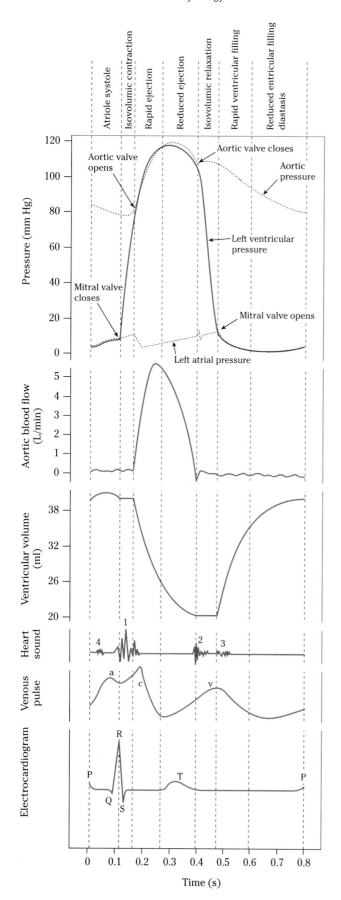

Figure 13.6 The cardiac cycle.

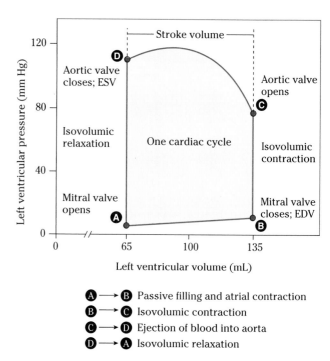

Figure 13.7 The cardiac cycle depicted as a pressure-volume loop. EDV, end-diastolic volume; ESV, end-systolic volume.

Systole The cardiac cycle consists of two phases, systole and diastole. **Systole** encompasses the time of ventricular contraction and can be audibly estimated as the period between the beginnings of the first and second heart sounds. The average systolic time is 0.28 second, and it accounts for about 35% of the cardiac cycle. As the ventricles begin to contract, an event coinciding with the *R wave* electrocardiographically, they very quickly achieve a ventricular pressure sufficient to force the atrioventricular valves shut. The vibrations produced by the closure of these valves and the turbulent flow resulting from their abrupt closure can be auscultated (heard through the stethoscope) on the chest wall as the **first heart sound**, known as **S₁**.

The interval of contraction between the AV valve closure and the opening of the semilunar valves is the period of **isovolumic contraction**, as the ventricle generates pressure without the expulsion of blood volume. Once the ventricular pressure exceeds that of the outflow tract (approximately 80 mm Hg for the aorta), the semilunar valves are forced open, and flow commences into the arterial tree.

Approximately 70% of the total ejected volume is expelled during the first third of the ejection interval, known as the period of **rapid ejection.** During this time the ventricular pressure continues to rapidly increase, and blood flow is maximal. As the displaced volume begins to redistribute further down the arterial system and the force of ventricular contraction decreases, ejection of the remaining 30% continues at a slower rate. This period, accounting for the last two thirds of the ejection time, is known as the **slow ejection phase** and is approximated electrocardiographically by the beginning of the **T wave.**

Although the LV and aortic pressure curves demonstrate a reversal of the pressure gradient immediately after the rapid ejection phase (with LV pressure falling slightly below aortic pressure), blood continues to flow from the ventricle to the aorta as a result of fluid momentum generated during ejection. As the ventricle begins to relax, its pressure eventually falls to a level insufficient to maintain the opening of the semilunar valves. Closure of these valves produces the **second heart sound, S_2,** and marks the end of systole. Examination of the atrial pressure curve during systole reveals an initial pressure increase, the *c wave*, during isovolumic contraction reflecting "bulging" of the AV valve leaflets into the atrial chambers. This is followed by a steady increase in atrial pressure, the *v wave*, reflecting the collection of venous return into the closed atrial chambers.

Diastole Diastole, encompassing the period of ventricular relaxation, begins with S_2. The interval between the closure of the semilunar valves and the opening of the AV valves, during which the ventricles relax, is known as the period of **isovolumic relaxation** as the ventricular chamber volume remains constant but chamber pressure drops. There is a brief positive deflection in the aortic pressure tracing at the start of this phase as the aortic valve closes and the elastic recoil of the aorta begins to squeeze the aortic blood. This is called the **dicrotic notch.**

The ventricular pressure continues to fall until it dips below the atrial pressure. At this time, the mitral and tricuspid AV valves open. The opening of the AV valves allows blood to once again flow freely into the ventricles, thereby releasing the pressure buildup represented by the atrial *v* wave. This initial flow of contents into the ventricles is known as the **rapid filling phase.** It makes up the first third of diastole and contributes the majority of volume to the ventricular chambers.

The second third of diastole, known as **diastasis**, represents effectively free flow from venous conduits to the ventricles; this period contributes minimally to the filling of the ventricles. Atrial contraction takes place during the last third of diastole and coincides with the **P wave** electrocardiographically, and the *a* wave on the atrial pressure tracing. While this **atrial kick** contributes only about 25% of the end-diastolic ventricular volume, it becomes a crucial event to a heart in which normal filling of the ventricle is compromised, such as rapid heart rate or severe AV valve stenoses (conditions that narrow the valve opening).

Normal Heart Sounds and Venous Pulsations A clinician relies on physical examination skills to appreciate the different periods and events of the cardiac cycle and to detect any abnormalities in the cycle. Two components of the cardiac clinical examination that pertain particularly to the cardiac cycle are heart sounds and venous pulsation. A brief overview of normal heart sounds and venous pulsation is therefore useful.

As mentioned above, systole begins with S_1. S_1 comprises two nearly superimposed sounds, the closure of the tricuspid and mitral valves, and its intensity is directly proportional to the distance between the valve leaflets as they begin close. The farther the leaflets must travel to close, the greater the intensity of vibration, and thus sound, that is produced. The first heart sound can be heard best over the auscultatory zones for each of the valves involved. Therefore, the mitral component, which provides the major contribution to S_1, is best auscultated over the fifth intercostal space at the cardiac apex, while the softer tricuspid component is heard best over the fifth intercostal space at the left border of the sternum.

The second heart sound, which marks the end of systole, is also a combination of two valve closures and can best be heard at the base (top) of the heart. The aortic valve closure, A_2, slightly precedes the pulmonic valve closure, P_2, owing to the greater pressure gradient between the aorta and LV versus the pulmonary trunk and the RV. During inspiration, the negative intrathoracic pressure produces increased venous return to the right heart (from extrathoracic sources via the superior vena cava and inferior vena cava) and also decreases venous return to the left heart (by pooling in the intrathoracic pulmonary venous tree). This change in ventricular volume prolongs ejection from the right heart, thereby delaying P_2, and shortens ejection from the left heart, thereby creating an earlier A_2. These slight changes in the timing of the two components of S_2 make them disparate enough to be audible as two distinct sounds by the human ear. This phenomenon is known as *physiological splitting of S_2.* Skilled auscultation can identify disturbances in physiological splitting, such as wide splitting or paradoxical splitting (splitting on expiration in place of inspiration), providing clues to the diagnosis of a variety of pathological conditions involving the structure of the valves or the pressures of the arterial roots. (See Clinical Application Box *S_3 and S_4 Heart Sounds.*)

The second observable event of the cardiac cycle is **venous pulsation.** The various stages of fluid collection and expulsion from the atria are manifested by the atrial *a* wave (**a**trial contraction), *c* wave (**c**ontraction of the ventricles), and *v* wave (**v**enous collection). Recall that there are no valves between the right atrium and the superior vena cava,

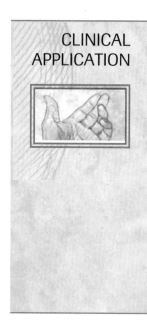

S_3 AND S_4 HEART SOUNDS

The S_3 heart sound is caused by vibration of the ventricle in early diastole, upon rapidly filling and suddenly reaching its elastic limits. An S_3 heart sound may be heard in healthy children and young adults, but in adults an audible S_3 is pathologic. An audible S_3 is heard in two conditions: overfilling and decreased cardiac compliance, as in constrictive pericarditis and cardiomyopathy. Overfilling occurs in congestive heart failure and valvular disease.

The S_4 heart sound is caused by vibration of the ventricle in late diastole, when atrial contraction causes an onrush of blood into the ventricle. The S_4 is heard in "high-output" states, which feature more vigorous atrial contractions. It is also heard in states of decreased cardiac compliance and in the arrhythmia called AV block (see Chapter 14), where conduction of the contractile signal is abnormal and contraction is uncoordinated. In this case, the atrium contracts against a closed mitral valve, drumming the blood on the roof of the sealed ventricle that should still be open but is not. S_4 is not heard in the arrhythmia called atrial fibrillation because there is no organized atrial contraction in atrial fibrillation.

or between the internal jugular (IJ) vein and the superior vena cava. The right atrium and IJ vein are therefore contiguous, and a clinician can gather information about the right atrium by examining the jugular veins. Distention of the jugular veins reflects the pressure in the right atrium, and venous pulsation in the IJ reflects the timing of the cardiac cycles. If the heart is not pumping adequately (e.g., owing to myocardial ischemia) and too much blood is left behind in the right atrium, the right atrial pressure will be elevated. This in turn will be reflected by the presence of *jugular venous distention (JVD).*

Oxygen Demand and Supply

As mentioned above, the heart has an enormous demand for oxygen, and it provides itself with a large flow of oxygenated blood through the coronary arteries. Flow through any circuit, in analogy to Ohm's law, is proportional to the pressure gradient and inversely proportional to resistance. Hence, blood flow (and oxygen supply) is increased by an increased pressure difference across the coronary arteries and reduced by an increased coronary resistance, as occurs in coronary atherosclerosis. Oxygen supply is a product of the blood flow and the arterial oxygen content. It is possible to have a high flow rate with decreased oxygen supply if the blood is hypoxic. The heart has a large arterial-venous oxygen difference, so the oxygen supply in a coronary capillary is rapidly consumed and exhausted of its oxygen content. Further oxygen consumption by the myocytes requires a fresh supply of oxygenated blood. Therefore, coronary blood flow is rate-limiting for cardiac oxygen consumption. This makes the myocardium particularly vulnerable to ischemia if the coronary blood flow is compromised.

The demand of O_2 by the myocardium is influenced by the work output of the muscle. The work output, in turn, is determined by heart rate, contractility, and wall tension. Increased heart rate increases metabolic demand by increasing contractions per unit time, while increased contractility increases ATP use through more rapid actin-myosin cross-bridge cycling. Finally, wall tension is a measure of afterload, representing the load against which the ventricles must contract. Wall tension of the ventricles is estimated by using **Laplace's law,** relating wall tension of a sphere to its dimensions and transmural pressure: $\sigma = Pr/2h$ where σ = wall tension, P = transmural pressure, r = sphere radius, and h = wall thickness. Therefore, wall tension (dynes/cm) increases with increased systolic ventricular pressure, increased chamber size, or decreased myocardial thickness. As this wall tension, or afterload, is increased, the myocardium must expend more energy per contraction. Wall tension is distinguished from wall stress, which is tension divided by wall thickness (dynes/cm^2).

The Regulation of Cardiac Output

The demand placed on the heart is enormous: it must maintain adequate systemic blood flow to meet the metabolic needs of all tissues of the body, at all times, under all conditions, ceaselessly for a lifetime. Fortunately, a healthy human heart is powerfully equipped to meet this demand with its unique physiology and regulatory mechanisms. This section focuses on the maintenance of adequate cardiac output (CO). As discussed in Chapter 12, however, CO is only one of the means by which perfusion of the tissues is regulated. The other means is the modification of systemic vascular resistance.

CO is routinely used as a measure of cardiac performance. It is the product of heart rate and SV. Thus, CO is regulated by alterations of SV and heart rate. Extrinsic regulatory systems, including the nervous system and reflex arcs, mediate adaptations in heart rate and in SV, while the primary intrinsic regulatory system, the Frank-Starling mechanism, mediates only SV changes.

Regulation of Stroke Volume The Frank-Starling mechanism helps to ensure that changes in preload lead to commensurate changes in SV and hence in CO. Changes in preload are changes in the LV end-diastolic volume and are caused by increases in cardiac filling (e.g., increased venous return as seen in exercise) or decreases in cardiac emptying (e.g., in aortic or mitral regurgitation). Owing to the Frank-Starling mechanism, however, this greater stretch of the myocardial fibers results in a stronger contraction, leading to the same LV end-systolic volume (FIGURE 13.8). Thus, increases in preload result in increases in SV. Without the Frank-Starling mechanism, increased venous return to the heart could not be met with increased CO, and the blood would back up in the veins. Inadequate CO with venous backup is what is known as congestive heart failure.

The Frank-Starling mechanism can also indirectly help the heart compensate for increased afterload. Increases in afterload, seen in situations such as hypertension or aortic stenosis, require the LV to attain a higher end-diastolic pressure before the aortic valve will open. The heart can sustain this pressure for a shorter period of time, so the valve shuts and the end-systolic volume is reached sooner, thereby reducing the SV. Importantly, however, this change in SV is rectified on the subsequent contraction. The decreased SV leads to a larger residual volume in the LV, to which the normal volume of blood from the right atrium will be added, thus increasing the LV end-diastolic volume. This increased LV end-diastolic volume (preload) will, by the Frank-Starling mechanism, proportionally increase the force of contraction and thus reestablish something close to the original SV. The reconstitution of SV, however, comes at the expense of higher end-diastolic filling volumes and pressures, which can have deleterious effects on long-term myocardial performance. Chronic changes in afterload are also compensated physically by structural changes of the heart, which may not be healthy in the long run. Since higher afterload means the LV must attain higher maximal pressures, the ventricle wall is subjected to higher transmural pressures. From Laplace's law, this means the wall tension is higher and the metabolic demand is higher. To compensate for the increased wall stress, the heart manipulates other variables in Laplace's law because it cannot modify the transmural pressure. It increases its wall

thickness (hypertrophy) and reduces its chamber size (concentric hypertrophy), thereby combating the increased wall stress of increased afterload.

Contractility is adjusted by regulatory systems extrinsic to the heart. Regardless of preload or afterload, if contractility is increased, the SV is increased. The body makes use of increases in contractility to boost the systemic blood pressure when its baroreceptors detect that blood pressure is low. Epinephrine and norepinephrine (sympathetic output) increase the contractility of the heart. Baroreceptor regulation of cardiac output is covered in Chapters 12 and 22.

In summary, SV, and thus CO output, are increased with increased preload and contractility and decreased by increased afterload (which is corrected at the expense of increased ventricular filling pressures and volumes [i.e., increased preload]).

Regulation of Heart Rate Heart rate, the second component of CO, is regulated in parallel with con-

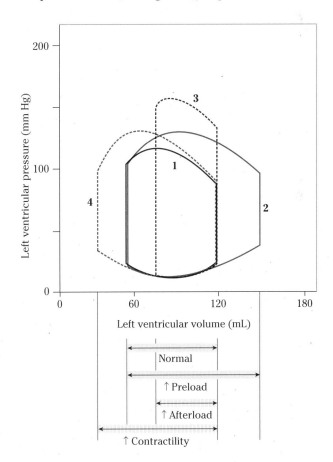

Figure 13.8 The effect of altered preload, afterload, and contractility on SV. Alterations in these parameters are depicted with pressure-volume loops to illustrate their effects on the entire cardiac cycle. Loop 1 represents the normal cardiac cycle. Loop 2 represents increased preload at the same afterload and contractility as loop 1 (which increases the SV by the Frank-Starling mechanism). Loop 3 represents increased afterload with the same preload and contractility as loop 1. Loop 4 represents increased contractility with the same preload and afterload as loop 1. Stroke volumes are shown below the pressure-volume graph.

tractility by the sympathetic and parasympathetic nervous systems. The heart is thus richly and strategically innervated by both divisions of the autonomic nervous system (ANS). The ANS can alone produce a twofold to threefold increase in CO or bring CO nearly to a halt. Parasympathetic control is mediated through the vagus nerve. The preganglionic cells arise in the medulla oblongata and synapse with postganglionic cells on or in the surface of the heart. Vagal innervation predominantly involves the **sinoatrial node** (containing "pacemaker" cells) and **atrioventricular node** and primarily affects heart rate through the release of acetylcholine.

Sympathetic innervation arises from spinal levels C7 through T6. The preganglionic fibers synapse in the stellate and cervical ganglia with postganglionic fibers, which then directly innervate the heart. The sympathetic nervous system predominantly innervates the ventricular tissue, with a lesser presence in nodal tissue. Stimulation of the sympathetic system leads to the activation of β-adrenergic receptors and primarily affects the contractility of the myocardium. Both divisions of the autonomic nervous system exhibit a tonic and antagonistic stimulation of the heart, allowing for precise manipulation of the heart rate and contractility by stimulation, attenuation, or both. Parasympathetic tone (vagal tone) predominates at the sinoatrial node and is therefore the major determinant of resting heart rate. Sympathetic input is also necessary, however, for the heart rate to increase significantly above 100 bpm. Therefore, the sympathetic nerves are very important for increasing heart rate as well as contractility.

Centers of heart rate control have been identified in the cerebral cortex and diencephalon. These centers are thought to be responsible for emotionally and thermally driven changes in heart rate. However, the medullary baroreceptor reflex is the most important regulatory system governing heart rate. It responds to changes in arterial pressure with changes in heart rate in parallel with changes in contractility. Decreased blood pressure leads to increased contractility (increased sympathetic tone) and increased heart rate (decreased parasympathetic tone). Increased blood pressure leads to decreased contractility and decreased heart rate.

Measuring Cardiac Output

The **Fick principle** was the first method described for estimating CO in a living animal. The method invokes the law of conservation of mass and uses O_2 flow to determine the flow of blood. Essentially, the Fick principle states that the mass of O_2 in the pulmonary artery plus the mass of oxygen added to the blood in the alveoli must equal the mass of O_2 in the pulmonary vein. (However, the equation is written with all of the above masses expressed as mass/time [i.e., flow].)

The flow of O_2 to the alveoli in the pulmonary artery (q_1) is calculated as the product of pulmonary arterial O_2 content ($[O_2]_{pa}$) and pulmonary arterial blood flow ($\dot{Q}$). The flow of O_2 from the alveoli in the pulmonary vein (q_3) is calculated as the product of systemic arterial O_2 content ($[O_2]_{pv}$) and systemic arterial blood flow ($\dot{Q}$). To calculate the flow of O_2 into the capillary bed from the alveoli (q_2), it is assumed that at equilibrium this flow equals O_2 consumption of the body. It is further assumed that blood flow in the pulmonary circulation and systemic circulation is equal and represents CO. Thus, algebraic manipulation, as shown below, yields an equation for cardiac output using measurable quantities. The O_2 content of the deoxygenated blood ($[O_2]_{pa}$) is measured in catheter-retrieved samples from the pulmonary artery, while that of oxygenated blood ($[O_2]_{pv}$) is measured in samples of systemic arterial blood acquired through needlestick. Finally, O_2 consumption (q_2) is measured by analyzing the volume and O_2 content of expired air.

$$q_1 = [O_2]_{pa}\dot{Q}$$
$$q_2 = O_2 \text{ consumption}$$
$$q_3 = [O_2]_{pv}\dot{Q}$$

The law of conservation of mass states:

$$q_1 + q_2 = q_3.$$

Therefore,

$$[O_2]_{pa}\dot{Q} + q_2 = [O_2]_{pv}\dot{Q}$$
$$[O_2]_{pa}\dot{Q} - [O_2]_{pv}\dot{Q} = -q_2$$
$$\dot{Q}([O_2]_{pa} - [O_2]_{pv}) = -q_2$$
$$\dot{Q} = q_2 / ([O_2]_{pv} - [O_2]_{pa}).$$

See Clinical Application Box *Thermodilution: The Modern Method of Assessing Cardiac Output.*

PATHOPHYSIOLOGY: HEART FAILURE

The primary consequence of disordered heart pumping is **congestive heart failure (CHF)**. In CHF, not enough blood is driven from the low-pressure venous system to the high-pressure arterial system, and blood accumulates in the venous system. Accumulation of blood in the pulmonary veins increases the hydrostatic pressure of the pulmonary vessels, which are in close contact with the low (atmospheric) pressure of air in the lungs. This pressure gradient thus leads to the expression of fluid into the pulmonary alveoli, a condition known as *pulmonary edema*. When fluid covers the gas-exchanging membranes, oxygenation becomes a problem, and the sensation of *dyspnea* (shortness of breath) ensues. When CHF is more se-

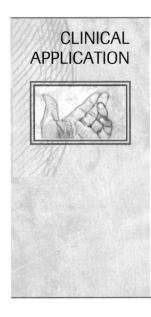

THERMODILUTION: THE MODERN METHOD OF ASSESSING CARDIAC OUTPUT

The *thermodilution* method for assessing cardiac output combines solid-state circuitry with catheter technology. A catheter is inserted into the venous system. The catheter is equipped with a proximal port, through which cold saline can be injected into the bloodstream, and a distal thermistor, which responds to changes in temperature with changes in its resistance. A constant voltage is applied across the thermistor, and changes in current are recorded as a function of time as cold saline is injected. The temperature curve over the distal thermistor will exhibit an exponential decay profile, the parameters of which are a function of the speed with which the saline reaches the thermistor. Knowing the distance between the port of injection and the thermistor, and the resistance changes with time, a computer can estimate the rate at which the saline is traveling, or the cardiac output. This catheter-based method requires only a venous puncture for measurement and is therefore the most commonly used method to estimate cardiac output in the hospital setting.

vere, the backup of fluid can go beyond the lungs and increase hydrostatic pressures in the systemic veins. Elevated hydrostatic pressures in the systemic veins lead to the expression of fluid into the interstitial tissues, called *peripheral edema*. Peripheral edema tends to affect the lower extremities in particular because gravity causes pooling there. Similarly, the lower portions of the lung are more strongly affected. The inferior parts of the body or of the lungs where fluids accumulate are termed the *dependent* areas.

There are two basic types of cardiac dysfunction that lead to CHF, and they correspond to the two basic phases of cardiac pumping: filling (diastole) and contraction (systole). **Systolic dysfunction** describes any situation in which the heart cannot pump effectively. **Diastolic dysfunction** describes any situation in which the heart cannot relax and fill effectively.

The most common cause of systolic dysfunction is ischemic injury to the myocardium due to **coronary artery disease (CAD)**. CAD often injures the myocardium in an acute event called a **myocardial infarction (MI)**, or *heart attack*, where a blood clot on a coronary atherosclerotic plaque interrupts blood flow to the myocardium. Ischemic injury to the myocardium results in decreased inotropy (decreased contractility). Decreased contractility means the heart cannot achieve its usual end-systolic volume, and the SV and ejection fraction accordingly fall. Diastolic filling now begins at a higher end-systolic volume and end-diastolic volume is therefore increased. Over time, the increased filling gradually increases the heart's size. This increases its preload and, by the Frank-Starling mechanism, helps to boost its SV. An enlarged ischemic heart is said to suffer from *dilated cardiomyopathy*. (See Clinical Application Box *What Is a Myocardial Infarction?*)

Diastolic dysfunction is often caused by hypertension. After chronically working against the increased afterload of elevated aortic pressure, the heart wall changes to relieve wall stress, as described above. It thickens so that the intraventricular volume is smaller, and it loses some of its compliance (its capacity to expand). A smaller amount of blood can enter the ventricle during diastole, so a smaller amount of blood can be pumped from the venous system into the arterial system. This is *hypertrophic cardiomyopathy*. Other diseases affecting the myocardium, such as amyloidosis, may decrease the compliance of the heart without hypertrophy. This is called *restrictive cardiomyopathy*.

The treatments for chronic CHF depend to some extent on whether the cause is systolic or diastolic dysfunction. They include (1) drugs to reduce afterload (i.e., antihypertensive [blood pressure-lowering] medications like ACE inhibitors); (2) drugs to reduce preload (i.e., diuretics such as furosemide [Lasix], which relieve the venous system of its congestion by purging fluid in the urine); and (3) drugs that increase contractility, such as digoxin. Irreversible cardiomyopathies can be treated by heart transplantation. Diuresis is typically not used in hypertrophic cardiomyopathy because in diastolic dysfunction, the heart is already troubled by underfilling and needs whatever preload it can get. The β-blocking drugs may also help the heart relax and hence to fill in diastolic dysfunction.

Valvular disorders are another group of maladies affecting the heart's pumping action. The four major valvular disorders are mitral stenosis, mitral regurgitation, aortic stenosis, and aortic regurgitation. *Stenosis* is a narrowing of the valve opening due to thickening of the valve. *Regurgitation* is a retrograde

WHAT IS A MYOCARDIAL INFARCTION?

A 57-year-old man with a history of angina and a 40-year history of smoking reports severe substernal chest pain, chest pressure, and shortness of breath. An electrocardiogram (ECG) reveals ST-segment elevation consistent with myocardial ischemia. The patient is administered propranolol (a β-blocker), aspirin, intravenous nitroglycerin, and heparin. An elevated creatine kinase (CK) level on blood chemistry later supports the diagnosis of **myocardial infarction (MI)**.

Coronary artery disease (CAD) is caused by injury to the coronary artery endothelium with subsequent invasion by cholesterol-storing macrophages. When the plaques grow large enough, they can rupture and a thrombus (blood clot) can further constrict or completely occlude the coronary artery. There are three main coronary arteries: the **right coronary artery (RCA)**, the **left anterior descending (LAD) artery**, and the **left circumflex (LCX) artery.** The artery affected by stenosis determines which area of the heart will be injured, and thus what sort of systolic dysfunction will ensue. The LAD is the main supply to the left ventricle, so CAD in the LAD can be a serious danger to cardiac function.

Angina is substernal (midline) chest pain and pressure attributed to cardiac ischemia. **Ischemia**, a reversible hypoperfusion of the myocardium, may lead to **infarction** (tissue death) when severe. Ischemia and infarction manifest with changes in the ECG tracing such as ST elevation and depression, T-wave inversion, and peaked T waves. Each of these findings is unreliably associated with certain patterns of injury and with injuries of a certain age (hours, days, older). The death of myocardial tissue also releases intracellular enzymes, such as CK.

The drugs mentioned above treat myocardial ischemia in the following ways. *β-blockers* inhibit sympathetic stimulation of heart rate and contractility, thereby decreasing myocardial workload and demand for oxygen that is in short supply. *Nitroglycerin* is a vasodilator that drops afterload (by arteriodilation), drops preload (by venodilation), and increases perfusion of the heart (coronary vasodilation). Decreased preload and afterload decrease cardiac workload and metabolic demand. *Aspirin* and *heparin* combat the development of any thrombus in the coronary arteries.

The mnemonic "BATH" may be useful in the treatment of unstable angina or acute MI: B for β-blocker, A for aspirin, T for trinitroglycerin (the IV preparation of nitroglycerin, trade name Tridil), and H for heparin. *Unstable angina* is angina that raises concern about an impending MI. It is identified by its divergence from previous patterns of angina in frequency, duration, and severity.

---

flow of blood through the valve due to valvular incompetence. Valvular disorders do not lead to CHF in the short term, but they can in the long term.

Summary

- Three variables affect SV: preload, afterload, and contractility.
- Stroke volume (SV) is the amount of blood expelled from the ventricle during one systolic contraction. The percentage expelled from the ventricle by each stroke is the ejection fraction (normal is >50%). What remains is the end-systolic volume.
- The cardiac preload is the degree of stretching of the ventricular myofibrils prior to systolic contraction. It is related to the end-diastolic volume.
- As the LV end-diastolic volume increases, the force generated by the LV will also increase, leading to a proportional increase in the SV. This is known as the Frank-Starling relationship.
- The afterload is the force opposing myocardial contraction. For the LV, this is primarily the aortic pressure.
- Afterload limits the end-systolic volume because when the aortic pressure is high, the LV must generate higher pressures to keep the aortic valve open and it cannot do this for as long as it does when working against a smaller afterload. The aortic valve shuts sooner.

- Contractility is the force generated by the myocardium under conditions of fixed preload and afterload. It is increased by adrenergic (sympathetic) nervous or hormonal stimulation.

- The Fick principle is a method of calculating cardiac output from the oxygen content of the pulmonary artery and vein and from oxygen consumption:

$$\dot{Q} = q_2 / ([O_2]_{pv} - [O_2]_{pa}).$$

- The primary consequence of disordered heart pumping is congestive heart failure (CHF). Two basic types of cardiac dysfunction lead to CHF, corresponding to the two basic phases of cardiac pumping: diastolic dysfunction corresponds to filling, and systolic dysfunction corresponds to contraction.

- The most common cause of systolic dysfunction is ischemia, or injury to the myocardium due to coronary artery disease (CAD).

Suggested Reading

Brutsaert DL, Sys SU. Relaxation and diastole of the heart. Physiol Rev. 1989;69(4):1228–1315.

Fuster V. The pathogenesis of coronary artery disease and the acute coronary syndromes (1). N Engl J Med. 1992; 326(4):242–250.

Jessup M, Brozena S. Heart failure. N Engl J Med. 2003; 348(20):2007–2018.

Shoucri RM. Theoretical study of pressure-volume relation in left ventricle. Am J Physiol. 1991;260(1 Pt 2): H282–291.

REVIEW QUESTIONS

Directions: Each of the numbered items or incomplete statements in this section is followed by answers or by completions of the statement. Select the ONE lettered answer or completion that is BEST in each case.

1. A 33-year-old woman reporting exertional chest pain undergoes a Doppler echocardiogram, which shows concentric thickening of the left ventricle, thickened aortic valve leaflets, and a 67-mm Hg pressure gradient from the left ventricle to the aortic root. Which of the following descriptors could best be applied to her cardiac dysfunction?

    (A) High preload
    (B) Mitral stenosis
    (C) Low contractility
    (D) Aortic regurgitation
    (E) Low ventricular compliance

2. A 70-year-old man with a history of coronary artery disease arrives in the emergency room unresponsive and hypotensive. His respirations are 35/min and his heart rate is 140/min. If he has had a massive MI, the primary cause of his hypotension is:

    (A) Dehydration
    (B) Peripheral edema with "third-spacing" of fluid
    (C) Decreased afterload
    (D) Decreased preload
    (E) Decreased contractility

3. Total occlusion of the left anterior descending (LAD) artery will have particularly devastating consequences for which part of the heart?

    (A) Right ventricle
    (B) Left ventricle
    (C) Right atrium
    (D) Left atrium
    (E) Sinoatrial node

ANSWERS TO REVIEW QUESTIONS

1. **The answer is E.** The patient has aortic stenosis, which has created a chronic obstruction to left ventricular outflow. This in turn has caused hypertrophy of the left ventricle, which decreases its compliance. Low compliance interferes with diastolic filling of the ventricle, leading to low preload, not high.

2. **The answer is E.** Myocardial infarction lessens the inherent strength (i.e., contractility) of the myocardium. With significantly reduced contractility, the left ventricle cannot sustain the pressure necessary for adequate SV, and the cardiac output falls. In accordance with the analogy to Ohm's law, which says that mean arterial pressure equals cardiac output times systemic vascular resistance, a drop in cardiac output means a drop in blood pressure (hypotension). CHF due to ischemic heart disease does cause peripheral edema and sequestration of fluid in the interstitial tissues does reduce intravascular volume, which in turn reduces preload, which in turn does reduce cardiac output. It is not known in this case whether the patient has CHF, but the primary cause of hypotension is decreased contractility due to MI. If the patient does have CHF with low preload, the original cause of the CHF is still likely to be systolic dysfunction with low contractility due to ischemic heart disease. Finally, low afterload is synonymous with low blood pressure, not the cause of the low blood pressure.

3. **The answer is B.** The LAD provides the main blood supply to the left ventricle.

14

The Electrical Activity of the Heart

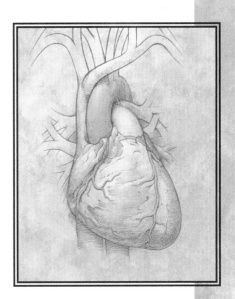

INTRODUCTION

In Chapter 13, we explored the mechanical properties of the heart pump and began with the principle of excitation-contraction coupling. This principle says that cellular action potentials lead to muscular contraction and, together with other mechanisms, determine the mechanical characteristics of the heart. In this chapter, we will delve into the genesis and transmission of excitatory action potentials through the myocardium. The heart contains specialized tissue for generating its own rhythmic action potentials (and hence, its own rhythmic contraction) independently of outside influences. It also contains specialized tissue for conducting those action potentials to the right places at the right times. The heart thereby ensures the correct delay between atrial and ventricular contraction, as well as the appropriate coordination of wall motion within the ventricles.

SYSTEM STRUCTURE

Under normal circumstances, cardiac excitation begins with the transmission of an action potential from the **sinoatrial (SA) node**, the natural pacemaker region of the heart. It then proceeds through the atrial muscle and through specialized atrial tracts to the **atrioventricular (AV) node.** From the AV node, excitation spreads through specialized conducting tissues within the *interventricular septum* and *moderator band*: the **His bundle, bundle branches**, and the network of **Purkinje fibers.** Finally, the impulses reach the ventricular muscle to initiate ventricular contraction (FIGURE 14.1).

Coordinated muscular contraction requires the rapid transmission of electrical impulses, which is facilitated by the *gap junctions* between myocardial cells; these junctions make the myocardium a functional *syncytium* (many cells that make the heart function as though it were a single continuous unit of cytoplasm). Consequently, a stimulus arising at any one point within the ventricle leads to the contraction of both ventricles; likewise, a stimulus arising within the atria leads to the contraction of both atria.

Normally, the SA node is the functional pacemaker of the heart, but under certain pathologic conditions, cells outside the sinus node (within the atria, the AV junction, or the ventricles) may act as independent pacemakers and generate their own intrinsic rhythm for the heart. The capacity to generate electrical impulses spontaneously, whether innate as in the SA node or acquired as in pathologic states, is called **automaticity. Ectopic automaticity** (misplaced automaticity) is important to understanding some of the common cardiac **arrhythmias** (rhythm disturbances) and electrocardiographic abnormalities seen in clinical practice.

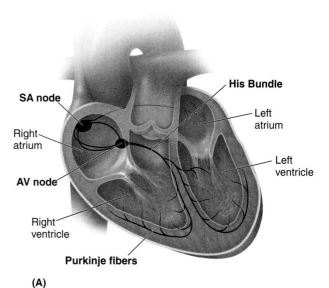

(A)

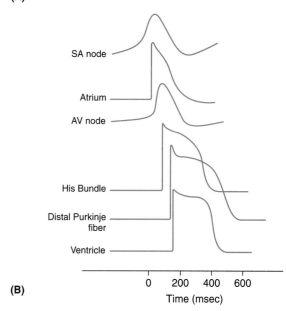

(B)

Figure 14.1 Pacemaker and conductive tissues of the myocardium. **A.** Anatomic locations of the various conductive tissues. **B.** Action potentials in the various tissues.

Conduction, the capacity to generate action potentials cell to cell at regular intervals, is another property of myocardial tissue that varies throughout the transmission pathway. Conduction is slow through the AV node and fast through the Purkinje fibers. Slow conduction at the AV node ensures that the ventricles have adequate time to fill before the signal for ventricular contraction arrives. As discussed below, these differences in conduction in the various parts of the heart are determined by differences in the type of the action potentials arising there.

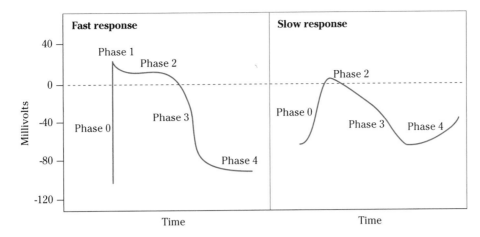

Figure 14.2 Fast and slow action potentials. Notice the automatic upturn in electrical potential in phase 4 of the slow response.

SYSTEM FUNCTION

This section has two main parts. The first, Cardiac Action Potentials, describes the ionic basis of the electrical activity in the heart. The second, Cardiac Conduction, moves from this cellular-level view to a description of the natural excitation of the heart as a whole, with attention to the surface electrocardiogram.

Cardiac Action Potentials

The notion of a muscle action potential was introduced in Chapter 6. Two principal types of action potentials are observed in the heart. The first is the so-called **fast response** observed in conductive cardiac tissue—that is, the myocardial fibers in the atrium, ventricles, His bundle, and Purkinje fiber network. The second is the **slow response**, distinguished by a more prolonged upstroke in electrical potential, seen in the pacemaker fibers of the SA and AV nodes (FIGURE 14.2). Only the slow fibers possess automaticity. The action potentials at various locations within each subgroup (SA versus AV node, atria versus ventricles) depart somewhat from the illustrated prototypes, but these variations are relatively unimportant. In the figure, notice that the slow response is distinguished by a smaller amplitude as well as a slower upstroke (phase 0). These features account for the lower conduction velocity relative to the fast-response fibers. In the following discussion, the ionic basis of the resting potential and both the fast and slow cardiac action potentials will be addressed.

The Resting Potential   The various phases of the cardiac action potential in both slow-response and fast-response fibers can be explained by changes in the permeability of the cell membrane to various ions—primarily sodium, potassium, and calcium.

These variations in permeability are accomplished through variations in the configuration and conductance of specialized transmembrane proteins known as **ion channels.**

Ion channels have two important functional properties: selectivity and gating. **Selectivity** is the ability of different channels to be selective for specific ions, such as Na^+ or K^+. **Gating** is a property that makes ion channels fluctuate between "open" and "closed" states, often in a voltage-sensitive fashion (i.e., the channel state depends on the electrical potential across the cell membrane at any given time). The total ionic current that flows through the channel is determined by the proportion of time spent in the open versus the closed state.

Myocardial cells, like other cells in the body, are highly permeable to K^+ in their resting state. This permeability to K^+ creates a resting membrane potential in the following way. The Na^+/K^+ ATPase in the cell membrane pumps Na^+ out of cells and K^+ into cells, accumulating K^+ inside the cells. This creates a strong chemical gradient for the diffusion of K^+ from inside the cell to outside. Because of high permeability to K^+, K^+ can flow down its concentration gradient out of the cell. This passage of cations out of the cell renders the inside of the cell electronegative, however. As more and more K^+ ions flow down the K^+ concentration gradient out of the cell, the inside of the cell becomes more and more electronegative, and eventually this negative charge begins to slow the efflux of K^+.

As the efflux of K^+ continues, the electrostatic force rises until it equals the driving force of the chemical gradient. At this point, the forces (chemical and electrical) are equal and opposite and said to be in equilibrium. The greater the permeability to K^+, the greater the flow down the chemical gradient and the more charge separation across the membrane is possible per unit of time; thus, the high K^+ permeability means that at equilibrium, K^+ has

Table 14.1   ION DISTRIBUTIONS AND INDIVIDUAL EQUILIBRIUM POTENTIALS

Ion	Extracellular Concentration	Intracellular Concentration	Equilibrium Potential
Na^+	145 mM	10 mM	70 mV
K^+	4 mM	135 mM	−94 mV
Ca^{2+}	2 mM	0.0001 mM	132 mV

flowed out of the cell, and the membrane possesses a negative charge (or potential) on the inside. The electrical potential inside the cell membrane at this point is known as the **equilibrium potential.** If the membrane is permeable only to K^+ and no other ions, the resting membrane potential of the cell is the K^+ equilibrium potential (E_K).

The *Nernst equation* relates the equilibrium potential for an ion to the concentrations of the ion outside versus in:

$$E_K = RT/zF \ln [K^+_o]/[K^+_i],$$

where $[K^+_o]$ is the concentration of K^+ outside the cell, $[K^+_i]$ is the concentration inside, and E_K is the electrical potential inside the cell. (The other terms of the equation are R, the ideal gas constant, 8.314 J/mol K; T, the absolute temperature in degrees Kelvin; z, the valence of K^+; and F, the Faraday constant, 9.648×10^4 C/mol; ln signifies the natural log function.) Note that there is no term for permeability in the Nernst equation, since equilibrium is independent of permeability for a single ion, given enough time for the ion to diffuse down its chemical gradient. Algebraic manipulation of this equation yields:

$$E_K = 61.5/z \log [K^+_o]/[K^+_i].$$

The *Goldman equation* is a variation of the Nernst equation that calculates the equilibrium concentration of a membrane with permeabilities to many ions (K^+, Ca^{2+}, Na^+, Cl^-) and that factors in the degree of permeability for each ion.

TABLE 14.1 shows the distribution of Na^+, K^+, and Ca^{2+} across cardiac cell membranes and the equilibrium potentials that would exist for each if each were the only ion permeability in the membrane. Positive potential indicates a net influx of that ion owing to concentration gradient, while negative potential (as in the case of K^+) indicates a net efflux. The true resting potential of the cardiac cell membrane, reflecting the resting permeability to these three ions, is −90 mV, close to the Nernst potential for K^+, which reflects the fact that at rest, the cell membrane is permeable primarily to K^+ ions and not Na^+ or Ca^{2+}. The slight variation between the measured resting poten-

tial and E_K reflects the fact that at rest, the cell membrane has a slight permeability to Na^+ ions as well. The slow leak inward of sodium ions slightly depolarizes the membrane, making the resting potential slightly more positive.

The negative overall potential inside the cell membrane with high K^+ permeability is the state in which cardiac cells are found before an action potential reaches them from a conduction pathway. When an ion flux renders the inside of the cell more negative, this is called **hyperpolarization**, as it exaggerates the charge difference (polarization) already present in the resting state. When an ion flux renders the inside of the cell more positive, this is called **depolarization**, as it partially abolishes the charge difference present in the resting state.

The Ionic Basis of the Fast Response   The action potential in myocardial cells is an all-or-nothing response, which requires initiation by a stimulus that raises (depolarizes) the resting membrane potential to a critical value called the **threshold potential** (roughly −65 mV). Stimulation below this threshold value results in no response, while stimulation at or above this value results in the propagation of a normal action potential. The contour of the fast-response action potential is illustrated in FIGURE 14.3. In cells exhibiting the fast response, depolarization of the resting membrane to the threshold value causes an increase in the membrane permeability to sodium. This change in permeability is effected by the activation (opening) of so-called fast sodium channels in the cell membrane, which then permit the rapid influx of sodium ions down their concentration and electrostatic gradient, further depolarizing the cell and accounting for the rapid upstroke (phase 0) of the fast action potential.

Sodium channel activation is effected by a *dual gating mechanism* (see FIGURE 14.4). The combined position of the two gates (the primary "sliding doors" gate and the secondary "ball-and-chain" gate) determines the state of the sodium channel: closed, open, or inactivated. The positions of the two gates are in turn dependent on the voltage applied across them. The primary gate is *closed* at a membrane potential of −90 mV, so net sodium flux across the fast sodium

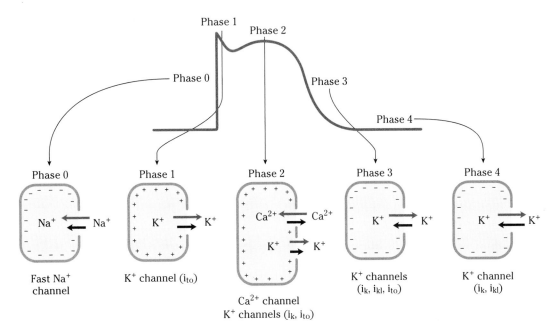

Figure 14.3 Phases of the fast-response action potential. The red arrow represents the chemical gradient and the black arrow represents the electrostatic gradient. i_{to}, i_k, i_{k1} represent currents through various types of K^+ channels.

channel is zero at rest. The ball-and-chain gate is open at rest, but both gates must be open for flux to occur. With depolarization to the threshold potential, the primary gate opens. For a brief time after threshold stimulation, both gates are *open*, allowing a rapid influx of sodium ions.

Gradually, however, the ball-and-chain gate begins to swing closed, obstructing the further influx of sodium, and the channel is *inactivated*, even though the primary gate remains open. This transition from "open" to "inactivated" accounts for the rapid changes in sodium conductance across the cell membrane and the brief duration of the action potential upstroke. In the inactivated state, the sodium channels are unavailable for recruitment for a second action potential; they are said to be refractory to another threshold-level stimulus. The duration of time spent in the inactivated state determines the cellular excitability. In nerve and muscle cells, this *refractory period* is very short—that is, cells recover from the inactivated to the closed (resting) state quickly—whereas in cardiac cells, this period is

more prolonged. This difference prevents tetany in the myocardium, as discussed below.

In actuality, membrane voltage does not have total control over the sodium channels. They open, close, and inactivate all the time at random. It is clear from patch-clamp experiments (techniques that investigate the dynamics of individual ion channels under various electrochemical conditions) that depolarization affects the *probability* that any given sodium channel will be open or closed.

In general, as seen in FIGURE 14.5, when the membrane potential is more negative than −80 mV, most sodium channels are not inactivated and therefore available for recruitment during a normal fast action potential. At membrane potentials more positive than −65 mV, nearly 75% of the sodium channels are inactivated, and this leaves too few sodium channels for the generation of an action potential. *Partial depolarization of the membrane can retard the effects of a subsequent threshold stimulus.* At potentials between −80 and −65 mV, 65% to 35% of channels may be available, resulting in abnormally slow conduction of the action potential. (See Clinical Application Box *Partial Depolarization As a Mechanism of Arrhythmia.*)

As shown in Figure 14.3, once sodium channels are activated by a threshold-level stimulus, they rapidly inactivate, transmembrane conductance of sodium falls off, and phase 0 ends. Phase 1 of the action potential marks a gradual increase in the transmembrane conductance of potassium, and an initial **repolarization** of the action potential. Complete repolarization of the membrane is prevented by the activation

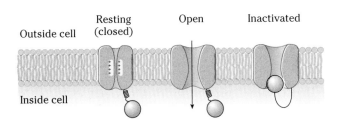

Figure 14.4 The dual gating of the sodium ion channel.

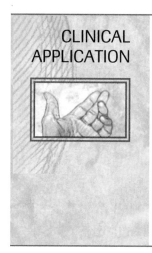

CLINICAL APPLICATION

PARTIAL DEPOLARIZATION AS A MECHANISM OF ARRHYTHMIA

Under conditions of poor blood flow to the myocardium, impaired delivery of oxygen and glucose prevents an adequate local generation of ATP. Inadequate supplies of ATP result in underfunctioning of the Na^+/K^+ ATPase pump. Without the ATPase to maintain intracellular K^+ stores, the concentration gradient for K^+ extrusion erodes, less K^+ efflux occurs, and the membrane depolarizes in its resting state. It does not depolarize to the threshold level, but rather to a level that causes significant sodium channel inactivation. The net result is a tendency toward slowed conduction in areas of the myocardium that are poorly perfused, a circumstance that predisposes to the development of abnormal heart rhythms. (Aberrant conduction through the heart is discussed further in the Pathophysiology section of the chapter.)

of calcium channels in the cell membrane, which promotes the influx of positive Ca^{2+} ions in accordance with calcium's chemical gradient from out to in. The simultaneous efflux of potassium and influx of calcium in phase 2 tend to balance each other, leading to a transient stabilization of the membrane potential and a plateau phase in the contour of the action potential.

The final repolarization of the membrane occurs at the end of phase 2, when the potassium efflux begins to exceed the influx of sodium and calcium ions. This happens because the calcium channels that opened near the end of phase 1 automatically begin to deactivate after a time, allowing the unopposed efflux of positive charges through open potassium channels. The duration of the phase 2 plateau varies between myocytes largely because of variations in the magnitude of potassium efflux during repolarization. The net outward potassium current is larger in atrial than in ventricular myocytes, and this is reflected in a more rapid repolarization in the atrial action potential.

The above description is an oversimplification of the action potential. In reality, several different types

of channels for each ion contribute to the net flux of ions across the cell membrane; for instance, there are at least three or four distinct K^+ channels that contribute to the observed contour of the action potential. This basic explanation of the action potential, however, is sufficient to understand the mechanism of action of several of the antiarrhythmic drugs, and to explain the genesis of the most common types of cardiac arrhythmias observed in the clinical setting. (See Clinical Application Box *Hyperkalemia.*)

The Ionic Basis of the Slow Response   As described above and illustrated in Figure 14.2, the fast action potential comprises five phases. The first three are an initial rapid upstroke and decline (phases 0 and 1, respectively); a plateau phase (phase 2); and a repolarization phase (phase 3). Phase 4 is the resting potential. In cells that exhibit the slow response, such as those in the pacemaker regions of the heart (SA/AV nodes), the rapid upstroke is absent, largely owing to the absence of the fast sodium channels that are responsible for the phase 0 depolarization. In the slow response, the upstroke is gradual and due to the influx of sodium and calcium ions through the nonspecific cation channels that are active during the plateau phase of the fast response. By blocking the fast sodium channels responsible for the phase 0 upstroke (using tetrodotoxin) in vitro, a fast action potential can be made to resemble the slow response.

The crucial difference between pacemaker cells and fast conduction fibers, however, is in phase 4 of the action potential. The specialized cells of the cardiac pacemaker regions possess a class of specialized sodium channels that gradually allow sodium ions to leak inward following repolarization. This phase 4 inward leak of sodium ions during diastole, called the **pacemaker sodium current**, leads to a gradual depolarization of the cell to the threshold value, with eventual activation of calcium channels and the generation of a new action potential. The

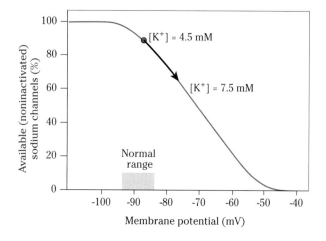

Figure 14.5 Na^+ channel inactivation versus membrane potential.

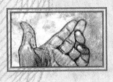

HYPERKALEMIA

Electrolyte disturbances may cause life-threatening cardiac complications by interfering with normal myocardial electrophysiology. **Hyperkalemia**, for example, a state of elevated serum potassium, is a medical emergency because it can generate lethal cardiac rhythm disturbances and sudden death. Why should this be so? As predicted by the Nernst equation, the elevation of extracellular potassium will alter the resting potential of the cardiac myocyte. Calculating E_K using a serum potassium level of 7.5 mM (normal is 4.0 mM) yields:

$$E_K = 61.5 \log [7.5 \text{ mM}]/[135 \text{ mM}] = -76.9 \text{ mV}.$$

Comparing this to the baseline value for E_K from Table 14.1 (-94 mV), we see that a mere 3.5-mM change in the extracellular potassium concentration raises the resting membrane potential by nearly 20 mV. This depolarization of the resting cell membrane changes the excitability of the cell (see Figure 14.2). Recall that the initial phase of the ventricular action potential (phase 0) depends on the rapid influx of sodium into the cell through fast sodium channels. The rate of phase 0 depolarization (i.e., the slope, dV/dt) is proportional to the number of sodium channels that are open during phase 0, since more open channels allow for more rapid sodium influx. The number of sodium channels available for recruitment during phase 0, however, varies with changes in the resting membrane potential.

At a membrane potential of -94 mV, a large fraction of the sodium channels are in the non-inactivated (closed) state and therefore can be opened with a threshold-level stimulus. When the resting potential is raised to -77 mV as in our example, however, the proportion of sodium channels in the inactivated state is increased. Since these inactivated channels are refractory to stimulation, the cell has become less excitable—that is, a threshold-level stimulus will activate fewer sodium channels, and lead to a smaller amplitude and slower upstroke during phase 0.

Clinically, this manifests as a prolongation of the action potential duration and a slowing of ventricular contraction (reflected on the surface ECG as a broadening of the QRS complex). This alteration in cellular excitability increases the likelihood of breakdown in the normal sequence of cardiac conduction and the likelihood that aberrant cardiac rhythms can arise.

Hyperkalemia is employed to the patient's benefit during cardiac surgery. During coronary artery bypass, surgeons employ cardioplegia to temporarily stop the beating heart and facilitate the attachment of vessels to the myocardial surface. The solution used to effect cardioplegia is nothing more than a high-potassium buffer containing 20 to 30 mM potassium, which depolarizes the cell to -50 to -35 mV. At this resting membrane potential, nearly all sodium channels are in the inactivated state, and a normal action potential therefore cannot occur, leaving the heart in a "plegic" or paralyzed state. The treatment of acute hyperkalemia is discussed in Chapter 24.

phase 4 pacemaker sodium current confers automaticity upon the SA and AV nodes.

Cardiac Conduction

Having explored the ionic basis of conduction, we can now look at the big picture: myocardial contraction, the underlying basis for many cardiac arrhythmias, and the varying sites of action of the panoply of antiarrhythmic drugs that are commercially available.

Under normal circumstances, the initial impulse for cardiac contraction begins in the SA node, which depolarizes spontaneously in a rhythmic fashion based on the action of the pacemaker sodium currents described above. The rate of this depolarization is influenced by the balance between adrenergic (sympathetic) and cholinergic (parasympathetic) tone in the body. During periods of stress, for example, adrenergic tone is high and the rate of sinus node depolarization increases. Under the influence of drugs or physiologic maneuvers (such as carotid massage, discussed in Chapter 12) that increase vagal tone, however, the sinus rate is suppressed. Since the upstroke of the action potential in these cells is primarily dependent on the influx of calcium (not sodium) during phase 0, calcium-channel blocking agents (e.g., verapamil and diltiazem) also have the effect of slowing nodal conduction, thereby reducing the heart rate.

From the SA node, the cardiac impulse spreads rapidly through the atria, whose cells exhibit characteristics of the fast response. The rate of impulse spread is enhanced by the presence of gap junctions between myocardial cells that connect them into an electrical unit. Atrial conduction proceeds in an organized fashion through well-defined pathways from the SA to the AV node in the right atrium and via Bachmann's bundle (anterior interatrial myocardial band) from the SA node to the left atrium. Conduction is then slowed through the AV node, which has similar electrical characteristics to the tissue of the SA node.

In the AV node, depolarization proceeds through the activation of calcium channels. Calcium channel-blocking agents, therefore, decrease the amplitude and duration of action potentials through this region, slowing atrioventricular conduction and blocking the transmission of impulses to the ventricles.

Because the AV node is the final common pathway (in the normal heart) for atrioventricular conduction, it is the primary pharmacologic target for the management of abnormal, rapid heart rhythms (tachyarrhythmias) originating within the conduction system above the AV node. (Such arrhythmias are called supraventricular because they originate above the ventricle.) Nodal blocking agents, such as calcium channel antagonists, β-blockers, and digoxin, all exert their antiarrhythmic effects primarily through their actions at the AV node and are therefore useful agents in the acute management of *supraventricular tachyarrhythmias (SVTs)*.

Having filtered through the AV node, impulses proceed down the right side of the interventricular septum through the His bundle. In turn, the His bundle divides rapidly into right and left bundle branches, which conduct impulses simultaneously to the right and left ventricles. These divisions give rise to a complex network of Purkinje fibers that conduct impulses through the remainder of the myocardial syncytium. Conduction through the Purkinje fibers is exceptionally fast, allowing rapid, nearly simultaneous activation of the entire endocardial surface of the heart, and thereby allowing coordinated ventricular contraction. Ventricular depolarization is not truly simultaneous, however, because of the order of impulse spread. Rather, the septum depolarizes first,

from left to right, simultaneously with the papillary muscles. Subsequently, impulses spread along the epicardial surface through the thickness of the myocardium of both ventricles, completing depolarization of the thinner right ventricle prior to the left. This pattern of depolarization is clearly reflected in the shape of the surface electrocardiogram.

Surface Electrocardiography   The pattern of normal impulse spread through the heart can be observed clinically through the use of the scalar **electrocardiogram (ECG)**. Using 12 standard electrodes, or leads, placed at well-defined points on the body surface, one can generate an electrical image of cardiac conduction that exposes the pattern and timing of depolarization and repolarization of the various portions of the heart. Each lead serves as a slightly different vantage point from which to view conduction through the heart. The standard positions of the leads can be divided into two groups. The first group includes the limb leads (I, II, III, aVL, aVR, aVF), which record depolarization of the heart in the frontal plane—that is, in a coronal plane cutting the body from head to foot (FIGURE 14.6A). The second group includes the precordial leads (V1 to V6), which record myocardial depolarization in the horizontal (or axial) plane (see Figure 14.6B). In this way, the 12-lead ECG gives the clinician a three-dimensional view of the process of depolarization in the heart.

What is actually recorded by the ECG leads are positive and negative deflections from a preset (isoelectric) baseline. *When depolarization proceeds in the direction of a given lead, a positive (upward) deflection is recorded on the tracing, and when it proceeds away from a given lead, a negative (downward) deflection is recorded.* The standard pattern seen on the ECG tracing during each cardiac cycle takes the form shown in FIGURE 14.7. Each deflection from the baseline represents a distinct event in cardiac conduction. FIGURE 14.8 shows an example of a normal surface ECG as recorded in a clinical setting.

The first hump, or **P wave**, represents atrial depolarization. This is normally recorded as a positive deflection in leads I, II, and aVF and a negative deflection in lead aVR, since atrial depolarization normally proceeds from the SA to the AV node (roughly in a line from the right shoulder to the left foot) in the direction of lead II and opposite that of lead aVR. Following the P wave, there is a short isoelectric segment representing the conduction of impulses from the AV node to the ventricle. The **PR interval**, measured from the onset of the P wave to the beginning of the QRS complex (see below), represents the time it takes for a stimulus initiated in the atrium to proceed through the AV junction to the ventricle. When conduction through the AV node is prolonged, cardiac events from the left side of the heart, septal depolarization is seen as a small deflection away from V6 (a negative Q wave). Compare this with the lead V1, which views the right side of the heart and therefore records septal depolarization as a positive deflection instead, recognizing depolarization toward its electrocardiographic vector. There is therefore no downward Q wave on a normal V1 tracing.

Conduction then proceeds down the right and left bundle branches, and there is simultaneous activation of the right and left ventricles. The electrically dominant event, however, is the depolarization of the larger, thicker left ventricle, and this is recorded as strong positive deflection (R wave) in the left-sided leads (V5/V6).

The precordial leads represent a series of snapshots of ventricular depolarization moving from right to left. As such, the R waves become progressively larger from leads V1 to V6 (representing the movement of the leads into the vectoral path of left ventricular depolarization). A loss of this progressive R-wave transition is seen in myocardial death, and therefore reduced magnitude of ventricular electrical depolarization and contraction. Hence, a loss of *R-wave progression* is one cardinal ECG manifestation of a heart attack in the anterior wall of the left ventricle, clinically termed a myocardial infarction. Recall that **myocardial ischemia** refers to a condition of impaired myocardial blood flow resulting in tissue hypoxia, while **myocardial infarction (MI)**, or *heart attack*, refers to dead, nondepolarizing myocardial tissue (often the result of prolonged ischemia).

Following ventricular contraction and the end of the QRS complex, there is a second isoelectric period

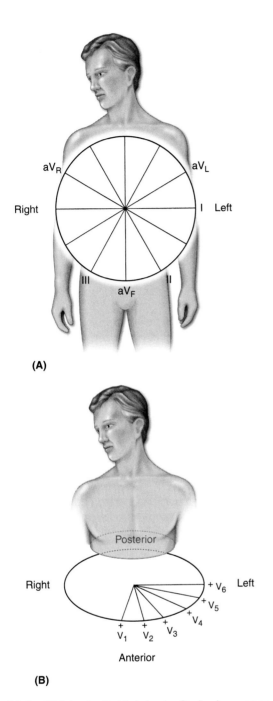

(A)

(B)

Figure 14.6 ECG leads. **A.** Limb leads. Six leads measure cardiac conduction in the frontal plane. **B.** Precordial leads. Six leads measure cardiac conduction in the horizontal plane.

the PR interval may also be prolonged, a condition known as *first-degree heart block.*

The **QRS complex** signifies ventricular depolarization. As noted previously, impulses arriving from the AV node pass into the ventricles via the His bundle. Since the His bundle travels down the interventricular septum, septal depolarization occurs first, with the left side of the septum being stimulated slightly before the right. Because of this left-to-right septal depolarization, and because V6 records

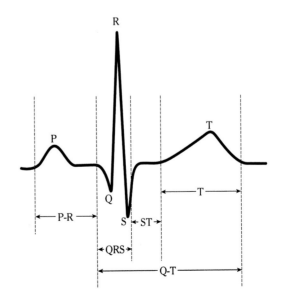

Figure 14.7 One cardiac cycle, traced by ECG. This schematic tracing shows the standard pattern of a cardiac cycle.

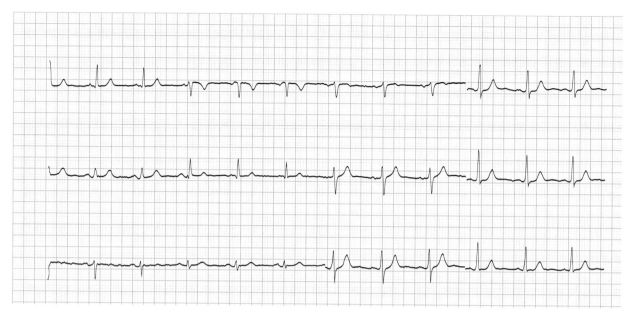

Figure 14.8   A normal 12-lead ECG. This is an actual ECG, recorded in the clinic.

known as the **ST segment** (measured from the end of the QRS complex to the beginning of the T wave). Deviations in this segment above or below baseline are seen in myocardial ischemia and infarction, and analysis of the ST segment forms the main basis for the ECG diagnosis of those two entities. The ECG cycle concludes with ventricular repolarization, recorded as the **T wave.** The duration of the electrical interval from the onset of the QRS complex to the end of the T wave is called the *QT interval,* a measure of the length of time required for the ventricles to return to their resting state.

The surface ECG reflects the summation of all the action potentials going on simultaneously in individual cells within the myocardium. The P wave represents the summation of atrial phase 0 and phase 1 depolarization. Atrial repolarization (phases 2 and 3 of the atrial action potential) happens simultaneously with ventricular depolarization and is therefore hidden in the QRS complex. For the ventricles, phase 0 and phase 1 of the action potential initiate ventricular contraction and are depicted in the QRS complex. The plateau phase (phase 2) is primarily expressed in the ST segment, and phase 3 (repolarization) is reflected in the T wave.

PATHOPHYSIOLOGY

Just as normal cardiac electrophysiology depends on the two functions of automaticity and conduction, arrhythmias arise from either faulty automaticity or faulty conduction. Both of these defects can result from a variety of insults to the myocardium.

Faulty Automaticity

Abnormal automaticity occurs when myocardial tissue outside the nodes begins to drive myocardial contraction. This can happen when the SA node's rhythm is slowed, allowing latent pacemaker tissue to escape from its control, or when ectopic automaticity arises with a rate greater than that of the SA node. One mechanism leading to ectopic beats is *after-depolarization,* in which an increase in Na^+ conductance in myocardial tissue allows depolarization to occur during the refractory period. This leads to extra beats.

Faulty Conduction

Conduction abnormalities include **slowed conduction** due to tissue injury and completely **blocked conduction** due to tissue injury; conversely, **bypass tracts**, which are alternative conductive pathways, may be present. A particular type of arrhythmia that can occur in the presence of blocked conduction is a *re-entrant rhythm.* In this situation, unidirectional blocked conduction leads to loops of excitation, mimicking an ectopic pacemaker.

Diagnosing Arrhythmias

The ECG is an important means of diagnosing cardiac arrhythmias. Under normal circumstances, as described, a P wave precedes each QRS complex, and a QRS complex follows every P wave. This pattern is called **normal sinus rhythm**, signifying impulses originating in the SA node and proceeding in the familiar fashion to the AV node and then to the ventricles to initiate myocardial contraction. When conduction begins lower down in the conduction system owing to ectopic or escape rhythms, however, the ECG will likely reflect this aberrant conduction. If impulses were to originate at the AV node rather than at the SA node, atrial depolarization would proceed in reverse, simultaneously with ventricular depolarization, and P waves would be hidden within the electrically dominant QRS complex. The ECG would thus display a *junctional rhythm*, with absent (or perhaps retrograde P waves) and regular QRS complexes.

Similarly, the duration of the various intervals on the ECG gives insight into potential defects in the conduction system. A prolonged PR signifies slowed conduction through the AV node, while a widened QRS complex is associated with defects in the ventricular conduction pathways, including the right and left bundle branches (or perhaps hyperkalemia, as noted in the prior discussion). Pharmacologic agents (e.g., sotalol or amiodarone) or metabolic abnormalities (e.g., hypercalcemia), which prolong phase 2 or phase 3 of the ventricular action potential, may affect the duration of ventricular repolarization, and this is reflected in prolongation of the QT interval. The ECG is thus a powerful tool in the clinical analysis of cardiac conduction and a window into the electrical events occurring at the cellular level in the myocardium.

Summary

- The rhythm of electrical discharge underlying cardiac contractions depends on two attributes of the myocardium: automaticity (the capacity to generate action potentials at regular intervals independent of outside influences) and conduction (the capacity to transmit action potentials along prescribed routes).

- The excitatory signal (action potential) for cardiac contraction begins in the sinoatrial (SA) node, passes to the atrial walls, and then reaches the atrioventricular (AV) node. The AV node possesses automaticity, but its intrinsic firing rate is slower than that of the SA node, so the SA node sets the pace of AV firing. From the AV node, the excitatory impulse moves into the His bundle in the interventricular septum and then into the Purkinje fibers, and finally into the whole ventricular myocardium.

- The equilibrium resting potential of myocardial cell membranes is -90 mV. The resting potential is determined by the diffusion of K^+ out of the cell, leaving behind negative charge inside the cell. The equilibrium resting potential reflects a balance of chemical and electrostatic forces.

- Conduction is effected by fast-response action potentials. Automaticity is affected by slow-response action potentials. Both types of action potentials proceed in phases.

  - Phase 0: Depolarization. In fast action potentials, massive Na^+ influx follows depolarization to threshold. In slow ones, Ca^{2+} influx follows threshold.

  - Phase 1: Repolarization begins as K^+ efflux increases.

  - Phase 2: Plateau. Na^+ channel inactivation begins and Ca^{2+} influx maintains depolarization.

  - Phase 3: Repolarization. K^+ efflux exceeds Ca^{2+} influx as Ca^{2+} channels inactivate.

  - Phase 4: In the fast action potential of conduction, this phase represents a return to resting potential. In the slow action potential of pacemaker tissue, phase 4 includes an automatic depolarization, by a Na^+ influx called the pacemaker sodium current, that will lead to threshold and another action potential.

- The electrocardiogram (ECG) measures cardiac conduction through 12 leads. When depolarization proceeds in the direction of a given lead, a positive (upward) deflection is recorded on the tracing, and when it proceeds away from a given lead, a negative (downward) deflection is recorded.

- The P wave is atrial depolarization, which normally initiates atrial contraction.

- The PR interval is transmission through the AV node.

- The QRS complex is ventricular depolarization, which normally initiates ventricular contraction. Atrial repolarization also occurs at this time, hidden in the QRS.

- The ST segment, if abnormally depressed or elevated, may reflect myocardial ischemia or infarction.

- The T wave is ventricular repolarization.

- Abnormal automaticity occurs when latent pacemakers escape from the control of a slowed SA node or when ectopic pacemakers outstrip the SA pace.

- Abnormal conduction may take the form of slowed conduction, blocked conduction, or bypass tracts. Unidirectional block may create a re-entrant arrhythmia.

Suggested Reading

Lee TH, Goldman L. Evaluation of the patient with acute chest pain. N Engl J Med. 2000;342(16):1187–1195.

Sonnenblick EH, Stam AC Jr. Cardiac muscle: activation and contraction. Annu Rev Physiol. 1969;31:647–674.

Spach MS, Kootsey JM. The nature of electrical propagation in cardiac muscle. Am J Physiol. 1983;244(1):H3–22.

Zimetbaum P, Josephson ME. Evaluation of patients with palpitations. N Engl J Med. 1998;338(19):1369–1373.

REVIEW QUESTIONS

Directions: Each of the numbered items or incomplete statements in this section is followed by answers or by completions of the statement. Select the ONE lettered answer or completion that is BEST in each case.

1. Which of the following drugs would prolong phase 0 of sinoatrial action potentials?
   (A) Sotalol
   (B) Amiodarone
   (C) Digoxin
   (D) Verapamil
   (E) Propranolol

2. The QT interval on the electrocardiogram reflects:
   (A) The duration of ventricular action potentials
   (B) Atrial repolarization
   (C) Atrial depolarization
   (D) Ventricular depolarization
   (E) Re-entry

3. A 54-year-old woman with renal failure is found to have a serum K^+ level of 8 mM. Her ECG shows wide QRS complexes. Cardiac conduction in this woman's heart is:
   (A) Fast, due to bypass tracts
   (B) Slow, due to high resting potential
   (C) Fast, due to low resting potential
   (D) Slow, due to Ca^{2+} channel blockade in the AV node
   (E) Slow, due to first-degree AV block

ANSWERS TO REVIEW QUESTIONS

1. **The answer is** D. Verapamil, a Ca^{2+} channel blocker, interferes with phase 0 depolarization in pacemaker tissue because phase 0 depolarization is dependent on Ca^{2+} influx.

2. **The answer is** A. The QT interval reflects the duration of ventricular depolarization and repolarization (i.e., the action potential duration).

3. **The answer is** B. The woman has hyperkalemia secondary to decreased renal clearance of K^+. Increased plasma K^+ prevents normal K^+ efflux and raises the resting potential of the myocardium. This inactivates Na^+ channels and impairs conduction, reflected in the long (slow) QRS ventricular depolarization. Slow conduction can lead to a variety of serious and unstable arrhythmias.

15

Exercise Physiology

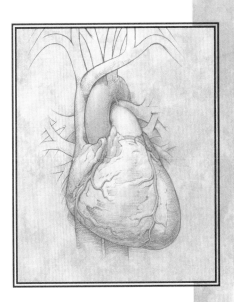

INTRODUCTION

If you've ever done even a small amount of exercise—run a marathon, for example, competed in an Olympic weightlifting competition, or carried your first-year medical school books up a couple of flights of stairs—then you're probably already familiar, in a general way, with how your body responds to the special demands exercise puts on it. Your heart beats harder and faster. Your respiratory rate increases. You sweat. The body maintains homeostasis when asked to run 26.2 miles, lift 600 pounds of iron, or drag around a hefty biochemistry text.

Of course, it's your muscles (and the parts of the brain that are controlling them) that are responsible for disturbing the pre-exercise equilibrium that your body had so elegantly created. During exercise, muscles become greedy for additional oxygen and nutrients to fuel their increased contraction. Increased muscular activity, in turn, produces more waste products of metabolism and more heat (see Chapter 6). The cardiovascular, respiratory, and temperature-related adaptations of the body attempt to meet the demands of exercising muscles.

SYSTEM FUNCTION

The cardiovascular system was covered in the previous three chapters (Chapters 12 to 14), and the respiratory system is covered in Part V (Chapters 16 to 19). Therefore, there is no System Structure section in this chapter. Function is addressed under the following three categories: cardiovascular adaptations, respiratory adaptations, and temperature adaptations.

Cardiovascular Adaptations

As it always does, the cardiovascular system functions during exercise to deliver oxygen and nutrients to muscles and to carry away metabolic by-products. In exercise, muscles have a greater need for the former, and they produce more of the latter. The cardiovascular system adapts to meet these needs in the following ways.

Cardiac Output   Cardiac output is the product of heart rate and stroke volume, both of which increase during exercise. The increase in heart rate results from diminished parasympathetic outflow to the sinoatrial (SA) node and increased sympathetic activity. The increase in stroke volume is primarily mediated by enhanced sympathetic stimulation of the ventricular myocardium, which boosts the heart's contractility; a modest increase in end-diastolic volume during exercise also contributes, via the Frank-Starling mechanism. These changes in parasympathetic and sympathetic tone during exercise are a function, in part, of central nervous system

(CNS) anticipation or awareness of exercise—an example of a feed-forward system (see Chapter 1). Further contributing to the altered neural tone is input from mechanoreceptors and chemoreceptors in muscles and from baroreceptors in the carotid sinus and aortic arch. During exercise, these baroreceptors are reset to a higher baseline pressure, so that despite an increase in mean arterial pressure over the resting pressure (see below), baroreceptor input to the CNS results in increased sympathetic and decreased parasympathetic tone (FIGURE 15.1).

Increased cardiac output during exercise is primarily a function of heart rate, which increases with exercise intensity until it reaches a plateau at around 180 bpm. While stroke volume can nearly double in extremely well-trained endurance athletes, in most people it increases only 10% to 35% and reaches its maximal level at a lower intensity of exercise than heart rate does (FIGURE 15.2).

Peripheral Resistance   Total peripheral resistance decreases during exercise (afterload reduction), contributing to the increase in stroke volume. Changes in peripheral resistance occur differentially throughout the body. Increased sympathetic tone causes vasoconstriction, and therefore increased resistance, in the splanchnic and renal vasculature as well as in blood vessels supplying inactive muscles. Despite an overall increase in cardiac output, blood flow to these areas actually decreases during exercise. Meanwhile, resistance in terminal arterioles supplying exercising muscles decreases markedly, in response to the release by exercising muscle of vasoactive substances. These vasodilators include potassium, adenosine (a

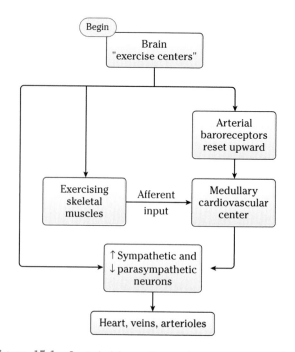

Figure 15.1 Control of the cardiovascular response to exercise.

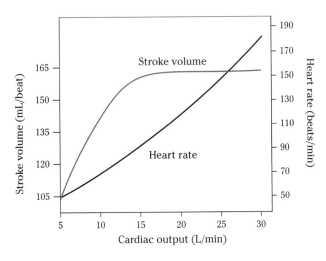

Figure 15.2 Increases in heart rate and stroke volume during exercise.

by-product of ATP metabolism), and lactic acid (a by-product of anaerobic glycolysis). Blood flow through these vessels can increase up to 25 times over the level at rest. In addition, through the phenomenon of capillary recruitment, blood flows through many muscle capillaries that are not perfused at rest. Blood flow to the brain does not change during exercise. Finally, blood flow to the skin initially decreases, owing to sympathetic vasoconstriction, and then increases as body temperature rises.

Arterial Pressure Arterial pressure is the product of cardiac output and total peripheral resistance. While total peripheral resistance decreases during exercise, the increase in cardiac output more than compensates, resulting in an increase of up to 30% in mean arterial pressure during exercise. Because of rapid left-ventricular contraction, systolic pressure increases more than diastolic pressure, resulting in an increased pulse pressure.

Venous Return To maintain an increased cardiac output during exercise, blood must return more rapidly from the venous circulation to the heart. This increased venous return is caused by four factors: (1) increased pumping of venous blood toward the heart from the contractions of exercising muscles compressing veins; (2) increased negative thoracic pressure caused by greater depth and frequency of inspiration, which draws blood back toward the thorax; (3) increased sympathetic nervous system tone, resulting in increased venoconstriction (i.e., venous tone); and (4) increased flow of blood from arteries to veins through dilated skeletal muscle arterioles. A failure to maintain sufficient venous return—in a case of dehydration, for example, when sufficient blood volume is simply lacking—can result in decreased delivery of blood to tissues, and therefore decreased exercise ability.

Isotonic Exercise **Isotonic exercise** occurs when contracting muscle shortens against a constant load. **Isometric exercise** occurs when contracting muscle increases tension while maintaining its length. Many common movements and exercises have both an isometric and an isotonic component. The mechanisms described above apply generally to dynamic exercise (e.g., marathon running) but not to isometric exercise (e.g., weight lifting). There is, however, one important difference. During sustained forceful isotonic muscle contraction, increased intramuscular pressure can exceed the systolic blood pressure, preventing adequate blood flow from reaching the exercising tissues. Despite the body's other cardiovascular adaptations, this roadblock to oxygen and nutrient delivery to tissues during isometric exercise quickly leads to muscle fatigue.

The Effects of Chronic Exercise Chronic endurance exercise results in enlargement of the chambers of the heart, hypertrophy of the myocardium, and a lower total peripheral resistance at rest. At rest, the cardiac output of a well-trained endurance athlete equals that of an untrained person; compared to the untrained person, however, the athlete can achieve this level with a lower heart rate and a greater stroke volume. Because chronic isometric exercise results in myocardial hypertrophy but not chamber enlargement, chronic isometric exercise does not lead to a change in resting heart rate and stroke volume.

Cardiovascular Limitations on Exercise Capacity During intense exercise, cardiac output rises to nearly 90% of its maximal level, with both heart rate and stroke volume increasing to nearly 95% of their maximal levels. At the same time, pulmonary ventilation increases to only just over half its maximal level. It is the cardiovascular system, therefore, rather than the pulmonary system, that limits the body's **maximal oxygen consumption ($\dot{V}_{O_2}$max)** and therefore its ability to exercise. This cardiovascular limitation on exercise ability holds true for both untrained people and trained endurance athletes, though for the latter the $\dot{V}_{O_2}$max can be significantly higher.

Respiratory Adaptations

During exercise, the respiratory system performs the same function—regulating levels of oxygen and carbon dioxide in the blood—as it does when the body is at rest. With exercise, however, the rate of blood flow through the lungs and the chemical composition of the blood change. The respiratory system copes with these changes in the following ways.

Increased Inspiratory Rate and Volume Input from the brain causes the respiratory rate and tidal volume to increase, preemptively preventing changes in blood

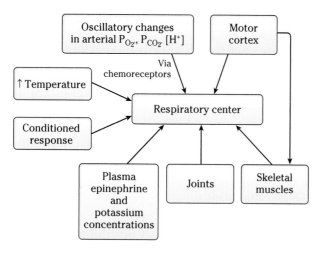

Figure 15.3 Control of the pulmonary response to exercise.

levels of oxygen and carbon dioxide as exercise begins and increases in intensity. This input from "central command" results from cognitive awareness of exercise, from the release of epinephrine and potassium, and from central and peripheral receptors sensitive to physical movement, temperature changes, blood flow, and blood gas concentrations in muscles and the mixed venous blood (FIGURE 15.3). As a result, total minute ventilation of the lungs increases abruptly with the onset of exercise and then increases in proportion to its intensity, up to 20 times that of resting levels. Since it is the cardiac output, not the lungs, that ordinarily limits exercise ability, the minute ventilation reaches a plateau as the body achieves $\dot{V}O_2$max.

Increased Pulmonary Blood Flow As cardiac output increases to meet the demands of exercising muscles, blood flow through the pulmonary vasculature increases. Owing to the low resistance and large capacitance of blood vessels in the lung, this increased flow is accomplished with only a modest increase in the pulmonary vascular pressure.

Blood Gases The oxygen-diffusing capacity (i.e., the rate at which oxygen can cross the alveolar walls into the blood) increases during exercise. This occurs as a result of the increase in pulmonary blood flow, which causes an increasing number of pulmonary capillaries to be perfused, diminishing ventilation perfusion ($\dot{V}/\dot{Q}$) mismatches present in the resting lung. The effect of exercise on blood gases is shown in FIGURE 15.4.

Alveolar PCO_2 determines arterial PCO_2. Furthermore, alveolar PCO_2 is itself a function of the ratio of CO_2 production to alveolar ventilation, which remains constant during moderate exercise. Therefore, while venous PCO_2 increases during exercise, alveolar and arterial PCO_2 levels change little. In fact, during intense exercise—when anaerobic metabolism results in the release of lactic acid into the bloodstream,

increasing H^+ and stimulating hyperventilation—alveolar and arterial PCO_2 levels decrease.

Arterial PO_2 remains constant during exercise, owing to increased alveolar ventilation, pulmonary blood flow, and oxygen diffusion capacity. Venous PO_2 decreases, however, as the exercising muscles and other tissues consume a greater amount of O_2 from the arterial blood in order to maintain ATP production necessary for continued exertion (i.e., the body approaches $\dot{V}O_2$max).

During intense exercise, the increased production of CO_2 and lactic acid by anaerobic metabolism results in an increase in arterial H^+ (i.e., a lower arterial pH). This surplus of arterial H^+ helps provoke the hyperventilation that accompanies intense exercise.

Temperature Adaptations

Heat is produced during exercise as a by-product of metabolic reactions, as well as the need to overcome forces of friction in muscles, joints, and the walls of blood vessels. All of this heat must be dissipated for the body to maintain thermal homeostasis. The body does this by sweating, a sympathetic-mediated process in which sweat glands actively secrete sweat to the skin surface. The subsequent evaporation of sweat causes the body to lose heat. In addition, the body recruits skin capillaries, perfusing

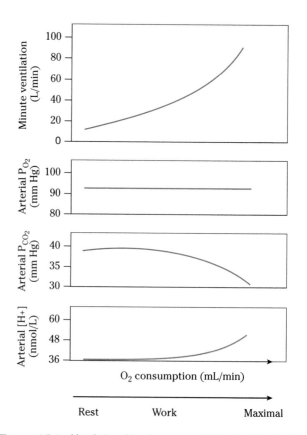

Figure 15.4 Ventilation, blood gases, and blood acidity during exercise.

them to allow heat to escape through the skin. A failure to dissipate heat adequately can lead to heat stroke, a pathologic condition of increased body temperature that can lead to death if untreated. Such a failure of homeostasis can occur in extremely hot or humid conditions, when too much clothing is worn, or when dehydration causes the body to vasoconstrict cutaneous blood vessels, leading to a decreased sweat output in order to preserve fluids.

PATHOPHYSIOLOGY

An understanding of exercise is important to clinical practice in three respects. One, patients with diseases such as congestive heart failure do not tolerate exercise because they cannot increase cardiac output and ventilation in the way that is necessary to meet muscular demand. Two, exercise puts stresses on the body that in some circumstances may lead to injury even without underlying chronic disease. Three, exercise is important to the treatment and prevention of illness. The importance of physical exercise to cardiovascular and general well-being is clear, but there is some controversy surrounding what type of exercise and how much is protective. Exercise limits weight gain, maintains bone strength, lowers the risk of atherosclerosis, and has many other benefits.

Summary

- The muscles' increased demand for oxygen and nutrients drives the cardiac and respiratory changes seen in exercise.
- Mechanoreceptors and chemoreceptors in muscles detect the increased muscular demand and communicate it to the brain, which increases sympathetic output and decreases parasympathetic output.
- Heart rate and stroke volume increase.
- Vascular resistance in skeletal muscle beds decreases owing to local factors that override the sympathetic activation (i.e., functional sympatholysis). Total peripheral resistance decreases.
- Venous return increases owing to increased venous pressure secondary to muscular flexion, among other causes.
- Isotonic exercise occurs when contracting muscle shortens against a constant load. Isometric exercise occurs when contracting muscle increases tension while maintaining its length.
- The cardiovascular system limits muscular oxygen uptake, not the pulmonary system.
- Data from peripheral chemoreceptors and from the cerebral cortex during exercise influence respiratory rate.
- Increases in body temperature associated with exercise eventually lead to vasodilation in the skin.

Suggested Reading

Erlichman J, Kerbey AL, James WPT. Physical activity and its impact on health outcomes. Obesity Rev. 2002;3:273–287.

Fletcher GF. Exercise standards for testing and training: a statement for healthcare professionals from the American Heart Association. Circulation. 2001;104:1694–1740.

Lee IM, Skerrett PJ. Physical activity and all-cause mortality: what is the dose-response relation? Med Sci Sports Exerc. 2001;33(6, suppl):S459–S471.

White RD, Evans CH. Performing the exercise test. Prim Care. 2001;28(1):29–53.

REVIEW QUESTIONS

Directions: Each of the numbered items or incomplete statements in this section is followed by answers or by completions of the statement. Select the ONE lettered answer or completion that is BEST in each case.

1. A 24-year-old woman suffers 3 days of watery diarrhea and then runs a marathon in very hot weather, during which she collapses. If she has collapsed from heat stroke, one reason might be:
   (A) She was unable to elevate cardiac stroke volume
   (B) She was unable to elevate her heart rate
   (C) She was unable to vasodilate the vascular beds in her skin
   (D) She was unable to vasodilate the vascular beds in her muscles
   (E) She was unable to conduct normal gas exchange

2. Patients with coronary artery disease may suffer angina during exercise because of:
   (A) Increased cardiac oxygen supply
   (B) Increased cardiac oxygen demand
   (C) Increased cardiac production of carbon dioxide
   (D) Pulmonary edema
   (E) Increased afterload

3. Blood pH may fall during intense exercise from:
   (A) Anaerobic metabolism
   (B) Aerobic metabolism
   (C) Gluconeogenesis
   (D) Sweating
   (E) Glycogenolysis

ANSWERS TO REVIEW QUESTIONS

1. **The answer is** C. Owing to dehydration, the woman was hypotensive. The baroreceptor reflex caused vasoconstriction in the vascular beds in her skin in order to preserve blood flow to the heart and brain. Vasoconstriction in the skin also had the undesirable effect of preventing cooling of the blood.

2. **The answer is** B. During exercise, increased muscular demand for oxygen leads to increased cardiac output (which in turn increases the flow of oxygenated blood to the muscles). Increased cardiac output requires an increased supply of oxygen to the myocardium. In coronary artery disease, the coronary arteries may not be able to supply the blood and oxygen needed by the myocardium, creating the sensation of angina.

3. **The answer is** A. When muscular demand outstrips the supply of oxygen, the muscles may turn to anaerobic metabolism for energy. Lactic acid is a by-product of anaerobic metabolism. It acidifies the blood, increases the PCO_2, and drives increased respiration by stimulating chemoreceptors.

Part V

PULMONARY PHYSIOLOGY

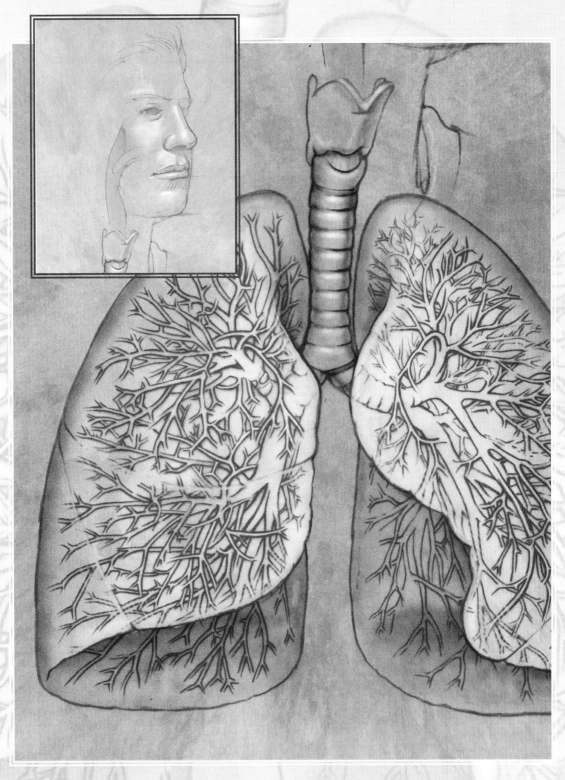

The Mechanics
of Breathing

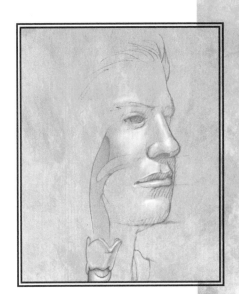

INTRODUCTION

Many species require oxygen in order to extract energy from their environment. The use of oxygen for energy extraction is called *aerobic respiration.* Aerobic organisms have varying methods for acquiring oxygen and eliminating carbon dioxide, the by-product of aerobic respiration. In some organisms, such as sea sponges, these molecules simply diffuse directly from cells to the environment or vice versa. In more complex organisms, a circulatory system and its red blood cells transport oxygen from a "gas exchanger" to the rest of the body and carbon dioxide from the body to the exchanger.

In all terrestrial (and some aquatic) vertebrates, gas exchange occurs in the air-filled lungs, which expose the blood of the circulatory system to the air. Oxygen in the air of the lungs diffuses into the blood. Carbon dioxide brought from the body tissues diffuses out of the blood into lung air. For this exchange to occur effectively, the air rich in carbon dioxide must be expelled and fresh air rich in oxygen must be brought into the lungs.

The movement of air in and out of the lungs is the process of **breathing** or **ventilation**, while **respiration** is the process by which our cells use oxygen to make ATP for energy. (However, in clinical settings, many physicians use "respiration" to refer to breathing.) Breathing makes the absorption of oxygen and elimination of carbon dioxide possible. The important components in this system are the airways (trachea and bronchial tree), the gas exchange area (alveoli), the bellows that provides the force to drive breathing (chest wall and diaphragm), and the control system (central nervous system and chemoreceptors). Interactions between these components enable adequate oxygenation and ventilation.

Animals possessing a rudimentary lung called an "air-bladder" first appeared in the Devonian period over 300 million years ago. By swallowing air into their air-bladders every 10 or 15 minutes like the lungfish of today, these early fishes enabled vertebrate life to migrate from the water into the mud flats and onward to the land. There, the more sophisticated air-breathing apparatus of higher animals would evolve.

SYSTEM STRUCTURE: THE THORAX

The system of air-conducting passages starts with the **trachea** and branches continually into smaller and smaller passages, resembling an upside-down tree. FIGURE 16.1 illustrates how the airways act as conduits that bring air from the environment into the lungs and down to the **alveoli**, the air sacs where gas exchange occurs. The upper airways consist of the nasopharynx, oropharynx, larynx, and trachea.

The trachea divides at the carina into the right and left mainstem **bronchi**, which extend into the lungs. The mainstem bronchi branch into sequentially smaller bronchi as follows: lobar bronchi, segmental bronchi, subsegmental bronchi, and smaller bronchioles. Eventually the airways become **terminal bronchioles**, which lead to **respiratory bronchioles, alveolar ducts,** and **alveolar sacs.** The terminal bronchioles are the smallest in diameter of the passages in the conducting portion of the bronchial tree. Distal to the terminal bronchioles, gas exchange begins to occur.

Histology

The histologic architecture of the bronchial tree remains relatively consistent from the trachea to the bronchioles. The trachea is a flexible tube of fibroelastic connective tissue that is lined by ciliated columnar epithelial cells. Mucus-producing *goblet cells* are also present. C-shaped rings of hyaline cartilage give the trachea semirigid support along its anterior and lateral surfaces (FIGURE 16.2). With this support system the trachea resists collapse, but it can accommodate changes in size, as can the more distal airways. An abundance of *elastin* provides the bronchial tree with the ability to expand during inspiration and to recoil during expiration. (See Clinical Application Boxes *Impaired Mucus Clearance in Smokers' Lungs* and *The Coughing Mechanism.*)

In the more distal conducting airways, the cartilage rings become less frequent and disappear completely in the bronchioles. The respiratory epithelium remains ciliated, but the cilia shorten and there are fewer goblet cells. The smooth muscle layer becomes especially prominent in the bronchioles and is arranged in a spiral manner, allowing for contraction in both length and diameter.

The lung parenchyma is composed primarily of alveoli. There are over 300 million alveoli in the adult lung, covering a total surface area approximately equal to the size of a tennis court. The lungs are divided into lobes. The right lung has upper, middle, and lower lobes, while the left lung only has upper and lower lobes. (A portion of the left upper lobe called the *lingula* corresponds anatomically to the middle lobe of the right lung.) The lungs are further divided into bronchopulmonary segments, which are shaped like pyramids with their apices pointing toward the hilum of the lung. Each bronchopulmonary segment is supplied by a segmental bronchus, segmental artery, and segmental vein. A state known as *atelectasis* results when one or more bronchopulmonary segments collapse. This might happen when a mucus plug obstructs a segmental bronchus, blocking the movement of air into that segment.

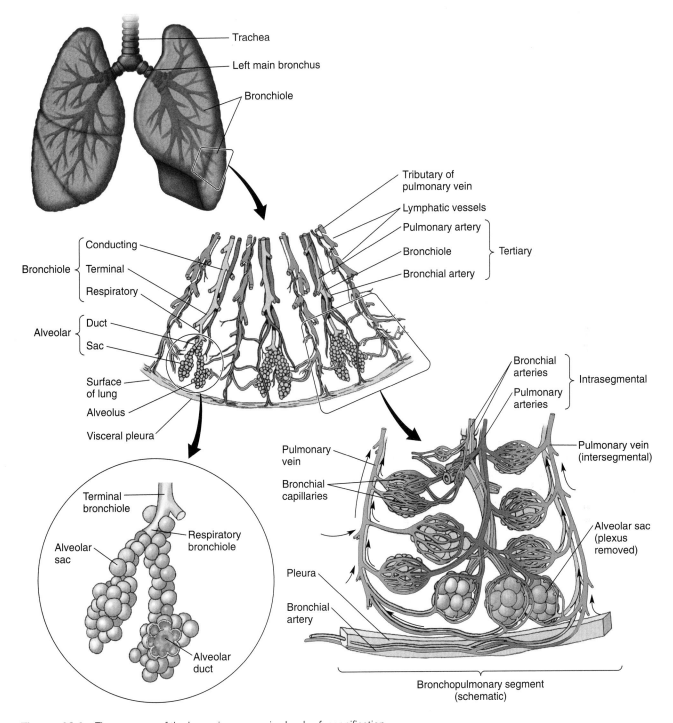

Figure 16.1   The structure of the lungs, in progressive levels of magnification.

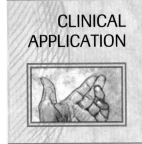

CLINICAL APPLICATION

IMPAIRED MUCUS CLEARANCE IN SMOKERS' LUNGS

Mucus helps trap debris and humidify air as it enters the lungs. Together the ciliated columnar epithelial cells and goblet cells form the mucociliary elevator, which continually moves glandular secretions and debris toward the pharynx to clear them from the lungs. Toxins from cigarette smoking impair the ciliated cells of this system, making it difficult to clear secretions and debris from the lungs.

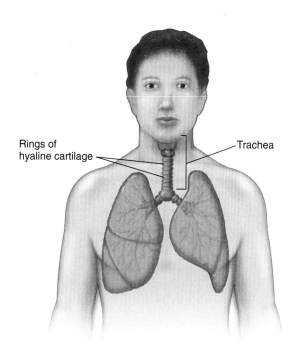

Figure 16.2 The trachea. The trachea is lined with C-shaped rings of hyaline cartilage.

The epithelium of the alveoli consists of type I and type II pneumocytes. **Type I pneumocytes** are large flat cells that are part of the thin gas-diffusion barrier. **Type II pneumocytes** are rounded and produce **surfactant**, a substance that reduces the surface tension in the alveoli, helping to prevent them from collapsing.

Gross Anatomy

There are no attachments between the lungs and the chest wall except at the *hilum*, where the lungs are suspended by the mediastinum, primary bronchi, pulmonary arteries, and pulmonary veins. The *pleura*, which has two layers, surrounds the lungs (FIGURE 16.3). The *visceral pleura* adheres to the lung and the *parietal pleura* adheres to the chest wall and diaphragm, the principal muscle of breathing. To visualize how the pleura enfold the lungs, imagine a fist pushing into the side of a large flat deflated balloon until the balloon completely encircles the fist in two layers. The fist is the lung, the wall of the balloon closer to the fist is the visceral pleura (attached to the lung), and the outermost wall of the balloon, which is not in direct contact with the fist, is the parietal pleura (attached to the inside of the chest wall). There is no air inside the balloon between the two walls, though there potentially could be.

In the lungs, this potential space between the two layers is called the **pleural space.** A small amount of *pleural fluid* in the pleural space lubricates the movements of the lungs inside the chest wall, but the space is otherwise empty, and the pleural surfaces are perfectly apposed with one another. The serous pleural fluid is secreted by the superficial mesothelium of the pleura. Lymph ducts continually drain the fluid from the pleural space into the hilar lymph nodes and from there convey it into the thoracic duct. This drainage keeps the pleural space a potential space—a near vacuum—so that during inhalation, when the diaphragm pulls down on the parietal pleura, the

---

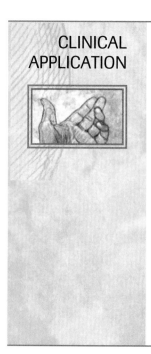

CLINICAL APPLICATION

THE COUGHING MECHANISM

Coughing is a matter of exhalation at high velocity. Coughs are initiated by irritant receptors in the large airways. They communicate with the medulla and cause a large inspiration of air. The epiglottis and vocal cords are sealed, abdominal muscles contract to generate high intrathoracic pressure, and the seal is abruptly released, driving air out at high velocity.

Tracheal contraction may add to the high velocity of exhalation. This part of coughing can be understood by applying Ohm's law, which states that flow (Q) equals the pressure gradient driving flow (ΔP) divided by the resistance (R): $Q = \Delta P/R$.

Smooth muscles connecting the open ends of the tracheal cartilage rings can contract and decrease the diameter of the trachea, thereby increasing tracheal resistance. Tracheal contraction with expiratory flow held constant requires the air to pass through a smaller diameter at higher speed, as when one partially occludes the nozzle of a hose to cause water to jet out at high speed. Increases in the force of diaphragmatic contraction and the contraction of the abdominal musculature together provide the added pressure gradient necessary to match the increased resistance and preserve flow. The higher speed of the expelled air mobilizes debris and helps clear phlegm or irritants from the throat.

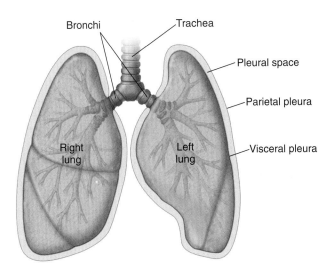

Figure 16.3 The pleura. Under physiologic conditions, the pleural space is only a potential space.

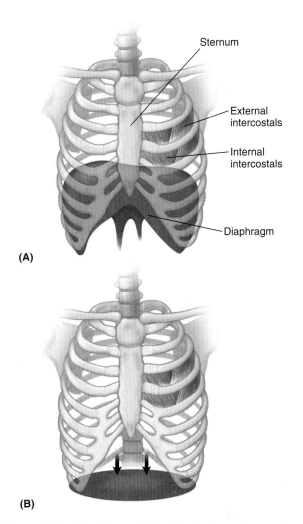

(A)

(B)

Figure 16.4 The chest wall. **A.** The diaphragm has a domed shape in its relaxed state. **B.** During inspiration, the diaphragm contracts and flattens, dropping the floor of the thoracic cavity and expanding the lungs.

parietal pleura cannot be pulled away from the visceral pleura. The diaphragm contracts and pulls the parietal pleura, which is vacuum-suctioned to the visceral pleura, and the lung is pulled open. (See Clinical Application Box *How Disease States Can Affect the Pleural Space.*)

The **chest wall** is a semirigid structure framed by bones (ribs, sternum, and spine) that protect and support the heart and lungs, and muscles that modify the volume of the thoracic cavity during breathing (FIGURE 16.4). The most important of these muscles is the dome-shaped **diaphragm**, which forms the floor of the thoracic cavity and contracts in a downward direction to expand the lungs during inhalation. The diaphragm is innervated by the *phrenic nerves*, which originate at cervical roots C3, C4, and C5. (See Clinical Application Box *Injuries to the Phrenic Nerves.*)

Accessory breathing muscles may assist the diaphragm during exercise or in disease states that compromise breathing function. The intercostal muscles extend between the ribs and can manipulate them to increase or decrease the dimensions of the thoracic cavity. The intercostal muscles include the external intercostals, internal intercostals, innermost intercostals, and the transversus thoracis muscle. Additional accessory muscles include the scalenes, sternocleidomastoids, anterior serrati, abdominal wall muscles (which push the abdomen in and diaphragm up during forced exhalation), and alae nasi (which flare the nostrils).

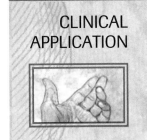

CLINICAL APPLICATION

HOW DISEASE STATES CAN AFFECT THE PLEURAL SPACE

Under pathological circumstances the pleural space can fill with air (*pneumothorax*), blood (*hemothorax*), or excess fluid (*pleural effusion*). A host of pathological events, including malignancy, infection, and trauma, may precipitate these conditions. The outcomes can range in severity from minor and self-healing to life-threatening emergencies.

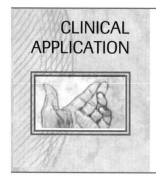

INJURIES TO THE PHRENIC NERVES

A cervical spinal injury at or above C3 often results in paralysis of the diaphragm, respiratory failure, and death. An injury from C3 to C5 may partially paralyze the diaphragm. Because cervical fracture and respiratory compromise are some of the most worrisome consequences of head and neck trauma, victims of such trauma should immediately have their cervical spine immobilized by a cervical collar. To remember the cervical roots of the phrenic nerve, use this mnemonic: "C3, 4, 5, keep the diaphragm alive."

SYSTEM FUNCTION: THE BELLOWS

The lungs are a bellows like the bellows used to blow air into a fireplace. When a bellows is drawn open, the pressure inside it drops and air rushes in to fill the expanded volume, as in **inspiration** (inhalation). When the bellows is compressed, the pressure rises inside and the air is expelled, as in **expiration** (exhalation).

Inspiration involves the contraction of the muscles of inspiration (primarily the diaphragm) and is thus considered an active process. Expiration occurs when these muscles relax. The recoil forces in the elastic lung tissue naturally contract the lung again when unopposed by the diaphragm, driving air back out of the lungs. Expiration is therefore a passive process, and takes about twice as long as inspiration. (During exercise or in disease states, the accessory breathing muscles may assist in expiration, actively supplementing the passive process.) (See Clinical Application Box *Accessory Breathing*.)

Transmural Pressure, Elastic Recoil Pressure, and Compliance

To understand how the body achieves breathing—the bellows effect—one must understand the forces that govern the expansion and contraction of a container. Understanding the forces at work in breathing is also key to understanding the consequences of pathologic derangements of the pulmonary system.

Transmural Pressure and Elastic Recoil Pressure   A container of air, such as a balloon or a lung, changes size because of a pressure gradient across the wall of the container, a **transmural pressure ($P_{transmural}$)**. (In Latin, *trans* means "across" and *murus* means "wall.") Transmural pressures are defined as the pressure inside the container minus the pressure outside the container:

$$P_{transmural} = P_{in} - P_{out}$$

A positive transmural pressure ($P_{in} > P_{out}$) works to expand a container. A negative transmural

pressure ($P_{in} < P_{out}$) works to collapse a container. During breathing, it is necessary for the container that is the lung to change size to allow inspiration and expiration. Therefore, a transmural pressure must occur across the lung, which is known as *transpulmonary pressure* ($P_{transpulmonary}$). In accordance with the definition of transmural pressure, transpulmonary pressure is defined as the pressure of air inside the lung (in the alveoli) minus the pressure of the space outside the lung (the pleural space):

$$P_{transpulmonary} = P_{alveoli} - P_{pleural\ space}$$

Transmural pressure is not the only factor determining the expansion or contraction of a container. The container wall also has innate properties that give it a tendency to collapse or expand. This tendency toward collapse or expansion is called **elastic recoil pressure (P_{el})**. For example, elastic recoil pressure in the wall of a balloon gives it a tendency to collapse. A positive transmural pressure (created by air blown into the balloon) would counter the innate recoil pressure. When the recoil pressure overcomes the positive transmural pressure, the net result is contraction and the air sputters out of the balloon. When the transmural pressure is higher than the recoil pressure, as occurs when one forcibly blows air into the balloon, the balloon expands. The **pressure of expansion or contraction ($P_{expansion\ or\ contraction}$)** for a container is thus the net result of recoil pressure and transmural pressure (FIGURE 16.5). If an expanding recoil pressure is defined as positive and a collapsing recoil pressure as negative, the following equation can be written:

$$P_{expansion\ or\ contraction} = P_{transmural} + P_{el}$$

When the container is neither expanding nor contracting, $P_{transmural}$ and P_{el} are equal and opposite and $P_{expansion\ or\ contraction}$ is zero.

The lungs, like a balloon, have a tendency to collapse. Connective tissues in the lung parenchyma, such as elastin and collagen, and the surface tension of the fluid that lines the alveoli give the lungs their collapsing tendency. Positive transpulmonary pressures

ACCESSORY BREATHING

During exercise and in some disease states, normal quiet breathing is not sufficient to move the necessary volume of air in and out of the lungs. In these cases, accessory muscles of breathing help expand and contract the thoracic bellows. During inspiration, the accessory muscles contract along with the diaphragm. The inspiratory accessory muscles include the external intercostal muscles, the sternocleidomastoids, the anterior serrati, and the scaleni muscles. When the accessory muscles contract, they elevate the ribs, causing them to pivot on their attachments with the spine and sternum. This pivoting increases the lateral diameter of the thorax, which assists the diaphragm in increasing the volume in the thoracic cavity. The accessory muscles also pull the sternum up, increasing the anteroposterior diameter of the thorax.

Although expiration is generally passive, the contraction of the rectus abdominis and internal intercostal muscles can actively assist in expiration. The rectus abdominis muscle pushes the abdominal contents (and hence the diaphragm) up and the internal intercostal muscles pull the ribs down, decreasing the anteroposterior diameter of the thoracic cavity and assisting the lungs' natural recoil in decreasing the volume of the thoracic cavity. The action of the external and internal intercostal muscles on the ribs during the breathing cycle is often referred to as the *bucket-handle effect* (FIGURE B16.1).

During an exacerbation of their disease, patients with chronic obstructive pulmonary disease (COPD) are sometimes found in the sitting position, leaning forward with their hands on their knees or grabbing a table. Called the *tripod position*, this pose optimizes the use of the accessory muscles to facilitate breathing.

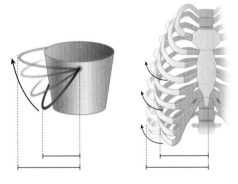

Figure B16.1 Accessory breathing muscles and the bucket-handle effect. Lifting the "bucket handle" of the ribs increases the lateral diameter of the thorax.

oppose the lungs' recoil pressure and must overcome this pressure to expand the lung. The recoil pressure of the lung drives contraction and exhalation.

The chest wall exerts a recoil pressure in the opposite direction of the lung; it has a tendency to expand or flare outward, increasing the volume of the chest cavity. Positive trans-chest wall pressures therefore supplement the expanding tendency of the chest wall. Negative trans-chest wall pressures oppose the recoil pressure of the chest wall and must overcome this pressure to reduce the volume of the chest wall container.

Compliance The shape of transmural pressure-volume curves for elastic containers like the lung is determined by the elastic recoil properties of the container walls. If recoil pressures were constant over all volumes, the transmural pressure-volume (PV) curve would be a straight line; that is, increases in transmural pressure against a constant recoil pressure would increase container volume in a direct proportion to those increases in transmural pressure (FIGURE 16.6). A container with a higher recoil force would have a PV curve with a decreased slope (tilted downward), as higher pressures would be required to overcome the recoil force and achieve the same volume. A container with a lower recoil force would have a PV curve with an increased slope (tilted upward), as less pressure is needed to expand the container to achieve the same volume.

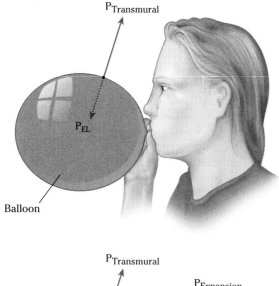

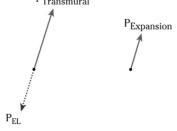

Figure 16.5 The pressures acting on the wall of a balloon. To inflate a balloon, transmural pressure to expand must exceed elastic recoil pressure to collapse, thereby providing a net pressure for expansion.

A container's compliance is one measure of its elastic recoil properties (FIGURE 16.7). **Compliance (C)** is defined as the change in volume (ΔV) that occurs for a given change in transmural pressure (ΔP):

$$C = \Delta V / \Delta P$$

Therefore, compliance is represented on the transmural PV curve as the slope of this curve. We saw in Figure 16.6 that the elastic recoil pressure determined the slope of the PV curve. *Recoil pressure and compliance are, in fact, inversely proportional.* Increased compliance (steep slope) reflects a lesser recoil force; the same increase in transmural pressure creates a larger increase in volume. Decreased compliance (flatter slope) reflects a greater recoil force; the same increase in transmural pressure creates a smaller increase in volume.

Recall that the linear relation between transmural pressure and volume implies a recoil force that is uniform over all volumes. What would the curve look like if the recoil forces were to change with respect to volume? The curves would not be linear. In fact, the transmural PV curves are not linear in the lung and chest wall (FIGURE 16.8). As the volume change goes farther against the natural tendency of the container,

the recoil force gets stronger. Similarly, a rubber band has a much greater recoil force the farther it is stretched. Thus, as the volume of the container gets larger against its collapsing recoil tendency, the recoil pressure gets stronger and the container becomes harder to expand. This effect progressively flattens the transmural PV curve. At high volumes, changes in pressure result in smaller changes in volume. One might expect this change in the slope after studying Figure 16.6. In that figure a container

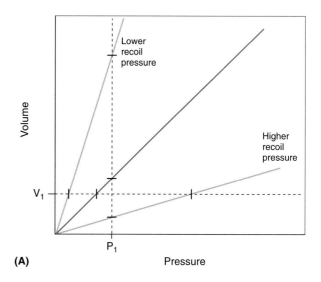

(A)

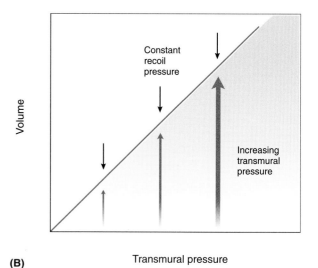

(B)

Figure 16.6 The pressure-volume (PV) curve for a container with a collapsing elastic recoil pressure that remains uniform at all volumes. **A.** A container with a lower recoil pressure requires less transmural pressure to sustain a given volume, V_1. A container with a higher recoil pressure requires more transmural pressure to sustain volume V_1. At a given transmural pressure, P_1, a container with lower recoil pressure has a higher volume. A container with a higher recoil pressure has a lower volume at P_1. **B.** Transmural pressure and recoil pressure push against one another to drive volume up or down.

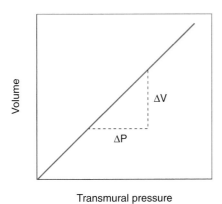

Figure 16.7 Compliance: the slope of the transmural PV curve. As a slope, compliance (C) is the rise, ΔV, over the run, ΔP. C = ΔV/ΔP.

with higher recoil pressure pushes the curve downward, reducing the slope of the curve.

FIGURES 16.9 and 16.10 depict the transmural PV curves for the lungs in isolation and for the chest wall in isolation. The compliance of the lungs has been measured experimentally by removing the lungs from the chest and measuring the changes in volume and pressure as they are artificially inflated. Similarly, the chest wall has been studied apart from the lungs and exposed to a range of transmural pressures. The recoil properties in these two physiologic containers determine the shapes of the curves.

There are two important features of the transmural PV curve of the isolated lungs (see Figure 16.9). First, isolated lungs have zero volume when transmural pressures are negative or zero. This is because

negative transmural pressures supplement the collapsing recoil tendency of the lungs; in this case, there is no force in support of lung expansion. With no transmural pressure present, the recoil force of the lung acts unopposed to collapse the lung. Second, at larger lung volumes the compliance is decreased, reflected by the slope of the curve approaching zero (i.e., recoil pressure is increased with increasingly positive transmural pressures). Further increases in transmural pressure cannot expand the lung, but would rupture them.

The shape of the transmural PV curve of the isolated chest wall is consistent with its known elastic recoil properties. The chest wall compliance is decreased (recoil pressure to expand is increased) over increasingly negative transmural pressures, and the transmural PV curve is nonlinear. Thus, the slope of the curve (the compliance) approaches zero as the

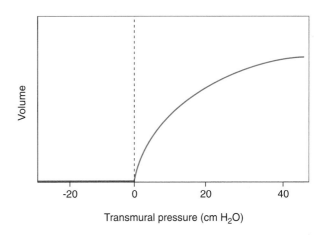

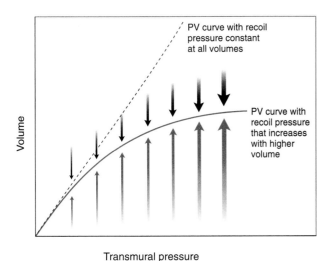

Figure 16.8 The PV curve for a container with a collapsing elastic recoil pressure that increases with increasing volume. Increased elastic recoil pressure at high volumes limits volume expansion and flattens the PV curve, lowering its slope.

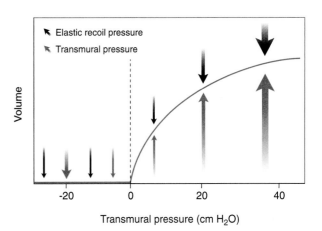

Figure 16.9 The PV curve for the lungs in isolation. The lung recoil pressure arrows always point down because they always favor volume contraction. When positive, transmural pressure favors volume expansion and the arrows point up. When negative, the transmural pressure arrows point down, driving contraction. The lungs in situ cannot achieve zero volume; this is possible only for lungs excised from the thoracic cavity.

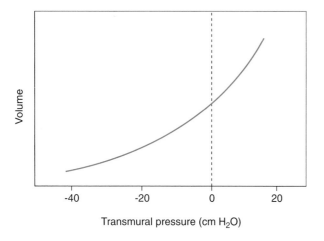

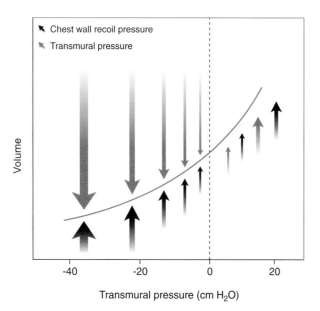

Figure 16.10 The PV curve for the chest wall in isolation. Chest wall recoil pressure arrows always point up, because they always favor volume expansion. Transmural pressure arrows point up when positive and down when negative. The figure does not show that at high volumes, this curve levels off. This is because after a certain volume, the chest wall resists expansion. At this point, the chest wall has a collapsing recoil force like the lung, and its recoil pressure arrows would point down.

transmural pressure becomes more negative. Any greater negative transmural pressure would damage or collapse the chest wall. Notice that the chest wall maintains a volume at zero transmural pressure. This is because the chest wall's recoil forces tend toward expansion; if unopposed by a negative transmural pressure, it will maintain a volume at about 60% of the thoracic capacity. Positive transmural pressures can increase the volume of the chest cavity even farther; however, at greater volumes, the chest wall's recoil force becomes negative, similar to the lung, and will resist more expansion.

The Lung/Chest Wall Counterbalance and the Breathing Cycle

Given the contrasting tendencies of the lung and chest wall, we can now understand the lung and chest wall as a unit. Recall that in a living person, the lungs and chest wall are in constant contact—held together by the pleural potential space—and therefore they must change volume as one. Combined, they create a new container wall (that of the entire chest wall/lung system) that has its own elastic recoil properties. These properties reflect the recoil forces of both the lungs and the chest wall. The interplay of these forces ultimately explains how breathing occurs.

The Counterbalance When the lungs are in the body, the force exerted by the lungs to collapse is countered by the force exerted by the chest wall to try to expand (FIGURE 16.11). Therefore, the lungs maintain a small volume even at negative transmural pressures, because the recoil force of the chest wall opposes the collapsing force of the negative transmural pressure. The chest wall in the combined respiratory system does not expand as much as the isolated chest wall with higher transmural pressures, because the recoil pressure of the lungs opposes the expanding force of the positive transmural pressure. At volumes >60% of capacity, the chest wall's recoil force changes direction to become a collapsing force like lung recoil. Therefore, at volumes >60% capacity, the combined system has a lower compliance than the lungs in isolation.

Figure 16.11 is a graph of the PV relationships of the chest wall/lung system in the absence of muscular exertion and with the pressure gradients adjusted by artificial means to obtain specific lung volumes and measure system compliance. The figure does not depict PV relationships of the chest wall/lung system during live breathing (i.e., when the diaphragm is at work). Note the point in Figure 16.11 where the transmural pressure from inside the lungs to outside the chest wall is zero. Without any muscular exertion, and with the epiglottis open so that alveoli and external atmosphere are in open communication, there is no pressure gradient between the outside and the inside of the chest wall/lung system. With no pressure gradient, the opposing recoil forces of lungs and chest wall are balanced, and the system settles into a resting state at a lung volume called the **functional residual capacity (FRC)** (FIGURE 16.12).

Inspiration A cycle of breathing entails changes in the counterbalance of forces that dictate thoracic volume. In a living person, the **breathing cycle** begins at FRC. With the glottis open, the lungs and chest wall are at a counterbalance, and pressure inside the lung is equal to the pressure outside the body (i.e., the

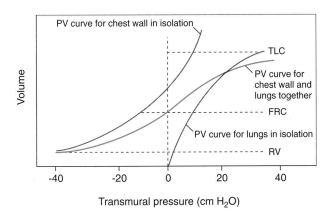

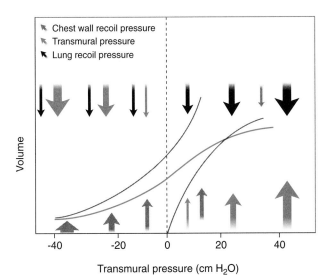

Figure 16.11 The PV curve for the lungs and chest wall together, connected by the pleural space. This curve reflects PV relationships over artificially introduced changes in transmural pressure. It does not show the PV relationships during the contraction of the diaphragm. TLC, total lung capacity; FRC, functional residual capacity; RV, residual volume. The chest wall recoil pressure arrow points down near TLC. This accounts for the fact that the chest wall/lung system is less compliant than the lungs alone at high lung volumes.

atmospheric pressure). The transmural pressure created by the respiratory muscles alters the balance of chest wall and lung forces. The contraction of the diaphragm or accessory muscles results in chest wall expansion by creating a bellows effect and drawing air into the lungs. As the lungs fill with air, the force of the muscular action on the chest wall overcomes the recoil force of the lungs and shifts the balance of the combined system toward expansion of the lungs to a larger volume. As the lung volume increases, lung compliance decreases and the lungs' recoil force increases, thereby progressively opposing further increases in lung volume. The maximum volume the lungs can achieve during inspiration is the *total lung capacity (TLC)*.

Expiration Once you have inhaled, the respiratory muscles can relax, shifting the balance of forces in favor of lung recoil. The chest wall/lung system will passively return to its resting state at FRC as air flows out of the lungs. Although expiration is a passive process, by contracting the abdominal muscles you can force air out of the lungs, driving lung volume down below FRC. However, the chest wall recoil force opposes this contraction of the chest wall/lung system below the system's resting state at FRC. Once the abdominal muscles relax, the system passively re-expands to FRC. The minimum volume the lungs can achieve is the *residual volume* (RV). Beyond this point, the abdominal muscles and lung recoil forces cannot overcome the recoil forces of the chest wall.

Transmural Pressures During the Breathing Cycle

We can translate the breathing cycle into more analytical language by considering the transmural pressures at each phase of the cycle.

At FRC At FRC, the pressure inside the alveoli of the lung, $P_{alveoli}$, and the pressure at the body surface, $P_{body\ surface}$, are equal to each other, at atmospheric pressure. Pulmonary physiologists call atmospheric pressure zero and measure all other pressures relative to the $P_{body\ surface}$ of zero. With $P_{alveoli}$ and $P_{body\ surface}$ both equal to zero at FRC, there is no transmural pressure gradient across the chest wall/lung system, and the system does not change in volume. The lung by itself, however, is not stable at a transmural pressure of zero; it collapses. Therefore, at FRC the lung's transmural pressure gradient cannot be zero. In fact, the transpulmonary pressure must be positive in order to keep the lung open. How can the transpulmonary pressure be positive when the transmural pressure across the chest wall/lung system is zero?

The answer is that the chest wall (lined by the visceral pleura) and the lung (lined by the parietal pleura) pulling away from each other creates a negative pressure in the pleural space relative to the $P_{body\ surface}$ and $P_{alveoli}$ of zero. Rather than create a positive transmural pressure by increasing P_{in} ($P_{alveoli}$), as when blowing up a balloon, the body lowers P_{out} ($P_{pleural\ space}$) to create a positive transpulmonary pressure, and the lungs inflate. This is similar to what happens to a helium balloon that escapes into the sky. As the balloon gains altitude, the pressure outside the balloon decreases, causing the balloon to expand and eventually burst. When patients cannot breathe for themselves and require a machine for ventilation, the positive transpulmonary pressure is generated by increasing $P_{alveoli}$ with respect to

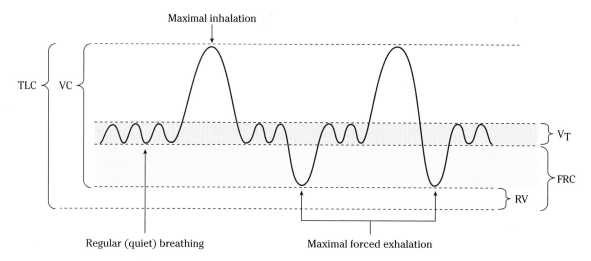

Figure 16.12 A spirogram of lung volumes. Functional residual capacity (FRC) is the relaxed lung volume at end-expiration/pre-inspiration. The tidal volume (V_T) represents the volume added to the FRC during a relaxed inhalation. Relaxed breathing shifts lung volume back and forth from FRC up to (FRC + V_T) and back again. The total lung capacity (TLC) represents the maximum lung volume attainable with forceful inhalation. The residual volume (RV) is the lung volume left over after the maximum amount of air has been forced from the lung. RV can never be zero, except in the case of total collapse of both lungs. The vital capacity (VC) is the volume between TLC and RV. The lung spaces are divided between air in the conducting airways and air in the alveolar spaces. Both spaces grow and shrink with inhalation and exhalation.

$P_{pleural space}$ and $P_{body surface}$. Because mechanical ventilation relies on *positive* $P_{alveoli}$, it is sometimes referred to as *positive-pressure ventilation*.

A similar situation occurs in the case of the chest wall. Figures 16.10 and 16.11 tell us that when the pressure across the chest wall alone is zero, the chest wall expands to a larger volume than FRC. Therefore, the transmural pressure for the chest wall alone cannot be zero when the transmural pressure for the chest wall/lung system as a whole is zero. The pressure across the chest wall is equal to P_{in} ($P_{pleural space}$), which is negative, minus P_{out} ($P_{body surface}$), which is zero. This negative transmural pressure keeps the chest wall slightly compressed.

During Inspiration During inspiration, the respiratory muscles supplement the chest wall's tendency to expand the thoracic cavity (FIGURE 16.13). The pressure in the pleural space drops even lower, changing the transmural pressures across the chest wall and across the lung. The transmural pressure across the chest wall is more negative. Does the contraction of the diaphragm paradoxically collapse the thoracic cavity? No, the expanding force of the muscles, combined with the expanding recoil force of the chest wall, overcomes the collapsing negative trans-chest wall pressures. Meanwhile, the even more positive transpulmonary pressure overcomes the lung's recoil pressure, and the chest wall/lung system expands. The increase in alveolar volume drops the $P_{alveoli}$ with respect to the $P_{body surface}$, and air rushes into the lungs. The lungs have been opened like a

bellows to draw in air. The volume drawn in during normal breathing is the *tidal volume (V_T)*.

At End-Inspiration (FRC + V_T) At end-inspiration, the rush of air into the lungs has raised the $P_{alveoli}$ back up to the atmospheric pressure of zero. The transmural pressure across the chest wall is more negative than at FRC (but the muscles resist this collapsing force), and the transpulmonary pressure is more positive than at FRC, holding the lungs open. Then the muscles stop contracting.

During Expiration Without the force of the muscles acting to expand the chest wall, the negative $P_{pleural space}$ is now enough to cause the collapse of the chest wall, and the recoil force of the lungs now overcomes the reduced positive transpulmonary pressure. The contracting lungs squeeze the alveolar air and raise alveolar pressure, and the air rushes out of the mouth and nose. As the alveolar pressure drops back to zero, the lungs contract down to FRC. The breathing muscles no longer pull at the pleural space and the recoil force of the lung on the pleural space is less, because the lung is no longer as stretched and is more compliant. The pleural space pressure assumes the less negative value with which it began the breathing cycle at FRC.

What happens when you hold your breath at end-inspiration? At FRC + V_T, you close your epiglottis and relax your diaphragm. The lungs and chest wall are not passively counterbalanced at FRC + V_T. At this volume, a positive transmural pressure is and less compliance, it is harder to keep the epiglottis closed than at lower lung volumes.

Surface Tension

Surface forces in the alveoli account for a majority of the recoil force of the lungs, while the elastic properties of lung connective tissue account for the rest. Lung function therefore depends in large part upon alveolar **surface tension**, the especially strong adherence of water molecules to one another along the water's surface.

The polarized nature of water molecules leads to forces of attraction between them (*hydrogen bonding*), and the forces are particularly strong at the air/water interface (FIGURE 16.14). Deep water molecules (those away from the surface) are pulled by attractive forces in all directions. By contrast, water molecules at the surface are pulled by attractive forces in every direction but up. A lack of upward attractive forces on the molecules at the surface results in less dispersal of surface molecules and shorter-range, stronger hydrogen bonding. Stronger hydrogen bonds create a tighter, more strongly adherent layer of molecules at the surface. The surface tension is a force that contributes to holding raindrops together. Another way to conceptualize surface tension is by analogy to a film stretched across the surface of the water like a tight drum, capable of sustaining the weight of an insect or a paper clip.

In the lung, the alveoli are lined by molecules of water and exhibit surface tension. The contractile surface forces cause the alveoli (and hence the lung) to tend to collapse. **Laplace's law** describes the transmural pressure (P) needed to keep open a sphere with a given surface tension (T) and radius

$$(r): P = 2T/r$$

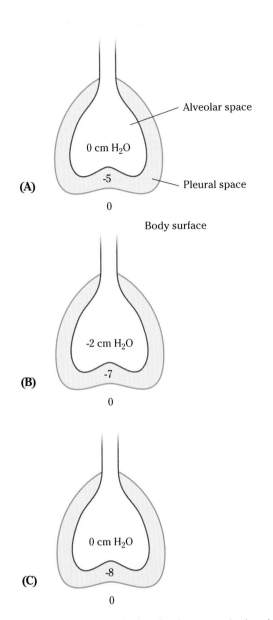

Figure 16.13 Pressures in the alveolar space, in the pleural space, and at the body surface during each phase of the breathing cycle. **A.** At FRC. **B.** During inspiration. **C.** At end-inspiration.

necessary to keep the system open. However, with the diaphragm relaxed, the transmural pressure across the system falls and the system contracts. As the system contracts against a lung volume sealed in by a closed epiglottis, $P_{alveoli}$ climbs. The system keeps contracting and $P_{alveoli}$ keeps going up until the trans-chest wall/lung system pressure is high enough to equal the system's recoil force and keep the lung open. If the lungs were less compliant, the greater recoil force would raise $P_{alveoli}$ even higher still, making it harder for the epiglottis to resist the transmural pressure across it. You can see this for yourself by comparing the sensations of holding a deep breath versus a small breath. At high lung volumes when the lung is more distended, having a greater recoil force

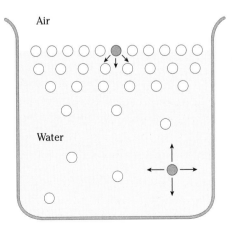

Figure 16.14 Surface tension. The circles represent water molecules. The *arrows* around the highlighted molecules depict forces of attraction toward other water molecules.

The transmural pressure (P) needed to keep the alveolus open is directly proportional to the surface tension (T) and inversely proportional to the radius (r) of the alveolus. The transmural pressure (P) is equal and opposite to the recoil pressure of the sphere.

A closer look at Laplace's law reveals that small alveoli (having small radii) require a higher transmural pressure to stay open and hence have a greater tendency to collapse. This means that a fully collapsed alveolus will require more pressure to inflate than a partially contracted alveolus. Lung compliance is lower at very low volumes where alveoli have a smaller radius (FIGURE 16.15). This explains why the transmural PV curve for the inflation of the isolated lung is actually somewhat flatter at the start of inflation in Figure 16.15 when compared to Figure 16.9. The true inflation curve has a slightly sigmoidal shape. However, the physiologic lung does not collapse at end-expiration but retains a residual volume, which means that the lung never shrinks down to those less compliant volumes. The maintenance of a residual volume thereby reduces the amount of transmural pressure needed for inflation and hence reduces the muscular work (pressure × volume) of breathing.

Not only does the lung make use of a larger alveolar radius (r) to reduce the transmural pressure (P) of inflation; it also has a means of lowering surface tension (T) to reduce transmural pressure. As mentioned earlier, type II pneumocytes produce surfactant in the alveolus. Surfactant consists primarily of the lipid *dipalmitoyl phosphatidylcholine (DPPC)*, whose hydrophobic nature interferes with the water–water hydrogen bonding that accounts for surface tension. Surfactant thereby decreases the surface tension of

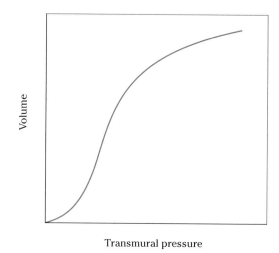

Figure 16.15   Low lung compliance at low lung volumes.

the alveoli, reduces the recoil force of the lungs, and makes inflation easier. (See Clinical Application Box *What Is Neonatal Respiratory Distress Syndrome?*)

Several other forces help stabilize the alveoli and prevent them from collapsing. The two most important of these are phenomena called interdependence and airway closure. *Interdependence* reflects the fact that alveoli, alveolar ducts, and other air spaces are adjacent to one another and mechanically dependent on each other. The collapsing force in one alveolus stents open adjacent alveoli. *Airway closure* refers to the fact that during late expiration, transmural pressures of the airways tend to collapse the airways. This traps some air distal to the area of collapse (i.e., in the alveoli) and helps keep the alveoli open at low lung volumes.

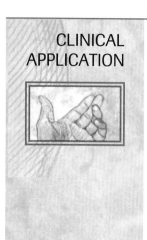

CLINICAL APPLICATION

WHAT IS NEONATAL RESPIRATORY DISTRESS SYNDROME?

A baby girl was delivered at 28 weeks after spontaneous premature labor. At delivery, the infant scored poorly on the Apgar test for neonatal distress. Soon afterward, she displayed significant respiratory distress (grunting, rapid breathing, nasal flaring) and showed an oxygen saturation of 83%, and her lips and nail beds were observed to be cyanotic (having a blue coloration). The neonatologist intubated the baby and began mechanical ventilation based on a diagnosis of neonatal respiratory distress syndrome (NRDS).

NRDS, a disease that affects premature infants, demonstrates the catastrophic effects of insufficient surfactant production. The lungs of these infants have not had time to develop completely and do not produce enough surfactant. The increased alveolar surface tension and very low lung compliance cause alveoli to collapse (atelectasis), making inflation of the lungs extremely difficult. This can lead to severe hypoxemia (low blood oxygen level) and death. However, if treated with aerosolized surfactant early, premature infants can improve dramatically.

Airway Flow and Resistance

Expansion and contraction of the thoracic cavity lead to pressure gradients (ΔP) that drive air flow (Q) from the body surface (i.e., mouth and nose) to the alveoli and back out again. The flow of air is directly proportional to ΔP and inversely proportional to resistance (R). This is analogous to **Ohm's law** in electricity: $Q = \Delta P / R$.

Holding the pressure gradient constant while increasing the resistance results in lower flow; holding resistance constant while decreasing the pressure gradient also results in lower flow.

If flow through the conducting airways is assumed to be laminar—nonturbulent and parallel to the walls of the airways—the airflow can be described by **Poiseuille's law**:

$$Q = \Delta P \pi r^4 / 8 \eta l$$

where r is the radius of the tube, η is fluid viscosity, and l is the length of the tube. If we combine Poiseuille's and Ohm's laws and solve for resistance, we find $R = 8 \eta l / \pi r^4$. Although flow through the airways is not truly laminar flow, this equation serves as a good approximation.

Note that resistance in Poiseuille's law is directly proportional to the viscosity of the air traveling through the tube and the length of the tube. More importantly, note that resistance is inversely proportional to the radius of the tube to the fourth power. This means small changes in the radii of the airways have a dramatic effect on the resistance and thus on the flow of air into and out of the lungs. This relationship between radius and resistance might suggest that the smallest airways, the bronchioles, have the greatest resistance. However, the greatest resistance is found in the medium-sized bronchi, because as the airways get smaller, more branching occurs. At the level of the bronchioles, there are so many small airways in parallel that the aggregate cross-sectional area of the smaller airways is actually greater than the aggregate of the medium-sized airways, leading to reduced resistance in the smaller airways. This is significant in certain disease processes. A substantial amount of damage to the smallest airways is necessary to change flow or resistance. Consequently, diseases such as bronchiolitis obliterans, chronic obstructive pulmonary disease (COPD), and asthma can progress fairly far in the small airways before the patient notices symptoms and before changes in the lungs are detectable.

The most important factors affecting the radius and hence the resistance of the conducting airways are bronchial smooth muscle tone and lung volume. The bronchioles are surrounded by spirally oriented smooth muscles, which decrease the radius and thus increase the resistance of the airways when they contract, resulting in partial obstruction of the airways. Several stimuli cause the bronchial smooth muscle to contract, including parasympathetic stimulation with acetylcholine by the autonomic nervous system, irritants, leukotrienes, low carbon dioxide levels, and histamine. Sympathetic stimulation, on the other hand, with epinephrine and norepinephrine, causes bronchial dilatation and lowers airway resistance. Drugs called *sympathetic agonists* interact with β_2 adrenergic receptors and may be used to induce bronchial dilatation. Albuterol is the most commonly used β_2 agonist. (See Clinical Application Box *What Is Asthma?*)

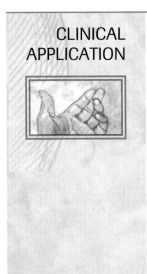

CLINICAL APPLICATION

WHAT IS ASTHMA?

Sally is a 25-year-old medical student with a history of childhood asthma who presents to her primary care physician with nonproductive cough, chest tightness, and exertional dyspnea (difficulty breathing). She reports that she was in her usual state of health until 3 days prior to presentation, when she developed nasal congestion, fatigue, and myalgias. Her initial symptoms were similar to those experienced earlier by her 4-year-old niece, with whom she had recent contact. On physical examination, Sally is afebrile, has tachypnea (rapid breathing), and demonstrates wheezes in all lobes on lung auscultation. Her physician treats her with inhaled β_2 agonists and corticosteroids, which alleviate her dyspnea, chest tightness, and coughing.

Asthma is an obstructive lung disease in which patients have an abnormal rise in smooth muscle tone when exposed to irritants, constricting air flow. Asthma exacerbations can be triggered by inflammation of the airways, as in an upper respiratory infection, and more commonly by exposure to environmental irritants, including allergens or cold air. Some patients can develop variants of asthma, such as exercise-induced asthma, where hyperventilation may trigger bronchospasm. Inhaled β_2 agonists are one form of treatment for this condition. Other treatments include anti-inflammatory agents, such as steroids, and leukotriene receptor antagonists.

Lung volume also has an important effect on airway resistance. Radial traction on the bronchi from surrounding lung tissue helps hold the bronchi open (recall the concept of interdependence from the discussion of surface tension). As lung volume increases, so does the recoil force of the stretched lung tissue, increasing this radial traction, which increases bronchial diameter and decreases resistance. Conversely, as lung volumes are reduced, airway resistance increases.

One physiologic situation in which airway resistance is important is that of **forced expiration.** Consider the transmural pressure across the airway walls during the breathing cycle. At end-inspiration, the pleural pressure is negative, the alveolar pressure is zero, and positive transmural pressure is holding the airways open. During forced expiration, the contraction of the abdominal wall muscles causes the pleural pressure and the alveolar pressure to become very positive, pushing air out of the lungs down a pressure gradient ($P_{alveoli} > P_{airways} > P_{mouth} = 0$). The high alveolar pressure in the parenchyma surrounding the airways creates a negative transmural pressure ($P_{airways} - P_{alveoli}$) across the airways, constricting them (FIGURE 16.16). The constriction and reduction in airway radius create resistance to outflow and impose limits on the velocity of flow achievable by forced expiration. The *equal pressure point theory* suggests that this outflow limitation occurs at a particular point. The theory posits a decrease in airway pressures from the alveoli to the mouth and defines the *equal pressure point (EPP)* as that point along the route where the pressure surrounding the airway (alveolar pressure) is equal to the pressure inside the

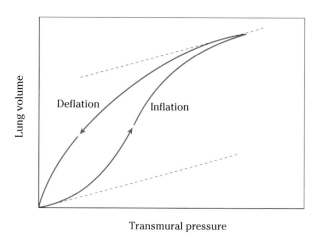

Figure 16.17 Hysteresis. On inflation, the lung shows decreased compliance at low lung volumes. On deflation, the lung shows decreased compliance at high volumes.

airway. Beyond this point, alveolar pressure exceeds airway pressure, causing dynamic compression of the airway and resistance to outflow.

The details of airway resistance are also important in explaining the phenomenon of hysteresis (FIGURE 16.17). **Hysteresis** refers to the differences in lung compliance during inflation versus deflation, reflected in distinct transmural PV curves. At low lung volumes, compliance is lower during inflation than in deflation. The reverse applies at high lung volumes: the lung is less compliant with deflation than inflation. It is widely believed that surfactant accounts for this difference, and it has been reported that at a given lung volume more alveoli are open in deflation than in inflation.

Another contributing factor may be airway resistance. While Poiseuille's law assumes no turbulence or friction, these effects are, in fact, present in the lung and affect the resistance to airflow. At low lung volumes, compliance may be lower with inflation than deflation because resistance is higher when air movement begins than when air has already been flowing. Think of the behavior of objects sliding on a surface: the coefficient of static friction exceeds the coefficient of kinetic friction. If airway friction is greater from rest, we would also expect decreased compliance in the deflation curve at high lung volumes compared to the inflation curve.

PATHOPHYSIOLOGY: DISORDERS OF PULMONARY MECHANICS

Pathologic changes in muscle tone, compliance of the respiratory system (chest wall and/or lung), architecture of the lung parenchyma, and airway resistance can create shifts in the balance of forces

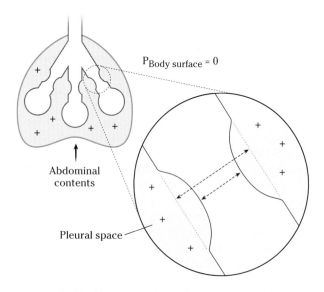

Figure 16.16 Airway constriction in forced expiration. Airway constriction decreases airway radius and increases resistance to airflow.

between lung and chest wall that govern the breathing cycle. There are two broad categories of ventilatory defects: restrictive and obstructive (FIGURE 16.18). Restrictive or obstructive lung diseases encompass not only diseases of the lung, but also diseases of the chest wall. (See Clinical Application Box *Pulmonary Function Tests.*)

Restrictive Lung Disease

In **restrictive lung disease**, a patient has a reduced lung volume. Lung volumes are decreased because of decreased compliance of the respiratory system or weakness of the respiratory muscles. The condition results from increased lung recoil force—for example, pulmonary fibrosis—or decreased thoracic expanding forces. Decreased forces of thoracic expansion fall into two main categories: weak inspiratory muscles, as in neurodegenerative diseases such as amyotrophic lateral sclerosis (ALS), or decreased chest wall compliance, as in obesity or kyphoscoliosis. Lung volumes are low and can result in decreased alveolar ventilation, which can lead to hypoxia. Space-occupying lesions such as tumors, pleural effusions, or pneumonia also have a restrictive pattern. Parenchymal abnormalities associated with some of these conditions can also contribute to hypoxia through $\dot{V}/\dot{Q}$ mismatch (see Chapter 17).

Pulmonary function tests typically reveal low vital capacity (VC), low TLC, and low RV. There is no problem with outflow in a purely restrictive defect; however, forced expiratory volume in 1 second (FEV_1), a measure of expiratory capability, may be low simply because VC is low. Therefore, it is important to look at the ratio of FEV_1 to forced vital capacity (FEV_1/FVC), which should be normal in restrictive defects, even if FEV_1 is low. FRC is usually low, but it may be normal in cases of muscle weakness.

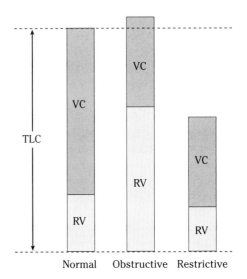

Figure 16.18 Physiologic and pathologic lung volumes. TLC and RV are increased in obstructive lung disease and decreased in restrictive lung disease. VC may be decreased in obstructive disease due to high RV.

Obstructive Lung Disease

In **obstructive lung disease**, a patient has impaired outflow, and lung volumes are typically high. The obstruction of flow is affected by two types of derangements. One is decreased lung recoil force—that is, increased lung compliance (as in emphysema, where inflammation destroys the lung's elastin and alveolar walls). Because lung volumes are high and forced expiration takes a long time, alveolar ventilation is decreased, which can result in hypoxia.

The other derangement that causes obstruction of outflow and increased lung volumes is increased airway resistance, which traps air in the lung (as in chronic bronchitis and asthma). *Air trapping* increases alveolar pressure, creating a more positive

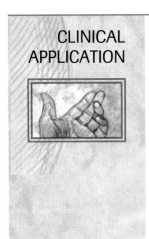

CLINICAL APPLICATION

PULMONARY FUNCTION TESTS

Pulmonary function tests (PFTs) are used to help differentiate the disorders of pulmonary mechanics. The tests are conducted by having a patient inhale maximally and exhale forcefully through a tube connected to a spirometer. The spirometer draws a chart of lung volume over time called a spirogram (see Figure 16.12). The physician is interested in five lung volumes: the *total lung capacity (TLC), residual volume (RV), vital capacity (VC), functional residual capacity (FRC),* and *forced expiratory volume in 1 second (FEV₁).* The patient blows down from maximal lung volume (TLC) to residual volume as hard and fast as possible. This volume is recorded as the *forced vital capacity (FVC).* The volume exhaled during the first second is the FEV_1. The FEV_1/FVC ratio is especially important in assessing lung function. Values that are 80% to 110% of predicted are generally considered normal.

transpulmonary pressure that favors expansion of the chest wall/lung system. Air trapping occurs because increased airway resistance hampers expiration more than it does inspiration. To produce flow into the lung across elevated resistance, the intrathoracic pressure must be made very low compared with the outside atmospheric pressure. A good inspiratory effort can usually accomplish this.

However, to produce flow out of the lung across elevated resistance, the intrathoracic pressure must be made very high compared with outside atmospheric pressure. Recall from the discussion of forced expiration that high intrathoracic pressure surrounding the airways leads to airway collapse, which further increases airway resistance. Efforts to increase outflow fail, and the end result of the airway collapse is increased airway resistance, and air trapping occurs, increasing RV. As in the overcompliant emphysematous lung, lung volumes are high (increased TLC). (Paradoxically, the VC may actually be low, because the RV is so high, foreshortening the volume of expiration.) The FEV_1 and more importantly the FEV_1/FVC ratio are low owing to outflow obstruction. Alveolar ventilation is decreased, and hypoxia can occur.

Gross Structural Disruptions of the Thoracic Bellows

Airway obstruction is one of the most common causes of death in trauma victims, which is why the airway is the first and most important component in the initial evaluation of a trauma patient (or any unconscious patient). The most common cause of airway obstruction in an unconscious patient is the tongue. When a person becomes unconscious, the tongue may relax back into the pharynx and obstruct the airway. A simple maneuver like a head tilt/chin lift or a jaw thrust (used when a cervical spine injury is suspected) will draw the tongue up out of the airway.

Airways may also become partially obstructed. Obstruction can be caused by swallowing foreign objects, tumors growing into the airway, and infections such as epiglottitis. Partial airway obstructions outside the lungs (in the trachea) manifest differently than partial airway obstructions inside the thoracic cavity. An understanding of transmural pressures makes it possible to predict which symptoms will occur in both cases. As a matter of normal physiology, negative intrathoracic pressure causes the trachea to decrease in diameter, since the pressure in the airway drops without an associated drop in the pressure outside the trachea. If there is a partial upper airway obstruction, this narrowing may hinder inspiratory flow (FIGURE 16.19). These patients exhibit

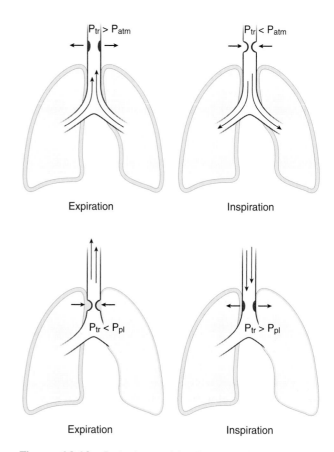

Figure 16.19 Expiration and inspiration with partial airway obstruction. The transmural pressures across the trachea inside the thoracic cavity are opposite those outside the thoracic cavity.

stridor, a prolonged high-pitched gasping sound heard during inspiration. During expiration, the positive pressure in the airway forces the airway open, and air is exhaled easily.

The opposite situation occurs when there is an intrathoracic airway obstruction. Airways within the thorax open during inspiration because of the negative intrathoracic pressure. During expiration, positive pressure pushing in on the airways will cause them to collapse, and audible expiratory wheezes will be heard. Patients with extra- or intrathoracic partial obstruction usually show evidence of respiratory distress, including increased respiratory rate and a complaint of shortness of breath.

An **open pneumothorax**, also called a sucking chest wound, occurs when there is a hole in the chest wall that connects the pleural space and the atmosphere (FIGURE 16.20). When this occurs, negative pleural pressure draws air into the pleural space. As the air rushes in, the chest wall expands slightly and the lung collapses. On each subsequent breath, air is drawn into the pleural space through the hole in the chest wall because it is the path of least resistance compared with the higher-resistance airways. A

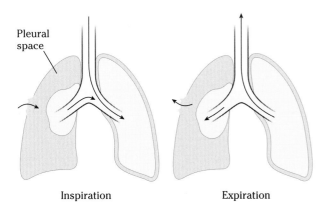

Figure 16.20 An open pneumothorax in inspiration and expiration.

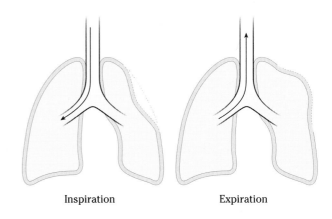

Figure 16.22 Flail chest in inspiration and expiration.

collapsed lung compromises ventilation and oxygenation. Emergency treatment consists of covering the hole in the chest wall with an occlusive dressing (air-tight and water-tight). Later the wound must be surgically closed and a chest tube placed in the pleural space to withdraw the air.

In a **tension pneumothorax**, there is a disruption in the visceral pleura, which connects the airways with the pleural space (FIGURE 16.21). During inspiration, air is drawn into the pleural space from the airways, but during expiration this air cannot escape because lung tissue surrounding the injury acts as a one-way valve. With each breath, more air is trapped in the pleural space, eventually leading to compression and collapse of the lung on that side. As the pressure continues to increase, the heart and the opposite lung are also compressed—an imminently life-threatening situation.

Signs of tension pneumothorax include decreased breath sounds on the side of the injury, massive jugular venous distention (because blood can

not return to the compressed heart), deviation of the trachea to the side opposite the injury, and severe shock. The treatment is decompression of the tension pneumothorax by inserting a chest tube through the chest wall into the pleural space and removing the air. Emergency decompression for a tension pneumothorax is also possible by putting a needle through the chest wall on the side of the pneumothorax. The needle is inserted in the second intercostal space in the mid-clavicular line.

Flail chest occurs when two or more adjacent ribs are broken in two places. This leads to a disruption in the integrity of the chest wall (FIGURE 16.22). During inspiration, the negative pressure created in the thorax will cause this disconnected section of the chest wall to be drawn inward. Likewise, the positive intrathoracic pressure during expiration will push this section of the chest wall out. Because these motions are the opposite of what normally occurs during breathing, they are termed *paradoxical chest wall motion*. The extreme pain of this condition hampers breathing.

AGING: ALTERED LUNG MECHANICS

Alterations in lung function also occur as part of the normal aging process. For reasons that are not well understood, lung compliance increases with age. This alters lung volumes and reduces outflow. The decreased lung recoil force results in decreased radial traction on the airways, leading to early airway closure and air trapping at end-expiration. The trapped air increases the FRC and RV. Because there is less room between FRC and TLC, the vital capacity is by definition lower. The decreased lung recoil and consequent decreased outflow also reduce the FEV_1. In addition, diffusing capacity and possibly chemoreceptor function (i.e., pCO_2, pO_2, or pH-sensing) decrease with age. Overall, oxygenation and exercise tolerance decline with age.

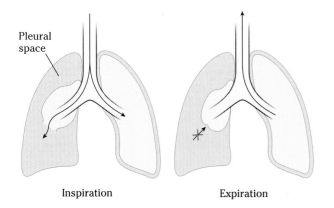

Figure 16.21 A tension pneumothorax in inspiration and expiration. The one-way valve effect leads to progressive inflation of the pleural space.

Summary

- The lungs and chest wall together function as a bellows that draws in and expels air. A potential pleural space connects the lungs to the chest wall.

$$P_{transmural} = P_{in} - P_{out}$$

$$P_{transpulmonary} = P_{alveoli} - P_{pleural\ space}$$

- The sum of transmural pressure and elastic recoil pressure determines whether a container like the lung will expand or contract.

$$P_{expansion\ or\ contraction} = P_{transmural} + P_{el}$$

- Compliance is a measure of the elastic recoil properties of a container. A high compliance means low elastic recoil pressure.

$$C = \Delta V/\Delta P$$

- The elastic recoil pressures of the lung and the chest wall are equal and opposite at functional residual capacity (pre-inspiration/end-expiration). Changes in transmural pressure, in the lung and chest wall elastic recoil pressures, and in the muscular force exerted by the chest wall shift this counter-balance toward expansion during inspiration or contraction during expiration and account for the bellows effect that is breathing.

- Surface tension gives alveoli a tendency to collapse. Surface tension accounts for a majority of the elastic recoil pressure of the lung; the rest is due to the elastic properties of lung connective tissue. The effects of surface tension are mitigated by surfactant, which is produced by type II pneumocytes.

$$P = 2T/r$$

- Airway flow is described by Ohm's law. Radius is the most important factor in determining airway resistance. Bronchial smooth muscle tone and lung volume are determinants of airway radius and hence resistance.

$$Q = \Delta P/R$$

$$Q = \Delta P\pi r^4/8\eta l$$

$$R = 8\eta l/\pi r^4$$

- Airway resistance can limit outflow velocity during forced expiration.

- The two broad categories of ventilatory defects are restrictive disease and obstructive disease. Restrictive conditions involve decreased lung volumes and are due to low respiratory compliance or muscle weakness. Obstructive conditions involve impaired outflow and increased lung volumes and are due to increased compliance or increased airway resistance.

- Pulmonary function tests help to differentiate between restrictive and obstructive ventilatory defects.

- Gross structural disruptions of the thoracic bellows—for example, airway obstruction, open pneumothorax, tension pneumothorax, or flail chest—may be life-threatening emergencies.

- Lung compliance increases with age.

Suggested Reading

Guyton AC. Measurement of the respiratory volumes of laboratory animals. Am J Physiol. 1947;147:70.

Guyton AC. Analysis of respiratory patterns in laboratory animals. Am J Physiol. 1947;147:78.

Rahn H, Otis AB, Chadwick LE, Fenn WO. The pressure-volume diagram of the thorax and lung. Am J Phys. 1946;146:161.

Thurlbeck WM, Henderson JA, Fraser RG, Bates DV. A comparison between clinical, roentgenologic, functional, and morphologic criteria in chronic bronchitis, emphysema, asthma, and bronchiectasis. Medicine. 1970;49:81.

REVIEW QUESTIONS

Directions: Each of the numbered items or incomplete statements in this section is followed by answers or by completions of the statement. Select the ONE lettered answer or completion that is BEST in each case.

1. A 68-year-old woman with pulmonary fibrosis presents with worsening exertional dyspnea. The mechanism of her pulmonary disease is consistent with which of the following pulmonary function test results?

    (A) FEV_1/FVC high, low VC, low TLC, low RV
    (B) FEV_1/FVC normal, low VC, low TLC, low RV
    (C) FEV_1/FVC normal, high VC, high TLC, high RV
    (D) FEV_1/FVC low, low VC, low TLC, low RV
    (E) FEV_1/FVC low, high VC, high TLC, high RV

2. A 3-year-old boy with dyspnea and wheezing is brought to the pediatric emergency room shortly after he swallowed a coin. His chest x-ray would be consistent with a partial airway obstruction at which of the following locations?

    (A) Alveolus
    (B) Bronchiole

(C) Larynx
(D) Oropharynx
(E) Trachea

3. A 28-year-old man presents with Guillain-Barré syndrome, an ascending polyneuropathy that may occur after a viral prodrome. He will need ventilatory assistance if his disease weakens muscles innervated by which of the following nerve root levels?

(A) C3, C4, C5
(B) C6, C7, C8
(C) T1, T2, T3
(D) T3, T4, T5
(E) L1, L2, L3

ANSWERS TO REVIEW QUESTIONS

1. **The answer is B.** Pulmonary fibrosis is a restrictive lung disease, in which decreased compliance of the respiratory system leads to decreased lung volumes. In the case of pulmonary fibrosis, this decreased compliance results from increased lung recoil force, while in a patient with neuromuscular weakness, it results from a decreased capability to expand the thoracic cavity. A patient with a restrictive lung disease will have no difficulty with the expiration of air, and consequently the FEV_1/FVC ratio should be normal. A pattern of high lung volumes and low FEV_1/FVC ratios would be more consistent with an obstructive pulmonary disease such as asthma or emphysema, with their characteristic difficulties with outflow of air.

2. **The answer is E.** Audible expiratory wheezes result from intrathoracic airway obstruction, such as in the trachea or a bronchus. The negative intrathoracic pressure of inspiration allows airways within the thorax to open, but the positive pressure against the airways during expiration will result in their collapse if an obstruction is present, resulting in a wheeze. An object the size of a coin is too large to pass through the branching bronchi to lodge in the small-diameter bronchioles. Alveoli lie distal to the bronchioles and are the sites of gas exchange. If an object were lodged in the larynx, inspiratory flow might be hindered, resulting in the high-pitched inspiratory gasps of stridor.

3. **The answer is A.** The most important muscle in the respiratory system is the diaphragm, which is innervated by the phrenic nerves from cervical roots C3, C4, C5. During inhalation, the diaphragm contracts, pulling down the floor of the thoracic cavity and allowing the lungs to expand. The accessory breathing muscles can assist the diaphragm in its work during exercise or some disease states, but none of them can fully substitute for the diaphragm. Involvement of the entire diaphragm by a disease process necessitates mechanical ventilation to help the patient breathe.

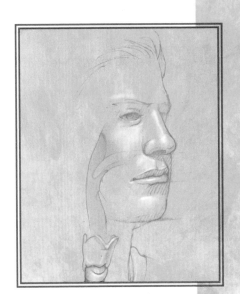

17

Gas Exchange in the Lungs

INTRODUCTION

The vital importance of breathing was clear even to the ancients who pondered the rush of air in and out of the body. *Pneuma*, in fact, was a Greek word both for breath and for spirit or soul: c. 300 B.C., Erasistratus, among other ancient Greeks, believed that the air we breathe, the *pneuma*, gives rise to the spirit. The lungs were the threshold between the world and the living being, the site of the spirit's mysterious dependence on the material world. About 500 hundred years later, Galen struggled to understand more fully the mechanisms that sustain life. He observed that for a fire to continue to burn, it required a supply of air and an outlet for the smoke it produced. He theorized that the lungs performed a similar function in sustaining the animal's "innate heat." He said, "[E]ven breathing out must be of no small use, in that it purges the smoky vapor, as it were, of the blood." The aptness of Galen's analogy is quite striking, especially given that it came so far in advance of modern chemistry. Indeed, the air's oxygen enables the release of energy that produces the light and heat of a fire and that drives the cell's work to maintain its structure and function.

If all organ systems ultimately maintain a biochemical milieu conducive to cell survival, the lungs have two essential projects in particular: (a) they provide oxygen to the cellular environment to enable energy release in oxidative phosphorylation; and (b) in conjunction with the kidneys, they help maintain the physiologically optimal pH by controlling the blood proportions of carbon dioxide, a constituent of the blood's bicarbonate buffer system and a waste product of cellular aerobic respiration. The lungs perform these tasks through passive gas exchange between the atmosphere and the blood, absorbing oxygen from air and releasing carbon dioxide into air. Breathing or ventilation—the mechanical function of the lung—makes effective gas exchange possible.

SYSTEM STRUCTURE: THE DISTAL RESPIRATORY TREE AND PULMONARY CIRCULATION

Lung structure was discussed in Chapter 16, but it is useful to review and expand upon some of this material with attention to pulmonary gas exchange. Recall that the trachea gives rise to large airways that progressively branch as they descend into the lungs, ultimately leading to the gas-exchanging tissues-the respiratory bronchioles and alveoli (FIGURE 17.1). The **large airways**, also known as the *conducting airways*, are passageways for air but do not perform gas exchange. (The air space in the lungs where no exchange occurs is called anatomic dead space.)

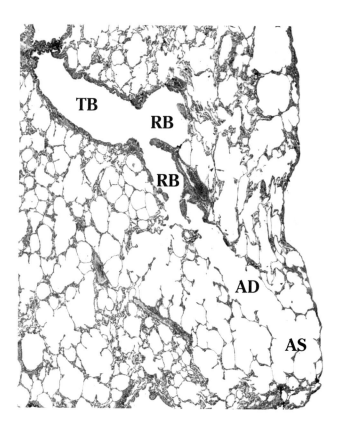

Figure 17.1   The respiratory bronchioles and alveoli. This photomicrograph shows a terminal bronchiole (TB), respiratory bronchiole (RB), an alveolar duct (AD), and an alveolar septum (AS). (×120)

The walls of the alveolar compartments, across which gas exchange occurs, are, in contrast with the large airways, only about two cells thick (FIGURE 17.2). The lumen of the alveolar pouch is lined by cells called **type I pneumocytes**, which are so flat and thin

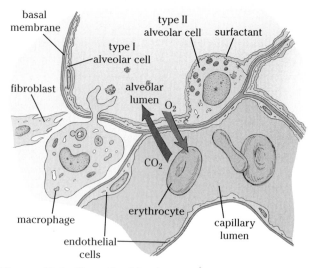

Figure 17.2   The walls of the alveoli. This drawing, adapted from an electron micrograph, shows the constituents of the alveolar wall. It also shows an erythrocyte in the capillary lumen.

as to be difficult to see even under a light microscope. The alveoli are enmeshed in an extensive plexus of capillaries, whose walls are formed by flat and thin endothelial cells. Between the type I pneumocyte and the capillary endothelial cell lies a common basement membrane of elastin and collagen.

If we were to traverse the barrier between one alveolus and another, we would first encounter a thin type I pneumocyte, then the basement membrane, then a capillary endothelial cell, then blood (this is as far as a molecule of oxygen would go before being swept away with the flow of blood), then the opposite wall of the capillary, formed by an endothelial cell, then basement membrane, then a type I pneumocyte, and finally the second alveolar space. Other cells appear intermittently in the alveolar walls but are not the main constituents of the blood/air barrier: type II pneumocytes that secrete surfactant, fibroblasts that lay down the basement membrane, macrophages, and Clara cells, which are the main secretory cell type in the distal conducting airways and are thought to play a role in defense against pollutants and in repair.

The right ventricle of the heart pumps deoxygenated blood to the pulmonary arteries, and from there to the capillaries surrounding the alveoli. From these capillaries, where gas exchange occurs, the oxygenated blood is carried into the pulmonary vein, which delivers the blood to the left ventricle of the heart for propulsion to the rest of the body. The pulmonary artery, capillaries, and pulmonary vein constitute the **pulmonary circulation.**

The lungs also contain arteries carrying oxygenated blood from the left heart, arteries that are part of the **systemic circulation** serving the rest of the body outside the lungs. One might think that the lung would need no supply of oxygenated blood. This is true in part; the alveolar tissues do not require a supply of oxygenated blood because they absorb oxygen directly from their immediate environment. The walls of the large airways, however, are too thick to rely on direct absorption of oxygen for the sustenance of all their cells. For this reason they receive oxygenated, systemic blood from the bronchial arteries, which in turn arise from the thoracic aorta or posterior intercostal arteries. The bronchial blood returns, however, by way of the pulmonary vein to the left heart and re-enters the systemic circulation. FIGURE 17.3 shows the functional units of the lung, including the two pulmonary arterial supplies.

SYSTEM FUNCTION: OXYGENATION AND THE CLEARANCE OF CARBON DIOXIDE

Our first consideration in understanding gas exchange is the behavior of gases in general. Therefore, we'll briefly review some introductory chemistry.

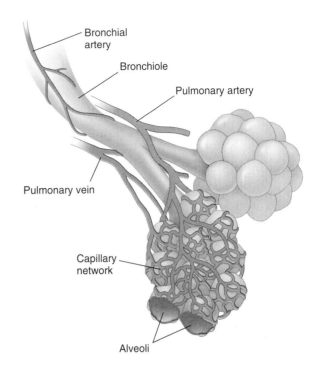

Figure 17.3 The functional units of the lung.

Gases

The relationships between the different quantitatively measurable aspects of a gas are expressed in the **ideal gas law:** PV = nRT, where P is the pressure the gas exerts, V is the volume the gas occupies, n is the number of moles of gas that are present (i.e., the number of molecules present), R is an empirically determined constant, and T is the temperature of the gas. This law applies for a gas of one molecular type or a gas composed of multiple molecular species all mixed together in the same space; our own atmosphere—air—is such a mixed gas.

In some situations, however, we might be interested in the amount of one particular molecular species in a mixed gas. How do we talk about the proportions of each gas in the total gas mixture or, in other words, about how much of each species of gas there is? One way to express the amount would be the *mol fraction* of gas 1, X_1, which is n_1/n_T, where n_1 is the moles of gas 1 and n_T is the total moles in the gas mixture. The mol fraction of oxygen is about 21% in atmospheric air. The mol fraction of carbon dioxide is negligibly small, and most of the rest of our atmosphere is nitrogen.

Another way to express the amount of one species of gas in a mixture is the **partial pressure.** The partial pressure of gas 1, P_1, is defined as the pressure gas 1 would exert if it were alone in the same space that the total mixture, gas T, occupied and at the same temperature as was gas T. The partial pressure of gas 1 is related to the total pressure of the gas mixture in proportion to the mol fraction; the more molecules of gas 1 there are bouncing around, the more gas 1 contributes pressure to the total pressure of the gas mixture. Stated mathematically, $P_1/P_T = n_1/n_T = X_1$; and $P_1 = P_T X_1$. This relation between partial pressure and mol fraction can be derived from the ideal gas law. Combine the ideal gas laws for gas T and for gas 1 in isolation:

$$P_T V_T = n_T R T_T$$

$$P_1 V_T = n_1 R T_T$$

and you get

$$P_1/P_T = n_1/n_T$$

This relationship also implies that since

$$n_T = n_1 + n_2 + n_3 + \ldots + n_n$$

therefore,

$$P_T = P_1 + P_2 + P_3 + \ldots + P_n$$

The last equation is the common form of **Dalton's law of partial pressures.**

Partial pressures are used by pulmonary physiologists to describe the quantity of a particular gas species in the gas mixture in the lungs. The term is also used to describe the quantity of a particular gas species that has dissolved into blood. Though it may seem counterintuitive to measure quantities of dissolved gas in pressures, we can better understand this convention by considering the following scenario.

Imagine a free gas collected over a liquid, as is the case in the alveolus, where air is collected over blood (FIGURE 17.4). The molecules in the free gas dissolve into the fluid through the chaotic motion of the gas molecules. Each individual molecular gas species in the total mixture dissolves into the fluid in proportion to the quantity in the free gas mixture. The greater the quantity (partial pressure) of gas 1 in the free gas mixture, the more molecules of gas 1 will dissolve into the fluid (see Figure 17.4A). Net dissolution of gas 1 into fluid goes on until an equilibrium of influx and efflux across the gas/fluid divide is reached (see Figure 17.4B).

Recall from basic chemistry how such an equilibrium occurs. Molecules continue to diffuse into the fluid until there are enough molecules in the fluid that some molecules randomly escape back out, and the process continues. As the number of dissolved molecules grows, the number of molecules going back out of the fluid grows and the net influx of molecules into fluid drops off. Finally, when there are enough molecules on both sides of the gas/fluid divide to drive molecular crossover at an equal rate in both directions, we have reached equilibrium.

A high P_1 in the free gas at equilibrium means there must be a large quantity of gas 1 dissolved in the fluid, countering the high influx of gas 1 from free gas with a high efflux from fluid. Accordingly, a low P_1 in the free gas at equilibrium means a small amount of 1 is being driven into fluid, and since the amount going in equals the amount going out, the amount going out of the liquid must be equally small. Therefore, a low P_1 in the free gas at equilibrium means that there is little of gas 1 in solution to drive efflux.

The quantity of gas 1 in the fluid is directly reflected by the equilibrium P_1 in the free gas mixture. That is why scientists can use the equilibrium P_1 as an index of the amount of gas 1 dissolved in a fluid. They say the quantity of gas 1 dissolved in a fluid accompanies an equilibrium vapor pressure P_1, and the equilibrium P_1 is the label for the amount of gas 1 dissolved in the fluid.

When pulmonary physiologists talk about the partial pressure of gas dissolved in blood, they use this concept of **equilibrium vapor pressure.** The PO_2 or PCO_2 of blood is defined as the **equilibrium partial pressure** of PO_2 or PCO_2 in gas collected over the blood in a chamber called a *tonometer*. In the hospi-

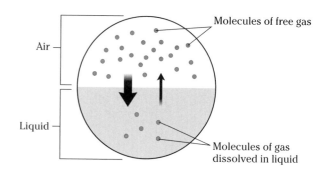

(A) Before equilibrium is achieved

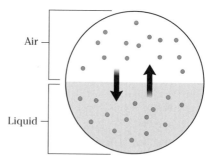

(B) At equilibrium

Figure 17.4 Equilibrium vapor pressure. **A.** The large amount of free gas and small amount of dissolved gas means more molecules randomly move into solution than come out. The amount of dissolved gas increases, which in turn increases the number of molecules coming out of solution. **B.** The amount of free gas depletes and the amount of dissolved gas increases until the rates of gas-liquid crossover become the same in both directions.

tal, when arterial (or sometimes venous) blood is submitted to *arterial blood gas (ABG)* testing, a tonometer in fact serves as a reference to produce a result in terms of partial pressure. Thus, an ABG measurement of PO_2 40 mm Hg in venous blood (P_vO_2) means that this blood has the same quantity of oxygen as blood in equilibrium with free air at PO_2 40 mm Hg in a tonometer. (See Clinical Application Box *How Blood Gas Analyzers Work*.)

By using this convention to describe the amount of blood gas, we can readily predict the direction of change of blood oxygen content when systemic venous blood (the same as pulmonary arterial blood), for example, is exposed to alveolar air. Since the venous blood would be at equilibrium exposed to air at 40 mm Hg PO_2, a higher alveolar PO_2 (P_AO_2) will drive more oxygen into solution until a new equilibrium is reached, with the blood and the alveolar air at the same PO_2. The equilibrium PO_2 is higher than blood's initial PO_2 and lower than alveolar air's initial PO_2 (FIGURE 17.5). For a list of some physiologically significant partial pressures, see TABLE 17.1.

Ventilation

While one is not breathing-in between breaths or while holding one's breath-the composition of the inspired air in the gas-exchanging portion of the lung, in the **alveolar gas**, will change. Since the peripheral tissues are continuously absorbing O_2 from the systemic blood and producing CO_2 into it, the blood returning to the lung from the body tissues is O_2-poor and CO_2-rich. In between breaths in the pulmonary capillaries, the O_2-poor and CO_2-rich blood continuously absorbs O_2 from the alveolar gas and deposits CO_2 into it. Therefore, O_2 levels in alveolar gas are continuously going down while CO_2 levels are going up. Simple diffusion accounts for this flow of molecules into and out of the body's cells in the periphery and across the lung membranes. Ventilation, or breathing, is an effort to keep alveolar gas high in O_2 and low in CO_2 by blowing off gas low in O_2 and high in CO_2 and replacing it with atmospheric gas, which has the opposite proportions. This maintains the alveolar gas to blood gas gradients necessary to promote continued clearance of CO_2 and absorption of O_2.

Before one inhales, the lung volume is sitting at a level called **functional residual capacity (FRC)**, as described in Chapter 16. The alveolar part of this initial lung volume is filled with low-O_2 and high-CO_2 gas-Galen's "smoky vapor." On inspiration, one adds a new volume, the tidal volume (V_T), to the pre-existing volume at FRC. As shown in FIGURE 17.6, two thirds of the tidal volume is added to the expanded alveoli; this added volume is called V_A. One third of the tidal volume is added to the expanded dead space; this added volume is called V_D.

$$V_A + V_D = V_T$$

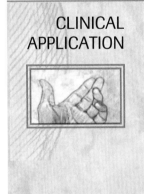

CLINICAL APPLICATION

HOW BLOOD GAS ANALYZERS WORK

The sensors in blood gas analyzers yield readings in partial pressure, but they do not measure partial pressure directly. When a blood sample (drawn by syringe, frequently from the radial artery) undergoes ABG testing, the analyzer takes a reading in millivolts. The millivolt reading comes from exposure of the sample to O_2, CO_2, and pH-sensitive electrodes that are covered with a gas-permeable membrane. The electrodes read a number of millivolts in proportion to the quantity of O_2 or CO_2 in solution. Finally, the millivolt reading must be converted to an equilibrium partial pressure using reference measurements from a tonometer.

These reference measurements derive from electrode sampling of blood from a tonometer with a known equilibrium partial pressure of O_2 or CO_2. By directing a constant flow of air whose partial pressure of O_2 or CO_2 is known into the air chamber of a tonometer, and allowing the air chamber to equilibrate with blood in the tonometer, one can establish with certainty the equilibrium partial pressure of the gas in that blood sample. A millivolt reading of blood O_2 by electrode at known tonometer PO_2 makes possible a correlation between millivolts and partial pressure. This correlation is the basis for a linear conversion from millivolts to equilibrium partial pressure in the analysis of a patient's blood sample.

The Clinical Laboratory Improvement Act of 1967, and more importantly the Clinical Laboratory Improvement Amendments of 1988 (CLIA 88), ensure that all clinical laboratories in the United States adhere to quality standards. According to CLIA 88, blood gas analyzers should be recalibrated to freshly tonometered blood samples every personnel shift.

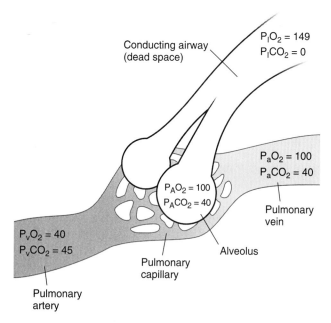

Figure 17.5 Equilibration of partial pressures between the alveolus and the blood. The partial pressures shown in the alveolus are those after inspired air has mixed with the "smoky vapor" and after this mixture has equilibrated with blood.

The added tidal volume mixes with the pre-existing FRC volume of gas. So, the added V_A will mix with the pre-existing alveolar volume of gas, filled with smoky vapor. In the new volume, composed of fresh air mixed with smoky vapor, the mol fraction and partial pressure of O_2 are higher than they were in the smoky vapor but lower than they were in fresh inspired air. Likewise, the mol fraction and partial pressure of CO_2 are lower than they were in

smoky vapor but higher than they were in fresh inspired air (where the PCO_2 is just about nil). Expiration blows off the same tidal volume and the same V_A with its new "smokier" composition and leaves the initial volume of alveolar gas at FRC with its new "less smoky" composition. Now there is a better gradient for O_2 absorption and CO_2 clearance (FIGURE 17.7).

The more time there is between breaths, the more time the alveolar gas at FRC will have to accumulate CO_2 and lose O_2. So at the end of a longer interval of not breathing, when a breath is finally drawn in and blown out, the mixed air left in the alveoli will be smokier. Taking shallow breaths at a normal rate (with CO_2 production held constant) would also likely result in smokier alveolar gas. This is because both infrequent breaths and normal-frequency small breaths add a smaller net V_A of inspired air to the alveolar gas over time. Breathing faster with CO_2 production held constant will allow less time for CO_2 to accumulate and O_2 to deplete in the alveolar gas at FRC, so the mixing will result in less smoky alveolar gas. Deep breaths at a normal rate will also likely result in less smoky alveolar gas. Deeper breaths add a larger-than-normal amount of inspired air over time.

Stated another way, the smaller the inspired V_A of fresh air over time, the larger the proportion of CO_2 in the resulting alveolar mixture and the smaller the proportion of O_2 in the mixture. The opposite holds for a large V_A. V_A and the amount of alveolar CO_2 (P_ACO_2) have an inverse relationship, while V_A and the amount of alveolar O_2 (P_AO_2) have a direct relationship. Thus, the partial pressures of O_2 and CO_2 in alveolar gas are a function of the net size of V_A's

Table 17.1   IMPORTANT PARTIAL PRESSURES (TYPICAL VALUES)

Partial Pressure	Symbol	Normal Value (mm Hg)
Alveolar partial pressure of oxygen	P_AO_2	100–105
Alveolar partial pressure of carbon dioxide	P_ACO_2	40
Arterial partial pressure of oxygen = PO_2 in pulmonary vein	P_aO_2	95–100
Arterial partial pressure of carbon dioxide = PCO_2 in pulmonary vein	P_aCO_2	40
Inspired partial pressure of oxygen	P_IO_2	149
Inspired partial pressure of carbon dioxide	P_ICO_2	0.3 (negligible)
Venous partial pressure of oxygen = PO_2 in pulmonary artery	P_vO_2	40
Venous partial pressure of carbon dioxide = PO_2 in pulmonary artery	P_vCO_2	45

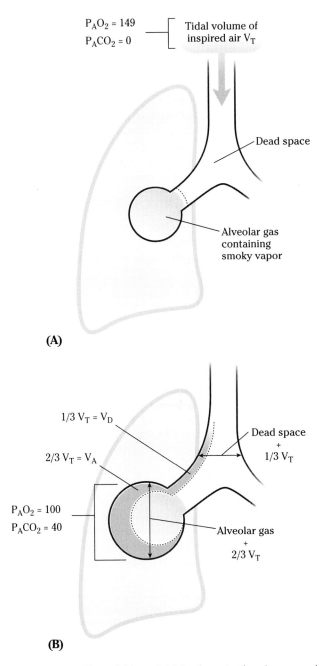

(A)

(B)

Figure 17.6 The addition of tidal volume to the airways and alveoli. Two thirds of the tidal volume is added to the gas exchanging alveolar space and one third to the dead space. For simplicity, the alveolar space is represented by one large schematic alveolus in one lung. **A.** At FRC: before the addition of a tidal volume V_T. **B.** At FRC + V_T: after the addition of a tidal volume V_T.

addition to alveolar gas per unit time, $\dot{V}_A$, which is the size of V_A multiplied by the frequency of $\dot{V}_A$'s addition to alveolar gas. In other words,

$$\dot{V}_A = V_A f$$

where V_A = the portion of the tidal volume added to alveolar gas, f = the frequency of breathing in breaths per minute, and $\dot{V}_A$ is the **alveolar ventilation.**

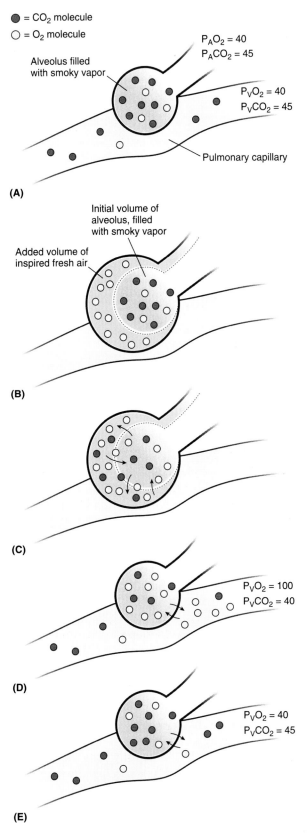

(A)

(B)

(C)

(D)

(E)

Figure 17.7 Gas exchange throughout the breathing cycle. **A.** At FRC, pre-inspiration, the alveolus filled with smoky vapor. **B.** At FRC + V_T, after inspiration, the added volume of inspired fresh air. **C.** At FRC + V_T, smoky vapor mixing with inspired fresh air. **D.** Back to FRC, after expiration. **E.** At FRC, after gas exchange has again created smoky vapor.

From the above relationships come the definitions of hyperventilation and hypoventilation. **Hyperventilation** refers to the situation where the elimination of CO_2 exceeds its rate of production, leading to a decreased pCO_2 in the blood (hypocapnia). An increased breathing frequency is known as *tachypnea*, and is not synonymous with hyperventilation. **Hypoventilation**, similarly, is not simply a decreased rate of breathing but a decrease in alveolar ventilation relative to CO_2 production. When the elimination of CO_2 is less than its production rate, the consequence is an increased arterial pCO_2 (hypercapnia).

The Alveolar Ventilation Equation The relationship between alveolar ventilation and P_ACO_2, described above, can be stated mathematically in the **alveolar ventilation equation**:

$$\dot{V}_A = (\dot{V}CO_2/P_ACO_2)(K)$$

where $\dot{V}CO_2$ is the rate of CO_2 production and K is a constant that includes conversion from standard to body temperature.

$\dot{V}CO_2$ represents the mass of CO_2 being constantly produced out of the blood in accordance with the cells' constant production into the blood. Unless the metabolic rate in the tissues changes, $\dot{V}CO_2$ remains constant. As $\dot{V}_A$ goes up and dilutes this constant amount of CO_2 production in the alveolar gas, the alveolar partial pressure of CO_2 (the P_ACO_2) goes down-an inverse relationship discussed above. $\dot{V}CO_2$ does not reflect some anatomic volume in the lungs; rather it is the volume per time that would be occupied by the mass of CO_2 produced if this CO_2 were at standard temperature and pressure in dry air (STPD).

One might at first think that the same sort of equation could be written for the relationship between $\dot{V}_A$ and P_AO_2, but it cannot. Whereas the relationship between $\dot{V}_A$ and P_ACO_2 is linear, the relationship between $\dot{V}_A$ and P_AO_2 is somewhat different. While increased $\dot{V}_A$ will increase P_AO_2, it does not do so in a linear relationship because unlike CO_2, there is a significant amount of O_2 in the inspired air.

Diffusion

The average distance between blood and alveolar air in the lung is less than 1.5 μm, making rapid diffusion possible. In the healthy lung, blood equilibrates with respect to O_2 and CO_2 after traveling about a third of the length of the pulmonary capillary. The equation that describes the determining factors for diffusion rate is **Fick's law**:

$$\dot{V}_G = (P_A - P_C)(A)(S)/(T)(\text{square root of MW})$$

where $\dot{V}_G$ = volume of gas transferred across membrane per unit time, P_A = partial pressure of the gas in the alveolus, P_C = partial pressure of the gas in the capillary, A = area of membrane of transfer, S = solubility of the gas in blood, T = thickness of membrane, and MW = molecular weight of the gas.

Because of the rapid diffusion rates of O_2 and CO_2, diffusion time creates no limit to the amount of O_2 and CO_2 exchange that may occur. If more CO_2 is delivered to the alveolar capillary per time or more O_2 is delivered to the alveolar air per time, the rate of diffusion will not stand in the way of increased exchange of O_2 and CO_2. The amount of blood flow to the alveoli, however, does set a limit to how much exchange of O_2 and CO_2 can occur. No matter how fast the diffusion time, if less blood is delivered per time to the alveolar capillary, less CO_2 will cross over into alveolar air and less O_2 will cross over into blood. Therefore, O_2 and CO_2 exchange is called **perfusion-limited gas exchange** in healthy lung tissue.

The exchange of other more slowly diffusing molecules, like CO, is known as **diffusion-limited gas exchange.** In the case of diffusion-limited molecules, blood might travel the whole length of the capillary before equilibrating (as opposed to equilibrating after one-third the length of the capillary, as do O_2 and CO_2), so a higher rate of blood flow would not increase the amount of gas exchanged. In fact, an increased rate of blood flow would decrease the amount of gas exchanged, as the blood would spend less time in the capillary before being swept downstream.

In perfusion-limited gas exchange, where the blood equilibrates with the air at the beginning of the capillary, the blood is "wasting its time" for the rest of its trip along the air-exposed capillary, with no more gas exchange occurring. Increasing the perfusion rate would expose new blood that could undergo gas exchange. The fact that O_2 exchange is perfusion-limited means increases in heart rate will increase oxygenation. Thickening of the exchange membranes in disease, such as pulmonary edema or fibrosis, can slow O_2 diffusion and make the exchange diffusion-limited, thereby compromising exercise tolerance.

Alveolar and Arterial Partial Pressures The rapidity with which alveolar gas equilibrates with blood has a fundamental implication for pulmonary physiology: the partial pressures of O_2 and CO_2 in the alveolus exactly match the partial pressures of O_2 and CO_2 in the blood leaving the alveolus. Recall that the partial pressure of a gas dissolved in a liquid is an equilibrium vapor pressure, meaning that the gas is dissolved to the same extent it would be if it were in equilibrium with a free gas at that partial pressure. Since gas exchange quickly reaches equilibrium, O_2 and CO_2's partial pressure in the blood leaving the alveolus must by definition equal the alveolar partial pressure of O_2 and CO_2. As shown in Table 17.1, the partial pressure of O_2 and CO_2 in the blood leaving the alveolus, heading for the pulmonary vein and then the systemic arteries, is written P_aO_2 and P_aCO_2, while the partial pressure of O_2 and CO_2 in the alveolus is written P_AO_2 and P_ACO_2. After rapid equilibration, $P_AO_2 = P_aO_2$ and $P_ACO_2 = P_aCO_2$. If all alveolar partial pressures of O_2 and CO_2 were the same in every alveolus, the arterial partial pressure would match that one number. However, as the following discussion will show, the alveolar partial pressures are not perfectly uniform across the entire lung.

Ventilation-Perfusion Relationships: $\dot{V}_A/\dot{Q}$ Mismatch

In the normal lung and in disease states, the alveolar ventilation $\dot{V}_A$ varies in different parts of the lung. In addition, the blood flow $\dot{Q}$ varies from one part of the lung to another. Consequently, some parts of the lung may have a higher **ventilation-perfusion ($\dot{V}_A/\dot{Q}$) ratio** and some a lower ratio. Imbalances in these ratios are called **$\dot{V}/\dot{Q}$ mismatches.**

Varying the regional $\dot{V}_A$ with respect to blood flow introduces regional variations in the alveolar partial pressures of O_2 and CO_2. Increasing the regional $\dot{V}_A$ is the same thing as creating regional hyperventilation, and has the same effects: an increase in the regional P_AO_2 and P_aO_2, and a decrease in regional P_ACO_2 and P_aCO_2. Decreasing the regional $\dot{V}_A$ is the same thing as creating regional hypoventilation, and has the same effects: a decrease in the regional P_AO_2 and P_aO_2, and an increase in regional P_ACO_2 and P_aCO_2.

Varying the regional $\dot{Q}$ with respect to alveolar minute ventilation also introduces regional variations in the alveolar partial pressures of O_2 and CO_2. Decreasing regional $\dot{Q}$ with respect to $\dot{V}_A$ has the same effect as increasing regional $\dot{V}_A$. With less blood flow there would be less net delivery of CO_2 to the alveoli (hence less dirtying of the alveolar air) and less net absorption of O_2 (hence less O_2 extraction from alveolar air). The P_AO_2 would be higher and the P_ACO_2 would be lower. The incoming blood would equilibrate with this higher P_AO_2 and lower P_ACO_2 and hence would have a higher regional P_aO_2 and a lower regional P_aCO_2. The alveolar ventilation equation predicts this. With a lower $\dot{V}CO_2$ in the alveolar ventilation equation and the same $\dot{V}_A$, P_ACO_2 would be lower and hence local P_aCO_2 would be lower as well. Meanwhile, in accordance with all the same principles, increasing regional $\dot{Q}$ with respect to $\dot{V}_A$ has the same effect as decreasing regional $\dot{V}_A$.

In summary: Given the effect of changes in $\dot{V}_A$ and $\dot{Q}$ described above, it is the $\dot{V}_A/\dot{Q}$ ratio that determines regional partial pressures. High $\dot{V}_A/\dot{Q}$ increases partial pressures of O_2 but decreases partial pressures of CO_2, and low $\dot{V}_A/\dot{Q}$ decreases partial pressures of O_2 but increases partial pressures of CO_2 (FIGURE 17.8).

The extreme $\dot{V}_A/\dot{Q}$ mismatches have special names. When $\dot{V}_A$ is zero and hence $\dot{V}_A/\dot{Q} = 0$, it is called a **shunt.** When $\dot{Q}$ is zero and hence $\dot{V}_A/\dot{Q} = \infty$, it is called **dead space.** The large airways are sites of dead space ventilation, since their surfaces are exposed to air with no blood supply for gas exchange; and they are also sites of shunt, since the bronchial arteries perfuse the deeper unventilated tissues of the large airways. Collapse of the alveoli in a part of the lung (*atelectasis*) creates shunt; so does filling of the alveoli in a part of the lung with inflammatory cells and exudate (*consolidation*), as happens in pneumonia.

Because $\dot{V}_A/\dot{Q}$ mismatches are regional, what effect do they have on the overall P_aO_2 and P_aCO_2- that is, on the pooled blood leaving the lungs in the pulmonary vein? Shunt or low $\dot{V}_A/\dot{Q}$ causes lower P_aO_2 and higher P_aCO_2 blood from these mismatched regions to mix with a larger amount of better-ventilated blood in the pulmonary vein. This drops the systemic P_aO_2 to some extent, but not significantly (in the healthy lung), and raises the systemic P_aCO_2 to some extent. Dead space makes no contribution per se to blood gas composition because by definition no blood ever sees this part of the lung. When higher P_aO_2 and lower P_aCO_2 blood from high $\dot{V}_A/\dot{Q}$ areas mixes with all the blood in the pulmonary vein, it will lower the P_aCO_2 some, but will not raise the P_aO_2 to any significant extent, as one might think it would.

The nature of the **oxyhemoglobin dissociation curve** (FIGURE 17.9) accounts for the way that regional changes affect overall values (see Chapter 18). The dissolved O_2 and CO_2 are not the only pools of O_2 and CO_2 in the blood. These gases are also bound to the protein hemoglobin, and high blood PO_2 or PCO_2 will drive more of these gases into association with hemoglobin. The vast majority of the total blood O_2 content is accounted for not by the dissolved O_2, measured in partial pressure, but in hemoglobin-associated O_2.

For a clearer picture of blood oxygen content, imagine that blood were a building with a small foyer and a large interior, and O_2 molecules were people

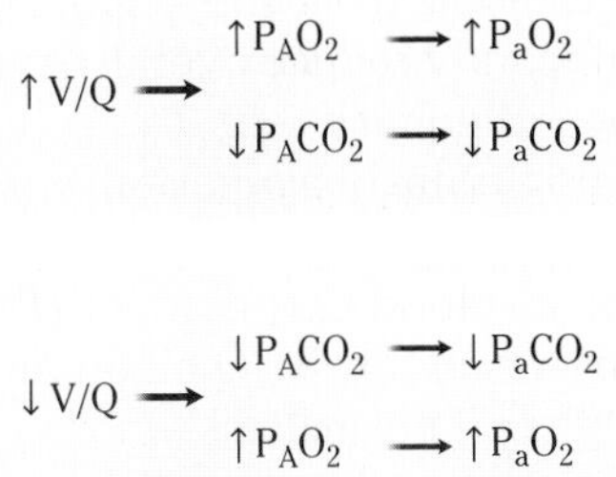

$$\uparrow V/Q \rightarrow \begin{array}{c} \uparrow P_AO_2 \rightarrow \uparrow P_aO_2 \\ \downarrow P_ACO_2 \rightarrow \downarrow P_aCO_2 \end{array}$$

$$\downarrow V/Q \rightarrow \begin{array}{c} \downarrow P_ACO_2 \rightarrow \downarrow P_aCO_2 \\ \uparrow P_AO_2 \rightarrow \uparrow P_aO_2 \end{array}$$

Figure 17.8 The effect of the $\dot{V}_A/\dot{Q}$ ratio on the partial pressures of O_2 and CO_2.

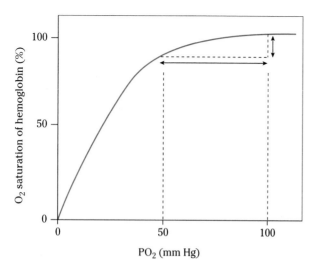

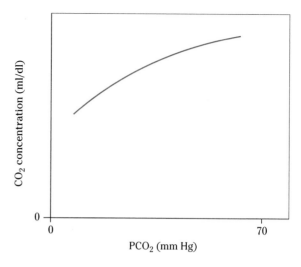

Figure 17.9 The oxyhemoglobin dissociation curve. A significant increase in PO_2 yields a much less significant increase in total O_2 content.

Figure 17.10 The CO_2 dissociation curve.

crowding into the building. At high P_AO_2, O_2 would pass through the foyer as dissolved O_2 and crowd into the large interior as hemoglobin-associated molecules until the interior were full, at which time the door to the interior would be sealed shut. With continued high P_AO_2, the O_2 would crowd into the foyer as high P_AO_2-dissolved O_2-but could not get into the interior. So, while the foyer would get more and more tightly packed, the overall number of people in the building would not be affected significantly.

In other words, at P_aO_2 values >50 mmHg (where hemoglobin is already nearly saturated with oxygen), increases in P_aO_2 do not produce significantly increased hemoglobin association and hence do not significantly elevate the total O_2 content. Therefore, the high P_aO_2 blood from the high $\dot{V}_A/\dot{Q}$ areas contributes little total O_2 content to the blood of the pulmonary vein and does not raise the overall P_aO_2 significantly.

On the other hand, at P_aO_2 values <50 mmHg (where hemoglobin is not near saturation), decreases in P_aO_2 do significantly reduce total oxygen content. Consequently, when blood from low $\dot{V}_A/\dot{Q}$ areas mixes with an equal amount of blood from high $\dot{V}_A/\dot{Q}$ areas, the blood from the regionally low $\dot{V}_A/\dot{Q}$ area does significantly reduce overall oxygen content and P_aO_2 in the pulmonary vein.

CO_2's hemoglobin dissociation curve is more linear; variations in P_aCO_2 are truer reflections of variations in total blood CO_2 content (FIGURE 17.10). For this reason, when low $\dot{V}_A/\dot{Q}$ blood and high $\dot{V}_A/\dot{Q}$ blood mix, the P_aCO_2 normalizes.

In summary: Low $\dot{V}_A/\dot{Q}$ lowers P_aO_2 and high $\dot{V}_A/\dot{Q}$ has a negligible effect on P_aO_2; high $\dot{V}_A/\dot{Q}$ can compensate for low $\dot{V}_A/\dot{Q}$ in the case of P_aCO_2 but not in the case of P_aO_2 (FIGURE 17.11).

The Alveolar Gas Equation   Low P_aO_2 is an important clinical sign. When a physician detects a low P_aO_2, he or she wants to know whether it has been caused by low $\dot{V}_A/\dot{Q}$ or by other pathologic means. The answer to this question is useful in the differential diagnosis because certain disease states lower P_aO_2 by low $\dot{V}_A/\dot{Q}$, while other disease states lower P_aO_2 by different means. The **alveolar gas equation**, or *alveolar air equation*, can be used by a physician at the bedside to determine whether a patient's low P_aO_2 is due to low $\dot{V}_A/\dot{Q}$. The alveolar gas equation provides this information by enabling physicians to calculate P_AO_2. Because average P_AO_2 is sometimes higher than P_aO_2 owing to low $\dot{V}_A/\dot{Q}$, as described above, we can compare our P_AO_2 value from the alveolar gas equation with measured P_aO_2. If there is a difference, which we term an **A-a gradient**, we know that low $\dot{V}_A/\dot{Q}$ exists.

The alveolar gas equation looks like this:

$$P_AO_2 = P_IO_2 - (P_ACO_2/R) + F$$

where P_IO_2 is the partial pressure of O_2 in inspired air, R is the respiratory exchange ratio equal to 0.8, and F is a correction factor that can be discounted

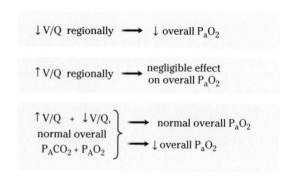

Figure 17.11 The effect of the $\dot{V}_A/\dot{Q}$ ratio on the overall partial pressures of O_2 and CO_2. Even if the overall P_AO_2 is normal, low $\dot{V}_A/\dot{Q}$ can decrease overall P_AO_2, creating an A-a gradient.

at an F_IO_2, or O_2 mol fraction, <50%, such as the atmospheric F_IO_2 of 21%. P_IO_2 is calculated for water-saturated air. PO_2 for dry air is (21%) (atmospheric pressure or 760 mm Hg) = 159 mm Hg. At normal body temperature of 37 degrees C, water vapor pressure at saturation is 47 mm Hg; PO_2 for air saturated with water vapor, as it is in the lung airways, is (21%) (760 − 47 mm Hg) = 149 mmHg. An R value of 0.8 means that 8 molecules of CO_2 are produced for every 10 molecules of O_2 consumed; that is, it is the ratio of the amount of CO_2 produced out of blood into alveolar air per amount of O_2 extracted from the alveolar air: $\dot{V}CO_2/\dot{V}O_2$. Another way to put this is that 1.2 mol of O_2 are extracted for every 1 mol of CO_2 produced.

What does the alveolar gas equation mean? Imagine a theoretical "first breath" that filled the entire space of the lungs with atmospheric air at P_IO_2 of 149 mm Hg. Now the alveolar gas is depleting in O_2 content and accumulating CO_2 content. According to R, we know that alveolar gas loses 1.2, or 1/0.8, mol O_2 for every 1 mol CO_2 produced. So we know that the amount that P_AO_2 has dropped from its initial P_IO_2 of 149 mm Hg is equal to the amount that P_ACO_2 has increased from its P_ICO_2 of 0 mm Hg multiplied by 1.2 mol of O_2 decrease per mol of CO_2 increase. Restated:

$$\Delta P_AO_2 = (\Delta P_ACO_2)(1.2 \text{ mol } O_2 \text{ consumed}/ \text{ mol } CO_2 \text{ produced})$$

or

$$P_IO_2[\text{initial } P_AO_2] - P_AO_2[P_AO_2 \text{ after exchange}]$$
$$= (P_ACO_2[P_ACO_2 \text{ after exchange}] - P_ICO_2$$
$$[\text{initial } P_ACO_2]) (1.2); \text{ with } P_ICO_2 = \text{ to } 0 \text{ mm Hg}$$

so

$$P_AO_2 = P_IO_2 - P_ACO_2 (1.2)$$

and

$$P_AO_2 = P_IO_2 - P_ACO_2/0.8$$

With P_ACO_2 we can now calculate P_AO_2. Because P_aCO_2 is not particularly sensitive to $\dot{V}_A/\dot{Q}$ mismatch, the average P_ACO_2 is considered always to be equal to P_aCO_2. Therefore, with an ABG test that gives us P_aO_2 and P_aCO_2, and with P_IO_2 known to be 149 mm Hg, we can calculate P_AO_2 and compare it to P_aO_2 to obtain our A-a gradient. (See Clinical Application Box $\dot{V}_A/\dot{Q}$ Mismatch and A-a Gradient as Synonyms on the Ward.)

The Physiologic A-a Gradient Even under normal physiologic conditions, there is a small A-a gradient of 5 or 10 mmHg. Several normal anatomic features that create shunts or low $\dot{V}_A/\dot{Q}$ account for this:

1. Some areas of high and low $\dot{V}_A/\dot{Q}$, which together result in decreased P_aO_2, are normally present in the lung. Following the lung from apex to base, blood flow increases and ventilation also increases. However, blood flow increases out of proportion to the increase in ventilation, resulting in lower $\dot{V}_A/\dot{Q}$ at the base and higher $\dot{V}_A/\dot{Q}$ at the apex. In other words, the gradient of increase of ventilation from the apex to the base of the lung is less than the gradient of increase of blood flow to the lung from the apex to the base. These regional differences in ventilation and blood flow in the healthy lung are in part determined by gravity. The *dependent* area of the lung (i.e., the inferior area or lung base) bears the weight of the lung tissues above it. This weight compresses the pleural space, making pleural pressure at the lung base less negative; this in turn reduces the transpulmonary pressure at the lung base. Recall that transpulmonary pressure is what causes the lung to open; lower transpulmonary pressures should mean reduced opening of the lung and a smaller alveolar ventilation volume per breath. However, compliance of the lung is greater at the lung base at FRC. Hence, alveolar ventilation at this level will in fact be greater than at the apex of the lungs. Gravity also causes blood to flow downhill to the lung base. Because the pulmonary vessels' smooth muscle tone is much lower than in the systemic vessels, the vessels accommodate this downhill flow in a way that systemic vessels would not. Pulmonary vessels in the dependent lung are more distended than those at the lung apex (FIGURE 17.12).

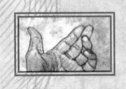

CLINICAL APPLICATION

$\dot{V}_A/\dot{Q}$ MISMATCH AND A-A GRADIENT AS SYNONYMS ON THE WARD

Any amount of low $\dot{V}_A/\dot{Q}$ in the lung means an A-a gradient is present. Since high $\dot{V}_A/\dot{Q}$ is not as important clinically, clinicians use the term $\dot{V}_A/\dot{Q}$ mismatch almost exclusively to mean low $\dot{V}_A/\dot{Q}$. When you hear low $\dot{V}_A/\dot{Q}$ or $\dot{V}_A/\dot{Q}$ mismatch, think A-a gradient.

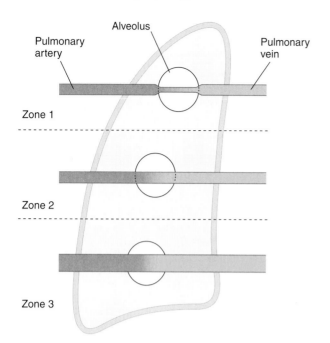

Figure 17.12 One cause of normal $\dot{V}_A/\dot{Q}$ mismatch: the distribution of ventilation and blood flow across the lung. Ventilation is higher at the apex of the lung, blood flow higher at the base. Gravity draws more blood flow to the bottom of the lung, and the weight of the superior lung tissue compresses the inferior lung tissue slightly, shrinking the alveolar spaces.

2. The bronchial arteries supply non–gas-exchanging tissues in the lung with oxygenated blood from the left heart. This blood then returns the left heart via the pulmonary vein, dumping its deoxygenated blood into the systemic arterial system without having first been ventilated. This constitutes an anatomic shunt-blood flowing through the lung returning to the left heart unventilated and deoxygenated.

3. The *thebesian veins* also create an anatomic shunt. They return used, deoxygenated blood from the coronary arteries directly into the left ventricle.

Pulmonary Blood Flow

It is well known that the pulmonary arteries carry deoxygenated blood and the systemic arteries carry oxygenated blood. The lung vessels represent a loop from right heart ventricle to left heart atrium, and the systemic vessels a loop from left heart ventricle to right heart atrium. There are, however, two other major differences between pulmonary arteries and systemic ones: blood pressure and the regulation of blood flow.

Pulmonary Blood Pressure   The pulmonary arterial blood pressure is much lower than the systemic

blood pressure. To understand why this must be so, consider the Starling forces at work on the pulmonary blood vessel (see Chapter 12). The pulmonary capillaries run very close to the outside atmosphere, and therefore the pressure surrounding the pulmonary capillaries is much lower than the pressure surrounding the systemic capillaries. Consequently, the pulmonary arterial system maintains a lower pressure than systemic blood pressure. If the pressure in the pulmonary capillaries were the same as the pressure inside systemic capillaries, there would be a large hydrostatic pressure gradient for fluid extravasation across the pulmonary capillary walls. The fluid would flow into the thin lung interstitium and then out into the alveolar spaces, covering the gas-exchanging surfaces. By keeping the pressure inside capillaries very low, the body avoids this large pressure gradient under normal circumstances (FIGURE 17.13). The body keeps pulmonary arterial pressure low by maintaining low muscle tone in the smooth muscles of the pulmonary arteries and with other structural differences from the systemic arterial vascular bed.

When cardiac output rises, as in exercise, and blood flow to the lung increases, the lung avoids high intravascular pressure by the process of **recruitment and distention.** Small, low-pressure pulmonary vessels that remain closed most of the time passively open during high blood flow. These recruited vessels increase the pulmonary vascular volume to accom-

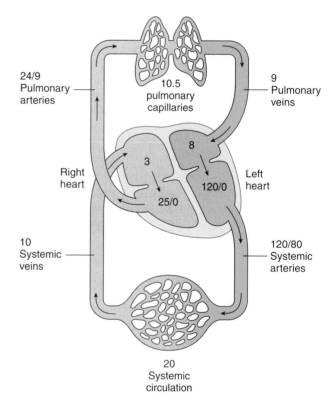

Figure 17.13 Blood pressures in the pulmonary circulation.

modate the increased blood volume, thereby keeping the pressure down. (The increased vascular area means a decrease in pulmonary vascular resistance, and in accordance with Ohm's law, $\Delta P = Q \times R$, less resistance at a given flow means less pressure.) When the pulmonary intravascular pressure rises owing to increased pulmonary venous pressure, however (as happens in *congestive heart failure*), recruitment and distention do not occur and fluid weeps easily from the lung membranes into the low-pressure alveolar spaces-*pulmonary edema*. Because there is more blood flow to the dependent lung, the pulmonary edema tends to collect at the lung bases.

The Regulation of Pulmonary Blood Flow The regulation of pulmonary blood flow is also much different from the regulation of systemic blood flow. Whereas hormones and the autonomic nerves predominantly govern the systemic arteries' tone, locally acting non-neurohumoral factors alone govern pulmonary vascular tone. The main factor is the P_AO_2. Low P_AO_2 causes constriction in the pulmonary arterioles neighboring those alveoli. This makes teleologic sense given the anatomy of the lung. A small pulmonary artery is surrounded by the alveoli it supplies. Under this anatomic set-up, the lung automatically reduces the blood flow to any alveoli that are not well ventilated and hence have a low P_AO_2. This regulatory process, known as **pulmonary hypoxic vasoconstriction**, combats $\dot{V}_A/\dot{Q}$ mismatching. (*Hypoxia* means low PO_2.)

In hypoxia that affects all alveoli uniformly-that is, global hypoxia, which takes place in hypoventilation or at high altitude-global hypoxic vasoconstriction ensues. This increase in vascular resistance across all pulmonary vascular beds results in pulmonary hypertension. Chronic pulmonary hypertension can lead to right-sided heart failure.

PATHOPHYSIOLOGY

Disorders of gas exchange consist of disorders of ventilation, disorders of diffusion, and disorders of $\dot{V}_A/\dot{Q}$ mismatching. All of these disorders can result in low P_aO_2, which is called **hypoxemia.**

Disorders of Ventilation

Recall that hypoventilation means a decreased $\dot{V}_A$ owing to decreased frequency of breathing and/or shallow breathing (small tidal volumes). The globally decreased $\dot{V}_A$ leads to a global decrease in P_AO_2 and hence a decrease in P_aO_2, or hypoxemia. As we will see below, hypoventilation also increases P_aCO_2, with important pathophysiologic consequences.

Hypoventilation can be caused by *primary respiratory depression,* a neurologic lack of respiratory drive, or by a *restrictive ventilatory defect* that limits the expansion of the lungs and hence reduces $\dot{V}_T$ and $\dot{V}_A$. *Obstructive ventilatory defects* can also cause hypoventilation. By impeding the expiration of air, they overfill the lung and make it difficult to get a good tidal volume of air in for exchange. *Upper airway obstruction* also produces hypoventilation by decreasing $\dot{V}_A$ with each breath.

Primary respiratory depression can be caused by narcotics or other derangements affecting the respiratory center in the medulla. Diseases that hamper the action of the respiratory muscles, such as neurodegenerative diseases like *amyotrophic lateral sclerosis*, or diseases that lower the compliance of the lung parenchyma, such as *pulmonary fibrosis*, cause restrictive ventilatory defects. *Asthma* and *chronic obstructive pulmonary disease* are obstructive pulmonary diseases. *Tumors* may cause upper airway obstruction.

Low atmospheric PO_2 at high altitudes has the same effect on P_AO_2 as does hypoventilation. It creates hypoxemia by a global, as opposed to regional, decrease in P_AO_2 (see Chapter 19). (See Clinical Application Box *Differential Diagnosis of Hypoxemia*.)

Respiratory Acidosis and Alkalosis Hypoventilation can cause not only hypoxemia, but also high P_aCO_2, which is called **hypercarbia**, or **hypercapnia.** Remember that CO_2 levels affect the bicarbonate buffer system in the blood through this relationship:

$$CO_2 + H_2O \leftrightarrow H_2CO_3 \leftrightarrow H^+ + HCO_3^-$$

Therefore, increased P_aCO_2 increases the concentration of H^+ in the blood; that is, it decreases blood pH. Hypoventilation and hypercarbia can therefore create *primary respiratory acidosis.* Conversely, disease that leads to proton wasting and metabolic alkalosis, such as vomiting or hyperaldosteronism, can cause a physiologic compensatory hypoventilation at the lungs to preserve blood CO_2 and hence keep down blood pH.

Hyperventilation, which is less common clinically as a primary cause of illness, yields increased P_aO_2 and decreased P_aCO_2. Decreased P_aCO_2 in turn creates alkalosis. The body consequently uses hyperventilation to combat nonrespiratory disease states that cause acidosis.

Disorders of Diffusion

Any thickening of the gas transfer membrane, as in pulmonary edema or fibrosis, can cause a diffusion defect, as discussed above. Recall that diffusion defects make O_2 transfer diffusion-limited rather than perfusion-limited, impeding oxygenation at an increased heart rate. Conditions that cause diffusion defects therefore result in poor exercise tolerance.

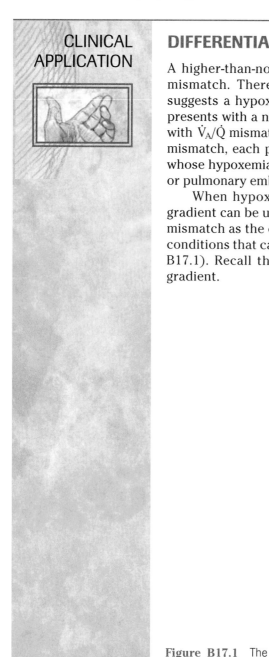

CLINICAL APPLICATION

DIFFERENTIAL DIAGNOSIS OF HYPOXEMIA

A higher-than-normal A-a gradient is the clinical sign of pathophysiologic $\dot{V}_A/\dot{Q}$ mismatch. Therefore, hypoxemia that presents with an elevated A-a gradient suggests a hypoxemic condition associated with $\dot{V}_A/\dot{Q}$ mismatch. Hypoxemia that presents with a normal A-a gradient suggests a hypoxemic condition not associated with $\dot{V}_A/\dot{Q}$ mismatch. Since neither hypoventilation nor high altitude involves $\dot{V}_A/\dot{Q}$ mismatch, each presents as hypoxemia without an elevated A-a gradient. Diseases whose hypoxemia is due to $\dot{V}_A/\dot{Q}$ mismatch—such as pneumonia, pulmonary edema, or pulmonary embolus—present as hypoxemia with an elevated A-a gradient.

When hypoxemia is detected, the presence or absence of an elevated A-a gradient can be used clinically to focus suspicion on either hypoventilation or $\dot{V}_A/\dot{Q}$ mismatch as the cause of the hypoxemia. This, in turn, focuses suspicion either on conditions that cause hypoventilation or on those that cause $\dot{V}_A/\dot{Q}$ mismatch (FIGURE B17.1). Recall that the alveolar gas equation can be used to calculate the A-a gradient.

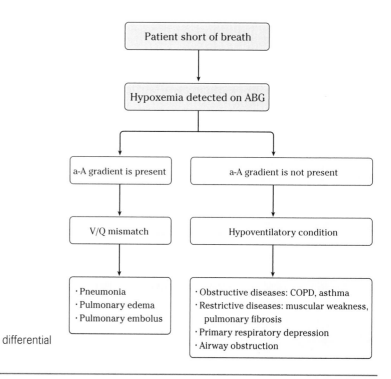

Figure B17.1 The differential diagnosis of hypoxemia.

Pathophysiologic $\dot{V}_A/\dot{Q}$ Mismatch

We have already touched on the physiologic A-a gradient due to low $\dot{V}_A/\dot{Q}$. Pathophysiology, however, can create larger A-a gradients whose associated hypoxemia may be life-threatening. *Pneumonia*, an infection of the distal lung tissues, can fill the alveoli with exudate, block local alveolar ventilation, and cause shunt. Pulmonary edema can also fill the alveoli with fluid, causing shunt in addition to hampering diffusion. Alveolar hemorrhage and *acute respiratory dis-*

tress syndrome (ARDS) will fill alveoli with fluid as well and create shunt.

A *pulmonary embolus*-an object such as a blood clot that clogs a pulmonary artery-also typically creates an A-a gradient. One might think otherwise because the embolus causes a dramatic decrease in perfusion to an area of the lung, thereby causing a high $\dot{V}_A/\dot{Q}$ ratio or creating dead space, and high $\dot{V}_A/\dot{Q}$ or dead space is not supposed to lower P_aO_2. It may be the low $\dot{V}_A/\dot{Q}$ indirectly created by a pulmonary embolus that leads to hypoxemia with A-a gradient. When blood that was perfusing well-ventilated areas of the lung gets blocked by an embolus, the blood flow gets diverted elsewhere. Since the lung has a finite reserve in well-ventilated lung areas, the blood will get diverted to more poorly ventilated lung, leading to low $\dot{V}_A/\dot{Q}$. With high enough right heart pressures, deoxygenated blood can even be diverted across a patent foramen ovale from right heart to left. The mechanisms for hypoxemia and an A-a gradient associated with pulmonary embolism remain controversial. (See Clinical Application Box *What Is Pneumonia?*)

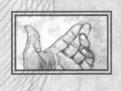

CLINICAL APPLICATION

WHAT IS PNEUMONIA?

A 70-year-old man comes into the emergency department with a complaint of shortness of breath. Over the last week, he has felt feverish with chills, had a cough productive of thick yellowish sputum, and had pain in his right upper chest that is worse during inhalation. His physical examination reveals crackles over the mid right lung and bronchial breath sounds over the lower right lung. Laboratory studies show a white blood cell count of 17,000/mm³ (normal 4,500 to 11,000) and ABG shows a pH of 7.4 (normal 7.4), a P_aCO_2 of 65 mm Hg (normal 40), and HCO_3^- of 34 mEq/L (normal 24). The chest x-ray, which shows right middle and lower lobe infiltrates, confirms the diagnosis of pneumonia.

Pneumonia is a common infection of the lower respiratory tract responsible for much morbidity and mortality worldwide; it is the leading killer among infectious diseases in the United States. It affects people of all ages and is caused by a wide variety of pathogenic microorganisms. Particular types of hosts are susceptible to their own particular groups of organisms; for example, *Pseudomonas aeruginosa* is common in hospital-acquired (nosocomial) pneumonias but not in community-acquired pneumonias.

Underlying the pathophysiology of pneumonia is an acute inflammatory response to either viral or bacterial infection. Local macrophages become immunologically activated upon phagocytosing foreign bacterial particles and secrete cytokines to draw neutrophils, which are another type of inflammatory cell. Bacterial chemoattractants also draw inflammatory cells. Injured local tissues and inflammatory cells release vasoactive substances that increase vascular permeability. The associated purulence (the gross appearance of the neutrophils) and leaking of fluid from capillaries both facilitate the immunologic attack on the pathogens; however, this process can cover the gas-exchanging membranes. This "filling in" of the alveoli and small airways is known as lung *consolidation*.

Most viral pneumonias are self-limiting and most bacterial pneumonias are treatable with antibiotics. If unusually severe or if left untreated, however, pneumonia can have serious consequences. The functional consequences of the acute inflammation include shunt and A-a gradient, which can proceed to respiratory failure, bacteremia (bacteria in the blood), and sepsis (bacteremia with shock). If the infection is not cleared but persists chronically, it can lead to abscess or scarring.

Pneumonias often manifest themselves with productive cough, fever, and chills following an upper respiratory infection. Other symptoms are dyspnea (shortness of breath) and pleurisy (chest pain upon breathing). The consolidated area transmits sound as a solid and may conduct large airway breath sounds (bronchial breath sounds) on auscultation or conduct voice vibrations better than normal lung; this finding is known as *increased tactile fremitus* on palpation. The area should also be dull to percussion. Very important to confirming a diagnosis of pneumonia is an infiltrate on chest x-ray, which is rarely absent in pneumonia. The CBC usually shows an elevated white count.

Management involves an attempt to identify the pathogen with a sputum culture, empiric administration of antibiotics chosen on the basis of the host setting, and supportive measures for hypoxemia or sepsis. With administration of the proper antibiotic, patients usually recover dramatically within several days.

Summary

- The partial pressure of a gas is proportional to its mol fraction in the gas mixture:

$$P_1/P_T = n_1/n_T = X_1$$

- The partial pressure of a gas collected over a liquid is its equilibrium vapor pressure. The gas contents of the blood are measured in equilibrium vapor pressures.

- Increases in the partial pressure (vapor pressure) of oxygen in the alveolus shift the equilibrium toward dissolution of oxygen into blood. Decreases in the partial pressure (vapor pressure) of carbon dioxide in the alveolus shift the equilibrium toward release of carbon dioxide out of blood and into alveolar air.

- Inspiration raises the alveolar partial pressure of oxygen and decreases the alveolar partial pressure of carbon dioxide.

- Inspiration adds a tidal volume, V_T, to the lung spaces. One third of V_T is added to the dead space in the conducting airways, and this portion of V_T is called V_D. Two thirds of V_T are added to the gas-exchanging alveolar space, and this portion of V_T is called V_A:

$$V_A + V_D = V_T$$
$$(1/3)\ (V_T) = (V_D)$$
$$(2/3)\ (V_T) = (V_A)$$

- Alveolar minute ventilation, s_A, is defined as V_A times f, where f is the frequency of breathing in breaths per minute.

$$\dot{V}_A = (V_A)(f)$$

- The larger the V_A added to the alveolar space per time, $\dot{V}_A$, the higher the P_AO_2 of alveolar air and the lower the P_ACO_2 of alveolar air.

- The alveolar ventilation equation describes the relationship between $\dot{V}_A$ and P_ACO_2:

$$\dot{V}_A = (\underline{V}CO_2/P_ACO_2)(K)$$

- Fick's law describes diffusion of gases between blood and air:

$$\dot{V}_G = (P_A - P_C)(A)(S)/(T)(\text{square root of MW})$$

- Rapid diffusion of O_2 and CO_2 makes the gas exchange of these molecules perfusion-limited. CO is a slow-diffusing molecule whose gas exchange is diffusion-limited. Diseases that thicken the gas-exchanging membranes can make O_2 and CO_2's exchange diffusion-limited.

- Rapid diffusion of O_2 and CO_2 means that the arterial blood leaving the alveoli shares the PO_2 and PCO_2 of alveolar air; that is, regionally:

$$P_AO_2 = P_aO_2 \text{ and } P_ACO_2 = P_aCO_2$$

- Here s_A may differ from place to place in the lung. $\dot{Q}$, the blood flow to the lung, may differ from one area to another as well. The ratio of $\dot{V}_A$ to $\dot{Q}$ in an area (the ventilation-perfusion relationship of that area) determines the regional alveolar and arterial partial pressures of O_2 and CO_2. When the $\dot{V}_A/\dot{Q}$ relationship is imbalanced, this is called $\dot{V}_A/\dot{Q}$ mismatch.

- Low regional $\dot{V}_A/\dot{Q}$ ratios decrease regional P_AO_2 and P_aO_2 and increase regional P_ACO_2 and P_aCO_2. High regional $\dot{V}_A/\dot{Q}$ ratios increase regional P_AO_2 and P_aO_2 and decrease regional P_ACO_2 and P_aCO_2. Very low regional $\dot{V}_A/\dot{Q}$ ratios ($= 0$) are called shunts.

- Low regional $\dot{V}_A/\dot{Q}$ ratios can have a significant lowering effect on systemic P_aO_2, even in the context of normal overall P_AO_2. Low regional $\dot{V}_A/\dot{Q}$ ratios do not significantly alter systemic P_aCO_2.

- A depressed P_aO_2 with a normal P_AO_2 is an A-a gradient. If a physician determines the P_aO_2 by ABG and calculates the P_AO_2, he or she can calculate the A-a gradient. An A-a gradient >5 to 10 mm Hg is indicative of a pathologic $\dot{V}_A/\dot{Q}$ mismatch.

- The alveolar gas equation is used to calculate P_AO_2 from P_IO_2 and P_ACO_2, which are always known or measured. At sea level, $P_IO_2 = 149$ mm Hg. $P_ACO_2 = P_aCO_2$, which is determined by drawing an ABG. R = 0.8.

$$P_AO_2 = P_IO_2 - (P_ACO_2/R)$$

- Imbalanced $\dot{V}_A/\dot{Q}$ ratios in normal lung create a physiologic A-a gradient. These imbalances are due to gravitational effects on blood flow and ventilation and to the anatomy of the bronchial and coronary vasculatures.

- Pulmonary blood pressures are lower than systemic to prevent fluid extravasation into the alveoli and are kept low through the mechanisms of recruitment and distention.

- Pulmonary blood pressure is regulated locally by pulmonary hypoxic vasoconstriction, which combats $\dot{V}_A/\dot{Q}$ mismatching. Chronic global hypoxia can lead to pulmonary hypertension.

- Diseases that affect gas exchange can lead to low P_aO_2, or hypoxemia. These diseases are divided into disorders of ventilation, disorders of diffusion, and disorders of low $\dot{V}_A/\dot{Q}$.

- Hypoventilation can lead to high P_aCO_2, or hypercarbia, and acidosis.

Suggested Reading

Galen. *On respiration and the arteries* [edited and translated by Furley DJ, Wilkie JS]. Princeton: Princeton University Press, 1984.

Kampelmacher MJ, van Kesteren RG, Winckers EK. Instrumental variability of respiratory blood gases among different blood gas analysers in different laboratories. Eur Respir J. 1997;10(6):1341–1344.

Milhorn HT, Pulley PE Jr. A theoretical study of pulmonary capillary gas exchange and venous admixture. Biophys J. 1968;8:337.

Paiva M, Engel LA. Theoretical studies of gas mixing and ventilation distribution in the lung. Physiol Rev. 1987;67(3):750–796.

Treacher DF, Leach RM. Oxygen transport 1. Basic principles. Br Med J. 1998;317(7168):1302–1306.

West JB, Dollery CT, Naimark A. Distribution of blood flow in isolated lung: relation to vascular and alveolar pressures. J Appl Physiol. 1964;19:713.

REVIEW QUESTIONS

Directions: Each of the numbered items or incomplete statements in this section is followed by answers or by completions of the statement. Select the ONE lettered answer or completion that is BEST in each case.

1. A 49-year-old man with pulmonary edema reports new-onset shortness of breath when walking upstairs. Thickening of the gas exchange membranes by his disease has resulted in which of the following?

   (A) Carbon monoxide exchange is now diffusion-limited.
   (B) Oxygen exchange is now diffusion-limited.
   (C) Carbon dioxide exchange is now perfusion-limited.
   (D) Carbon monoxide exchange is now perfusion-limited.
   (E) Oxygen exchange is now perfusion-limited.

2. A 72-year-old woman who recently underwent hip replacement surgery develops a large left lower lobe pulmonary embolus. The ventilation and perfusion status in the alveoli of her affected lobe could best be described by which of the following?

   (A) V_A is 0, Q is normal.
   (B) V_A is 0, Q is low.
   (C) V_A is normal, Q is high.
   (D) V_A is normal, Q is normal.
   (E) V_A is normal, Q is 0.

3. A 65-year-old woman has right middle lobe pneumonia. Her blood gas on room air indicates a P_aO_2 of 57 mm Hg and a P_aCO_2 of 32 mm Hg. If P_IO_2 on room air is 149 mm Hg, what is her A-a gradient?

   (A) 25 mm Hg
   (B) 52 mm Hg
   (C) 60 mm Hg
   (D) 92 mm Hg
   (E) 109 mm Hg

ANSWERS TO REVIEW QUESTIONS

1. **The answer is B.** In healthy lungs, the diffusion of carbon dioxide and oxygen across the alveolar membrane is rapid. In a healthy person, the degree of carbon dioxide and oxygen exchange is determined instead by the amount of blood flow to the capillary, which is perfusion-limited exchange. In diseased lung where the alveolar membranes are thickened, the diffusion of oxygen is slower, and oxygen exchange becomes perfusion-limited. During states of increased blood flow such as exercise, there is decreased oxygen exchange in the lung with thickened membranes, which can result in symptoms of exercise intolerance. Carbon monoxide has a slower diffusion rate, even in the healthy lung, and is consequently diffusion-limited in both normal and abnormal conditions.

2. **The answer is E.** In a pulmonary embolus, a blood clot blocks the flow of blood to a part of the lung, resulting in no perfusion to the affected area ($Q = 0$). The alveoli in the affected region are still exposed to air by ventilation, but there is no blood supply for gas exchange. The affected region is dead space. In situations where there is adequate blood flow but no ventilation ($V_A = 0$), this is called a shunt. A shunt exists both in pneumonia, where the alveoli are filled with inflammatory cells and exudate, and in the case of atelectasis, where the alveoli have collapsed.

3. **The answer is B.** The clinically useful form of the alveolar gas equation is as

follows:

$$P_AO_2 = P_IO_2 - P_ACO_2/0.8$$

The average P_ACO_2 is considered to be equal to P_aCO_2. With a P_aCO_2 of 32 mm Hg and a P_IO_2 of 149 mm Hg on room air, P_AO_2 will be 109 mm Hg. The P_aO_2 from the blood gas is 57 mm Hg. The difference between P_AO_2 and P_aO_2 yields an A-a gradient of 52. An A-a gradient of >5 to 10 mm Hg is abnormal. The acute inflammation and exudate of pneumonia typically causes both an A-a gradient and a shunt.

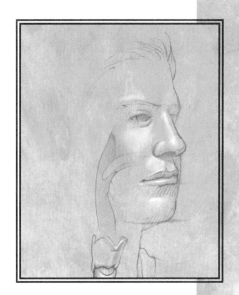

18

Gas Transport

INTRODUCTION

The lungs do not alone perform all the functions necessary for cellular respiration. The transport of oxygen and carbon dioxide between the lungs and the periphery relies on the critical participation of two other systems—the hematologic and cardiovascular systems. Blood carries oxygen from the lungs to the body tissues and carbon dioxide from the tissues to the lungs. The heart participates in gas transport by pumping the blood from the lungs to every cell in the body and back to the lungs. O_2 moves from alveolar gas into pulmonary capillaries and from systemic capillaries into the tissues by simple diffusion. CO_2 also moves by simple diffusion—from the tissues to the blood and from the blood to the alveolar gas.

SYSTEM STRUCTURE: OXYGEN RESERVOIRS AND HEMOGLOBIN

Each 100 mL of arterial blood contains a mass of oxygen equivalent to about 20 mL (if the oxygen were isolated and measured at standard temperature and pressure). With a cardiac output of 6 L/min, we can calculate that approximately 1,200 mL of oxygen is delivered to the body per minute. Of the 1,200 mL of O_2/min, the body consumes 300 mL/min and the remaining 900 mL flows back to the heart each minute in the venous blood. To keep up with this level of oxygen demand, a majority of blood oxygen content must be bound to **hemoglobin (Hb)** inside red blood cells, with only a small remainder dissolved in the plasma in free solution. (See Integrated Physiology Box *Oxygen Extraction*.)

Oxygen Reservoirs

If oxygen were carried in free solution only, the blood could not contain enough oxygen to deliver 300 mL of oxygen to the body per minute. **Henry's law** states that the amount of gas dissolved in any liquid is proportional to its partial pressure. There is 0.003 mL of dissolved O_2 per 100 mL of blood for each mm Hg of PO_2. At the normal arterial PO_2 of 100, 100 mL of blood contains only 0.3 mL of dissolved O_2, a small amount of O_2 that could not begin to match the body's metabolic demand.

To load the blood with the O_2 we need, the blood must contain an additional reservoir for O_2 storage. That reservoir is hemoglobin, a protein inside red blood cells that binds dissolved O_2 molecules and takes them out of free solution. When blood is exposed to alveolar gas, hemoglobin's binding of dissolved oxygen prevents plasma from reaching its saturation point of 0.3 mL O_2/100 mL blood. More O_2 can then diffuse out of alveolar gas into solution in blood, and that O_2 can in turn bind to hemoglobin. With hemoglobin, the O_2-carrying capacity of blood is increased over 60-fold.

Hemoglobin Structure and Cooperativity

The structure of hemoglobin enables it to bind O_2 and to undergo important conformational changes. Normal adult hemoglobin is a 65-kD protein made up of four subunits: two identical alpha chains and two identical beta chains (FIGURE 18.1). Each subunit contains a *heme group*, which is a porphyrin ring with an iron atom in the center. In the absence of oxygen, the four subunits are tightly bound to each other with electrostatic interactions into a tense (T) conformation. This T conformation, known as "reduced hemoglobin" or *deoxy-hemoglobin*, has a relatively low affinity for oxygen. The oxygen diffuses into the red blood cell from the pulmonary alveoli and noncovalently binds to the iron atom in the center of the porphyrin ring of one subunit. This binding induces a conformational change in that subunit into the relaxed (R) conformation.

Because the subunits are in close apposition, the change in one subunit to the R conformation induces all of the other subunits to change to the R form via

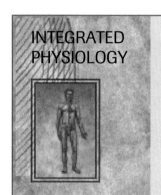

INTEGRATED PHYSIOLOGY

Oxygen Extraction

Oxygen extraction varies from organ to organ. As stated in the text, of the 1,200 mL O_2 delivered to the body each minute, the body consumes 300 mL and 900 mL remains in the venous blood. This 25% oxygen extraction rate is an average for the body. The heart, for example, extracts almost all of the oxygen it receives, while the kidneys extract a very small percentage of the oxygen they receive.

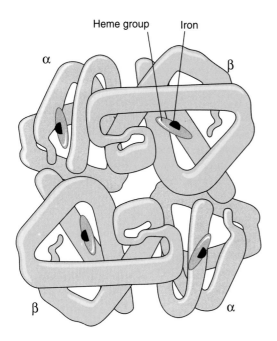

Figure 18.1 Hemoglobin. Hemoglobin is composed of four subunits. Each subunit contains a heme group.

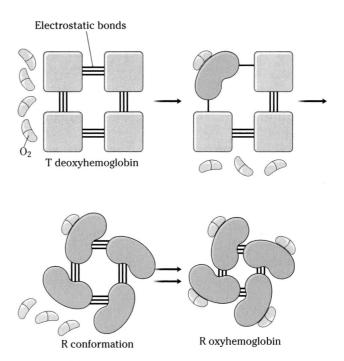

Figure 18.2 Changes in hemoglobin conformation and oxygen affinity. The T conformation has a low affinity for oxygen, and the R conformation has a high affinity for it. Oxygen binding promotes the R conformation and therefore more oxygen binding.

mechanical and electrostatic interactions (FIGURE 18.2). The R form has 500 times higher affinity for oxygen than the T form. Therefore, the remaining three subunits quickly pick up O_2 molecules. This is called **cooperativity**; the binding of one subunit to O_2 makes it easier for the other three subunits to bind O_2. This sequence essentially occurs in reverse when O_2 is unloaded in the periphery after being carried through the arterial system.

SYSTEM FUNCTION: OXYGEN AND CARBON DIOXIDE TRANSPORT

The presence of two oxygen reservoirs and the structure of hemoglobin have important functional consequences. They facilitate the loading of O_2 in the pulmonary capillaries, the unloading of O_2 at the tissues, and the adaptation of hemoglobin to meet changing metabolic demands.

The O_2-Hemoglobin Equilibrium Curve

The interaction between hemoglobin and O_2 at the molecular level is described by **the O_2-hemoglobin equilibrium curve.** The equilibrium curve is derived by taking a series of closed containers with a fixed quantity of blood and adding gas with varying partial pressures of O_2. After allowing time for equilibration, the total oxygen content of the blood and PO_2 of the blood are measured. Using Henry's law, we can calculate the amount of dissolved O_2 from the

PO_2 and subtract that value from the total O_2 content. The resultant value, the O_2 content of hemoglobin, can be plotted against PO_2 (FIGURE 18.3). The O_2 content of hemoglobin is expressed as a percentage of the maximum O_2 capacity, or *% O_2 saturation.*

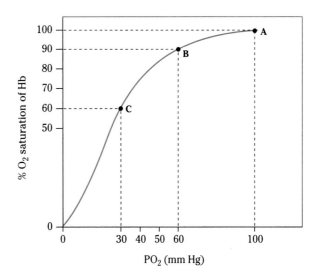

Figure 18.3 The O_2-hemoglobin equilibrium curve. From point A to point B, PO_2 drops by 40 mm Hg but O_2 saturation drops by only 10%. From point B to point C, O_2 saturation drops by about 30% and PO_2 drops by only 30 mm Hg. PO_2s of 40, 50, and 60 mm Hg correspond roughly to O_2 saturations of 70%, 80%, and 90%.

The O_2-hemoglobin equilibrium curve is sigmoid in shape. The allosteric properties of hemoglobin account for this shape. At low PO_2, the deoxyhemoglobin molecules begin to bind their first molecule of O_2 and the flat slope of the curve reflects the low affinity of the T conformation for O_2. After one O_2 molecule gets bound, the conformation of hemoglobin changes to the R conformation, making it much easier for the second, third, and fourth molecules of O_2 to bind. The slope of the curve rises rapidly to reflect the higher O_2 affinity of the R conformation. As hemoglobin becomes saturated, the curve flattens again. This is because even though there are many dissolved molecules of O_2 in competition for hemoglobin binding sites, there simply are not enough sites left to accommodate the O_2. Near the saturation point, therefore, large increases in the amount of dissolved O_2 (the blood PO_2) produce only small increases in the amount of O_2 loaded onto hemoglobin. (See Clinical Application Box *Pulse Oximetry*.)

This sigmoid relationship between PO_2 and hemoglobin O_2 saturation creates certain physiological advantages in the loading of O_2 in the lungs and unloading in the periphery. In the flat upper portion of the curve, when the PO_2 drops from the normal 100 mm Hg to 60 mm Hg (see Figure 18.3, A → B), the O_2 saturation drops only to 90%. This means that O_2 loading will not be compromised even if the PO_2 drops significantly owing to lung disease. In addition, the flat upper portion of the curve ensures that even when 90% of hemoglobin has become saturated, a large O_2 partial pressure difference between alveolar gas and blood still exists. The blood PO_2 is only at 60 mm Hg compared with the alveolar PO_2 of 100 mm Hg. This gradient of 40 mm Hg drives continued O_2 diffusion into blood even after hemoglobin is 90% loaded with O_2.

The steep portion of the O_2-hemoglobin equilibrium curve means that the peripheral tissues can remove a large amount of O_2 from hemoglobin (see Figure 18.3, B → C) in exchange for a small drop in capillary PO_2. The capillary PO_2 remains high, maintaining a high capillary to tissue PO_2 gradient. Even after the upstream tissues have removed a lot of O_2, there is still an adequate gradient to drive dissolved O_2 into the downstream tissues. The O_2-hemoglobin equilibrium curve shows that hemoglobin buffers O_2 content against pathologic falls in blood PO_2 and maintains favorable gradients for O_2 diffusion.

Hemoglobin's Adaptation to Changing Oxygen Requirements

Hemoglobin can also respond to the body's constantly changing need for oxygen. When metabolic activity increases and the demand for O_2 is high, hemoglobin responds by increasing its ability to unload O_2 at the tissues. The following markers of increased metabolic activity act on hemoglobin to produce this effect: heat, PCO_2, H^+ concentration, and *2,3-bisphosphoglycerate (2,3-BPG)* concentration. With high metabolic activity, body heat rises, as does the level of CO_2 production. Increased CO_2 levels drive increased carbonic acid production and raise the level of H^+, which is also boosted by the lactic acid produced with high metabolic demand. Finally, through an unknown mechanism, chronic hypoxemia or acidemia causes an increase in red blood cell 2,3-BPG concentration. Mature red blood cells have no mitochondria and thus depend solely on glycolysis for metabolism; 2,3-BPG is a normal intermediate in the glycolysis pathway.

These markers of oxygen demand affect the interaction of hemoglobin with O_2 in the following ways. The laws of chemical equilibrium dictate that

---

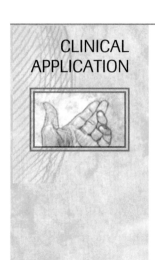

CLINICAL APPLICATION

PULSE OXIMETRY

Saturation of O_2 is measured clinically by a pulse oximeter. Through the fingertip, the probe transmits two wavelengths of light that are absorbed differently by oxyhemoglobin and deoxyhemoglobin. A photodetector measures the amount of each wavelength transmitted and a ratio of oxyhemoglobin to deoxyhemoglobin, and thus the O_2 saturation can be calculated.

A simple rule for remembering the O_2-hemoglobin equilibrium curve can help in interpreting pulse oximeter readings. The equilibrium curve can be committed to memory using the "40, 50, 60 for 70, 80, 90" rule. The PO_2s of 40, 50, and 60 mm Hg approximately correspond to O_2 saturations of 70%, 80%, and 90%, respectively. Pulse oximetry does not yield information about a possible A-a gradient, nor does it indicate the adequacy of alveolar ventilation. More information, if necessary, would require arterial blood gas determination.

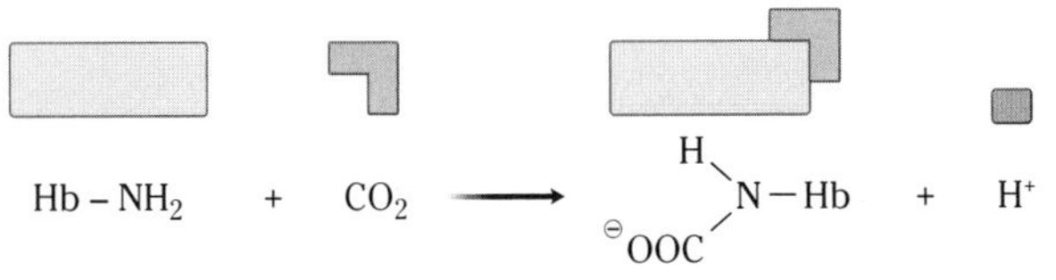

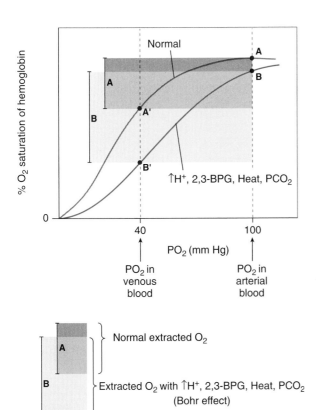

Figure 18.4 The formation of carbaminohemoglobin from CO_2 and hemoglobin.

Table 18.1	**THE BASICS OF THE BOHR AND HALDANE EFFECTS**
Bohr Effect	**Haldane Effect**
CO_2 and H^+ binding to Hb → decreased Hb affinity for O_2	Deoxygenation of Hb → increased Hb affinity for CO_2
Shifts O_2-hemoglobin curve RIGHT	Shifts CO_2-blood curve LEFT

increased temperature favors dissociation. Increases in body heat therefore lower the affinity of hemoglobin for O_2. Carbon dioxide covalently binds to the amino termini of the hemoglobin subunits and forms carbaminohemoglobin (FIGURE 18.4), which favors the T conformation. Hydrogen ion and 2,3-BPG both bind specific sites on the hemoglobin protein, also favoring the T conformation. Recall that the T conformation of hemoglobin has a lower affinity for oxygen.

Therefore, when the markers of oxygen demand are increased, hemoglobin will have a lower affinity for O_2. On the O_2-hemoglobin curve, O_2 saturation will be lower for a given PO_2 and, accordingly, for a given O_2 saturation, the PO_2 tension will be higher. This manifests as a rightward shift on the O_2-hemoglobin equilibrium curve (FIGURE 18.5). PCO_2 and H^+'s right-

ward effect on the curve is known as the **Bohr effect** (TABLE 18.1). The P50 (the PO_2 corresponding to 50% hemoglobin saturation) serves as an index of the position of the O_2-hemoglobin curve. Heat, CO_2, H^+, and 2,3-BPG all increase P50 and shift the O_2-hemoglobin curve to the right.

How does this shift of the O_2-hemoglobin curve correlate with increased oxygen delivery to the body? At high PO_2, a horizontal shift has a minimal effect on O_2 loading because the curve is relatively flat. However, at relatively low PO_2, the saturation is significantly lower on the rightward-shifted curve. This means that more O_2 will be unloaded in the tissues at low blood PO_2. Overall, more oxygen is extracted from hemoglobin because O_2 loading is largely unaffected, but O_2 unloading in the tissues is greatly increased.

Hemoglobin was recently discovered to have yet another mechanism for responding to physiologic oxygen needs: it promotes vasodilation and hence perfusion in hypoxic tissues by releasing **nitric oxide (NO)**, a potent vasodilator. Oxyhemoglobin binds NO tightly but deoxyhemoglobin does not. Oxyhemoglobin therefore serves to scavenge NO from blood. In hypoxic tissue, the oxyhemoglobin unloads oxygen and becomes deoxyhemoglobin. Because deoxyhemoglobin has a low NO affinity, NO is concurrently released. The release of NO leads to local vasodilation, helping to direct blood flow, and hence O_2, specifically to hypoxic tissue. (See Clinical Application Box *Carbon Monoxide Poisoning.*)

CO_2 Transport

Cellular metabolism in the tissues of a resting adult produces a mass of CO_2 equivalent to 200 mL per minute of CO_2 at standard temperature and pressure. Each 100 mL of venous blood contains about 50 mL of carbon dioxide. Therefore, 3 L of CO_2 is delivered to the lungs per minute (cardiac output of 6 L/min times 500 mL/L). Of the 3 L, however, only 200 mL is extracted by the pulmonary alveoli for excretion to maintain a steady state. The lungs excrete only a small amount of the CO_2 delivered to them

Figure 18.5 The Bohr effect. When the markers of increased metabolic demand are increased, decreases in hemoglobin's oxygen affinity lead to increased oxygen extraction from hemoglobin.

CLINICAL APPLICATION

CARBON MONOXIDE POISONING

Carbon monoxide (CO) is a colorless, odorless gas formed from the incomplete combustion of any carbon material. It is present in automobile exhaust fumes, cigarette smoke, and wood smoke, and is released by furnaces and gas stoves. At high concentrations, it can cause illness or even death.

Carbon monoxide interferes with tissue oxygenation in two ways. It binds hemoglobin with an affinity 250 times that of oxygen, thereby competitively inhibiting oxygen loading onto hemoglobin. CO also inhibits the unloading of oxygen because when CO binds hemoglobin, forming carboxyhemoglobin, it shifts hemoglobin into the R conformation, which increases hemoglobin's affinity for oxygen. For a given O_2 saturation, the blood now has a lower PO_2, reducing the gradient for O_2 diffusion into the tissues. In **CO poisoning**, not only does hemoglobin carry less oxygen to the tissues, it also cannot efficiently unload the oxygen it does carry (FIGURE B18.1).

Carbon monoxide poisoning is treated with administration of 100% O_2, which increases the PO_2 enough to overcome CO's competitive inhibition of oxygen loading.

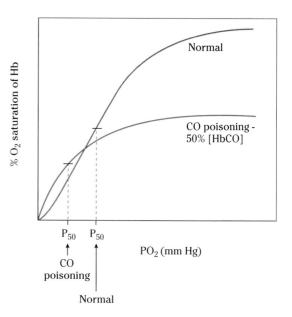

Figure B18.1   Carbon monoxide poisoning. The oxygen-carrying capacity of hemoglobin is drastically decreased and the curve is shifted to the left.

because (a) the kidneys share the burden of handling CO_2 produced by cellular metabolism, and (b) the brain and kidneys regulate CO_2 excretion so as to leave some in the blood at all times as part of the blood's bicarbonate buffer system:

$$CO_2 \leftrightarrow H_2CO_3 \leftrightarrow H^+ + HCO_3^-$$

The constant presence of bicarbonate in the blood buffers the acid load created by the metabolism of dietary carbohydrates and fats (see Chapter 25).

CO_2 exists in blood in three forms: 5% is dissolved in plasma, 5% is covalently bound to hemoglobin as carbaminohemoglobin, and 90% is bicarbonate. The amount of dissolved CO_2 is proportional to the PCO_2 in accordance with Henry's law. However, CO_2 is 20 times more soluble in plasma than

O_2. (At an equal level of PCO_2 and PO_2, there is much more dissolved CO_2 than there is dissolved O_2.) Therefore, dissolved CO_2 contributes to a significant proportion of the exhaled CO_2. Dissolved CO_2 is present in both plasma and red blood cells.

Carbaminohemoglobin is formed by the covalent binding of CO_2 to the terminal amine groups of the hemoglobin subunits, releasing H^+ as a by-product (see Figure 18.4). This reaction occurs spontaneously without enzymatic catalysis. This form of CO_2 is circulated strictly in the red blood cells.

Bicarbonate, the major form of CO_2, is carried mostly in plasma, but it is formed in the red blood cell. CO_2 from the tissues diffuses into the red cell, where it is hydrated by carbonic anhydrase to form carbonic acid. Carbonic acid then spontaneously dissociates into H^+ and bicarbonate. Bicarbonate moves out of the red cell into the plasma in exchange for chloride ions entering the cell from the plasma, thereby maintaining electroneutrality. This is known as the **chloride shift**; the protein carrier mediating this is a chloride-bicarbonate exchanger known as the band 3 protein. To buffer the red blood cell from increasing acidity, the H^+ ions are scavenged by hemoglobin (FIGURE 18.6). In the lungs, all of the above reactions occur in reverse to release CO_2.

The CO_2-Blood Equilibrium Curve   The CO_2-blood equilibrium curve relates total CO_2 content to PCO_2. It is derived in a fashion analogous to the derivation of the O_2-hemoglobin curve. In contrast to the O_2-hemoglobin curve, however, the relationship is essentially linear (FIGURE 18.7). This is so because (a) there is a lack of molecular cooperativity in CO_2 loading, and (b) over the range of PCO_2 values compatible with human life, blood has no saturation point for CO_2; that is, there is no ceiling for increases in CO_2 content that would flatten the curve. Notice that there are two lines drawn in Figure 18.7. The position of the CO_2-blood

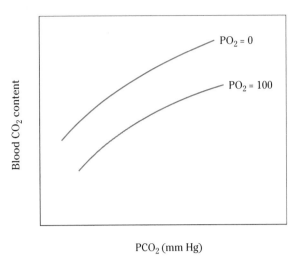

Figure 18.7   The CO_2-blood equilibrium curve. The two lines show the curve in oxygenated versus deoxygenated blood, illustrating the Haldane effect.

equilibrium line is shifted leftward when hemoglobin is less saturated with oxygen. For any given PCO_2, deoxygenated blood can carry more CO_2. For any given level of CO_2 content in blood, deoxygenated blood has lower PCO_2. This leftward shift of the CO_2-blood equilibrium curve when blood is deoxygenated is known as the **Haldane effect** (see Table 18.1).

The explanation for this phenomenon lies in the inherently different molecular properties of oxyhemoglobin versus deoxyhemoglobin. First, deoxyhemoglobin has a greater affinity for CO_2, binding it to form carbaminohemoglobin. Second, deoxyhemoglobin is a better proton acceptor than oxyhemoglobin. It scavenges H^+ ions formed when carbonic acid dissociates and when carbaminohemoglobin is formed. The removal of an end-product drives the two reactions to the right (Le Chatelier's principle), favoring the formation of more carbaminohemoglobin. These two properties result in a greater CO_2 content in deoxygenated blood for any given PCO_2—the Haldane effect.

Coupled CO_2 and O_2 Transport

The mechanisms involved in the transport of O_2 from the lungs to the periphery and CO_2 from the periphery to the lungs have been discussed as separate entities, but in fact the two processes are coupled and facilitate each other. The loading of CO_2 in the periphery promotes O_2 unloading, and the unloading of O_2 in the periphery promotes CO_2 loading. In the lung, O_2 loading promotes CO_2 unloading, which in turn promotes O_2 loading (FIGURE 18.8).

In the periphery, as blood passes through tissue capillaries, the uptake of CO_2 leads to an increase in

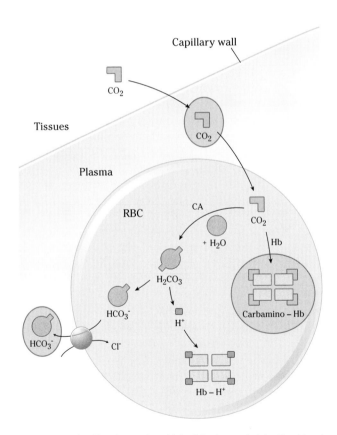

Figure 18.6   The forms in which CO_2 is carried in the blood. Once CO_2 enters the bloodstream, 5% of it remains as CO_2, 5% is converted to carbaminohemoglobin, and 90% of it is converted to bicarbonate. The transport of bicarbonate from the cell to the plasma occurs in exchange for chloride entry into the cell—the chloride shift.

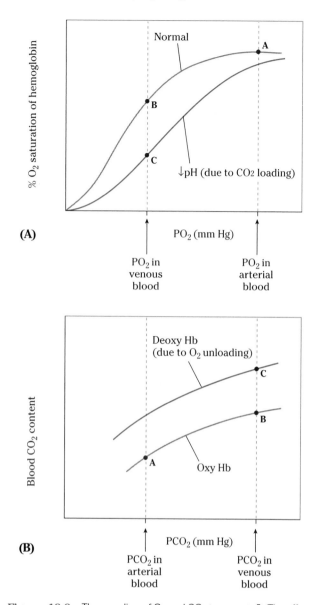

(A)

PO₂ in venous blood

PO₂ in arterial blood

(B)

PCO₂ in arterial blood

PCO₂ in venous blood

Figure 18.8 The coupling of O_2 and CO_2 transport. **A.** The effect of CO_2 loading on O_2 unloading. Without the Bohr effect, there would be less unloading of oxygen in the tissues (point A → point B). With the Bohr effect from CO_2 loading there is more unloading of oxygen in the tissues (point A → point C). **B.** The effect of O_2 unloading on CO_2 loading. Without the Haldane effect, there would be less CO_2 loading (A → B). With the Haldane effect from O_2 unloading, there is more CO_2 loading (A → C).

H^+ concentration in the red blood cells as CO_2 forms carbonic acid, which dissociates into H^+ and HCO_3^-. The O_2-hemoglobin curve is subsequently shifted to the right via the Bohr effect as the protons and CO_2 bind hemoglobin, inducing the T conformation, with its reduced O_2 affinity (FIGURE 18.9). The oxygen tension (PO_2) becomes higher for a given O_2 saturation, leading to a greater PO_2 gradient between the capillary and tissues, facilitating O_2 unloading. Also, at a given venous PO_2, the O_2 saturation decreases, reflecting greater O_2 unloading.

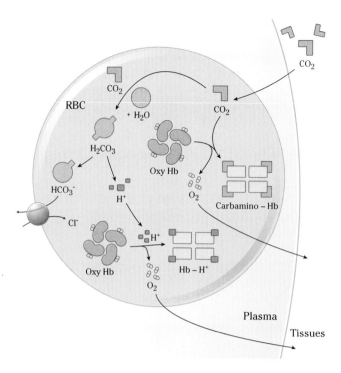

Figure 18.9 The effect of CO_2 on hemoglobin. By two distinct pathways, CO_2 promotes the T conformation of hemoglobin and thereby promotes unloading of O_2 into the tissues.

Conversely, the unloading of oxygen leads to the formation of deoxyhemoglobin. In accordance with the Haldane effect, the deoxyhemoglobin has an increased affinity for CO_2 and H^+, thus promoting the formation of bicarbonate and carbaminohemoglobin. This leads to a lower PCO_2 for a given CO_2 content, facilitating CO_2 loading by increasing the PCO_2 gradient between the capillary and tissues. Furthermore, at a given venous PCO_2, the CO_2 content is higher, reflecting greater CO_2 loading.

These steps occur in reverse for the unloading of CO_2 and loading of O_2 in the pulmonary capillaries. O_2 loading forms oxyhemoglobin, which dumps CO_2, raising PCO_2 for a given CO_2 content, and increasing the gradient for diffusion of CO_2 into alveolar gas. CO_2 unloading promotes the R conformation of hemoglobin (both directly and by raising the cellular pH, as the $CO_2 \leftrightarrow H_2CO_3 \leftrightarrow H^+ + HCO_3^-$ reaction is shifted to the left in the cell), and the R conformation promotes O_2 loading. This lowers PO_2 for a given O_2 content, increasing the gradient for diffusion of O_2 from gas to blood.

PATHOPHYSIOLOGY

Disorders of oxygen transport result in inadequate oxygen delivery to tissues—tissue **hypoxia.** Hypoxia means low PO_2. **Hypoxemia** is defined as a decreased PO_2 in arterial blood—that is, hypoxia in the blood. Hypoxemia has three causes: low atmospheric PO_2, hypoventilation, and most commonly, ς/Θ mismatch (or shunt). Low arterial oxygen tension (hypoxemia) can cause hypoxia in the tissues. However, hypoxemia and hypoxia are not strictly equivalent terms because disorders in gas transport can cause hypoxia in the tissues without causing hypoxemia. A clinical example (anemia) will help illustrate this point as well as help explain the difference between PO_2, O_2 saturation, and O_2 content.

Anemia, a reduction in the concentration of hemoglobin in blood, is diagnosed by a decreased hematocrit. The *hematocrit* is the percentage of blood composed of red blood cells (by volume) and can be determined by allowing the red cells to settle to the bottom of a column of blood. Anemia can be caused by acute or chronic blood loss, by decreased production of red cells (e.g., vitamin B_{12} or folate deficiency), or by increased destruction (e.g., immune-mediated hemolysis).

Anemia leads to hypoxia by reducing the oxygen-carrying capacity of blood. The normal hemoglobin concentration of blood is about 15 g/100 mL. Since 1 g of hemoglobin can carry 1.4 mL of O_2, the O_2 capacity of normal blood will be 21 mL O_2/100 mL blood. Accordingly, an anemic patient with a hemoglobin concentration of 7.5 g/100 mL will have an O_2 capacity of 10.5 mL/100 mL. He will have normal gas exchange, however, and therefore will not be hypoxemic (i.e., he will have a normal PO_2). He will also have normal O_2 saturation (amount of oxyhemoglobin expressed as a percentage of total hemoglobin). Therefore, the O_2-hemoglobin dissociation curve of this patient will be normal. However, if O_2 content, expressed as total mL O_2/100 mL blood, is plotted against PO_2, the curve of the anemic individual is very different (FIGURE 18.10). It is easy to appreciate that less O_2 will be delivered to the tissues per 100 mL of blood. Cardiac output is increased to compensate. Owing to this increased work and tissue hypoxia, patients develop fatigue and headaches.

Patients with anemia also develop skin pallor because hemoglobin imparts the red color to blood. Interestingly, if they happen to have respiratory compromise and desaturate, they are less likely to be *cyanotic*, characterized by a bluish appearance to the skin due to low oxygen saturation, as in respiratory disease. Oxyhemoglobin is bright red while deoxyhemoglobin is purple. Given a normal O_2 saturation, an anemic patient will have a less-than-normal absolute amount of purple deoxyhemoglobin and will therefore be less cyanotic. Accordingly, a person with an abnormally high hematocrit (polycythemia) will be more cyanotic at the same O_2 saturation. Anemia can be treated acutely with blood transfusions if severe. Otherwise, treatment is dictated by the primary cause.

Summary

- Given the relatively small amount of O_2 blood can carry in solution, O_2 in solution cannot alone meet tissue demand for O_2. A second reservoir for O_2 in the blood must be present.

- The two O_2 reservoirs are O_2 in solution and O_2 bound to the protein hemoglobin inside red blood cells. Ninety-six percent of total O_2 content in arterial blood is carried by hemoglobin.

- The PO_2 is directly proportional to the quantity of O_2 dissolved in blood. There is 0.003 mL of dissolved O_2 per 100 mL of blood for each mm Hg of PO_2.

- Hemoglobin is composed of four subunits, each containing an iron-based heme group. Each heme group can bind one O_2 molecule.

- Hemoglobin's subunits can be arranged in T conformation (tense) or R conformation (relaxed). The T conformation has a low affinity for O_2 and the R conformation has a high affinity for O_2.

- O_2 binding of one subunit in the T conformation shifts the other three subunits into R conformation. This property of hemoglobin, called cooperativity, means that O_2 binding

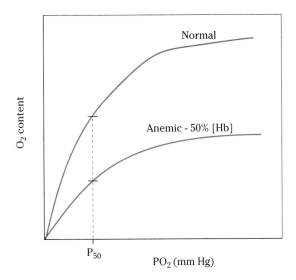

Figure 18.10 Anemia. The Y axis is total O_2 content, not percent saturation of hemoglobin as on the O_2-hemoglobin equilibrium curve. Note that the P50 of the patient with anemia remains the same.

promotes further O_2 binding. Conversely, dissociation of O_2 from hemoglobin promotes more dissociation of O_2 from hemoglobin.

- As PO_2 increases, more O_2 molecules associate with hemoglobin. The O_2-hemoglobin equilibrium curve precisely defines this relationship between PO_2 and hemoglobin saturation. Hemoglobin is 90% saturated at a PO_2 of roughly 60 mm Hg.

- CO_2 exists in blood in three forms: 5% is dissolved in plasma, 5% is covalently bound to hemoglobin as carbaminohemoglobin, and 90% is bicarbonate. The CO_2-blood equilibrium curve describes the relationship between total CO_2 content and PCO_2. Because there is no physiologic saturation point for CO_2 content, this curve is more linear than the O_2-hemoglobin equilibrium curve.

- CO_2 and H^+ interact with hemoglobin to shift it into T conformation and reduce its affinity for O_2. This is called the Bohr effect, and it manifests as a rightward shift of the O_2-hemoglobin equilibrium curve.

- Deoxyhemoglobin has a higher affinity for CO_2. This is called the Haldane effect, and it manifests as a leftward shift in the CO_2-blood equilibrium curve.

- The Bohr and Haldane effects account for the coupling of O_2 and CO_2 transport (in the lungs O_2 loading and CO_2 unloading promote each other; at the tissues O_2 unloading and CO_2 loading promote each other) and for increased O_2 delivery in the presence of high metabolic demand.

- In anemia, the amount of hemoglobin is decreased. This reduces total oxygen content without reducing PO_2 or hemoglobin saturation.

Suggested Reading

Geers C, Gros G. Carbon dioxide transport and carbonic anhydrase in blood and muscle. Physiol Rev. 2000;80(2):681–715.

Hsia CCW. Respiratory function of hemoglobin. N Engl J Med. 1998;338:239–247.

Treacher DF, Leach RM. Oxygen transport 1. Basic principles. Br Med J. 1998;317(7168):1302–1306.

REVIEW QUESTIONS

Directions: Each of the numbered items or incomplete statements in this section is followed by answers or by completions of the statement. Select the ONE lettered answer or completion that is BEST in each case.

1. A 9-year-old boy with a family history of a hemoglobinopathy is analyzed for hemoglobin mutations. He is found to have a mutation that decreases the oxygen affinity of his hemoglobin. The mechanism by which this happens might be which of the following?

   (A) The mutation enhances the binding of carbon monoxide to hemoglobin.
   (B) The mutation increases cooperativity between hemoglobin molecules.
   (C) The mutation decreases the binding of carbon dioxide to hemoglobin
   (D) The mutation inhibits the association of the subunits of hemoglobin.
   (E) The mutation decreases the binding of hydrogen ions to hemoglobin.

2. A 15-year-old girl with hemolytic anemia (increased destruction of red blood cells) reports fatigue and headaches. Her total oxygen content is reduced by which of the following mechanisms?

   (A) Decreased PO_2
   (B) Increased hemoglobin oxygen saturation
   (C) Increased amount of hemoglobin
   (D) Decreased amount of hemoglobin
   (E) Decreased hemoglobin oxygen saturation

3. A 37-year-old man is running the Marine Corps Marathon. The increased oxygen demand of his body is met by which of the following mechanisms?

   (A) Increased oxygen affinity of hemoglobin
   (B) Decreased oxygen affinity of hemoglobin
   (C) Acute increase in hemoglobin production
   (D) Increased oxygen loading in lungs
   (E) Decreased levels of carbon dioxide in blood

ANSWERS TO REVIEW QUESTIONS

1. **The answer is** D. The cooperativity of hemoglobin results from the association of its subunits. If one subunit binds oxygen and shifts to the higher-oxygen- affinity R conformation, it triggers shifts to the R conformation in the three other subunits. Mutations that prevent the close association of hemoglobin's subunits will result in the loss of this cooperativity and a decrease in oxygen affinity. The binding of carbon dioxide and hydrogen ions to hemoglobin stabilizes the low-oxygen-affinity T conformation of hemoglobin. The binding of carbon monoxide results in the formation of carboxyhemoglobin, which increases the oxygen affinity of hemoglobin by shifting it into the R conformation.

2. **The answer is** D. In anemia, the number of red blood cells is decreased, which results in a decreased amount of hemoglobin available to bind oxygen. A patient with anemia will have normal gas exchange in the lungs and will have a normal PO_2. Hemoglobin oxygen saturation is the amount of oxyhemoglobin expressed as a percentage of total hemoglobin. While this patient's total hemoglobin is decreased, her amount of oxyhemoglobin is decreased by a similar degree. Therefore, her oxygen saturation will be normal.

3. **The answer is** B. Increased metabolic activity results in elevated levels of heat, carbon dioxide, hydrogen ions, and 2,3-bisphosphoglycerate, all of which stabilize the low-oxygen-affinity T conformation of hemoglobin. During exercise, oxygen loading of hemoglobin in the lungs is relatively unchanged by these factors because of the high PO_2. However, in the tissues where PO_2 is low, the stabilization of hemoglobin's lower oxygen affinity by these factors results in greater unloading of oxygen to the tissues.

19

The Regulation of Breathing

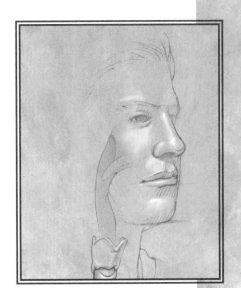

INTRODUCTION

The human respiratory system has the critical task of responding to the oxygen demands of the organism and maintaining a relatively constant range of oxygen and carbon dioxide in the blood. Unlike the heart, with its intrinsic pacemaker, the rhythmic action of the diaphragm and other muscles of respiration is governed by both voluntary and involuntary neural pathways. Thus, while the body regulates respiration automatically during every waking moment and throughout periods of unconsciousness such as sleep, one can voluntarily override this control for short periods of time, allowing activities such as talking, eating, and drinking. To maintain homeostasis, the neural pathways must be sensitive to changes in the oxygen, carbon dioxide, and H^+ content in the peripheral blood.

SYSTEM STRUCTURE AND FUNCTION

Breathing is governed by the nervous system. As with many other topics within neurophysiology, the function of respiratory regulation is inseparable from its neuroanatomy. Structure and function are therefore best discussed concurrently in this case.

The Initiation and Regulation of Breathing in the CNS

Like all skeletal muscles, the diaphragm and other muscles of respiration require *action potentials* to initiate contraction. During relaxed breathing, action potentials traveling along nerves to the inspiratory muscles initiate inspiration, and the cessation of those action potentials results in passive expiration as the inspiratory muscles relax and the elasticity of the lungs mandates their recoil. During active expiration, additional force augments lung recoil. This action is achieved by the stimulation of previously inactive expiratory muscles, including the abdominal recti and internal intercostal muscles.

The neurons responsible for the rhythmic stimulation of the respiratory cycle lie in the medulla and pons (FIGURE 19.1). Efferent nerves from these centers travel through spinal tracts to synapse on motor neurons in the cervical, thoracic, and lumbar spinal cord. These spinal neurons in turn innervate the diaphragm, the intercostal muscles, and the abdominal muscles, respectively. Efferent nerves from motor neurons in the cervical segments, C3 to C5, represent the *phrenic nerves*, which stimulate diaphragmatic contractions to drive relaxed tidal breathing. Damage to the spinal cord at this level, a dreaded sequela of traumatic head and neck injuries, can lead to diaphragmatic paralysis. This acutely life-threatening event often requires mechanical ventilation for survival.

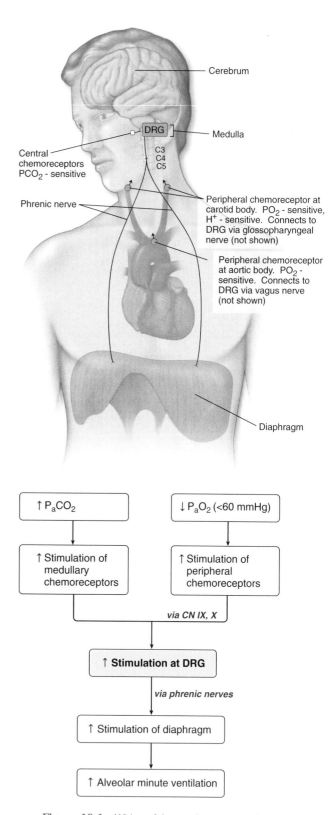

Figure 19.1   Wiring of the respiratory control system.

Anatomically, these tracts can be separated into voluntary and involuntary pathways. Nerve fibers supporting voluntary control of respiration are located in the dorsolateral corticospinal tracts, while involuntary nerve fibers lie ventrally in the cervical

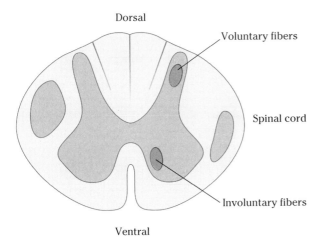

Figure 19.2 The location of voluntary and involuntary nerve fibers in the spinal cord.

spinal column in the medial portion of the anterior horn (FIGURE 19.2). This arrangement provides an anatomic basis for the ability of the CNS to voluntarily override the automatic regulation of respiration for short periods of time. Thus, one can voluntarily breathe above or below the normal rate of respiration, which is usually 12 to 20 breaths per minute for an adult.

Medullary Control The initiation and regulation of breathing in the medulla are mediated primarily by two distinct sets of neurons: the dorsal respiratory group and the ventral respiratory group (FIGURE 19.3).

The **dorsal respiratory group (DRG)** is a bilateral collection of neurons that is the inspiratory rhythm generator of respiration. The DRG lies within the *nuclei of the tractus solitarius*, where afferents of the *vagus nerve* (cranial nerve X) and the *glossopharyngeal nerve* (cranial nerve IX) synapse. These nerves carry information about peripheral changes in pH, PCO_2, and PO_2, enabling the DRG to be responsive to those parameters. In addition, alterations in the physical characteristics of the lungs and noxious stimuli in the airway are transmitted to the DRG and help modulate respiratory rhythm.

The signal generated by the DRG is commonly referred to as a **ramp signal**. Rather than releasing a single burst of action potentials to signal the onset of the respiratory cycle, the DRG initiates inspiration with a weak burst of action potentials that gradually increases in amplitude over the next few seconds. It then ceases for approximately 3 seconds until the cycle begins anew (FIGURE 19.4). The advantages of the generation of inspiration via a ramp signal are twofold. First, it provides for a gradual increase in lung volume during normal inspiration and avoids the gulps of air that would result from the instantaneous firing of all neurons within the DRG at the onset of inspiration. Second, it allows for the control of ventilation by altering either the rate of increase of action potential firing (changing the slope of the ramp) or by the set point at which the DRG ceases to fire (changing the height of the ramp).

The function of the **ventral respiratory group (VRG)**, located anterolaterally to the DRG in the *nucleus ambiguus* and *retroambiguus* of the medulla, is not as clearly defined. The VRG appears to exert its influence during labored respiration. As respiratory effort increases, action potentials from neurons within the VRG both augment the inspiratory ramp signal from the DRG and assist in the stimulation of the expiratory muscles of respiration.

Additional Respiratory Centers in the Pons Though the DRG within the medulla is generally accepted as

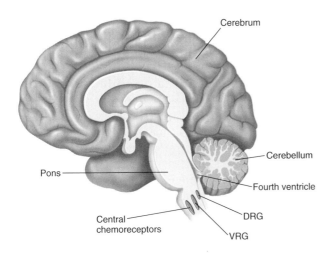

Figure 19.3 Respiration centers in the medulla. The dorsal respiratory group (DRG) is a bilateral collection of neurons within the nuclei of the tractus solitarius in the medulla. These neurons generate the ramp signal that initiates respiration. The ventral respiratory group (VRG), lying anterolaterally to the DRG in the nucleus ambiguus and retroambiguus of the medulla, augments the signal from the DRG during increased respiratory effort and stimulates the muscles of expiration.

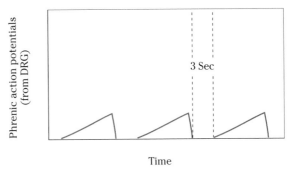

Figure 19.4 The inspiratory ramp signal. Neurons within the DRG initiate inspiration with a weak burst of action potentials that gradually increases in amplitude over the next few seconds and then ceases for approximately 3 seconds until the cycle begins anew.

the rhythm generator of respiration, centers within the pons act to modify both the rate and pattern of respiration. These include the pneumotaxic center, located rostrally in the pons in the nucleus parabrachialis, and the apneustic center, located caudally.

The major function of the **pneumotaxic center** is the regulation of the inspiratory volume and respiratory rate. Signals from this center control the cessation of the inspiratory ramp signal from the DRG, thus determining the length of inspiratory effort. If the pneumotaxic signals are weak, the ramp signal from the DRG continues for a longer period, increasing the duration of inspiration and the resultant tidal volume. Conversely, a strong pneumotaxic signal will stimulate an increased respiratory rate by lowering the set point for the termination of the ramp signal and shortening the respiratory cycle.

The **apneustic center** is a poorly defined group of neurons located in the caudal pons in proximity to both the DRG and the VRG. The function of the apneustic center is unclear, but it may assist in the regulation of the depth of lung inflation during inspiratory effort.

The Role of Central Chemoreceptors   Under normal conditions, central chemoreceptors lying just beneath the ventral surface of the medulla supply the most important sensory inputs to the medullary respiratory centers. Rather than relaying input from a peripheral source, they detect chemical changes in their immediate environment and transmit this information to the respiratory centers in the medulla and pons.

The central chemoreceptors react to the arterial partial pressure of carbon dioxide (P_aCO_2). As P_aCO_2 rises, the central chemoreceptors trigger an increase in ventilation (FIGURE 19.5). If ventilation were to decrease, the consequent rise in P_aCO_2 would drive a corrective increase in ventilation. Approximately 75% to 85% of respiratory drive under normal conditions is due to central chemoreceptor stimulation by CO_2. Thus, the CO_2 level drives the continued ventilation necessary to oxygenate the body tissues. The medullary chemoreceptor response to P_aCO_2 also represents homeostatic regulation of the P_aCO_2 level to keep it within narrow limits. P_aCO_2 homeostasis is critical to the maintenance of a stable blood pH, since P_aCO_2 and pH are related to one another by the **blood buffer equation** (see Chapter 25):

$$P_aCO_2 \leftrightarrow H_2CO_3 \leftrightarrow H^+ + HCO_3^-$$

A stable pH is in turn critical to the function of all the enzymes that constitute physiologic functioning. Obviously, the central chemoreceptors have a crucial physiologic role.

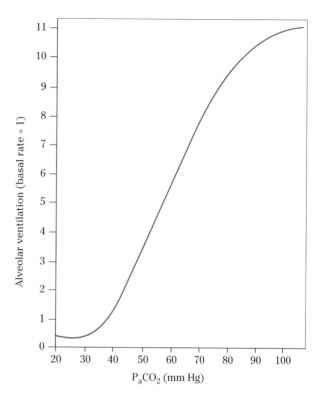

Figure 19.5   The effects of increased P_aCO_2 on respiration. Increased P_aCO_2 increases ventilation. Note that minute ventilation increases when the P_aCO_2 rises above 40 mm Hg.

P_aCO_2 affects the central chemoreceptors by increasing the cerebrospinal fluid (CSF) H^+ concentration, which stimulates the central chemoreceptive neurons. Since cationic H^+ ions do not cross the blood–brain barrier, this works in the following way. An increase in P_aCO_2 drives dissolved carbon dioxide across the blood–brain barrier and results in an increase in the CO_2 content of the CSF. This carbon dioxide is readily hydrated to carbonic acid, which then dissociates into bicarbonate and H^+ (FIGURE 19.6). These H^+ ions then signal the chemoreceptive center to stimulate an increase in respiratory drive through the respiratory centers to maintain normal P_aCO_2.

Given that the central chemoreceptors respond directly only to H^+, one might conclude that low arterial pH (high H^+ concentration) would stimulate the chemoreceptors. However, as noted, cationic H^+ ions cannot cross the blood–brain barrier and CSF pH is slow to change in response to altered blood pH. Studies have shown that it is the peripheral chemoreceptors that have the primary role in the acute respiratory response to acidic blood pH (acidemia). The central chemoreceptors may play a role in the chronic response to acidemia. (See Integrated Physiology Box *Collaboration Between the Lungs and Kidneys in the Regulation of P_aCO_2 and pH.*)

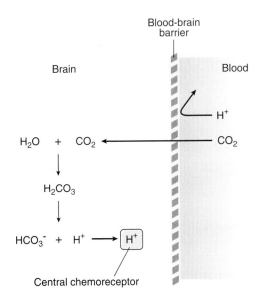

Figure 19.6 The stimulation of central chemoreceptors. Although chemoreceptors ventral to the medulla respond primarily to H$^+$, these charged molecules cannot cross the blood–brain barrier. Instead, carbon dioxide, which readily crosses this barrier, is hydrated in the CNS to H$_2$CO$_3$ that releases H$^+$ ions, which then stimulate the central chemoreceptors.

Peripheral Chemoreceptor Contribution to the Regulation of Breathing

Under normal conditions, changes in the arterial partial pressure of oxygen (P$_a$O$_2$) have a negligible influence on the central regulation of respiration. Teleologically, this may be explained by the flat portion of the O$_2$-hemoglobin equilibrium curve. Recall that in this part of the curve, oxygen saturation of hemoglobin remains within a narrow range over a wide range of P$_a$O$_2$ values. (P$_a$O$_2$ can vary from 60 to 100 mm Hg, while oxygen saturation remains within the 90% to 100% range.) Thus, it would not be advantageous for the body to make P$_a$O$_2$ the primary stimulus for fine control of respiratory drive. This role

has been reserved for P$_a$CO$_2$, which is a direct reflection of blood CO$_2$ content. However, in cases of pathologically low P$_a$O$_2$, peripheral chemoreceptors can respond to changes in P$_a$O$_2$ with an increase in respiratory drive.

Anatomy of the Peripheral Chemoreceptors In humans, the most physiologically studied peripheral chemoreceptors lie in the **carotid bodies**, small paraganglia lying at the bifurcation of the common carotid arteries, bilaterally (FIGURE 19.7). The carotid bodies comprise *glomus cells* that contain oxygen-sensitive potassium channels. Afferent nerves from the carotid bodies travel through *Hering's nerves* to the glossopharyngeal nerves, which synapse in the nuclei of the tractus solitarius at the site of the DRG. These afferent nerves are thus in a position to allow stimuli from the chemoreceptors within the carotid bodies to influence the DRG and contribute to the regulation of respiration. The **aortic bodies** are located at the arch of the aorta and contain chemoreceptors that send afferent signals through the vagus nerves to synapse in the vicinity of the DRG.

The anatomy of the carotid and aortic bodies is designed to maximize the ability of the peripheral chemoreceptors to respond to changes in the P$_a$O$_2$. Located at sites of high arterial blood flow, these specialized bodies receive >2,000 mL/100 g of tissue per minute. Therefore, they remove only an insignificant fraction of oxygen from their blood supply. The result is that the chemoreceptors avoid a false interpretation of decreased P$_a$O$_2$ due to their own oxygen extraction, and they can respond to true changes in P$_a$O$_2$.

Responses to Decreased P$_a$O$_2$ As stated above, changes in P$_a$O$_2$ under normal conditions have a negligible effect on the respiratory centers of the CNS. However, the peripheral chemoreceptors in the

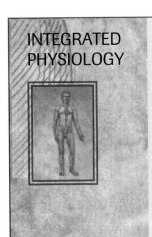

INTEGRATED PHYSIOLOGY

Collaboration Between the Lungs and Kidneys in the Regulation of P$_a$CO$_2$ and pH

While the central chemoreceptors are primarily responsible for governing the P$_a$CO$_2$ level, what happens when a disease state impairs the lungs' capacity to ventilate? In such a case, the P$_a$CO$_2$ climbs because of hypoventilation and, despite increased ventilatory drive, ventilation obviously cannot be increased. The increased P$_a$CO$_2$ lowers the blood pH through the blood buffer equation.

Fortunately, the kidney tubular cells also respond to pH. Acid pH prompts the kidney to excrete H$^+$ ions and to generate more bicarbonate, thus reversing the acidity. The kidney thereby compensates for one of the sequelae of a pathologic deficiency in ventilation (*respiratory acidosis*). The kidney cannot, however, compensate for decreased oxygenation as a result of hypoventilation.

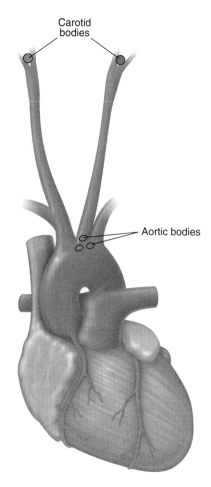

Figure 19.7 Anatomy of the peripheral chemoreceptors. Chemoreceptors located in the carotid bodies (at the bifurcation of the common carotids) and in the aortic bodies (along the arch of the aorta) play an integral role in stimulating an increase in ventilation in response to hypoxemia.

influx of calcium ions through calcium channels, leading to increased cell excitability and transmission of the signal to the DRG through pathways noted above.

However, not all causes of a decrease in the oxygen content of the blood will lead to an increase in respiratory drive via the peripheral chemoreceptors. The carotid chemoreceptors are designed to detect changes in the amount of dissolved O_2 (the PO_2) in the arterial blood supply. In cases of low oxygen content due to insufficient amounts of functional hemoglobin (as occurs in anemia, carbon monoxide poisoning, and methemoglobinemia), the amount of dissolved O_2 remains within normal limits, and the carotid chemoreceptors do not stimulate an increase in ventilation. Meanwhile, the aortic chemoreceptors do appear to respond to anemia by prompting an increase in cardiac output; however, this is not thoroughly understood.

The importance of the peripheral chemoreceptors can be directly observed in animal models in which the carotid bodies are experimentally removed. In such cases, hypoxia paradoxically inhibits respiration by two mechanisms. First, hypoxemia depresses neuronal activity in the respiratory centers in the CNS. Second, the response of the cerebral vasculature to hypoxemia is to reflexively vasodilate to increase cerebral blood flow. This has the effect of lowering the PCO_2 in the CSF, resulting in a decrease in the CO_2-mediated stimulus for ventilation from the central chemoreceptors. Thus, without the peripheral chemoreceptors, the body would fail to adapt to conditions of hypoxemia and would indeed hypoventilate in response to hypoxemia.

carotid and aortic bodies have an important role in the response to hypoxemia because they alone can increase ventilation when arterial hypoxemia occurs. They override the normal P_aCO_2-mediated regulation of respiration and stimulate a maximal increase in respiratory drive when the P_aO_2 decreases to <50 mm Hg (FIGURE 19.8). The peripheral chemoreceptors do not begin to fire until the P_aO_2 drops to <100 mm Hg; however, they do not attain >25% of maximal response until the P_aO_2 falls to <50 mm Hg, the point at which oxygen saturation of hemoglobin begins to drop below 90%—and the point at which oxygen delivery to the tissues is threatened. However, below this point, a further decrease in P_aO_2 has a very potent stimulatory effect on the peripheral chemoreceptors.

In the carotid bodies, decreased P_aO_2 appears to cause a decrease in K^+ influx through oxygen-sensitive K^+ channels in the glomus cells. The drop in P_aO_2 also stimulates adenylate cyclase, leading to an increase in cyclic AMP that further inhibits the K^+ channels. The resultant change in the membrane potential causes an

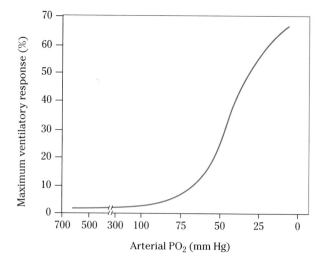

Figure 19.8 The response of peripheral chemoreceptors to hypoxemia. The peripheral chemoreceptors are designed to sense drops in P_aO_2 to <50 mm Hg, the point at which the hemoglobin buffer system begins to fail to adequately oxygenate peripheral tissues. Below this critical set point, the activity of these receptors increases at a rapid rate to stimulate an increase in ventilation.

***Peripheral Responses to Changes in P_aCO_2 and H^+
Concentration*** Like the central chemoreceptors, the
peripheral chemoreceptors respond to elevated
P_aCO_2 by stimulating an increase in ventilation from
the DRG in the medulla. The resultant increase in ventilation, though less potent than that mediated
through the central chemoreceptors, occurs more
rapidly, thereby enabling the body to react quickly to
changes in P_aCO_2, such as during exercise. In addition,
the peripheral chemoreceptors have a very important
role in the response to blood pH. Acid pH stimulates
these receptors, prompting an increase in ventilation
through the DRG. This increase in ventilation drops
the P_aCO_2, shifting the blood buffer equation to the
left, which correctively raises the pH. In disease states
where the blood pH is decreased, as in *metabolic acidosis*, the peripheral chemoreceptors thereby mediate the respiratory compensation (see Chapter 25).

For a summary of central and peripheral regulation of breathing, refer to Figure 19.1.

Other Contributors to the Regulation
of Breathing

Though respiration is primarily regulated by the
CNS response to changes in P_aCO_2, other mechanical
and physical stimuli may modulate the rate and pattern of breathing via the stimulation of peripheral
receptors.

The Hering-Breuer Reflex The **Hering-Breuer reflex** is mediated by **stretch receptors** found within
the smooth muscles of the small airways. Stimulated
by an increase in transmural pressure accompanying
the physical stretching of the lung parenchyma during inflation, these mechanoreceptors send inhibitory signals via afferent fibers in the vagus nerve
to the respiratory centers in the medulla and pons.
The stimulation of these stretch receptors causes
contraction of the expiratory muscles and produces
a period of *apnea* (termination of breathing after end-
expiration). The Hering-Breuer reflex is prominent in
newborns but plays a lesser role in the regulation of
respiration in adults.

Hering and Breuer's paper was one of the first
demonstrations of an autonomic feedback system in
mammals. Josef Breuer is even more famous for the
foundational discovery in the field of psychoanalysis;
he co-authored *Studies in Hysteria* with Sigmund
Freud in 1895.

J Receptors Named for their location in juxtaposi-
tion with capillaries in the pulmonary interstitium, **J
receptors** are thought to mediate *tachypnea* (rapid
breathing) and the sensation of *dyspnea* (shortness
of breath) in certain pathophysiologic states. They

are stimulated both by toxins in the pulmonary circulation and by the distention of the pulmonary vessels, as can occur in pulmonary edema secondary to
heart failure.

Irritant Receptors **Irritant receptors** and **C-fiber receptor** neurons are located in the epithelium of the
large airways (trachea, bronchi, and bronchioles).
They are stimulated by various noxious agents and
result in diverse reflexive responses, including
coughing, sneezing, mucus secretion, and bronchoconstriction. The *cough reflex* is an example of
how irritant receptors function to clear the airways of
debris. When irritant receptors are exposed to noxious stimuli, vagal afferent nerves signal the CNS respiratory centers to direct the inspiration of a large
volume of air. The epiglottis and vocal cords are then
closed to seal this inspired volume within the lungs.
The muscles of expiration contract against this seal
to generate extraordinarily high intrapulmonary
pressures. When the seal is broken as the epiglottis
and vocal cords are reopened, this pressure expels
the air and ideally the source of the initial noxious
stimulus from the lungs. This reflex is inhibited by alcohol, which may account in part for the prevalence
of aspiration pneumonia in alcoholics.

Chest Wall Receptors As with all skeletal muscles,
the muscles of inspiration contain receptors that relay information pertaining to *preload* (stretch before
contraction) and *afterload* (force opposing contraction) to the CNS. For a detailed review of the function
of these receptors, which include the joint, tendon,
and muscle spindle receptors, see Chapter 6. In brief,
they serve to dampen changes in ventilation that
would otherwise result from changes in preload and
afterload through reflexes occurring at the level of the
spinal cord. Afferents from spindle receptors also signal the CNS when afterload becomes excessive, as can
occur in restrictive lung disease or with increased airway resistance, resulting in the sensation of dyspnea.

Sleep

Sleep, defined as the state of unconsciousness
during which an individual can be aroused by stimuli,
is marked by alterations in respiratory drive with resultant changes in the patterns of respiration. Sleep is
generally divided into two major stages: **slow-wave
sleep**, named for the brain waves that predominate
during this stage, and **rapid-eye-movement (REM)
sleep**, a type of sleep marked by prominent brain activity. Disturbances in breathing that can occur during
these stages may have long-term deleterious effects on
several organ systems. (See Clinical Application Box
What Is Sleep Apnea?)

WHAT IS SLEEP APNEA?

A 55-year-old obese man is admitted to the internal medicine service with a complaint of swollen legs and shortness of breath, which has come on gradually over many months. His wife reports no other health problems except for a long history of sleepiness during the day. An EKG is unremarkable except for sinus tachycardia (normal rhythm with increased heart rate) and findings suggestive of an enlarged right atrium. Chest x-ray reveals an enlarged heart, with prominent pulmonary vasculature. After ruling out imminently life-threatening conditions that can cause shortness of breath, the medical resident recommends a sleep study on suspicion of sleep apnea.

Two main types of apnea are observed during sleep: central and obstructive sleep apnea. **Central sleep apnea**, presumed to result from an abnormality in respiratory drive, is characterized by intermittent cessation of the rhythmic activity of the central respiratory centers, resulting in a loss of respiratory muscle activity. Individuals may exhibit hundreds of apneic periods during the night, each potentially lasting up to 1 minute, resulting in significant drops in arterial oxygen saturation and recurrent micro-arousals from sleep to stimulate ventilation. The cause of central sleep apnea is unclear, but the syndrome has been associated with obesity, CNS malformations, and cases of pseudotumor cerebri.

Obstructive sleep apnea, on the other hand, is a disorder related to body mechanics, classically observed in obese individuals with "bull" necks. A decrease in skeletal muscle tone normally occurs during sleep; however, some individuals exhibit such a marked loss of tone in their upper airways during sleep that they intermittently obstruct their pharynx on inspiration. Obesity contributes added bulk to the relaxed airway and predisposes toward obstruction. Upon obstruction, the individual experiences a brief arousal from sleep—frequently unbeknownst to him or her—that restores tone to the upper airway. This cycle may repeat itself hundreds of times throughout the night.

The sequelae of central and obstructive sleep apnea can be severe. Due to the hundreds of micro-arousals that occur during sleep, the apneic individual may suffer marked *hypersomnolence* (sleepiness) that interferes with activities of daily life. These individuals may also be at increased risk for motor vehicle accidents and work-related injuries secondary to hypersomnolence. The long-term sequelae of severe sleep apnea can lead to significant morbidity. The response of the pulmonary vasculature to hypoxemia is to vasoconstrict, and after years of nightly desaturation, the apneic individual may develop pulmonary hypertension and edema.

Fortunately, sleep apnea is a treatable condition. *Polysomnography*, a study that tracks respiratory patterns and blood oxygen content during sleep, is essential in diagnosing and characterizing the degree and type of apnea. Many apneic individuals who require therapeutic intervention benefit from supplemental nighttime oxygen and/or *continuous positive airway pressure (CPAP)* to stent the airway open and maintain favorable oxygen saturations.

Normal Mechanisms of Breathing During Sleep A significant difference between the waking and the sleeping individual lies in the tone of skeletal muscles. In the waking individual, the muscles of the upper airway (nasopharynx, oropharynx, and larynx) are tonically active and maintain the patency of the upper airway. As the diaphragm contracts and the intrapleural and alveolar pressures drop below that of the atmosphere to initiate inspiration, pressure in the upper and lower airways also decreases to subatmospheric levels. Thus, without the contribution of the upper air-

way muscles, tissues of the upper airway tend to collapse, increasing airway resistance and the work of respiration. In the case of obstructive sleep apnea, occlusion of the airway occurs with relaxation of the upper airway musculature. Arousal is necessitated to increase upper airway tone and allow the passage of air.

The regulation of breathing by the respiratory centers in the CNS also differs in the sleep state. Respiratory drive is suppressed in sleep by a decrease in neural activity within the respiratory centers in the medulla. This results primarily from a loss of excitatory influences from other brain centers, such as the *reticular activating system (RAS)*, which are inhibited during sleep. In slow-wave sleep, P_aCO_2 increases in proportion to the decrease in alveolar ventilation. In addition, the drive for respiration in response to increased P_aCO_2 is blunted, permitting this rise in P_aCO_2 to occur without a subsequent increase in ventilation. The P_aCO_2-mediated drive for respiration is further attenuated during REM sleep, and the hypoxemia-stimulated increase in respiratory drive via peripheral chemoreceptors becomes important in maintaining the oxygen saturation of arterial blood. (Without P_aCO_2-mediated drive, some individuals with intrinsic lung disease, such as chronic obstructive pulmonary disease, can experience hypoxemia, with P_aO_2 levels <60 mm Hg.) During REM sleep, irregular patterns of breathing are observed, resulting from the influence of increased brain activity on the normal rhythmic pattern of respiration originating in the medullary and pontine respiratory centers.

Responses to High Altitude

Atmospheric pressure at a given height is simply a function of how much gas bears down from above. At sea level there is considerably more air pushing down from above (>14 pounds per square inch) than in the Himalayas. While the fractional concentration (or mol fraction) of oxygen remains constant at 21% at all altitudes, the partial pressure of oxygen, PO_2, declines with higher altitudes. PO_2 at sea level is 21% of 760 mm Hg, or 160 mm Hg, while PO_2 on Mt. Everest might be 21% of 250 mm Hg, or 53 mm Hg. Physiologically, decreased atmospheric pressure decreases the partial pressure of inspired oxygen (P_IO_2), lowering the partial pressure of oxygen in the alveolus (P_AO_2) and in arterial blood (P_aO_2).

The responses of the lungs to high altitude may be acute or chronic. Acutely, the lungs respond to hypoxemia as described above: the hypoxemia drives hyperventilation through stimulation of the peripheral chemoreceptors. Hyperventilation partially reverses the low alveolar P_AO_2 to maintain favorable gradients for the diffusion of O_2 into the blood. The central chemoreceptors do not contribute to increased ventilation because the P_aCO_2 is low at high altitude; the hypoxia-driven hyperventilation eliminates more CO_2 than usual, dropping P_aCO_2 in the blood and creating a respiratory alkalosis (see Chapter 25). In addition, the cardiac output rises to increase total oxygen delivery to the tissues at lower P_aO_2. Beyond a certain altitude, even very high alveolar minute ventilation cannot produce adequate oxygenation, and respiratory failure ensues. This is why mountain climbers wear oxygen masks and airplanes are equipped with supplemental oxygen in the event of cabin depressurization.

At a habitable high altitude, however, these acute responses attenuate over a period of days as the body makes adjustments to life at a slightly lower P_aO_2. Hypoxia stimulates *erythropoietin* production in the kidneys by an uncertain mechanism—possibly through *hypoxia-inducible transcription factor (HIF-1)*, an enzyme produced in all cells. Erythropoietin causes the bone marrow to produce more red blood cells, increasing the hematocrit and raising the oxygen-carrying capacity of the blood. Thus, even though P_aO_2 is lower and hemoglobin is less saturated with oxygen, there is more total hemoglobin available, ensuring adequate delivery of oxygen to the tissues. (See Clinical Application Box *What Is High-Altitude Pulmonary Edema?*)

PATHOPHYSIOLOGY: ABNORMAL PATTERNS OF BREATHING

A myriad of respiratory patterns is observed in the context of dysfunction in respiratory control. These pathophysiologic states may result from structural changes in the CNS, respiratory abnormalities, behavioral disorders, or cardiovascular disease.

Cheyne-Stokes Breathing

Cyclic waxing and waning of tidal volume separated by periods of apnea is characteristic of **Cheyne-Stokes breathing** (FIGURE 19.9). This periodic pattern of respiration represents an instability of respiratory control that may be observed in association with hypoxia, CNS disease, congestive heart failure, drug overdose, and occasionally sleep. In some cases, Cheyne-Stokes breathing is thought to be caused by a delay in feedback to central and peripheral chemoreceptors secondary to an increase in circulatory transit time. Thus, in conditions such as congestive heart failure, where circulatory time is markedly delayed, changes in respiratory drive from the respiratory centers in the CNS lag behind changes in arterial blood gases originating from the lungs, leading to periodic Cheyne-Stokes breathing. A separate mechanism accounts for such breathing in the case of CNS injury. When CNS injury occurs at the level of the brain stem, there can be a delay in response to information from peripheral and central chemoreceptors, producing periodic breathing, as seen with Cheyne-Stokes breathing.

Biot's Breathing

The pattern of respiration in **Biot's breathing** is characterized by prolonged periods of apnea interrupting normal respiratory cycles. Though the mechanism of Biot's breathing has not been eluci-

CLINICAL APPLICATION

WHAT IS HIGH-ALTITUDE PULMONARY EDEMA?

A 30-year-old man who has been skiing in the Rocky Mountains at 3,500 m collapses on a trail. Upon examination, a doctor at the mountaintop clinic finds the man suffering from dyspnea (shortness of breath), cough, headache, and extreme fatigue. The doctor draws an arterial blood gas (ABG), which reveals a pH of 7.6, a P_aCO_2 of 19, and a P_aO_2 of 38 mm Hg. He then administers oxygen at 6 L by nasal cannula and calls for helicopter evacuation in a portable hyperbaric chamber. The diagnosis is **high-altitude pulmonary edema**.

High-altitude pulmonary edema occurs in some otherwise healthy individuals who rapidly ascend to high altitude. It is a condition where the lungs' vasoconstrictive mechanisms for adapting to low P_AO_2 end up worsening oxygenation instead of improving it. Recall that the pulmonary arteries constrict in parts of the lung that have low P_AO_2 (*pulmonary hypoxic vasoconstriction*). This is an effort to divert blood flow to better-ventilated portions of the lung. At high altitude, however, the reduced P_IO_2 reduces P_AO_2 across the entire lung. Because the vasoconstriction is uniform across all pulmonary vascular beds, it leads to pulmonary hypertension. Finally, high pulmonary pressure produces clinically observable pathology at the level of the capillary. Here, high microvascular pressure leads to stress failure of the pulmonary capillary walls and flooding of the alveoli with fluid exudate.

With many alveoli flooded and unavailable for gas exchange—a state of low; $\dot{V}_A/\dot{Q}$—hypoxemia is the result, as is apparent in this patient's P_aO_2 of 38 mm Hg. At the same time the hypoxemia drives hyperventilation through stimulation of the peripheral chemoreceptors, the P_aCO_2 drops, and pH rises (*alkalosis*). Patients are whenever possible treated with oxygen administration and may also be treated with a hyperbaric chamber and/or descent to lower altitude. Each of these treatments serves to raise P_AO_2 and alleviate the pulmonary hypoxic vasoconstriction that is behind the alveolar flooding.

---

dated, it is thought to represent a form of Cheyne-Stokes breathing, resulting from CNS disease.

Kussmaul Breathing

An increase in the rate of ventilation along with an increase in tidal volumes is observed in **Kussmaul breathing**. Seen most commonly in the setting of diabetic ketoacidosis, this is an attempt to compensate for metabolic acidosis by blowing off carbon dioxide, thereby raising the pH of the blood. However, with prolonged metabolic acidosis, tissues become depleted of bicarbonate and the inspiratory muscles become fatigued, leading to severe acidosis and death.

Summary

- The DRG, located in the medulla, is the primary control center in the regulation of respiration.

- The DRG generates rhythmic ramp signals that connect to the diaphragm via the phrenic nerves. The signals lead to rhythmic diaphragmatic contraction and relaxation, the basis of breathing.

- The DRG emits its rhythmic signal by default and involuntarily, but it is possible temporarily to make voluntary alterations in the ramp signal.

- The VRG assists in the coordination of labored breathing involving forced expiration.

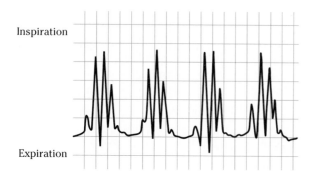

Figure 19.9 Cheyne-Stokes breathing. Note the episodic periods of hyperventilation and apnea. The periods of apnea are associated with a decrease in arterial O_2 saturation.

- The pneumotaxic and apneustic centers influence inspiratory volume and respiratory rate.

- The central chemoreceptors in the ventral medulla prompt the DRG to increase ventilation in response to elevated P_aCO_2. The CO_2 level is the primary driver of respiration under normal circumstances.

- The peripheral chemoreceptors in the carotid bodies and the aortic bodies prompt the DRG to increase ventilation in response to decreased P_aO_2. Peripheral respiratory drive becomes especially significant when P_aO_2 falls to <60 or 50 mm Hg.

- The peripheral chemoreceptors also prompt the DRG to increase ventilation in response to decreased pH (increased H^+ concentration). This is important in the respiratory compensation for metabolic acidosis.

- Other receptors influence breathing through reflex arcs. These include stretch receptors in the smooth muscles of small airways, J receptors in the pulmonary interstitium, and irritant receptors in the epithelium of the large airways.

- Breathing patterns change during sleep: respiratory drive decreases (and P_aCO_2 consequently increases) and pharyngeal muscle tone decreases. In predisposed individuals, the latter may occlude the airway, requiring arousal for recovery of muscle tone and successful inspiration. This is called sleep apnea.

- High altitude can create hypoxemia and hyperventilation via the peripheral chemoreceptors. Adaptation to chronic habitation at high altitude involves increased erythropoietin production, which increases hemoglobin production and in turn the oxygen-carrying capacity of the blood.

- Disease states may lead to abnormal breathing patterns. Examples are Cheyne-Stokes breathing, seen in CNS injury and congestive heart failure, and Kussmaul breathing, seen in diabetic ketoacidosis.

Suggested Reading

Cohen, MI. Central determinants of respiratory rhythm. Annu Rev Physiol. 1981;43:81.

Hackett PH, Roach RC. High-altitude illness. N Engl J Med. 2001;345(2):107–114. Review.

Long S, Duffin J. The neuronal determinants of respiratory rhythm. Prog Neurobiol. 1986;27:101.

Mitchell RA, Burger AJ. Neural regulation of respiration. Am Rev Respir Dis. 1975;111:206.

Rausch SM, Whipp BJ, Wasserman K, Huszczuk A. Role of the carotid bodies in the respiratory compensation for the metabolic acidosis of exercise in humans. J Physiol. 1991;444:567–578.

Richter DW. Generation and maintenance of the respiratory rhythm. J Exp Biol. 1982;100:93.

REVIEW QUESTIONS

Directions: Each of the numbered items or incomplete statements in this section is followed by answers or by completions of the statement. Select the ONE lettered answer or completion that is BEST in each case.

1. A 52-year-old man with a history of alcoholism develops aspiration pneumonia several days after a prolonged drinking binge. Alcohol inhibits the cough reflex, which involves which of the following receptors?

   (A) J receptors
   (B) Irritant receptors
   (C) Carotid body chemoreceptors
   (D) Aortic body chemoreceptors
   (E) Stretch receptors

2. A 26-year-old man who lives at sea level travels to Colorado for a ski trip. Upon arrival at high altitude, he experiences dyspnea. The mechanism by which he adjusts acutely to high altitude includes which of the following?

   (A) Hyperventilation via hypercarbia-driven stimulation of J receptors
   (B) Hyperventilation via stimulation of peripheral chemoreceptors by low arterial pH
   (C) Increased hematocrit via hypoxia-driven stimulation of erythropoietin production
   (D) Hyperventilation via hypercarbia-driven stimulation by central chemoreceptors
   (E) Hyperventilation via hypoxia-driven stimulation by peripheral chemoreceptors

3. A 42-year-old man with severe hypertension has a cerebrovascular accident localized to his medulla and requires mechanical ventilation. The nuclei of the tractus solitarius, the home of the dorsal respiratory group (DRG), appear to be involved. Involvement of the DRG is most likely to obliterate which function of respiratory control?

   (A) Stimulation of expiratory muscles
   (B) Regulation of rate of respiration
   (C) Management of depth of lung inflation
   (D) Stimulation of inspiration via a ramp signal
   (E) Regulation of inspiratory lung volume

ANSWERS TO REVIEW QUESTIONS

1. **The correct answer is B.** Noxious agents stimulate the activity of irritant receptors, which subsequently trigger reflexive responses such as coughing and sneezing in an attempt to remove the noxious stimulus. Alcohol inhibits the cough reflex. J receptors can be stimulated by the distention of pulmonary vessels or by toxins, and mediate tachypnea and dyspnea. Carotid body and aortic body chemoreceptors sense the presence of arterial hypoxemia and stimulate respiratory drive when that is detected. Stretch receptors detect physical stretching of the lung parenchyma and are involved in the Hering-Breuer reflex.

2. **The correct answer is E.** At high altitude relative to sea level, the decreased atmospheric pressure results in lower P_aO_2 and lower P_aCO_2. Peripheral chemoreceptors in the carotid and aortic bodies are stimulated by low P_aO_2, triggering hyperventilation. Peripheral chemoreceptors are also activated by low arterial pH (high H^+ concentration). At high altitude, a respiratory alkalosis (high arterial pH) exists because more CO_2 than usual is eliminated by hypoxia-induced hyperventilation. Central chemoreceptors are activated by increased levels of P_aCO_2 and thus are not involved in the acute adjustment to high altitude. Stimulation of erythropoietin production by hypoxia is part of the chronic response to high altitude. J receptors are thought to mediate tachypnea in certain pathophysiologic states, but by either toxins or distention of pulmonary vessels, not by hypercarbia.

3. **The correct answer is D.** The DRG acts to generate the rhythm of respiration, which it does via initiation of a series of weak action potentials that gradually increase in amplitude, known as a ramp signal. The ventral respiratory group (VRG) in the medulla helps stimulate the muscles involved in expiration under conditions of labored respiration. The pneumotaxic center in the pons regulates both inspiratory volume and respiratory rate. The apneustic center of the pons is thought to manage the depth of lung inflation in inspiration.

RENAL PHYSIOLOGY

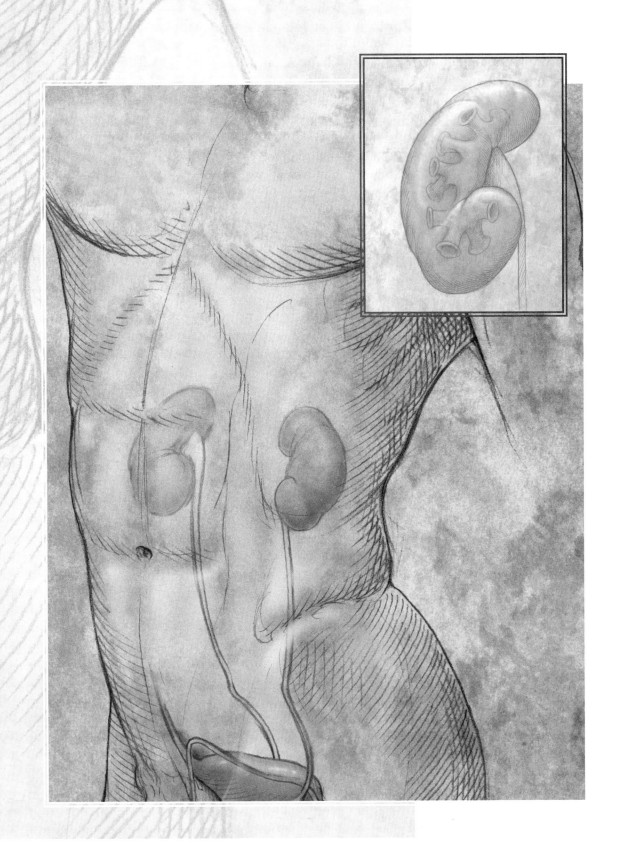

Renal Functions, Renal Circulation, and Glomerular Filtration

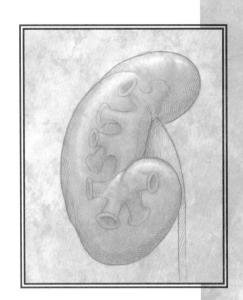

INTRODUCTION

In the most literal sense, the function of the kidney is to filter the blood and produce urine, but its role far transcends this description. The kidney is the principal organ of homeostasis. The second law of thermodynamics states that matter proceeds toward a low-energy equilibrium in which particles are distributed evenly throughout space. Life opposes entropy, or disorder, and it is defined by the energy-requiring organization of matter into stable structures that differ from their surroundings and resist dissipation. The kidneys ensure that despite entropy and changing outside conditions, the inside conditions that maintain the order required for life vary only within a small range. Thus, our evolutionary ancestors were able to migrate from the sea to the land; the kidney has ensured that we carry in our veins the life-supporting ingredients of the sea of our origin.

The kidney's filtration of blood, and modification of that filtrate by epithelial transport, produces urine in order to accomplish the following functions:

1. Control of the composition of body fluids, the concentration of electrolytes, and the excretion of metabolic waste products and foreign substances.

2. Control of body fluid volume and osmolality.

3. Regulation of the acidity of the blood.

The kidney also performs hormonal and metabolic functions, including the production and secretion of erythropoietin, the activation of vitamin D, and the performance of gluconeogenesis. **Gluconeogenesis**, which also occurs in liver and muscle tissue, is the synthesis of glucose from amino acids and other noncarbohydrate precursors.

Part VI (Chapters 20–26) will outline the various functions of the kidney. In this chapter, we focus on the initial step in urine formation, the production of a plasma ultrafiltrate by the process of glomerular filtration.

SYSTEM STRUCTURE: THE KIDNEY

The kidneys are retroperitoneal organs, lying alongside the vertebral column at the level of the T12-L3 vertebrae. Each adult kidney weighs between 115 g and 170 g and is approximately the size of the human hand made into a fist. FIGURE 20.1 shows the urinary system and the gross anatomical features of the human kidney. The medial side of the kidney has an indentation, the *hilum*, where the renal artery and nerves enter the kidney and the renal veins exit. The funnel-shaped *renal pelvis* also exits at the hilum. It then connects to the *ureter*, forming a contractile conduit that pushes the urine from the kidney to the bladder.

The kidneys are covered by a fibrous capsule. On bisecting a kidney, we encounter two layers of tissue, an outer region called the **cortex** and an inner region called the **medulla**. The medulla forms 10 to 18 cone-shaped structures, the *renal pyramids*. The apex of each pyramid, called the *papilla*, projects into the urinary collection space. Urine expressed from each papilla is collected by a *minor calyx*, the smallest

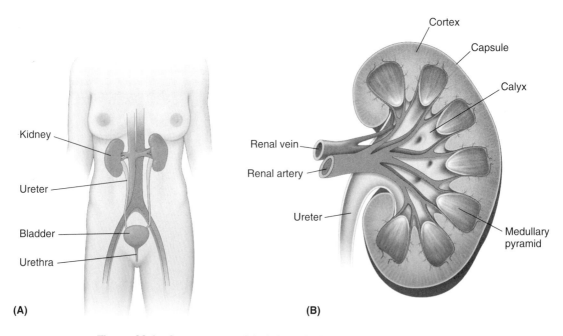

(A)

Kidney
Ureter
Bladder
Urethra

(B)

Cortex
Capsule
Calyx
Renal vein
Renal artery
Ureter
Medullary pyramid

Figure 20.1 Gross anatomy of the kidney. **A.** The urinary system. **B.** The kidney.

branch of the urinary collection system. The minor calyces coalesce to form *major calyces*, which in turn coalesce to form the renal pelvis.

The Vasculature

The kidney is one of the most well-perfused tissues in the human body. Although the kidneys make up less than 0.5% of total body weight, they receive 20% to 25% of total cardiac output; that is, about 1.25 liters per minute. This disproportionately large amount of blood flow enables the kidney to excrete large quantities of nitrogenous waste products while at the same time requiring the kidney mechanisms to avoid excessive losses of fluid and nutrients. It is important that the kidney has the ability to regulate renal blood flow and glomerular filtration rate independently, and in some disorders of reduced blood volume or increased osmolarity, the kidney has the ability to compensate through mechanisms that reduce renal blood flow.

The renal vascular system is illustrated in FIGURE 20.2. The **renal artery** enters the kidney at the hilum. It branches into *interlobar arteries* that run between the renal pyramids. At the junction between the cortex and the medulla, the interlobar arteries form arching branches, the *arcuate arteries*. The arcuate arteries, in turn, give off perpendicular branches that rise toward the capsule, the *interlobular arteries*. From the interlobular arteries arise the **afferent arterioles**, which supply blood to the **glomerular capillaries**. The glomerular capillaries coalesce to form the **efferent arterioles**, which then supply the **peritubular capillaries**, a capillary network surrounding the renal tubules. Each glomerulus is a discrete functioning unit connected to its own afferent and efferent arteriole. A subset of the peritubular capillaries called the **vasa recta** supplies the tubules in the medulla. As blood exits the peritubular capillaries, it enters the venous system, which follows approximately the same course as the arteries.

Note that the renal circulation has two sets of capillary beds in sequence: glomerular and peritubular. Blood exiting the glomerular capillaries remains in the arterial system and passes through the peritubular capillaries before entering the venous system. The kidney is one of a few organs with this unusual circulatory anatomy (another is the pituitary gland). Why does the renal circulation have such an unusual design? Each of the kidney's two capillary beds has a specialized function: The glomerular capillaries filter large volumes, while the peritubular capillaries reabsorb fluid and solute. Flow regulation through each of these capillary beds is critical to kidney function. As we will see, the structure allows for integration of filtration and reabsorption.

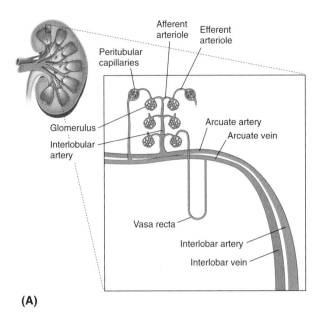

(A)

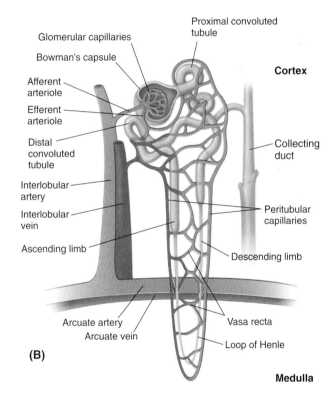

(B)

Figure 20.2 The vascular system of the kidney. **A.** The vasa recta are extended peritubular capillaries that come from the efferent arterioles in the renal cortex. The vasa recta loop down into the medulla and then empty into the arcuate vein. **B.** Details of the vasculature of the renal tubules.

The Nephron

The functional unit of urine formation in the kidney is the **nephron** (FIGURE 20.3). Each kidney contains approximately 1 million nephrons (range of approximately 600,000 to 1.2 million). The kidney

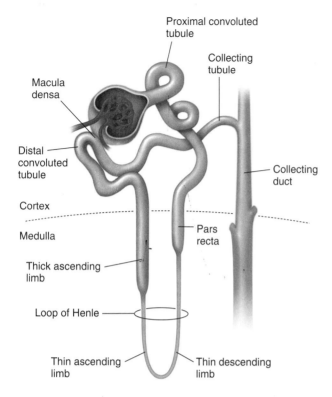

Figure 20.3   Basic components of the nephron.

cannot regenerate nephrons. When nephrons are lost from disease or by normal aging, the kidneys compensate with adaptive changes in the remaining nephrons.

The initial part of the nephron, located in the cortex, is the **glomerulus**, the network of capillaries just described. The glomerulus filters plasma into the urinary space of a surrounding pouch called **Bowman's capsule** (the parietal epithelium of the glomerulus and its basement membrane). The filtrate then flows into the **proximal tubule**, which forms several coils before dipping toward the medulla. From there, the fluid flows into the **medullary proximal straight tubule** and the **loop of Henle**, a hairpin-shaped structure divided into the **thin descending limb**, the **thin ascending limb**, and the **thick ascending limb**. The fluid continues to the **distal tubule**. A specialized segment of the distal tubule, at a point where the tubule passes between the afferent and efferent arterioles, makes up the **macula densa**. Distal tubules from several nephrons empty into a **cortical collecting duct**. Cortical collecting ducts then become **medullary collecting ducts** in the outer medulla. The medullary collecting duct descends to the tip of the renal papilla (inner medulla), emptying into the collecting system.

Although all nephrons share the same general features, they exhibit some structural variation depending on their location within the kidney. Nephrons can be broadly divided into two groups: cortical nephrons

and juxtamedullary nephrons. **Superficial nephrons** have glomeruli in the outer regions of the cortex and short loops of Henle, which lack a thin ascending limb and barely dip into the medulla. Their peritubular capillaries form extensive networks surrounding the tubules, allowing for an efficient exchange of substances and water between the tubules and the circulation. In contrast, **juxtamedullary nephrons** have glomeruli near the medulla, and their loops of Henle travel deep into the medulla. Note that all glomeruli are in the cortex. Juxtamedullary nephrons have vasa recta. These long, thin peritubular capillaries travel alongside the loops of Henle into the medulla and then loop back toward the cortex. The vasa recta play an important role in the concentration of urine and in nature, mammals that must excrete concentrated urine have the longest nephron loops.

The Glomerulus

During development, the glomerular capillaries push into the closed end of the proximal tubule, like a fist pressing into a balloon (FIGURE 20.4). This invagination forms Bowman's capsule (the punched-in "balloon"), made up of two epithelial layers—the visceral layer tightly enveloping the "fist" of glomerular capillaries, and the parietal outer layer. The space between these two layers (the inside of the balloon), which remains connected to the lumen of the proximal tubule, forms the urinary space, or **Bowman's space.** The visceral epithelial cells, or *podocytes*, tightly envelope the capillaries, adhering to them with foot processes. The histology of the glomerulus is illustrated in FIGURE 20.5.

FIGURE 20.6 is a closer view of the layers that substances must cross in traveling from the blood into Bowman's space. These layers make up the **filtration barrier.** The first layer is the capillary endothelium. The endothelium has many holes, or *fenestrations*, that make it highly permeable to water and also allow small molecules, including many plasma proteins, to pass freely. Covering the endothelium is a basement membrane containing collagen type IV and negatively charged proteoglycans. The basement membrane provides a charge barrier for the negatively charged plasma proteins. The third layer is the visceral epithelium. In the visceral epithelium, small spaces between the podocytes, called **filtration slits,** are bridged by a thin diaphragm. The filtrate passes through the filtration slits and flows around the foot processes into Bowman's space.

The Juxtaglomerular Apparatus

As shown in Figure 20.5, the region where the distal tubule passes between the afferent and efferent arterioles contains a set of structures, the macula

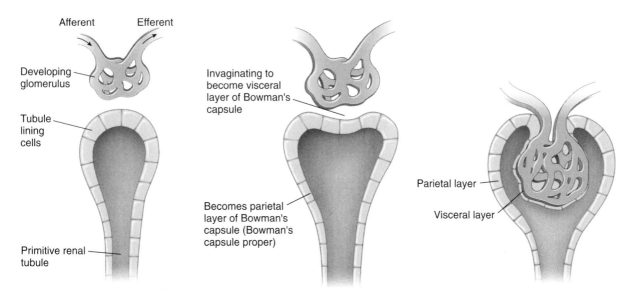

Figure 20.4   Development of the glomerulus. The invagination of the glomerular capillaries into the closed end of the proximal tubule forms Bowman's capsule.

densa, and the **juxtaglomerular cells**, known together as the **juxtaglomerular apparatus.** The epithelial cells of the distal tubule in this region form the macula densa. The juxtaglomerular cells are modified smooth muscle cells in the arteriolar walls adjacent to the macula densa. They secrete the enzyme renin, stored in intracytoplasmic granules. The important role these structures play in the autoregulation of renal blood flow will be discussed later in this chapter.

SYSTEM FUNCTION: THE KIDNEY

To produce urine, the kidney first generates a cell-free and protein-free ultrafiltrate by glomerular filtration. The urine then continues from Bowman's space into the tubular system. In the tubules, the quantities of particular substances in the urine are modified by further exchange between the tubules and the peritubular capillaries. Thus, three processes determine

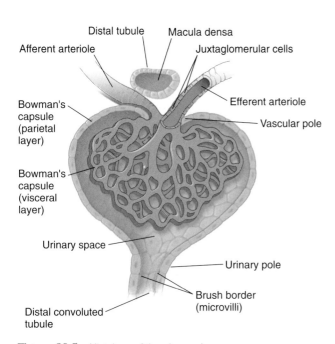

Figure 20.5   Histology of the glomerulus.

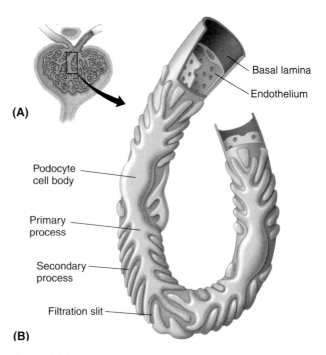

Figure 20.6   The glomerular filtration barrier. **A.** Podocytes and fenestrations. **B.** A closer view of the same.

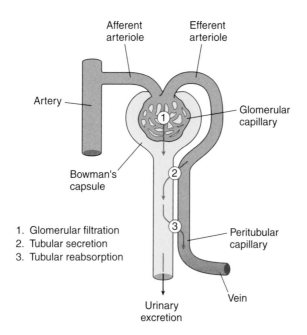

Figure 20.7 Three essential renal mechanisms. The general processes in the nephron that determine urine composition are glomerular filtration, reabsorption, and secretion.

the amount of a substance excreted in the urine: (1) glomerular filtration, (2) reabsorption from the tubule lumen back into the peritubular capillaries, and (3) secretion from the peritubular capillaries into the tubule lumen (FIGURE 20.7). The processes are related in the following mass balance equation:

Amount of substance excreted
= amount of substance filtered
+ amount secreted − amount reabsorbed

Glomerular Filtration

The initial step in urine formation is the generation of a plasma ultrafiltrate by the process of **glomerular filtration**. As mentioned previously, substances traveling from the glomerular capillaries into the urinary space must traverse the filtration barrier, composed (sequentially) of a fenestrated capillary endothelium, the negatively charged basement membrane, and the filtration slits between podocytes. Because of its physical characteristics, the filtration barrier allows large amounts of water to pass through, and it sorts other molecules by size and charge. The fenestrations in the endothelium allow water and most molecules to pass through, but they are too small for cells to penetrate. The basement membrane, with its meshwork of connective tissue, provides a barrier for larger molecules. In addition, because of its negative charge, the basement membrane is particularly impermeable to negatively charged macromolecules, such as plasma albumin.

More cationic proteins, like immunoglobulins, are not freely filtered because of their larger size. Small-molecular-weight solutes, whether positively or negatively charged, are freely filtered (e.g., sodium, chloride, bicarbonate). The diaphragms across the filtration slits between podocytes provide an additional filter. Nephrin, a protein associated with the diaphragms, is thought to be important in blocking the filtration of proteins in the blood. The podocyte cytoskeleton also plays a role in preventing protein filtration. In all, the normal adult may filter only 1 g of albumin a day, although an amount approximately equal to 35,000 g is delivered to the kidney in 24 hours. Because albumin is reabsorbed by the renal tubules, less than 25 mg may be lost in the urine.

The filtration of molecules on the basis of size and charge is demonstrated by an experiment measuring the filtration of dextrans—polysaccharides that can be synthesized with varying charges and molecular weights (FIGURE 20.8). The larger the dextran molecule is, the smaller the fraction that is filtered into the urinary space will be. Moreover, for any given molecular weight, a smaller fraction of negatively charged (anionic) dextrans is filtered compared to their neutral or positively charged (cationic) counterparts. TABLE 20.1 lists the filterability of various plasma molecules according to molecular weight, with "filterability" representing how fast a given molecule is filtered compared to water filtration. As might be expected from these data, the ultrafiltrate generated by glomerular filtration has approximately the same concentration as the plasma of electrolytes, glucose, and other small molecules, but it is largely cell-free and protein-free. Note, however, that some small molecules, such as calcium and free fatty acids, travel in the plasma mostly

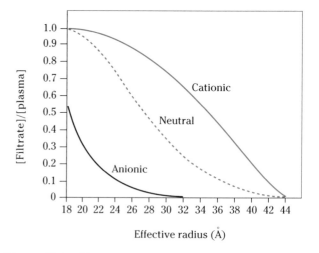

Figure 20.8 Filtration rates of dextrans. Larger molecules and negatively charged molecules are less freely filtered. A filterability value of 1 indicates that the molecules are filtered as freely as water; a value of 0 implies that they are not filtered at all.

Table 20.1 THE FILTERABILITY OF PLASMA MOLECULES

Substance	Molecular Weight	Filterability
Water	18	1
Glucose	180	1
Myoglobin	17,000	0.75
Hemoglobin	68,000	0.03
Albumin	69,000	<0.01

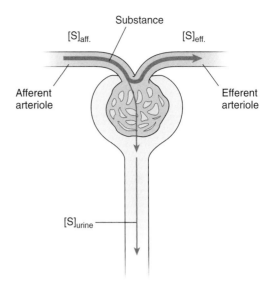

$$(\dot{V}_{aff})([S]_{aff}) = (\dot{U})([S]_{urine}) + (\dot{V}_{eff})([S]_{eff})$$

Figure 20.9 The excretion of a substance S into the urine. We can write a mass balance equation between the amount of substance coming into the glomerulus per unit time: [(volume of plasma entering in afferent arteriole) × (concentration of S in afferent plasma)] and the amount leaving the glomerulus, which equals the amount excreted in urine [(volume of urine) × (concentration in urine)] plus the amount in efferent arteriole [(volume of efferent plasma) × (concentration of S in efferent plasma)].

bound to proteins. These bound molecules are also largely excluded from the ultrafiltrate. For example, only about 50% of plasma calcium is filterable; the remaining component is bound to albumin.

In some renal diseases, the glomerular basement membrane is damaged and loses its negative charge. The consequences of this injury are predictable. The filtration barrier becomes more permeable to the negatively charged plasma proteins, and large amounts of protein (mostly albumin) are lost in the urine where it can be measured clinically, a condition called **proteinuria**. Extreme losses of albumin from the plasma can lead to a shift in fluid from the blood vessels to the extracellular spaces due to decreased oncotic pressure, leading to edema. Severely low albumin due to heavy proteinuria is one of the causes of edema in the condition called **nephrotic syndrome** (see Chapter 22).

Measuring GFR Glomerular filtration rate (GFR) is the volume of plasma that is filtered in the glomeruli per unit time, usually reported in mL/min. For adults, the GFR averages 125 mL/min, or 180 L/day. This tremendous filtration rate is the first step in a process that allows the kidneys to regulate the composition and volume of body fluids. It is important to note that the GFR is only a fraction of the blood flow through the glomerular capillaries (about 20%); that is, most of the fluid and substances passing through the glomerular capillaries remain in the glomerular capillaries and are not filtered (FIGURE 20.9).

The plasma volume that leaves the capillary to enter Bowman's space per unit time (e.g., 1 minute) is the GFR. Estimating a patient's GFR has several important clinical applications, from assessing the degree of damage to the kidneys to determining appropriate doses of medications (because many medications are excreted in the urine). We can measure GFR by using substances that are freely filtered in the glomerulus but are neither secreted nor reabsorbed in the tubules. ("Freely filtered" means that filtered plasma holds the same concentration of a substance as unfiltered plasma.) One such substance is a polyfructose called **inulin** (different from insulin) that is found in dahlia roots and the Jerusalem artichoke. Because inulin is neither secreted nor reabsorbed, all the inulin that is filtered by the glomerulus is excreted in the urine (FIGURE 20.10). We can state this concept as a mass balance equation:

Filtered inulin = Excreted inulin

Recall that the mass of a solute equals the concentration of the solute times the volume of the solution. Thus, the amount of inulin filtered per minute equals the volume of plasma filtered per minute—the GFR—times the plasma inulin concentration, $[inulin]_P$. Similarly, the amount of excreted inulin equals the urine flow volume per minute ($\dot{V}$) times the concentration of inulin in the urine, $[inulin]_U$. We can then rewrite the mass balance equation as:

$$GFR \times [inulin]_P = \dot{V} \times [inulin]_U$$

(Filtered inulin = Excreted inulin)

Solving for GFR, we come up with:

$$GFR = \dot{V} \times [inulin]_U / [inulin]_P$$

Thus, if we infuse inulin into a patient so that it reaches a steady-state plasma concentration, we can measure the volume of urine and the inulin

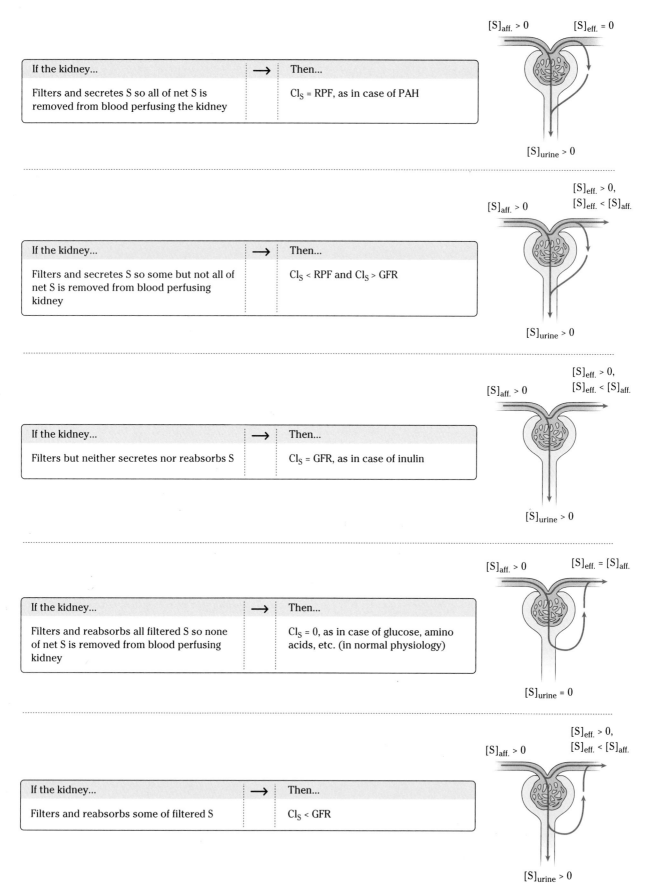

If the kidney...	$\rightarrow$	Then...
Filters and secretes S so all of net S is removed from blood perfusing the kidney		$Cl_S = RPF$, as in case of PAH

$[S]_{aff.} > 0$ $\quad\quad\quad [S]_{eff.} = 0$

$[S]_{urine} > 0$

If the kidney...	$\rightarrow$	Then...
Filters and secretes S so some but not all of net S is removed from blood perfusing kidney		$Cl_S < RPF$ and $Cl_S > GFR$

$[S]_{aff.} > 0$ $\quad\quad\quad [S]_{eff.} > 0,$ $[S]_{eff.} < [S]_{aff.}$

$[S]_{urine} > 0$

If the kidney...	$\rightarrow$	Then...
Filters but neither secretes nor reabsorbs S		$Cl_S = GFR$, as in case of inulin

$[S]_{aff.} > 0$ $\quad\quad\quad [S]_{eff.} > 0,$ $[S]_{eff.} < [S]_{aff.}$

$[S]_{urine} > 0$

If the kidney...	$\rightarrow$	Then...
Filters and reabsorbs all filtered S so none of net S is removed from blood perfusing kidney		$Cl_S = 0$, as in case of glucose, amino acids, etc. (in normal physiology)

$[S]_{aff.} > 0$ $\quad\quad\quad [S]_{eff.} = [S]_{aff.}$

$[S]_{urine} = 0$

If the kidney...	$\rightarrow$	Then...
Filters and reabsorbs some of filtered S		$Cl_S < GFR$

$[S]_{aff.} > 0$ $\quad\quad\quad [S]_{eff.} > 0,$ $[S]_{eff.} < [S]_{aff.}$

$[S]_{urine} > 0$

Figure 20.10 The clearance of S under different types of renal handling.

concentrations in the plasma and urine to obtain an estimate of the patient's GFR.

When physicians want to estimate GFR, they use another method that is somewhat less accurate but simpler than the inulin method. The common clinical technique for estimating GFR entails measuring levels of **creatinine**, a product of creatine phosphate hydrolysis in skeletal muscle. It enters the plasma from muscle at a relatively fixed rate determined by the muscle mass of the individual. In the kidney, creatinine is filtered by the glomerulus and is secreted to a small extent but not reabsorbed. Thus, measuring plasma and urine creatinine levels and urine volume per time (a standard is 24 hours) allows us to estimate GFR in a manner analogous to the inulin method. Urea, a product of protein metabolism, is also freely filtered but is not a good quantitative marker of GFR because it is significantly reabsorbed by the tubules. Both creatinine and urea rise in the blood when GFR is reduced in kidney failure. The blood concentration of creatinine is equal to the production rate of creatinine divided by the clearance of creatinine. The blood concentration of urea (usually given as the blood urea nitrogen, or BUN) is equal to the production rate of urea divided by the clearance of urea. The concept of clearance is discussed later in this chapter.

Measuring RPF Renal plasma flow (RPF) is the volume of plasma that enters the kidney per minute. This is different from GFR, the number of milliliters per minute that is _filtered_. GFR is always a small fraction (about 20%) of RPF. Measuring RPF requires a substance that is completely eliminated from the plasma entering the kidney, and thus it is completely excreted in the urine. No substance can be completely filtered because not all plasma water is filtered, and the concentration of solutes in the filtered quantity cannot exceed the concentration in the unfiltered quantity. Therefore, to eliminate an amount of a solute in excess of that filtered requires a secretory mechanism. Note from Figure 20.10 that to eliminate all of the substance (S) from the plasma entering the kidney, all of S passing through the peritubular capillaries would have to be secreted into the urine, with no reabsorption into the circulation downstream. A commonly used substance that approximates these characteristics at low concentrations is **para-aminohippurate (PAH)**. At low PAH plasma concentrations, all the PAH delivered to the kidney is excreted in the urine. Consequently, we can state:

Mass of PAH entering kidney = Mass of PAH excreted in urine

The mass of PAH entering the kidney per minute equals the plasma volume entering the kidney per minute—the RPF—times the concentration of PAH in

the plasma, $[PAH]_P$. The mass of PAH excreted in the urine per minute equals the urine flow rate ($\dot{V}$) times the concentration of PAH in the urine, $[PAH]_U$. Thus:

$$RPF \times [PAH]_P = \dot{V} \times [PAH]_U$$

Solving for RPF:

$$RPF = \dot{V} \times [PAH]_U / [PAH]_P$$

This equation lets us estimate RPF by using an infusion of PAH and measuring the urine output and the concentrations of PAH in the plasma and urine. Other methods that do not require complete elimination of the solute into the urine can be used to measure renal plasma flow, and these will be discussed in Chapter 21.

Measuring RBF The renal plasma flow can be used to derive the **renal blood flow (RBF)**. Recall that hematocrit (HCT) equals the percentage of blood volume occupied by red blood cells (e.g., an HCT of 40% indicates that a fraction of 0.4 of total blood volume is made up of red blood cell mass). Everything else is the plasma; thus, $(1 - HCT)$ represents the fraction of blood volume occupied by plasma. In the example of a HCT of 40%, the fraction of blood that is plasma is 0.6. Consequently,

$$RPF = (RBF)(\text{fraction of blood that is plasma})$$

$$RPF = (RBF)(1 - HCT)$$

$$RBF = RPF/(1 - HCT)$$

If we measure the RPF, we calculate RBF. By determining the RBF and with knowledge of the cardiac output, we can assess what percentage of the cardiac output is headed for the kidneys.

Filtration Fraction The **filtration fraction** represents the fraction of renal plasma flow that is filtered through the glomerulus. This can be stated mathematically as:

$$\text{Filtration fraction} = GFR/RPF$$

Normally, this fraction is approximately 20%. In other words, of the plasma entering the kidney, 20% is filtered through the glomerular capillaries and the other 80% exits the glomeruli via the efferent arterioles and continues on to the peritubular capillaries.

Renal Clearance The concept of clearance focuses on the excretory function of the kidney. **Clearance** of a particular substance is defined as the volume of incoming plasma from which all substance is removed and excreted into the urine per minute. We have already seen two special examples of clearance measurements. For inulin, the clearance equals the GFR, because all the inulin in the volume of plasma filtered by the glomerulus each minute (GFR) ends up in the urine. For PAH, the clearance equals the RPF, and therefore, all the plasma entering the kidney per minute is completely cleared of PAH (Figure 20.10). When a solute is only handled by filtration (and not by secretion or reabsorption), as in the case of inulin, the value of clearance actually corresponds to a real value of plasma volume filtered. This is not the case in the clearance of a solute such as PAH, which is so readily secreted that none of the solute reaches the renal vein. Although the solute was fully cleared from plasma, the total renal plasma volume never left the circulation.

Note that the value for the clearance of any specific substance S is a *calculated* number used to describe the way the kidney handles substance S. The kidney may leave some of S in the blood, but we still say there was clearance of S. The clearance of S is a calculated theoretical number answering this question: Given the amount of S excreted by the kidney (amount filtered + amount secreted − amount reabsorbed), what volume of incoming plasma per minute would have to be totally cleared of S to surrender that amount of excreted S?

It may help to imagine that the plasma flowing through the kidney comes in two volume compartments: one containing the S that will not be excreted after filtration, secretion, and reabsorption; and one containing the S that will be excreted after filtration, secretion, and reabsorption (FIGURE 20.11). This imagined volume containing the S that is destined for excretion is the volume that is "cleared" of S. Then, imagine that the two compartments coalesce upon leaving the kidney in the veins, after being worked on by filtration, secretion, and reabsorption. Imagine that the S from the nonexcreted compartment

diffuses into the cleared compartment. That is how we can have a clearance for S without removing *all* of S from the RPF.

We can derive a general formula for clearance by beginning with a **mass balance** equation for hypothetical substance S. As before, $[S]_P$ and $[S]_U$ represent the concentrations of S in the plasma and urine, and $\dot{V}$ represents the volume of urine produced per minute. Now, we will denote the clearance of S as Cl_S, the volume of plasma per minute from which S has been removed and excreted into the urine. Using the concept of mass balance, we write:

$$\text{Mass cleared from the plasma/time}$$
$$= \text{Mass found in the urine/time}$$

Because mass/time equals concentration times volume/time, we find that:

$$[S]_P \times Cl_S = [S]_U \times \dot{V}$$

Solving for clearance yields:

$$Cl_S = [S]_U \times \dot{V}/[S]_P$$

We can verify now, looking back to our earlier equations, that the clearance of inulin equals the GFR and the clearance of PAH equals the RPF. We can also verify that the units of clearance are mL/min (the units for concentration cancel out and $\dot{V}$, the urine flow rate or volume of urine per minute, can be measured in mL/min). These units are in accordance with our definition of clearance as the volume of plasma being cleared of a substance per minute. Although we have only discussed renal clearance, the concept of clearance has multiple applications beyond renal physiology; for example, the clearance of toxins and drugs from the plasma is important in hepatic physiology.

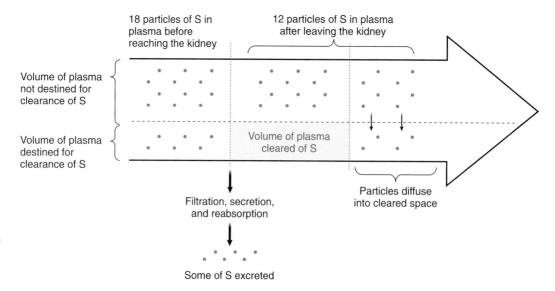

Figure 20.11 Two imaginary compartments of plasma laden with substance S. Each dot represents a particle of substance S. One compartment is destined for renal clearance of S and one is not.

Determinants of GFR and RBF

As in other capillary beds, the rate of fluid filtered by the glomerulus is determined by the balance of oncotic and hydrostatic forces. These forces are illustrated in FIGURE 20.12. The balance of forces is summarized in the Starling relationship. According to the Starling relationship, flow is proportional to a permeability coefficient and the driving forces that apply:

$$GFR = K_f [(P_G - P_B) - (\Pi_G - \Pi_B)]$$

The **filtration coefficient (K_f)** is the product of the hydraulic conductivity of the glomerular capillary and the surface area available for filtration. The hydraulic conductivity, in turn, represents the flux of water per unit time for a defined pressure gradient and surface area. As we saw earlier, the physical properties of the glomerular filtration barrier, particularly the fenestrations in the endothelium, make it highly permeable. Consequently, in the kidney, the hydraulic permeability is more than 50 to 100 times greater than many other peripheral capillary beds, accounting in large part for the high filtration rate in the glomeruli. Another factor in sustaining high filtration is the extremely large total filtration surface area, which may be as much as $0.3 \ m^2$.

The **hydrostatic pressure in the glomerular capillary (P_G)** favors filtration, while the **hydrostatic pressure in Bowman's space (P_B)** opposes it. Normally, the glomerular capillary pressure is significantly greater than the pressure in Bowman's space. Thus, the net hydrostatic force, $P_G - P_B$, favors filtration. In fact, the hydrostatic gradient for filtration is especially favorable in the glomerular capillary bed compared to other beds in the body; so the high GFR is not only attributable to high K_f. An anatomic characteristic that most distinguishes glomerular filtration from filtration in other beds (e.g., skeletal muscle), is that glomerular filtration occurs into an interstitial space (i.e., Bowman's space), that is infinitely compliant by virtue of being connected to the outside world. Bowman's space can accommodate 180 L/day and can remain at a pressure of about 12 mm Hg.

The **oncotic pressure in the glomerular capillaries (ΠG)** opposes filtration. Because the glomerular ultrafiltrate is nearly protein-free, the oncotic pressure in Bowman's space, Π_B, is close to zero. Therefore, the net oncotic pressure favors absorption into the glomerular capillaries. (See Clinical Application Box *Dialysis*.)

FIGURE 20.13 shows the dynamics of the Starling forces along the glomerular capillary. The net hydrostatic pressure remains fairly constant because the capillaries, with their large cross-sectional area, provide little resistance to flow. In the initial portions of the glomerular capillaries, the glomerular oncotic pressure (keeping fluid in) is significantly lower than the net hydrostatic pressure (pushing fluid out), so the balance of forces favors filtration. As the blood travels along the capillary, protein-free fluid is filtered into the urinary space, making the proteins remaining in the capillaries more and more concentrated, thereby raising the glomerular oncotic pressure. The oncotic pressure continues to increase

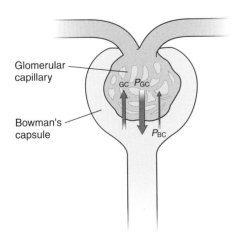

Figure 20.12 Starling forces in the glomerulus. P_G = hydrostatic pressure in glomerulus, P_B = hydrostatic pressure in Bowman's capsule, Π_G = oncotic pressure in the glomerulus. (The oncotic pressure in Bowman's capsule, Π_B, is close to zero.)

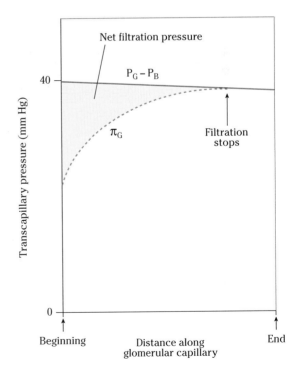

Figure 20.13 Changes in Starling forces along the glomerular capillary. The solid line is net hydrostatic pressure and the dotted line is net oncotic pressure. The net hydrostatic pressure remains fairly constant, while the net oncotic pressure increases as the proteins in the glomerular capillary become increasingly concentrated.

CLINICAL APPLICATION

DIALYSIS

When the kidneys fail to regulate the composition of the blood, whether acutely or chronically, it is sometimes necessary to restore the blood composition to desired levels by machine. This process is called **dialysis**, and there are two forms: hemodialysis and peritoneal dialysis. In *hemodialysis*, the patient's blood is circulated through an extracorporeal circuit, where it is pumped through selectively permeable synthetic capillary tubing (the dialysis membrane) bathed in an electrolyte solution similar in osmotic concentration to that of normal plasma, but devoid of urea and creatinine and with desired concentrations of solutes such as potassium and bicarbonate (the dialysate). Because the dialysate is low in substances that accumulate in the blood during kidney failure, the dialysate provides a favorable gradient to remove unwanted solutes from the blood by passive diffusion into the dialysis solution. The mechanism responsible for the movement of fluid from the blood to the dialysate is similar to the Starling factors that govern glomerular filtration. The membrane has intrinsic parameters of surface area and hydraulic conductivity, and pressure gradients favoring ultrafiltration are achieved through the use of blood and dialysate pumps.

In *peritoneal dialysis*, dialysate fluid is infused by catheter into the patient's abdominal cavity where the peritoneal membrane provides the surface for unwanted solute removal (by diffusion) and ultrafiltration. The peritoneum provides a large surface area, and the pressure gradients that drive ultrafiltration from body fluids to intraperitoneal space are osmotic gradients achieved by infusing concentrated glucose solutions into the abdomen. In a diabetic, this could result in hyperglycemia. Unwanted substances diffuse into the fluid, which is withdrawn through the catheter. In many cases, chronic kidney disease leads to dialysis. Renal transplantation is also used to treat advanced renal failure. Usually, kidney function declines to nearly 10% of normal before dialysis is indicated.

until it may become as strong as the net hydrostatic pressure. At this point, the forces for and against filtration balance out, and filtration ceases (filtration pressure equilibrium). Filtration pressure equilibrium, however, is not inevitable. At high plasma flow rates, a balance of pressures favoring and opposing filtration will not be achieved, because there will be less of an increase in plasma oncotic pressure, despite high filtration. In the situation of very high plasma flow rates, GFR will become a maximum value. At low renal plasma flow, equilibrium is more likely to be achieved. The K_f is not a determinant of GFR under conditions of filtration pressure equilibrium.

Figure 20.14 graphs the hydrostatic pressures along the renal arterial system. Observe that the greatest drops in pressure occur along the afferent and efferent arterioles. Note also that in the peritubular capillaries, the hydrostatic pressure is much lower than in the glomerular capillaries. In the peritubular capillaries, consequently, the oncotic forces favoring reabsorption are greater than hydrostatic forces favoring filtration, and net reabsorption takes place. On the whole, efferent arteriolar resistance plays a particularly important role in determining the

Starling relationships in the glomerulus and the peritubular capillary. It maintains P_G, and therefore GFR, with consequent increase in Π_G. In addition, downstream from the efferent arteriole, the peritubular capillary hydrostatic pressure will be decreased by the arteriolar resistance. Thus, we see an important role of efferent resistance on both glomerular filtration and tubular reabsorption.

Renal blood flow is governed by the same variables that determine flow through any organ, namely:

$$\text{Flow} = (\text{Arterial pressure} - \text{venous pressure})/\text{Total renal vascular resistance}$$

This is the Ohm's law analogy:

$$Q = \Delta P / R \text{ or } \Delta P = Q \times R$$

Thus, changes in systemic blood pressure would tend to affect renal blood flow. The kidney, however, has precise mechanisms for autoregulation of flow, changing its vascular resistance mainly in the afferent and efferent arterioles, in response to changes in systemic blood pressure. These mechanisms maintain relatively constant RBF and GFR when the systemic blood pressure ranges from approximately 80 to 170 mm Hg (Figure 20.15).

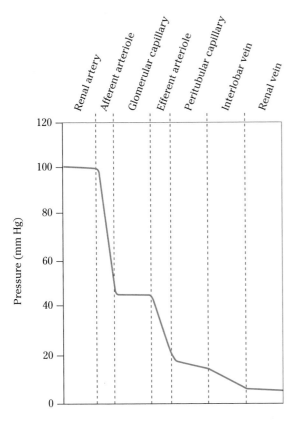

Figure 20.14 Hydrostatic pressures along the renal arterial system. Note the pronounced drops in pressure along the efferent and afferent arterioles and the difference in pressures in the glomerular and peritubular capillaries.

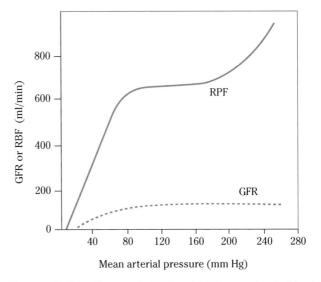

Figure 20.15 Changes in RBF and GFR as systemic blood pressure changes. Note that RBF and GFR remain relatively constant at systemic blood pressures between 80 and 170 mm Hg.

The Effects of Changes in the Starling Relationship on GFR

The determinants of GFR are the renal plasma flow, the K_f, and the Starling driving forces. These variables can be affected by physiological and pathological processes. From the principles of capillary flow we have outlined, we can predict how these changes would affect GFR. It is important to think of GFR as a continuous function of its determinants.

Changes in K_f The filtration coefficient, K_f, depends on both the permeability of the filtration barrier and the total surface area available for filtration. Various disease processes can affect these parameters. For example, in glomerulonephritis, the glomerular capillary basement membrane can become thickened or damaged, reducing its permeability. Eventually, glomeruli can become entirely nonfunctional, reducing the total filtration area of the kidney. These chronic changes eventually lead to a decreased K_f, and (from the Starling equation) to a decreased GFR. K_f can also be decreased by constriction of mesangial cells within the glomerular tuft. Hormones such as angiotensin-II and high levels of blood calcium can cause this constriction, which decreases filtration surface area.

In pregnancy, GFR is increased by as much as 50%, largely owing to increased renal plasma flow, but the K_f may be increased as well, contributing to the GFR rate normally seen.

Changes in P_B Normally, the hydrostatic pressure in Bowman's space is low. When the flow of urine is completely blocked downstream, however, such as with a kidney stone lodged in the ureter, the urine backs up and the pressure in Bowman's space builds. This increase in P_B opposes glomerular filtration, so the GFR decreases.

Changes in Π_G We noted earlier that as protein-free plasma filters out of the glomerular capillaries, the remaining proteins become more concentrated, increasing glomerular oncotic pressure (Figure 20.13). As the renal blood flow increases, however, the amount of plasma filtering out represents a smaller fraction of the total amount of plasma passing through the capillaries. Consequently, the oncotic pressure in the capillaries increases less rapidly. By this mechanism, increases in RPF decrease the average glomerular oncotic pressure. Decreased glomerular oncotic pressure favors increased filtration, thereby increasing the GFR. Thus, increasing RPF tends to increase GFR. In individuals given saline infusions, GFR increases due to increased P_G but more importantly, decreased Π_G (due to dilution).

Changes in P_G The glomerular hydrostatic pressure depends on the arterial pressure and the resistance of the afferent and efferent arterioles. Greater arterial pressure increases the glomerular hydrostatic pressure, thus increasing the GFR. Increased afferent arteriolar resistance decreases the hydrostatic pressure and the GFR, while increased efferent arteriolar resistance increases the GFR. To visualize these effects, we can think of glomerular filtration as water leaking through a hole in a hose. If we increase the pressure in the hose by opening up the faucet, more water will leak. If we squeeze the hose prior to the hole (i.e., if we increase the resistance in the afferent vessel), less water will leak out. Conversely, if we squeeze the hose past the hole (increasing the resistance of the efferent vessel), the flow through the hole will increase.

One factor complicates this analysis, however. When the resistance of the efferent arterioles increases, not only do we increase the hydrostatic pressure in the glomerulus (increasing GFR), but we also increase the total renal vascular resistance. The increased vascular resistance decreases renal blood flow. A smaller amount of blood can course through the glomerular capillary per unit time. Remember from the previous example that lower RBF leads to *decreased* GFR because of a higher net oncotic pressure in the glomerulus. Thus, the net effect on GFR of efferent arteriolar constriction depends on the balance of changes in RBF and glomerular hydrostatic pressure. In hypotension or when the major renal arteries narrow due to atherosclerosis (renal artery stenosis), renal plasma flow is decreased, P_G is also decreased, and GFR is reduced. This reduction in P_G and GFR can be minimized by an increase in efferent arteriolar resistance, due to angiotensin-II vasoconstriction.

P_G can be increased in states of plasma volume expansion, as well as in the case of loss of one kidney. In the latter situation, the remaining kidney undergoes enlargement, with increased renal plasma flow, P_G, and GFR.

The Regulation of RBF and GFR

When we analyzed the effects of Starling force changes on GFR, we ignored the kidney's ability to compensate for such changes. In fact, the kidney actively regulates RBF and GFR. Furthermore, long-term compensatory mechanisms exist that alter overall renal function. For example, we would predict that a loss of nephrons would lead to decreased surface area for filtration and thus to decreased GFR. In reality, however, the kidney has a tremendous ability to compensate for nephron loss, with the remaining nephrons adjusting their perfusion, function, and size. For example, if a healthy adult donates a kidney to a sibling with kidney failure, overall GFR in the donor may fall only by 20% instead of 50% (a value predicted by a loss of one-half the renal mass). It is not until the kidney's compensatory abilities are exceeded that we notice larger decreases in GFR. This is a common theme in many organ systems,

known as *physiologic reserve*. We turn next to some of the regulatory mechanisms the kidney uses in the short term to control RBF and GFR.

Autoregulation We have already observed that the kidney maintains relatively constant flow despite wide fluctuations in systemic blood pressure. Two mechanisms play a role in this autoregulation of flow: myogenic autoregulation and tubuloglomerular feedback. **Myogenic autoregulation** involves the constriction of afferent arterioles in response to wall stretch. The stretching of smooth muscle cells in the walls of arterioles is thought to open calcium channels in their membranes, increasing the influx of calcium ions and thereby triggering contraction. Accordingly, when a rise in arterial pressure stretches the afferent arteriole, the arteriole contracts. The increase in afferent arteriolar resistance offsets the pressure increase, maintaining constant RBF and GFR. This myogenic mechanism operates in many arterioles throughout the body.

Tubuloglomerular feedback involves structures in the juxtaglomerular apparatus. The anatomical arrangement of the juxtaglomerular apparatus provides an ideal setting for interaction between distal tubule flow and glomerular vascular tone (Figures 20.3 and 20.5). Tubuloglomerular feedback works in the following manner. An increase in arterial blood pressure increases renal blood flow and GFR. An increased GFR leads to a greater amount of fluid delivered to the distal tubule. Evidence indicates that the macula densa senses the chloride concentration in the tubular fluid. When the macula densa senses this increase in concentration, it activates an effector mechanism that increases resistance in the afferent arteriole. Adenosine mediates the constriction of the afferent arteriole. Increased afferent arteriolar resistance decreases RBF and GFR, returning them to their initial levels. The converse sequence of events ensues with decreases in arterial blood pressure. Note that in the afferent arteriole adenosine is a vasoconstrictor, an action opposite to its vasodilating effects on cardiac arterioles.

In addition to its role in tubuloglomerular feedback, the macula densa is involved in the release of renin by the juxtaglomerular cells, as discussed later in this chapter.

Regulation by the Sympathetic Nervous System
The sympathetic nervous system innervates the afferent and efferent arterioles. Firing of these nerves causes the arterioles to constrict, decreasing RBF and GFR. Epinephrine, released from the adrenal medulla into the circulation, has similar effects. Sympathetic inputs are also involved in releasing renin, with the subsequent formation of angiotensin I from angiotensinogen.

Angiotensin II The renin-angiotensin system plays an important role in regulating RBF and GFR. In response to a drop in systemic blood pressure (hypotension), signals from the macula densa and from sympathetic nerves induce the juxtaglomerular cells to release renin. As discussed in more detail in Chapter 22, renin initiates a catalytic cascade that results in the generation of angiotensin II. Angiotensin I is converted to angiotensin II by angiotensin-converting enzyme. Angiotensin II has vasoconstrictive effects on both afferent and efferent arterioles, but it constricts the efferent arteriole to a greater extent. The constriction of the arterioles leads to decreased renal blood flow. Because the efferent arteriole is constricted more than the afferent arteriole, however, the glomerular hydrostatic pressure is increased, and the GFR is relatively preserved.

One might assume that angiotensin II "squeezes" the kidney arteries in response to hypotension to drop the GFR and prevent the loss of intravascular volume to the urine. In fact, angiotensin II preserves GFR and urine output in humans by supplying some of the hydrostatic force for filtration lost in hypotension and addresses hypotension in a different way. Angiotensin II counters hypotension by (1) triggering sodium reabsorption and (2) diverting blood flow away from the kidneys and other organs so that systemic blood pressure is higher. When RBF is reduced and GFR is relatively preserved under the influence of angiotensin II, the filtration fraction rises. Only in severe hypotension does angiotensin's reduction of RBF (along with the drop in RBF due to the hypotension itself) overwhelm angiotensin's buoying effect on GFR. With severe drops in RBF, the GFR does fall. Angiotensin's role in the regulation of blood pressure and extracellular fluid volume is examined more closely in Chapter 22.

A relatively common cause of hypertension is **renal artery stenosis**, a partial blockage of the arteries to the kidneys. In patients with this condition, the kidneys maintain adequate GFR in response to low renal blood flow by using the renin-angiotensin system. Angiotensin-converting enzymes (ACE) inhibitors, a class of antihypertensive medications, work by blocking the formation of angiotensin II. If patients with renal artery stenosis receive ACE inhibitors, they can suffer from a severe decrease in GFR, leading to acute renal failure. (See Clinical Application Box *The Effect of an ACE Inhibitor on a Patient with Volume Depletion*.)

Prostaglandins and Other Mediators Several prostaglandins produced within the kidney cause dilatation of the afferent and efferent arterioles,

---

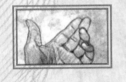

CLINICAL APPLICATION

THE EFFECT OF AN ACE INHIBITOR ON A PATIENT WITH VOLUME DEPLETION

A 59-year-old man has congestive heart failure, and his medications include an ACE inhibitor. He was doing well until he developed severe diarrhea after dining at an all-you-can-eat buffet. He presented to his primary care physician, having lost 10 pounds in 2 days. His diarrhea is resolving, but he is concerned because he has not urinated since the previous day. On examination, his oral mucosa is dry, his skin turgor is poor, and he has orthostatic hypotension, all of which are physical signs of volume depletion.

He is admitted to the hospital for rehydration and further management. His admission serum creatinine is 3 mg/dL, which is elevated from his baseline of 1 mg/dL. He is rehydrated with intravenous fluids, and his ACE inhibitor is stopped. Over the next several days, his weight returns to his baseline, his urine output increases, and his serum creatinine decreases to 1.5 mg/dL.

This scenario illustrates the importance of the renin-angiotensin system in maintaining adequate GFR in a state of volume depletion. ACE inhibitors block the formation of angiotensin II and therefore block the blood pressure-raising effects of angiotensin II. ACE inhibitors also block angiotensin II's autoregulatory function, whereby GFR is preserved even as RBF is decreased. The patient's diarrhea-induced volume depletion would normally trigger an increase in the level of angiotensin II, but his ACE inhibitor prevents that. Consequently, he cannot as effectively restore lost blood volume and his GFR is not preserved in the event of decreased RBF. Urine output falls and serum creatinine rises, although he has no glomerular or tubular damage. Once the ACE inhibitor is stopped, his renin-angiotensin system can respond appropriately, and with rehydration, his kidney function returns to normal.

increasing renal blood flow. *Prostaglandins* are released in response to norepinephrine or angiotensin II. As a result, they temper the vasoconstriction caused by sympathetic activation and angiotensin II, protecting against excessive decreases in RBF. Dopamine, (NO), and atrial natriuretic peptide are examples of other vasodilators in the kidney, whereas endothelin has been shown to be vasoconstrictive.

Synthetic Functions

Although most of the energy consumed by the kidney is directed toward solute transport by specialized epithelial cells, renal cells perform some very important synthetic functions.

Erythropoietin Erythropoietin is the hematopoietic growth factor that is produced primarily in renal tissue (and to a lesser degree, in the liver). It acts in the bone marrow to stimulate the production of new red blood cells, and its production in the kidney is increased when oxygen levels in the blood are chronically depressed. It is not surprising that cells in the interstitium of the kidney, situated largely at the cortical-medullary border, contain a heme-like protein that acts as an oxygen sensor. In hypoxic conditions, this sensor leads to an increase in a hypoxia-inducible transcription factor, which induces the erythropoietin gene to produce more hormone. It has been suggested that the sensing mechanism governing erythropoietin production resides in renal tissue because oxygen tension decreases as blood enters the medulla from the cortex, thus sensitizing this region in particular to hypoxic conditions. Another possible advantage of renal erythropoietin production may be that regulation of the hematocrit is determined both by red cell mass and plasma volume, and the renal tubules are important in sensing and responding to changes in body fluids.

Metabolic Synthetic Functions The cells of the renal proximal tubule are the only renal cells that are gluconeogenic, and during a fast, they contribute significant amounts of glucose to the circulation. Renal gluconeogenesis is under hormonal control (by glucagon, corticosteroids, epinephrine) and is also increased in metabolic acidosis in concert with the production of alpha ketoglutarate and $2NH_3$ from glutamine. Metabolic acidosis will be discussed in Chapter 25. The proximal tubule cells are specialized not only for gluconeogenesis, but also to donate the newly made glucose to the circulation. The activity of hexokinase (the enzyme catalyzing the first step in glycolysis) is lowest in proximal tubule cells and highest in the distal nephron where energy is derived from glycolysis. As a result, glucose reabsorbed by proximal tubule cells (approximately 900 mmol per day) or made by gluconeogenesis does not undergo glycolysis, but rather is available for transport back to the circulation.

The kidney, when functioning normally, is the major source of arginine for the body, and in renal failure, the renal synthesis of arginine may falter. Under such conditions, arginine must be absorbed through the diet, making it an essential amino acid. The kidney takes up citrulline from the circulation to produce arginine.

The mitochondria of the proximal tubule are the site of activation of 25-OH D3 to the active form, 1,25 OH D3. Vitamin D metabolism will be discussed in Chapter 35.

PATHOPHYSIOLOGY

Renal dysfunction, or renal failure, is typically classified according to the duration of the pathological process. **Acute renal failure** describes a rapid and frequently reversible deterioration of renal function, marked by a drop in GFR. **Chronic renal failure**, in contrast, is a more sustained, often progressive and irreversible decrease in renal function. Both can result from a wide variety of causes. The list of the kidney's functions (with which we began this chapter) gives us an idea of the kinds of clinical consequences of either acute or chronic renal failure. For instance, we might predict that renal failure will cause derangements in electrolyte concentrations, accumulations of metabolic toxins, volume overload, or acid-base imbalances. As we acquire a more sophisticated understanding of the various functions of the kidney in the following chapters, we can make more detailed predictions regarding the precise consequences of renal dysfunction. Because of the kidneys' great ability to compensate, a disease process generally has to affect both kidneys before any clinical findings arise.

Types of Acute Renal Failure

For now, we will focus on acute renal failure to illustrate the physiological principles we have discussed in this chapter. A useful framework for categorizing the many causes of acute renal failure divides them according to the location of the primary disease process. In this classification, the causes of acute renal failure fall into the following three categories:

- *Prerenal*: Decreased GFR owing to compromise in the blood flow to the kidney.

- *Intrinsic*: Disease involving any of the various components of the kidney—the glomerulus, the tubules, the interstitium, or the microvasculature—leading to decreased GFR.

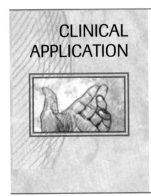

NONSTEROIDAL ANTI-INFLAMMATORY DRUG INTERFERENCE WITH RBF PRESERVATION

As RBF falls, resulting in the release of angiotensin II and norepinephrine, the release of prostaglandins is also stimulated. Those prostaglandins counter excessive renal arteriolar constriction and preserve RBF. Because *nonsteroidal anti-inflammatory drugs)*, such as aspirin, block the synthesis of prostaglandins, they interfere with the preservation of RBF. If nonsteroidal anti-inflammatory drugs are taken in the setting of decreased RBF, the compensatory prostaglandin response is thwarted. The resulting excessive vasoconstriction can lead to acute renal failure.

- *Postrenal*: Obstructions of the urinary tract, anywhere from the renal pelvis to the urethra, resulting in kidney dysfunction by increasing hydrostatic pressure in Bowman's space, impeding glomerular filtration.

Prerenal Failure   Normal fluctuations in fluid intake, heart rate and contractility, and vascular tone produce daily changes in blood flow to the kidney. It is only when pathologic decreases in RBF exceed the kidney's ability to compensate that GFR falls far enough to be classified as prerenal failure. Anything that causes a drop in cardiac output can cause acute prerenal failure, from myocardial infarction to hemorrhage to vomiting and diarrhea. Some conditions and clinical scenarios can also selectively decrease RBF relative to overall cardiac output. If prerenal causes are repaired, the kidney returns to normal function. (See Clinical Application Box *Nonsteroidal Anti-Inflammatory Drug Interference with RBF Preservation*.)

Intrinsic Renal Failure   **Glomerulonephritis** refers to a group of autoimmune disorders that involve inflammation in the glomerular capillaries. Inflammatory cells or proliferating glomerular cells interfere with the passage of filtrate out of the glomerular capillary, and these cells may therefore acutely re-duce the GFR. They reduce the K_f by decreasing the surface area of filtration. Other glomerular conditions, such as **diabetic nephropathy**, may result in chronic reductions in GFR (chronic renal failure).

Tubular and renal interstitial disease can also reduce GFR and cause acute renal failure. The most common variety of tubulointerstitial disease is **acute tubular necrosis.** Acute tubular necrosis may result from drug toxicity (e.g., due to the administration of certain antibiotics) or severe renal ischemia.

Tubular pathology decreases GFR independently of glomerular pathology through two mechanisms. The first is the autoregulatory mechanism, tubuloglomerular feedback. With tubular pathology and impaired proximal reabsorption, heavier flow may reach the distal tubule. As occurs in tubuloglomerular feedback under normal conditions, the macula densa then senses the increased flow and triggers vasoconstriction of the afferent arteriole, lowering blood flow to the glomerulus and decreasing GFR. The second mechanism is increased pressure in the tubule, similar to postrenal failure. Poor absorption of fluid and cellular debris associated with tubular disease may block tubular outflow and, in turn, create an unfavorable hydrostatic gradient for glomerular filtration. There may also be a backleak of tubular fluid, a mechanism not seen in the normal tubule. (See Clinical Application Box *An Example of Glomerulonephritis*.)

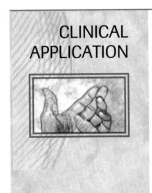

AN EXAMPLE OF GLOMERULONEPHRITIS

Goodpasture's disease is an autoimmune condition in which the body forms antibodies against collagen type IV, a major component of the glomerular basement membrane. The deposition of antibodies in the basement membrane begins an inflammatory process that destroys the integrity of the filtration barrier. Red and white blood cells can thus penetrate the glomerulus. The inflammatory cells can also block the glomerular capillary lumens, decreasing the total area available for filtration and thereby reducing the GFR. As discussed in later chapters, one of the consequences of reduced GFR is hypertension. The clinical findings of red blood cells in the urine and hypertension are features of the nephritic syndrome.

Postrenal Failure We noted earlier that blockage of a ureter by a renal stone can increase the pressure in Bowman's space and decrease the GFR in the kidney. If only one ureter is blocked, the other kidney is able to compensate, and the overall GFR is generally unaffected. When urine flow from both kidneys is blocked, however, renal failure can ensue. One common cause of bilateral urinary flow obstruction in men is **benign prostatic hyperplasia**, a condition in which the prostate enlarges, compressing the urethra as the urethra passes through the prostate. In addition to reducing the GFR, the increased pressure in the urinary space can eventually damage the kidneys, resulting in permanent injury. This condition of urinary "backup" is known as *obstructive nephropathy*. **Hydronephrosis** is the anatomic appearance of a dilated collecting system, the consequence of obstruction.

Summary

- The initial step in urine formation by the kidneys is the generation of a plasma ultrafiltrate by glomerular filtration.
- The glomerular filtration barrier filters substances by size and charge, eliminating large, negatively charged molecules, and generating a largely protein-free ultrafiltrate.
- The glomerular ultrafiltrate is further modified by exchange between the tubules and the peritubular capillaries; that is, by reabsorption and secretion.

The amount of substance excreted = the amount of substance filtered + the amount secreted − the amount reabsorbed

- Knowledge of how particular substances (e.g., inulin, creatinine, and PAH) are handled by the kidney allows us to measure GFR, RPF, and RBF, and to understand clearance.

$$\text{Filtered inulin} = \text{Excreted inulin}$$

$$GFR = \dot{V} \times [\text{inulin}]_U / [\text{inulin}]_P$$

$$RPF = \dot{V} \times [PAH]_U / [PAH]_P$$

$$RBF = RPF/(1 - HCT)$$

$$\text{Filtration fraction} = GFR/RPF$$

$$Cl_S = [S]_U \times \dot{V}/[S]_P$$

- GFR is determined by the balance of oncotic and hydrostatic forces.

$$GFR = K_f\,[(P_G - P_B) - (\Pi_G - \Pi_B)]$$

- GFR and RBF are actively regulated by autoregulatory mechanisms that seek to maintain constant flow and by neural and hormonal mechanisms that respond to changing physiological demands.
- Autoregulatory mechanisms protecting GFR are myogenic autoregulation and tubuloglomerular feedback.
- Preferential efferent vasoconstriction by angiotensin II helps to preserve GFR when renal plasma flow is decreased.
- Prostaglandins and nitric oxide are vasodilators in the renal microcirculation, whereas the sympathetic nervous system and endothelin are examples of vasoconstrictors.
- Renal failure means a drop in GFR. The three categories of acute renal failure are prerenal, intrinsic, and postrenal.

Suggested Reading

Briggs JP, Schnermann J. The tubuloglomerular feedback mechanism: functional and biochemical aspects. Ann Rev Physiol. 1987;49:251–273.

Shannon JA, Smith HW. The excretion of inulin, xylose, and urea by normal and phlorinized man. J Clin Invest. 1935;14:393–401.

Shipley RE, Study RS. Changes in renal blood flow, extraction of inulin, glomerular filtration rate, tissue pressure and urine flow with acute alterations of renal artery blood pressure. Am J Phys. 1951;167:676.

Wright FS, Briggs JP. Feedback control of glomerular blood flow, pressure, and filtration rate. Physiol Rev. 1979;59(4):958–1006 (Oct).

REVIEW QUESTIONS

Directions: Each of the numbered items or incomplete statements in this section is followed by answers or by completions of the statement. Select the ONE lettered answer or completion that is BEST in each case.

1. A 39-year-old man with insulin-dependent diabetes mellitus demonstrates thickened glomerular capillary basement membranes on renal biopsy. The decreased GFR resulting from his diabetic nephropathy is caused by which of the following?

   (A) increased hydrostatic pressure in Bowman's space
   (B) decreased glomerular oncotic pressure
   (C) increased total filtration area of kidney
   (D) decreased permeability of filtration barrier
   (E) decreased oncotic pressure in Bowman's space

2. A 63-year-old man with a history of urinary hesitancy is found to have a large asymmetric mass in his prostate gland. Upon biopsy, he is diagnosed with prostate cancer. His disease places him at risk for which of the following mechanisms of renal failure?

(A) prerenal failure secondary to hemorrhage

(B) prerenal failure due to tubular damage

(C) intrinsic renal failure due to glomerular damage

(D) postrenal failure due to renal artery stenosis

(E) postrenal failure due to increased pressure in the urinary space

3. A 3-year-old male child has a condition that leads to an absence of charge on the proteoglycans in his glomerular basement membrane. An investigation of his urine might reveal which of the following?

(A) increased amounts of negatively charged small molecules

(B) increased amounts of negatively charged large molecules

(C) increased amounts of positively charged small molecules

(D) increased amounts of positively charged large molecules

(E) no discernible difference from a normal child's urine

ANSWERS TO REVIEW QUESTIONS

1. **The answer is** D. By the Starling equation {GFR = $K_f[(P_G - P_B) - (II_G - II_B)]$}, we can predict that the GFR is decreased by decreases in the filtration coefficient, K_f. The thickened glomerular capillary membranes characteristic of diabetic nephropathy have two effects on K_f. The thickening of the membrane itself reduces its permeability. Once the disease progresses far enough, entire glomeruli can become nonfunctional, which would reduce the total surface area available for filtration. Either of these effects can reduce K_f. The pressure in Bowman's space (P_B) is typically low, except in situations when the outflow of urine is obstructed, such as by a urinary calculus. Decreased glomerular oncotic pressure (II_G) would actually increase GFR. The oncotic pressure in Bowman's space (II_B) is usually close to zero in a healthy individual with protein-free urine.

2. **The answer is** E. In this patient, the prostate tumor is likely placing increased pressure on his urethra, making it more difficult for him to void his bladder. This can result in bilateral urinary flow obstruction and hydronephrosis with a subsequent decrease in GFR because of the increased pressure in Bowman's space. The patient has no history of hemorrhage, making that an unlikely cause of prerenal failure. *Intrinsic renal failure* is a term used to describe disease processes that affect the kidneys directly, such as autoimmune disorders or drugs that damage the glomeruli or tubules themselves. Renal artery stenosis is a cause of prerenal failure.

3. **The answer is** B. The loss of negative charge will not result in increased amounts of negatively charged small molecules in the urine because in all situations, small molecules are freely filtered. Negatively charged large molecules, such as albumin, will be more likely to traverse the filtration meshwork of the glomerular basement membrane. Each 10 g/L of plasma albumin has approximately 2.5 mEq/L negative charge. A neutral charge to the basement membrane instead of a negative charge might decrease the filtration of positively charged macromolecules.

21

Tubular Transport

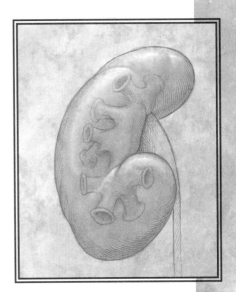

INTRODUCTION

As we began to see in the previous chapter, the processes of glomerular filtration, tubular reabsorption, and tubular secretion determine the composition of the urine and the blood leaving the kidney. The kidney modulates tubular reabsorption and secretion to maintain blood volume and solute composition at the levels necessary for physiologic functioning. Even as the body's interactions with its external environment produce changes in the blood volume and solute levels, the kidney makes ongoing corrections, keeping internal conditions stable. Homeostasis is achieved through regulated tubular transport of solutes in both directions (reabsorption and secretion), as well as reabsorption of water.

This chapter will describe reabsorption and secretion in general, the specialization of different parts of the tubule for transporting various substances, and the cellular transporters that convey substances across the tubule walls. Chapters 22–25 will describe the homeostatic mechanisms governing each element of blood: volume, salt content, potassium, and pH.

SYSTEM STRUCTURE: FUNCTIONAL ANATOMY OF THE KIDNEY TUBULE

Recall that the **nephron** is the functional unit of the kidney. It contains a glomerulus, where the initial filtration of blood occurs, and a **tubule**, where reab-

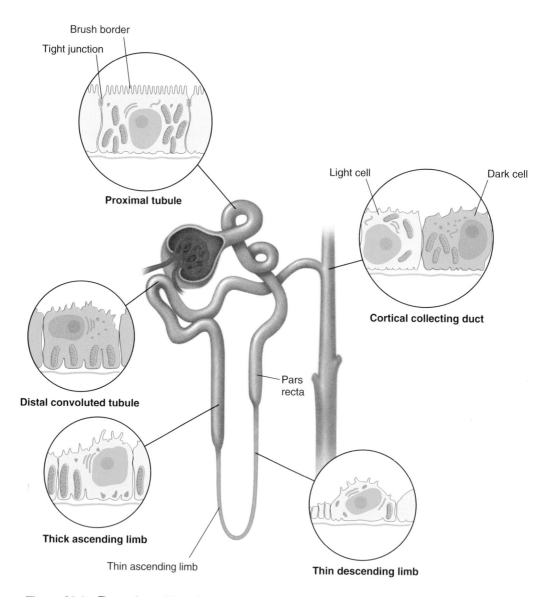

Figure 21.1   The nephron. Although only depicted on the proximal tubule cell, tight junctions and the lateral intercellular space are present in the epithelium in all parts of the tubule. The pars recta is the straight portion of the proximal tubule.

sorption and secretion occur (FIGURE 21.1). The tubule's parts have separate names: the *proximal tubule, loop of Henle, distal tubule, collecting duct,* and a regulatory structure called the *juxtaglomerular apparatus.* Transport takes place in every part of the tubule.

The epithelial cells are connected to each other along the entire tubule by *tight junctions,* which separate the cell surface into an *apical-luminal side* facing the tubule lumen, and a *basolateral side* facing the interstitium and the peritubular capillaries (FIGURE 21.2). Between the cells, yet still on the basolateral side of the tight junction, is an area known as the *lateral intercellular space.* The lateral intercellular space and the *basal space* are divided from the interstitium by the tubular basement membrane, but the basolateral spaces exchange contents freely with the interstitium.

The **proximal tubule** is located in the cortex of the kidney along with the glomerulus. Ultrafiltrate from the glomerulus flows directly into the proximal tubule, which is initially convoluted and then straight. The differences between the convoluted and straight portions demonstrate the way that tubule structure reflects its function. The *proximal convoluted tubule*

has more surface area for transport than the straight portion; accordingly, the straight portion—the *pars recta*—conducts less transport (Figure 21.1).

Different cell types are found in each portion, reflecting the greater transport function of the proximal convoluted tubule. The cells of the proximal convoluted tubule (S1 and S2 cells) are cuboidal epithelial cells, which have a distinct brush border on the apical-luminal side, consisting of microvilli that help provide a large surface area for transport. Each of these cells also has a highly invaginated basolateral cell membrane, thereby increasing the surface area for transport on the other side of the cell and a large number of basal mitochondria to supply added power for transport. Another distinguishing characteristic of cells in the proximal convoluted tubule is interdigitation of cell surfaces. S3 cells, which are found in the pars recta, are very similar to S1 and S2 cells but have a less-prominent brush border and fewer basal mitochondria, as less transport occurs in that area. After passing through the proximal convoluted tubule and then the pars recta, the filtrate moves into the loop of Henle.

The **loop of Henle** is a U-shaped structure that dips into the medulla of the kidney (Figure 21.1). The filtrate in the lumen encounters the three sections of the loop of Henle in the following order: the thin descending limb, the thin ascending limb, and the thick ascending limb. The *thin descending limb* consists of a low cuboidal or squamous epithelium. The thin descending limb is permeable to water but impermeable to salt. In the *thin ascending limb,* the reverse is true: It is impermeable to water, but the passive permeability to salt is high. (These features of the loop of Henle also have important consequences for kidney function.) The *thick ascending limb* differs from the thin ascending limb only in that the thick limb actively rather than passively transports salt out of the lumen into the interstitium. These thick ascending limb cells have marked basal striations due to the presence of invaginated basolateral membranes housing mitochondria for the active pumps. Unlike cells of the proximal convoluted tubule, which undertake a great deal of reabsorption, they have no brush border. As the filtrate passes through the thick ascending limb, sodium is pumped out, the fluid becomes hypotonic, and it eventually passes into the distal tubule.

The **distal convoluted tubule** is located in the cortex of the kidney. Its cellular architecture is similar to that of the thick ascending limb of the loop of Henle. Cells located in the distal tubule are cuboidal and have extensive infoldings of the basolateral membranes and numerous mitochondria. Multiple neighboring distal convoluted tubules empty into a common collecting duct.

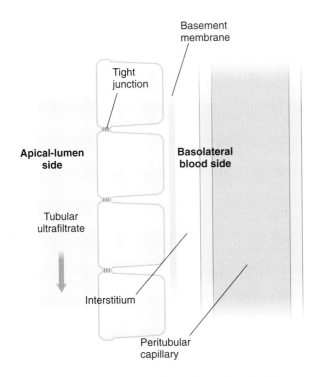

Figure 21.2 Two distinct surfaces of tubular cells. The apical-luminal side refers to the inside of the tubule, where the ultrafiltrate flows. The basolateral side constitutes the outside of the tubule and faces the peritubular capillaries. The tight junctions in between the epithelial cells separate the tubule lumen from the outside.

Collecting ducts receive fluid from distal convoluted tubules in the cortex and transport the fluid through the medulla. The portion of the duct that receives fluid from the distal tubule is known as the *cortical collecting duct*, which becomes the *medullary collecting duct* as it passes into the medulla. The cortical collecting duct has a large lumen and is composed of two main cell types, the principal cells and intercalated cells, with distinct roles that will be discussed later in the chapter. These cuboidal cells are large and pale. They lack a brush border but have very distinct lateral borders. The intercalated cells have a high density of mitochondria, but the principal cells have very few. Cells of the inner medullary collecting duct have few mitochondria and lack specialization of either the basolateral or apical surface.

SYSTEM FUNCTION: REABSORPTION AND SECRETION

To understand the epithelial secretion and reabsorption that are critical to the homeostasis of the body, we must first review the concept of mass balance, introduced in Chapter 20. This concept, which relates to the *net results* of secretion and reabsorption, prepares the way for a discussion of the more minute *mechanisms* of secretion and reabsorption and the specialization of transport in the different segments of the tubule.

Mass Balance

Mass balance is a straightforward and intuitive principle: what goes in must come out. "What goes in" is the blood supplied to the kidney by the renal artery. This blood contains plasma, which consists of water, ions, proteins, and other solutes. "What comes out" is twofold: that which leaves the kidney via the renal vein and that which leaves the kidney via the urine (for the moment, we will assume no production or metabolism of a given solute). The Fick equation is one way to express mass balance for any specific substance S:

$$(\dot{Q}_{renal\ artery})([S]_{arterial\ blood}) = (\dot{V})([S]_{urine})$$
$$+ (\dot{Q}_{renal\ vein})([S]_{venous\ blood})$$

The first term in the equation is the incoming mass of S: $\dot{Q}$, the flow per minute through the renal artery, multiplied by the concentration of S in the artery. The terms on the other side of the equation represent the outgoing mass of S: the mass of S in urine plus the mass of S in the vein. (An equivalent mass balance equation may be written for a single nephron by substituting into the above equation the flow through the afferent arteriole and efferent arte-

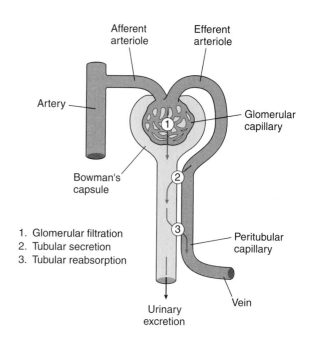

Figure 21.3 The division of filtrate between urine and venous blood. Filtration, reabsorption, and secretion determine how much of each substance ends up in the urine and how much is in the venous blood.

riole.) The distribution of renal output between the vein and urine is determined by glomerular filtration, reabsorption, and secretion (FIGURE 21.3).

Tubular **secretion** refers to the transport of substances from the peritubular capillaries to the tubular lumen via the nephron's epithelial cells. Tubular **reabsorption**, the opposite of secretion, refers to the transport of substances from the tubular lumen to the interstitium. It is important to remember the direction of solute movement attached to these terms. Secretion means transport *to* the lumen, and reabsorption implies reabsorption *from* the lumen.

Filtration and secretion can also be confused. Although they both refer to adding to the tubular lumen, filtration only describes the bulk-flow process in the glomerulus. Secretion can and does happen all along the rest of the tubule. Be aware, too, that some substances (such as K^+ and uric acid) are both secreted into and reabsorbed from the lumen during their journey through the nephron, but these terms usually refer to *net* secretion or *net* reabsorption. Although a substance may be reabsorbed overall, it may have been both reabsorbed and secreted at different points along the nephron.

Finally, a note of qualification about the mass balance equation: The equation assumes no consumption or creation of substances in the kidney, but consumption (metabolism) and creation of substances do occur in some cases. To account for this, the mass balance equation can be rewritten:

$$(\dot{Q}_{renal\ artery})([S]_{arterial\ blood})$$
$$+\ mass\ of\ S\ produced\ by\ the\ kidney$$
$$=(\dot{V})([S]_{urine})+(\dot{Q}_{renal\ vein})([S]_{venous\ blood})$$
$$-\ mass\ of\ S\ consumed\ by\ kidney.$$

Epithelial Transport

Recall that tight junctions separate the cell surface into an apical-luminal side and a basolateral side that faces the interstitium. To secrete or reabsorb, the nephron must convey substances across this boundary from lumen to interstitium or vice versa. It does so by various forms of epithelial transport, and there are two basic routes this transport can take. Solutes and ions can pass through the tight junctions if their electrochemical gradient allows it; this is known as the **paracellular route** of solute transport, as the solutes cross near (but not through) the cell (FIGURE 21.4). The other route of reabsorption, the **transcellular route**, is through the cell via specific transporter proteins on the apical and basolateral membranes of the epithelial cells. These transporters and channels convey substances across the apical membrane, through the cell, then across the basolateral membrane and vice versa. Both routes of transport can accommodate movement in either direction, thus accounting for both reabsorption and secretion.

Most solute transport is essentially driven by the **Na⁺/K⁺-ATPase** in the basolateral membrane. Although this pump works directly only to move Na⁺

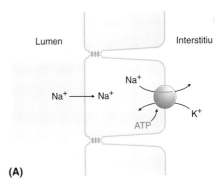
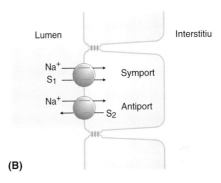

Figure 21.5 Transcellular active transport. **A.** Primary active transport of Na⁺ by the basolateral Na⁺/K⁺-ATPase. **B.** Secondary active transport of a solute S₁, coupled to Na⁺ movement by a symporter, and another solute S₂, coupled to Na⁺ movement by an antiporter. S₁ is actively reabsorbed, and S₂ is actively secreted.

and K⁺, it is ultimately responsible for the reabsorption and secretion of other ions as well. When the ATPase pumps Na⁺ out toward the interstitium in exchange for potassium and at the expense of ATP, it is conducting **primary active transport** (FIGURE 21.5A). Specialized proteins then couple this Na⁺ transport to the transport of other solutes. This process works in the following manner: first the primary active transport of Na⁺ out of the cell creates a low intracellular [Na⁺], which in turn provides a driving force for Na⁺ entry down a favorable electrochemical gradient. Na⁺ ions flow into the cell through apical Na⁺ channels. Apical *symporters* couple solutes to Na⁺ movement and drag the solutes in the same direction as Na⁺. *Antiporters* in the apical membrane couple solutes to Na⁺ movement but push the other solutes in the opposite direction from Na⁺. If the energy available in the sodium gradient is large enough to move the coupled solute against its own electrochemical gradient, then the coupled solute can reach concentrations that indicate active transport (additional energy added). This process, which couples Na⁺ transport to the symport or antiport of another solute, is termed **secondary active transport** because there is an indirect requirement for ATP (Figure 21.5B). Once the symporter has compelled the movement of a solute into the cell across the apical membrane, the

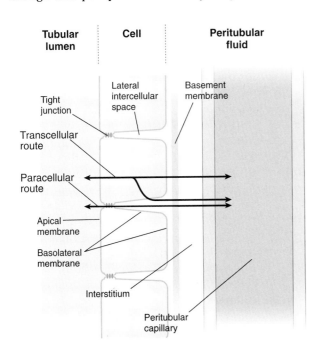

Figure 21.4 Paracellular and transcellular transport routes across the wall of the renal tubule.

solute can then diffuse across the basolateral membrane into the interstitium via specific channels or carriers. Similarly, once the antiporter has extruded a solute into the tubule lumen, the intracellular concentration of that solute falls, and more of that solute will diffuse into the cell across the basolateral membrane. The principal antiporter in the kidney is the proximal tubular Na^+/H^+ exchanger or NHE3, and the solute it secretes (a proton) is replaced by dissociation of water.

Transcellular transport may, in turn, drive paracellular transport. Transcellular translocation of cations and anions can create electrical and osmolar gradients across the tight junction that promote the movement of ions and water. For instance, if mostly cations have crossed transcellularly, an electrical gradient is set up that promotes the movement of anions (such as Cl^- or HCO_3^-) across the tubular epithelium via the paracellular route. Also, as solutes cross the membrane, they establish an osmolar gradient; water then crosses the epithelium paracellularly.

While the entire tubule makes use of the transport mechanisms mentioned previously, each epithelial segment of the nephron has unique transport properties. This is because different parts of the tubule have various types of pumps and channels. In addition, as proximal parts of the tubule modify the tubule contents, the distal elements receive different luminal compositions from those that entered proximally. The mechanism of transport that occurs in the distal segments may differ from mechanisms occurring in the proximal segments, even for the same solute. A good example of this is the varying mechanisms of apical Na^+ reabsorption along the tubule and the transporters that mediate proton secretion.

Reabsorption

Reabsorption is the transport of substances from the tubule lumen to the interstitium and peritubular capillary. Owing to the large rate of filtration, there is a burden on the tubule to prevent valuable solutes from becoming lost in the urine. Consequently, the tubule must perform a large amount of reabsorption and must expend a great deal of energy doing so. As a rule, solutes are initially reabsorbed in bulk, followed by a regulated titration, to achieve the urinary excretion required to maintain balance.

An important aspect of bulk reabsorption is the concept of **transport maximum (T_m)**. Simple diffusion across a membrane obeys the electrochemical gradient without limitation. Carrier-mediated diffusion of the sort that takes place on the apical tubular membrane, however, is limited by the capacity of the carrier proteins (transporters). As the concentration of a substance climbs, the transport rate for that sub-

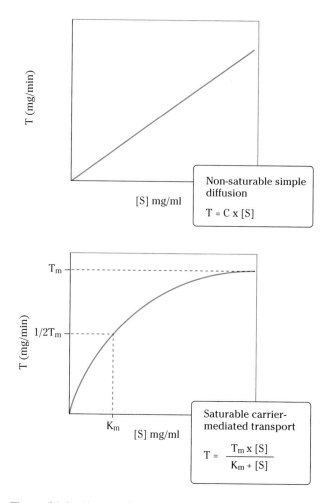

Figure 21.6 Nonsaturable and saturable transport. T = transport rate. T_m = maximum transport rate for substance S. [S] = the concentration of substance S in the compartment from which S is being transported (e.g., the tubule lumen). C = a constant. K_m = the concentration of S at which the transport rate is half-maximum.

stance climbs until the substance saturates its transport proteins, at which point the transport rate reaches its maximum, T_m (FIGURE 21.6). A substance's K_m is the concentration at which the transport rate is half-maximum.

D-glucose is a valuable solute that is almost completely reabsorbed under normal circumstances (zero clearance). In a person with a normal plasma glucose level, the amount of glucose filtered does not elevate the tubular glucose concentration high enough to saturate the glucose transporters; the tubular glucose transport rate is below T_m, and nearly all the glucose is reabsorbed. A patient with diabetes mellitus, however, has an abnormally high plasma glucose concentration, which leads to more filtered glucose, and a tubular glucose concentration that exceeds capacity; the transporters become saturated and cannot reabsorb all of the glucose. As a result, some glucose is excreted. The plasma concentration of glucose (holding GFR constant) in which sugar first appears in the urine is known as the *renal threshold for glucose*.

Although the appearance of large amounts of glucose in the urine depends mainly on the T_m, it should also be noted that a trace amount of glucose does appear in the urine before the T_m is reached. This premature spilling of glucose, known as **splay**, probably happens because the nephrons are heterogeneous, and not all of them have the exact same *single nephron glomerular filtration rate (snGFR)*. A higher snGFR would result in a greater amount of glucose filtered, which results in more glucose in the tubular lumen and therefore a greater likelihood of saturating the transporters and exceeding the single nephron T_m, resulting in premature spillage of glucose from this nephron. Furthermore, not all nephrons have the same T_m for glucose. In general, it is very unusual for an elevated overall GFR to lead to *glucosuria* (glucose in the urine) at a normal blood sugar. In pregnancy, however, a normal state in which GFR may be increased by 50%, a small amount of glucose may spill into the urine.

Whether a substance has a high or a low T_m may reflect whether the kidney regulates the level of that solute in the blood. For instance, phosphate has a lower T_m that is easily reached if plasma phosphate rises just slightly above normal. This creates de facto regulation of phosphate, for when plasma levels rise too high, transport capacity is exceeded and the excess phosphate is excreted into the urine. The T_m for phosphate is regulated by hormones such as parathyroid hormone PTH and vitamin D. Furthermore, in the growing child, the T_m for phosphate is higher than for the adult, allowing the blood level of phosphate to rise in a way optimal for the growth of the skeleton. By contrast, the kidneys are not the primary regulator of glucose levels in the blood (that is accomplished by pancreatic insulin-secreting cells); however, they do contribute to the blood sugar through the process of gluconeogenesis during an overnight fast, and also offset severe hyperglycemia in the diabetic patient, whose blood sugars rise above the threshold for excretion. Although this could be construed as a regulatory mechanism, the osmotic diuresis that ensues leads to disruption of body fluid volume and a loss of calories from the body. At normal glomerular filtration, spillage of glucose into the urine does not occur until the blood sugar exceeds approximately 180 mg/dL, a higher-than-normal fasting value.

Secretion

Secretion is the process of transport of substances from the peritubular capillaries to the tubular lumen. Many substances that are freely filtered by the glomeruli—organic anions and metabolic products (such as choline and creatinine)—are also eliminated from the body by this route. Because substances that are highly protein-bound in the plasma will not be freely filtered by the glomerulus, these solutes need to be secreted to be cleared. In order to be filtered or secreted, protein-bound solutes must coexist with an unbound or "free" component in the plasma. The kidney also secretes H^+, K^+, and foreign compounds such as drugs. Most substances, including H^+, are secreted in the proximal tubule, whereas H^+ and K^+ are secreted in the distal tubule and collecting ducts (information to follow).

One example of an exogenous substance that is actively secreted in the proximal tubule is the organic anion *para-aminohippurate (PAH)*. Like glucose reabsorption, PAH secretion has a T_m. As long as T_m is not reached, virtually all PAH that reaches the kidney is secreted and thus excreted. Therefore, the amount of plasma cleared of PAH is a good estimate of the renal plasma flow, as all the blood that passes through the kidney is cleared of PAH.

The Proximal Tubule

Now we will consider the specialized reabsorptive and secretory functions of each tubule segment. Our journey begins in the proximal tubule, where two-thirds of Na^+ and H_2O reabsorption takes place. Different types of ion transport take place in the early and late proximal tubule subsegments.

Reabsorption in the Early Proximal Tubule   In the early proximal tubule, Na^+ reabsorption is coupled with the reabsorption of glucose, amino acids, lactate, and phosphate by apical symporters (also known as *cotransporters*). Like glucose, the other solutes are almost completely reabsorbed from the lumen during the first half of the proximal tubule. Na^+ reabsorption is also coupled to bicarbonate reabsorption in the early proximal tubule in a slightly more complex way. Although Na^+ reabsorption is accomplished by the symporters mentioned previously, Na^+ is primarily reabsorbed in the early proximal tubule across an apical antiporter that secretes H^+ ions from inside the cell to the tubular lumen (Na^+/H^+ exchange or NHE). Once the H^+ is inside the tubular lumen, it can combine with filtered bicarbonate to form H_2CO_3 and then CO_2 and H_2O, facilitated by the carbonic anhydrase enzyme located on the apical brush border of the epithelium. CO_2 can now readily diffuse into the cell. When inside the cell, CO_2 once again recombines with H_2O to form H^+ and bicarbonate via carbonic anhydrase. The bicarbonate can cross the basolateral membrane by secondary active transport, usually via a Na^+/bicarbonate cotransporter. The energy driving this transport is the net electrochemical gradient, as the basolateral Na^+/K^+ ATPase and the cell membrane's permeability to K^+ render the inside of the cell electronegative with a low Na^+ concentration. As described previously, this draws Na^+ across the apical membrane and the cell's electronegativity then propels $3\ HCO_3^-$ with $1\ Na^+$ across the basolateral membrane. Thus, the net effect is the reabsorption of $NaHCO_3$ (FIGURE 21.7A AND B).

Water reabsorption occurs via water channels on the apical and basolateral membranes, paracellularly across the tight junctions, and is driven by an osmotic gradient between the lumen and interstitium (that is, by luminal hypotonicity created by active Na^+ transport). Because proximal water permeability is high, water follows the solute reabsorption freely, so the reabsorbed fluid is isosmotic to the filtrate. By the end of the early proximal tubule, a significant portion of water has been reabsorbed. This osmotic flow of water (both transcellular and paracellular) results in a **solvent drag**, in which additional solutes such as Na^+, Cl-, K^+, Ca^{2+}, and Mg^{2+} are carried by water flow into the interstitium.

Reabsorption in the Late Proximal Tubule In the late proximal tubule, the main salt reabsorbed is NaCl via both transcellular and paracellular pathways (Figure 21.7C). In the lumen of the late proximal tubule there is little glucose, amino acids, lactate, and a relatively low $[PO_4^{3-}]$ and $[HCO_3^-]$—due to the reabsorption of these solutes in the early proximal tubule. (The stoichiometry of the glucose transporter changes from 1 Na^+ to 1 glucose in the early proximal tubule, to 2 Na^+ to 1 glucose in the late tubule; the energetics of 2 to 1 coupling allow for complete glucose reabsorption as luminal concentrations fall.) The amount of water is significantly reduced in the lumen of the late proximal tubule because water has osmotically followed the proximal reabsorption of solutes, while the amount of Cl^- has remained constant because it has not been reabsorbed. Thus, $[Cl^-]$ is higher in the late proximal tubule lumen. This rise in $[Cl^-]$ creates a chemical gradient to drive Cl^- across the tight junctions and into the interstitium, where the chloride concentration approximates that of plasma. Because Na^+ has been reabsorbed in the early proximal tubule with HCO_3^-, allowing the Cl concentration to rise, there is also an HCO_3^- gradient in the late proximal tubule such that interstitial HCO_3^- concentration exceeds the luminal concentration. The reflection coefficient for HCO_3^- exceeds that for Cl^-, such that Cl^- preferentially moves from the lumen to the interstitium. It is notable that all nerves and hormones that affect proximal Na^+ and Cl^- reabsorption do so by impinging on the proximal Na^+/H^+

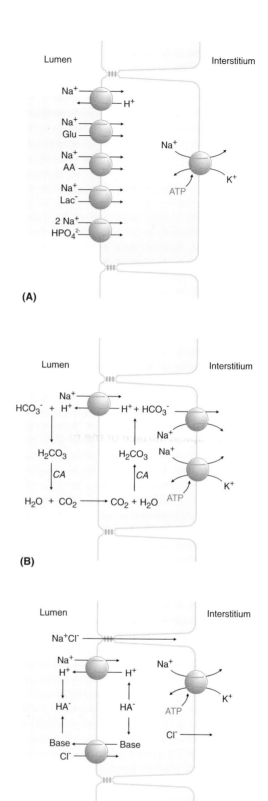

Figure 21.7 Solutes transported in the proximal tubule. **A.** Early proximal tubule: glucose (Glu), amino acids (AA), lactate (Lac$^-$), and phosphate (HPO_4^{2-}) reabsorbed by Na^+ symporters and extrusion of H^+ by a Na^+ antiporter. **B.** Early proximal tubule: bicarbonate (HCO_3^-) reabsorbed via the Na^+/H^+ antiporter and carbonic anhydrase (CA). **C.** Late proximal tubule: chloride (Cl^-) reabsorbed transcellularly via Cl^-/anion (A^-) antiporter and paracellularly by a chemical gradient.

exchanger (NHE3), which serves to lower the luminal HCO_3^- and increase the luminal Cl^-. Because the chemical gradient is large enough to drive the movement of Cl^- against its electrical gradient, the movement of Cl^- lowers the electrical potential of the interstitium and Na^+ is drawn into the interstitium, restoring electroneutrality.

Transcellular Cl^- crossing in the late proximal tubule is possible via parallel operation of Na^+/H^+ and Cl^-/A^- antiporters, where A^- represents anions such as OH^-, oxalate, or formate (HCO_2^-). The secreted H^+ and A^- combine in the tubular lumen to reform the weak acid (e.g., formic acid), and re-enter the cell by diffusion, so the net effect is the reabsorption of NaCl into the cell. Na^+ leaves the cell by the basolateral Na^+/K^+-ATPase pump, and Cl^- leaves by Cl^- channels along a favorable chloride concentration gradient.

Reabsorption of Proteins in the Proximal Tubule

The glomerular filtration of proteins is normally small, but in toto, it adds up to a significant daily filtered load. If the tubule were unable to reabsorb the filtered protein, the body would lose a considerable amount of it. Enzymes including peptidases and proteinases on the apical surface of the proximal tubule lumen can partially degrade these polypeptides and proteins, which are then taken up by endocytosis and digested into amino acids, which diffuse back to the bloodstream via basolateral channels. This protein catabolic mechanism is easily saturated, so protein can appear in the urine if there is an increased amount of protein in the tubular lumen, as in the case where damage to the glomeruli allows too much protein to leak through, or as is sometimes seen in increased protein intake.

Secretion in the Proximal Tubule

The proximal tubule also secretes organic anions and cations, especially those that are bound to plasma proteins and are thus not easily filtered by the glomerulus. The secretion rates of these substances are high, as indicated by the fact that the kidney can completely clear many organic ions and some drugs from the plasma. Organic anion secretion is best illustrated by the secretion of PAH. PAH crosses the basolateral membrane against its chemical gradient by a PAH-dicarboxylate (such as alpha-ketoglutarate) and tricarboxylate antiporter. The dicarboxylates and tricarboxylates are recycled back into the cell via a basolateral di/tricarboxylate-Na^+ symporter. These combined actions result in a high intracellular concentration of PAH, which can now drive PAH across the apical membrane into the tubular lumen via a PAH/A^- antiporter. This organic anion transport system is not specific, so many organic anions compete for these transporters; increasing the plasma concentration of a single one can inhibit the secretion of all other anions. For instance, aspirin can increase the blood concentration of uric acid, an important metabolic waste product secreted in this way. Use of the antituberculosis drug, pyrazinamide, also increases blood uric acid levels. In a similar competition, administering an inhibitor of organic anion transport, such as the drug probenecid, will decrease the secretion of penicillin, thereby mitigating the loss of penicillin by the kidneys.

For organic cations, there is also an active secretory pathway that has a T_m and is nonspecific. Organic cations enter the cell across the basolateral membrane via facilitated diffusion and exit across the apical membrane via an organic cation/H^+ antiport.

The Loop of Henle

Whereas the proximal tubule reabsorbs water and NaCl simultaneously as an isosmotic fluid, the loop of Henle splits the reabsorption of water and NaCl. This is critical for generating the salt gradient in the kidney, where osmolality increases with descent into the renal medulla. Recall that the descending limb of Henle is permeable to water but not to NaCl. As the filtrate passes down the descending limb, water is reabsorbed (another 20% on top of the proximal tubule's 67%), and the filtrate becomes concentrated in salt. The thin ascending limb is impermeable to water but permeable to NaCl. This allows the thin ascending limb to gradually unload its concentrated salt into the medullary interstitium, maintaining the medullary salt gradient. This salt gradient, along with a urea gradient, is necessary for the regulated reabsorption of water from the collecting duct, a topic to which we will return.

Upon reaching the thick ascending limb (also permeable to salt but not water), approximately 25% more of the filtered Na^+, K^+, and Cl^- load is actively reabsorbed. The main energy source is the basolateral Na^+/K^+-ATPase pump, which establishes a low intracellular $[Na^+]$, rendering the filtrate that leaves the loop hypo-osmotic to plasma. In the thick ascending limb, the Na^+ is reabsorbed across the apical membrane by a $Na^+/K^+/2Cl^-$ symporter—different from the symporters found in the proximal tubule. Cl^- ions leave passively via a basolateral Cl^- channel, whereas K^+ ions can leave via K^+ channels located on both the apical and the basolateral sides. Because intracellular K^+ and Cl^- both leave via the basolateral side, but only K^+ can exit the apical side, the tubular lumen becomes positively charged relative to the interstitium. This positive electrical potential drives paracellular diffusion of Na^+, K^+, Ca^{2+}, and Mg^{2+}. Na^+ also enters the cell via a Na^+/H^+ antiporter, which results in the ultimate reabsorption of HCO_3^- across the basolateral

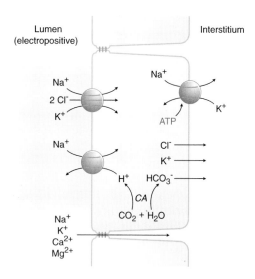

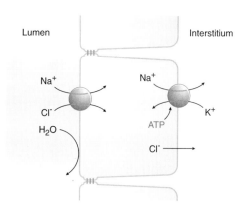

Figure 21.9 Reabsorption in the early distal tubule. Salt (but not water) is reabsorbed, similar to the situation in the ascending limb of the loop of Henle.

Figure 21.8 Reabsorption in the thick ascending limb of the loop of Henle. Salt is actively reabsorbed without water, unlike the isosmotic reabsorption in the proximal tubule. Bicarbonate is reabsorbed here as well. Na^+, K^+, Mg^{2+}, and Ca^{2+} are reabsorbed paracellularly by electrical gradient.

duct and is morphologically and functionally similar to the collecting duct.

The Early Distal Tubule The early distal tubule is impermeable to water. It can reabsorb Na^+, Cl^-, and Ca^{2+}, thereby further diluting the tubular fluid. Na^+ and Cl^- enter the cell across the apical membrane via the Na^+/Cl^- cotransporter. Once in the cell, Na^+ exits to the blood via the $Na^+/K^+ATPase$, and Cl^- diffuses across the basolateral membrane via a Cl^- channel. Thiazide diuretics, such as hydrochlorothiazide, can block this Na^+/Cl^- cotransporter (FIGURE 21.9; see also Clinical Application Box *Loop Diuretics*).

membrane (FIGURE 21.8). The diuretic furosemide inhibits one of the Cl^- sites on the $Na^+/K^+/2Cl^-$ cotransporter, which in turn decreases K^+ uptake and therefore recycling of K^+ back to the lumen. As a result, the lumen is less positively charged and Ca^{2+} and Mg^{2+} reabsorption is diminished. Furosemide therefore has an effect to increase Ca^{2+} excretion. In another setting, when blood Ca^{2+} is high, Ca^{2+} binds to a basolateral membrane Ca^{2+} receptor, which leads to an inhibition of apical $Na^+/K^+/2Cl^-$ transport and decreased Ca^{2+} reabsorption.

The Late Distal Tubule and Collecting Duct The late distal tubule or connecting tubule and the collecting ducts have two types of cells: intercalated cells and principal cells. The alpha-intercalated cells secrete H^+ and reabsorb HCO_3^- independently of Na^+ transport, which is important in the regulation of blood pH. The beta-intercalated cells secrete HCO_3^- ions into the lumen. Intercalated cells also reabsorb K^+ by a mechanism involving $H^+/K^+-ATPase$. These transporters will be discussed in subsequent chapters.

The Distal Tubule and Collecting Duct

The distal tubule is divided into two segments with very different properties. The early distal tubule extends from the juxtaglomerular apparatus to the middle of the distal convolution. The late distal tubule continues from there to the cortical collecting

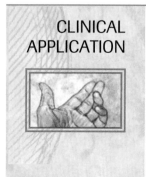

CLINICAL APPLICATION

LOOP DIURETICS

Diuretics are drugs that can increase urine output, usually by blocking Na^+ reabsorption. One class of diuretics is the *loop diuretics*, such as furosemide and bumetanide, which work by directly inhibiting the $Na^+/K^+/2Cl^-$ symporter in the thick ascending limb of the loop of Henle. This keeps the medullary interstitium less hypertonic and thus prevents water reabsorption in the collecting ducts, leading to a large diuresis. Proximal tubule diuretics do not work as well, because there is some reserve capacity of the thick ascending limb to reabsorb more Na^+ to compensate when proximal Na^+ reabsorption is blocked.

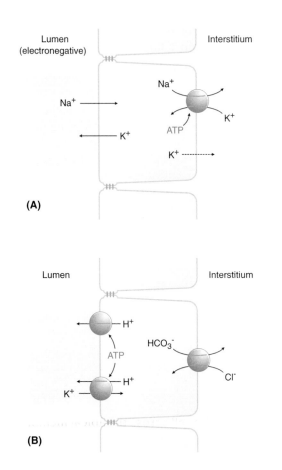

(A)

(B)

Figure 21.10 Reabsorption and secretion in the late distal tubule and collecting duct. **A.** Transport in a principal cell. **B.** Transport in an intercalated cell.

Principal cells contain the widespread basolateral Na^+/K^+-ATPase pump, reabsorb Na^+, and secrete K^+ across the apical membrane through protein channels in the membrane. K^+ also flows out of the cell down its chemical gradient via channels on the basolateral membrane (FIGURE 21.10). Basolateral flux exceeds apical flux, as demonstrated by the following observations. Principal cells reabsorb about 5% of the filtered Na^+, or about 1,200 mmol/day.

Based on the 3:2 stoichiometry of the Na^+/K^+-ATPase, 800 mmol of K^+ ions must enter principal cells each day via the Na^+/K^+-ATPase. This same number of K^+ ions must also leave the cell each day via K^+ channels. The typical diet contains about 80 mmol of K^+/day, which is the same amount that must appear in the urine. Therefore, basolateral exit of K^+ must exceed apical exit by tenfold in principal cells.

When Na^+ is reabsorbed across the apical membrane, a negative charge is left in the lumen, which creates an electrical gradient favorable to K^+ secretion. In addition, the passage of tubular fluid through the collecting duct has the effect of sweeping away the K^+ secreted by the principal cell. This keeps the luminal $[K^+]$ low outside the principal cell and maintains a favorable chemical gradient for K^+ secretion. Together, these processes allow K^+ secretion to take place. The principal cells also reabsorb Cl-, but the mechanism is unclear. Aldosterone acts on the basolateral Na^+/K^+-ATPase of principal cells to increase its activity, but its primary effect is to increase the activity of the apical Na^+ channels (ENaC). (See Clinical Application Box *Potassium-sparing Diuretics*.)

Water channels called *aquaporins* are thought to be present in all cell types that routinely conduct osmosis. The collecting duct, however, does not express aquaporins on its surface until stimulated to do so by antidiuretic hormone (ADH). In the presence of ADH, water is passively reabsorbed from the collecting duct, owing to the medullary osmotic gradient created by the loop of Henle.

Fractional Excretion

The **fractional excretion (FE)** of a solute can tell us to what extent a solute has been reabsorbed or secreted. Fractional excretion equals the quantity of solute excreted divided by the quantity of solute filtered:

$$FE = \text{amount in urine} / \text{amount filtered}$$
$$= \{[\text{solute}]_{urine} \times \dot{V}\} / \{[\text{solute}]_{plasma} \times GFR\}$$

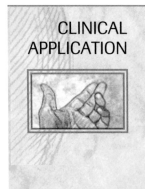

CLINICAL APPLICATION

POTASSIUM-SPARING DIURETICS

The apical Na^+ channels found on principal cells are blocked by diuretics such as amiloride and triamterene. These drugs are not as effective at increasing natriuresis as diuretics that work on earlier segments of the nephron, because most of the Na^+ has already been reabsorbed by the time the filtrate has reached the late distal tubules and collecting ducts. By blocking the reabsorption of Na^+, these diuretics reduce the negative charge in the lumen, which decreases the electrical driving force for the secretion of K^+. Thus, they are known as *potassium-sparing diuretics*. Spironolactone is another potassium-sparing diuretic that acts on the principal cell of the collecting duct. It inhibits the action of aldosterone and therefore on ENaC and the Na^+/K^+-ATPase, preventing both Na^+ reabsorption and K^+ secretion.

As explained in Chapter 20, GFR is equal to the clearance of creatinine.

GFR = clearance of creatinine

$$= \dot{V} \times [\text{creatinine}]_{\text{urine}} / [\text{creatinine}]_{\text{plasma}}$$

We can substitute the clearance of creatinine into the equation for FE to come up with the following equation for FE.

$$FE = \{[\text{solute}]_{\text{urine}} \times [\text{creatinine}]_{\text{plasma}}\} /$$
$$\{[\text{solute}]_{\text{plasma}} \times [\text{creatinine}]_{\text{urine}}\}$$

$$\text{or, } FE = \{[\text{solute}]_{\text{urine}} / [\text{solute}]_{\text{plasma}}\} /$$
$$\{[\text{creatinine}]_{\text{urine}} / [\text{creatinine}]_{\text{plasma}}\}$$

(The latter expression of FE reveals an important clinical feature of FE—namely, that it describes the renal handling of a solute more specifically than does a simple measurement of solute concentration in urine. A solute concentration in the urine can be affected by reabsorption of the solute and by the reabsorption of water. The denominator of FE corrects for water reabsorption, which is the only factor that alters the urine-to-plasma [creatinine] ratio.)

The FE of Na^+, called **FeNa** in clinical contexts, is a clinically relevant calculation in patients who have a low urine output and acute renal failure. A patient with renal failure owing to volume depletion but intact tubular function would have a high fractional reabsorption of Na^+—usually greater than 99%. This means that less than 1% of filtered Na^+ would be excreted (FeNa < 1%). In acute tubular necrosis (ATN), another cause of renal failure in which tubular function is abnormal, Na^+ reabsorption is impaired and a value for FeNa would be greater than 2%. In the context of a normal individual with high GFR, however, a low FeNa does not indicate an abnormality. For example, in someone in balance on a 100 mEq/day Na^+ intake (or 100 mEq/day Na^+ excretion) who has a GFR of 180 L/day and a plasma Na^+ of 140 mEq/L, the FeNa is 100 divided by the product of 180 times 140, or 0.4%.

Glomerular-Tubular Balance

Recall from Chapter 20 that tubuloglomerular feedback is a form of autoregulation that stabilizes GFR and RBF through compensatory mechanisms. **Glomerular-tubular balance (G-T balance)** refers to the relationship between the load delivered to a tubule segment and reabsorption by that segment. (You can keep the two straight by remembering that the first term in each phrase names the site of initial change, the second the site of compensatory reaction.) Without G-T balance, an increase in GFR would result in large volumes of water loss and solute loss in the urine because an increase in GFR means that more solute, such as Na^+, and more water are filtered

into the tubule lumen. If the proximal tubules merely reabsorbed a fixed amount of Na^+ under these circumstances, there would be a greater than normal excretion of Na^+. The proximal tubules do not reabsorb a constant amount of Na^+ and other solutes, however. Instead, they reabsorb a fairly constant *percentage* of the filtered load. A higher GFR meets with more tubular reabsorption of solute and water. There are probably two mechanisms for G-T balance.

The first mechanism for G-T balance is due to changes in pressure in the efferent arteriole and peritubular capillaries. A higher GFR means more plasma water will be filtered, leaving behind a higher oncotic pressure in the efferent arteriole and peritubular capillary. If the rise in GFR is due to increased resistance in the efferent arteriole (relative to the resistance in the afferent arteriole), then the peritubular capillary downstream of the arteriole will also have lower hydrostatic pressure. The combination of increased oncotic "pull" and decreased hydrostatic pressure in the peritubular capillary shifts the Starling forces in favor of an increased reabsorption of Na^+ and water from the lumen of the proximal tubule (FIGURE 21.11).

The second mechanism follows from the fact that flow rate and reabsorptive rate are linked. An increased GFR results in a greater filtered load not only of Na^+ but also of all other normally filtered substances. Many of these substances cotransport with Na^+ in the proximal tubule, and this increased delivery

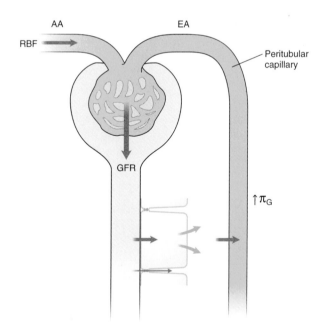

Figure 21.11 Starling forces and glomerular-tubular balance. AA is the afferent arteriole, EA is the efferent arteriole, and Π_{pc} is the oncotic pressure in the peritubular capillary.

of cotransported solutes increases the amount of Na^+ that can be cotransported across the membranes.

PATHOPHYSIOLOGY OF THE KIDNEY TUBULE

An understanding of the consequences of renal disease follows logically from an understanding of the normal physiology of the kidney and the normal functions of the nephron. Because the nephron performs essential homeostatic functions, including electrolyte and water balance, nitrogenous waste removal, and reabsorption of valuable substances, it therefore follows that disorders of the tubule compromise these homeostatic functions. Disorders can lead to retention of unwanted substances and fluid or the loss of valuable substances.

Kidney disease specific to the tubule falls into two broad categories: disorders that adversely affect the tubular transport proteins without killing the tubule cells and disorders that kill the tubule cells, leading to a specific scenario known as ATN, which is the common terminus of many sorts of acute insults to the kidney.

Disorders of the Tubular Transport Proteins

Disorders that affect the tubular transport proteins without causing acute cell death may result from hereditary factors, toxicity, endocrine abnormalities, inflammation, or ischemia. There are many inherited disorders of renal transport, although they are generally low in incidence. Toxicity is a more common cause of tubular dysfunction. The renal tubule is particularly vulnerable to toxins because many of these substances are transported by the tubular epithelium. While ischemia often leads to ATN, it may also impair transport without causing cell death by splitting the tight junctions. The kidney is highly sensitive to ischemia, possibly because the oxygen tension in the medulla is quite low. This sensitivity is due to the medulla's lesser degree of perfusion and the anatomy of the vasa recta, which is not favorable to oxygen delivery. The outer medulla, particularly the late proximal tubule, is most susceptible to ischemic injury because the proximal tubule cannot perform anaerobic glycolysis. Tubular dysfunction can also occur secondary to chronic glomerular disease, as the excess protein filtered in glomerular disorders over years can cause tubular injury.

Since each part of the tubule has a distinct function, pathological transport has different sequelae depending on the tubule segment affected. We will discuss examples of transport derangements in each one, proceeding from the proximal tubule onward.

Disorders of Transport in the Proximal Tubule   A host of rare genetic disorders disrupt the proximal tubule's capacity to reabsorb many small molecules, such as glucose, amino acids, phosphate, and bicarbonate. Renal glucosuria is a benign tubular disorder that is characterized by normal levels of glucose in the blood, but high levels of glucose in the urine. It results from faulty glucose transport mechanisms, resulting in impaired glucose reabsorption. Defects in amino acid transport systems may result in a generalized *aminoaciduria*, where all amino acids are not reabsorbed, or in failure to reabsorb specific amino acids such as cysteine and glycine. **Gout**, a common disease of increased plasma urate level, may be caused by an inherited defect that increases proximal tubular reabsorption of urate by acquired renal disease or by nonrenal factors. (See Clinical Application Box *What Is Gout?*)

We mentioned previously that the nephron is vulnerable to toxic injury. As the proximal tubule is located next to the glomerulus, where plasma is filtered and because of its extensive reuptake of filtered substances, the proximal tubule is particularly susceptible to this type of injury. In **lead nephropathy**, a condition in which lead toxicity impairs proximal tubular reabsorption, loss of glucose in the urine (*glucosuria*) and loss of amino acids in the urine (aminoaciduria) occurs. In addition, because the proximal tubule is responsible for reabsorbing phosphates, low levels of phosphates are found in the serum (*hypophosphatemia*). Another important function of the proximal tubule is to reabsorb bicarbonate. When this function is compromised, the serum pH decreases; therefore, lead toxicity may lead to acidosis. Such clinical findings of general proximal tubule failure are described as **Fanconi's syndrome**. Fanconi's syndrome may also be inherited or may be caused by toxic exposure to other agents.

Disorders of Transport in the Loop of Henle   Recall that the loop of Henle is essential for the concentration of urine and the reabsorption of water from the collecting duct. It also reabsorbs the majority of the sodium, potassium, and chloride not reabsorbed in the proximal tubule. In an uncommon genetic disorder known as **Bartter's syndrome**, sodium, potassium, and chloride are not reabsorbed, and the ability of the kidney to concentrate urine and reabsorb water in the collecting duct is consequently impaired. As a result, large volumes of urine are formed. The patient develops thirst, takes in more fluids, and as a result, may maintain a high urine output. Because of the resultant volume depletion, the renin-angiotensin-aldosterone system is activated, resulting in an increase in Na^+ reabsorption and increased H^+ and K^+ excretion. The ultimate result is severe volume deple-

WHAT IS GOUT?

A 69-year-old man calls his internist complaining that he was awakened at night by severe hot pain in his left big toe. The toe has been so painful it will not tolerate even the pressure of a bed sheet. In the office, the patient reports he has never suffered joint pain and has never been diagnosed with arthritis. History reveals a diet high in meat and daily light alcohol consumption (one beer with dinner). Aspiration of the left first metatarsal-phalangeal joint relieves the pain to some extent, and examination of the aspirate under the microscope reveals abundant urate crystals. The internist administers a corticosteroid shot in the affected joint, prescribes indomethacin, a NSAID, and recommends the reduction of meat and beer intake. The diagnosis is gout.

Uric acid is a nitrogenous end-product of purine metabolism that cannot be further catabolized by the body. Consequently, uric acid accumulates if the kidney is unable to excrete it in amounts that match production. In **gout**, either an overproduction of uric acid or decreased renal excretion of uric acid leads to a high level of uric acid in the plasma (hyperuricemia). In cases when the kidney fails to excrete uric acid, the problem seems to be in the proximal tubule. For reasons that are not well understood, the proximal tubule has the ability to both actively secrete and reabsorb urate, the anion of uric acid, and in some individuals, the reabsorption of urate by the proximal tubule is excessive. Various types of intrinsic renal disease and some drugs such as pyrazinamide can decrease urate excretion. Other drugs are uricosuric, for example, probenizid, which inhibits uric acid reabsorption.

As the concentration of urate in the plasma reaches the limits of its solubility, uric acid crystals begin to precipitate, forming inflammatory deposits, usually in the joints. Gout attacks tend to be sudden in onset and frequently affect a peripheral joint in the lower extremities, often in the big toe. Treatment includes corticosteroids, NSAIDs, colchicine (which inhibits neutrophils' phagocytosis of urate crystals), and dietary modification. Underlying causes of hyperuricemia should be addressed, and drugs are also available to decrease the plasma urate level. Uricosuric drugs increase renal excretion of urate, and xanthine oxidase inhibitors block the final step in the production of urate.

---

tion, low serum concentrations of potassium (*hypokalemia*) and chloride (*hypochloremia*), and oversecretion of acid, which creates a metabolic alkalosis.

Disorders of Transport in the Distal Tubule and Collecting Duct   The distal tubule normally reabsorbs Na^+ and Cl^-. Although infrequently observed clinically, mutations can occur in the Na^+/Cl^- cotransporter located in the distal tubule. In that case, Na^+, Cl^-, and consequently, water, are wasted in the urine, and volume depletion can occur. Toxins such as lithium can impair the response to ADH in the distal tubule and collecting duct by an unknown mechanism, leading to failure to concentrate the urine (i.e., failure to reabsorb water) and wasting of water.

In addition to regulating water reabsorption, the distal tubule and collecting duct fine-tune the amount of Na^+ reabsorbed by the kidney and secrete K^+ and H^+. When the transport capabilities of the collecting duct are impaired, Na^+ wasting, hyperkalemia, and acidosis can occur. When transport in the distal

tubule and collecting duct is overactive, just the opposite occurs. Under conditions in which too much aldosterone is secreted (e.g., by an adrenal tumor), then too much Na^+ is reabsorbed and too much K^+ and H^+ are secreted, resulting in mild hypernatremia, hypokalemia, and alkalosis.

Under the control of ADH, water reabsorption also occurs in the collecting duct. If ADH is not secreted or if the tubules are not responsive to ADH, as in *diabetes insipidus*, water will not be reabsorbed properly. Conversely, if excess ADH is inappropriately secreted, then the collecting duct will reabsorb too much water, lowering the concentration of the serum electrolytes.

Acute Tubular Necrosis

Acute tubular necrosis (ATN) may result from ischemic, toxic, or inflammatory injury. Severe hypotension—as seen in septic shock, hemorrhage, or shock during major surgery—causes insufficient perfusion of the tubules and is the predominant cause of ischemic tubular injury and ischemic ATN. The ischemic insult to the tubules can also be exacerbated by toxic mediators that are present because of tissue damage or sepsis. As alluded to previously, the outer medulla is especially susceptible to ischemic injuries.

Because toxins can reach high concentrations in the tubular epithelial cells, the kidney is also very susceptible to damage by a broad range of toxins, including both exogenous and endogenous substances. Exogenous substances frequently implicated in nephrotoxic ATN include antibiotics such as aminoglycosides or amphotericin B, chemotherapeutic agents like cisplatin, heavy metals, or radiocontrast agents. Endogenous toxins include myoglobin, which is released after muscle breakdown due to crush injuries or pressure sores, and hemoglobin in the context of a transfusion reaction.

Whatever the cause, the common pathway of ATN starts with a depletion of tubular cell ATP and damage to the tubular cell membranes. This leads to increasing intracellular calcium, activation of proteases and lipases, and eventual cell death. The dead tubular cells slough off, form aggregates called *casts*, and block the tubules. Blockage of the tubules ultimately results in a decrease in GFR and backup of filtered fluid. ATN is therefore classified as a major cause of intrinsic renal failure (i.e., acute renal failure originating within the renal parenchyma).

Because ischemia often causes ATN, the prerenal failure of ischemia and the intrinsic renal failure of ATN are often seen together. Furthermore, given that they both reduce the GFR, they share certain clinical signs, such as elevated plasma creatinine and urea. Many clinical signs differentiate the two, which is important in the differential diagnosis of acute renal failure. For example, the ratio of plasma urea to creatinine is higher in prerenal failure, the fractional excretion of sodium (FeNa) is elevated only in intrinsic renal failure, and muddy granular casts are not seen in the urine unless ATN is present (Table 21.1).

The prognosis for patients who have had ATN without any other serious medical problems is good and the tubular cells regenerate; however, these patients may have some degree of prolonged renal impairment. For patients with preexisting renal disease or serious comorbid conditions, such as sepsis, the mortality rate can be high.

Summary

- The renal tubule has three main parts: the proximal tubule, where the bulk of salt, water, and other solutes are reabsorbed; the loop of Henle, where salt is concentrated in the medulla; and the distal tubule and collecting duct, where water reabsorption is regulated to control serum osmolality.

- Tight junctions divide the tubule cells into an apical-luminal side and a basolateral side that faces the interstitial fluid and the peritubular capillary.

- A mass balance equation describes the allocation of renal arterial contents between the urine and the renal vein:

$$(\dot{V}_{renal\ artery})([S]_{arterial\ blood}) = (\dot{V}_{urine})([S]_{urine}) + (\dot{V}_{renal\ vein})([S]_{venous\ blood})$$

- The processes of filtration, reabsorption, and secretion determine how a given substance will be divided between urine and venous blood.

- Solutes and water may cross from tubule lumen to the interstitium by a transcellular route or a paracellular route.

Table 21.1   **A COMPARISON OF LAB VALUES IN PRERENAL FAILURE AND INTRINSIC RENAL FAILURE**

	Prerenal Failure	Intrinsic Renal Failure
Fractional excretion of sodium (%)	<1	>1
Urine sodium concentration (mmol/L)	<10	>20
Urine creatinine to plasma creatinine ratio	>40	<20
Urine-specific gravity	> 1.018	<1.015
Urine osmolality (mOsm/kg H_2O)	>500	<300
Plasma BUN/creatinine ratio	>20	<10–15
Urinary sediment	Hyaline casts	Muddy brown granular casts

- The Na^+/K^+-ATPase pump drives all reabsorption and secretion across the tubule wall. Na^+ is reabsorbed by primary active transport, whereas other solutes are moved by secondary active transport; that is, they are indirectly coupled to the movement of sodium.

- Reabsorption and secretion of certain solutes by transporter proteins are saturable processes and consequently have a transport maximum T_m. Spilling of a solute in urine before the tubular solute concentration has saturated the transporters is called *splay*.

- The tubule reabsorbs 99% of Na^+, 100% of glucose, and the majority of Mg^{2+}, Ca^{2+}, K^+, phosphate, and amino acids. The bulk (about two-thirds) of the reabsorption takes place in the proximal tubule, but the "fine-tuning" of the amounts of each solute to be conserved or excreted takes place in the distal portions of the nephron. Thus, the percentages reabsorbed in the distal portions will change depending on dietary intake and other mechanisms.

- Na^+ reabsorption in the early proximal tubule takes place via cotransport with glucose, amino acids, lactate, phosphate, and bicarbonate and in the late proximal tubule with Cl^-.

- Because water osmotically follows these solutes, 67% of water is reabsorbed iso-osmotically in the proximal tubule; solvent drag also contributes to the reabsorption of Na^+, Cl^-, K^+, Ca^{2+}, and Mg^{2+}.

- Substances that require elimination but could not be filtered are often secreted. Many organic anions and cations are completely cleared via proximal tubule secretion.

- Overall, the loop of Henle reabsorbs 20% of the filtered load of Na^+, Cl^-, Ca^{2+}, and Mg^{2+}. It also reabsorbs about 20% of the filtered water, which occurs in the descending limb of Henle. The active pumping of salts along the thick ascending limb makes the tubular fluid hypo-osmotic, with an osmolarity less than 150 mOsm/kg H_2O.

- In the late distal tubule and collecting duct, principal cells actively reabsorb Na^+ and secrete K^+. Intercalated cells secrete H^+ and reabsorb bicarbonate.

$$FE = \text{amount in urine/amount filtered}$$
$$= \{[solute]_{urine} \times [creatinine]_{plasma}\}/$$
$$\{[solute]_{plasma} \times [creatinine]_{urine}\}$$

- G-T balance yields proportional changes in Na^+ reabsorption with changes in GFR.

- Tubular dysfunction may disrupt transport without killing tubular cells or may involve ATN.

- ATN is caused by ischemia or toxicity and results in derangements of tubular transport and decreased GFR.

Suggested Reading

Emmerson BT. The Management of gout. N Engl J Med. 1996;334:445–451.

Esson ML, Schrier RW. Diagnosis and treatment of acute tubular necrosis. Ann Intern Med. 2002;137:744–752.

Klahr S, Miller SB. Acute oliguria. N Engl J Med. 1998;338:671–675.

Thadhani R, Manual P, Bonventre JV. Acute renal failure. N Engl J Med. 1996;334:1448–1460.

REVIEW QUESTIONS

Directions: Each of the numbered items or incomplete statements in this section is followed by answers or by completions of the statement. Select the ONE lettered answer or completion that is BEST in each case.

1. A 65-year-old man underwent surgery for the repair of an abdominal aortic aneurysm. In the postoperative period, he was noted to have decreased urine output. His BUN and creatinine were 29 and 1.9 mg/dL, indicating a decreased GFR. His fractional excretion of sodium was 4.2%. Muddy brown granular casts were observed on urinalysis, indicating tubular necrosis. His increased fractional excretion of sodium is likely due to:

   (A) increased filtration of sodium
   (B) increased filtration of glucose
   (C) decreased reabsorption of sodium
   (D) increased secretion of chloride
   (E) increased secretion of sodium

2. A 34-year-old woman being treated for a urinary tract infection is diagnosed with diabetes mellitus after urinalysis shows glucose in her urine and blood tests confirm hyperglycemia. The likely cause of her glucosuria is:

   (A) a decreased glucose T_m in the proximal tubule
   (B) saturation of the Na^+/glucose cotransporters
   (C) severely decreased Na^+ reabsorption
   (D) an elevated GFR
   (E) backflow of glucose across faulty tight junctions

3. A 72-year-old man with congestive heart failure due to idiopathic dilated cardiomyopathy was placed on furosemide to help alleviate his peripheral edema. Which of the following electrolyte abnormalities may result from his use of this drug?

   (A) hyponatremia
   (B) hypocalcemia
   (C) hypermagnesemia
   (D) hypokalemia
   (E) two of the above

ANSWERS TO REVIEW QUESTIONS

1. **The answer is C.** The renal tubule normally reabsorbs 99% or more of the filtered sodium, but in this patient, ATN has interfered with the tubule's ability to reabsorb sodium, leaving excess sodium in the urine and increasing the FeNa above its normal limit of 1%. Although increased filtration of sodium would increase the tubular sodium load, we know that in this case, the GFR is low and that sodium filtration is actually *decreased*; furthermore, a normally functioning tubule would still reabsorb the increased load of sodium. Increased filtration of glucose is not present because GFR is decreased; moreover, increased filtration of glucose *promotes* sodium reabsorption—this is one of the mechanisms of G-T balance. The kidney does not secrete either sodium or chloride; it only reabsorbs them.

2. **The answer is B.** In diabetes mellitus, a high serum glucose level (hyperglycemia) leads to an abnormally high filtered load of glucose. The Na^+/glucose transporters become saturated and cannot reabsorb all the filtered glucose; the rest is lost to the urine. Normally, all the glucose is reabsorbed. An inherited disorder can lower the glucose transport maximum (T_m) and can cause glucosuria in the context of normal serum glucose, but the patient's serum glucose is not normal in this case. Severely decreased Na^+ reabsorption would decrease glucose reabsorption because glucose is cotransported with Na^+, but this is not the cause of glucosuria in diabetes mellitus. Increased GFR can contribute to splay and faulty tight junctions would interfere with solute reabsorption, but these are not contributors to diabetic glucosuria.

3. **The answer is D.** Furosemide can cause hypokalemia because inhibition of salt reabsorption in the thick limb results in increased delivery of Na^+ to the collecting duct, where K^+ is secreted. That is why potassium-sparing diuretics are useful adjuncts in the treatment of the edematous patient. Although furosemide increases urinary calcium and magnesium excretion, hypocalcemia is unusual because the blood calcium is closely regulated by hormonal influences. Hypomagnesemia, on the other hand, is not unusual. *Hyper*magnesemia is not a feature of furosemide treatment. The drug causes diuresis through the inhibition of the $Na^+/K^+/2Cl^-$ reabsorptive symporter in the thick ascending limb of the loop of Henle. This prevents dilution of the tubular fluid, which is necessary for water reabsorption in the collecting duct, and induces a higher urine volume. Inhibition of K^+ reabsorption may lead to hypokalemia as a side effect. Under normal circumstances, the $Na^+/K^+/2Cl^-$ symporter and the distribution of ion channels in the thick ascending limb also lead to an electropositive tubule lumen that drives the paracellular reabsorption of Ca^{2+} and Mg^{2+}. Inhibition of the symporter disrupts the establishment of a net positive charge on the inside of the tubule lumen and the driving force for reabsorption of Ca++ and Mg++ is diminished, resulting in hypercalcuria and magnesuria. Loop diuretics do not usually create hyponatremia, despite decreased water reabsorption unless the patient is not drinking (see Chapter 23).

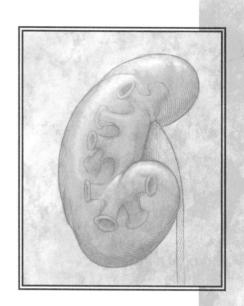

22

The Regulation of Blood Pressure and Extracellular Fluid Volume

INTRODUCTION

Don't be fooled. This chapter is essentially about blood pressure. The cardiovascular system does not govern blood pressure by itself; equally important to the regulation of blood pressure is the kidney's control over the volume of the extracellular fluid. Recall that systemic blood pressure (SBP) equals cardiac output (CO) times systemic vascular resistance (SVR). Note that this is a restatement of Ohm's law: pressure equals flow times resistance.

$$SBP = CO \times SVR$$

The cardiovascular system affects BP by adjusting CO and SVR at the level of the heart and the arterioles, respectively. The kidney affects BP by adjusting the size of the extracellular fluid compartment. The intravascular volume, part of the extracellular space, in turn affects the heart's preload and CO. The cardiovascular and renal effectors of blood pressure homeostasis act in concert, and the nervous system coordinates their efforts.

The kidneys control volume in the same way that they control the level of solutes in the bloodstream—by modifying the reabsorption of solutes and water filtered into the tubule. In the case of extracellular volume control, the kidney adjusts the reabsorption of isotonic fluid.

SYSTEM STRUCTURE: BODY FLUID COMPARTMENTS

Recall that body fluid is divided into two spaces, extracellular and intracellular. **Extracellular fluid (ECF)** is divided into intravascular and interstitial compartments that are separated by capillary endothelium, which is freely permeable to water and small ions but not to proteins. **Intracellular fluid (ICF)** is the fluid contained inside all the cells of the body.

Also remember from previous chapters that Na^+ (sodium) is the major cation of the ECF, and K^+ (potassium) is the major cation of the ICF (FIGURE 22.1). The Na^+/K^+-ATPase pump that operates in all body tissues segregates Na^+ and K^+ to the outside and the inside of cells, respectively. Na^+ is therefore primarily responsible for creating the osmotic pressure that holds water (and volume) in the extracellular space, whereas K^+ is primarily responsible for the osmotic pressure that holds water in the intracellular space. (See Chapter 23 for more discussion of osmotic pressure and fluid shifts.) Changes in the Na^+ concentration of the ECF alter the osmotic pressure of the ECF. If Na^+ is added to the ECF—for example, by eating a salty meal and absorbing salt into the blood from the intestines—the osmotic pressure of the ECF will increase, and

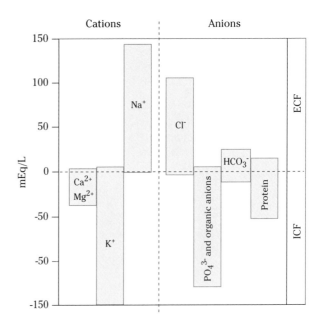

Figure 22.1 Major cations and anions of the ECF and ICF. Na^+ and Cl^- are the major ions of the ECF. K^+ and a variety of anions, including PO_4^{3-}, are the major ions of the ICF.

water will move from the ICF into the ECF, thereby increasing the ECF volume.

The kidney makes use of this principle when it alters the volume of the ECF. By adjusting the amount of Na^+ reabsorbed from the nephron tubule, the kidney adjusts the osmotic gradient for water reabsorption from the tubule, and thereby adjusts the amount of water and volume reabsorbed from the tubule back into the bloodstream. The point here is not that water reabsorption always follows salt reabsorption in the kidney; in fact, in certain parts of the tubule, salt reabsorption without water is essential to kidney function. The kidney does not control ECF volume by hydrostatically pumping filtered water back into the bloodstream; instead, it does so by creating osmotic gradients with Na^+, the major ECF cationic osmole (FIGURE 22.2).

SYSTEM FUNCTION: BLOOD PRESSURE HOMEOSTASIS

Chapter 5 lists the basic components of regulatory homeostatic systems in the body (see Figure 5.1). They are:

- Sensors that collect data about some parameter of physiological functioning.
- Afferent transmission pathways that carry the data from the sensors to a control center.
- A control center that compares the actual level of the parameter with the desired level.

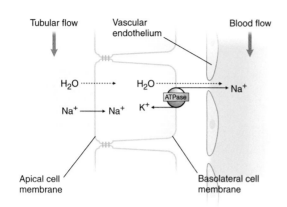

Figure 22.2 Water and salt reabsorption in the kidney. Water follows salt.

- Efferent transmission pathways that carry signals from the control center to the effectors.
- Effectors that restore the actual level of the parameter back to the desired level.

With all of these homeostatic elements, the kidneys maintain blood pressure and perfusion pressure

by increasing the ECF volume when perfusion pressure is low and decreasing ECF volume when perfusion pressure is high. FIGURE 22.3 breaks down renal and cardiovascular regulation of perfusion pressure into homeostatic elements.

Perfusion pressure refers to the local arterial blood pressures at particular organs, such as the brain or the kidneys, as opposed to the average systemic blood pressure. Because sensors of blood pressure must reside in one local area of the vasculature, sensors actually measure local perfusion pressures as indicators of the average systemic blood pressure.

The Two Homeostatic Systems That Regulate Blood Pressure

The two regulatory systems governing BP, cardiovascular and renal, share similar sensors but employ different effector mechanisms. As we shall see, renal and cardiovascular regulation are intimately connected. In both systems, BP regulation begins with the **baroreceptors**, which sense changes in perfusion pressure. The term *baroreceptor reflex* is used to describe the feedback loop by which the

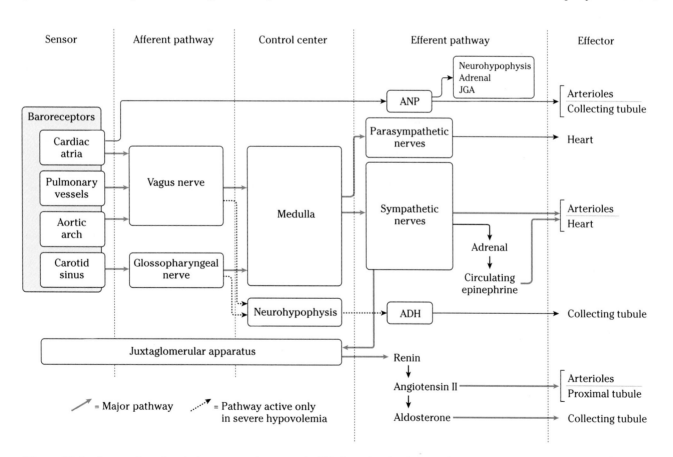

Figure 22.3 An overview of perfusion pressure homeostasis. This figure breaks down perfusion pressure homeostasis into the classic homeostatic elements: sensors, afferent transmission pathways, control centers, efferent transmission pathways, and effectors.

nervous system responds to changes in perfusion pressure.

Cardiovascular Cardiovascular regulation is initiated by baroreceptors in the heart, lungs, and carotid arteries. On the basis of information it receives from the baroreceptors, the brain discharges impulses through the *sympathetic nervous system* and *parasympathetic nervous system* to control heart rate, heart contractility, and resistance of the blood vessels. The sympathetic outflow also impinges on the kidney to regulate proximal reabsorption, renin secretion, and renal vascular resistance. More sympathetic output raises BP and less lowers it. More parasympathetic output slows the heart rate and less increases the heart rate.

Renal Three main feedback loops constitute the renal regulation of BP:

1. Just as baroreceptors activate the cardiovascular response to pressure changes in the larger arteries, such pressure changes within the renal microcirculation stimulate the vascular component of the juxtaglomerular apparatus (JGA) associated with the afferent arterioles in the kidney. Directly and through sympathetic nerve activity, the JGA in turn elevates or reduces the level of renin secretion, leading to increased or decreased production of angiotensin II. Elevated circulating angiotensin II then results in adrenal release of aldosterone (the renin-angiotensin-aldosterone [RAA] hormonal cascade). Angiotensin II and aldosterone increase the reabsorption of isotonic fluid from the renal tubules. Angiotensin II also increases vascular resistance throughout the body so that it affects blood pressure by changing both intravascular volume and systemic resistance.

2. Atrial and ventricular receptors sense stretch and alter the release of atrial natriuretic peptide (ANP), a 28-amino acid peptide stored in granules of the myocytes and brain natriuretic peptide (BNP). These peptides are systemic vasodilators, act on the kidney to raise glomerular capillary pressure, and reduce tubular salt and water reabsorption.

3. When pressure is extremely low, the baroreceptors stimulate the secretion of antidiuretic hormone (ADH), which increases the reabsorption of water from the tubule.

FIGURE 22.4 provides an overview of the homeostatic responses to changes in perfusion pressure.

Sensors of Perfusion Pressure

BP changes throughout the day in accordance with stress, exertion, variations in dietary salt and water intake, and fluid losses. BP also changes in many pathologic states, such as hemorrhage. Sensors of perfusion pressure detect both physiologic and pathologic challenges to normal BP and trigger homeostatic correction.

Baroreceptors signal the brain in response to stretch in blood vessel walls. When increased perfusion pressure distends the vessel wall, the baroreceptor increases its rate of firing. The stretch of these specialized cells is due to the transmural pressure gradients felt across the vessel wall. For example, the myocytes containing ANP and BNP stretch in response to a pressure gradient between the atrial cavity and the intrathoracic space. As mentioned in Chapter 12, a **perfusion pressure** or **driving pressure** is the gradient of pressures between two places within the circulation. The actual pressure at one site in the circulation contributes both to the transmural pressure and the driving pressure forward through the circulation. Therefore, the actual pressure at a site in the circulation where the peripheral or atrial mechanoreceptors exist contributes to a transmural distending pressure.

There are two baroreceptors in low-pressure areas of the vascular tree and three in high-pressure areas. The first group is located in the low-pressure cardiac atria and pulmonary vessels. The second group of receptors is found in the high-pressure aortic arch, carotid sinus, and in the JGA in the afferent arterioles of the kidney. In addition to serving as baroreceptors, the cells of the JGA produce, store, and secrete renin.

In some pathologic conditions, the ECF volume may be high (hypervolemia) while the perfusion pressures are low. An example is congestive heart failure (CHF), when fluid pools in the veins and CO falls owing to poor heart pumping ability. Because the homeostatic sensors respond to perfusion pressure, which will be low in the poor CO state, they trigger changes in ECF volume. The kidneys add to the ECF volume to boost the blood pressure, although the ECF volume is already expanded. (Most of this volume is in the venous side of the circulation.) This added fluid collects in the high-capacitance veins and eventually leaks out into the interstitium from the peripheral capillary, causing swelling in the tissues. The driving forces for the movement of fluid from vascular to interstitial compartments are the Starling forces that include capillary hydrostatic pressures in excess of interstitial hydrostatic pressures. Therapeutic intervention with *diuretics* removes the excess fluid and swelling, and other drugs can improve the performance of the heart. (See Clinical Application Box *Diuretics*.)

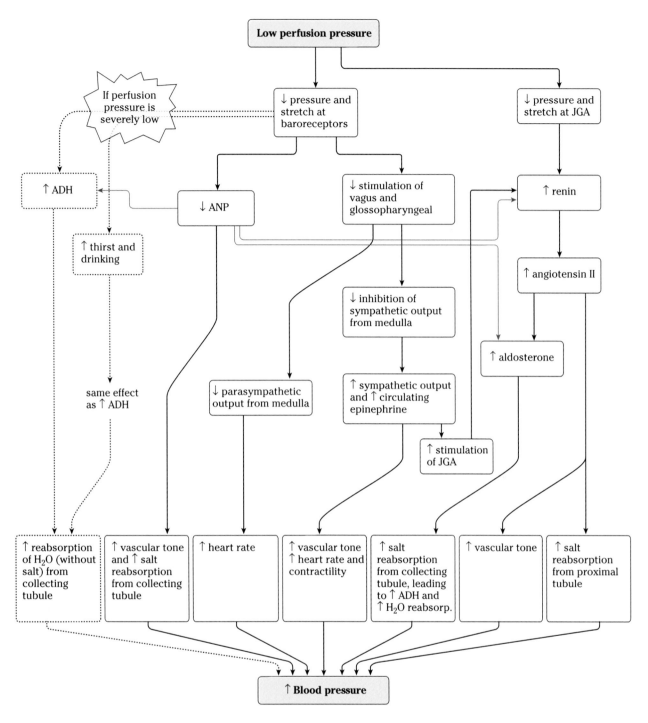

Figure 22.4 Homeostatic responses to changes in perfusion pressure. This chart shows all the parallel pathways that are activated in the response to changes in perfusion pressure, as well as the horizontal interactions between pathways. As we discuss each individual efferent pathway, we will reproduce this figure with the relevant pathway highlighted. Note that only the response to low perfusion pressure is depicted in this figure and in each of the related highlighted figures. High perfusion pressure produces effects through the exact same pathways and with all the same interactions, but the changes are in the opposite direction. The baroreceptors detect *increased* stretch, ANP AND BNP secretion goes *up*, vagal stimulation goes *up*, sympathetic inhibition goes *up*, renin secretion goes *down*, etc., and finally, blood pressure is *decreased*.

DIURETICS

Diuretics are drugs used to elevate urine volume and decrease ECF volume. They are most often used to treat hypertension or CHF. There are four kinds of diuretics: loop diuretics, thiazide-type diuretics, K^+-sparing diuretics, and carbonic anhydrase inhibitors (FIGURE B22.1). Loop diuretics inhibit the Na/K/2Cl cotransporter in the loop of Henle, impeding salt reabsorption. Thiazide diuretics bind the Na/Cl cotransporter in the distal tubule, inhibiting salt reabsorption there. Loop and thiazide diuretics can promote K^+ wasting because they increase tubular flow to the K^+ secretion site in the collecting duct. Increased flow keeps the tubule $[K^+]$ down and improves the gradient for K^+ secretion. K^+-sparing diuretics inhibit salt reabsorption where salt reabsorption is coupled with K^+ secretion (i.e., they inhibit aldosterone), thereby preserving serum K^+. Carbonic anhydrase inhibition in the proximal tubule cells inhibits bicarbonate reabsorption and thereby osmotically promotes diuresis.

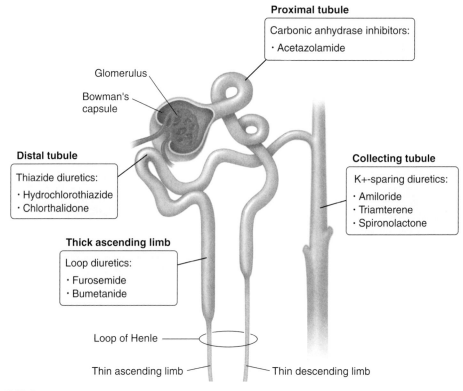

Proximal tubule
Carbonic anhydrase inhibitors:
· Acetazolamide

Glomerulus

Bowman's capsule

Distal tubule
Thiazide diuretics:
· Hydrochlorothiazide
· Chlorthalidone

Collecting tubule
K+-sparing diuretics:
· Amiloride
· Triamterene
· Spironolactone

Thick ascending limb
Loop diuretics:
· Furosemide
· Bumetanide

Loop of Henle

Thin ascending limb   Thin descending limb

Figure B22.1   Diuretics and their sites of action along the nephron.

Therefore, it is important to remember that although ECF volume and perfusion pressure are related, they are not the same, and despite the fact that the kidney affects perfusion pressure by altering ECF volume, the kidney senses only arterial perfusion pressure. Many texts use the term *effective circulating volume (ECV)* in addressing pathologic situations such as the one just described. The idea is that only some of the high fluid volume in the body is "effective"; that is, only some of the volume is actively perfusing the tissues while the rest remains pooled in the veins or sitting in the interstitium, effectively out of circulation. Only the ECV, not the ECF volume, affects perfusion pressure. Therefore, alterations in ECV, not total ECF volume, drive the baroreceptor reflex. Note that in the heart failure patient, there can simultaneously be increased stretch of atrial myocytes, releasing ANP and BNP, and decreased arterial pressure, stimulating Na^+-retaining nerves and hormones. The net effect may be vasoconstriction and Na^+ retention, rather than vasodilation and natriuresis (Na^+ excretion).

Afferent Pathways of Transmission and Control Centers

The baroreceptors in the low-pressure atria and pulmonary vessels communicate with the control center, the **medulla** in the brain, via the **vagus nerve** (cranial nerve X). To some extent, the atrial and ventricular receptors also function as their own control center, secreting the hormones ANP and BNP directly when stimulated. The aortic arch and carotid sinus baroreceptors transmit information to the medulla as well—the aortic arch through the vagus nerve and the carotid sinus through the **glossopharyngeal nerve** (cranial nerve IX). Higher perfusion pressure leads to more stimulation from peripheral baroreceptors, which in turn signals the body to lower the blood pressure through its effector mechanisms. Lower perfusion pressure and less stimulation of the baroreceptors and medulla tells the body's effectors to do the opposite.

The JGA is its own control center. It alters its renin secretion in direct response to stimulation by changes in stretch at the afferent arteriole of the nephrons.

Efferent Pathways of Transmission

In general, the efferent pathways are neural or hormonal. The sympathetic nerves are a major route of efferent transmission, extending from the medulla to peripheral arterioles throughout the body. The sympathetic nerves also synapse with the adrenal gland and help to govern the secretion of *epinephrine* from the adrenal gland into the bloodstream. Circulating epinephrine is a hormonal efferent pathway that reinforces the effects of stimulation by the sympathetic nerves. The medulla also sends out signals along the parasympathetic efferent fibers in the vagus nerve. Under normal circumstances, there is always some amount of output from the medulla along sympathetic and parasympathetic nerves. This output is called *sympathetic tone* and *parasympathetic tone*. When the body makes changes using these pathways, it increases or decreases sympathetic and parasympathetic tone. Parasympathetic output works reciprocally with sympathetic output; that is, when perfusion pressure is high, the body decreases sympathetic tone and increases parasympathetic tone. As we will see in the information to follow, reduced sympathetic tone decreases the blood pressure and the ECF volume. Increased sympathetic tone raises the blood pressure and the ECF volume. In response to increased perfusion pressure, the parasympathetic tone acts mainly as a negative chronotrope at the heart (meaning it lowers the heart rate) to reduce CO and BP. Sympathetic nerves also

synapse with the JGA, augmenting the stimulation from the JGA's own sensors (FIGURE 22.5).

The JGA transmits information to the effectors of the **RAA system**. When perfusion pressure is low, the JGA senses this directly through its own baroreceptors and indirectly through the body's other baroreceptors, which tell the JGA through increased sympathetic input to the JGA. The JGA then secretes more renin. When perfusion pressure is high, the JGA secretes less renin. **Renin** converts *angiotensinogen* (produced in the liver) to *angiotensin I*, and angiotensin I is converted in the lung to its active form, angiotensin II, with the help of *angiotensin-converting enzyme (ACE)* (FIGURE 22.6). ACE is found in large quantities on the endothelial surfaces of the pulmonary vasculature. Because angiotensinogen and ACE are readily available in high concentrations, renin secretion yields rapid production of angiotensin II. **Angiotensin II** acts directly on the kidney and blood vessels to increase blood volume and pressure, and also acts on the zona glomerulosa of the adrenal cortex, promoting the aldosterone secretion. **Aldosterone** is a steroid hormone (a mineralocorticoid as opposed to a glucocorticoid) that acts on the kidney to increase blood volume by means that will be discussed later in this chapter. FIGURE 22.7 highlights the role of the RAA system in responding to changes in perfusion pressure.

The RAA system is a vital component of the rapid response to depleted intravascular volume and pressure, as might occur with hemorrhage. The result is prevention of excess urinary losses of fluid and vasoconstriction of vessels to maintain pressure. In some disease states, however, the RAA system may act to increase blood pressure and blood volume inappropriately. This situation can occur with tumors of the kidney that secrete renin or of the adrenal gland where aldosterone is overproduced.

The atrial baroreceptor, in addition to transmitting information via the autonomic nerves, also secretes the hormone **ANP**. In contrast to the RAA system, more ANP is secreted in response to *high* perfusion pressure. ANP acts to decrease the blood volume by means that will be discussed later, and decreases systemic vascular resistance (SVR), thereby lowering blood pressure. FIGURE 22.8 summarizes the role of ANP in responding to changes in perfusion pressure.

Finally, **ADH** is secreted from the posterior pituitary as an agent of efferent transmission. The baroreceptors send signals directly to ADH secretory cells in the neurohypophysis. This process is known as **baroreceptor control of ADH**, in contrast to osmoreceptor control of ADH, the usual mode of ADH control. Normally, ADH's role is in connection with regulating plasma osmolality (see Chapter 23). When plasma osmolality is high, ADH acts at the kidney to promote the

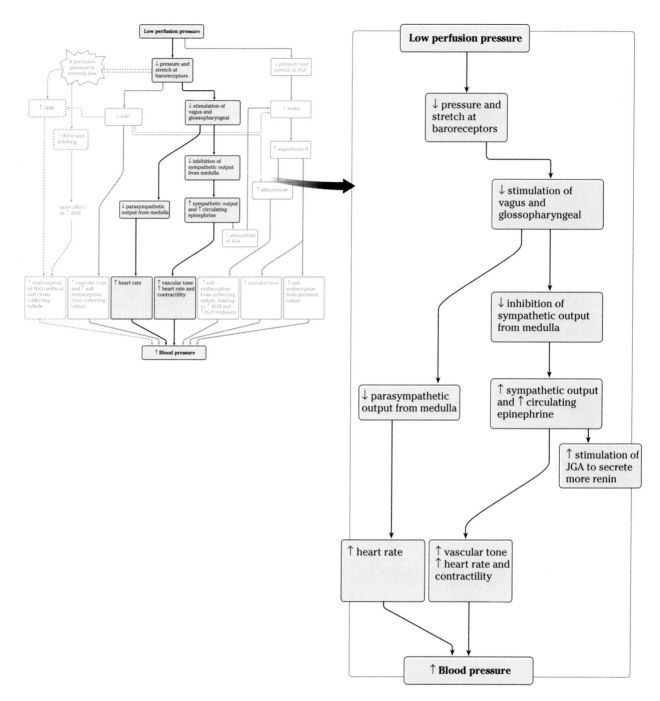

Figure 22.5 Sympathetic and parasympathetic responses to changes in perfusion pressure. This auto-nomic pathway represents the sum total of cardiovascular responses to changes in perfusion pressure. It is also a major contributor to the renal response by way of its stimulation of the JGA and RAA system.

reabsorption of water without solute, thereby reduc-ing the plasma osmolality. In severe blood volume depletion, however, the baroreceptors stimulate ADH secretion (FIGURE 22.9). The baroreceptor system is less sensitive than the osmoreceptor system for ADH secretion, and the baroreceptors require a 5% to10% reduction in blood pressure before inducing ADH se-cretion. In contrast, the sympathetic nerves and RAA system respond to smaller decrements of pressure

and volume. Once the less sensitive baroreceptor control of ADH is activated, however, baroreceptor control overrides osmoreceptor control. In the case when large volumes of water are ingested at a time of extreme hypotension, the baroreceptor-mediated in-crease in ADH predominates over the osmoreceptor-mediated decrease. The result is water retention and a low body fluid osmolality until the intravascular vol-ume is replenished.

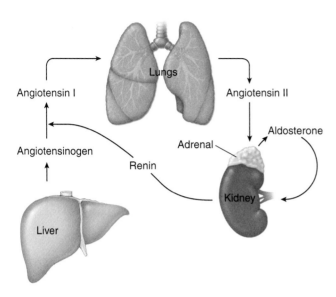

Figure 22.6 Components of the RAA system. The liver produces angiotensinogen in order to maintain a constant level of it in the bloodstream. The liver does not participate in the homeostatic response to changes in perfusion pressure.

Not only does reduced baroreceptor stimulation lead to the hypothalamic production of ADH; it also contributes to the thirst response, which will be described in more detail in Chapter 23. Also, baroreceptor input to the hypothalamus can reduce the hypothalamic set point for osmotic ADH secretion. The consequence is that in hypotensive patients, lower levels of plasma osmolality will stimulate ADH, and, in fact, such patients may become severely hyponatremic.

Effector Mechanisms in the Regulation of Perfusion Pressure

Once the sensors have detected a change in perfusion pressure and the control center has sent out signals along the efferent pathways, it is finally up to the effectors to do the work of returning perfusion pressure to its desired level. The effectors are best discussed by grouping them under the efferent pathway that triggers them.

The Effects of the Sympathetic Nerves The sympathetic nerves employ as their effectors the heart and arterioles throughout the body. Most important to renal function, the sympathetic nerves also indirectly stimulate angiotensin II through sympathetic stimulation of the JGA. Sympathetic constriction of vascular beds throughout the body increases SVR and raises BP. (See Chapter 12 for more information on how increased SVR affects BP.) The nerves achieve this through direct synaptic secretion of norepinephrine onto blood vessels and through stimulat-

ing the adrenal medulla to produce circulating epinephrine. It should be noted, however, that arterioles supplying active skeletal muscle beds do not constrict. When exercised, active muscle, in fact, produces local vasodilation and blood flow increases to the active muscle. This is because local vasodilating metabolites override the sympathetic vasoconstriction. Resting muscle during exercise maintains vasoconstrictor tone, allowing active muscle to receive greater blood flow. Thereby, sympathetic vasoconstriction does not impede muscular action during the "fight-or-flight" response.

Constriction of the afferent and efferent arterioles at the kidney nephrons has special consequences. Not only does this contribute to the increase in SVR, but it also decreases renal blood flow (RBF), which reduces the glomerular filtration rate (GFR). In turn, decreased GFR means a slightly higher percentage of plasma volume and salt is retained in the blood vessels. It is a common misconception among students, however, that GFR reduction is an important means of increasing the ECF volume. Although GFR reduction does conserve water and volume in some fishes like eels and salmon, and in marine mammals, it is not a means of protecting the ECF volume in humans. First, remember that the human body has autoregulatory mechanisms in place to *preserve* GFR, even in the face of decreased RBF (see Chapter 20). Second, remember that blood composition after passing through the kidney is determined by the combination of filtration, reabsorption, and secretion. *Tubular reabsorption of salt is the most important determinant of ECF volume, not filtration.* A slightly decreased GFR does reduce the amount of salt and water delivered to the tubule, making it somewhat easier for the tubule to prevent the loss of salt, water, and volume from the body, but other mechanisms are far more important to the preservation of blood volume.

At the heart, sympathetic stimulation increases the heart rate and contractility, which increases stroke volume. Stroke volume times the heart rate equals cardiac output (CO). Increased CO means increased BP, according to the Ohm's law analogy. When perfusion pressure is low and sympathetic tone is high, parasympathetic tone is conversely low, lessening the inhibition of the heart rate.

The Arteriolar Effects of Angiotensin II on Perfusion Pressure The RAA system's effectors are the body's arterioles and the renal tubule. When low perfusion pressure stimulates the JGA, renin is released, yielding angiotensin II and aldosterone, as described previously (Figure 22.6). Angiotensin II has two direct effects on perfusion pressure. It acts as a vasoconstrictor on arterioles throughout the body, raising the SVR, and it stimulates increased salt reabsorption in the proximal tubule.

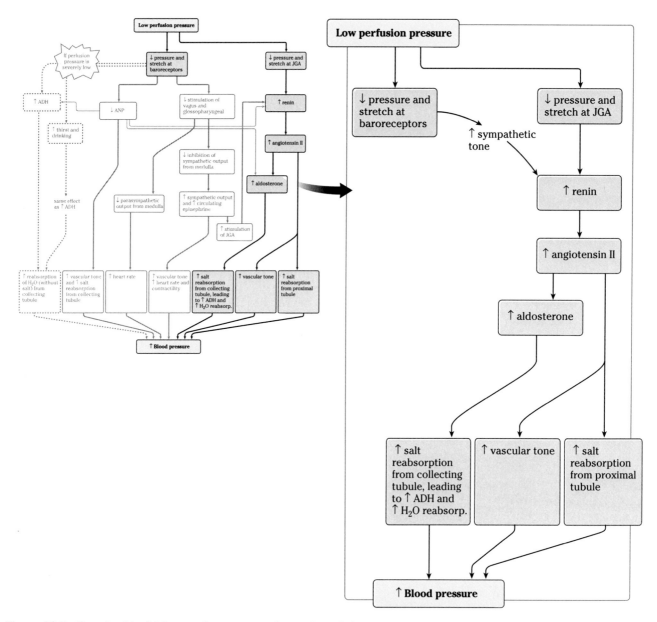

Figure 22.7   The role of the RAA system in response to changes in perfusion pressure.

In discussing sympathetic constriction of the arterioles, we noted that autoregulatory mechanisms preserve GFR even as the renal blood flow is reduced. Recall that angiotensin II actually creates a drop in RBF and accomplishes autoregulation at the same time. It constricts the efferent arteriole more than the afferent, increasing the hydrostatic pressure in the glomerulus to favor filtration (FIGURE 22.10). This rises the GFR as the RBF drops, thus raising the filtration fraction (FIGURE 22.11).

This efferent arteriolar constriction not only preserves GFR but also augments fluid reabsorption into the peritubular capillaries by lowering the hydrostatic pressure in the peritubular capillary. Also, because the filtration fraction has gone up, the oncotic

pressure in the peritubular capillaries is greater. Both of these changes favor the reabsorption of fluid from tubule to capillary (FIGURE 22.12).

How Angiotensin II Expands Extracellular Fluid Volume   To understand how angiotensin II's increased salt reabsorption in the proximal tubule expands the ECF volume, we must first understand the features of the proximal tubule wall and its contents. The proximal tubule wall is permeable to water and salt and contains basolateral Na^+/K^+-ATPase pumps that drive Na^+ reabsorption (FIGURE 22.13). The proximal tubule contents are isotonic to plasma, because the glomerulus filters solution isotonic to plasma. Therefore, when the proximal tubule pumps Na^+ out

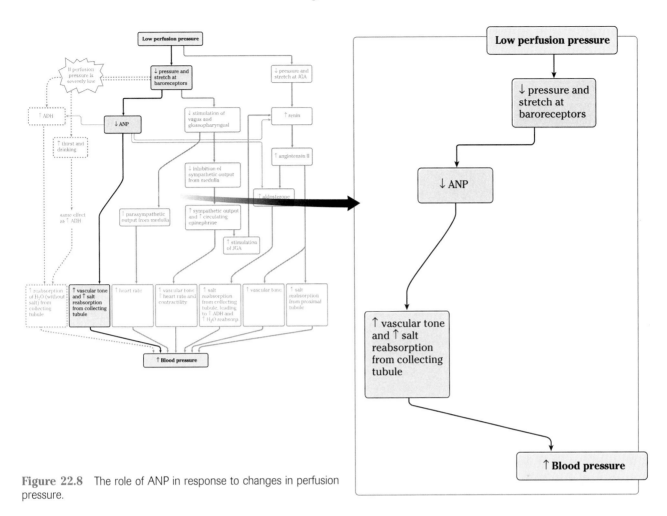

Figure 22.8   The role of ANP in response to changes in perfusion pressure.

of the tubule lumen and into the interstitium, water passively follows by osmosis, and a saltwater solution isotonic to plasma is reabsorbed and added back to the plasma of the peritubular capillary.

Why is it important that the kidney add *isotonic* fluid back to the bloodstream in its efforts to boost ECF volume? If it added hypotonic fluid, much of the added fluid would osmotically redistribute into the ICF space, thus failing to raise ECF volume as much. Why is it important that the proximal tubule reabsorb an isotonic *sodium* salt solution? Na^+ is the major effective osmole in the ECF space. The proximal tubule reabsorbs K^+ in proportion to Na^+, but because reabsorbed Na^+ stays in the ECF space as an effective osmole, the water (and hence, the volume) stays in the ECF space.

Given the information in the previous paragraph, we should not be surprised that when angiotensin II prompts increased activity of the apical Na^+/H^+ antiporter, the ECF expands. Increased activity of the Na^+/H^+ antiporter drives more Na^+ into the cell, in turn driving more Na+ across the basolateral membrane by the Na^+/K^+-ATPase—that is, driving more salt reabsorption—and adding more isotonic fluid to the ECF space.

The Indirect Effects of Angiotensin II on Perfusion Pressure   In addition to its two direct effects, angiotensin II has two indirect effects on perfusion pressure. It stimulates aldosterone secretion from the adrenal gland, and, alongside the baroreceptor control of ADH, it also stimulates the secretion of ADH at very low blood volumes. Finally, angiotensin II has a negative-feedback effect on renin, inhibiting its secretion from the JGA.

The Effects of Aldosterone   Aldosterone acts on the principal cells of the cortical collecting tubule (FIGURE 22.14A). Here, it transduces its signal like all steroids, by binding to an intracellular receptor that turns on protein synthesis. This protein synthesis yields more Na^+/K^+-ATPase and more Na^+ channels, increasing salt reabsorption. As in the proximal tubule, the reabsorption of salt leads to expansion of the ECF volume. The expansion due to aldosterone action is not a simple case of adding isotonic saline solution to the ECF, however. Fluid in the collecting duct is not isotonic to plasma, and the collecting duct is not permeable to water unless ADH is present. Aldosterone may prompt the reabsorption of Na^+ without water, and the water may follow only after osmoreceptors in the

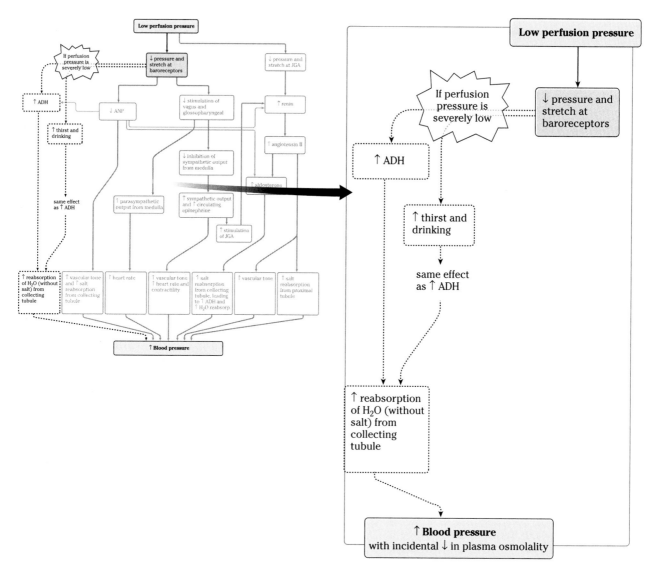

Figure 22.9   The role of ADH in response to very low perfusion pressure. ADH is the critical hormone in renal osmoregulation and is not a participant in the regulation of perfusion pressure unless perfusion pressure drops significantly. ADH is not an important constituent of the response to high perfusion pressure.

brain have detected an increase in osmolality and prompted the secretion of ADH. Then, water can be osmotically reabsorbed after the salt, producing a net effect of salt, water, and hence volume addition to the ECF (Fig. 22.14B). (See Integrated Physiology Box *How Aldosterone Links ECF Volume, K⁺, and H⁺ Balance.*)

The Effects of ANP   The effector mechanisms employed by ANP and BNP are different from those employed by the RAA system; whereas the RAA system signals to increase perfusion pressure, ANP and BNP signal to decrease perfusion pressure. As one might predict, this means that different stimuli prompt ANP and BNP secretion. Low pressure at the baroreceptors yields higher sympathetic tone and renin release; high pressure and stretch at the atrial baroreceptors leads to ANP and BNP secretion directly from the atria.

ANP and BNP achieve salt excretion in three ways: they directly inhibit salt reabsorption in the collecting duct, they inhibit the release of aldosterone from the adrenal gland, and they inhibit renin release from the JGA. The consequent decrease in reabsorption of saltwater from the tubule increases the percentage of the filtered volume that is lost to urine and therefore subtracts from the ECF volume. ANP and BNP also promote the loss of water without salt to some degree, by inhibiting the secretion of ADH from the posterior pituitary and inhibiting ADH action on the collecting duct. Finally, ANP and BNP act on the arterioles throughout the body to vasodilate, thus lowering systemic vascular resistance. ANP and BNP reduce ECF volume in concert with the lowering of sympathetic tone and the reduction of renin output.

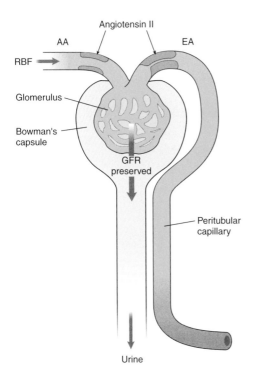

Figure 22.10   The effect of angiotensin II on the renal arterioles. Angiotensin II decreases renal blood flow while preserving GFR.

The Effects of ADH   ADH's main effector is the collecting duct in the nephron. ADH promotes water reabsorption without solute. As stated previously, adding pure water to the ECF is not as effective as adding isotonic saline; furthermore, under normal circumstances, the body deploys ADH to lower plasma osmolality and not to correct low perfusion pressure.

ADH secretion in response to baroreceptor stimulation is a type of last resort for raising perfusion pressure in very low volume states. At very high levels, ADH also has a systemic vasoconstrictive effect, which accounts for its alternate name, *vasopressin*. In fact, vasopressin infusions are used clinically to raise blood pressure in critically ill patients with hypotension.

Other Mediators

Whereas the sympathetic nerves, the RAA system, ANP, BNP, and ADH are the main efferents involved in the regulation of perfusion pressure, there are other mediators that act systemically to help maintain vessel tone and BP. Although these mediators are not involved with the homeostatic response to changes in BP, disturbances in their secretion can have dramatic effects on BP. **Glucocorticoids** from the zona fasciculata of the adrenal cortex are critical to the maintenance of normal blood pressure. Cortisol potentiates the constrictive action of catecholamines, decreases the permeability of the vascular endothelium to keep fluid inside the vascular tree, and enhances myocardial function. Cortisol generates a constant level of vessel tone, and, once again, *does not* respond to changes in BP. Estrogen has a number of less critical effects on BP. It is thought to raise BP by increasing salt retention and RAA activity from an increased production of angiotensinogen and to have a vasodilatory effect through the stimulation of nitric oxide (NO) synthase.

In addition to the systemically acting mediators, there are vasoactive mediators produced by endothelial cells that act locally—in other words, at or near their site of origin. Mediators acting at their site

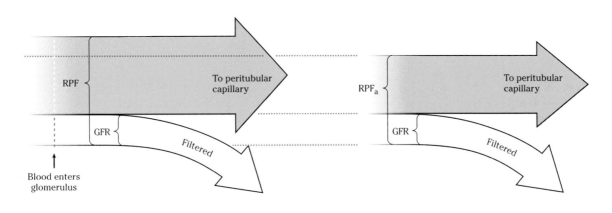

RPF = Volume of plasma entering glomerulus per unit time

GFR = Volume of blood filtered per unit time

GFR/RPF = Filtration fraction

RPF_a = Volume of plasma entering glomerulus per unit time **under the influence of angiotensin II**

GFR/RPF_a = Filtration fraction **under the influence of angiotensin II**

Figure 22.11   The effect of angiotensin II on filtration fraction. Under the influence of angiotensin II, the volume of plasma entering the glomerulus per unit time falls while GFR remains roughly the same. Therefore, $GFR/RPF_a > GFR/RPF$; the filtration fraction rises under the influence of angiotensin II.

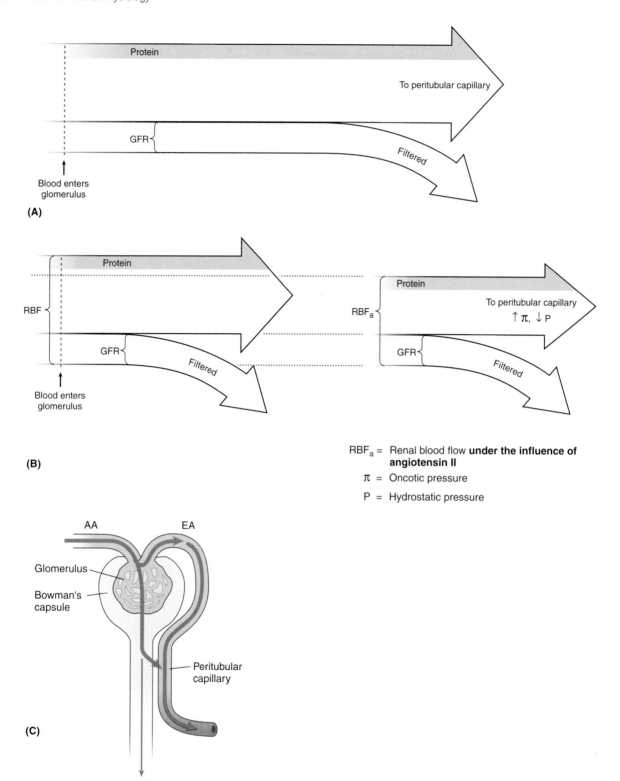

Figure 22.12   The impact of increased filtration fraction on peritubular reabsorption. **A.** The oncotic pressure goes up in the postfiltration fluid of the efferent arteriole. Owing to the lower fluid volume in the efferent fluid, there is also less hydrostatic pressure. **B.** Increased filtration fraction under the influence of angiotensin II results in an even higher oncotic pressure in the efferent peritubular fluid. **C.** This increased peritubular oncotic pressure and decreased hydrostatic pressure under the influence of angiotensin II means that there will be more fluid reabsorption by the peritubular capillary.

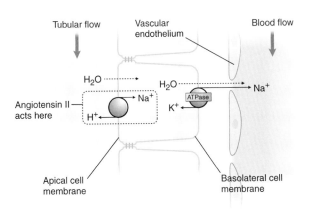

Figure 22.13 Angiotensin II action in the proximal tubule. Angiotensin II increases the activity of the apical Na^+/H^+ antiporter.

of origin are called *autocrine*; mediators acting near their site of origin are called *paracrine*. In response to a variety of stimuli, endothelial cells produce vasodilators such as *NO* and *prostaglandin*, and vasoconstrictors such as *endothelin*. Nitric oxide's potent vasodilatory effect works through a cyclic GMP mechanism. Many vascular beds can synthesize NO locally for regulation of blood flow. The kidney is an important site of NO synthesis because the kidney is an arginine producer for the body, and arginine can be converted to NO. (Intestinal citrulline is taken up by proximal tubule cells and converted to arginine. Due to the absence of the urea cycle enzyme, arginase, arginine is not recycled into urea and ornithine.) Locally produced renin and angiotensin act independently of the renal RAA system. The vasodilatory effects of some prostaglandins serve to dampen the response to low perfusion pressure.

PATHOPHYSIOLOGY

Dietary variations in salt and water intake produce daily fluctuations in ECF volume. These fluctuations must be corrected in order to keep ECF volume high enough for adequate perfusion and to keep ECF volume low enough to avoid edema and hypertensive complications. Normally, the kidneys can handle these fluctuations in salt and water intake without difficulty. In fact, on average, Americans consume more than 20 times the salt they need every day, and the majority stay free of hypertension as long as they have normal renal function. Various conditions may either overwhelm or impair the kidney's ability to maintain normal ECF volume, however.

Although this chapter discussed homeostatic regulation of blood pressure in general, the pathophysiology section is limited to derangements of fluid volume. It does not discuss the very important topic

of essential hypertension—that is, hypertension at normal fluid volumes.

Disorders of Extracellular Fluid Volume

There are three main types of disorders of ECF volume: hypovolemia with low intravascular volume and therefore low perfusion pressure, hypervolemia with normal or high intravascular volume and therefore high perfusion pressure, and hypervolemia with low intravascular volume and therefore low perfusion pressure (Table 22.1). Hypovolemia with high perfusion pressure is infrequent. In cases of malignant hypertension (extreme hypertension due to factors other than ECF volume), hypovolemia and hypertension may be seen together.

Hypovolemia Causes of **hypovolemia**, or low ECF volume, include hemorrhage, vomiting, diarrhea, poor fluid intake, and many conditions that lead to polyuria (diabetes mellitus, diabetes insipidus, iatrogenic overtreatment with diuretics, and hypercalcemia). In these situations, the baroreceptors sense low perfusion pressure, sympathetic tone increases,

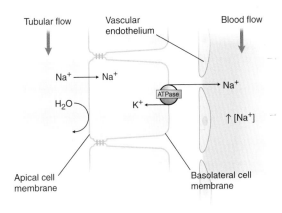

(A)

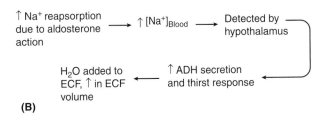

(B)

Figure 22.14 Aldosterone action in the cortical collecting duct. **A.** Aldosterone increases the number of Na^+/K^+-ATPases on the basolateral membrane and the number of Na+ channels on the apical side. Water cannot directly follow salt here. **B.** Aldosterone-mediated increases in Na^+ reabsorption alter osmolality and lead to ADH secretion. Aldosterone can raise the ECF volume only through ADH secretion.

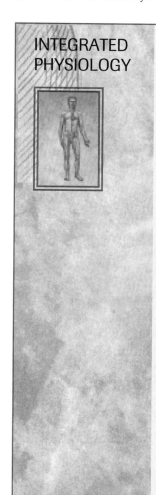

INTEGRATED PHYSIOLOGY

How Aldosterone Links ECF Volume, K⁺, and H⁺ Balance

In addition to its effects on ECF volume, aldosterone governs K^+ balance and affects acid-base balance. As aldosterone upregulates the activity of the Na^+/K^+-AT-Pase to pump Na^+ into the interstitium from the tubule lumen, it concurrently pumps K^+ from the blood and interstitium into the lumen for excretion. Not only does this occur as an incidental result of efforts to restore ECF volume; the adrenal gland actually senses the plasma $[K^+]$ and releases aldosterone in response to high $[K^+]$. Aldosterone also has an effect on acid excretion because it stimulates the activity of the H^+-ATPase in the intercalated cells of the collecting duct, thereby increasing acid excretion in urine. As a result of these multiple roles, ECF volume status, K^+ balance, and acid-base balance are interrelated. Decreases in perfusion pressure that prompt the release of aldosterone may also drive down the plasma $[K^+]$ and raise the plasma pH. (The latter situation is sometimes called a *contraction alkalosis* because *contracted* ECF volume drives aldosterone release and consequent H^+ excretion). Increases in $[K^+]$ that prompt the release of aldosterone may promote salt reabsorption and volume expansion, although this relationship is less clinically important than the one between ECF volume and plasma pH, for reasons discussed in Chapter 24.

Why should one hormone, aldosterone, participate in more than one homeostatic system? One possible reason is that this situation creates negative feedback to avoid either too much volume expansion or too much K^+ secretion. When a lot of volume has been added, the adrenal gland will sense low $[K^+]$ and scale down its production of aldosterone, preventing further volume expansion and hypokalemia from aldosterone. Both the homeostatic system governing ECF volume and that governing $[K^+]$ employ other, more important, sources of negative feedback; however, the body typically involves redundant systems as backup mechanisms.

Table 22.1 DISORDERS OF ECF VOLUME

Disorder	Causes

Hypovolemia	Hemorrhage
	Vomiting
	Diarrhea
	Poor fluid intake
	Polyuria
	  Diabetes mellitus
	  Diabetes insipidus
	  Iatrogenic overtreatment
	    with diuretics
	  Hypercalcemia

Hypervolemia with normal or high perfusion pressure	Advanced renal failure Nephrotic syndrome
Hypervolemia with low perfusion pressure	Congestive heart failure Cirrhosis Nephrotic syndrome with severe proteinuria

renin is released, and the body attempts to reverse the low blood pressure. Signs and symptoms of hypovolemia may include dry mucous membranes (such as inside the mouth), fainting (syncope), orthostatic hypotension, and an elevated blood urea nitrogen (BUN)/creatinine (Cr) ratio. BUN and Cr are routine lab values.

All of these signs and symptoms reflect inadequate perfusion; in syncope, it is a case of poor perfusion of the brain. In people with hypovolemia, venous return to the heart drops when they change from a sitting or lying position to a standing position. The drop in venous return to the heart causes a decrease in blood pressure and a compensatory rise in heart rate (tachycardia). Measuring blood pressure and heart rate in the supine position and then in the standing position (sometimes referred to in the hospital as performing "orthostatics") is often a part of assessing a patient with syncope. (See Clinical Application Box *The Vasovagal Response.*)

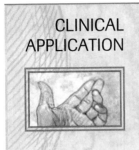

THE VASOVAGAL RESPONSE

CLINICAL APPLICATION

People with no disturbance of their ECF volume can faint from low blood pressure, too. In the vasovagal response, anxiety may trigger vigorous sympathetic-mediated ventricular contraction leading to parasympathetic output, which decreases cardiac output and causes syncope. *Micturition syncope* is another form of vasovagal response. In this case, the parasympathetic output associated with urination decreases cardiac output and causes syncope.

The elevated BUN/Cr ratio in hypovolemia reflects the way that urea and creatinine are cleared from the blood. Creatinine is filtered, but not reabsorbed and secreted only to a small extent. Urea is filtered and reabsorbed. The increased tubular reabsorption of fluid associated with hypovolemia (affected by the mechanisms described previously) increases the reabsorption of urea in the proximal tubule and medullary collecting duct, but not that of creatinine.

Hypovolemia with poor renal perfusion is one cause of acute prerenal failure. Thus, an elevated BUN/Cr ratio (usually > 20:1) is sometimes called a "prerenal" condition.

Hypervolemia with Normal or High Perfusion Pressure **Hypervolemia** is high ECF volume. Diseases that significantly decrease renal Na+ excretion lead to significant water retention, hypervolemia, and generalized edema. The two major examples are advanced renal failure and many cases of nephrotic syndrome. In advanced **renal failure** when the GFR is very low, little salt and water are delivered to the tubule to allow excretion. **Nephrotic syndrome** refers to a group of disorders that increase glomerular permeability to protein. For reasons not well understood, an increase in collecting duct reabsorption of salt is associated with the nephrotic syndrome, which expands the ECF volume. (Increased glomerular permeability leads to a loss of albumin, the major protein in the blood, to urine; if the proteinuria is severe enough, it can create cases of nephrotic syndrome in which the hypervolemia is associated with low perfusion pressure.) Volume expansion due to increased salt reabsorption can also be seen in cases of acute *glomerulonephritis*, a group of inflammatory disorders of the glomerulus. When salt and water retention expand the ECF volume, the hydrostatic pressure created in the capillaries by the volume expansion leads to leakage from the capillaries into the interstitium. This is *generalized edema*, a general swelling of the tissues. (See Clinical Application Boxes *What Is Nephrotic Syndrome?* and *Causes of Edema in Nephrotic Syndrome.*)

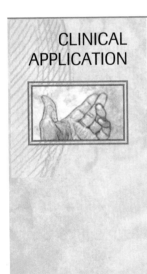

WHAT IS NEPHROTIC SYNDROME?

CLINICAL APPLICATION

A 15-year-old boy goes to see the pediatrician with a complaint of swelling around the ankles of several months' duration. Aside from some pitting edema of the lower extremities, he has a normal physical exam and a blood pressure of 130/80 mm Hg. Lab tests reveal 3.5 g of albumin in the 24-hour urine (normally < 30 mg per day) and a low serum albumin of 3.0 g/dL (normal is 3.5 to 5 g/dL). The pediatrician suspects nephrotic syndrome.

Nephrotic syndrome is caused by damage to the glomerulus and is characterized clinically by heavy proteinuria, hypoalbuminemia, and edema. The most common underlying pathology in children is *minimal change disease*, but this disease also affects adults. Other causes include focal and segmental glomerular sclerosis, membranous glomerulonephritis, diabetic nephropathy, amyloidosis, and preeclampsia. In these conditions, the glomerulus becomes permeable to protein macromolecules. Damage to the renal tubule leads to salt retention and hence edema. When the hypoalbuminemia associated with the disease is more severe, the oncotic gradient decreases between the intravascular space and the interstitium, promoting more edema. Minimal change disease responds very well to treatment with glucocorticoids and rarely progresses to renal failure.

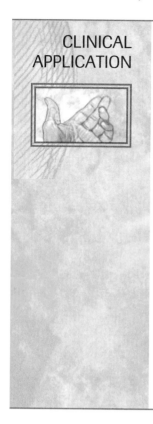

CAUSES OF EDEMA IN NEPHROTIC SYNDROME

As explained in the text, some cases of nephrotic syndrome lead to hypervolemia with high perfusion pressure, and some lead to hypervolemia with low perfusion pressure. When should we expect normal or high pressure with edema from salt and water retention (*overflow edema*), and when should we expect normal or low pressure with edema from proteinuria and low oncotic pressure (edema from *underfilling* of the vasculature)?

When hypoalbuminemia is less severe, we should expect to see hypervolemia with high intravascular volume and pressure. Even though proteinuria has decreased the intravascular oncotic pressure, why does the oncotic pressure gradient not favor extravasation of fluid from the vessels? The hypoalbuminemia has caused the oncotic pressure of the interstitium to drop in proportion to that of the vessels. Remember that it is the oncotic pressure of the vessels relative to the interstitium, the oncotic *gradient*, which drives the movement of fluid. In this case, there is no oncotic gradient.

When the hypoalbuminemia becomes more severe (e.g., less than 2.5 g/dL), however, the oncotic pressure gradient does begin to favor extravasation of fluid. The protein level of the interstitium reaches a minimum below which it cannot sink. As the intravascular protein level continues to fall, its oncotic pressure falls relative to the interstitial oncotic pressure. The vessels lose fluid to the interstitium, creating edema from underfilling of the vascular space, and as in cirrhosis and CHF, hypervolemia with low pressure ensues. The baroreceptors worsen the problem by signaling the kidneys to hold onto more salt and fluid, which is immediately third-spaced.

Hypervolemia with Low Perfusion Pressure In some states of increased ECF volume (often referred to clinically as *volume-expanded* states), the volume and pressure in the arterial system may be low. Important examples are congestive heart failure (CHF), cirrhosis, and some cases of nephrosis. In **CHF**, the heart's failure to pump blood from the low-pressure veins into the higher-pressure arteries leads to venous pooling. Hydrostatic pressure builds in the veins and fluid leaks from the veins into the interstitium, causing edema. In **cirrhosis** (liver failure), the liver's failure to produce albumin lowers the oncotic pressure of the plasma, and fluid is lost from the intravascular space to the interstitium. Also, scarring in the liver obstructs the passage of plasma through the portal venous system. Hydrostatic pressure builds in the liver and in the portal system (portal hypertension), and fluid leaks into the peritoneum. The accumulation of fluid here is known as *ascites*. In severe cases of nephrosis, or nephrotic syndrome, the loss of albumin (the major protein in blood) to the urine from damaged glomeruli may also lower oncotic pressure and cause a loss of fluid to the interstitium, leading to generalized edema with low perfusion pressure.

When fluid builds up in the ECF space but outside of the vasculature, clinicians sometimes call this *third-spacing* because the fluid is not in the vessels and not in the cells, but in a third space—the interstitium, or a potential space similar to the peritoneum that is not normally filled with fluid. When a large amount of extracellular fluid is sequestered in a third space and the intravascular volume and blood pressure are low, the baroreceptors cause more salt and water reabsorption. Much of the added fluid is merely lost to the third space, however, worsening the edema and/or ascites.

Why is interstitial swelling (third-spacing) a problem? First, third-spacing means fluid is being lost from the intravascular volume, and the patient may be hypotensive. Second, third-spacing leads to organ dysfunction. In CHF, fluid backup in the venous system congests the organs. Congestion in the lungs—pulmonary edema—compromises respiratory function. Congestion of the liver farther down the venous circuit can lead to liver dysfunction. Generalized edema is also extremely uncomfortable, as is ascites, and the ascites fluid can become infected, leading to peritonitis.

The BUN/Cr ratio will also be elevated in hypervolemia with low perfusion pressure. This is because the BUN/Cr ratio reflects the adequacy of kidney perfusion rather than reflecting the ECF volume.

Summary

- Because Na^+ is the major cation of the ECF, and because water osmotically follows salt, the volume of the ECF is controlled by the renal handling of Na^+.

- The cardiovascular and renal organ systems together accomplish the baroreceptor reflex, which ensures blood pressure homeostasis.

- In response to baroreceptor detection of changes in perfusion pressure, the cardiovascular organ system alters SVR and CO through the autonomic nervous system.

- In response to baroreceptor detection of changes in perfusion pressure, the renal organ system alters SVR through the RAA system, and alters ECF volume (which in turn alters CO) through the RAA system, ANP, BNP, and ADH.

- The baroreceptor reflex may be broken down into the classic homeostatic elements. The sensors of perfusion pressure are the baroreceptors and JGA.

- The afferent pathways of transmission are the vagus and glossopharyngeal cranial nerves.

- The control centers are the medulla and JGA.

- The efferent pathways of transmission are the neural and hormonal activation of effectors—sympathetic nerves, circulating epinephrine and parasympathetic nerves, RAA system, ANP, BNP, and ADH.

- The effectors in the regulation of perfusion pressure are the systemic arterioles, the heart, and the salt-reabsorbing elements in the nephron tubule.

- A wide array of other mediators affects blood pressure without participating directly in its homeostasis. These mediators are important to consider when evaluating derangements in blood pressure.

- Disorders of ECF volume fall into one of three categories: hypovolemia, hypervolemia with normal or high intravascular volume, and hypervolemia with low intravascular volume.

Suggested Reading

Cowley AW Jr. Long-term control of arterial blood pressure. Physiol Rev. 1992;72(1):231–300 (Jan).

DiBona GF, Kopp UC. Neural control of renal function. Physiol Rev. 1997;77(1):75–197 (Jan).

Hall JE. Control of sodium excretion by angiotensin II: intrarenal mechanisms and blood pressure regulation. Am J Physiol. 1986;250(6 Pt 2):R960–872 (Jun).

Hamlyn JM, Blaustein MP. Sodium chloride, extracellular fluid volume, and blood pressure regulation. Am J Physiol. 1986;251(4 Pt 2):F563–575 (Oct).

Reid IA. Interactions between ANG II, sympathetic nervous system, and baroreceptor reflexes in regulation of blood pressure. Am J Physiol. 1992;262(6 Pt 1):E763–778 (Jun).

Skott O. Body sodium and volume homeostasis. Am J Physiol Regul Integr Comp Physiol. 2003;285(1):R14–18 (Jul).

REVIEW QUESTIONS

Directions: Each of the numbered items or incomplete statements in this section is followed by answers or by completions of the statement. Select the ONE lettered answer or completion that is BEST in each case.

1. An 84-year-old man is admitted to the intensive care unit with a mean arterial blood pressure of 60 mm Hg and a pulse of 130 beats per minute. A Swann-Ganz catheter is placed, and his cardiac output is determined to be 2 L/min. The right atrial pressure is 20 mm Hg. His total peripheral resistance is:

   (A) 20 mm Hg/L per min
   (B) 30 mm Hg/L per min
   (C) 200 mm Hg/L per min
   (D) 300 mm Hg/L per min
   (E) 2,000 mm Hg/L per min
   (F) 3,000 mm Hg/L per min

2. A 28-year-old woman is involved in a motor vehicle accident and suffers serious blood loss. With activation of the compensatory mechanisms to maintain her blood pressure, which of the following serum factors is likely to be LOW?

   (A) natriuretic peptides
   (B) renin
   (C) angiotensin II
   (D) aldosterone
   (E) antidiuretic hormone (ADH)

3. A patient with primary aldosteronism (excess serum concentrations of aldosterone) will have which of the following?

   (A) hypotension (low blood pressure)
   (B) bradycardia (low heart rate)
   (C) hyponatremia (low serum sodium concentration)
   (D) hypokalemia (low serum potassium concentration)
   (E) hypovolemia (low extracellular fluid volume)

ANSWERS TO REVIEW QUESTIONS

1. **The answer is** A. Mean systemic blood pressure is the product of the cardiac output (CO) in liters per minute and the systemic vascular resistance (SVR), expressed as a restatement of Ohm's law: SVR = (MAP − RAP)/CO, where MAP = mean arterial pressure (in mm Hg) and RAP = right atrial pressure (in mm Hg). SVR in units of mm Hg/L per min may be converted to a standard unit of measurement of resistance in dynes $\times$ cm^{-5} by multiplying by 80.

$$(60 - 20) \text{ mm Hg}/2 \text{ L per min} = 20 \text{ mm Hg/L per min,}$$
$$\text{or } 1{,}600 \text{ dynes} \times \text{cm}^{-5}$$

This patient has a low systemic blood pressure and a low cardiac output, consistent with a number of diseases. Because the heart rate (pulse) is elevated and the cardiac output is low, the stroke volume must also be small: (2,000 mL/min)/(130 beats/min) = 15.4 mL/beat. The situation reflects profound intravascular volume depletion with an elevated SVR.

2. **The answer is** A. With the rapid loss of ECF (and intravascular) volume from hemorrhage, the baroreceptors throughout the vascular tree signal to the kidneys to conserve volume and to the brain to increase volume intake and maintain blood pressure, respectively. The kidneys activate the RAA system, so all of these factors should increase in concentration. Likewise, the production and release of ADH should increase in order to (1) promote thirst so the patient will drink (if able), (2) retain free water at the kidney, and (3) vasoconstrict. (Recall that ADH is also called *vasopressin* for its vasoconstrictive effects, which increase SVR and, thus, blood pressure.) Concentrations of ANP and BNP, however, should drop because this agent causes the kidneys to decrease sodium reabsorption and decrease ECF volume, which would be maladaptive in these circumstances.

3. **The answer is** D. Excess aldosterone causes the kidney to reabsorb more sodium from the renal tubule than is necessary. Because water follows sodium in this case, the ECF volume increases (hypervolemia, not hypovolemia), and with the increase in intravascular volume, the blood pressure increases (hypertension, not hypotension). A typical cardiac response to hypervolemia is an increase in heart rate (tachycardia, not bradycardia). The serum sodium does not drop profoundly unless extenuating circumstances (such as increased free water intake) intervene, but aldosterone causes the kidney to save sodium by exchanging it for potassium. Thus, the kidneys excrete large amounts of potassium, and the serum potassium drops (hypokalemia).

23

Osmoregulation

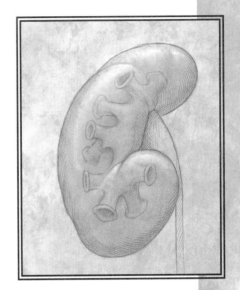

INTRODUCTION

The **osmolality**—or concentration of the solutes in the body fluids—is critical to organ function and must be closely regulated. As we shall see, disturbances in the osmolality of the body fluids arise from the gain or loss of water, or from the gain or loss of osmoles (glucose, urea, salts). Accordingly, normal plasma osmolality is restored by the excretion of extra water, the replenishment of lost water, or by the restoration of normal amounts of solutes in the body.

SYSTEM STRUCTURE: BODY FLUID COMPARTMENTS

Osmoregulation shares its anatomic terrain with the regulation of blood pressure; that is, it acts upon the body fluid compartments. Instead of modulating the volume of the extracellular fluid (ECF) through variations in Na^+ reabsorption, however, the osmoregulatory apparatus modulates the Na^+ *concentration* in the ECF by varying the amount of water within the total body water space. Recall that in the adult, approximately 50% to 60% of body weight is water and that two-thirds of the water is within cells (the intracellular water), while one-third is in the ECF. For the purposes of osmoregulation, the total body water is the compartment of interest, because water can freely move between cells and the ECF.

The anatomic elements that constitute the homeostatic feedback loop are fewer than those in the loop that controls ECF volume and blood pressure; the organs involved in osmoregulation are the brain and the kidney, and to a lesser extent, the intestines and the circulatory system, which act as conduits. In osmoregulation, the hypothalamus and neurohypophysis play the most important roles in the brain, and the loop of Henle and the collecting duct effect regulation in the kidney tubule.

SYSTEM FUNCTION: HOMEOSTASIS OF SODIUM CONCENTRATION

Before detailing the governance of Na^+ concentration, it is first necessary to establish the physiological importance of a stable Na^+ concentration and the challenges to the stability of plasma $[Na^+]$. In order to do that, we should review the concept of osmolality and re-examine the constitution of the body fluid compartments.

Osmolality, Osmosis, and Fluid Shifts Between Body Fluid Compartments

Recall that both **molarity** and **molality** describe the concentration of solute in a solution; however, they do so in different units of measurement. The units of molarity are mol solute/L solution. The units of molality are mol solute/kg solvent. Because volume changes with temperature, molarity is temperature-dependent. Molality is independent of temperature because it is relative to mass of solvent. *Osmolarity* and *osmolality* reflect the number of moles of *solute particles* in a solution, as opposed to moles of compound in a solution. So, if a solution contained 140 mmol NaCl per 1 kg water, its molality would be 140 mmol/kg. Its *osmolality* would be 280 mOsm/kg because we would count the free-floating ions Na^+ and Cl^- separately.

Also, recall that **osmosis** is the diffusion of water (as solvent) across a membrane from an area of low-solute concentration to an area of high-solute concentration (i.e., along a concentration gradient). It is a passive process that occurs only in liquids, not gases, and obeys the second law of thermodynamics, the law of entropy. The random molecular motion of the water molecules causes them to traverse the membrane in both directions. Molecules starting on the high-solute concentration side of the membrane and moving toward the membrane for crossover are obstructed in their progress by their "sticky" interactions with the excess solute. Fewer water molecules make it across from the high-solute concentration side than do molecules from the low-solute concentration side. A net influx of water molecules onto the high-solute concentration side occurs. The influx of water from the high-solute concentration side stops when the solute concentrations on each side are equal—that is, when the amount of solute obstructing water efflux is equal on both sides. The rate of efflux is the same on both sides, and osmotic equilibrium is reached.

Osmotic Pressure   The osmolarity or osmolality of the compartments on either side of a membrane is what determines the compartments' **osmotic pressure,** which is a reflection of how much water that compartment will draw into it through osmosis. With 1 mmol/kg of glucose on one side of a membrane and 1 mmol/kg NaCl on the other, water will diffuse into the NaCl side because that side's osmolality is twice as high. Osmosis is sensitive to the number of free dissolved particles and does not distinguish between different molecular species like Na^+ and Cl^-.

Effective Osmoles   Note that in the situations considered in the preceding paragraph, the osmoles of solute may or may not be able to cross the membrane. If the osmoles of solute could cross the membrane freely, as water does, the solute would distribute evenly, and there would no longer be a concentration gradient to drive osmosis. Such solutes—for example, ethanol and urea—are not effective osmoles because they do not create osmotic pressure. Effective osmoles cannot freely diffuse across membranes; their movement is determined by the presence of pumps and the distribution of channels. Examples of effective osmoles are the solutes Na^+, K^+, and Cl^-. The pumps and channels keep Na^+ mostly outside of cells and K^+ mostly inside of cells as effective osmoles (see Figure 22.1). In a diabetic patient, when glucose cannot freely enter cells because of low insulin levels, glucose becomes an effective osmole, attracting water from cells to the ECF.

Aquaporins It is also important to note that just as the body limits the diffusion of solutes, in some cases, it can limit the diffusion of its primary solvent; although water freely crosses most cell membranes in the body, it does not cross all membranes as easily. In fact, the default state of the cell membrane is relatively low permeability to water. Recall that the interior of the cell membrane phospholipid bilayer is nonpolar and hydrophobic. Consequently, ions can cross membranes only via channels, and a polar molecule like H_2O only crosses the membrane to a limited extent without a channel. The permeability of cells to water is greatly increased, however, by water channels called **aquaporins** in the membrane. Permeability to water increases in proportion to the number of these channels. Different tissues have various densities of aquaporins, so their cells may be more or less water permeable than others. Some tissues are practically impermeable to water, and some have variable permeability that is regulated by hormonal control over the insertion and removal of aquaporins. As most body tissues are significantly water permeable, and because an absence of aquaporins confers water impermeability upon a tissue, it is probable that most tissues express aquaporins to some degree.

Fluid Shifts What are the implications of the fact that the body fluid compartments (ECF and ICF; Figure 23.1) are in general freely permeable to water and contain effective osmoles Na^+ in the ECF and K^+ in the ICF? First, the free movement of water means that the ECF and ICF always come to osmotic equilibrium and achieve equal osmolality, because when the osmolality changes on one side of the membrane, water shifts until the solute concentrations are equal. Second, the presence of effective osmoles means that osmotic pressure can be created on one side of the membrane. An increase or decrease in $[Na^+]$ in the ECF will cause fluid shifts between ECF and ICF. Ingesting a salty meal adds salt to the ECF, raising the ECF osmolality. Fluid moves from the ICF into the ECF, shrinking the ICF volume and expanding the ECF volume. Adding isotonic saline to the ECF (i.e., adding

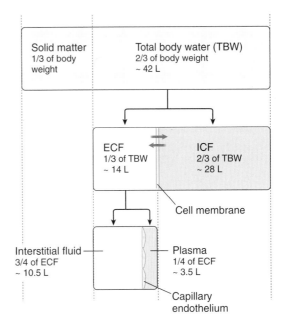

Figure 23.1 Extracellular fluid compartments in a 70-kg individual. The red arrows denote the free movement of water across the cell membranes that divide the ECF from the ICF. Because the plasma is a subsegment of the ECF space and shares its osmolality, the terms *plasma (or serum) osmolality* and *ECF osmolality* are often used interchangeably.

NaCl in solution with the same osmolality as the ECF) will increase the size of the ECF but no fluid shift will occur, so ICF volume will stay the same. Drinking water adds pure water to the ECF, dropping the ECF osmolality, so some fluid will shift from the ECF to the ICF. The ECF volume expands some and the ICF volume expands some (in proportion to the relative volume of ICF and ECF). Because only changes in the level of effective osmoles in the ECF can produce such fluid shifts, fluid shifts do not necessarily correlate with the total osmolality of the ECF, but only with the osmolality of the effective osmoles, most importantly Na^+. **Tonicity** refers to the effect that a particular solute concentration has on cell volume. A hypertonic ECF will lead to cell shrinkage, an isotonic ECF no change at all in ICF, and a hypotonic ECF will expand cell volume.

The Physiologic Importance of Maintaining Constant Plasma Osmolality The body encounters daily changes in ECF osmolality relative to ICF as a consequence of variations in water elimination and intake. If the body had no means of regulating the plasma osmolality, fluid shifts would occur unopposed between the ECF and ICF. The body, however, would not be able to tolerate those fluid shifts, which create swelling or shrinkage of the ICF volume and hence, of the cells. Neither ICF swelling (in the context of plasma hypo-osmolality) nor shrinkage (in plasma hyperosmolality) is good for physiologic functioning, especially in the brain. Thus, when the body's sensors detect that a fluid shift has begun to occur, which indicates a change in ECF osmolality, effector mechanisms restore normal ECF osmolality, thereby reversing the fluid shift and protecting the ICF from expansion or contraction.

Physiologic Challenges to Osmolality Homeostasis

Many disease states threaten the constancy of the plasma osmolality, but as mentioned previously, so does normal physiology. In the normal state, fluids lost from or added to the ECF are usually hypotonic. When hypotonic fluid is lost, water is lost in excess of solute and the plasma solute concentration increases. When hypotonic fluid is added to the plasma, its solute concentration decreases. The osmoregulatory apparatus of the kidney and brain modulates water elimination and intake to maintain constant osmolality.

A variety of physiologic processes involve exchanges of hypotonic fluid with the external environment (TABLE 23.1). Water may be lost in excess of solute in the stool, in evaporation from the respiratory tract (in this case, the loss is all water and no solute), and in the hypotonic fluid of sweat, which is produced in connection with the hypothalamic regulation of body temperature. Finally, excretion of nitrogenous wastes requires a minimal level of urinary water loss that concentrates the plasma.

Unregulated additions of water to the ECF occur dietarily through social or habitual drinking and through the ingestion of food, which has a water content that can approach 1 L per day. The water inside dietary food is sometimes called **preformed water**. Unregulated additions of water to the ECF also occur metabolically. Recall from biochemistry that *oxidative phosphorylation* is the means by which the reduced cofactors of the citric acid cycle are aerobically transduced to ATP. This process consumes oxygen and yields H_2O on an ongoing basis in every aerobic cell. Water produced from oxidative phosphorylation is sometimes called **metabolic water**. Approximately 20 mol of water (and CO_2) may be produced per day normally in an adult. Because water is 55 mol/L, water production is approximately 20/55 of a liter, or close to 400 mL per day.

Obligatory Water Loss in the Excretion of Nitrogenous Wastes

It may not seem immediately obvious why urinary excretion of nitrogenous wastes causes an obligatory concentration of the plasma. If the urine is even more concentrated than the blood (plasma osmolality is around 280 mOsm/kg, whereas maximum urine concentration is around 1,200 mOsm/kg), in what sense is hypotonic fluid being lost in the urine? To understand this better, we must first understand the obligation to excrete nitrogenous wastes. The di-

---

Table 23.1 PHYSIOLOGIC CHALLENGES TO OSMOLALITY HOMEOSTASIS[a]

Source of Unregulated Water Loss From ECF		Volume
Stool		200 mL/day
Respiratory tract		400 mL/day
Urine		500 mL/day is the minimum loss of water to urine for excretion of nitrogenous wastes.
Skin	Evaporation	500 mL/day evaporates from skin and mucous membranes under any circumstances.
	Sweat	Under circumstances of elevated body temperature, up to 7,000 mL water/day or more can be lost to sweat.
Source of Unregulated Water Addition to ECF		**Volume (mL/day)**
	Eating (preformed water)	850

[a] The table does not include urinary losses of hypotonic fluid that occur as a part of osmoregulation, as those losses respond to the unregulated additions of water to the ECF. The table also does not include ADH-mediated additions to the ECF, or water ingested due to thirst, because these additions respond to, and should be differentiated from, the unregulated losses from the ECF.
[b] Obviously, habitual and social water ingestion is highly variable from person to person. It is also difficult to distinguish habitual drinking from osmoregulatory (thirst-stimulated) drinking quantitatively. BD Rose and TW Post estimate total average water consumption at 400 to 1,400 mL/day. The figure 7,000 mL/day comes from H Smith.

gestion of dietary proteins yields amino acids. Some of these amino acids are used in protein synthesis, while others are metabolized to nitrogen-free compounds (such as pyruvate) that may yield energy through the citric acid cycle. Hence, metabolism of amino acids requires their deamination and yields the toxic substance, ammonia (NH_3). The liver combines NH_3 with CO_2 to make the less-toxic substance, **urea** (NH_2-CO-NH_2), but urea must also be eliminated, lest it have toxic effects, particularly on the brain. One of the kidney's important functions is to excrete urea.

If urea is to be carried out of the body in solution, it must be carried out in a certain amount of water donated from the plasma. (To conserve water, chickens excrete nitrogen in stool in the solid form of uric acid.) The plasma must donate a hypotonic volume of water for this purpose so that this volume of water can be loaded with osmoles of urea. If the plasma donated an isotonic volume of water, the body would face the problem of wasting excess salt in urea excretion and compromise extracellular fluid volume. Also, because the maximal osmolality of human urine is about 1,200 mOsm/kg, only 600 mOsm can be excreted in a half liter of water. About half of this amount of normal osmole excretion is urea. To excrete the same amount of urea with additional salt, more water would be required. Although the American kangaroo rat, a desert animal, can concentrate its urine with 70 times the efficiency of the human kidney, most mammals face much lower limits to the concentration of urine they can achieve. The reasons for this lie in the urinary concentrating mechanism, which will be discussed later in this chapter. Thus, the plasma must donate a minimum level of hypotonic fluid to urine in order to excrete urea in solution. Around 10 mL of water is required for every gram of metabolized protein, meaning that a minimum of approximately 500 mL water/day must be lost to the urine. Low-protein diets can help reduce this obligatory urinary water loss. Even on a protein-free diet, however, the kidney has excretory duties that require water to transport wastes from the body. The absolute lower limit of obligatory water loss on a protein-free diet is about 300 mL water/day.

Control of ECF Osmolality

Together, the brain and kidney maintain a steady plasma osmolality through two effector mechanisms. The principal one involves a hormone introduced in Chapter 22, **antidiuretic hormone (ADH)**, also known as *vasopressin*. An increased level of ADH increases the reabsorption of water without solute in the kidney (thus lowering urine volume, i.e., opposing diuresis). This in turn dilutes ECF Na^+ and lowers plasma osmolality. A decreased level of ADH decreases reabsorption of water without solute in the kidney (thus increasing the urine volume, i.e., creating a diuresis). This excretion of water without solute drains the pool of water around the Na^+ and raises plasma osmolality. The second important homeostatic response to plasma osmolality is **thirst**. The higher the plasma osmolality is relative to the ICF, the greater the perception of thirst will be, which in turn, leads to behavior (drinking) that will add water to the ECF. Recall that regulating ECF osmolality is in turn a regulation of total body fluid osmolality because osmotic equilibrium is achieved between the ECF and ICF.

Like other homeostatic systems, the osmoregulatory system is composed of sensors, a control center, and effectors. The ADH and thirst mechanisms for altering ECF osmolality share a similar sensor and control center, which we will now consider.

Osmoreceptors The sensor and the control center involved in the regulation of ECF osmolality are located in the diencephalon in the brain (FIGURE 23.2). When changes in osmolality drive fluid shifts, **osmoreceptor cells** in the hypothalamus and in related structures swell or shrink. Just like many other cells in the body, they swell in response to decreased plasma osmolality and shrink in the presence of increased plasma osmolality. Unlike other cells, however, osmoreceptor cells yield a particular response to changes in volume. Shrinkage depolarizes the cells by stimulating mechanosensitive channels in the cell membrane. The stimulation results in an increased cationic conductance, cations rush into the cell, and the cations raise the intracellular electrical potential, thus initiating an action potential or predisposing the cell toward an action potential. Conversely, swelling

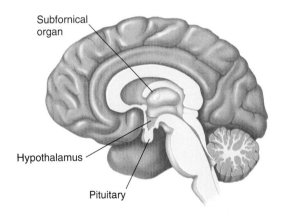

Figure 23.2 The hypothalamus and pituitary. Osmoreceptors in the hypothalamus project their axons into the posterior pituitary, also known as the neurohypophysis. The termini of these axons secrete ADH. Circumventricular organs such as the subfornical organ also participate in osmoreception and thirst generation.

inhibits these channels, decreasing cationic conductance and hyperpolarizing the cell, thus inhibiting action potentials.

Some of the osmoreceptor cells are magnocellular neurons located in the supraoptic and paraventricular nuclei of the hypothalamus, and the axons of these cells project directly into the posterior pituitary. Action potentials traveling down these axons to their termini in the pituitary then cause Ca^{2+}-dependent release of ADH into the bloodstream by exocytosis of ADH granules. Other osmoreceptor cells are thought to exist in *circumventricular organs* nearby: the subfornical organ (SFO), the organum vasculosum of the lamina terminalis (OVLT), and others. These centers may augment or modulate the excitement of the magnocellular osmoreceptors. Some investigators refer to the entire group as an **osmoreceptor complex**. Although the neurophysiology is incompletely understood, it is clear that the osmoreceptor complex not only drives increased ADH secretion, but it also helps generate the thirst sensation and drinking behavior.

While one might think that osmoreceptors respond directly to the total osmolality of the ECF, they cannot and do not. Only a change in the level of *effective* osmoles in the ECF relative to the ICF can swell or shrink cells, and osmoreceptors are no different in this respect from other cells. They respond to changes in the effective osmolality of the plasma. Accordingly, the ineffective osmoles of solutes that can pass freely from ECF to ICF, such as urea, cannot affect the osmoreceptors, so a high plasma urea concentration (uremia) does not drive an osmoregulatory response. The hypothalamus is, however, quite sensitive to changes in effective osmolality, with changes as small as 1% producing a secretory response (Figure 23.3A).

Recent research suggests that **peripheral osmoreceptors** located in the oropharynx may also contribute to the ADH response. Evidence indicates that oropharyngeal exposure to hypertonic fluid may increase the ADH level independent of any increase in plasma osmolality. These oropharyngeal receptors are thought to be NaCl-sensitive. Thirst is also stimulated by oropharyngeal receptors.

Baroreceptors Recall from Chapter 22 that in addition to osmoreceptor control of ADH secretion, the baroreceptors also exert some influence over ADH secretion. Under circumstances of severe volume depletion, baroreceptors trigger the secretion of ADH in order to raise ECF volume. (Keep in mind that an addition of water without solute raises both ECF and ICF volume.) Secretion of ADH for the purposes of ECF volume control means that the baroreceptors can cause dilution of the plasma regardless

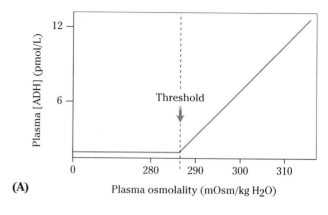

(A)

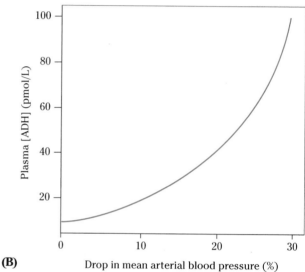

(B)

Figure 23.3 Correlations between ADH secretion and its provoking factors. **A.** Osmoreceptor control of ADH. Although the graph does not reflect it, regulation occurs by increasing or decreasing ADH levels, not by turning ADH secretion completely on or completely off. **B.** Baroreceptor control of ADH. Severe decreases in blood volume and pressure prompt ADH secretion. ADH secretion in response to hypovolemia is not significant until a 10% drop in blood pressure has occurred.

of plasma osmolality. If the plasma osmolality is normal and the blood volume is extremely low, the baroreceptors' invocation of ADH secretion may cause an undesired hypo-osmolality in the plasma, if dilute fluids are ingested (Figure 23.3B). This is important clinically when evaluating possible causes of low plasma $[Na^+]$. The baroreceptors also stimulate the hypothalamus to produce a thirst response in severe volume depletion.

The baroreceptors appear to influence the osmoreceptor complex via the vagus nerve, which synapses in the medulla. Neurons in that area project into the hypothalamus. Another possible point of connection between the regulation of blood pressure and osmoregulation is angiotensin II. Angiotensin II, which increases blood pressure and ECF volume, is thought to stimulate thirst.

The Set Point The hypothalamus functions as a control center in osmoregulation. The afferent data from the osmoreceptors are subject to processing before the efferent signals are released and ADH is secreted. In fact, osmoreceptor data undergo processing of the sort typical of homeostatic control centers; that is, the hypothalamus compares an observed level of osmolality with a desired level. The maximum level of osmolality tolerated before ADH is secreted is known as the osmolal **set point**. Beyond this threshold of approximately 280 or 285 mOsm/kg H_2O, the hypothalamus discharges its efferent signals. (Note that some ADH is present in the bloodstream below threshold. Osmoregulation is not effected through the presence or absence of ADH, but rather through the increase or decrease in ADH.) The osmolal setpoint for thirst is higher than that for ADH secretion by about 10 mOsm/kg. Thus, the usual plasma Na^+ concentration is closer to the ADH set point, which gives humans the ability to concentrate urine without thirst. This ability is well adapted to life without constant drinking behavior.

The set point can be lowered under certain circumstances, such as under baroreceptor stimulation or during pregnancy. A lowered set point means ADH will start being secreted at a lower plasma osmolality. Consequently, when the baroreceptors respond to severe volume depletion by stimulating the osmoreceptors, not only do they promote ADH secretion per se, but they also lower the threshold for ADH secretion in response to plasma osmolality.

Thirst as an Effector Mechanism Physiologists and neuroscientists still have much to learn about how increased osmolality leads to thirst and drinking behavior, but it is clear that thirst serves, along with ADH, to decrease plasma osmolality and increase ECF volume. The absorption of ingested water from the intestines adds this water without solute to the ECF in the same way that the kidney adds water under the influence of ADH. Thirst, like ADH, thereby expands ECF volume and dilutes the plasma osmoles, which in turn reverses the fluid shift caused by high plasma osmolality and prevents shrinkage of the ICF.

Both central and oropharyngeal osmoreceptors trigger thirst through stimulation of the osmoreceptor complex. The more recently described oropharyngeal pathway may be of added importance, however, because it tallies especially well with two aspects of thirst. First, the thirst sensation is associated with "dry mouth," a possible indicator that thirst arises from oropharyngeal stimulation. Second, the oropharyngeal pathway would help explain the mystery of thirst termination.

The thirst sensation may arise in connection with increased plasma osmolality, but it dissipates long before normal plasma osmolality is restored. It takes only a short time to consume the appropriate amount of water to correct plasma osmolality. It takes longer for the plasma osmolality to actually correct, as the water must first be absorbed from the intestines and distributed into the ECF. If thirst and drinking were only to stop when plasma osmolality had corrected, one would overshoot one's water needs and become hypo-osmolar. The body possibly avoids such a dysfunctional means of thirst termination through the oropharyngeal osmoreceptors. The application of water to the oropharynx may relieve the peripheral receptors of salt stimulation and help abolish thirst long before the intestines absorb the water and the plasma osmolality is corrected. (See Integrated Physiology Box *Alternatives to Thirst in the Animal Kingdom.*)

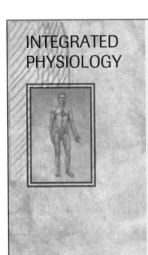

INTEGRATED PHYSIOLOGY

Alternatives to Thirst in the Animal Kingdom

Thirst is not universal in the animal kingdom. All animals do require a supply of water without solute in order to correct increases in plasma osmolality (if dilution is unneeded or if concentration of plasma is needed, free water can then be purged in urine); however, evolution has devised myriad strategies in addition to drinking for the acquisition of free water. The cartilaginous marine fish maintain a high urea level in the blood to extract free water osmotically from the sea. In arid climates, preformed water and metabolic water may be the only sources of solute-free water. Some moths and beetles subsist wholly on metabolic water and can live in a nearly anhydrous environment. Finally, marine mammals do not drink either, as highly concentrated seawater is the only water supply available to them and would leave them unable to dilute their plasma effectively. Marine mammals derive all their water from preformed sources (i.e., food) and from metabolism.

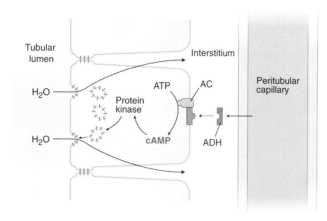

Figure 23.4 Cyclic-AMP-mediated insertion of vesicles carrying aquaporins. ADH triggers a cAMP-mediated signal transduction cascade. R = ADH receptor. AC = adenylyl cyclase. For simplicity, the diagram shows adenylyl cyclase directly attached to the ADH receptor. In fact, adenylyl cyclase is a membrane-bound enzyme and is dependent on a G protein for connection with the receptor and for signal transduction from receptor to adenylyl cyclase.

ADH Action as an Effector Mechanism Once secreted, ADH travels via the blood circulation to the kidney. ADH diffuses out of the peritubular capillary to act on the basolateral side of the tubule. It acts in two places: at the thick ascending limb, where it promotes salt reabsorption, and at the collecting duct, where it increases permeability of the duct to water, facilitating water reabsorption. The mechanism of ADH action in the thick ascending limb is unclear; however, the activity of the $Na^+/K^+/2Cl^-$ symporter is known to increase in animals in the presence of ADH. In the collecting duct, ADH binds membrane-bound receptors that trigger a cAMP-mediated signal transduction cascade. The end result is the insertion of aquaporins in the otherwise poorly permeable collecting duct apical surface (FIGURE 23.4). The effect of ADH is to increase water permeability approximately 100-fold. Now we turn to the following question: How exactly do the actions of ADH account for the tubular reabsorption of water and its subsequent addition to the ECF?

Countercurrent Multiplication in the Loop of Henle

We established earlier that water moves passively across tubule walls only in accordance with osmotic gradients. Consequently, without an osmotic gradient favoring the reabsorption of water, the ADH-dependent increase in the water permeability of the collecting duct would not move any water

by itself. In the proximal tubule, water reabsorption occurs through an active pumping of solute, causing water to follow solute out of the tubule and into the interstitium. In the collecting duct, however, water reabsorption can far exceed the level accounted for by its reabsorption of solute. Thus, in order to reabsorb water in this part of the tubule, the kidney must use a different mechanism to create an osmotic gradient that would cause water to flow out of the collecting duct and into the surrounding tissue in the presence of aquaporins.

That mechanism is called **countercurrent multiplication** in the loop of Henle, a system that maintains high solute concentration in the renal medulla. Countercurrent multiplication requires a particular tubular anatomy and special tubular transport properties. The loop of Henle is a U-shaped segment of the nephron composed of the thin descending limb, which is permeable to water but has low permeability to salt; the thin ascending limb, which is permeable to salt but not to water; and the thick ascending limb, which reabsorbs salt by active transport and is impermeable to water. This arrangement generates an increasing salt concentration with descent into the medullary interstitium (FIGURE 23.5).

Countercurrent Multiplication as a Form of Countercurrent Exchange Although the concentrating function of the loop of Henle is called *countercurrent multiplication*, it is, underneath, just a slightly more complicated form of **countercurrent exchange**. A simpler example of countercurrent exchange is that of heat exchange between arteries and veins in the extremities (FIGURE 23.6). Because the arteries carry blood from the heart, they also consequently carry heat away from the body core. Veins, by contrast, carry blood from the less well-insulated and hence cooler extremities. Because the arteries and veins of the extremities run in parallel, they are subject to transverse heat exchange from hot artery to cool vein. For example, the artery is hottest in the proximal extremity, and delivers heat to the veins as they ascend, which brings the heat immediately back to the body core. As the arterial blood passes farther down the arm, it continues to unload heat into the vein, and the vein carries the heat back to the body core. By the time the arterial blood has reached the tip of the extremity, it has already lost much of its heat and therefore has less heat to give; both arteries and veins are cooler here than proximally. In this way, heat is recycled to the body core, maintaining a high core body temperature.

The physiology of the loop of Henle is analogous to heat exchange in an extremity. The hairpin turn at the bottom of the loop is similar to the body core and salt concentration is like heat (FIGURE 23.7A). The fluid

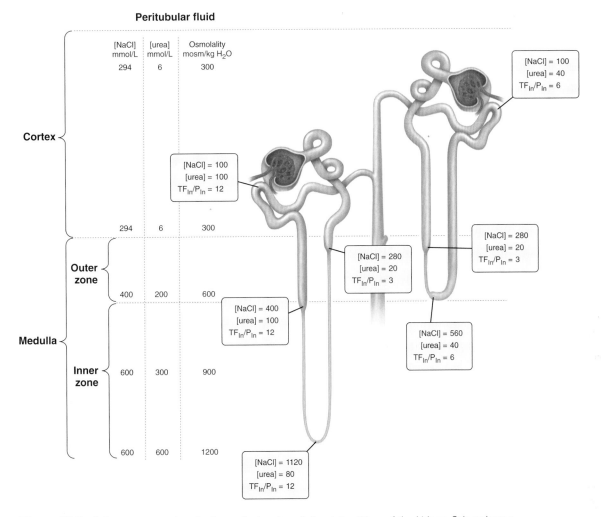

Figure 23.5 Solute concentrations in the cortical and medullary interstitium of the kidney. Salt and urea concentrations rise with descent into the medulla. Urea accounts for a larger percentage of total osmolality deep in the inner medulla.

entering the descending limb is isotonic to plasma (less salt-concentrated than the base), so the descending limb is like the cool vein. The ascending limb, loaded with high salt concentration (for reasons we will discuss later), is like the hot artery. NaCl in the ascending limb is reabsorbed transversely (without water), and the salt concentration rises in the fluid of the descending limb. The fluid of the descending limb acquires a higher salt concentration through the descending limb's reabsorption of water. Salt concentration is thus recycled to the inner medulla, maintaining a high inner medullary salt concentration. When ADH increases the water permeability of the collecting duct, water can flow down its osmotic gradient into the medullary interstitium.

One matter complicating the analogy to heat exchange in the extremities is that although salt is reabsorbed by the ascending limb, salt is not secreted into the descending limb in the same way that heat is transferred directly into the vein. Rather, the fluid of

the descending limb acquires a higher salt concentration through the descending limb's reabsorption of water. First, the ascending limb reabsorbs salt without water into the interstitium, raising the osmolality of the interstitium. Then the increased osmolality of the interstitium draws water without salt from the tubule lumen, concentrating the fluid of the descending limb. Thus, while salt itself does not pass all the way from the ascending limb to the descending limb, *salt concentration does* in a manner analogous to heat exchange (Figure 23.7B).

The difference between heat transfer and the flow of salt concentration does, however, have a critical functional ramification. In heat exchange, an absolute quantity is passed transversely, whereas in the exchange of salt concentration, only a ratio (mOsm of salt to kilograms of water) is passed transversely. Consequently, the interstitium is not just a passageway for small amounts of salt; rather, the interstitium acquires a high salt concentration. The

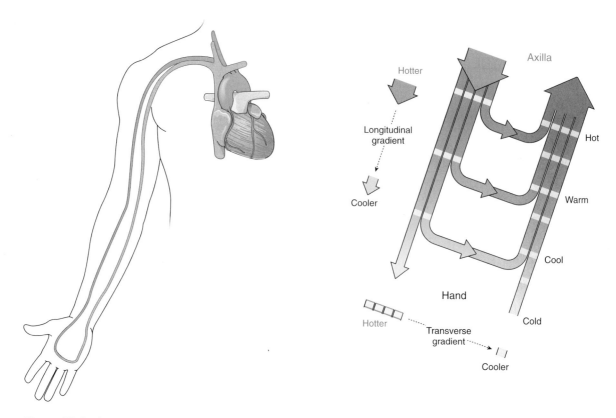

Figure 23.6 Countercurrent heat exchange in the upper extremity. Heat flows along a transverse heat gradient from artery to vein to create a longitudinal heat gradient from axilla to hand. The process is analogous to countercurrent multiplication in the loop of Henle.

high salt concentration of the interstitium is necessary osmotically to draw water from the descending limb. Furthermore, a high salt concentration in the interstitium is necessary to compel water reabsorption from the collecting duct, which is the purpose of the apparatus. *The transverse flow of salt concentration in the loop of Henle accounts for the high interstitial salt concentration of the medulla.* FIGURE 23.8 amends Figure 23.7 to reflect the fact that the interstitium shares the same high salt concentration as the tubular fluid.

The Ultimate Origin of the High Salt Concentration Entering the Ascending Limb: The Na⁺/K⁺-ATPase? Urea?

The Ultimate Origin of the High Salt Concentration Entering the Ascending Limb: The Na^+/K^+-ATPase? Urea?   A final matter complicating the analogy between heat exchange and countercurrent multiplication is that of origins. Heat in the artery comes from metabolism in the body core, a process external to heat exchange. In the loop of Henle, however, the high salt concentration entering the ascending limb appears to depend on the function of the loop itself.

The ascending limb receives tubular fluid high in salt concentration from the descending limb. The descending limb in turn has a high salt concentration because water has diffused out of the tubule into the interstitium, which is highly concentrated in salt. Meanwhile, the interstitium is highly concentrated in salt because of salt reabsorption from the highly

concentrated ascending limb. Werner Kuhn, who proposed the countercurrent multiplication hypothesis in 1942, believed that active transport of Na^+ from the ascending limb into the interstitium was the point of origin in the cycle that creates high interstitial salt concentration. By actively pumping salt into the interstitium, the descending limb could be secondarily concentrated through water reabsorption, thus delivering highly concentrated fluid to the ascending limb. This would enable the ascending limb to deliver even more solute to the interstitium in a self-amplifying process. The theoretically self-amplifying character of the process is what led Kuhn to give it the name *multiplication.*

The mechanism for active Na^+ reabsorption in the thick ascending limb of Henle is the Na^+/K^+-ATPase on the basolateral membrane and the apical $Na^+/K^+/2Cl^-$ cotransporter. However, while the *thick* ascending limb does have Na^+/K^+-ATPase pumps, the *thin* ascending limb does not appear to have these pumps. Thus, how the inner medullary interstitium acquires its high salt concentration remains an unsolved problem. One possible explanation is that much of the interstitial osmolality at the base of the loop of Henle is accounted for by urea and not salt. If the descending limb were largely impermeable to urea, the interstitial urea concentra-

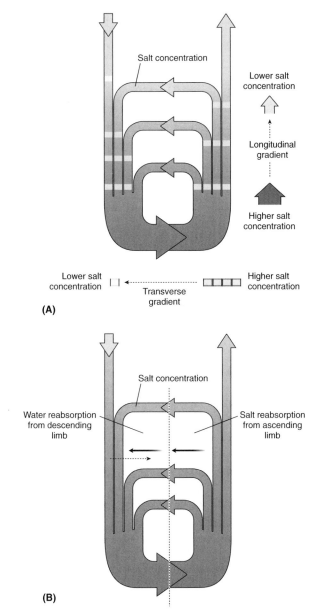

(A)

(B)

Figure 23.7 Flow of salt concentration in the loop of Henle. **A.** The recycling of salt concentration to the base of the loop. The flow of salt concentration along transverse concentration gradients from ascending to descending limb creates a longitudinal concentration gradient from renal cortex to inner medulla. **B.** Two constituents of the leftward flow of salt concentration. Salt reabsorption to the left and water reabsorption to the right both affect salt concentration flow to the left.

within the inner medulla. Consequently, urea remains trapped deep in the medullary interstitium in steady concentrations. This phenomenon is known as **urea trapping**.

On the whole, it can be safely stated that recycling of salt and urea through the medullary interstitium accounts for the high osmolality of the inner medulla, and that the thick ascending limb Na^+/K^+-ATPase and luminal $Na^+/K^+/2Cl^-$ cotransporter render the fluid entering the distal tubule and collecting duct hypotonic (FIGURE 23.9). Central to this concept is the fact that the thick limb is highly impermeable to water.

Given the high medullary salt concentration, the hypotonic solution that enters the collecting duct can be dealt with in either of two ways. It can pass out of the body as dilute urine, or, if plasma dilution is needed, water can be reabsorbed through ADH action. The ADH will insert aquaporin water channels, and water will flow osmotically from low tubular solute concentration to high interstitial solute concentration. ADH acts in the cortical collecting duct and in medullary collecting duct cells. When ADH is present, cortical water reabsorption renders the tubular fluid isosmotic to plasma as it enters the medulla. Further concentration of the urine takes place in the medullary collecting duct.

Countercurrent Exchange in the Vasa Recta   Once ADH has enabled the reabsorption of water into the salty interstitium, the water must find its way back into the bloodstream if it is to help reduce plasma

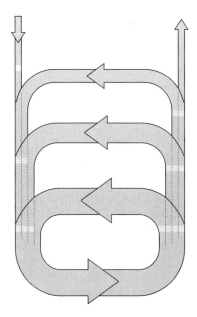

Figure 23.8 Interstitial salt concentration as a result of salt flow concentration in the loop of Henle. Unlike in heat exchange, a flow of salt concentration means that the interstitium must acquire the same salt concentration as the ascending limb, and the descending limb must acquire the same salt concentration as the interstitium.

tion could draw water from the descending limb, thus delivering fluid high in salt concentration to the thin ascending limb. Then, the high luminal NaCl could passively be reabsorbed in this segment. The question then remains, of course, where did the medullary urea come from?

An incomplete answer is that urea is reabsorbed from the medullary collecting duct and secreted in the loop of Henle; urea thereby follows a circular path through the nephron and the interstitial tissue

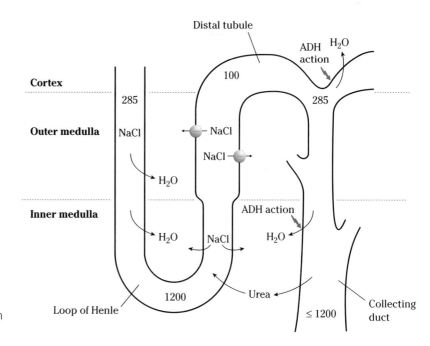

Figure 23.9 Handling of salt, water, and urea in the loop of Henle and collecting duct.

osmolality. How does it do so? Recall that the peritubular vasa recta has a high oncotic pressure owing to the previous loss of protein-free fluid to glomerular filtration. The high oncotic pressure of the vasa recta reabsorbs this water, and carries it away into the renal vein. The vasa recta also absorbs some solute; this way, countercurrent multiplication does not accumulate salt and water indefinitely in the interstitium, and a steady state is achieved.

Why doesn't the vasa recta completely dissipate the salt gradient concentrated here by the loop of Henle? The vasa recta runs in parallel to the loop of

Henle and shares its U-shape (Figure 23.10). As the vasa recta runs down into the increasingly salty medulla, it loses water and absorbs solute, gaining in osmolality. It seems counterintuitive that the descending vasa recta (DVR), with its high oncotic pressure, would actually lose some of its water to the surrounding interstitial fluid (ISF). As the DVR enters the high salt environment of the medullary ISF, however, the driving force for osmotic water flow from the capillary into the high NaCl ISF exceeds the oncotic forces favoring water moving into the capillary. (This is the only place in the body where

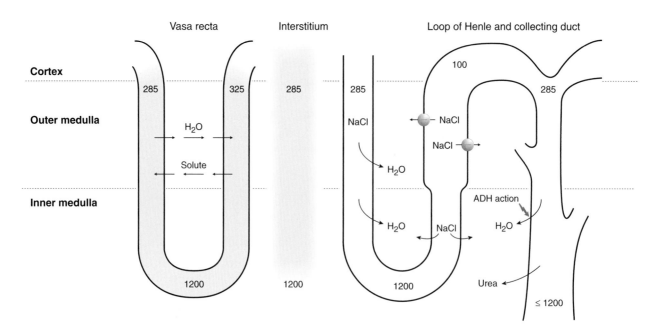

Figure 23.10 The vasa recta.

osmotic pressure overpowers oncotic pressure.) As the ascending vasa recta (AVR) flows into the less-concentrated portions of the medullary interstitium, it gains water and loses solute. If the vasa recta took a straight path through the medulla, it would certainly dissipate the gradient. With its U-shape, however, it keeps the medullary salt gradient intact and absorbs any excess water or solute. The volume flow of the AVR exceeds that of the entering DVR by the amount of volume reabsorbed by the descending limb and the collecting duct. Once again, this is a form of countercurrent exchange; the vasa recta transversely cycles solute from ascending to descending limb, thereby conserving osmolality in the inner medulla.

The vasa recta capillaries also bring with them red blood cells (RBCs). The RBCs play an important role in the ability to concentrate urine. Given the fact that the inner medulla has a high urea concentration, RBCs in the DVR could potentially lose enough water to shrink to the point of hemolysis. An RBC membrane urea transporter with high capacity ensures the rapid equilibration of urea into the RBC, preventing this shrinkage. The transporter also allows the rapid efflux of urea. If that urea could not exit the AVR rapidly as it flows toward the cortex, the RBC would swell to the point of hypotonic lysis. Furthermore, it would be impossible to excrete urea because the RBC would carry urea that came from filtration back to the renal vein.

Urine Osmolality When ADH enables water reabsorption back into plasma, and the dilution of plasma, it consequently leaves the fluid of the collecting duct concentrated with solute. Normally, when plasma osmolality rises, urine osmolality rises, and vice versa. The urine, however, can never be more concentrated than the medullary interstitium, because water diffuses through aquaporins until osmolality is equal on both sides of the tubule membrane. Urine osmolality peaks, therefore, around 1,200 mOsm/kg, the maximum osmolality achieved in the medullary interstitium. It is interesting to recall that ADH stimulates NaCl reabsorption in the thick ascending limb, as well as inserts aquaporin channels into the collecting duct apical membrane. In this sense, ADH enhances ISF osmolality as well as water permeability.

The minimum urine osmolality is 50 to 75 mOsm/kg. It is less than the 100 mOsm/kg leaving the loop because some salt reabsorption does occur in the collecting duct. (Recall that this aldosterone-influenced Na^+ reabsorption is one of the means of governance over the ECF volume.) The removal of this salt can further dilute the tubular fluid. Decreased ADH is required to dilute the urine. As a

peptide hormone, ADH can disappear from the circulation in a matter of minutes, another factor giving great flexibility to the handling of water.

Medullary Osmolytes Part of the teleological reason for osmoregulation is that a hypertonic ECF space leads to fluid loss from the ICF space and therefore shrinkage of cells. With a highly salty medullary interstitium, what prevents the cells of the medulla from suffering terrible shrinkage? The answer is that the medullary cells manufacture their own internal effective osmoles to match the osmolality of the medullary ECF. Such solutes, which serve an osmotic function, are known as **osmolytes**. They include methylamines, sorbitol, and inositol. As we will discuss later, in certain disease states, neurons manufacture their own osmolytes to counteract shrinkage due to chronic plasma hypernatremia (high $[Na^+]$). The renal medullary osmolytes are permanent, however, because the medullary salt gradient is always present, unlike plasma hypernatremia.

Free Water Clearance

Free water clearance (C_{H2O}) is an index of how much water free of solute has been cleared from the body. The free water clearance is normally only a positive number in hypo-osmotic situations (for example, after one drinks water), when the suppression of ADH causes "free water" to be excreted from the tubule in hypo-osmotic urine, thus returning the plasma osmolality to normal. In a disorder known as *diabetes insipidus*, however, free water clearance is positive even without drinking, leading to an increased body fluid osmolality. When ADH causes free water to be reabsorbed and added to plasma, there is either no free water clearance or there may be a negative C_{H2O}. Free water clearance is a different concept from urine osmolality, as the former is quantitative rather than qualitative.

The calculation of free water clearance is relatively straightforward. Free water clearance equals the urine volume per time, V, minus the **osmolar clearance (C_{osm}):**

$$C_{H2O} = \dot{V} - C_{osm}$$

C_{osm} is defined in accordance with the standard clearance equation:

$$C_{osm} = (U_{osm})(\dot{V})/P_{osm}$$

Total osmolar clearance equals urine osmolality times the urine flow rate divided by the plasma osmolality. Putting the two equations together, we have an equation for free water clearance as follows:

$$C_{H2O} = \dot{V} - (U_{osm})(\dot{V})/P_{osm}$$

In accordance with the definition of *clearance* and *mass balance* (see Chapter 20), the osmoles in the volume of plasma cleared must equal the osmoles that show up in the urine. Filtration at the glomerulus is isoosmotic. If the tubule did not alter the tubular fluid solute concentration, the urine volume would equal the volume of plasma cleared of solute. In that case, the plasma volume cleared would have been filtered and excreted with no net reabsorption of water or secretion of solute. If the urine volume carrying the excreted solute is larger than the volume of plasma cleared, we know that there was a net "addition" of free water to the tubular fluid before it left the collecting duct and entered the urinary collecting space. Therefore, the free water added to the tubule for excretion—the free water clearance—is defined as the urine volume minus the volume of plasma cleared of solute. Because water is not secreted, this "additional" free water could only be formed from reabsorption of solute without water. This ability to dilute the tubular fluid is a property of the thick ascending limb of Henle and the cortical distal tubule. The process is known as *separation* and requires impermeability of the cells to water. The impermeability is always present in the thick limb, but in the distal tubule and collecting duct it is only present when ADH is decreased. It may be useful to calculate free water clearance in the evaluation of **polyuria,** increased urine volume.

Sometimes it is also clinically useful to use the *electrolyte-free water clearance* instead of the osmolar-free water clearance described previously. The expression has a similar form to that for osmolar-free water clearance:

$$C_{H20} = \dot{V} - (U_{Na} + U_K)(\dot{V})/P_{Na}$$

This expression ignores the nonelectrolyte osmoles, most importantly urea. For somewhat complex reasons, the calculation of urea clearance does not help to quantify the amount of water added or lost to the body fluids that will have an impact on body fluid osmolality. Urea, which is excreted in a concentrated small volume of urine, will in fact, require a net amount of water to be reabsorbed; but in a steady state, hepatic urea synthesis adds an equal amount of urea to the body fluids, so that the blood urea concentration does not change and there is no net gain of free water to the body.

In order to produce maximum amounts of dilute urine, three aspects of integrated tubular function are required. First, there must be adequate *delivery* of isotonic fluid from the proximal tubule. Second, the thick ascending limb and distal tubule, as diluting segments, must be able to reabsorb NaCl: the *separation* step. Third, ADH must be low, so that water is not reabsorbed with NaCl in the distal tubule, and the collecting duct remains relatively impermeable to

water: the *regulation* step. In order to maximally absorb water while concentrating the urine, that is, to achieve negative free water clearance, three tubular functions are also required. There must be adequate *delivery* of isotonic fluid from the proximal tubule, allowing maximum NaCl accumulation in the medulla, concentrating the ISF (*separation*). The *regulation* step involves the presence of ADH to allow water movement across the collecting duct.

Synthesis of Volume and Osmolality Control

Now that we have been introduced to the body's interrelated mechanisms for ECF volume and osmolality homeostasis, we can predict the body's response to a number of different homeostatic challenges (TABLE 23.2). The osmolality of fluids added to or lost from the ECF affects the ECF volume. Likewise, the regulation and treatment of ECF volume has implications for the plasma osmolality. (See Clinical Application Box *Fluid Management.*)

PATHOPHYSIOLOGY: DISORDERS OF SERUM OSMOLALITY AND THEIR SEQUELAE

Plasma osmolality, or serum osmolality, may be calculated using the following equation:

$$P_{osm} = 2 ([Na^+]) + [glucose]/18 + BUN/2.8$$

The term *2 ([Na⁺])* represents Na^+ and its anions, primarily Cl- and HCO_3^-. These are the major extracellular ions. The divisors for glucose and urea (BUN) are conversions from mg/dL to mmol/L. Normally, P_{osm} = 280 mOsm/kg to 290 mOsm/kg. Remember that even though urea contributes to the plasma osmolality, it does not create osmotic pressure as Na^+ and glucose do. This is because urea is freely permeable across the cell membranes; that is, it is an ineffective osmole.

Disorders That Affect Plasma Osmolality

Various conditions may cause abnormal deviations from the normal P_{osm}. Most of these conditions do so by disturbing the body's osmoregulatory function and causing the kidney to reabsorb too much or too little water, lowering or raising the plasma $[Na^+]$. Thus, **hyponatremia,** low plasma Na^+, and **hypernatremia,** high plasma Na^+, are the common endpoints of osmoregulation disorders, and we will discuss their consequences shortly. First, we'll briefly summarize how some conditions derange plasma osmolality. (See Clinical Application Box *The Osmolal Gap.*)

Table 23.2 **RESPONSES TO PHYSIOLOGIC AND PATHOPHYSIOLOGIC CHALLENGES TO OSMOLALITY HOMEOSTASIS**

Challenge	Δ in ECF/ICF Vol.	Δ in Plasma Osmolality	Main Homeostatic Response
Addition of isotonic saline to ECF	↑ ECF volume No Δ in ICF	No Δ in Plasma osmolality	↓ Salt and water reabsorption ↑ Iso-osmotic urine output ↓ ECF volume
Addition of water or hypotonic fluid to ECF	↑ ECF volume, then shift into ICF Net Δ: some ↑ ECF, some ↑ ICF	↓ Plasma osmolality	↑ Free water clearance (i.e., ↑ hypo-osmotic urine output) ↑ Plasma osmolality ↓ ECF volume
Addition of salt to ECF	Fluid shifts from ICF to ECF, ↑ ECF, ↓ ICF	↑ Plasma osmolality	↓ Free water clearance (i.e., ↓ urine volume) ↑ Urine osmolality ↓ Plasma osmolality ↑ ECF volume
Loss of isotonic fluid, as in hemorrhage	↓ ECF No Δ in ICF	No Δ in plasma osmolality	↑ Salt and water reabsorption ↓ Iso-osmotic urine output ↑ ECF volume
Loss of hypotonic fluid, such as sweat	↓ ECF ↓ ICF as fluid shifts from ICF to ECF	↑ Plasma osmolality	↑ Salt and water reabsorption ↓ Free water clearance ↓ Urine volume ↑ Urine osmolality ↓ Plasma osmolality ↑ ECF volume

Diabetes Mellitus In **diabetes mellitus (DM),** the plasma glucose concentration is abnormally elevated, which directly raises the plasma osmolality by the equation shown previously. Glucose, acting as an effective osmole, causes water to leave cells and enter the ECF. The result will be a dilution of the serum sodium concentration despite the high osmolality. Elevated plasma glucose concentration also raises the osmolality in another way—by creating an **osmotic diuresis**. The high plasma glucose concentration overwhelms the reabsorptive capacity of the tubule and the intratubular glucose concentration goes up. This increases the osmotic pressure in the tubule and impairs water reabsorption. ADH is unable to successfully increase water reabsorption and correct the hyperosmolality. The plasma $[Na^+]$ therefore begins to rise, and eventually, hypernatremia may be observed. The osmotic diuresis accounts for the

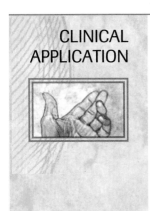

CLINICAL APPLICATION

FLUID MANAGEMENT

With an understanding of what happens in the body in response to various homeostatic challenges, we can make more informed clinical decisions regarding the appropriate fluids for treating patients. By considering volume status, blood pressure, and plasma osmolality in the context of the disorder present, we can best judge whether the patient needs volume added or subtracted from the ECF—and whether this fluid should be hypotonic or isotonic. In cases of dramatic hypotension, as in hemorrhage or shock, 1 to 2 L of isotonic saline or Ringer's lactate (which is also isotonic to plasma) may be administered rapidly through a large bore catheter. The choice of isotonic fluids avoids changes in body fluid osmolality. One of the reasons paramedics and physicians are so quick to establish an IV line in emergency situations is to gain control over the ECF volume and thereby over the perfusion pressure.

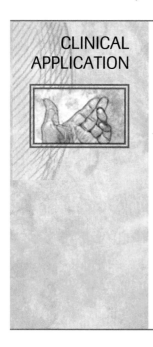

CLINICAL APPLICATION

THE OSMOLAL GAP

The equation for calculating plasma osmolality describes the main physiologic contributors to plasma osmolality: Na^+, Cl^-, glucose, and urea. In some conditions, such as methanol intoxication, the concentration of other solutes not included in the equation rises, thus contributing to plasma osmolality. In such cases, P_{osm} measured by freezing point depression will differ from the calculated P_{osm}:

$$P_{osm} = 2\,([Na^+]) + [glucose]/18 + BUN/2.8$$

The difference between measured and calculated P_{osm} is called the **osmolal gap.**

In many instances of osmolal gap, an acidosis or other more prominent findings lead the way to the diagnosis. An **anion gap** is created not by *osmoles* unaccounted for in physiologic calculation but by *anions* unaccounted for by physiologic calculation. Many acidoses create an anion gap, and many neutral solutes can cause an osmolal gap and an anion gap because of the presence of anionic metabolites. Ethanol is one substance that can create an osmolal gap without creating an anion gap. Methanol intoxication creates an osmolal gap and an anion gap, as it is metabolized to the anion formate.

---

increased urination (polyuria) observed in DM, and the hyperosmolality accounts for the thirst and increased drinking (polydipsia).

Diabetes Insipidus Diabetes insipidus (DI) is a disorder in which the brain produces too little ADH (*central diabetes insipidus*) or when the kidney fails to respond to circulating ADH (*nephrogenic diabetes insipidus*). Central DI may be caused by damage to the pituitary or hypothalamus, as in head trauma, surgery, or global chemical derangements that affect the brain, such as hypoxia. Nephrogenic DI is associated with chronic lithium use (for bipolar disorder) or hypercalcemia. When ADH cannot act, water cannot be reabsorbed normally to correct hyperosmolality, and hypernatremia and polyuria ensue.

Syndrome of Inappropriate Secretion of ADH Like central DI, the **syndrome of inappropriate secretion of ADH (SIADH)** appears in connection with disorders that affect the pituitary and hypothalamus. In this case, the problem is too much ADH action, as opposed to too little. The kidney absorbs excess water (decreased or negative free-water clearance), and hyponatremia follows. One of the most common causes of this syndrome is the secretion of ADH by tumors, particularly certain lung cancers. Hypoxia and pulmonary infections can also cause ADH secretion.

ECF Volume Depletion As described previously and in Chapter 22, very low intravascular pressures trigger the baroreceptors to signal ADH release from the brain, regardless of the plasma osmolality. The kidney reabsorbs more water than the plasma os-

molality requires, the plasma osmolality drops, and hyponatremia follows.

Consequences of Osmolar Disturbances: Hypernatremia and Hyponatremia

Earlier, we stated that osmoregulation is necessary to prevent the fluid shifts associated with changes in ECF osmolality. Thus, we should expect that hypernatremia (e.g., due to DM or DI) causes fluid to shift from ICF to ECF, shrinking the cells. Likewise, hyponatremia causes fluid to shift from ECF to ICF, swelling the cells. See Clinical Application Box *Pseudohyponatremia*.)

Cellular shrinkage and swelling are particularly dangerous for the brain. Cerebral shrinkage and cerebral edema may lead to altered mental status, seizures, or coma. These symptoms occur only in acute cases of hypo- or hypernatremia (within a day or two). When plasma osmolality changes gradually, brain tissue adapts to minimize fluid shifts. It does so by modulating the level of intracellular organic solutes, such as inositol, glutamine, and taurine. The concentrations of these organic osmolytes are reduced in the case of hyponatremia, and are increased in the case of hypernatremia, to lessen the osmotic pressure gradient that drives a fluid shift. Recall that the cells of the renal medulla make use of osmolytes to prevent cell shrinkage in instances of very high ECF salt concentrations.

Because of adapted osmolyte levels in chronic hypo- or hypernatremia, cell volume is normal despite the abnormal osmolality. Therefore, it is im-

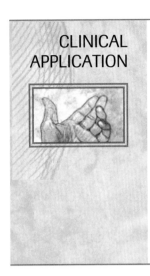

CLINICAL APPLICATION

PSEUDOHYPONATREMIA

In some disease states, *hyperlipidemia*, excess lipids, or *hyperproteinemia*, excess proteins, can reduce the percentage of plasma that is water. Recall that blood is composed of red blood cells and plasma. Plasma is composed of plasma water and solids. Plasma is 93% water. Hyperlipidemia or hyperproteinemia, the excess solids can drive plasma water down below 75%. In such a case, lab tests will reveal hyponatremia because they measure the $[Na^+]$ in the plasma, not just in the plasma water. The osmolality and $[Na^+]$ of the plasma water remains normal, however, and the tissues are not exposed to any osmotic stress. The appropriate treatment would focus on the hyperlipidemia or hyperproteinemia and not the hyponatremia, because it is a false finding (thus the name *pseudo*hyponatremia). Multiple myeloma is a common cause of hyperproteinemia and pseudohyponatremia. A direct measurement using an ion-selective electrode in an undiluted plasma sample will get around this artifact.

portant *not* to try to rapidly reverse the chronic disturbance in plasma osmolality. A rapid reversal of chronic hyponatremia causes cell shrinkage from the reduced osmolyte levels. Likewise, a rapid reversal of hypernatremia causes cerebral edema. As water is added, it will enter the brain cells, which will expand starting from an adapted normal volume.

The Contribution of Potassium to Body Fluid Osmolality Because one observes solute concentrations through routine blood tests in practice, the window into body fluid osmolality is the extracellular fluid; therefore, sodium is of major importance. If one were to sample intracellular water, the major osmolyte would be potassium, with its accompanying anions. In fact, in determining the total body osmolality, both Na^+ and K^+ are important. Consider a loss of K^+ from the body, as might occur in diarrhea or in the urine. As cells become depleted in K^+, Na^+ may enter cells and give the appearance of hyponatremia. Similarly, if a concentrated KCl solution were given, K^+ would move into cells with water, resulting in hypernatremia. For these reasons, it is necessary to consider the osmotic impact of both Na^+ and K^+ in intravenous fluids and when assessing urinary free-water clearance.

Summary

- Na^+ is the major cation of the ECF. Therefore, $[Na^+]$ is the main determinant of ECF osmolality.

- Na^+ is an effective osmole, meaning that it cannot freely diffuse out of the ECF, and that it creates osmotic pressure in the ECF.

- Changes in ECF $[Na^+]$ relative to the ICF osmolality cause fluid shifts between ECF and ICF, leading to cellular swelling or shrinkage.

Cellular swelling and shrinkage are unfavorable for physiologic functioning.

- The brain and kidney regulate the ECF $[Na^+]$ to protect the ICF from fluid shifts.

- Osmoreceptors in the hypothalamus and circumventricular organs shrink and swell like other cells in response to changes in the effective osmolality of the ECF. In addition, osmoreceptors respond to shrinkage and swelling by modulating ADH secretion and thirst.

- During severe volume depletion, baroreceptors will trigger the hypothalamus to release ADH, thus boosting ECF volume at the expense of strict osmoregulation.

- Baroreceptors can also lower the hypothalamic set point, or the threshold for ADH secretion. Pregnancy is also known to lower the osmoregulatory set point.

- Thirst termination may occur via oropharyngeal afferents synapsing in the hypothalamus. This mechanism prevents overcorrection of hyperosmolality by drinking.

- ADH promotes the insertion of aquaporins in the collecting duct, increasing its permeability to water. Signal transduction is cAMP-mediated.

- Increased water permeability in the collecting duct can only promote water reabsorption, given a favorable osmotic gradient for water reabsorption in this part of the nephron. The favorable gradient is established by countercurrent multiplication in the loop of Henle, which maintains a high solute concentration in the renal medulla.

- Water reabsorption without solute in the descending limb of the loop of Henle concentrates the solute in the descending limb. NaCl reabsorption without water in the ascending limb concentrates the medullary interstitium and renders the tubular fluid low in solute concentration. These properties, plus the U shape of the loop of Henle, lead to recycling of NaCl in the medullary interstitium.

- Urea trapping contributes to the high medullary osmolality that enables water reabsorption from the collecting duct.
- When ADH prompts the reabsorption of water into the interstitium, the vasa recta are responsible for absorbing this water into the bloodstream. The vasa recta avoid dissipating the medullary solute gradient by countercurrent exchange.
- When plasma osmolality goes up and the ADH adds water to the ECF, urine osmolality goes up. When plasma osmolality goes down and excess water is excreted from the ECF, urine osmolality goes down. The maximum urine osmolality = medullary interstitial osmolality = 1,200 mOsm/kg.
- Medullary osmolytes avoid cellular shrinkage in the hypertonic interstitial environment.
- Free water clearance equals the urine volume per time,

$\dot{V}$, minus osmolar clearance (C_{osm}):
$$C_{H20} = \dot{V} - C_{osm}$$

- C_{osm} is defined in accordance with the standard clearance equation:
$$C_{osm} = (U_{osm})(\dot{V})/P_{osm}$$

- Plasma osmolality, or serum osmolality, may be calculated using the following equation:

$$P_{osm} = 2\,([Na^+]) + [glucose]/18 + BUN/2.8$$

- DM causes osmotic diuresis and may cause hypernatremia.
- DI causes increased free water clearance and may cause hypernatremia.
- SIADH and ECF volume depletion may cause hyponatremia.
- Hypernatremia causes shrinkage of brain cells, and hyponatremia causes swelling. Osmolyte levels in the brain are increased in response to chronic hypernatremia and are decreased in response to chronic hyponatremia. A rapid reversal of chronic hypernatremia or hyponatremia thus poses a threat to the patient.

Suggested Reading

Jamison RL, Bennett CM, Berliner RW. Countercurrent multiplication by the thin loops of Henle. Am J Physiol. 1967;212:357–366.

Jamison, RL, Maffly RH. The urinary concentrating mechanism. N Engl J Med. 1976;295:1059–1067.

Kuramochi G, Kobayashi I. Regulation of the urine concentration mechanism by the oropharyngeal afferent pathway in man. Am J Nephrol. 2000;20(1):42–47 (Jan-Feb).

Oliet SH, Bourque CW. Osmoreception in magnocellular neurosecretory cells: from single channels to secretion. Trends Neurosci. 1994;17(8): 340–344 (Aug).

Verney EB. The antidiuretic hormone and the factors which determine its release. Proc R Soc (Biol). 1947;135:25–106.

Wells T. Vesicular osmometers, vasopressin secretion and aquaporin-4: a new mechanism for osmoreception? Mol Cell Endocrinol. 1998;136(2):103–107 (Jan15).

REVIEW QUESTIONS

Directions: Each of the numbered items or incomplete statements in this section is followed by answers or by completions of the statement. Select the ONE lettered answer or completion that is BEST in each case.

1. A 25-year-old psychiatric patient drinks huge quantities of water because he is worried that he is losing excessive fluid from his body. Drinking large amounts of water may result in which of the following acute changes?

    (A) hyperosmolality in ECF
    (B) hypo-osmolality in ECF
    (C) decreased ECF volume
    (D) decreased ICF volume
    (E) no change in ICF volume

2. A 15-year-old boy has a mutation that interferes with the action of ADH in the collecting duct. If he feasts on a salty meal, he might have difficulty with hypernatremia for which of the following reasons?

    (A) enhanced urea reabsorption
    (B) failure of salt reabsorption
    (C) enhanced salt reabsorption
    (D) failure of water reabsorption
    (E) enhanced water reabsorption

3. A 65-year-old man with a pituitary tumor is found to be hyponatremic. His hyponatremia may be the result of which of the following?

    (A) elevated plasma glucose
    (B) cerebral edema
    (C) central diabetes insipidus
    (D) nephrogenic diabetes insipidus
    (E) excess secretion of ADH

ANSWERS TO REVIEW QUESTIONS

1. **The answer is B.** Drinking excessive quantities of free water, as might occur in a patient such as this with psychogenic polydipsia, leads to the addition of water to the ECF. This leads to a drop in ECF osmolality, which will then trigger a fluid shift of water from the ECF to the ICF, expanding the ICF volume, until the ECF and ICF are isotonic once more.

2. **The answer is D.** The action of ADH in the collection duct results in the insertion of aquaporins into the apical surface of the collecting duct. This results in enhanced water reabsorption, which would increase ECF fluid levels and act to decrease plasma osmolality. ADH enhances salt reabsorption in the thick ascending limb, which functions as part of the loop of Henle's counter-current multiplication system to enhance the reabsorption of pure water.

3. **The answer is E.** Pituitary pathology may lead to central DI or SIADH. We know that SIADH (excess secretion of ADH) is present because of the hyponatremia. In patients with excess secretion of ADH, excessive water reabsorption by the kidney dilutes the ECF fluid and leads to hyponatremia. Hyponatremia, in turn, may lead to cerebral edema by the shift of fluid from the ECF to the ICF; the edema is therefore not the cause but the effect of the hyponatremia. Elevated plasma glucose, as seen in DM, would result in impaired water reabsorption and hypernatremia. Likewise, in either central or nephrogenic DI, there is inadequate water reabsorption, and *hyper*natremia can occur.

The Regulation of Potassium Balance

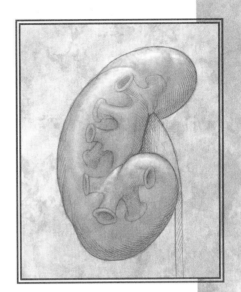

INTRODUCTION

In the previous two chapters, we made several observations about extracellular fluid (EFC) volume and osmolality: (1) the stability of these parameters is critical for normal physiologic functioning; (2) these parameters are subject to daily changes; and (3) the kidney counters these changes in order to preserve stable ECF volume and osmolality. In this chapter and the next, we will see that the same principles apply to two other critical physiologic parameters: the plasma $[K^+]$ and the plasma acidity or pH.

K^+ is present in human tissues at an overall concentration of about 50 mEq/kg body weight. Because plant and animal cells are filled with K^+, it is also ingested daily in dietary vegetables, fruits, and meats, which adds K^+ to the plasma through the intestines, raising plasma $[K^+]$ (FIGURE 24.1). The kidney modulates excretion of this daily K^+ load in order to keep the plasma $[K^+]$ stable, which in turn, maintains the special distribution of K+ between the intracellular fluid (ICF) and the ECF. Without this special distribution of K+, the basic functions of most tissues would not be possible.

SYSTEM STRUCTURE: THE DISTRIBUTION OF POTASSIUM

Just as Na^+ is the major cation of the ECF, K^+ is the major cation of the ICF. Roughly 98% of total body K^+ resides in the ICF, with 2% in the ECF. In absolute terms, this represents a total of 3,500 mEq of potassium in the ICF and 70 mEq in the ECF in the average person (TABLE 24.1). The Na^+/K^+-ATPase pumps that drive Na^+ out of cells and K^+ into cells create this distribution.

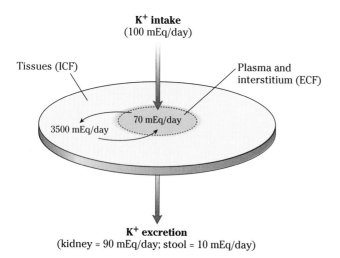

K⁺ intake
(100 mEq/day)

Tissues (ICF)

Plasma and interstitium (ECF)

70 mEq/day

3500 mEq/day

K⁺ excretion
(kidney = 90 mEq/day; stool = 10 mEq/day)

Figure 24.1 Potassium intake, excretion, and body stores. The values are totals, not concentrations, and are meant to represent averages for a 70-kg person. The arrows reflect the fact that K⁺ moves across the cell membranes.

Table 24.1 THE NORMAL DISTRIBUTION OF POTASSIUM

	ICF	ECF
Total value	~3,500 mEq	~70 mEq
Percentage of total	98%	2%
$[K^+]$	140 mEq/L	4 to 5 mEq/L

The two basic homeostatic elements in the regulation of the potassium distribution are the sensors of plasma $[K^+]$ and the effectors of regulatory K^+ reabsorption and secretion. The K^+ sensors are thought to be located in the adrenal gland, perhaps in the zona glomerulosa, where aldosterone is secreted. The regulated reabsorption and secretion of K^+ takes place in the late distal tubule and collecting duct. (The proximal tubule conducts a great deal of K^+ reabsorption on an unregulated basis, i.e., it reabsorbs a majority of K^+ regardless of the plasma $[K^+]$.) When $[K^+]$ rises or falls in the ECF, this homeostatic system accelerates or slows the elimination of K^+ from the ECF. There are other mechanisms for regulating potassium distribution, but they are not associated with distinct anatomical entities, as we shall see.

SYSTEM FUNCTION: POTASSIUM HOMEOSTASIS

Why is a stable distribution of potassium physiologically important? There are two reasons, one specific and one more general. To understand the more specific reason, recall that the segregation of K^+ inside cells is the chief determinant of the resting cell membrane potential, and that the resting membrane potential accounts for the excitability of nervous and muscle tissue. Without the potassium distribution, muscles could not contract, and neurons could not generate or transmit action potentials.

The distribution of potassium accounts for tissue excitability in the following way. First, the Na^+/K^+-ATPase pump creates a large $[K^+]$ gradient between the inside of cells and the outside. In addition, the high density of K^+ channels in most cell membranes (high K^+ permeability) allows K^+ to flow down that concentration gradient. The migration of positively charged K^+ ions out of the cell renders the intracellular side of the membrane electronegative (polarized). When a neurotransmitter stimulates an influx of Na^+ down its concentration gradient, the electrical potential inside of the cell increases (depolarizing the cell), and this change in transmembrane voltage triggers the opening of more Na^+ channels. As the membrane depolarizes, more K^+ channels also open, leading to an efflux of K^+. If the initial neurotransmitted stimulus is strong enough, the influx of Na^+ continues to depolarize the cell, which opens more Na^+ channels. The Na^+ influx continues to build until the Na^+ influx surpasses the K^+ efflux, giving the inside of the cell a positive electrical potential, or **action potential**. The **threshold potential** is the minimum initial depolarized potential that the neurotransmitter must achieve in order to send the cell into the self-amplifying ascent toward action potential. The K^+ distribution thus establishes the electrophysiological ground upon which action potentials can occur. More generally, a high intracellular $[K^+]$ is necessary for a wide variety of enzymatic cell functions, including the regulation of protein synthesis, cell growth and division, and glycogen synthesis.

Just as the distribution of Na^+ binds water into the ECF, the K^+ distribution binds negative potential and a milieu conducive to protein function into the ICF. Disturbances in K^+ distribution, reflected in high or low plasma $[K^+]$, therefore threaten vital tissue functions. Consequently, many mechanisms are brought to bear upon the plasma $[K^+]$ to keep it within tight bounds.

Challenges to Stable Transmembrane Potassium Distribution

The main source of increased plasma $[K^+]$ is the diet (TABLE 24.2). Cellular breakdown on a massive scale, as in crush injuries, can also release potassium into the bloodstream in significant amounts. Unregulated potassium losses occur in the stool and in a variety of disease states, as will be discussed later. Increased cellular production, which traps large amounts of potassium inside cells, can also result in increased uptake of potassium, which lowers the plasma $[K^+]$. When vitamin B_{12} is used to treat anemia, the resultant increase in cellular production has been observed to drop the plasma $[K^+]$. Pregnant mothers may also experience a drop in their plasma $[K^+]$ as the growing fetus traps potassium inside its cells.

Table 24.2 SOURCES OF UNREGULATED POTASSIUM ADDITIONS AND LOSSES[a]

Factors That ↑ plasma $[K^+]$	Factors That ↓ plasma $[K^+]$
Diet	Losses in stool
Cellular breakdown	Cellular uptake

[a]This table does not include disturbances in the mechanisms that regulate $[K^+]$, although such disturbances are the most common causes of derangements in plasma $[K^+]$. Rather, the table is meant to show the types of challenges that may confront the physiologic regulatory apparatus.

Because the precise transmembrane potassium gradient is so critical to neuromuscular function, disturbances in the distribution can create life-threatening cardiac arrhythmias. Consequently, dietary loads of potassium must be removed from the ECF immediately. The renal excretion of dietary potassium takes place over hours—a time frame that is too slow to protect cardiac functioning. That is why the body has evolved other first-line defenses to dispose of dietary potassium. These rapid defenses rely on intracellular storage of the potassium absorbed from the intestines as a temporary measure until renal mechanisms are able to eliminate the excess potassium.

Intracellular Storage: The Rapid Phase of Normalization

Within minutes of an increase in plasma $[K^+]$, K^+ is stored inside cells. Without storage, one meal's addition of 50 mEq of K^+ to the roughly 14 L ECF would double the normal plasma $[K^+]$ of 4 mEq/L. This change in plasma $[K^+]$ would significantly alter the resting membrane potential. Two factors promote intracellular storage to alleviate this disturbance: the plasma $[K^+]$ itself and hormone action. The plasma pH may promote or impede intracellular storage.

Plasma Potassium Concentration The problem of increased plasma $[K^+]$ is partly self-correcting, as some of the K^+ storage occurs unassisted. This is because the increased ECF $[K^+]$ favors K^+ entry into the cell and opposes its egress. Some of the added K^+ is pumped into the cells as the altered gradient facilitates the work of the Na^+/K^+-ATPase. The proportionate distribution of some of the added K^+ between the ICF and ECF thus preserves the membrane potential in part and mitigates the problem of increased plasma $[K^+]$. The Na^+/K^+-ATPase appears not to be able to normalize the potassium distribution (and hence the tissue membrane potential) by itself; therefore, other rapid defenses are in place in addition to slow renal excretion to lower the plasma $[K^+]$ by intracellular storage.

Insulin and Catecholamines The body also assists potassium storage with two types of hormones: insulin and the catecholamines. The main function of **insulin** is to store glucose inside cells in response to high glucose levels and to promote anabolic pathways for the cellular storage of carbohydrate energy. It is a matter of controversy whether insulin is secreted in direct response to plasma $[K^+]$. If it were, it would be part of homeostatic regulation of plasma $[K^+]$, as opposed to influencing plasma $[K^+]$ as an incidental effect of glucose regulation. Nevertheless, whether or not insulin release is directly linked to increases in plasma $[K^+]$, it is indirectly linked to

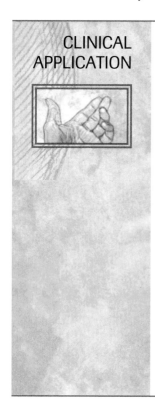

EXERCISE AND β-BLOCKADE

In addition to the primary factors mentioned in the text, secondary factors affect the plasma [K$^+$]. Two examples are exercise and drugs called **β-blockers.** Such factors do not normally cause pathogenic disturbances in the plasma [K$^+$], but they can do so in the context of another underlying disturbance in potassium homeostasis. Therefore, they can be important clinical considerations.

Exercise may transiently increase the plasma [K$^+$]. The ATP depletion that occurs during exercise and muscle contraction may open ATP-dependent potassium channels, increasing permeability to potassium in the muscle cells. Given that efflux of potassium follows muscular contraction in the repolarization period, one might think that muscular action potentials themselves would contribute to the increased plasma [K$^+$]. This is not the case, because the number of mEq of K$^+$ exchanged during and after the action potential is extremely small and does not affect the overall plasma [K$^+$].

β-2-blockers like propanolol are competitive antagonists for adrenergic β-receptors. They inhibit the binding of epinephrine and norepinephrine and interfere with the actions of those hormones, such as increasing heart rate and cardiac output. They are therefore used to treat hypertension. Because the catecholamines also promote the cellular uptake of K$^+$, these drugs may also increase the plasma [K$^+$]. When these drugs are administered in the context of another aggravating factor, they may cause **hyperkalemia**—pathologically high plasma [K$^+$], > 5 mEq/L. Hyperkalemia may have very serious consequences for cardiac function if left untreated.

such increases through its governance of the blood glucose level. After a meal, intestinal absorption of foodstuffs yields a load of both glucose and potassium together. Insulin's linkage with the blood glucose level therefore indirectly yokes the hormone's secretion to the K$^+$ level. Insulin is sometimes administered therapeutically to lower the plasma [K$^+$].

The **catecholamines** (the most important examples outside the brain are *epinephrine* [adrenalin] and *norepinephrine*) are secreted at a basal level and are increased in response to stress. They have a wide variety of effects, including an increase in cardiac output and blood pressure. The catecholamines are not thought to regulate plasma [K$^+$] but only to lower it as an incidental effect. Although the physiologic importance of catecholamine-mediated potassium uptake is uncertain, the therapeutic blockade of adrenergic hormone action can have incidental consequences for the plasma [K$^+$]. β-adrenergic agonists, such as salbutamol, can also be used in the treatment of high plasma [K$^+$]. (See Clinical Application Box *Exercise and β-Blockade*.)

Plasma pH Whereas potassium storage is critical to handling potassium loads, the cellular uptake and release of potassium is also important for the rapid handling of acid loads. When the [H$^+$] rises in the blood—for example, due to the metabolism of digested proteins—H$^+$ diffuses into cells. The migration of the positive charge inward results in an efflux of positively charged Na$^+$ and K$^+$ and the plasma [K$^+$] rises (FIGURE 24.2). In fact, 60% of acid loads are "buffered" by cellu-

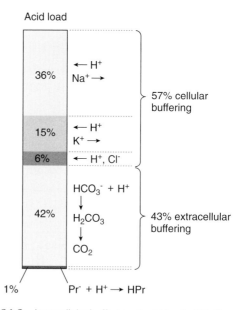

Figure 24.2 Intracellular buffering of acid loads. This figure shows that in addition to the exchange of H$^+$ for Na$^+$ and K$^+$, H$^+$ migration into cells draws a small amount of Cl-. Pr = plasma protein. The protonation of plasma proteins is a minimal contributor to buffering. These data are derived from experiments in which HCl was infused intravenously into nephrectomized dogs.

lar uptake. The rest of the load is buffered by bicarbonate in solution in the blood (see Chapter 25).

The reverse is also true but not to the same degree. When the [H⁺] falls, H⁺ migrates out of the cell, and K⁺ shifts inward toward the negative charge left behind by the H⁺. The plasma [K⁺] therefore falls. The rise in pH, however, does not lower the [K⁺] to the same extent that low pH raises the plasma [K⁺]. The reasons for this are not entirely clear.

Renal Handling: The Slow Phase of Normalization

Whereas intracellular storage takes place in minutes, it represents only a temporary solution to the problem of excess K⁺. Without actual elimination of K⁺ from the body, the plasma [K⁺] would continue to rise and the transmembrane distribution (and potential) would be increasingly disturbed. Consequently, renal excretion of K⁺ is critical to avoid life-threatening increases in the plasma [K⁺]. (A small amount of K⁺ is excreted in the stool, but it is not enough to match daily potassium intake and is not subject to homeostatic regulation.) When plasma [K⁺] is low, nearly all filtered K⁺ may be reabsorbed, but the kidney always excretes some K⁺ in the urine—regulation simply determines how much is excreted. As with other parameters under renal control, the kidney adjusts excretion or clearance (and hence the plasma [K⁺]) through adjustments in tubular reabsorption and secretion. Under normal circumstances of adequate amounts of dietary potassium, secretion predominates and can lower the plasma

[K⁺] in a time frame of hours. In order to understand the renal regulation of plasma [K⁺], we must first review the tubular transport of K⁺.

Renal Potassium Transport   The renal handling of potassium follows that of many solutes: It is reabsorbed in bulk in the proximal tubule and loop of Henle, while regulation of K⁺ balance takes place in the late distal tubule and collecting duct. In these late tubule segments, smaller amounts of K⁺ are reabsorbed or secreted under the control of regulatory mechanisms. Roughly 65% of K⁺ is reabsorbed in the proximal tubule, 25% is reabsorbed in the loop of Henle, and the remainder of the filtered amount is usually excreted along with additional K⁺ secreted in the late tubule segments (FIGURE 24.3). Although the thick ascending limb of Henle may reabsorb 25% of the filtered K⁺, a significant amount of K⁺ crossing the apical membrane into the cell via the NaK2Cl cotransporter is recycled back to the lumen, a process that maximizes NaCl reabsorption in that segment.

While the proximal tubule cells are rich with basolateral Na⁺/K⁺-ATPases that drive K⁺ from the interstitium *into the cells*, most of renal K⁺ reabsorption occurs here. How can this be, given the ATPase-governed movement of K⁺ *away from* the interstitium? One answer is that proximal tubular K⁺ reabsorption is thought to be mainly paracellular. Two forces may drive paracellular K⁺ reabsorption. Recall that the large proximal tubular flow of water from lumen to interstitium drags solutes with it. This first means of K⁺ reabsorption is known as **solvent drag**, and it occurs not through the genesis of an

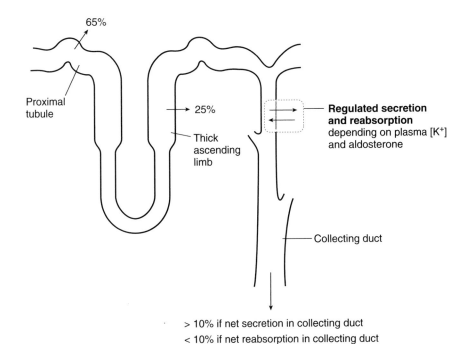

Figure 24.3   Potassium transport along the renal tubule. Reabsorption in the proximal tubule and loop of Henle are obligatory. Net excretion is determined by regulated reabsorption and secretion in the late distal tubule and collecting duct.

electrical or chemical gradient for K$^+$ but merely because the flowing water imparts kinetic energy to the K$^+$ ions. A second driving force is the electropositivity of the late proximal tubule lumen. Recall that the cotransport of Na$^+$ with a variety of non-Cl$^-$ anions in the early proximal tubule raises the [Cl-] in the luminal fluid. This action creates a concentration gradient for paracellular Cl- reabsorption in the late proximal tubule, and the migration of negatively charged Cl- anions from lumen to interstitium raises the electrical potential of the lumen. This, in turn, may provide an electrical driving force for the paracellular reabsorption of K$^+$ (as it does for Na$^+$). Some investigators believe proximal tubular K$^+$ reabsorption also occurs by means of a transcellular pathway, mediated by an unknown mechanism.

The reabsorption of K$^+$ in the thick ascending limb of the loop of Henle also occurs paracellularly due to a positively charged tubule lumen. Recall that the Na$^+$/K$^+$-ATPase drives Na$^+$ across the basolateral and hence the apical membrane of the tubule cells. The apical translocation of Na$^+$ across the Na$^+$/K$^+$/2Cl$^-$ symporter drives the reabsorption of K$^+$ and Cl-. Chloride is reabsorbed across the basolateral membrane into the interstitium. Potassium, which is also driven inside the cell by the Na$^+$/K$^+$-ATPase, can escape either through basolateral channels into the interstitium or through apical channels back into the tubule lumen. Apical recycling of the K$^+$ *without Cl$^-$* renders the tubule electropositive and drives the paracellular reabsorption of K$^+$ and other cations.

Potassium may be either reabsorbed or secreted by the late distal tubule and collecting duct (FIGURE 24.4). In some types of intercalated cells, the H$^+$/K$^+$-ATPase may drive transcellular K$^+$ reabsorption in exchange for H$^+$ secretion.

Potassium secretion takes place in principal cells of the late distal tubule and collecting duct and is driven by the Na$^+$/K$^+$-ATPase. The basolateral Na$^+$/K$^+$-ATPase pumps Na$^+$ from inside the cell to the interstitium and K$^+$ from the interstitium into the cell. The high intracellular [K$^+$] causes K$^+$ to flow down its concentration gradient across apical and basolateral K$^+$ channels. At the same time, the low intracellular [Na$^+$] causes Na$^+$ reabsorption across the apical membrane from lumen to cytosol. Sodium reabsorption in excess of anions leaves the lumen negatively charged, however. Consequently, the electronegative tubule lumen favors net diffusion of K$^+$ across its apical channels and hence net secretion of K$^+$. The end result is that the Na$^+$/K$^+$-ATPase drives K$^+$ secretion in this part of the nephron.

Tubular flow promotes increased K$^+$ secretion by sweeping away luminal potassium in its forward flow and reducing the luminal [K$^+$]. This augments the concentration gradient for potassium diffusion into

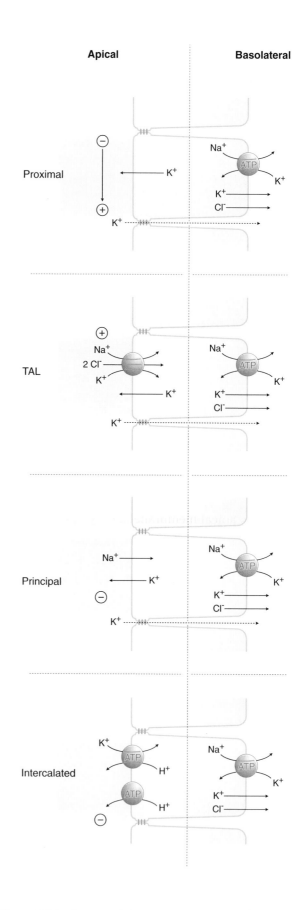

Figure 24.4   Pumps and channels participating in K$^+$ transport.

the tubule lumen. Increased tubular flow therefore increases potassium secretion and excretion. Another mechanism by which increased flow increases potassium excretion is that of increased sodium delivery to the distal tubule. Increased sodium delivery increases sodium reabsorption here, which drives potassium secretion by the mechanisms described previously. Increased tubular flow in this region of the tubule is sometimes called **distal flow**.

Regulatory Factors in Renal Potassium Excretion

There are two main regulators of renal K^+ excretion: aldosterone and the plasma $[K^+]$ per se. **Aldosterone** is a steroid produced in the zona glomerulosa of the adrenal gland. It promotes K^+ secretion from principal cells in the late distal tubule and collecting duct. It does so by diffusing out of the peritubular capillaries and acting on the nuclei of principal cells to modulate DNA transcription, producing several end results via messenger proteins. Primarily, aldosterone enhances the performance of the Na^+/K^+-ATPase in the basolateral membrane. This increases the tubular intracellular $[K^+]$, but more importantly, it stimulates increased Na^+ uptake from the tubule lumen. (Recall that aldosterone is also an important hormone in the regulation of Na^+ reabsorption and ECF volume.) Increased Na^+ uptake increases the electronegativity of the tubule lumen and promotes paracellular K^+ secretion by electrostatic force. Aldosterone also increases the apical permeability to Na^+ by causing the principal cell to insert more channels into its apical membrane and by opening silent Na^+ channels. This further increases Na^+ uptake and hence K^+ secretion (FIGURE 24.5).

Aldosterone has a cytoplasmic receptor that also recognizes cortisol, which is in greater concentration, yet has little effect on potassium, sodium, and hydrogen transport. The reason is that the collecting duct cell has an enzyme, 11-beta OH steroid dehydrogenase, which converts cortisol to inactive cortisone. There is an ingredient of natural licorice that inhibits the enzyme, causing hypertension (Na^+ retention), hypokalemia (K secretion), and alkalosis (H^+ secretion).

Aldosterone secretion is thought to be controlled by two different homeostatic systems: that for regulating blood pressure and that for regulating plasma $[K^+]$. Recall that low blood pressure stimulates aldosterone secretion through the renin-angiotensin-aldosterone system. High plasma $[K^+]$ stimulates the secretion of aldosterone, perhaps by stimulating K^+ sensors in the zona glomerulosa.

Increased plasma $[K^+]$ is also thought to act independently of aldosterone on the principal cells and to reproduce the same effects as aldosterone does, although to a lesser degree. This hypothesis is supported by experiments with adrenalectomized dogs. FIGURE 24.6 summarizes the hormonal influences on plasma $[K^+]$, on both intracellular storage and renal excretion. (See Integrated Physiology Box *Potassium and ECF Volume Homeostasis*.)

PATHOPHYSIOLOGY: DISORDERS OF PLASMA [K⁺] REGULATION

Because the regulatory apparatus is equal to the task of handling most additions and losses of plasma K^+, pathologic derangements in plasma $[K^+]$ are usually due to defects or alterations in the regulatory apparatus itself. **Hyperkalemia** is pathologically high plasma $[K^+]$, and it is usually defined as a plasma $[K^+] > 5.5$ mEq/L. **Hypokalemia** is pathologically low plasma $[K^+]$, and it is usually defined as a plasma $[K^+] < 3.5$ mEq/L.

Membrane excitability is determined by the difference between the negative resting potential and the less-negative threshold potential. (Recall that the threshold potential is the minimum depolarizing potential that is necessary from a synaptic stimulus to trigger an action potential.) If the resting potential (e.g., -70 mV in most neurons) is close to the threshold potential (e.g., -60 mV), a smaller stimulus may bump up the electrical potential inside the cell enough to achieve the threshold potential of -60 mV and send the cell over the edge to an eventual action potential. If the resting potential (again, suppose -70 mV) is farther from the threshold potential (e.g., -50 mV), a larger amount of depolarization is necessary to reach the threshold potential. When the resting and threshold potentials are close together and action potentials are achievable with smaller stimuli, the membrane is considered more excitable. When the membrane requires larger stimuli for an action potential, the membrane is said to be less excitable.

Because the plasma $[K^+]$ determines the resting potential, alterations in plasma $[K^+]$ alter the resting potential, and consequently can alter membrane

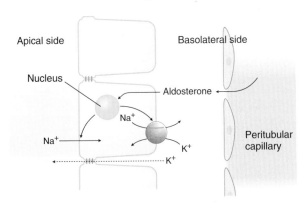

Figure 24.5 Aldosterone action in the principal cell. Aldosterone stimulates the production of proteins that stimulate the basolateral Na^+/K^+-ATPase and that upregulate the number and the activity of apical Na^+ channels.

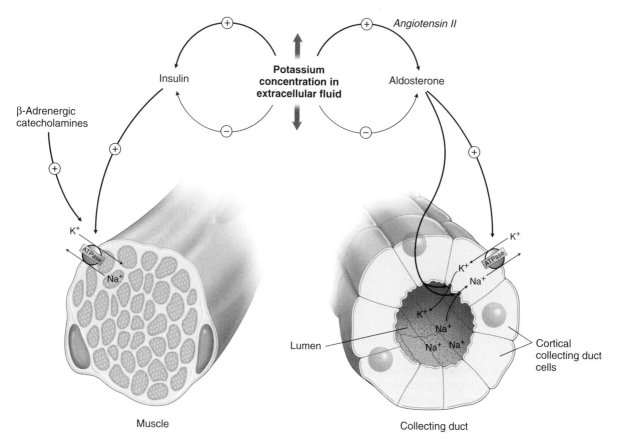

Figure 24.6   A summary of hormonal influences on plasma [K$^+$]. Although the figure suggests insulin secretion is promoted by high plasma [K$^+$] and vice versa, this is a matter of controversy. Some investigators believe catecholamine-stimulated K$^+$ uptake to be mediated by β-receptors.

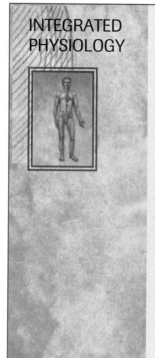

INTEGRATED PHYSIOLOGY

Potassium and ECF Volume Homeostasis

Because aldosterone helps regulate both plasma [K$^+$] and ECF volume, how does the body avoid disturbing plasma [K$^+$] when it seeks to correct ECF volume? How does it preserve ECF volume when aldosterone is being secreted to correct plasma [K$^+$]? The answer is distal flow.

When ECF volume is decreased, the RAA system stimulates increased aldosterone secretion. In turn, the increased aldosterone secretion promotes increased Na$^+$ reabsorption in the distal tubule by enhancing the activity of the basolateral Na$^+$/K$^+$-ATPase. Enhanced activity of the basolateral Na$^+$/K$^+$-ATPase, however, also means increased secretion of K$^+$. If this were the whole story, ECF volume depletion would lead to potassium wasting and **hypokalemia,** or low plasma [K$^+$].

Potassium wasting does not occur owing to the effects of decreased ECF volume on distal flow. When decreased ECF volume stimulates the RAA system, not only do aldosterone levels increase, but so do angiotensin II levels. Angiotensin II promotes proximal tubular Na$^+$ reabsorption by stimulation of the apical Na$^+$/H$^+$ antiporter. This, in turn, leads to increased water reabsorption in the proximal tubule. Consequently, distal flow is reduced. With less distal flow, secreted potassium is not swept away as fast, the tubular [K$^+$] is higher, and the gradient for potassium secretion is less favorable. Distal flow thereby serves as an autoregulatory mechanism protecting potassium balance from the RAA system.

excitability. Hyperkalemia will impede the resting efflux of potassium and render the resting potential less negative, or closer to threshold. Hypokalemia does the reverse. Therefore, hyperkalemia should render cell membranes more excitable and hypokalemia less excitable. The actual situation is slightly more complicated, however. Although the previously mentioned prediction is true initially, prolonged exposure to disturbances in plasma [K⁺] may actually produce the opposite effects, with hyperkalemia leading to *decreased* excitability and hypokalemia to *increased* excitability. This may occur through effects on Na+ channel inactivation. Both hyperkalemia and hypokalemia may lead to serious cardiac arrhythmias and muscle weakness.

Hyperkalemia

Hyperkalemia is not particularly common outside of patients with renal failure, but when severe (> 6 or 7 mEq/L), this condition is more imminently life-threatening than hypokalemia. *There is one principal cause of hyperkalemia: decreased renal excretion.* Two other causes—increased dietary intake and increased release from cells—are mainly significant in the context of decreased renal excretion.

The two main causes of decreased renal excretion are decreased filtration and decreased secretion. Decreased glomerular filtration is called **renal failure**. Acute renal failure is probably the most common cause of hyperkalemia. Whereas 90% of filtered K⁺ is usually reabsorbed, decreased glomerular filtration rate (GFR) prohibits the elimination of the remaining 10% and also interferes with secretion. Secretion depends on a good distal flow rate and when GFR is reduced, the distal flow rate is reduced. Decreased secretion may occur independently of decreased GFR in the case of hypoaldosteronism and as a side effect of some medications. *Hypoaldosteronism* is decreased aldosterone secretion, which may occur in Addison's disease (primary adrenal insufficiency), in hyporeninemia secondary to various types of kidney disease, or as an idiopathic effect (having an unknown cause). A variety of drugs impair K⁺ secretion, including potassium-sparing diuretics and nonsteroidal anti-inflammatory drugs.

In the context of renal failure, a large dietary potassium load may overwhelm whatever secretory capacities remain in the kidney, thereby leading to hyperkalemia. (Administering potassium to treat *hypo*kalemia is a common cause of hyperkalemia in hospitals.) Likewise, an increased release of K⁺ from cellular breakdown in the context of renal failure may cause persistent hyperkalemia. If renal failure is not present, these conditions may cause transient hyperkalemia. Three examples of such increased cellular breakdown are *tumor lysis syndrome,* wherein cancer chemotherapy leads to widespread cell death; *rhabdomyolysis,* massive tissue breakdown, as in crush injuries; and *hemolysis,* the rupture of red blood cells, as in transfusion reactions or vasculitis, where inflammation in the blood vessels damages the red blood cells. The release of potassium from cells by way of transmembrane shifting may also cause hyperkalemia. Metabolic acidosis and the administration of β-blockers may create hyperkalemia this way, especially in the context of renal failure. (See Clinical Application Box *What is Rhabdomyolysis?*)

The signs and symptoms of hyperkalemia include cardiac arrhythmias (and accompanying abnormalities on electrocardiogram), muscle weakness or paralysis, paresthesias (tingling or other unusual peripheral sensations), and metabolic acidosis. For plasma [K⁺] values of < 7 mEq/L, treatment with Kayexalate (sodium polystyrene sulfonate) may be sufficient. Kayexalate is an orally administered ion exchange resin that draws excess K⁺ into the intestinal lumen. Hyperkalemia of > 7 mEq/L should be treated with intravenous calcium gluconate, which helps restore the normal level of excitability of the myocardium. Glucose and insulin may be administered together—the insulin to shift the K⁺ rapidly inside the cells, and the glucose to prevent hypoglycemia (low blood sugar) due to the insulin. Salbutamol, a β-adrenergic agonist, may also be administered to shift K⁺ rapidly into cells. Finally, dialysis may be used to reverse hyperkalemia.

Hypokalemia

In 1998, the *New England Journal of Medicine* reported that hypokalemia may be the electrolyte abnormality most commonly seen in clinical practice. Hypokalemia is, however, not as life threatening as hyperkalemia. When mild, it may in fact, produce no symptoms at all; when more severe, it may cause muscle weakness, paresthesias, muscle necrosis, a variety of impairments in renal function, and cardiac arrhythmias—although this is more common in patients with preexisting cardiac disease or taking cardiotoxic medication, such as digoxin.

Hypokalemia is caused by excess losses in the urine, excess losses in the stool, shifting of K⁺ into cells, and increased cellular uptake. Thiazide and loop diuretics cause excess K⁺ secretion by increasing distal flow, and they are the most common cause of hypokalemia. Other causes of increased tubular flow may lead to potassium wasting as well. For example, glucosuria in diabetes mellitus causes an osmotic diuresis that can result in excess K⁺ secretion in the distal nephron. Hyperaldosteronism, which occurs in some adrenal tumors, may lead to an excess loss of K⁺.

WHAT IS RHABDOMYOLYSIS?

A 19-year-old male is rushed by ambulance from the scene of a motor vehicle accident. He has sustained massive crush injuries to his lower extremities, but he is breathing, has a pulse of 130 bpm and a BP of 80/50, is alert and oriented, and his pupils are equally round and reactive to light. History taking reveals the boy was trapped in his car for over an hour. Shortly after arrival in the ER, the patient develops a cardiac arrhythmia with QRS complexes that are wide and low in amplitude. He loses consciousness and goes into cardiac arrest. After CPR and an IV push of calcium gluconate, he recovers. He receives IV glucose, insulin, and salbutamol. Lab values show an initial serum K^+ of 10 mEq/L, confirming the diagnosis of hyperkalemia secondary to rhabdomyolysis.

Rhabdomyolysis is widespread breakdown of muscle tissue. It may occur in crush injuries, due to large pressure sores from immobility, in circumstances of heat and exertion, in the context of illicit drug use, including cocaine and ecstasy, and in other scenarios. In addition to releasing large amounts of potassium into the bloodstream, rhabdomyolysis also dumps large amounts of myoglobin (a protein that serves as an oxygen reservoir in muscle tissues) into the bloodstream. When myoglobin is filtered in the kidney, it can cause intrinsic renal failure. The combination of acute renal failure and release of K^+ from the cells makes rhabdomyolysis especially predisposing toward hyperkalemia.

Immediate treatment should be directed at the respiration and circulation, including hemostasis, if hemorrhaging is present; the administration of calcium gluconate should be provided to stabilize the membrane potential of excitable tissue exposed to hyperkalemia; and drugs such as insulin and β-2 agonists should be used to reduce the plasma $[K^+]$ if hyperkalemia and cardiac arrhythmias are present. Treatment should next focus on preserving renal function with IV hydration and, if necessary, dialysis.

Any cause of diarrhea may lead to hypokalemia. In patients with eating disorders, for example, chronic diarrhea due to laxative abuse may lead to hypokalemia. This may be worsened by decreased dietary intake of potassium. Starvation by itself may or may not cause hypokalemia, as wasting of body tissues releases potassium into the ECF. Gastrointestinal losses are especially threatening in the context of renal potassium wasting, as the kidney can usually compensate for losses with increased reabsorption.

An increased plasma pH will cause H^+ to shift out of cells and K^+ into cells, leading to decreased plasma $[K^+]$. β-adrenergic agonists, which are used in treating asthma to dilate the bronchioles, may also shift potassium into cells by mimicking the action of catecholamines. Vitamin B_{12} therapy for anemia may promote cell growth and trap potassium inside cells. Other conditions of rapid cell growth, such as pregnancy, may drop the plasma $[K^+]$.

The treatment for hypokalemia, in addition to addressing the underlying cause, is repletion of body K^+. Repletion should be done slowly, preferably with oral KCl supplements. Among naturally occurring foods, dried figs, molasses, and seaweed have the highest concentration of potassium.

Summary

- Body potassium is 98% intracellular and 2% extracellular.
- This distribution is critical to establishing the resting membrane potential in excitable cells, such as muscle and nervous tissue. It is also important to the performance of many internal cell functions.
- The body faces constant challenges to the physiologic distribution of potassium between the ICF and ECF, including dietary intake and the loss of K^+ in the stool.
- The body normalizes the plasma $[K^+]$ after a dietary load with rapid mechanisms and slower mechanisms.

- The rapid mechanisms for normalizing plasma $[K^+]$ after a dietary load involve intracellular storage of K^+. The slower mechanisms involve increased renal excretion of K^+.

- The factors promoting intracellular potassium storage are high plasma $[K^+]$ and the secretion of insulin and catecholamines.

- Low plasma pH (high $[H^+]$) causes H^+ to shift inside body cells in exchange for potassium, raising the plasma $[K^+]$.

- About 65% of filtered K^+ is reabsorbed in the proximal tubule, and another 25% is reabsorbed in the loop of Henle; the remaining 10% is usually excreted.

- Under normal circumstances, in addition to excreting 10% of filtered potassium, the distal tubule and collecting duct secrete potassium to eliminate the rest of the excess plasma potassium.

- Regulatory factors control potassium secretion in the distal segments of the tubule. High plasma $[K^+]$ and aldosterone promote distal potassium secretion.

- Increased distal flow promotes potassium secretion.

- Disorders of potassium level are almost always due to disturbances in renal secretion. Other causes of high or low plasma $[K^+]$ become more important when they are present alongside an exacerbating disturbance in renal secretion.

- Hyperkalemia, high plasma $[K^+]$, is most often caused by decreased renal secretion of potassium due to renal failure. It causes life-threatening cardiac arrhythmias and is treated with calcium gluconate, Kayexalate, glucose and insulin, salbutamol, and dialysis.

- Hypokalemia, low plasma $[K^+]$, is most often caused by excess potassium secretion in the distal nephron due to the administration of diuretics. It is associated with less morbidity and mortality than hyperkalemia but is far more common. It is treated with potassium repletion, usually oral KCl.

Suggested Reading

Gennari FJ. Hypokalemia. N Engl J Med. 1998;339(7): 451–458 (Aug 13).

Giebisch G. Renal potassium channels: function, regulation, and structure. Kidney Int. 2001;60(2):436–445 (Aug).

Giebisch G. Renal potassium transport: mechanisms and regulation. Am J Physiol. 1998;274(5 Pt 2):F817–833 (May).

Mandal AK. Hypokalemia and hyperkalemia. Med Clin N Am. 1997;81(3):611–639 (May).

Sauret JM, Marinides G, Wang GK. Rhabdomyolysis. Am Fam Physician. 2002;65(5):907–912 (Mar 1).

Ten S, New M, Maclaren N. Clinical review 130: Addison's disease 2001. J Clin Endocrinol Metab. 2001;86(7): 2909–2922 (Jul).

REVIEW QUESTIONS

Directions: Each of the numbered items or incomplete statements in this section is followed by answers or by completions of the statement. Select the ONE lettered answer or completion that is BEST in each case.

1. An 80-year-old woman is treated for congestive heart failure with the loop diuretic, furosemide. After complaining of fatigue, she is found to have a low serum K^+ level of 2.6 mEq/L. Her hypokalemia is due to which of the following mechanisms?

   (A) increased activity of the distal Na^+/K^+-ATPase
   (B) increased glomerular filtration
   (C) increased distal flow
   (D) decreased proximal K^+ reabsorption
   (E) decreased K^+ reabsorption in the loop of Henle

2. A 28-year-old HIV-positive man with a recent history of pulmonary tuberculosis presents with loss of energy and a dark pigmentation to his skin. He is found to have low blood pressure, low blood glucose, and an elevated plasma $[K^+]$. Further lab studies are likely to show:

   (A) low serum $[Na^+]$
   (B) low serum ACTH
   (C) low serum renin
   (D) low hematocrit
   (E) low serum aldosterone

3. A 45-year-old woman with a long history of asthma runs a 10 km race on a cold October morning and has to stop several times to use her albuterol inhaler (a β2-adrenergic agonist). If she has inadvertently dropped her serum $[K^+]$, the reason could be:

   (A) exercise
   (B) transmembrane K^+ shift
   (C) osmotic diuresis
   (D) hyperaldosteronism
   (E) inhibition of the $Na^+/K^+/2Cl^-$ symporter

ANSWERS TO REVIEW QUESTIONS

1. **The answer is** C. The loop diuretic furosemide (Lasix) can cause hypokalemia by increasing tubular flow. It does so by inhibiting Na^+ reabsorption in the loop of Henle (which in turn, inhibits water reabsorption from the collecting duct). Increased flow in the distal segments of the tubule washes away tubular K^+ and creates a favorable gradient for potassium secretion. Increased Na^+ delivery results in more Na^+ reabsorption here and an electrical gradient for paracellular potassium secretion. Although increased activity of the distal Na^+/K^+-ATPase would result in increased potassium secretion, the scenario stated that the drug in question acts in the loop of Henle and not distally; furosemide does not act in the distal segments. Furthermore, increased Na^+/K^+-ATPase activity would have an *anti*diuretic effect. Spironolactone, a "potassium-sparing" diuretic that acts on the distal Na^+/K^+-ATPase, *inhibits* this ATPase and conserves potassium. Increased GFR could increase potassium secretion by increasing tubular flow, but there is no reason to suspect an increased GFR. In a patient with congestive heart failure, in fact, the GFR would likely be normal or low due to decreased renal blood flow, but likely not high. Decreased proximal reabsorption would also lead to potassium wasting, but neither congestive heart failure per se nor furosemide action in the loop of Henle cause decreased proximal tubular reabsorption. Finally, furosemide does inhibit the $Na^+/K^+/2Cl^-$ symporter in the loop of Henle and may impede potassium reabsorption here, but this is not the direct mechanism of potassium loss with loop diuretics. If potassium loss in the loop of Henle were the only mechanism of excess potassium excretion, the distal segments of the tubule could make up for it with increased reabsorption. Because increased distal flow accelerates distal potassium secretion, no such compensation can occur.

2. **The answer is** E. The patient has Addison's disease, probably due to a tubercular infection of the adrenal glands. Addison's disease is primary adrenal failure, in this case, due to infectious destruction of the glands. Addison's disease results in a failure to secrete glucocorticoids and the mineralocorticoid, aldosterone. (Failure of the adrenal medulla may also occur, but this does not produce significant symptoms, as the sympathetic nervous system compensates.) Lack of glucocorticoids results in hypoglycemia and low blood pressure, and lack of aldosterone results in decreased distal Na^+ and water reabsorption (leading to low blood pressure) and decreased K^+ secretion (leading to hyperkalemia). Although less Na^+ is reabsorbed distally in the absence of aldosterone, this would not decrease the plasma $[Na^+]$. Remember that the amount of distal free water reabsorption determines the $[Na^+]$ and that free water reabsorption is determined by ADH, not aldosterone. Adrenocorticotropic hormone (ACTH) is not low but high in Addison's disease. With no negative feedback from adrenal hormone secretion, the pituitary secretes more ACTH, not less. If the problem were a lack of central endocrine stimulation to the adrenal from the pituitary (hypopituitarism), we might still expect aldosterone secretion to occur as part of the RAA system and in response to high plasma $[K^+]$, because neither plasma $[K^+]$ nor blood pressure is regulated through the pituitary. Hyperpigmentation can occur in Addison's disease because of the increased levels of ACTH and melanocyte-stimulating hormone MSH. Low renin would explain the hypoaldosteronism and low blood pressure but not the other clinical signs. In fact, in Addison's disease, renin is likely to be high to counteract the low blood pressure. Low hematocrit can be associated with transient hyperkalemia if the hyperkalemia is due to hemolysis. There is nothing to suggest hemolysis in this case, nor would hemolysis explain the other findings.

3. **The answer is** B. The woman has suffered a transmembrane shift of potassium cations from ECF to ICF from her use of a β2-agonist with sympathomimetic effects (i.e., effects mimicking the sympathetic catecholamine neurotransmitters, epinephrine and norepinephrine) that shift potassium intracellularly. Exercise does not decrease plasma $[K^+]$ but transiently *increases* it by opening ATP-dependent potassium channels and enabling more potassium flow out of cells. An osmotic diuresis, if it occurred, could cause distal potassium wasting by increasing distal flow, but osmotic or any other diuresis is not relevant to this scenario. Hyperaldosteronism would increase potassium secretion and decrease the plasma $[K^+]$, but again, it is not relevant to this case. Inhibition of the $Na^+/K^+/2Cl^-$ symporter would, like osmotic diuresis, increase potassium secretion by increasing distal flow. This is the mechanism of action of loop diuretics such as furosemide, but it has nothing to do with this case.

25

Acid-Base Homeostasis

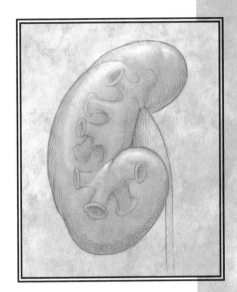

INTRODUCTION

Bodily processes are sensitive to pH. Deviations from the normal range of blood pH of 7.35 to 7.45 may have serious consequences. A drop in pH below 7.2 causes significant clinical manifestations including impaired growth, decreased cardiac output, decreased blood pressure, insulin resistance, and hyperkalemia. High pH (>7.6) is equally destructive, producing disturbances in heart rhythm and tetany from low free calcium. This pH sensitivity reflects the chemical reactivity of free protons. Inappropriate protonation and deprotonation of proteins caused by abnormal pH can dramatically alter protein structure and render the proteins less functional. Because biochemical processes cannot tolerate marked changes in pH, the body has an elaborate system to ensure pH regulation.

Most of our view of acid base balance pertains to the blood and thus extracellular fluid (ECF), but also important is the regulation of pH by various cells of the body and the brain. The brain utilizes sensitive transport and metabolic mechanisms to closely maintain its pH. Intracellular pH is usually more acid than the ECF because the cells are electronegative with respect to the ECF. Most cells have H^+ secretory mechanisms such as H^+-ATPases and Na^+/H^+ exchangers NHE that provide the housekeeping function of pH regulation for the metabolically active cell.

SYSTEM STRUCTURE: COMPONENTS OF THE pH REGULATORY APPARATUS AND THE DISTRIBUTION OF BODY ACID

The components of the acid-base homeostatic system include the body fluid buffers, chemosensors in the circulation and brain, the brain, the kidneys, and the lungs. Carbonic acid (H_2CO_3) and its two sets of breakdown products constitute the most important buffer in the blood. These breakdown products exist in relationship to one another in the blood, as described by the following equation:

$$CO_2 + H_2O \leftrightarrow H_2CO_3 \leftrightarrow H^+ + HCO_3^-$$

The HCO_3^- buffer opposes dramatic changes in the concentration of H^+ (denoted $[H^+]$) by titrating acid loads added to the blood. The HCO_3^- cannot work alone to keep pH stable, however. Although the HCO_3^- lessens the change in $[H^+]$ caused by acid loads, it does not eliminate the change. Therefore, the lung and the kidney modulate the elements of the buffer equilibrium to oppose the changes in $[H^+]$. The lungs eliminate CO_2, lowering PCO_2 to shift the reaction to the left, thus reducing the $[H^+]$. The kid-

neys excrete protons and make new bicarbonate to reduce the $[H^+]$. When the arterial PCO_2 rises above about 40 mm Hg, the respiratory centers drive more ventilation to drop the arterial PCO_2. The kidneys respond directly to increases in $[H^+]$ (decreases in pH), and when the blood pH dips under 7.4, the kidneys eliminate acid in the urine and manufacture new bicarbonate.

Neural Structures in the Regulation of Acid-Base Balance

The central nervous system (CNS) is responsible for the total body content of CO_2, achieved as a result of the modulation of both voluntary and involuntary respiration. Voluntary respiration and the hyperventilation seen in anxiety and certain primary CNS lesions are determined by higher cortical centers. Involuntary respiration is controlled by areas in the brain stem and depends on input from both central and peripheral sensory receptors that respond to the concentrations of hydrogen ion, PCO_2, and PO_2 of the blood and CSF.

The central component in involuntary ventilatory control is the respiratory control center in the medulla oblongata, composed of several nuclei that both create and modify the respiratory pattern. The best understood of these centers is the family of medullary centers, consisting of the dorsal and ventral respiratory groups of neurons. This area is responsible for establishing the basic respiratory pattern and integrates input from multiple sources, including higher brain centers, central and peripheral chemoreceptors, and baroreceptors.

Input from these peripheral and central sensors allows this center to modify respiration based on the acid-base status of the blood. Central chemoreceptors are distinct from the respiratory control center but are located adjacent to it at the ventrolateral surface of the medulla. Two areas of chemosensation have been identified in this region, one caudal and one rostral, which sense changes in the pH and PCO_2 of the brain stem ISF. Gap junctions in the pia may permit mixing of the brain ISF and cerebrospinal fluid (CSF), allowing the chemosensitive areas to sense changes in the pH, PCO_2, and bicarbonate concentrations of the CSF.

The central chemoreceptors have been shown to be exquisitely sensitive to changes in hydrogen ion concentration; PCO_2 is also a potent stimulus for these cells, although the response to PCO_2 diminishes with age. The central chemoreceptors are relatively insensitive to changes in PO_2 except in cases of severe hypoxia.

Peripheral sensory input is contributed by pulmonary stretch receptors and carotid sinus and aortic arch chemo- and baroreceptors. The most important of these for maintenance of systemic acid-base balance is the carotid chemoreceptor, although the aortic appears to play a minor role.

The carotid bodies, surrounded by a capillary plexus affording close proximity to systemic blood, respond to hypercapnia and hydrogen ion concentrations. Their response to both PCO_2 and to hydrogen ion concentration is virtually linear in the range of PCO_2 from 25 to 65 mm Hg and a hydrogen ion concentration of 25 to 60 mEq/L. The carotid chemosensor is less sensitive to hypoxia with a PO_2 of less than 60 mm Hg required for stimulation. Recall that at these PO_2 levels, hemoglobin desaturation becomes significant. The carotid chemoreceptors' sensitivity to combined hypoxia and hypercapnia exceeds the additive effect of the response to each stimulus individually: hypoxia renders the chemoreceptors more sensitive to hypercapnia, and vice versa. It has been suggested that the effect of hydrogen ion concentration is independent of hypercapnia or hypoxemia, increasing the chemoreceptors' sensitivity to hypercapnia at any PCO_2 concentration.

An important concept in understanding the regulation of ventilation is that CO_2 permeates into the CNS across the blood brain barrier more quickly than HCO_3^-. Therefore, sudden increases in PCO_2 peripherally will cause CO_2 to enter and acidify the brain interstitial fluid and promote hyperventilation. A sudden decrease in PCO_2 will allow CO_2 to leave the CNS, giving a transient alkalinization of the brain interstitial fluid, depressing ventilation.

Acids in the Body

There are two common physiologic sources of acid inputs to the blood, known as volatile (gaseous) and nonvolatile acid loads. **Volatile acid** is the CO_2 produced by the metabolism of dietary carbohydrates and fats as a part of the citric acid cycle in aerobic respiration. This CO_2 production is occurring in almost all body tissues nearly all the time. (Erythrocytes are an exception; they are anaerobic, and in oxygen debt, such as during extreme exertion, the muscles may also rely on anaerobic respiration.) The CO_2 acidifies the blood because it is hydrated to carbonic acid, which in turn, partly dissociates into bicarbonate and a proton, in accordance with the bicarbonate buffer equilibrium equation. The more CO_2, there is, the higher the $[H^+]$ will be. **Nonvolatile acid** comes from the metabolism of amino acids, which yields HCl and H_2SO_4, strong acids that deposit protons into solution in the blood, thus raising $[H^+]$, and in turn, lowering HCO_3^- by pushing the reaction to CO_2.

SYSTEM FUNCTION: THE VARIATION AND CONTROL OF pH

Before beginning to learn more about the acid loads that vary the plasma pH and about the mechanisms that counter those variations to serve homeostasis, it is first necessary to have a good understanding of the physiologic buffers. The simplest way to understand physiologic buffers is to review the basic chemistry.

A Review of Chemical Equilibria and Buffers

When we first learn about chemical reactions, we hear about reactants and products, and we learn that some reactions can proceed in reverse as well as forward. If the energetics of the reactants heavily favor product formation, this does not necessarily mean that all the reactants disappear and reappear as products. Rather, it means that the forward reaction between molecules of reactants occurs much more easily and frequently than the reverse reaction between molecules of products (FIGURE 25.1). The reverse reaction may still occur on a smaller scale and does so at the same time that the forward reaction proceeds. In this equation, the two-way arrow denotes reversibility.

$$A + B \leftrightarrow C + D$$

Also recall that in first-order kinetics, the rate of the forward reaction is proportional to the concentration of the reactants in solution; conversely, the rate of the reverse reaction is proportional to the concentration of the products. The more reactant molecules there are, the more reaction occurs between them per unit time. In a forward reaction that is energetically favorable, the reactants convert to products until the reactant concentrations have dropped considerably. In turn, the product concentrations have risen. The rate of the forward fast reaction decreases along with the dropping reactant concentration, and the rate of the reverse slow reaction climbs along with rising product concentration. When the forward and reverse rates meet and become equal, the concentrations of reactants and products can no longer change, and chemical **equilibrium** is reached. Most metabolic reactions and drug metabolic processes occur with first-order kinetics, but recall that in some cases, the rate of product formation is independent of reactant concentration, and therefore linear (zero order, as in the case of alcohol metabolism when excess alcohol has saturated the enzyme alcohol dehydrogenase), and in other cases, the reaction rate is related to the square of the reactant concentration (second-order kinetics).

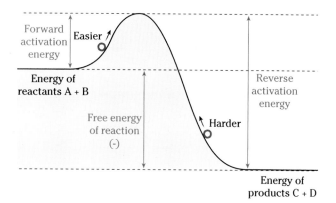

Figure 25.1 Forward and reverse activation energies. A ball rolling up the curve toward the right is the forward reaction, and the reverse reaction is a ball rolling up the curve toward the left. The forward reaction requires less kinetic energy to make it over the hump from reactants to products than the reverse reaction requires to clear the hill from products to reactants. Because of the greater energy requirement for the reverse reaction, if reactant and product concentrations are equal, fewer reverse balls will clear the hill and go to reactants. The reverse rate will therefore be slower than the forward rate. The passage of balls (reactions) over the hill will be net in a forward direction. Once the number of product molecules becomes large enough, however, the rate of passage over the hill from right to left will grow. The energy requirement has not changed; the number of molecules (balls) attempting the hill from right to left has increased. Even if the same low percentage of balls clears the hill, the total number of balls clearing the hill has risen. When the rate of passage of balls (reactions) is equal in both directions, equilibrium has been reached. The longer the ascent is from right to left, the more products there will have to be before the rate of passage from right to left increases. This means K as a ratio of products over reactants will be larger. Therefore, a larger K means a more favorable forward reaction.

If the energetics favor the forward reaction, the equilibrium is pushed "to the right," toward the products. The rate of reaction is determined by the reactant concentration (determines the frequency of molecular collisions), the temperature and environmental factors such as catalysts, enzymes and pH. When the forward reaction is very energetically favorable and thus very fast (implying that the reverse reaction is unfavorable and very slow), the reactant concentration must drop very low, and the product concentration must build up quite high before forward and reverse reactions have an equal rate. Thus, the more favorable the forward reaction is, the larger the ratio of products to reactants at equilibrium will be. This equilibrium ratio of products to reactants is described by the **equilibrium constant** expression:

$$K = [C][D]/[A][B]$$

K is the equilibrium constant, which reflects the ratio of forward to reverse rate constants of the reaction. The more favorable the forward reaction is, the higher K will be. The opposite holds for a reaction in which the energetics are more favorable to the re-

verse reaction. Then the equilibrium is pushed "to the left," toward the reactants, and the K ratio of products to reactants at equilibrium must be lower. An irreversible reaction is one in which the reactants completely disappear as products appear; consequently, the K is infinite.

Adding to or subtracting from the concentrations of the reactants or products in equilibrium will cause a shift in the concentrations of reactants and products until they again reach equilibrium, where the ratio of products to reactants is again, K. In Figure 25.1, if more A is added, for example, the forward reaction rate climbs, and more product is made. The forward rate then falls, and the reverse rate climbs, until equilibrium ratio K is again achieved. If D is subtracted (e.g., by reaction with another chemical species), the reverse reaction rate falls, and net product is made until the forward and reverse rates are again equal. At constant temperature, the equilibrium constant K does not change but instead dictates the proportion of changes in reactant and product concentration after additions and subtractions of those chemicals.

Equilibrium equations are also written for **dissociation reactions**, such as when an acid HA (considered the reactant) dissociates into products H^+ and an anionic **conjugate base** A^-:

$$HA \leftrightarrow H^+ + A^- \qquad K = [H^+][A^-] / [HA]$$

Acids are defined as **strong acids** or **weak acids**, depending on their tendency to dissociate into H^+ and A-; stronger acids are more inclined toward dissociation and therefore have larger Ks, and weaker acids are less inclined toward dissociation and have smaller Ks.

Buffer solutions are solutions in which a weak acid (reactant) and conjugate base (product) are present together in similar concentrations at equilibrium. This kind of buffer equilibrium can neutralize additions of either acid or base. When a strong base is added, swallowing up protons, more net weak acid dissociates, producing more H^+ and A^- until the equilibrium ratio of products to reactants is recovered, and the weak acid therefore acts as a reservoir for protons to restore the $[H^+]$. When a strong acid is added, raising $[H^+]$, the conjugate base associates with added free H^+, producing more HA until recovery of the equilibrium ratio, and the conjugate base thus acts as a sponge for protons. In an unbuffered solution, adding acid will increase the free proton concentration dramatically, causing a steep drop in the pH. Adding base to an unbuffered solution will decrease the free proton concentration dramatically, causing a steep rise in pH.

It is important to understand that buffers lessen changes in pH but do not eradicate them. For example, an addition of H^+ to the buffer equilibrium results in a redistribution of the protons. Some of the added H^+ is free, and some is moved into association with A^- as HA on the other side of the reaction equation. To reiterate, the products-to-reactants ratio is shifting back toward K, the equilibrium ratio.

The Bicarbonate Buffer in the Blood

The most important extracellular buffer in body fluids is the bicarbonate/CO_2 system.

$$CO_2 + H_2O \leftrightarrow H_2CO_3 \leftrightarrow HCO_3^- + H^+$$

The buffer is composed of a weak acid, carbonic acid (H_2CO_3), and a conjugate base, bicarbonate (HCO_3^-). In addition, H_2CO_3 exists in a chemical equilibrium with the CO_2. This latter reaction is greatly accelerated in many tissues by an enzyme called *carbonic anhydrase (CA)*. HCO_3^- also exists in equilibrium with carbonate, CO_3^{2-}, a reaction favored at an alkaline pH, as is found in bone. These dual reactions to form CO_2 or CO_3^{2-}, make HCO_3 an ampholyte (a substance than can act as either an acid, in the presence of a strong base, or a base, when in the presence of a strong acid).

Because of the rapid interconversion of CO_2 and HCO_3^-, we sometimes ignore the presence of H_2CO_3 in the reaction sequence shown previously, and instead write:

$$CO_2 + H_2O \leftrightarrow HCO_3^- + H^+$$

The equilibrium equation is the following, with α equal to 0.03 mmol/L per mm Hg, the constant that accounts for dissolved CO_2 and H_2CO_3 in solution:

$$K = 1 \times 10^{-6.1} = [HCO_3^-][H^+]/\alpha PCO_2$$

The bicarbonate buffer behaves in accordance with the description of buffers just shown. Adding or subtracting products or reactants drives the reaction either forward or backward, until the equilibrium ratio of products to reactants is restored. When protons are added, most of them will react with bicarbonate to form CO_2, as dictated by the buffer's equilibrium constant. In this way, changes in pH are minimized. Some added protons do remain, however, and the pH does drop slightly, as discussed. On the other hand, losses of H^+ will cause CO_2 to combine with water, and then break down into HCO_3^- and H^+, thus restoring some of the lost H^+ and preventing a severe change in pH. Increases in bicarbonate consume some protons and raise the pH to a limited extent. Loss of bicarbonate will cause a shift to the right in the reaction. More CO_2 will dissociate into H^+ and HCO_3^-, and the increase in H^+ means a drop in pH. Because it is a buffer system, the equilibrium constant dictates that much of the acid (CO_2) stays as

CO_2, and therefore the pH drop is limited. Increases in CO_2 will also shift the reaction to the right, elevating the free $[H^+]$, but again, the equilibrium constant dictates that much of the added CO_2 stay as CO_2. Decreases in CO_2 cause protons and bicarbonate to react to replace the lost CO_2, raising the pH to a limited extent. All of these changes are important for understanding how acid loads affect the blood and how the lungs and kidneys modulate pH.

In considering the bicarbonate buffer relationships, physiologists use a more convenient form of the equilibrium equation, called the **Henderson-Hasselbalch equation.** It relates pH directly to the PCO_2 and $[HCO_3^-]$, mathematically summarizing the notion that increases in CO_2 drop the pH (and vice versa) and decreases in $[HCO_3^-]$ drop the pH (and vice versa):

$$pH = 6.1 + \log \{[HCO_3^-]/[0.03] \text{ X } [PCO_2] \}$$

By measuring arterial PCO_2 and serum bicarbonate level and inserting them into this simple equation, we can rapidly calculate the pH of the blood. Under normal physiologic conditions, with $[HCO_3^-] = 24$ mmol/L and arterial $PCO_2 = 40$ mm Hg, the ratio of $HCO_3^-/0.03(PCO_2)$ is 20/1:

$$pH = 6.1 + \log [24/(0.03) \text{ X } (40)] = 7.4$$

The normal physiologic pH of the blood is thus in the range of 7.40.

Because the best buffers are those that have a pK close to the pH of body fluids (ratio of base-to-acid close to 1), one might expect the HCO_3^-/CO_2 buffer pair *not* to be a good buffer with its pK of 6.1, far from the normal pH of 7.4. The reason that HCO_3 is considered a good buffer at physiological pH is because the system works in an "open" fashion in which CO_2 is allowed to escape from the system via ventilation (as opposed to a "closed" container). The lungs prevent buildup of acid and CO_2 when an excess of H^+ is added to the body. (See Integrated Physiology Box *Derivation of the Henderson-Hasselbach Equation.*)

Other Buffers in the Body

In addition to the bicarbonate buffer system, there are other buffers in the ECF and the intracellular fluid (ICF). The same body fluid H^+ concentration is simultaneously in equilibrium with multiple buffer pairs, the importance of each depending on their pK and the amount of buffer present. This isohydric principle allows for the acid base status to be examined by close evaluation of a single buffer pair, such as HCO_3^-/PCO_2. Protein and phosphates both act as weak acid buffers inside and outside of cells. Buffering inside cells by protein and phosphate takes place when an increase in the extracellular $[H^+]$ leads to the diffusion of

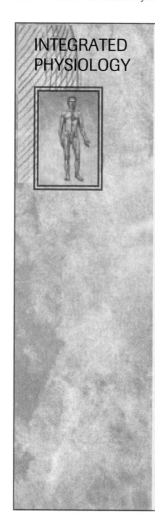

INTEGRATED PHYSIOLOGY

Derivation of the Henderson-Hasselbalch Equation

Recall that log (x) = y when 10^y = x; so, roughly speaking, log (x) is x's exponent, or order of magnitude.

$$\log (ab) = \log a + \log b$$

$$\log (a/b) = \log a - \log b$$

Add exponents when multiplying and subtract when dividing. And, by definition:

$$-\log[H+] = pH$$

$$-\log[K] = pK$$

$$K = [H+][A-]/[HA]$$

$$[H+] = K\,[HA]/[A-]$$

$$\log [H+] = \log K + \log ([HA]/[A-])$$

$$-\log[H+] = -\log K - (\log[HA]/[A-])$$

$$-\log[H+] = -\log K - (\log[HA] - \log[A-])$$

$$-\log[H+] = -\log K - \log[HA] + \log[A-]$$

$$-\log[H+] = -\log K + (\log[A-] - \log[HA])$$

$$-\log[H+] = -\log K + \log ([A-]/[HA])$$

$$pH = pK + \log ([A-]/[HA])$$

For the bicarbonate buffer specifically, where pK = $-\log K = -\log 10^{-6.1}$ = 6.1:

$$pH = 6.1 + \log ([HCO_3^-]/\alpha PCO_2)$$

protons into cells. (In red blood cells, hemoglobin is a protein that buffers $[H^+]$ changes intracellularly.) Bone mineral appears to be an important site of acid buffering through H^+ absorption. In fact, patients who are unable to excrete the daily, nonvolatile acid load (e.g., in certain renal diseases) may maintain a constant serum HCO_3^- level despite the daily acid retention: the source of HCO_3^- that replaces lost blood HCO_3^- is bone carbonate salts. Therefore, these patients may suffer bone demineralization.

Intracellular buffering may account for half or more than half of the buffering of acid loads (see Figure 24.2). When increased plasma $[H^+]$ shifts from the ECF to the ICF, important changes occur in the levels of other cations in the blood. When the protons diffuse into the cell, there is an increase in the positive charge inside the cell, slightly depolarizing the membrane, reducing the resting negative transmembrane electrical potential, and thus reducing the electrical gradient that opposes K^+ efflux from the cell. The net result is that H^+ enters the cell and K^+ leaves, raising the plasma $[K^+]$. This is why *acidemia* (low

serum pH) is often associated with *hyperkalemia* (high serum $[K^+]$), as discussed in Chapter 24.

Acid Loads

Metabolically generated acid can be divided into two main groups: gaseous or volatile acid (CO_2) and nongaseous or nonvolatile acids, as mentioned earlier. Acid loads are buffered, but they still acidify the blood to some extent. The increase in $[H^+]$ signals the kidney to excrete protons and make bicarbonate; to some extent, the acidity drives the respiratory centers to increase ventilation, dropping CO_2, which in turn, drops $[H^+]$. The increase in $[H^+]$ also drives up the PCO_2, which stimulates more ventilation at the lung (see Chapter 19).

Volatile Acids Oxidative metabolism of carbohydrates and fats produces large amounts of CO_2, on the order of 15,000 to 20,000 mmol/day. The production of CO_2 raises PCO_2, raises $[H^+]$, and lowers blood pH, in accordance with the equilibrium equation described previously. The kidneys respond to the acidity, and the lungs respond to the increased CO_2 (and to the acidity) to counter the drop in pH. CO_2 accounts for the vast majority of acid produced by the body. Because the end product of metabolic reactions of carbohydrates and fats is CO_2 and water, it follows that the production of 20 mol of CO_2 would also produce 20 mol of water. The molecular weight of water is 18 g/mol, and there are 1,000 grams of water in a liter (density is 1,000 g/L), so the molarity of water is 55 mol/L. Therefore, the production of 20 mol of water (with the 20 mol of CO_2) adds about 364 mL of water daily to the body fluids. Still, this is less than the water lost in sweat and via the respiratory tree, so that there is a net loss of water per day amounting to about 500 mL.

Nonvolatile Acids The metabolism of amino acids, nucleic acids, and other compounds releases acidic and alkaline byproducts that are not gaseous (nonvolatile), sometimes called **fixed acids** and **bases**. The breakdown of sulfur-containing amino acids such as cysteine and methionine yields acid sulfates, whereas lysine, arginine, and histidine are often hydrochlorides. The digestion of organic phosphorus-containing compounds gives rise to acid phosphates. Alkaline byproducts come from the metabolism of anionic amino acids such as aspartate and glutamate with accompanying strong cations such as Na^+, K^+, and Ca^{2+}. The normal, high-protein American diet yields a greater quantity of acid than base. On average, a net of 1 mEq/kg per day of nonvolatile organic and inorganic acids is produced.

The addition of H^+ to the blood raises $[H^+]$, lowers pH, and raises PCO_2 in accordance with the equilibrium equation. The kidneys respond to the acidity, and the lungs respond to the increased CO_2 (and to the acidity) to counter the drop in pH.

The Reabsorption of Filtered HCO_3^-

Before we consider the kidney's response to acid loads, we should consider the consequences of the fact that bicarbonate is freely filtered across the glomerulus. The daily filtered HCO_3^- (about 4,320 mEq of HCO_3^-, the product of a glomerular filtration rate of 180 L/day and an $[HCO_3^-]$ of 24 mEq/L) is presented to the tubules. Clearly, the first critical step confronting the tubule is to reabsorb this enormous filtered quantity, because loss of even a small fraction of that amount would result in severe acidosis. Therefore, the kidney not only responds to acid loads by creating new bicarbonate and excreting acid, but must also first reabsorb all of the bicarbonate in the tubular filtrate in order to maintain the blood pH at normal levels.

How does the reabsorption of bicarbonate take place? Renal tubule cells do not have any apical transporters to reabsorb bicarbonate directly. Instead, the cells along the nephron use a more complex series of reactions to reabsorb the bicarbonate (FIGURE 25.2). Although the actual reabsorption reactions are more involved than direct transport of bicarbonate, the end result is that bicarbonate is translocated from the tubule lumen into the bloodstream at the expense of adenosine triphosphate (ATP).

The Transport of Bicarbonate in the Proximal Tubule
The majority of bicarbonate reabsorption occurs in the proximal tubule. Note in Figure 25.2 that the familiar reactions interconverting CO_2 and HCO_3^- recur. After passing through the glomerulus into the

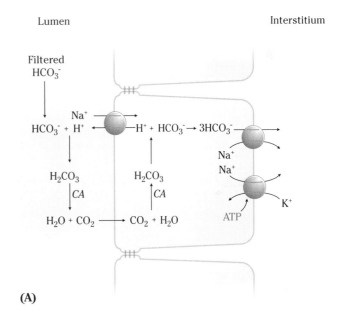

(A)

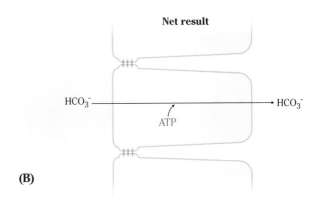

(B)

Figure 25.2 The reabsorption of bicarbonate in the early proximal tubule. CA = carbonic anhydrase, the enzyme that facilitates interconversion between H_2CO_3 and CO_2 and H_2O.

tubular fluid, the HCO_3^- molecule combines with H^+, which is continuously secreted by the proximal tubular cell. The H^+ secretion is driven by the basolateral Na^+/K^+-ATPase, which provides a gradient for apical Na+ reabsorption across a Na^+/H^+ antiporter. An apical H^+-ATPase may have a lesser role here, as well. The continual secretion of H^+ raises the tubular $[H^+]$ and helps drive the reaction of H^+ and HCO_3^-, which produces water and CO_2. The presence of carbonic anhydrase in the luminal membranes greatly accelerates this reaction, keeping the luminal $[H^+]$ depressed and avoiding an unfavorable gradient for H^+ secretion into the lumen. Once formed, CO_2 rapidly diffuses into the cell, with a membrane that is highly permeable to the dissolved gas.

Inside the cell, the reverse reaction takes place, again catalyzed by carbonic anhydrase: CO_2 and H_2O combine to form HCO_3^- and H^+. The bicarbonate exits the basolateral membrane into the peritubular blood across an $Na^+/3HCO_3^-$ symporter, driven in part by the intracellular electronegativity created by the basolateral Na^+/K^+-ATPase and K^+ permeability. (The stoichiometry of the pump—$2 K^+$ enter the cell for every $3 Na^+$ that leave—renders the inside of the cell electronegative and the K^+ permeability allows accumulated intracellular K^+ to diffuse out of the cell down its concentration gradient, causing a separation of charge across the membrane and negative potential inside the cell.)

The proportion of bicarbonate reabsorbed in each segment of the nephron is shown in FIGURE 25.3.

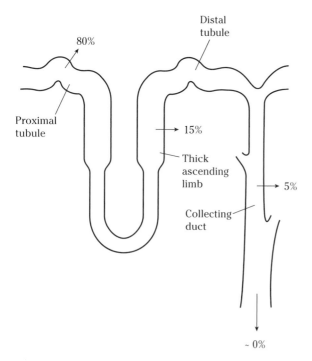

Figure 25.3 The reabsorption of bicarbonate along the nephron. The majority of HCO_3^- reabsorption occurs in the proximal tubule.

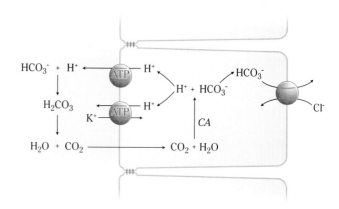

Figure 25.4 The reabsorption of bicarbonate in the intercalated cell of the collecting duct. Bicarbonate reabsorption in this part of the tubule does not occur via Na^+ reabsorption but by active H^+ secretion and HCO_3^-/Cl^- antiport driven by Cl^- diffusion down its concentration gradient.

The proximal tubule accomplishes 80% to 90% of HCO_3^- reabsorption. The next 5% to 15% is reabsorbed in the thick ascending limb of the loop of Henle by the same mechanism as in the proximal tubule. The collecting duct reclaims the remaining 5%. Nearly all filtered bicarbonate is reabsorbed under normal conditions when the urine pH is < 6.0. The range of urine pH is between 5.0 and 8.0, so that in circumstances when the more alkaline pH is reached, bicarbonate is present in the urine.

The Transport of Bicarbonate in the Collecting Duct

Reabsorption in the collecting duct takes place through the intercalated cells in a manner slightly different from HCO_3^- reabsorption in earlier tubule segments (FIGURE 25.4). First, there is no luminal carbonic anhydrase in the collecting duct, so the dehydration reaction of H_2CO_3 to CO_2 and water proceeds more slowly. This is in keeping with the decreased amount of HCO_3^- reabsorbed in these segments. Second, the transporters that secrete protons differ. The Na^+/H^+ exchanger of the proximal tubule is replaced by two types of active transporters. One type, the H^+-ATPase, pumps out protons using energy from ATP hydrolysis. The other type, the H^+/K^+-ATPase, uses energy from ATP to secrete a proton for a potassium ion reabsorbed. Finally, the bicarbonate exits the cell into the blood using a different transporter: an HCO_3^-/Cl^- exchanger in the basolateral membrane. The basolateral reabsorption may result from the movement of Cl^- into the cell down a concentration gradient, extruding HCO_3^- via antiport. In the collecting duct, where Na^+ concentration is less than that of the proximal tubule and pH is lower in the lumen compared to the proximal tubule, the driving forces available for an Na^+/H^+ exchange mechanism may not be adequate to accomplish acid secretion.

Under such circumstances, the ATP-dependent proton-secreting mechanisms have added importance. The predominant intercalated cell (alpha) has an apical H^+-ATPase and basolateral Cl^-/HCO_3^- exchanger, which functions in the setting of acid loads in need of excretion. An intercalated cell of reverse polarity (beta) in the cortical collecting duct, with basolateral H^+ pumps and apical Cl^-/HCO_3^- exchangers, is primed to secrete bicarbonate in the setting of an alkaline load. The number of each cell type may be dictated by the acid-base needs of the individual.

Although the individual transporters differ in the earlier and later segments of the nephron, the principles for HCO_3^- reabsorption are similar. In all locations, a secreted proton combines with a luminal HCO_3^-, converting it into CO_2, which diffuses into the cell; the bicarbonate is then reconstituted and passes across the basolateral membrane into the interstitium and on into the peritubular blood.

The Regulation of Acidity

In the absence of an acid load in the plasma, an amount of H^+ is secreted across the apical membranes. This H^+ escorts filtered HCO_3^- into the cell, is secreted again, escorts more HCO_3^- into the cell, is secreted again, and so on; acidity is cycled back and forth across the apical membrane in the transcellular reabsorption of HCO_3^- back to the bloodstream. The kidney thus saves all the bicarbonate that had entered the tubule by filtration.

When the average daily acid load of 70 mEq H^+ acidifies the blood, chemical events change in the bicarbonate-reabsorbing cells of the proximal tubule and collecting duct. Instead of reabsorbing filtered HCO_3^- with no net secretion or reabsorption of H^+, the tubule cells secrete net H^+ and generate new HCO_3^- in addition to the HCO_3^- reabsorbed from the tubule lumen. The clearance of H^+ from the blood and the addition of HCO_3^- to the blood reverse the impact of the acid load on the blood buffer and on the blood pH. In order to understand these events more clearly, we will proceed sequentially from introduction of the acid load to correction of the blood pH.

Acidification of the Blood and the Tubular Cells

When protons are added to the blood, some of them remain free, which drops the pH, and others react with bicarbonate, which drops the $[HCO_3^-]$ and increases the PCO_2. These changes in the ECF pH then cause changes in the renal tubular intracellular pH. Increased PCO_2 leads to diffusion of CO_2 from the peritubular capillaries across the gas-permeable cell membranes of the tubule cells and increases PCO_2 in the cells. Decreased peritubular and interstitial $[HCO_3^-]$ alters the basolateral transmembrane

$[HCO_3^-]$ gradient in favor of reabsorption of HCO_3^- into the interstitium. Increased reabsorption of HCO_3^- drops the intracellular $[HCO_3^-]$. Increased PCO_2 and decreased $[HCO_3^-]$ in the tubule cells pushes the buffer reaction rightward, leading to an increase in $[H^+]$ and therefore a drop in intracellular pH. Under normal dietary conditions, changes in ECF pH are minimal.

Pathologic conditions may also add nondietary acid loads to the blood, may directly increase the PCO_2, or may directly decrease the $[HCO_3^-]$, all of which drop the plasma pH and the tubular ICF pH by the mechanisms just described. Unless the secretory and reabsorptive functions of the cell are impaired, the renal tubular cells will respond to pathologic increases in acidity in the same way that they respond to physiologic acid loads. Only when an acid load exceeds the capacity of the kidney to excrete that load does systemic pH noticeably change.

Renal Acid Secretion

In both the proximal tubule and the collecting duct, increased intracellular acidity stimulates an increase in H^+ secretion through active and passive mechanisms. In the proximal tubule cell, the increased intracellular $[H^+]$ drives more H^+ down its concentration gradient across the apical Na^+/H^+ exchanger and into the tubule lumen. The performance of the exchanger is also enhanced by low pH, as is that of the proximal tubular H^+-ATPase. In the collecting duct, more H^+-ATPase is inserted into the apical membrane by a process of exocytosis, thereby increasing H^+ secretion.

With increased H^+ secretion, H^+ is now secreted in excess of the amounts required for complete bicarbonate reabsorption. Remember that the binding of secreted H^+ and filtered HCO_3^- to form CO_2 was ultimately necessary for HCO_3^- reabsorption, and this still occurs. In fact, increased H^+ secretion accelerates HCO_3^- reabsorption as luminal CO_2 is produced at a higher rate. The H^+ secreted in excess of luminal HCO_3^-, however, has no HCO_3^- to bind with and remains in the urine where it will be excreted after combining with the urinary buffers, particularly ammonia (NH_3) and phosphate.

Why does much more of this excess H^+ secretion take place in the distal tubule segments than in the proximal tubule? Consider how acidification of the tubular cell occurs in the presence of an acid load. Excess CO_2 in the blood diffuses into the tubular cell, and the HCO_3^- deficit in the blood leads to increased basolateral HCO_3^- reabsorption. Because of the high basal level of HCO_3^- reabsorption in the proximal tubule, however, the PCO_2 of the proximal tubular cells is higher than other parts of the tubule. Less CO_2 can diffuse out of the blood and into the tubular cell here. Because basolateral HCO_3^- reabsorption is already high from reabsorption of filtered HCO_3^-, the level of basolateral HCO_3^- reabsorption can perhaps only be increased so much before approaching maximum capacity. The proximal tubular cell is therefore less easily acidified by acid loads than is the distal tubular cell, which is not engaged in as much basal HCO_3^- reabsorption.

Moreover, to the extent that the proximal tubular cell is acidified, this increase in H^+ secretion does not result in H^+ excretion to the same extent it does in the distal tubule segments. The high luminal $[HCO_3^-]$ in the proximal tubule means that increased H^+ secretion mainly serves to accelerate the formation of luminal CO_2 and thus accelerate the reabsorption of filtered HCO_3^-. In addition, the proximal tubule faces several other limiting factors in its ability to acidify tubular fluid: the proximal epithelium contains a leaky tight junction that does not withstand much of a pH gradient, and Na^+/H^+ exchangers cannot generate much of a gradient in the first place. For example, if the Na^+ gradient from lumen to cell was tenfold favoring Na^+ entry, the maximal gradient of H^+ secretion would be ten times the H^+ concentration in the lumen compared to the cell. This would mean that if the cell pH were approximately 7.2, the limiting luminal pH would be 6.2. In reality, proximal tubule luminal pH does not even approach that value.

The Generation of New Bicarbonate

When an acid load in the plasma acidifies the tubular cells—by increased PCO_2 and decreased intracellular $[HCO_3^-]$—this pushes the buffer reaction rightward, yielding new intracellular H^+ *and new HCO_3^-*. As mentioned earlier, the increased $[H^+]$ leads to increased H^+ secretion, which exceeds the amount required for HCO_3^- reabsorption. The new HCO_3^- replaces that which was lost from the cell when the bicarbonate-poor plasma in the peritubular capillary absorbed more HCO_3^- across the basolateral membrane. With intracellular $[HCO_3^-]$ partially replenished, the bicarbonate-poor blood can continue to extract increased amounts of HCO_3^- from the tubular cells. H^+ secretion in excess of luminal HCO_3^- increases the generation of new HCO_3^- because secreting H^+ keeps the buffer relation at a rightward tilt, which generates more HCO_3^-. (If the renal tubular cell were acidified without increased H^+ excretion—for example, if all the H^+ came right back in with reabsorption of filtered bicarbonate—the buildup of $[H^+]$ would stop the buffer relation's movement to the right, toward products, and no more HCO_3^- could be produced.) For new bicarbonate to be generated, the secreted H^+ combines in the lumen with phosphate and NH_3 buffers rather than filtered bicarbonate.

To the extent that the proximal tubular cell is less acidified to begin with than the distal tubular cell, the proximal tubular cell makes less new HCO_3^- by this mechanism. To the extent that the proximal tubular cell is acidified but does not achieve much net H^+ excretion—increasing HCO_3^- reabsorption instead—this also limits the formation of new HCO_3^-. The distal tubule cells, which are more acidified and which achieve more net H^+ excretion, also produce more new HCO_3^-.

The Restoration of Normal Plasma Acidity: Effects of the Kidneys and Lungs

The peritubular capillaries are the site where the acid load's alterations in the blood buffer are relieved. Excess CO_2 diffuses out of the blood, more HCO_3^- than usual diffuses into the blood, and the kidney takes on the acidic burden that formerly belonged to the blood. The tubular cells finally dispense with this burden through increased H^+ secretion and generation of new HCO_3^-. The ability of renal tubular cells to secrete and excrete H^+ and to generate new HCO_3^- without increasing their own acidity, allows the peritubular blood to continue to deliver CO_2 and to reabsorb HCO_3^- from the kidney. The decrease in plasma PCO_2 and increase in plasma $[HCO_3^-]$ reverses the changes imposed by the acid load.

The lungs, meanwhile, contribute to handling of the acid load as well. They detect increased PCO_2 at the central chemoreceptors and increased acidity (decreased pH) at the peripheral chemoreceptors. In response, they increase lung ventilation to reduce the plasma PCO_2, shifting the buffer relation leftward and consuming H^+. Through pulmonary regulation of ventilation, renal modulation of acid excretion, and new bicarbonate formation, all acting in concert, the body counters changes in blood pH.

A simple stoichiometric way to think about renal handling of acid loads is to focus on what happens to CO_2 in the kidney. Just as CO_2 is cleared from the lungs, the renal response to acid pH is also a type of elimination of CO_2. In the reabsorption of filtered HCO_3^-, no net CO_2 is consumed. The intracellular CO_2 that is hydrated and breaks down to give H^+ and HCO_3^- was first created in the tubule lumen by H^+ secretion. The net effect is the translocation of HCO_3^- from the tubule lumen to the blood with no net increase or decrease in the PCO_2 of the tubular cell. When an acid load acidifies the tubular cell, however, CO_2 is hydrated and broken down to H^+ and HCO_3^- in excess of the CO_2 delivered from luminal HCO_3^- reabsorption. The new H^+ is excreted, and the HCO_3^- is transferred to the blood—a new HCO_3^- at the cost of a CO_2.

There are two possible sources of net consumed CO_2, depending on the source of acidity. Consider the case in which decreased lung ventilation (hypoventilation) has acidified the blood by increasing blood

PCO_2. The excess PCO_2 diffuses into the tubule cell and yields increased intracellular $[H^+]$ and $[HCO_3^-]$. The excess H^+ is excreted, and the HCO_3^- is reabsorbed. In this case, consumed CO_2 comes from the blood.

On the other hand, when HCO_3^- is lost from the plasma due to diarrhea, an acid pH can develop with a decreased PCO_2. In this example, it is the loss of HCO_3^- from the tubular cell that creates new H^+ and HCO_3^-. Now the CO_2 comes from the tubular cell's own reservoir of CO_2, produced by the citric acid cycle in the mitochondria. Continued secretion of excess H^+ (and hence H^+ excretion) consumes more CO_2 from the metabolic reservoir and gives more new HCO_3^-. When an acid load has acidified the tubular cell with increased PCO_2 *and* decreased HCO_3^-, some of the net consumed CO_2 comes from the plasma and some comes from the cell's own stores.

Urinary Titration of Excreted Acid

We established that when H^+ is secreted in excess of luminal HCO_3^-, it remains in the urine, where it will be excreted. This is because there is not enough HCO_3^- to react with the H^+ in the tubule lumen. Although the protons lost in the urine do not react with bicarbonate, they cannot remain free in the tubular fluid. If the protons remained free in the lumen, the luminal pH would rapidly drop, and the high concentration of luminal protons would produce a large lumen-to-cell proton gradient. At a certain point, the pumps responsible for secreting protons would not be able to function against this gradient. This point corresponds to a urinary pH of around 4.5, or a free proton concentration of 0.03 mEq/L. The limitation of the pumps would create a discrete limit to the amount of free acid that could be excreted in a given volume of urine. Also, the backleak of H^+ would prevent such a low urine pH. To excrete enough free protons to counter the daily acid load and still keep the urine pH above 4.5, the kidney would have to produce more than 2,000 L of urine a day! Instead, the kidneys overcome this problem in a familiar fashion: they use buffers to avoid a luminal buildup of H^+ and maintain the luminal pH above 4.5. The two most important urinary buffers are phosphate and ammonia (FIGURE 25.5). NH_3 is not actually a urinary buffer per se, because the pK of the reaction $NH_3 + H^+ \rightarrow NH_4^+$ (ammonium) is 9.1, well above the urine pH. Rather, it acts like a urinary buffer because of the different permeabilities of the tubule for NH_3 and NH_4^+, as we will discuss. The availability of these buffers determines the capacity for urinary acid excretion and bicarbonate creation. Recall that the nonvolatile acids produced were in association with anions that need to be excreted in the urine. These anions, such as Cl-

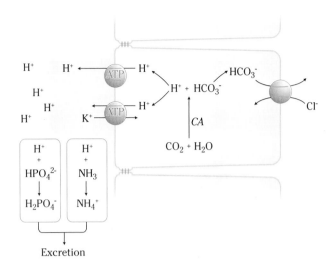

Figure 25.5 Urinary buffering of secreted protons in the distal tubule segments. Some buffering by phosphate also occurs in the proximal tubule.

and PO_4^{3-}, balance the charge of the protons added to the urinary buffers.

The Phosphate Buffer: $HPO_4^{2-}/H_2PO_4^-$ The phosphate available for buffering depends primarily on the dietary intake of phosphate-containing compounds. Phosphate is filtered through the glomerulus and then partially reabsorbed proximally. The remaining 10% to 20% of the phosphate serves to buffer urinary protons. Because the pK for the reaction $HPO_4^{2-} + H^+ \rightarrow H_2PO_4^-$ is 6.8, phosphate is a good urinary buffer. Two-thirds of the phosphate buffer is consumed by acidity due to HCO_3^- reabsorption and excess H^+ secretion in the proximal tubule. Because most of the excess H^+ secretion takes place distally, the quantity of phosphate buffer is clearly insufficient by itself to handle excreted protons. Furthermore, phosphate is not regulated to maintain acid-base balance as much as it is to maintain phosphorus homeostasis.

The Ammonia Buffer: NH_3/NH_4^+ The most important urinary buffer is **NH_3/NH_4^+**. NH_3 is produced by the metabolism of amino acids, purines, pyrimidines, and other nitrogen-containing compounds in many body tissues, especially the liver and kidney. Because NH_3 reacts with an intermediate in the citric acid cycle, it impedes ATP production and is toxic to the tissues. The liver fixes NH_3 in urea to prevent ammonia toxicity. The kidney has a special use for NH_3, and therefore must produce it in large amounts. Fortunately, the renal use of NH_3 is as a urinary buffer, so that the NH_3 formed in the kidney is excreted in the urine.

The primary site of ammonia production is the proximal tubule mitochondria. The proximal tubule cells express high levels of the enzyme *glutaminase*, which helps convert *glutamine* to *glutamate*, liberating an NH_4^+. The enzyme *glutamate dehydrogenase* converts glutamate to *α-ketoglutarate* and a second NH_4+ (FIGURE 25.6). The consumption of glutamine by this pathway leads to increased uptake of glutamine from the bloodstream, which supplies the pathway with constant substrate. Under conditions of increased acid loads, more glutamine is transported into the proximal cell and the glutaminase activity is increased. (See Integrated Physiology Box *The Role of Metabolism in the Regulation of Acidity.*)

Once produced, the NH_4^+ is secreted into the proximal tubule lumen, putatively across the Na^+/H^+ antiporter, with NH_4^+ in place of H^+ (FIGURE 25.7). NH_4^+ cannot leave the lumen, which is impermeable to this cation, until it reaches the thick ascending limb of the loop of Henle. NH_4^+ is then actively reabsorbed in the thick ascending limb, via the K^+ locus in the $Na^+/K^+/2Cl^-$ symporter. The H^+ is secreted into the loop of Henle tubule lumen in exchange for Na^+, where it serves HCO_3^- reabsorption. Meanwhile, the NH_3, to which only the basolateral membrane is permeable, diffuses into the interstitium. In this way, through *countercurrent exchange*, a medullary interstitial NH_3 gradient is maintained and ammonia is prevented from reaching the highly vascular renal cortex, where it could diffuse into the systemic blood.

The high medullary interstitial NH_3 drives the diffusion of NH_3 into the collecting duct. If an acid load has acidified the tubular intercalated cells, the cells are secreting acid in excess of HCO_3^- reabsorption. The NH_3 binds this excess H^+, keeping the luminal $[H^+]$ low so that H^+ secretion can continue unopposed. Once the NH_3 has bound H^+ and formed NH_4^+, it is trapped in the lumen because the cell membranes are less permeable to it. This is known as **ammonium trapping**, and results in excretion of excess acid in the titrated form of NH_4^+. Another mechanism for entry of NH_3 into the collecting duct lumen involves recently discovered Rh factor glycoproteins that mediate an exchange of NH_4^+ for H^+. These ammonium transporters exist on both the apical and basolateral membranes of collecting duct cells.

Not only does ammonium account for the majority of urinary H^+ excretion, but it is also another means of regulating H^+ excretion. Whereas the phosphate buffering capacity of the urine is relatively fixed and largely determined by body phosphate balance, the amount of ammonia available can be regulated by the kidney to match demands for acidification. *Increased NH_3 production is a major regulatory response to increased plasma acidity alongside increased H^+ secretion/HCO_3^- creation.* When NH_4^+ production goes up, more NH_3 accumulates in the interstitium and more NH_3 diffuses into the collecting

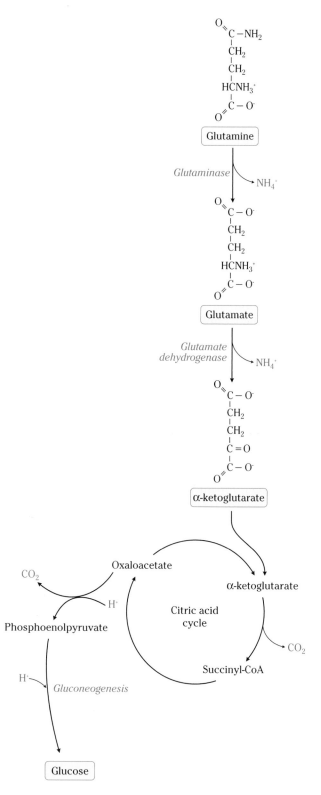

Figure 25.6 The metabolism of glutamine to ammonium in the proximal tubule cell. Increased $NH4^+$ production helps to buffer urinary H^+, thereby increasing the amount of H^+ that may be secreted and excreted. This diagram also shows the fate of α-ketoglutarate.

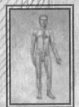

The Role of Metabolism in the Regulation of Acidity

Some researchers heavily emphasize that when glutamine is metabolized to α-ketoglutarate and NH_4^+, new HCO_3^- is also produced. They argue that glutamine metabolism and its regulation is a significant, even central, means of producing new bicarbonate and therefore, of handling the acid load. This approach to understanding acid-base homeostasis is interesting, but perhaps misleading.

Although the metabolism of one molecule of α-ketoglutarate does yield two molecules of HCO_3^-, this pathway is not a particularly good way to alkalinize the proximal tubule cell or the blood. The proximal tubular cell handles α-ketoglutarate in more than one way, but the high level of gluconeogenic enzymes in the kidney means that much of the α-ketoglutarate will pass through the citric acid cycle and into gluconeogenesis, where its carbon skeleton contributes to a molecule of glucose (see Figure 25.6). The α-ketoglutarate is an anion with two negatively charged carboxyl groups. In the process of conversion to glucose, which is an electrically neutral molecule, the α-ketoglutarate acquires two protons.

The acquisition of two protons is the reason some investigators assert that H^+ is consumed and new HCO_3^- is formed. During conversion from the five-carbon α-ketoglutarate to the three-carbon phosphoenolpyruvate (two molecules of which will go on to form the six-carbon glucose), α-ketoglutarate is also *twice decarboxylated*. That is, the metabolism of α-ketoglutarate consumes two protons, *but it also yields two molecules of CO_2*. The subtraction of H^+ from the cytosol may reduce intracellular $[H^+]$, but the addition of CO_2 will raise $[H^+]$.

The net effect of α-ketoglutarate metabolism is thus not alkalinization of the cell, and is not a strict stoichiometric addition of HCO_3^-. The formation of NH_4^+ is not a source of H^+ consumption and HCO_3^- production, either. The two protons consumed in conversion from $2NH_3$ to $2NH_4^+$ are cancelled out by the donation of two protons in the deaminations of glutamine and glutamate.

What does create new HCO_3^- is the net secretion of H^+ in excess of that required for luminal HCO_3^- reabsorption—that is, net H^+ excretion. This controversy underlines the dangers of looking at acid-base homeostasis as a molecule-for-molecule accounting of total body protons. When trying to understand the impact of acid loads on the plasma, the impact of acid plasma on tubular cells, and the homeostatic means of reversing cellular and plasma acidity, *always consider what changes have been introduced to the bicarbonate buffer, whether in the blood or in the renal tubular cell.* In general, cellular metabolism in the tubular cells is a source of CO_2, the production of which does not by itself govern cellular or plasma acidity. Metabolic CO_2 can provide a source of new HCO_3^- under circumstances of increased peritubular absorption of HCO_3^- and increased H^+ secretion.

That is not to say that regulation of metabolic pathways plays no role in the regulation of plasma acidity. Some investigators have shown that endogenous acid production (in the form of lactic acid and ketoacids) may be up- or down-regulated by changes in blood pH. These changes in metabolism may contribute to the regulation of blood pH.

duct. This lowers the luminal $[H^+]$ and allows more H^+ secretion and excretion and hence more HCO_3^- production. Recent studies also suggest that NH_3 directly stimulates distal H^+ secretion in intercalated cells of the collecting duct by promoting the insertion of H^+/K^+-ATPase into the apical membrane of these cells. Acid loads, both nonvolatile and due to elevated PCO_2, increase ammonia production. Another regulator of ammoniagenesis is hypokalemia, which may be associated with intracellular acidosis. The advantage of increased NH_4^+ production in hypokalemia could be the provision of an expendable cation, NH_4^+, for excretion with waste anions while enabling the kidney to preserve Na^+ and K^+.

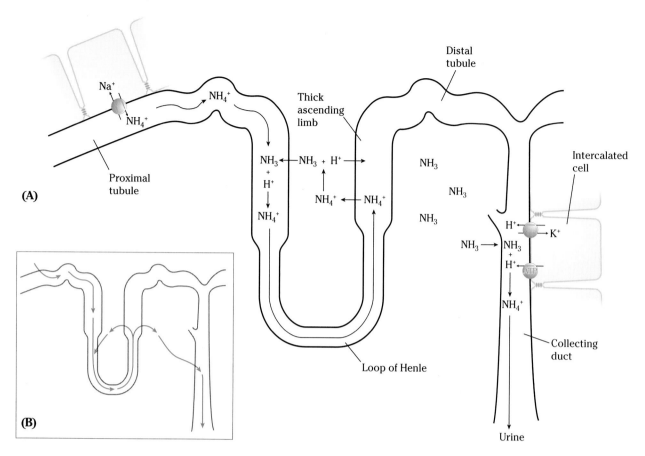

Figure 25.7 Ammonia secretion and excretion in the renal tubule. **A.** Ammonia transport and trapping. **B.** The overall pathway of ammonia through the tubule.

The Influence of Volume and Potassium Homeostasis on Renal Acid Excretion

We have already seen that the intracellular pH of the renal tubular cells is the most important afferent input in the homeostatic regulation of renal acid excretion. Because H^+ transport involves the antiport and symport of other ions, the homeostatic governance of transport of these other ions has a nonhomeostatic effect on H^+ secretion and HCO_3^- generation.

When blood pressure is low and *angiotensin II* stimulates increased proximal Na^+ (and hence water) reabsorption, the activity of the Na^+/H^+ exchanger is enhanced. More H^+ is secreted. HCO_3^- reabsorption is enhanced, and proximal H^+ excretion is increased. As a result, low blood volume and pressure (hypovolemia) can perpetuate an underlying alkalosis by preventing decreased HCO_3^- reabsorption and decreased H^+ excretion. This condition is sometimes called a **contraction alkalosis** because the alkalosis is maintained by contracted blood volume.

Aldosterone also contributes to this phenomenon by increasing the activity of the distal apical Na^+ channel and Na^+/K^+ exchanger in principal cells, thereby increasing distal Na^+ reabsorption. This leaves the tubule lumen more electronegative and promotes H^+ secretion from the intercalated cells. Furthermore, aldosterone stimulates the H^+-ATPase. *Overall, through the actions of angiotensin II and aldosterone, low blood volume increases bicarbonate reabsorption and may increase acid excretion.*

Low plasma $[K^+]$ (hypokalemia) may lead to alkalosis. This relationship is due to transmembrane shifting of H^+ and K^+ in the periphery and increased H^+ secretion in the proximal and distal tubule segments. Low $[K^+]$ causes K^+ to shift out of cells, making the cell interior more negative, which draws in H^+, alkalinizing the blood pH. In the proximal tubule, there is increased Na^+/H^+ exchange activity and Na^+-HCO_3^- cotransport at the basolateral membrane. Hypokalemia also increases proximal ammonium production. In the collecting duct, increased K^+ reabsorption across the H^+/K^+-ATPase may drive excess H^+ secretion. The decreased K^+ secretion in the collecting duct may also fail to raise the electrical potential of the tubule lumen, creating an increased electrical gradient for H^+ secretion. *Overall, hypokalemia leads to or maintains metabolic alkalosis.*

PATHOPHYSIOLOGY: ACIDOSIS AND ALKALOSIS

Many disease states can cause derangements in blood pH. Such conditions alter the PCO_2, the $[H^+]$, or the $[HCO_3^-]$, pushing the pH out of normal bounds. A condition that lowers the pH level is classified as an **acidosis**. One that elevates the pH is classified as an **alkalosis**. The terms *acidosis* and *alkalosis* are technically distinct from *acidemia* and *alkalemia*. *Acidemia* and *alkalemia* refer only to the blood pH. If the pH of the blood falls below the normal range (7.35 to 7.45), this condition is called **acidemia**. Conversely, if the pH is above the normal range, the condition is called **alkalemia**. The terms *acidosis* and *alkalosis*, on the other hand, refer to *processes* that tend to lower or raise the blood pH. This is relevant when two processes are working at the same time to raise and/or to lower the blood pH. Both acidoses and alkaloses are divided into two major subcategories: respiratory and metabolic. Processes that affect pulmonary ventilation and skew the PCO_2 are labeled *respiratory*. Processes that alter the $[H^+]$ or the $[HCO_3^-]$ are called metabolic. There are four main types of acid-base disorders: respiratory acidosis, respiratory alkalosis, metabolic acidosis, and metabolic alkalosis.

Respiratory Acidosis

A **respiratory acidosis** is an acidosis that derives from decreased pulmonary ventilation. Any condition that limits the ability of the lungs to ventilate will cause an accumulation of CO_2 in the blood. This leads to a fall in blood pH—an acidemia. Some of this extra CO_2 can be buffered by the bicarbonate system and by intracellular buffers, such as hemoglobin. In addition, when the lungs are unable to fully accomplish their task, the kidneys can partially compensate. By increasing the proton excretion and bicarbonate generation, the kidneys can oppose the pH change produced by the rising PCO_2. The kidney will also begin to increase NH_4^+ production in the proximal tubule, which will promote distal H^+ secretion by buffering more tubular acid and by direct stimulation of H^+ secretion.

An example of respiratory acidosis is decreased central respiratory drive. The lungs regulate PCO_2 by adjusting alveolar ventilation to keep arterial PCO_2 at about 40 mm Hg. This requires intact central neurologic input to the pulmonary system. If the respiratory center is damaged by stroke or suppressed by drugs such as opioids, ventilation will be inadequately stimulated and hypoventilation will set in. When ventilation falls, CO_2 will not be eliminated at a sufficient rate. This accumulation of CO_2 will lower the pH. The kidneys will compensate by eliminating protons and making more bicarbonate.

Respiratory Alkalosis

A **respiratory alkalosis** is an alkalosis that derives from increased pulmonary ventilation. If ventilation increases above the level necessary to keep CO_2 at 40 mm Hg, the PCO_2 will fall, and the pH will rise. In this case, to offset the decrease in PCO_2, the kidneys will effect a decrease in plasma bicarbonate concentration. This is accomplished by both a reduction in bicarbonate reabsorption and actual bicarbonate secretion. Bicarbonate secretion occurs in certain subtypes of intercalated cells in the collecting duct. These subtypes have H^+-ATPases on their basolateral side and HCO_3^-/Cl- antiporters on their apical side (i.e., their transporters are reversed with respect to the usual intercalated cell to conduct HCO_3^- in the opposite direction).

An example of respiratory alkalosis is any cause of pulmonary V/Q mismatch where oxygenation is inadequate, but the exchange of CO_2 remains adequate (which can occur because of the differences between the oxygen-hemoglobin equilibrium curve and the carbon dioxide-blood equilibrium curve; see Chapters 17 and 18). Conditions such as pneumonia and pulmonary edema can cause oxygen desaturation and hyperventilation, driving down the PCO_2. Respiratory alkalosis also occurs in the context of increased central respiratory drive. Some common causes are anxiety, fever, and pregnancy. In pregnancy, the high levels of progesterone stimulate the respiratory center to increase ventilation. Respiratory alkalosis is the most common acid-base disorder and is frequently benign.

Metabolic Acidosis

Metabolic acidosis refers to nonrespiratory causes of acidemia. Three types of processes result in metabolic acidosis: increased nonvolatile acid loads in the blood, decreased renal acid excretion, and loss of bicarbonate in urine or stool (TABLE 25.1). The lowered pH in any of these situations will stimulate the respiratory center to increase ventilation, which in turn lowers PCO_2. This shifts the buffer reaction to the left, consuming H^+ and opposing the drop in pH. The deep hyperventilatory breathing sometimes observed in patients with metabolic acidoses is called *Kussmaul's respiration*. The kidneys also make adjustments in response to increased acidity. In the absence of primary kidney pathology (i.e., not in cases of decreased renal acid excretion), the kidneys will increase H^+ secretion and the generation of new bicarbonate, shifting the buffer reaction to the left. Prolonged metabolic acidosis will promote increased NH_4^+ production in the proximal tubule.

Metabolic acidosis is further subcategorized as an **anion gap acidosis** or a **normal anion gap/hyper-**

Table 25.1   **CAUSES OF METABOLIC ACIDOSIS**

	Increased Nonvolatile Acid Load in Blood	Decreased Renal Acid Excretion	Loss of Bicarbonate
Increased Anion Gap	• Poisoning (aspirin, ethylene glycol, methanol, etc.) • Ketoacidosis and lactic acidosis	• Renal failure	
Normal Anion Gap		• Type 1 (distal) renal tubular acidosis (RTA)[a] • Type 4 RTA (hypoaldosteronism)	• Diarrhea • Type 2 (proximal) RTA[a]

[a] Type 3 RTA is a rare combination of types 1 and 2.

chloremic acidosis. Cases of increased nonvolatile acid loads are anion gap acidoses. Some cases of decreased renal acid excretion are anion gap and some present (manifest clinically) with a normal anion gap. All cases of lost bicarbonate present with a normal anion gap.

What is an anion gap? The total number of cations and anions in the ECF must be equal because the blood is electrically neutral. Most of the cations in the ECF are sodium. The anions are bicarbonate, chloride, plasma proteins (mainly albumin), and to a lesser extent, phosphate, sulfate, and organic acid ions. Sodium, bicarbonate, and chloride are measurable ions. The other anions are not usually measured. Therefore, the sodium level minus bicarbonate and chloride levels yields a number equal to the concentration of unmeasured anions; this is the *anion gap*. The anion gap is present even under normal circumstances due to albumin and other unmeasured anions normally present in the blood.

$$\text{Anion gap} = [Na^+] - ([Cl^-] + [HCO_3^-])$$

Plugging in the normal values, $[Na^+] = 140$ mEq/L, $[Cl^-] = 106$ mEq/L, and $[HCO_3^-] = 24$ mEq/L, we can calculate the normal anion gap to be about 6 to 10 mEq/L. Normal dietary nonvolatile acid loads and their unmeasured anionic conjugate bases do not cause significant increases in the anion gap under normal conditions.

Pathologic acid loads and their anionic conjugate bases can raise the anion gap to a significant extent, however. Ethylene glycol is a poison that can cause an anion gap acidosis. The ethylene glycol is metabolized to glyoxalate and oxalic acid in the liver, lowering pH, and these anions account for the increased anion gap. Two very clinically relevant examples of anion gap acidosis owing to the body's own pathological products are ketoacidosis and lactic acidosis. Ketoacidosis follows from starvation metabolism, which occurs not only in starvation but also in diabetes mellitus. Starvation metabolism yields acid metabolites that have unmeasured anionic conjugate bases (such as β-hydroxybutyrate and acetoacetate). Lactic acidosis may occur in circulatory or respiratory failure, when the tissues are deprived of oxygen. Anaerobic metabolism of carbohydrates in the tissues yields lactic acid, and lactate is the unmeasured anion associated with the acidosis. In renal failure, the kidney fails to excrete acid, owing to decreased NH_3 production, and to make bicarbonate, and at the same time, fails to clear the sulfate and phosphate that are the unmeasured anionic conjugate bases of dietary nonvolatile acid.

Cases of decreased acid excretion other than renal failure—as in *renal tubular acidosis*—present with a normal anion gap. Inherited defects in tubular pumps and transporters, autoimmune injury to these membrane proteins, hormone deficiencies, drug effects, and so on, can impair $H+$ secretion and hence HCO_3^- reabsorption. Impaired HCO_3^- reabsorption acidifies the plasma, and, unlike anion gap acidosis, represents a subtraction of bicarbonate, rather than an addition of H^+. This failure to reabsorb anionic HCO_3^- results in a charge separation that causes Cl- to increase in place of HCO_3^-. This is why normal anion gap acidoses are also called *hyperchloremic*, because the plasma chloride level is high in these conditions. Diarrhea is another form of normal anion gap/hyperchloremic acidosis—in this case, due to a loss of HCO_3^- through the intestines. The loss of Na$^+$

with the HCO_3^- leaves relatively more Cl^- behind in the ECF, giving a hyperchloremic acidosis.

Metabolic Alkalosis

Metabolic alkalosis refers to nonrespiratory causes of alkalemia. An excessive loss of acid, as in vomiting and in the use of loop or thiazide diuretics, or an excessive intake of alkali, predisposes to an increase in bicarbonate and therefore an increase in pH. (Vomiting leads to the loss of acid because of the HCl lost from the stomach.) The lungs will respond to elevated pH by decreasing ventilation. This compensatory mechanism is greatly limited by the need to ventilate in order to take up oxygen. The kidneys also react to an increase in bicarbonate by reducing bicarbonate reabsorption along the nephron. In fact, the kidneys have an enormous capacity to excrete filtered bicarbonate in the urine. Therefore, metabolic alkalosis requires situations that specifically limit this compensatory ability of the kidney.

The two factors that interfere with renal correction of metabolic alkalosis are ECF volume depletion (hypovolemia) and hypokalemia. In hypovolemia, angiotensin II stimulates the reabsorption of Na^+ via the Na^+/H^+ antiporter in the proximal tubule, and aldosterone stimulates H^+ secretion by the H^+-ATPase in the cortical collecting duct. The increased acid excretion and bicarbonate reabsorption perpetuate the alkalosis—so-called contraction alkalosis, as just mentioned. Recall that hypokalemia also drops the plasma $[H^+]$ because K^+ shifts out of cells and H^+ shifts into them. Hypokalemia also stimulates distal H^+ secretion. Therefore, hypokalemia exacerbates alkalosis.

Blood Gas Analysis

In medical practice, we use laboratory values as a window into physiologic processes. The information needed to analyze a patient's acid-base disorder can be obtained from a sample of arterial blood called an *arterial blood gas (ABG)*. The blood is typically drawn from the radial artery near the wrist. In this sample, we can measure the three parameters critical to acid-base balance: pH, PCO_2, and HCO_3^-. Typical normal ranges for these tests are pH: 7.35 to 7.45, PCO_2: 38 to 42 mm Hg, and HCO_3^-: 22 to 28 mmol/L.

A systematic approach to the results of arterial blood gases is diagrammed in FIGURE 25.8 and outlined in the following list.

1. Determine the pH. If the pH is below 7.4, there is an acidemia. If it is above 7.4, an alkalemia exists.

2. Determine what type of process produced the observed pH change. To develop

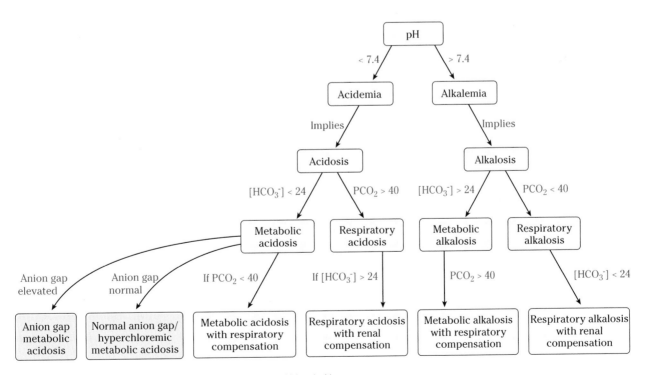

Figure 25.8 A flow chart for the analysis of disturbances of blood pH.

acidemia, an acidosis must be present. Likewise, the creation of alkalemia requires an alkalosis. We must determine which type of alkalosis or acidosis is present.

    a. Acidemia: If the PCO_2 is elevated—greater than 40 mm Hg—there must be a respiratory acidosis. If the HCO_3^- is depressed—less than 24 mEq/L—there is a metabolic acidosis.

    b. Alkalemia: If the PCO_2 is decreased—less than 40 mm Hg—a respiratory alkalosis is present. If $[HCO_3^-]$ is increased—greater than 24 mEq/L—a metabolic alkalosis is present.

3. Determine whether there are any compensatory changes. We expect that any primary acid-base disturbance will induce compensatory alterations. Therefore, if we determined that a respiratory acidosis was present, we would predict that the bicarbonate concentration would also be elevated. This reflects the renal compensation for the respiratory disorder. A respiratory alkalosis should be accompanied by a drop in $[HCO_3^-]$. If there is no compensation—that is, if both PCO_2 and $[HCO_3^-]$ push the blood pH in the same direction, then the patient may have a "mixed disorder," combining respiratory and metabolic etiologies. (See Clinical Application Box *A Sample Analysis of an Acid-Base Disorder.*)

One point of potential confusion is the fact that an uncompensated metabolic acidosis is *not* associated with an increased PCO_2. When acid is added to the blood buffer and the H^+ is bound by HCO_3^-, it should

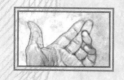

CLINICAL APPLICATION

A SAMPLE ANALYSIS OF AN ACID-BASE DISORDER

A 12-year-old boy has had recent polyuria (increased urine volume) and polydipsia (increased thirst). He suddenly developed nausea, lethargy, weakness, and shortness of breath and was found to have hyperglycemia (high blood sugar), a blood pH of 7.25, a PCO_2 of 25 mm Hg, and a serum HCO_3^- of 10 mEq/L. The $[Na^+]$ was 140 mEq/L (normal); $[K^+]$ 3.5 mEq/L (normal); $[Cl^-]$ 100 mEq/L (normal). The anion gap was increased to 30 mEq/L.

If we submit this case to the guidelines for the analysis of an acid-base disorder, we begin with inspection of the blood pH. It is less than 7.4, which is acidemic, implying the presence of an acidosis. Next, we examine the PCO_2 and $[HCO_3^-]$. The PCO_2 is low (< 40 mm Hg), which argues against a respiratory acidosis. The $[HCO_3^-]$ is also low (< 24 mEq/L), which supports the diagnosis of a metabolic acidosis. In addition to excluding a respiratory acidosis, the low PCO_2 also suggests that the metabolic acidosis is being partially compensated for by hyperventilation. Finally, the increased anion gap suggests this is an **increased anion gap metabolic acidosis** (sometimes called an *anion gap acidosis*, for short). From Table 25.1, we might conclude that the patient has one of the following disorders: poisoning, ketoacidosis, lactic acidosis, or renal failure.

The answer comes from integrating the lab findings with the history. The polyuria, polydipsia, and hyperglycemia are highly suggestive of diabetes mellitus. In diabetes, a lack of insulin results in failure to transport glucose into cells. The liver is driven into a starvation metabolism in which it breaks down fats and proteins to make ketone bodies. **Ketone bodies**, namely β-hydroxybutyric acid and acetoacetic acid, accumulate in the blood until a gradient is established for continued diffusion of the ketone bodies into the starved body tissues. There, the ketones yield acetyl-CoA and provide an alternative source of energy to the citric acid cycle in the context of diminished glucose availability. The accumulation of these acids in the blood also drops the blood pH, binds HCO_3^- (dropping the $[HCO_3^-]$), and contributes unmeasured anions to the blood (β-hydroxybutyrate and acetoacetate), creating an increased anion gap. This condition is called **diabetic ketoacidosis,** and it is a medical emergency requiring intravenous insulin.

not only decrease the $[HCO_3^-]$ but also produce more CO_2 and thus elevate the PCO_2. The "uncompensated" condition is something of a misnomer; it is a more clinically useful category than a purely physiologic one. When acid is added to the blood, the PCO_2 does go up, and even before clinically defined "compensation," the lungs do increase ventilation to get rid of this PCO_2 and bring the PCO_2 down to 40 mm Hg. This response is mediated by the peripheral chemoreceptors and it does help mitigate plasma acidity. The lung response is not called true compensation, however, until the peripheral chemoreceptors drive the PCO_2 below 40 mm Hg in response to rising $[H^+]$. In any case, uncompensated respiratory acidosis and uncompensated metabolic acidosis are not only separated by their differing PCO_2 levels but by their differing $[HCO_3^-]$ levels. The $[HCO_3^-]$ in uncompensated metabolic acidosis is low, and the $[HCO_3^-]$ in uncompensated respiratory acidosis is slightly high.

To summarize, respiratory compensation occurs in metabolic disorders such that a change in bicarbonate concentration is met with a change in PCO_2 in the same direction (e.g., decreased bicarbonate leads to decreased PCO_2). Note that this brings the ratio of HCO_3^-/PCO_2 back toward normal. From the Henderson-Hasselbalch relationship, normalization of the ratio brings the pH toward normal. Likewise, in primary respiratory disorders, changes in PCO_2 are met with changes in HCO_3^- concentration via renal mechanisms, in the same direction to partially correct the pH. Generally, pH does not completely correct through compensation, and the degree of compensation is predictable.

Summary

- Stable pH is critical to physiological functioning because protonation or deprotonation of proteins alters their charge, shape, and therefore, their function.
- The first line of defense against changes of pH inside the body is the bicarbonate buffer. The following three equations describe the bicarbonate buffer equilibrium.

$$CO_2 + H_2O \leftrightarrow H_2CO_3 \leftrightarrow HCO_3^- + H^+$$

$$K = 1 \times 10^{-6.1} = [HCO_3^-][H^+]/\alpha PCO_2$$

$$pH = 6.1 + \log \{[HCO_3^-]/[0.03] \times [PCO_2]\}$$

- The last of the above equations is called the Henderson-Hasselbalch equation.
- When the PCO_2 rises, more HCO_3^- and H^+ are formed. When H^+ is added to the buffer equilibrium, some of it reacts with HCO_3^-, driving $[HCO_3^-]$ down and PCO_2 up. When HCO_3^- is lost, the equilibrium shifts to the right; PCO_2 goes down, $[H^+]$ goes up, and some of the lost HCO_3^- is replenished.
- When H^+ is added to the blood, more than half of it is initially buffered by intracellular proteins such as hemoglobin. The H^+ influx is associated with a K^+ efflux, raising the plasma $[K^+]$.
- The kidney filters more than 4,000 mEq/L HCO_3^- per day into the nephrons. About 99% of it must be reabsorbed in order to maintain the basal $[HCO_3^-]$ and hence the basal blood pH of 7.4.
- HCO_3^- reabsorption takes place predominantly in the proximal tubule. Na^+-coupled H^+ secretion binds HCO_3^- in the proximal tubule lumen, forms CO_2 (expedited by carbonic anhydrase), and the CO_2 diffuses into the tubule cells, where it is rehydrated and dissociates into H^+ and HCO_3^-. The HCO_3^- is reabsorbed across a $Na^+/3\ HCO_3^-$ symporter, and the H^+ is secreted.
- This shuttling of acid back and forth across the proximal tubule membrane accounts for HCO_3^- reabsorption.
- The body encounters daily acid loads. It confronts a volatile acid load in the form of metabolically produced CO_2, which shifts the buffer equilibrium to the right. It confronts a nonvolatile acid load in the form of HCl and H_2SO_4, which are derived from the metabolism of dietary amino acids, and H_3PO_4, which is derived from phosphorus-containing foodstuffs.
- Acid loads add H^+ to the blood buffer, which drops the blood pH, consumes HCO_3^-, and produces CO_2. The buffer mitigates the acidification, but the disturbance in blood pH must still be corrected. If it were not corrected, the acidification would worsen with the next acid load because the first acid load has consumed some of the HCO_3^- and hence some of the buffering power of the blood.
- In order to reverse this disturbance in the blood pH, the lungs increase ventilation to blow off more CO_2, and the kidneys increase H^+ excretion.
- Acid pH in the blood acidifies the cytosol of the tubular cells in the kidney through diffusion of CO_2 into the cell and basolateral transport of HCO_3^- out of the cell.
- Intracellular acid pH promotes H+ secretion by active and passive mechanisms in the proximal and distal segments of the tubule.

- The response to acid pH in the proximal tubule is increased gradient for H^+ secretion across the Na^+/H^+ exchanger and H^+-ATPase, enhanced activity of the Na^+/H^+ antiporter, of the H^+-ATPase, and of the $Na^+/3\ HCO_3^-$ symporter, and finally, increased NH_4^+ production from glutamine.

- Those proximal responses all increase H^+ secretion, which accelerates HCO_3^- reabsorption, and which leads to some H^+ secretion in excess of luminal HCO_3^-. The excess H^+ is titrated by HPO_4^{2-}, and is ultimately excreted as $H_2PO_4^-$.

- The response to acid pH in the distal tubule and collecting duct is increased gradient for H^+ secretion across the intercalated cells' H^+-ATPase and H^+/K^+ exchanger and increased recruitment of the H^+-ATPase into apical membranes.

- The distal responses also increase H^+ secretion in excess of luminal HCO_3^-. The excess H^+ binds to the remaining HPO_4^{2-} and to NH_3 and is ultimately excreted as $H_2PO_4^-$ and NH_4^+, accompanied by the acid anions such as Cl^-.

- Renal acid excretion also achieves the generation of new bicarbonate. The excess H^+, destined for excretion, is formed alongside HCO_3^- from intracellular CO_2. When the H^+ is excreted rather than bound to luminal HCO_3^-, the intracellular HCO_3^- is left behind as "new" bicarbonate. Thus, renal acid excretion consumes intracellular CO_2, excretes the proton, and makes new HCO_3^-, which is then reabsorbed.

- Renal acid excretion and new bicarbonate production allows the blood to keep delivering its excess H^+ to the tubule cells through the peritubular capillary and to keep absorbing HCO_3^- in excess of the amount reabsorbed from filtered HCO_3^-. This replenishes the HCO_3^- lost owing to the acid load.

- Net peritubular loss of H^+ and gain of HCO_3^- restores normal plasma pH after the disturbance of the acid load.

- Much more net acid excretion and HCO_3^- production occurs in the distal tubule segments. Even under circumstances of increased acidity, the proximal tubule serves primarily to reabsorb HCO_3^- and only secretes a proportionally small amount of excess H^+.

- Proximal NH_4^+ production from glutamine results in countercurrent exchange of NH_3/NH_4^+ and a medullary interstitial NH_3 gradient. High interstitial $[NH_3]$ leads to NH_3 secretion in the collecting duct, where it titrates secreted H^+ and promotes insertion of the H^+/K^+ ATPase into the apical cell membrane.

- Hypovolemia and hypokalemia can be associated with alkalosis. Hypovolemia's effects on H^+ balance are partly mediated by angiotensin II and aldosterone.

- There are four types of pathophysiologic derangements in pH: respiratory acidosis, respiratory alkalosis, metabolic acidosis, and metabolic alkalosis.

- The respiratory disorders alter pH through primary disturbances in ventilation and hence PCO_2. The metabolic disorders alter pH through primary disturbances in $[H^+]$ or $[HCO_3^-]$. Metabolic acidosis may be due to added acid, retained acid, or lost bicarbonate; metabolic alkalosis may be due to added bicarbonate or lost acid.

- The lungs can partially compensate for metabolic disturbances with changes in ventilation, and the kidneys can partially compensate for respiratory disturbances with changes in acid excretion and bicarbonate reabsorption.

- The normal anion gap, which reflects the presence of unmeasured anions in the blood (like albumin), is defined by the following equation:

$$\text{Anion gap} = [Na^+] - ([Cl^-] + [HCO_3^-])$$

- Some metabolic acidoses are associated with an increased anion gap. The excess unmeasured anions are the conjugate bases of the acids that have caused the metabolic acidosis.

Suggested Reading

Alpern RJ. Cell mechanisms of proximal tubule acidification. Physiol Rev. 1990;70(1):79–114.

Aronson PS. Mechanisms of active H+ secretion in the proximal tubule. Am J Physiol. 1983;245(6):F647–659.

Cogan MG, Alpern RJ. Regulation of proximal bicarbonate reabsorption. Am J Physiol. 1984;247(3 Pt 2): F387–395.

Knepper MA, Packer R, Good DW. Ammonium transport in the kidney. Physiol Rev. 1989;69(1):179–249.

Levine DZ, Jacobson HR. The regulation of renal acid secretion: new observations from studies of distal nephron segments. Kidney Int. 1986;29(6): 1099–109.

Seifter JL, Aronson PS. Properties and physiologic roles of the plasma membrane sodium-hydrogen exchanger. J Clin Invest. 1986;78(4):859–864.

REVIEW QUESTIONS

Directions: Each of the numbered items or incomplete statements in this section is followed by answers or by completions of the statement. Select the ONE lettered answer or completion that is BEST in each case.

1. A 21-year-old heroin addict overdoses and is found unresponsive and barely breathing at four breaths per minute. His body attempts to compensate for his acid-base imbalance by which of the following methods?

   (A) decreased proton secretion by the kidneys
   (B) decreased CO_2 exhalation by the lungs
   (C) increased CO_2 exhalation by the lungs
   (D) increased renal bicarbonate production
   (E) decreased renal bicarbonate reabsorption
   (F) decreased NH_4^+ production

2. A 3-year-old boy is found unresponsive in his parents' garage, and an empty bottle of antifreeze (ethylene glycol) is beside him. He is breathing with deep and long inspirations. Which of the following clinical observations are likely to be made in this case?

   (A) increased plasma $[Cl^-]$
   (B) $PCO_2 > 40$ mm Hg
   (C) increased anion gap
   (D) $[HCO_3^-] > 24$ mEq/L
   (E) normal blood pH

3. A 14-year-old girl with violent bacterial food poisoning is found to have a metabolic alkalosis. Her acid-base disorder might result from which of the following?

   (A) decreased H^+ production
   (B) increased ventilation due to fever
   (C) compensatory hypoventilation
   (D) diarrhea
   (E) increased oral alkali intake
   (F) increased H^+ loss

ANSWERS AND EXPLANATIONS

1. **The answer is D.** This patient's decreased central respiratory drive results in the accumulation of CO_2, which lowers blood pH, resulting in a respiratory acidosis. To compensate, the kidneys increase the production of bicarbonate and the excretion of protons. NH_4^+ production would be increased, not decreased, to further promote H^+ excretion.

2. **The answer is C.** A patient with ethylene glycol toxicity has an anion gap metabolic acidosis. The lowered pH stimulates increased respiratory drive to lower PCO_2 and consume H^+ by shifting the buffer reaction to the left, which will oppose the decreased pH. The kidneys will also increase bicarbonate reabsorption and production in an attempt to shift the buffer reaction to the left. The plasma $[HCO_3^-]$ will be low, however, due to the titration of the HCO_3^- buffer by added H^+ from the ethylene glycol. The plasma $[Cl^-]$ is elevated in normal anion gap/hyperchloremic acidosis, not in conditions like this one, in which the anion gap is elevated by the unmeasured anion, oxalate, derived from the ethylene glycol. *Kussmaul's respiration* is the term applied to the deep, rapid breathing observed in patients with metabolic acidosis.

3. **The answer is F.** Her metabolic alkalosis likely results from an increased loss of H^+, most likely secondary to vomiting, and a loss of HCl from her stomach as a result of her food poisoning. Although the central respiratory drive and hyperventilation can be caused by fever, the question states that the girl has a *metabolic* alkalosis. Febrile hyperventilation is a cause of primary respiratory alkalosis. Respiratory compensation does not cause metabolic alkalosis; rather, metabolic alkalosis causes compensatory decreased ventilation, which raises the blood PCO_2 and shifts the buffer reaction to the right, yielding H^+ and lowering pH. Diarrhea is often associated with food poisoning, and if Cl-rich, it may cause metabolic alkalosis, but more often it is a cause of metabolic acidosis owing to increased HCO_3^- loss in the stool. Increased alkali intake would cause metabolic alkalosis by elevating the $[HCO_3^-]$ in the plasma, but the patient's history is not suggestive of increased intake of alkali or any food. Although this girl does have an elevated $[HCO_3^-]$, the reason is likely to be vomiting and loss of H^+, shifting the buffer relation to the right.

Micturition

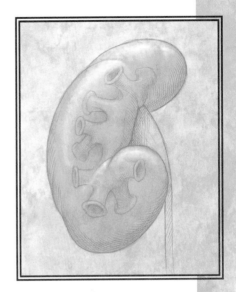

INTRODUCTION

Micturition is the process by which the urinary bladder empties its contents, and it is more commonly known as *urination*. This process involves two steps: (1) the bladder fills until wall tension exceeds a certain threshold level and (2) a nervous reflex known as the *micturition reflex* occurs, and the bladder empties. The **micturition reflex** is an autonomic spinal cord reflex, occurring independently of signals higher up in the central nervous system. Micturition can be inhibited or facilitated by centers in the cerebral cortex or the brain stem. An individual may consciously suppress the desire to urinate created by the micturition reflex or may attempt to urinate even without such a feeling of urgency.

SYSTEM STRUCTURE: ANATOMY OF THE URINARY SYSTEM

The fluid that pools in the renal calyces is the same urine that exits the body during micturition. No further reabsorption or secretion of solutes, and no further transport of water across cell membranes, occurs once the urine passes through the collecting ducts of the kidney. Urine is transported from the kidneys to the urinary bladder via two muscular tubes known as **ureters** (FIGURE 26.1). The bladder is a smooth muscle chamber that has two main parts. The body, also known as the *fundus*, is the main part of the bladder and acts as a storage chamber for the urine. The **bladder neck**, also known as the *posterior urethra*, is a funnel-shaped extension of the body of the bladder. This extension continues as the urethra, which opens to the outside of the body.

The smooth muscle of the bladder is known as the **detrusor muscle**. These muscle fibers extend in all directions around the bladder—longitudinally, radially, and spirally—without distinct layers, and the muscle cells themselves are fused together, similar to the syncytium of cardiac muscle. These muscle patterns create low-resistance electrical pathways between the cells and allow for a given action potential to spread quickly throughout the entire detrusor muscle, thereby producing a synchronous bladder contraction for micturition.

The mucosa of the bladder consists of a transitional epithelium, which includes basal columnar cells on the outside, intermediate cuboidal cells, and superficial squamous cells on the inside (FIGURE 26.2A). When the bladder is empty or underfilled, even the superficial cells are slightly rounded. These cells actually bulge into the lumen of the bladder, leaving room for chamber expansion as the superficial cells stretch and flatten into the classic squamous shape. In addition to this distensibility at the histologic level, the bladder mucosa also maintains

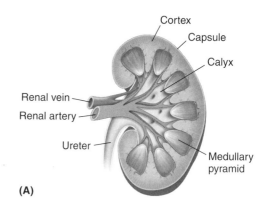

(A)

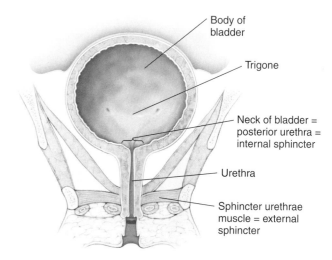

(B)

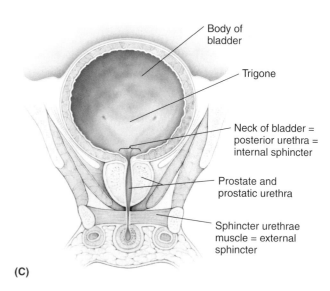

(C)

Figure 26.1 Gross anatomy of the urinary collecting system, the ureters, and the bladder. **A.** A cross-sectional view of the kidney. **B.** The female bladder. **C.** The male bladder.

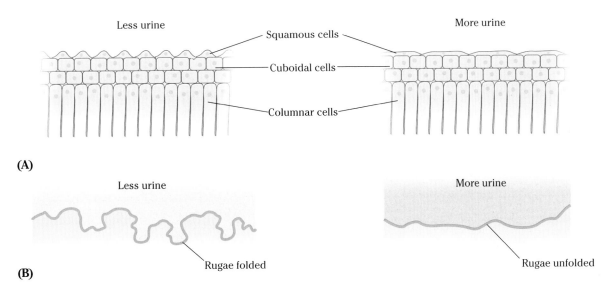

Less urine

More urine

— Squamous cells —

— Cuboidal cells —

— Columnar cells —

(A)

Less urine

More urine

Rugae folded

Rugae unfolded

(B)

Figure 26.2 Accommodating increased bladder volume. **A.** On the histologic level, the squamous cells flatten out to accommodate increased urine volume (bladder filling) and relieve tension in the bladder wall. **B.** On the anatomic level, the rugae flatten out to accommodate increased urine volume (bladder filling) and relieve tension in the bladder wall.

an anatomic level of distensibility (Figure 26.2B). The mucosal surface at rest is grossly folded into *rugae*, similar to that of the stomach, and can also stretch and flatten to accommodate increases in urine volume. These two levels of distensibility enable the bladder to expand in volume without significantly increasing the pressure inside.

Urine enters the bladder through two ureters and leaves through a single **urethra**. These three ports make up the angles of the **trigone,** a small triangular area on the posterior wall of the bladder immediately above the neck (Figures 26.1B and C). The mucosa of the trigone is distinct from that of the rest of the bladder. Whereas the majority of the bladder mucosa is folded into rugae, the trigone mucosa is smooth, regardless of the volume of urine. The ureters enter obliquely through the detrusor muscle, coursing one to two centimeters beneath the bladder mucosa before emptying into the bladder along the two upper angles of the trigone. This oblique extended course through the bladder wall helps prevent *vesicoureteral reflux*, the retrograde flow of urine from the bladder into the ureters. The posterior urethra constitutes the lowermost apex of the trigone. In the female, the urinary tract nearly ends with the posterior urethra as it leads almost directly to the outside of the body. In the male, the posterior urethra leads to the anterior urethra, which extends through the penis before opening to the outside of the body at the external meatus.

The bladder neck consists of the inferior two to three centimeters of the bladder. Its wall, like the wall of the bladder body, comprises the detrusor muscle;

however, the muscle here is organized into distinct layers to form the **internal sphincter** of the bladder. Sympathetic tone supplied to the internal sphincter through the hypogastric nerve keeps the internal sphincter tonically contracted. Additional control of micturition is located beyond the bladder neck as the urethra passes through the urogenital diaphragm. Here, the **external sphincter** of the bladder, a voluntary muscle layer as opposed to the smooth muscle of the body and neck of the bladder, can be consciously controlled to prevent or interrupt urination.

Innervation of the Bladder

The bladder is innervated by the **pelvic nerves**, the **hypogastric nerves**, and the **pudendal nerves** (FIGURE 26.3). These nerves provide parasympathetic, sympathetic, and somatic innervation, respectively. As a whole, they include afferent as well as efferent fibers, and impart voluntary as well as involuntary control of micturition. The nerves are wired to the spinal cord to participate in spinal reflex arcs. The spinal neurons receive input from the **pontine micturition center** in the brain stem, which in turn, receives higher inputs from the diencephalon and cerebral cortex.

The pelvic nerves are the primary nerve supply of the bladder. Arising from the sacral spinal cord at levels S2, S3, and S4, the pelvic nerves contain both sensory and motor parasympathetic fibers. The sensory fibers detect the degree of stretch in the bladder wall, and the motor fibers return the reflex signal and stimulate the bladder wall to contract for micturition.

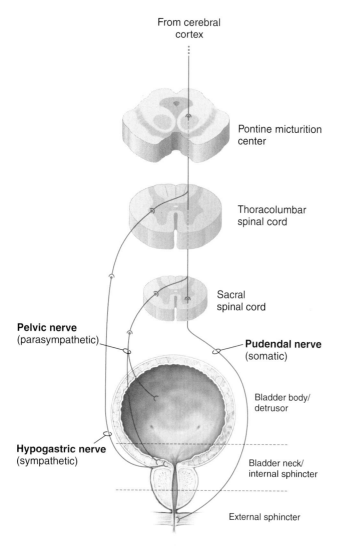

From cerebral
cortex

Pontine micturition
center

Thoracolumbar
spinal cord

Sacral
spinal cord

Pelvic nerve
(parasympathetic)

Pudendal nerve
(somatic)

Bladder body/
detrusor

Hypogastric nerve
(sympathetic)

Bladder neck/
internal sphincter

External sphincter

Figure 26.3 Innervation of the bladder. The hypogastric nerve is symphathetic, the pelvic nerve is parasympathetic, and the pudendal nerve is somatic. The pudendal nerve alone stimulates the contraction of skeletal muscle. Afferent pathways are not shown in this figure.

The hypogastric nerves arise from the spinal cord mainly at L2 and pass through the sympathetic chain. These nerves then send sympathetic innervation to the bladder neck and induce closure of the internal sphincter, which facilitates urine storage in the bladder body and seals off the urinary tract during ejaculation. They play little role in the actual contraction of the bladder body for micturition. The hypogastric nerves also contain some sensory fibers, which sense fullness as well as pain.

The pudendal nerves innervate the skeletal muscle of the external sphincter. The somatic motor fibers provide the signals for the sphincter to contract; thus, cortical inhibition of the pudendal nerve leads to a voluntary relaxation of the external sphincter, allowing the bladder to empty.

SYSTEM FUNCTION: THE TRANSPORT OF URINE AND ITS NEURAL CONTROL

Urine from the collecting ducts of the kidneys is ready for elimination by the body. The basic function of the rest of the urinary tract is to transport the urine from the kidneys to the bladder and ultimately outside the body. Spinal reflexes and their conscious and unconscious modulation by the brain control this final step of voiding the bladder of urine.

The Transport of Urine from Kidney to Bladder

Whereas the hydrostatic pressure of filtration drives the urine into the renal calyces, from that area, urinary flow is assisted by the elasticity of the urinary conduit. As the urine pools in the renal calyces, the walls are stretched, initiating a series of peristaltic smooth muscle contractions, which spread to the renal pelvis and down the ureter. These contractions force the urine in the calyces toward the bladder for temporary storage before micturition.

For urine to enter the bladder, the pressure generated by the peristaltic wave in the ureter must exceed the pressure on the ureter caused by the inherent tone of the detrusor muscle of the bladder wall. This high pressure in the ureter pushes open the **intravesical ureter** and allows the urine to drain into the body of the bladder. (*Vesical* comes from the Latin *vesica* for bladder, and *intravesical* means inside the bladder.) Remember that the ureters normally course at an oblique angle through the wall of the bladder. The bladder wall compresses the ureters and acts as a valve to prevent the backflow of urine. This mechanism is important when the pressure in the bladder increases with micturition or external compression. In fact, during bladder contraction, the detrusor muscle further compresses the intravesical ureters and occludes them to prevent the backflow of urine. Note that if the distance that one (or both) of the ureters courses through the bladder wall is less than normal (i.e., if the ureter courses at a less oblique, more direct angle), bladder contraction becomes less efficient at completely occluding that ureter and preventing backflow. The "valve" becomes leaky.

Vesicoureteral reflux is the pathologic backflow of urine and pressure. Chronic reflux can lead to enlargement of the affected ureter or ureters. If severe, it can lead to increased pressure in the renal calyces and ultimately damage the structures of the renal medulla.

The renal medulla is also protected from excess backflow by a reflex originating in the ureter. When an obstruction is sensed in the ureter, such as a kidney stone, the ureter undergoes an intense reflex constriction. This reflex is also associated with intense pain, because the ureters are well supplied with pain fibers by the pelvic nerves. This pain impulse precipitates a sympathetic reflex at the level of the kidney, decreasing urine output from the affected kidney (by increasing salt and water reabsorption), and minimizing the backflow of urine and pressure into the renal medulla. This protective reflex at the ureteral level is known as the *ureterorenal reflex*.

The Spinal Micturition Reflex

Remember that the bladder wall contains many folds known as *rugae*, thus creating a very distensible chamber. As the bladder fills with urine, the rugae smooth out and allow the volume inside the chamber to increase without increasing the pressure inside the chamber. Thus, a normal bladder can fill to a volume of about 300 mL with only a small increase in intravesical pressure. Once this volume is reached, the inner wall of the bladder is smooth, and subsequent increases in total urine volume stretch the bladder wall like air blown into a balloon. Then, after the body of the bladder is expanded, urine begins to fill the neck of the bladder. (Imagine that the neck of the bladder is equivalent to the tip of a balloon. The tip fills last; first the larger part of the balloon, which is nearer to the air inlet, fills and builds up a good deal of air under pressure.)

As the bladder continues to fill, sensory stretch receptors in the bladder wall are stimulated, sending signals along the pelvic nerves to the spinal cord. Such stretch receptors are especially numerous in the bladder neck, making the neck more sensitive to filling than the body. Similar to the patellar stretch reflex, this bladder stretch reflex returns to the bladder from the spinal cord via parasympathetic fibers of the pelvic nerve, resulting in an intense stimulation and contraction of the bladder wall's detrusor muscle. Remember that the individual muscle cells of the bladder wall are joined as a syncytium, and any stimulation for the contraction of a muscle fiber will cause the entire bladder to contract. The micturition reflex is initiated upon reaching threshold pressure.

When the bladder is only partly filled, the micturition contraction acutely increases the pressure inside the bladder and then spontaneously relaxes after a few seconds. The pressure inside the bladder subsequently falls back to the baseline tonic pressure from the total urine volume. This completes a single cycle of the micturition reflex (FIGURE 26.4). The frequency of the micturition reflex increases with an increase in total urine volume (and increase in tonic pressure). Also, the reflex may be self-regenerative in that the micturition contraction also increases the pressure inside the bladder and stimulates additional

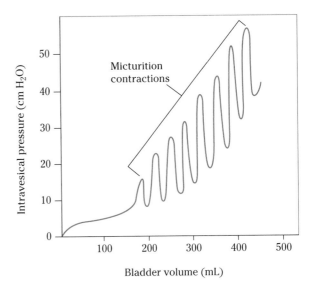

Figure 26.4 Pressure in the bladder during filling. The micturition reflex creates spikes in pressure once the urine volume and pressure pass a certain threshold.

sensory stretch receptors. As the bladder continues to fill, these reflexes increase in frequency and the micturition contractions increase in power and duration until a voluntary decision to urinate intervenes, allowing the micturition reflex to go uninhibited and the internal and external sphincters to relax. The voluntary decision inhibits the firing of the motor fibers in the pudendal nerve, eliminating its tonic contraction of the external sphincter, thereby relaxing it (FIGURE 26.5; see also Clinical Application Box *What is Benign Prostatic Hyperplasia?*).

PATHOPHYSIOLOGY: URINARY INCONTINENCE

Urinary incontinence, the loss of voluntary bladder control, affects millions of Americans of all ages. Approximately 50% of women experience occasional urinary incontinence. The incidence of urinary incontinence increases with age and its accompanying increase in pelvic relaxation. Urinary continence is possible because the intraurethral pressure exceeds the intravesical pressure. Tonic contraction of the internal and external sphincters are crucial mechanisms for preserving continence. The submucosal vasculature of the urethra also plays a role in maintaining urinary continence. Through a mechanism known as *mucosal coaptation*, the vasculature complex fills with blood, thus further increasing intraurethral pressure. In women, this mechanism is estrogen-sensitive, which partly explains why urinary incontinence occurs more frequently in postmenopausal women (FIGURE 26.6).

Urinary incontinence can be categorized into four subgroups: stress incontinence, urge

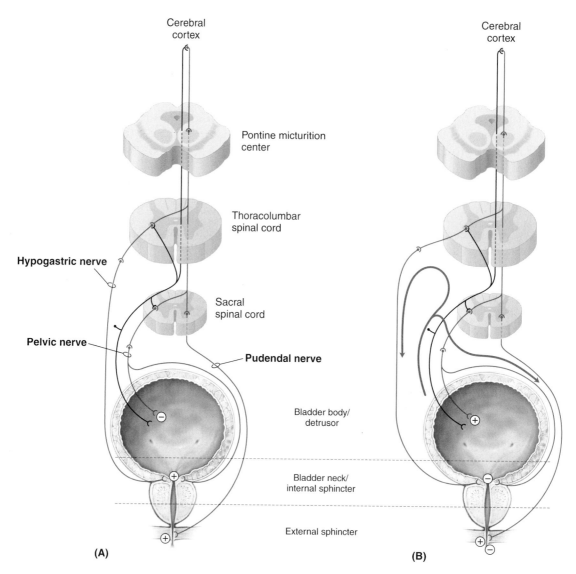

Figure 26.5 The spinal micturition reflex. **A.** Tonic muscle contraction during urine storage and prior to initiation of the reflex. The plus signs denote tonic contraction of the sphincters, and the minus sign denotes inhibition of detrusor contraction. The black line denotes the afferent neural pathway ascending to the spinal cord through the pelvic nerve. **B.** During the micturition reflex. The plus signs denote contraction of the detrusor, and the minus signs denote relaxation of the sphincters. (The plus/minus sign indicates that the external sphincter may be contracted or relaxed during the reflex, depending on cortical signals.) The black line denotes the afferent neural pathway ascending to the spinal cord through the pelvic nerve. The thick red arrows indicate the spinal sympathetic and parasympathetic micturition reflexes. The sympathetic reflex (afferent: pelvic, efferent: hypogastric) relaxes the internal sphincter. The parasympathetic reflex (afferent: pelvic, efferent: pelvic) contracts the detrusor and relaxes the internal sphincter. Cortical signals tonically inhibit the spinal micturition reflex. Conscious removal of this inhibition increases the strength of the spinal reflex and relieves the contraction of the external sphincter so that urination may begin.

incontinence, total incontinence, and overflow incontinence. **Stress incontinence** involves the loss of urine with increased straining, usually in the setting of increased pelvic relaxation. The straining from activities such as coughing, laughing, or exercising increases abdominal pressure and allows the intravesical pressure to exceed the intraurethral pressure, resulting in stress incontinence.

Urge incontinence involves urine leakage due to uninhibited, involuntary bladder contraction, which increases intravesical pressure. This heightened micturition reflex overwhelms voluntary control. Such detrusor instability can result from urinary tract infections, bladder stones, cancer, diverticula, or neurologic disorders causing hyperreflexia, although many cases are idiopathic. Common urinary com-

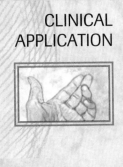

CLINICAL APPLICATION

WHAT IS BENIGN PROSTATIC HYPERPLASIA?

A 56-year-old man complains to his primary care physician that he is awakened several times a night with the need to urinate. Upon further questioning, he indicates that he often must strain slightly by tensing his abdominal muscles in order to initiate urination. He believes his urinary stream is "weaker than it used to be" and complains of a sensation of incomplete voiding after urination. He does not experience any burning sensation or pain during urination, and he has not noticed any blood or other discoloration of his urine. On conducting a rectal exam, the doctor finds an enlarged prostate.

As the name would suggest, **benign prostatic hyperplasia (BPH)** is a nonmalignant growth of the male prostate gland. Because of the prostate's anatomic location, it may create a urethral obstruction to outflow. This obstruction has several physiologic consequences. First, the obstruction means that higher intravesical pressures are necessary to drive the urine through the urethra. Patients may consequently complain of an inability to generate as strong a urinary stream as in their youth and may feel the need to push or strain to begin urination. Second, the higher pressure necessary for urination may lead to incomplete bladder emptying. Normal micturition usually leaves no more than 5 to 10 mL of urine remaining in the bladder; this volume is known as the *postvoid residual (PVR)*. In BPH, the PVR is typically elevated. One can imagine that a high PVR decreases the interval of time that it takes the bladder to refill and therefore increases the frequency of urination.

Men with BPH often complain of *nocturia* (the need to urinate at night) as well as an increased frequency of urination throughout the day. They may notice that they void smaller amounts each time, and may complain of a feeling of incomplete voiding (urinary retention). Many of these symptoms are at least partially relieved when the obstruction is reduced. For well over 50 years, a surgical procedure known as a *transurethral resection of the prostate* has been the mainstay of treatment, although medical therapy has been assuming increasing importance.

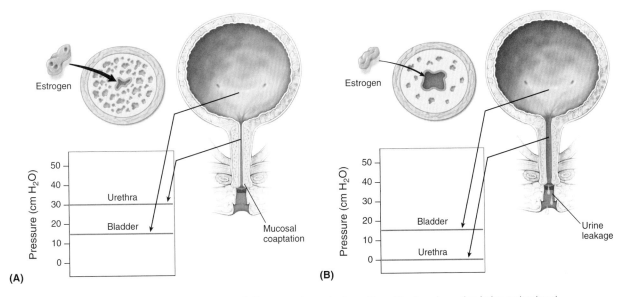

Figure 26.6 Mucosal coaptation. **A.** Estrogen-dependent swelling of the female urethra helps maintain urinary continence by increasing urethral pressure. **B.** Estrogen deficiency results in decreased urethral pressure.

plaints in this setting include urgency and frequency. (See Clinical Application Box *What Is a Urinary Tract Infection?*)

The uninhibited *neurogenic bladder* is an example of how partial damage to the spinal cord or brain stem interrupts cortical inhibitory signals. Remember that these cortical signals keep the external sphincter voluntarily contracted, as well as curb the micturition reflex until micturition is voluntarily desired. Without these cortical signals, the sacral centers of micturition become overexcitable, such that even small amounts of urine in the bladder can elicit micturition reflexes and result in urinary frequency. Sometimes after spinal cord damage, *spinal shock* occurs, in which even the micturition reflex is suppressed. After a few days, and assuming that the bladder is protected from overstretching with artificial emptying—that is, catheterization—the micturition reflex gradually returns and at this point may become hyperreflexic due to lost inhibition from upper motor neurons. This condition is similar to the initial hyporeflexia or even areflexia followed by hyperreflexia of the patellar reflex with proximal spinal cord damage.

The restoration of the micturition reflex occurs without any voluntary control or sensation, thus resulting in periodic but unannounced bladder emptying. Some patients are able to learn new stimuli for the micturition reflex so that they can bring it on themselves and preempt unannounced micturition reflexes. Patients learn to associate local skin stimuli (i.e., scratching, tickling) with the micturition reflex. By stimulating their skin in the genital region, these patients are able to elicit an involuntary micturition reflex and empower themselves with a simulated voluntary control of micturition.

Total incontinence, in which urine leaks from the body as soon as it is delivered from the ureters, is typically the result of a urinary fistula. Connections between the bladder or urethra and the intestines are possible, as well as between the bladder or urethra and the vagina. Causes of these fistulae include pelvic radiation, pelvic surgery, and gastrointestinal diseases such as diverticulitis, colon cancer, and Crohn's disease. Treatment is typically surgical separation.

Overflow incontinence results from weak or absent bladder contractions, leading to urinary retention and overdistension of the bladder. The bladder empties only when its capacity is exceeded. Patients may present with a complaint of constant dribbling. This atonic bladder may result from afferent nerve fiber destruction, resulting in the lack of transmission of stretch signals from the bladder wall. Other causes include certain medications, outflow obstruction (as in benign prostatic hyperplasia [BPH]), or even postoperative overdistension. Self-catheterization may be necessary if medical management is not sufficient.

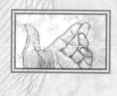

CLINICAL APPLICATION

WHAT IS A URINARY TRACT INFECTION?

Melissa, age 30, has no significant past medical history. She lives alone and does not smoke or drink. She reports to her doctor that she's been feeling "this burning when I go to the bathroom all day." The discomfort has worsened, and Melissa has also experienced increased urinary frequency and very small urine volumes. She complains of a vague discomfort in her lower abdomen immediately after she finishes urinating. She has no fever or chills and no tenderness at the costovertebral angles on the back (location of the kidneys). Examination of the urine reveals a high white blood cell count. The doctor prescribes a sulfa antibiotic for acute uncomplicated **urinary tract infection (UTI)**.

A UTI is a bacterial infection of the urethra that spreads to the bladder, where it causes inflammation. (Inflammation of the bladder is called *cystitis*.) These infections may be complicated by ascent of the infection to the kidneys (*pyelonephritis*), and they may be chronic or recurring. Most often, they are acute and uncomplicated. The cystitis causes increased detrusor contraction, leading to increased frequency and urgency. Urethritis and cystitis cause a burning sensation upon urination and pain in the area of the bladder.

Treatment is with antibiotics and sometimes with phenazopyridine, an analgesic that distributes well to the urinary space. Prophylaxis should address the risk factors for UTI. UTIs are often caused by *E. coli* bacteria from the rectum. Consequently, women should wipe from front to back to avoid contaminating the urethra with rectal *E. coli*. Urination shortly after sexual intercourse may also decrease the risk of infection. Some studies indicate that drinking cranberry juice may help prevent UTIs.

Summary

- Urine is ready for excretion once it leaves the renal tubular collecting ducts. From the collecting ducts, it flows into the renal calyces, the renal pelvis, the ureter, and into the bladder.

- The calyces, pelvis, and ureter help push the urine down the ureter through elastic and peristaltic contraction. The muscular wall of the bladder compresses the ureters and acts as a one-way valve to prevent urinary backflow.

- The detrusor muscle in the bladder wall squeezes the urine during urination but is normally relaxed. The internal and external sphincters open during urination but are normally contracted.

- Three nerves mediate the spinal micturition reflex: hypogastric (sympathetic), pelvic (parasympathetic), and pudendal (somatic).

- Afferent signals detect stretch in the bladder walls when the bladder fills with urine. These signals travel via the pelvic nerve to the spinal cord and return efferents via the hypogastric and pelvic nerves. The efferent signals trigger detrusor contraction and sphincter relaxation.

- The reflex occurs intermittently, leading to spikes in intravesical (intrabladder) pressure. The spikes increase in amplitude and frequency as urine volume climbs.

- Firing from upper motor neurons inhibits the spinal micturition reflex and keeps the external sphincter contracted. The conscious reduction of upper motor neuron inhibition allows the micturition reflex to occur unimpeded, and urination occurs. Loss of upper motor neurons due to neurologic injury or disease can result in a hyperactive micturition reflex.

- Incontinence and other difficulties with urination may arise from neurologic or structural factors.

- The four varieties of incontinence are stress incontinence, urge incontinence, total incontinence, and overflow incontinence.

Suggested Reading

Chai TC, Steers WD. Neurophysiology of micturition and continence. Urol Clin N Am. 1996;23(2):221–236.

Fihn S. Clinical practice. Acute uncomplicated urinary tract infection in women. N Engl J Med. 2003;17;349(3):259–266.

Oesterling JE. Benign prostatic hyperplasia: medical and minimally invasive treatment options. N Engl J Med. 1995;332(2):99–108.

Shefchyk HJ. Spinal cord neural organization controlling the urinary bladder and striated sphincter. Prog Brain Res. 2002;137:71–82.

REVIEW QUESTIONS

Directions: Each of the numbered items or incomplete statements in this section is followed by answers or by completions of the statement. Select the ONE lettered answer or completion that is BEST in each case.

1. A 25-year-old man is stabbed multiple times in the lower back and pelvis, damaging one of the nerves that innervate the bladder. If he goes on to develop an atonic bladder and overflow incontinence, he is likely to have damaged neurons in which location?

    (A) pelvic nerves
    (B) hypogastric nerves
    (C) pudendal nerves
    (D) pontine micturition center
    (E) cerebral cortex

2. A 64-year-old postmenopausal woman with two grown children, both delivered vaginally, reports occasional incontinence after coughing or laughing. Her incontinence likely results from which of the following mechanisms?

    (A) involuntary bladder contraction
    (B) increased pelvic relaxation
    (C) neurogenic bladder
    (D) leakage from a urinary fistula
    (E) urinary retention due to obstruction

3. A 72-year-old man reports increased frequency of urination but decreased amounts of urine relative to several years ago. On urinary catheterization, he is found to have an increased postvoid residual, which might result from which of the following?

    (A) Crohn's disease
    (B) urinary tract infection
    (C) increased pelvic relaxation
    (D) history of diverticulitis
    (E) prostate cancer

ANSWERS TO REVIEW QUESTIONS

1. **The answer is** A. The primary nerve supply of the bladder, the pelvic nerves, arises from the sacral plexus. Damage to these nerves would result in difficulty stimulating the contraction of the bladder wall for micturition. The hypogastric nerves are responsible for closure of the internal sphincter, which facilitates urine storage. The pudendal nerves are responsible for contracting the external sphincter. The cortex and pontine micturition center normally inhibit the micturition reflex and maintain contraction of the external sphincter. Voluntary removal of these inhibitory signals allows urination to occur.

2. **The answer is** B. This patient suffers from stress incontinence, which involves the leakage of urine in situations of increased straining or abdominal pressure. This often occurs in the setting of increased pelvic relaxation, which is a consequence of vaginal deliveries. Urge incontinence, which involves leakage secondary to uninhibited, involuntary bladder contraction, causes urinary urgency and increased frequency. Total incontinence is characterized by leakage of urine as soon as it enters the bladder, and typically results from a urinary fistula. Overflow incontinence may lead to constant urinary dribbling due to overdistention of the bladder, and may result from obstruction.

3. **The answer is** E. This patient's increased postvoid residual results from outflow obstruction, which might occur with prostate cancer in a male. Crohn's disease and diverticulitis might predispose a patient to develop urinary fistulas, which would lead to urinary leakage, not retention. A urinary tract infection would be likely to result in frequent bladder emptying, not increased urinary retention. Increased pelvic relaxation is likely to result in stress incontinence, and is more frequent in women.

Part VII

GASTROINTESTINAL PHYSIOLOGY

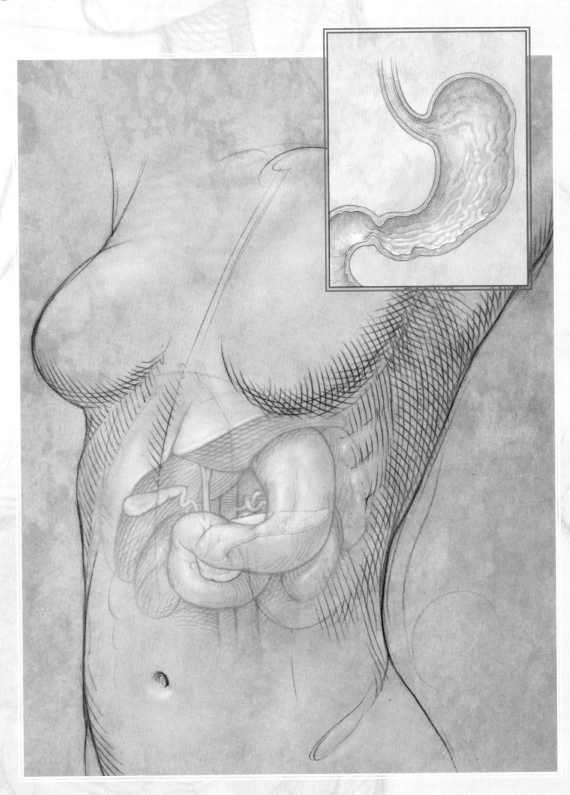

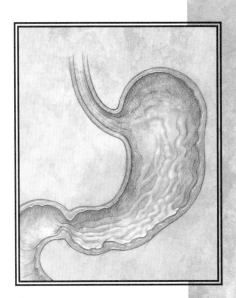

27

Nutrition, Digestion, and Absorption

INTRODUCTION

The gastrointestinal (GI) system supplies the fuel and the building blocks for the functioning of the body through the digestion and absorption of nutrients. Its machinery for doing so is the **alimentary canal**, also called the *gastrointestinal tract*, a highly specialized long tube that connects the mouth and the anus. Food and water enter the tract at the mouth and are propelled forward by muscular action. The food is digested and absorbed along the path to the anus and indigestible materials are expelled. The tube is subdivided into successive functional units: the mouth, pharynx, esophagus, stomach, small intestine (duodenum, jejunum, and ileum), large intestine, and anus. Muscular sphincters and one-way valves open and close portals between many of the units. The ducts of various secretory organs also open onto the lumen of the gut along the way. Associated organs include the salivary glands, the liver (and the gallbladder), and the pancreas.

The GI system provides the body with the water, vitamins, minerals, carbohydrates, proteins, and lipids (fats and cholesterol) essential for the maintenance of homeostasis. These substances are the body's structural materials and energy sources. They maintain the delicate internal milieu and are the reactants for the myriad biochemical reactions of metabolism. In addition, the GI system handles and eliminates many of the biochemical waste products of metabolism. While providing for the absorption of essential nutrients, the GI tract must also serve a critical barrier function, protecting the components of the body fluids from loss into the intestinal lumen, and at the same time preventing entry of toxic substances and organisms found in the environment (and therefore in the lumen of the digestive tract).

SYSTEM STRUCTURE

In general, the GI tract can be viewed as a hollow tube surrounded by a wall consisting of four layers. Starting from the inside, they are the mucosa, submucosa, muscularis, and serosa (FIGURE 27.1). The *mucosa* consists of an epithelial lining, a lamina propria (loose connective tissue, blood vessels, lymphatics), and a muscularis mucosae. The *submucosa* is like the lamina propria but its connective tissue is denser and it contains nerves. The *muscularis* contains two layers of smooth muscle. The inner layer of smooth muscle is circular (muscle fibers running around the circumference of the gut) and the outer layer of smooth muscle is arranged longitudinally (muscle fibers running along the length of the gut). Interposed between these two layers is the myenteric nerve plexus. The *serosa* is a thin layer of connective tissue

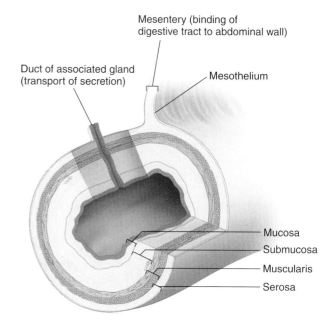

Figure 27.1 Cutaway view of a segment of the GI tract. The GI tract is essentially a hollow tube surrounded by a wall consisting of four main layers: from inside to out, the mucosa, submucosa, muscularis, and serosa.

consisting of blood vessels, lymphatics, adipose tissue, and a simple squamous epithelium, sometimes called a mesothelium. The neural innervation of the GI tract will be discussed in detail in Chapter 28.

In the intestine, the epithelial cells of the mucosa are called **enterocytes**. Enterocytes have a **luminal (or apical) membrane**, which faces the alimentary lumen, the hollow in the center of the digestive tract, and a **basolateral membrane**, which faces the interstitial lamina propria and the blood supply. Factors that aid in digestion are secreted across the luminal membrane, and foodstuffs are absorbed by facilitated diffusion and active transport across the luminal and then the basolateral membrane. Then they move on into the bloodstream for distribution to the tissues. This division of the intestinal epithelium into apical and basolateral membranes (with differing transporters on each side) is found in the epithelia of many organ systems. Other examples are the epithelium of the thyroid follicles and the epithelium of the renal tubules.

The abdominal portions of the digestive tract are supplied by the celiac and mesenteric arteries; venous blood collects into the **portal vein**, which then branches into a venous capillary bed within the liver. This is the portal circulation, where two capillary beds are arrayed in sequence—first the capillaries supplying arterial blood to the digestive tract, then the capillaries distributing the blood to the hepatic tissues for metabolism.

The Oral Cavity

Digestion begins in the **oral cavity**, which contains the tongue, teeth, and **salivary glands** (FIGURE 27.2). Three paired salivary glands are associated with the oral cavity—the *parotid, submandibular,* and *sublingual glands*—and smaller salivary glands are scattered throughout the mouth. Within the glands are two types of secretory cells, the serous (protein-secreting) and mucous (mucus-secreting) cells, and an associated duct system leading from the glands to the oral cavity.

The Stomach

The pharynx is a transitional zone conveying food from the oral cavity to the esophagus. Food leaves the esophagus, passes through the **lower esophageal sphincter**, and enters the stomach. The **stomach** consists of four main regions (in proximal to distal order): the cardia, fundus, body, and pylorus. On the macroscopic level, the stomach's mucosa is bunched into *rugae* (similar to the bladder), which increase the surface area of the stomach and allow for expansion and filling. On a microscopic level, the surface mucosa of the stomach invaginates to form *gastric pits*.

Emptying into the gastric pits are branched tubular *gastric glands*, whose function is different in each region of the stomach. The *cardia*, a narrow (<3 cm) band at the junction of the distal esophagus and stomach, contains glands that secrete mucus and *lysozyme* (which hydrolyzes bacterial cell walls). The glands of the *fundus* and *body* contain most of the stomach's *parietal cells*, which secrete hydrochloric acid. Parietal cells populate the upper half of the gastric glands, while chief cells populate the lower half. *Chief cells* produce and secrete enzymes for the

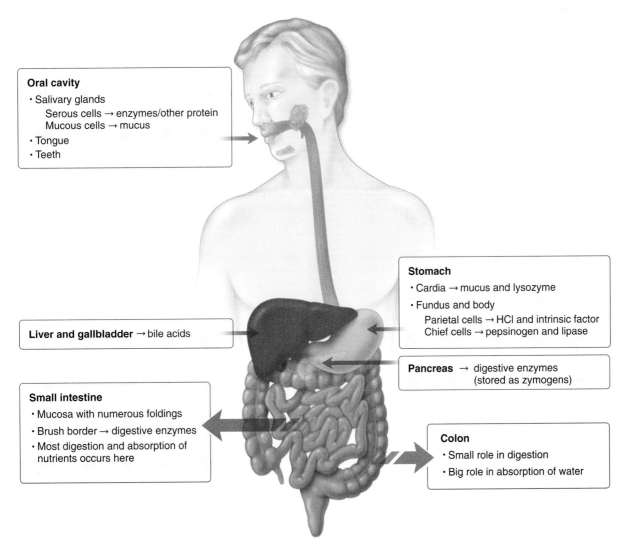

Oral cavity
- Salivary glands
    Serous cells → enzymes/other protein
    Mucous cells → mucus
- Tongue
- Teeth

Liver and gallbladder → bile acids

Small intestine
- Mucosa with numerous foldings
- Brush border → digestive enzymes
- Most digestion and absorption of nutrients occurs here

Stomach
- Cardia → mucus and lysozyme
- Fundus and body
    Parietal cells → HCl and intrinsic factor
    Chief cells → pepsinogen and lipase

Pancreas → digestive enzymes (stored as zymogens)

Colon
- Small role in digestion
- Big role in absorption of water

Figure 27.2   Overview of the GI tract organs and their roles.

digestion of protein and fat. Specifically, they contain cytoplasmic granules full of pepsinogen and lipase.

A small amount of absorption takes place in the stomach (fat only). However, most absorption of nutrients takes place after the partially digested food, or *chyme*, passes beyond the **pyloric sphincter**, which divides the stomach from the small intestine.

The Small Intestine

The **small intestine** is the last and most important site of food digestion and food absorption (but not the last site of water absorption). It consists of three segments (in proximal to distal order): the **duodenum**, **jejunum**, and **ileum**. These segments are coiled and tethered to the posterior wall of the abdominal cavity by the fatty *mesentery*, which contains the intestinal blood vessels.

The structure of the small intestine is well suited for digestion and absorption. Its great length (approximately 5 m) permits prolonged contact between food and enzymes and between digested foodstuffs and the absorptive lining. The small intestine also has a large surface area for digestion and absorption, achieved through numerous folds in the mucosa (FIGURE 27.3). The folds of the mucosa and submucosa are visible to the naked eye and are called *plicae circulares*. The plicae circulares are in turn ruffled into finger-shaped outgrowths of mucosa called **villi**, which are around 1 mm long. Finally, *microvilli* are located on the luminal (apical) surface of absorptive cells in the small intestine. Each microvillus (1 μm tall by 0.1 μm in diameter) is a cylindrical protrusion of apical cytoplasm and cell membrane-enclosing actin filaments. Each absorptive cell bears about 3,000 microvilli. The plicae circulares are most prominent in the jejunum, and their presence triples the surface area of the intestine. The villi increase the surface area by approximately 10-fold and the microvilli by 20-fold.

Microvilli bear enzymes bound to their membranes. These enzymes hydrolyze complex carbohydrates and peptides into simple sugars and amino acids. In between the villi, tubular glands (also called the crypts of Lieberkuhn) open onto the intestinal lumen. The glands consist of primarily of stem cells that divide and replace lost epithelial cells and the other intestinal cells found on the villi: mucus-producing cells (goblet cells), lysozyme-producing cells (Paneth cells), and enteroendocrine cells.

Carrier molecules are present in the apical membrane of intestinal enterocytes. These proteins enable specific substances in the lumen to be absorbed into the enterocyte. Also, Na$^+$/K$^+$-ATPase molecules, which utilize energy from the hydrolysis of ATP to pump Na$^+$ ions out of the enterocyte, are located on

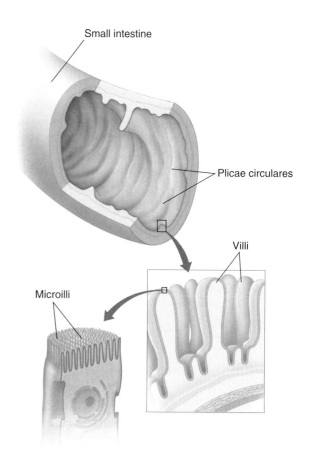

Figure 27.3 Folds of the small intestine. The folds are shown at progressive levels of magnification.

the basolateral membrane of the absorptive cell. The absorption of certain nutrients, such as sugars and amino acids, is directly linked to the Na$^+$ gradients that are established by this ion pump. In addition to absorption through the various carrier mechanisms, some molecules can be absorbed through the **tight junctions** between epithelial cells.

The blood vessels that remove the products of digestion from the small intestine penetrate the muscularis to form a submucosal capillary network. From there, branches of the plexus penetrate the muscularis mucosae and lamina propria to supply the villi. At the tip of each villus is a capillary network that drains into veins of the submucosal plexus (FIGURE 27.4). (These veins drain into the mesenteric veins, which in turn empty into the portal vein that carries blood to the liver.) **Lymphatics** (lymph vessels), which are important for the absorption of lipids, are also located in each villus. Lymphatics begin as blind-ended vessels within the villus. These vessels join and are known as *lacteals*. Lacteals anastomose to form the lymphatic drainage of the intestine, which eventually drains into the thoracic duct. The thoracic duct empties into the systemic venous circulation at the left subclavian and brachiocephalic veins.

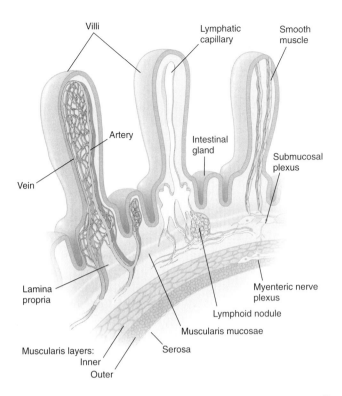

Figure 27.4 Structure of the villi. Nutrients absorbed by the villi pass directly into the plasma through capillaries or into the lymphatic system, which empties its contents into the thoracic duct. The thoracic duct in turn empties into the subclavian vein.

The Pancreas, Liver, and Gallbladder

The pancreas and liver are important secretory organs that empty their products into the duodenum. The **pancreas** is both an *exocrine organ* (secreting substances out of the body, into the GI lumen) and an *endocrine organ* (secreting hormones into the body via the bloodstream). It is the exocrine portion of the pancreas that participates in digestion by producing and secreting a host of important enzymes. Like the parotid gland, the exocrine pancreas is organized into *acini*, which are small groups of serous (protein-secreting) cells clustered around a secretory duct. Pancreatic acinar cells contain granules loaded with inactive digestive enzyme precursors called **zymogens**. When stimulated, the acini dump their zymogens into the **pancreatic duct**, which empties into the **ampulla of Vater**. The ampulla in turn leads directly to the duodenum.

The **liver** also plays a key role in digestion, mainly through its production of *bile acids*, which are essential for the digestion of lipids. Once bile is produced, the **gallbladder**, a hollow pear-shaped organ on the undersurface of the liver, concentrates and stores it. The gallbladder empties 30 to 50 mL of bile when activated. Mucus-secreting cells are also present in the gallbladder and produce the mucus found in bile. Bile is collected from the liver into the *common hepatic duct*, which communicates with the gallbladder via the *cystic duct*. At the point where the cystic and hepatic ducts join, they are called the **common bile duct**. The common bile duct joins the pancreatic duct at the ampulla of Vater, which conducts bile and pancreatic secretions into the duodenum. Some of the other critical roles of the liver will be discussed in Chapter 29.

The Large Intestine

When all the foodstuffs the body requires have been digested and absorbed, the remaining water, salt, and solids pass through the **ileocecal valve** into the large intestine. The main function of the **large intestine**, also called the *colon*, is to absorb water and ions (Na^+, Cl^-) that escape absorption in the small intestine. Once the process of absorption of salt and water is complete, **feces** are formed from dietary residua. Unlike the small intestine, the colonic mucosal membrane has no folds or villi except in the rectum. However, like the small intestine, the large intestine contains a large number of absorptive cells that contain Na^+/K^+-ATPase molecules on the basolateral membrane, as well as carrier molecules on the apical surface for ion absorption.

SYSTEM FUNCTION

A typical diet consists of carbohydrates, fats, and proteins, which are used to meet the maintenance, growth, and energy needs of the body. However, before the body is able to absorb and utilize what is ingested, these nutrients must first be broken down from macromolecules into their component building blocks. The process of breaking down ingested nutrients is called **digestion**. In the case of carbohydrate digestion, polysaccharides and disaccharides are processed into monosaccharides. Triglycerides are digested into glycerol and fatty acids. Protein is digested into its component amino acids. Nucleic acids (DNA and RNA) are degraded into their constituent bases, which in some cases are further modified.

While different enzymes and different intestinal locations are involved in the digestion of the various classes of nutrients, one basic chemical process is used in the digestion of all the major types of food: **hydrolysis**. Its general formula is as follows, where R represents an undefined organic group:

$$R''-R' + H_2O \rightarrow R''OH + R'H$$

During this process, substrate-specific enzymes catalyze the addition of water to a macromolecule, leading to its breakdown. Hydrolysis is the opposite of *condensation*, which forms larger molecules from smaller building blocks. FIGURE 27.5 shows the chemical structure of macromolecules and the process of hydrolysis to building blocks.

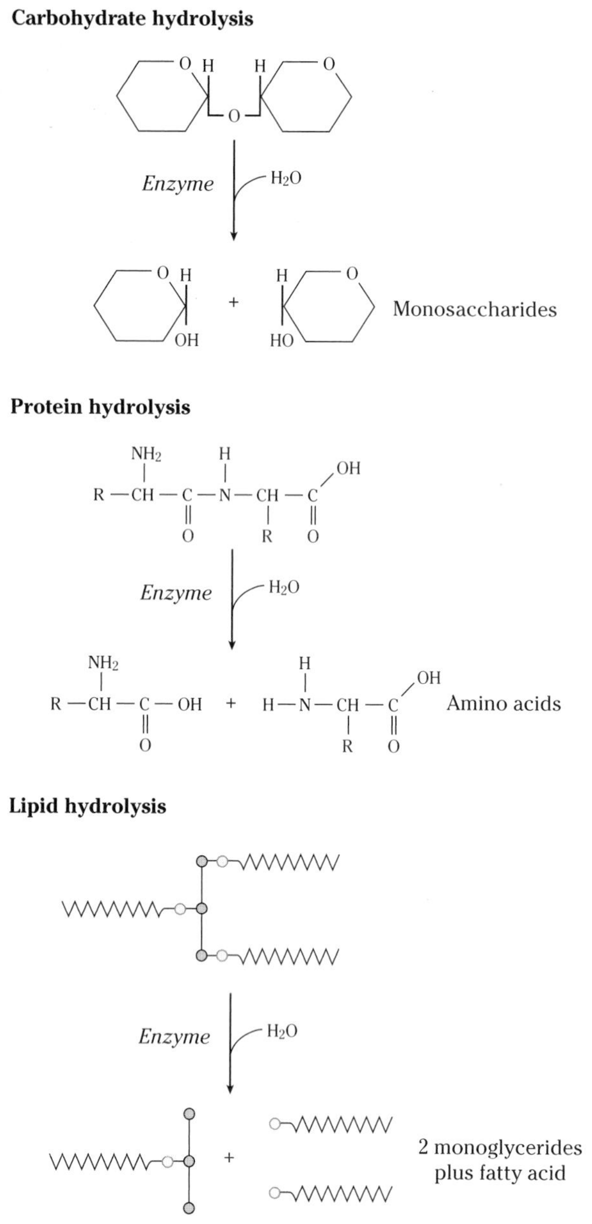

Carbohydrate hydrolysis

Protein hydrolysis

Lipid hydrolysis

Figure 27.5 Hydrolysis of macronutrients. Hydrolysis degrades the macronutrients into their building blocks.

Digestion is followed by **absorption**, wherein nutrients are transferred from the intestinal lumen into the bloodstream for delivery to the periphery. Absorptive processes, like digestive ones, vary from one nutrient class to another. However, there are several recurring absorptive mechanisms, including active transport, diffusion, and solvent drag. *Active transport* is an energy-requiring process in which a substance is usually transported against its concentration gradient. *Diffusion* occurs when a substance is transported along its concentration gradient, thus requiring no energy expenditure. *Solvent drag* occurs when water (the primary physiologic solvent) is absorbed in bulk quantities, "dragging" with it the solutes in the water.

We will consider, in turn, the mechanisms of digestion and absorption for each class of nutrients, along with the importance of nutrients to physiological functioning and their sources in the diet. At least 6 of the 10 leading causes of death in the United States (heart disease, cancer, hypertension, stroke, diabetes, and liver disease) are related to the American diet. Thus, understanding **nutrition**—the relationship of diet to health and disease—is critical for a well-educated physician.

Metabolism: The Reason We Eat

A few biochemical definitions are useful in considering the nutritional value of substrates in the diet. **Metabolism** encompasses the sum of all the energy transactions by which living tissues are produced and maintained. Metabolic processes are divided into two main categories: **anabolic reactions**, the synthesis of macromolecules from building blocks, a process requiring energy, and **catabolic reactions**, the breakdown of macromolecules into simpler substances, thereby releasing energy. The catabolism of energy-storing molecules from outside the body is necessary to conduct the anabolic reactions of life, such as replacing old tissues with new, the growth of new tissue, and the healing of damaged tissue. Catabolic reactions are also necessary for the transduction of *chemical energy* into other forms of energy the body needs. Chemical energy is transduced into *mechanical energy* in muscles, into *electrical energy* in muscles and nerves, and into *heat energy* in all body tissues. Because the forms of energy are interchangeable, dietary energy is expressed in terms of heat—calories or kilocalories—even though most of that dietary chemical energy will be put to other uses. A **calorie** is defined as the amount of heat required to raise 1 gram of water 1 degree Celsius in temperature. A **kilocalorie (kcal)** is defined as the amount of heat needed to raise 1 kilogram of water 1 degree Celsius in temperature.

All the chemical energy stored in food derives ultimately from nuclear fusion and fission in the sun. These reactions cast *photoenergy* onto Earth that is captured in chemical bonds by the anabolic process of photosynthesis in algae and plants. Animals eat the plants; they oxidize the plants' carbohydrates, fats, and proteins; and they thereby extract the energy for their own anabolism. Human beings eat animal products and plants to capture this photoenergy.

All organisms invest captured energy in storage forms (in animals, glycogen and fat). If the diet does not provide enough calories to fuel metabolism, the body will catabolize these internal energy stores. When the internal energy stores are exhausted, metabolism will require catabolic breakdown of tissues that are not meant to store energy but nevertheless contain energy, such as the protein in muscle. Organic molecules yield energy in the following amounts:

- 1 gram of protein yields 4 kcal
- 1 gram of carbohydrate yields 4 kcal
- 1 gram of fat yields 9 kcal
- 1 gram of alcohol yields 7 kcal

Basal metabolic rate (BMR) refers to the rate of catabolism necessary to sustain the vital functions of life. In a subject at rest, BMR can be measured by either the heat generated or the amount of oxygen consumed by the body per unit time. The metabolic rate may be lifted above its basal level during exercise and in a host of other physiologic and pathologic states. The hormones epinephrine and thyroxine influence the metabolic rate. BMR can be determined by measuring the *resting energy expenditure (REE)* at least 12 hours after a meal. The *Harris-Benedict equations* are one way to estimate the REE:

$$66 + 13.7 \text{ (weight in kg)} + 5 \text{ (height in cm)}$$
$$- 6.8 \text{ (age)} = \text{REE in kcal/day, men}$$

$$655 + 9.6 \text{ (weight in kg)} + 1.7 \text{ (height in cm)}$$
$$- 4.7 \text{ (age)} = \text{REE in kcal/day, women}$$

These equations are consistent with a caloric requirement of around 1,500 kcal/day in the average adult. Such calculations are useful in the hospital, especially during the delivery of parenteral nutrition (i.e., intravenous nutrition that is *para*, alongside, the intestinal or *enteral* route).

When enough energy is captured in the diet, that energy is invested in anabolism, but it is not the only dietary ingredient invested in anabolism. *Food provides not just energy but also raw materials for anabolism.* The organic molecules consumed in the diet are literally incorporated into the organism that has consumed them. Various enzymes help convert one form of organic nutrient into another, but some nutrients cannot be manufactured from other ones and hence must be present in the diet. Most vitamins and minerals are required elements of the diet. Vitamin deficiencies may lead to a wide array of disease states.

Carbohydrates

Carbohydrates are a class of organic compounds made of carbon, hydrogen, and oxygen with hydrogen and oxygen present in the ratio of water (two atoms of hydrogen for each atom of oxygen). Carbohydrates are made from various species of **monosaccharides**, which often have six carbons and

form a ring, as glucose does. Chains of monosaccharides are called **polysaccharides**.

Carbohydrates in the Diet Carbohydrates are the major source of calories in a typical diet. The monosaccharide glucose is the sole source of energy for the brain, and the oxidation of carbohydrates is the preferred mode of energy extraction all over the body. Carbohydrates are not essential to the diet, however, as they can be manufactured in the body when they are scarce in the diet. This is called *gluconeogenesis*: the manufacture of glucose from noncarbohydrate organic compounds.

There are both digestible and nondigestible carbohydrates. The digestible dietary carbohydrates are starches, monosaccharides, and disaccharides (two monosaccharides linked together). Most dietary carbohydrate is starch. **Starches** are complex polysaccharides composed of long chains of glucose molecules linked by α-1,4 glycosidic bonds. Side branches of glucose are connected to the main chain via α-1,6 glycosidic bonds. The most abundant starch is *amylopectin*, a plant starch. Another dietary starch is *glycogen*, an animal starch. Bread and pasta, which contain flour, are major sources of starch. Flour is milled from wheat—a cereal grain (type of grass). Corn and rice are other grasses that are major sources of starchy fuel for the world's population.

The main monosaccharides in the diet are *glucose* and *fructose*, found in honey and fruit. Important examples of **disaccharides** are *lactose* (found in dairy products), *maltose* (found in beer), and *sucrose* (table sugar). Sucrose is harvested from sugar cane and sugar beets.

Nondigestible carbohydrates, referred to collectively as **dietary fiber**, include *cellulose*, a β-1,4-linked glucose polymer. Cellulose is a major source of dietary fiber found in grasses and leaves. It is not digestible because the enzyme capable of hydrolyzing β-1,4 glucose linkages is not present in the human intestine. Species that can digest cellulose, such as horses and other grazing herbivores, play host to symbiotic gut bacteria that make *cellulase* for them. (Only a few animals can make cellulase themselves; one example is the insect commonly known as the silverfish.)

Carbohydrate Digestion The digestion of carbohydrates is critical because the intestines can absorb only monosaccharides such as glucose, galactose, and fructose. Carbohydrate digestion begins in the mouth, where food is ground into smaller pieces by the action of the teeth and tongue. Here it is also mixed with saliva. Salivary secretions contain **salivary α-amylase**, an enzyme that hydrolyzes α-1,4 bonds (but not α-1,6 branchpoint linkages). The main products of digestion by α-amylase are maltotriose (three glucose molecules joined by α-1,4 bonds), maltose (two glucose molecules joined by an α-1,4 bond), and α-limit dextrins (two or three glucose molecules joined by α-1,4 bonds with a glucose side-chain of two of three molecules joined to the main chain by an α-1,6 bond). FIGURE 27.6 summarizes the digestion of carbohydrates by α-amylase. Before swallowing occurs, approximately 5% of dietary starch is digested.

Carbohydrate digestion continues in the stomach until salivary α-amylase is inactivated by the stomach's acidic environment. It is estimated that 30% to 40% of dietary starch is digested before food leaves the stomach. After leaving the stomach, the acidic and partially digested food and enzyme mixture called *chyme* enters the small intestine and mixes with pancreatic secretions containing **pancreatic α-amylase**. This α-amylase is much more powerful than the salivary form. Soon after entering the intestines nearly all the starch is digested. At this point, carbohydrate is in the form of maltose, maltotriose, α-limit dextrins, and other small glucose polymers.

Digestion to monosaccharides occurs in the duodenum and jejunum, which contain **intestinal disaccharidases** in the brush border of the epithelial membrane. The major brush border enzymes are α-dextrinase, maltase, sucrase, and lactase, which hydrolyze disaccharides to glucose, fructose, and galactose (FIGURE 27.7). Once digested to these monosac-

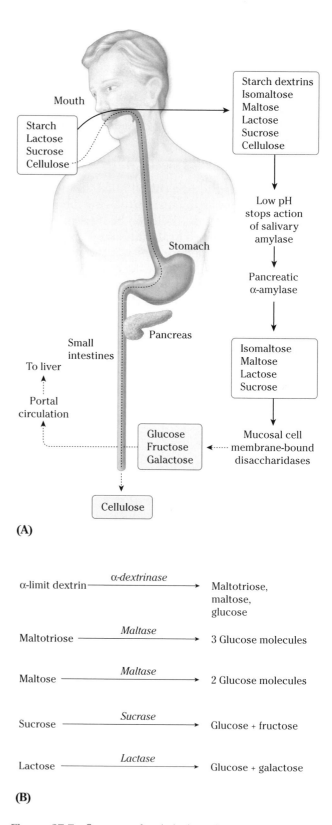

(A)

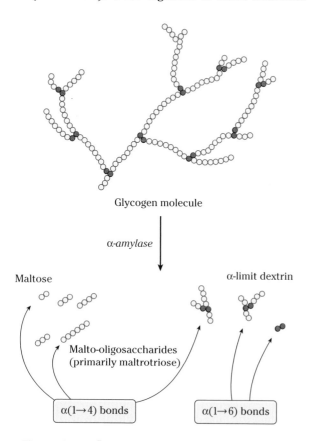

Figure 27.6   Digestion of carbohydrates by α-amylase.

(B)

Figure 27.7   Summary of carbohydrate digestion. **A.** Carbohydrate digestion at each location in the GI tract. **B.** Hydrolytic reactions involved in carbohydrate digestion.

charides, absorption is possible. About 80% of ingested carbohydrate is digested to and absorbed as glucose. Most carbohydrate absorption occurs in the upper small intestine (duodenum and upper jejunum).

Carbohydrate Absorption   The absorption of glucose and galactose occurs via a *cotransport* (or symport) mechanism linked to the absorption of sodium (FIGURE 27.8). This is a form of *secondary active transport*. The process is considered "secondary" because the absorption of the sugars is dependent on a sodium gradient established by the Na⁺/K⁺ pump, rather than ATP directly. The process is considered "active" since ATP is required to fuel the pump that generates the Na⁺ gradient.

The absorption of sodium, to which the absorption of glucose and galactose is linked, can be thought of as occurring in two stages. First, before apical sodium can be absorbed, an electrochemical gradient favoring absorption must first be established. This is accomplished through the active transport of sodium from the enterocyte cytoplasm through the basolateral membrane and into interstitial fluid and the paracellular spaces by **Na⁺/K⁺-ATPase** molecules located in the basolateral membrane of the enterocyte. After this transport process has occurred, the intracellular concentration of sodium is less than that in the lumen. This gradient favors the movement of sodium from the lumen into the cell.

The second stage of intestinal glucose or galactose absorption involves the absorption of sodium from the lumen via *facilitated diffusion*. This process is termed "facilitated" because it involves a carrier protein. The movement is considered "diffusion"

since it occurs in a direction *along* the concentration gradient for sodium. The process begins when sodium binds to a transport protein located in the brush border of the enterocyte. However, before the carrier changes configuration and allows the sodium into the cell, another substance, such as glucose or galactose, must bind to the protein as well. Once both the sugar and the sodium have bound to their appropriate sites on the Na⁺/monosaccharide symporter also known as the Na⁺/glucose cotransporter (SGLT1), they are simultaneously transported into the enterocyte. Sodium travels in a direction along its concentration gradient, while the sugar molecule travels in a direction opposite to its gradient. The concentrations of glucose and galactose increase within the enterocyte as transport continues. A gradient favoring the movement of the sugars into the interstitial space and then into the blood is eventually established. This final phase of glucose and galactose absorption is accomplished via passive or facilitated diffusion through a non- Na⁺-dependent glucose transporter (GLUT).

The absorption of fructose differs from that of glucose and galactose. It occurs by facilitated diffusion but does not involve a sodium cotransport mechanism. In addition, once fructose is present within the enterocyte, some of it is phosphorylated. This form of fructose can be used to generate ATP for cellular activities. It also can be converted to glucose, which is then absorbed along with other glucose molecules into the paracellular spaces.

Glucose may be produced in the intestinal lumen, by the action of disaccharidases such as maltase. If glucose is highly concentrated in the intestinal lumen, absorption can also occur via a solvent drag mechanism in addition to the Na⁺-cotransport process. When the concentration of glucose in the lumen is especially high, absorption by solvent drag can be double or triple that absorbed via sodium cotransport. However, it is the sodium cotransport that enables solvent drag to take place. As glucose is absorbed by Na⁺-cotransport, its concentration grows in the paracellular space. This increases the osmotic pressure in the paracellular space, which causes water to move from the intestinal lumen into the paracellular space. This movement of water occurs directly through intercellular junctions, bypassing the interior of the enterocyte. As fluid moves, glucose is "dragged" along with it. (See Integrated Physiology Box *Transcellular and Paracellular Transport*.)

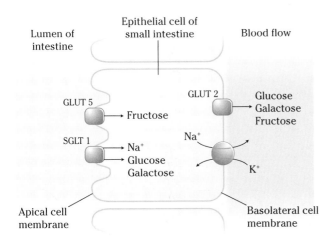

Figure 27.8 Absorption of glucose, galactose, and fructose. The absorption of glucose and galactose is sodium-coupled. The absorption of fructose is independent of sodium. SGLT, sodium glucose transporter.

Proteins

Proteins are critical structural and functional units in living things. They bind cells together in the extracellular matrix and compose the filaments of the

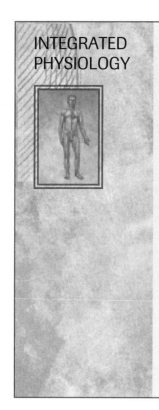

INTEGRATED PHYSIOLOGY

Transcellular and Paracellular Transport

Glucose transport in the intestines exemplifies the two general mechanisms of transepithelial transport in the body, transcellular and paracellular, and demonstrates the roles, regulation, and coordination of these forms of transport. Transcellular pathways depend on specialized, selective, and saturable transporters within the cell membranes. The paracellular pathway, with the rate-limiting step of transport across the barrier located at the tight junction (zona occludens), is the pathway of least resistance and greater capacity. The paracellular pathway is less specific in that small molecules are generally permeable, although cations are more permeant than anions. The paracellular pathway provides for intestinal barrier functions and helps the cell maintain its polarity for vectorial transport (directional movement across the cell). The cellular mechanisms of transport are regulated by neurohumoral (cell signaling pathways) as well as luminal influences such as solute concentrations. The paracellular pathways are influenced by the enteric nervous system (especially acetylcholine, which decreases paracellular conductance) and the nutritional state (decreased transport with fasting).

An example of the coordination of cellular and paracellular transport is observed when SGLT1 is activated. There follows an increase in tight junction permeability mediated by a contraction of cytoskeletal elements known as the actomyosin ring. The contraction is mediated by phosphorylation of myosin-regulating light-chain proteins.

---

cytoskeleton. They make up enzymes, intra- and extracellular signals, receptors, ion pumps, and ion channels, and they conjugate with other molecules to form compounds such as lipoproteins. Like the genetic code or written words, proteins are composed of just a small number of subunits—**amino acids**—lined up in a row. The chain of amino acids making up a protein is called a **peptide**. With different linear combinations and permutations of amino acids, different protein structures and functions are possible, just as different arrangements of letters or base pairs make different words or codons. While there are several hundred naturally occurring amino acids, mammals possess just 20.

Proteins in the Diet Proteins are necessary for growth to occur. In addition, the continuous breakdown of proteinaceous tissue in the body necessitates a fresh supply of amino acids to rebuild those tissues. This supply must come from the diet, because while amino acids can be metabolized to carbohydrates and fat, the reverse is not true. Carbohydrates and fats do not contain nitrogen, so they cannot alone generate protein. The nitrogen must come from dietary amino acids (and a few other nitrogen-containing biomolecules), which in turn owe their nitrogen content to the Earth's atmosphere. Inert N_2 composes 79% of dry air. Microorganisms, many of them living in symbiotic relationships with plants, make this inert nitrogen available to the biosphere for incorporation into amino acids. In the

process called **nitrogen fixation**, they transform inert N_2 into the reactive species ammonia (NH_3), thus acquiring for the global biosphere an annual supply of nearly 200 million metric tons of nitrogen.

Once some amino acids are ingested, providing a source of nitrogen, others can be generated from the nitrogen and carbon substrates. However, there are nine **essential amino acids** that cannot be synthesized by the human body; they must be consumed directly. The remaining 11 are the **nonessential amino acids**. These two demands—total amino nitrogen and essential amino acids—necessitate an average protein intake of 1 gram per kilogram of body weight per day. Poor caloric intake or high caloric expenditure can also influence protein needs. Such states result in the wasting of energy stores and the diversion of body protein to meet energy needs. Finally, anabolic states of growth (e.g., puberty, pregnancy, or wound healing) demand increased protein consumption. *Kwashiorkor* and *marasmus* are wasting syndromes that result from dietary protein and total energy deficiency, respectively. Major sources of protein in the diet include meat, fish, eggs, dairy, and vegetables. The intestines must also handle proteinaceous secretions from the intestine itself (mucin, digestive enzymes), sloughed epithelial cells, and bacteria.

Protein Digestion The digestion of protein begins in the stomach. Chief cells in the stomach secrete *pepsinogen*, which is converted to the active enzyme

WHAT IS PEPTIC ULCER DISEASE?

A 35-year-old man complains of "stomach pain" of several months' duration. The pain is described as a nagging ache or a burning sensation below the sternum. It is transiently relieved by taking Tums (a calcium carbonate antacid). The gastroenterologist performs an endoscopy with biopsy of the gastric and duodenal mucosa. The pathology reveals gastric metaplasia, ulceration of the duodenal epithelium, and colonization with the bacterium *Helicobacter pylori*. The diagnosis is peptic ulcer disease.

Peptic ulcer disease (PUD) affects 4 million Americans and costs the U.S. economy $20 billion annually. It can affect the gastric mucosa or the duodenal mucosa. In the United States duodenal ulcers are more common, but in Japan, the reverse is true. Peptic ulcers represent breakdowns in the intestinal epithelium that result from excess secretion of acid and a failure of the barriers that normally protect the mucosa from acid injury.

Two major causes of weakened mucosal defenses against acid are infection with *H. pylori* and the use of nonsteroidal anti-inflammatory drugs (NSAIDs). *H. pylori* is a bacterium that is adapted to life at low pH, such as in the human stomach. (It survives by hydrolyzing urea into ammonia to buffer the acidity.) Its presence causes inflammation that breaks down the protective mucosal barrier in the stomach. Injury to the duodenal wall (by acid hypersecretion) results in transformation of the duodenal epithelium into gastric mucosa (gastric metaplasia). This allows *H. pylori*, which is trophic for gastric tissue, to colonize the duodenum, worsening the duodenal injury.

NSAIDs interfere with prostaglandin-mediated defense mechanisms against gastric acidity: mucus production, bicarbonate secretion, and others. The most serious complications of PUD are hemorrhage and perforation of the digestive tract.

---

pepsin by gastric hydrochloric acid (HCl). As mentioned above, the principal reaction of protein digestion into constituent amino acids is enzymatic hydrolysis of peptide bonds, and pepsin catalyzes this hydrolysis. HCl is secreted by parietal cells in the stomach by an H^+/K^+-ATPase pump. (Activation of pepsinogen is one of the two major functions of acidity in the stomach. The other is protection against microbial pathogens in food; many bacteria cannot survive the acidity of the stomach. See Clinical Application Box *What Is Peptic Ulcer Disease?*)

There are several different kinds of **proteases** (enzymes that break down proteins). Pepsin is an *endopeptidase*, meaning it can cleave peptide bonds in the middle of (*endo-*, inside of) a peptide polymer. An enzyme that can cleave only a terminal peptide bond (i.e., one at the end of a polypeptide polymer) is called a *carboxypeptidase* (C-terminal) or an *aminopeptidase* (N-terminal). (Recall that amino acids are so named because they have an amino group on one side and an acidic carboxyl group on the other; thus, peptide chains must also have an amino group on one end and a carboxyl group on the other.) The actions of these enzymes are illustrated by the following equations, where A represents an amino acid with its amino terminus on the left:

$$A\text{-}A\text{-}A\text{-}A\text{-}A \xrightarrow{\text{endopeptidase}} A\text{-}A + A\text{-}A\text{-}A$$

$$A\text{-}A\text{-}A\text{-}A\text{-}A \xrightarrow{\text{aminopeptidase}} A + A\text{-}A\text{-}A\text{-}A$$

$$A\text{-}A\text{-}A\text{-}A\text{-}A \xrightarrow{\text{carboxypeptidase}} A\text{-}A\text{-}A\text{-}A + A$$

Approximately 10% to 20% of total protein is digested in the stomach by pepsin. Most protein digestion occurs in the duodenum and jejunum, catalyzed by proteases secreted by the exocrine pancreas. The pancreas secretes the inactive **zymogens** (proenzymes) *trypsinogen*, *chymotrypsinogen*, *procarboxypeptidases A* and *B*, and *proelastase* into the pancreatic duct. These forms are activated when they enter the intestine, and the mucosa of the duodenum and jejunum secretes the enzyme **enterokinase**. Enterokinase converts trypsinogen to *trypsin*. Trypsin then activates the other zymogens as well as more molecules of trypsinogen. Both trypsin and *chymotrypsin* contribute to protein digestion by cleaving internal peptide bonds. *Carboxypeptidase* cleaves C-terminal amino acids from the ends of protein molecules. *Elastase* digests elastin fibers in the connective tissues of ingested animal flesh.

The pancreas secretes the proenzymes that digest most dietary protein and the small bowel activates those enzymes. The combined actions of the pancreas and small bowel break the polypeptides into shorter chains. Digestion continues in the small intestine with the action of peptidases on the brush border. These enzymes cleave the peptide fragments into smaller and smaller bits until they are single amino acids, dipeptides, and tripeptides. All three of these peptide species are absorbed into the enterocytes, the mucosal cells lining the intestinal wall. Within the enterocyte cytosol, additional peptidases digest the di- and tripeptides to amino acids, which then pass into the bloodstream. The steps in protein digestion are summarized in FIGURE 27.9.

Protein Absorption Like the absorption of glucose, the absorption of amino acids, dipeptides, and tripeptides occurs through sodium-dependent secondary active transport (FIGURE 27.10). Na^+/K^+-

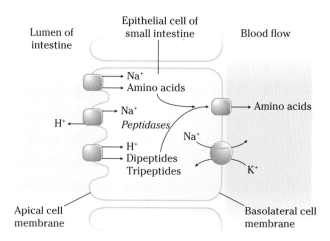

Figure 27.10 Absorption of amino acids, dipeptides, and tripeptides. Sodium-dependent active transport facilitates the absorption of these molecules.

ATPase pumps located in the basolateral membrane of enterocytes lower the intracellular concentration of sodium by transporting sodium into the paracellular spaces. This mechanism establishes a gradient favoring the transport of sodium from the intestinal lumen into the enterocytes. Sodium binds to a carrier protein located on the brush border of the enterocyte. However, before the carrier changes configuration, a peptide or amino acid molecule must bind to the carrier as well. Once both molecules have bound to the appropriate sites on the carrier, they are transported into the enterocyte. Four different carriers for amino acid transport are located in the intestinal brush border, each one specific for neutral, acidic, basic, or imino amino acids.

Small peptides are absorbed through a transporter protein with broad specificity. They are absorbed in a manner that also depends on the Na^+/K^+-ATPase but that is distinct from the mechanism of amino acid absorption. In the first phase, the Na^+/K^+-ATPase drives an influx of Na^+ across a Na^+/H^+ antiporter, which builds the luminal concentration of H^+ and leads to a flow of H^+ back into the cell. The movement of H^+ into the cell is coupled by a symporter to the movement of the small peptides, causing them to be absorbed. Once inside the enterocyte, cytoplasmic proteases digest the peptides to amino acids.

The second phase of protein absorption involves the transfer of amino acids through the basolateral membrane into the interstitial space and then into the mesenteric-portal venous system. This process occurs via both simple diffusion and facilitated diffusion. Up to 5% of dietary protein (1 to 3 g/day) is not absorbed from the small intestinal lumen, but rather passed on to the large intestine.

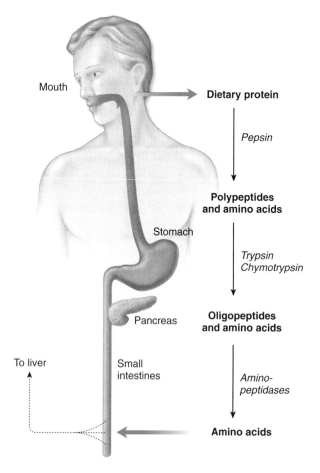

Figure 27.9 Summary of protein digestion.

In the adult minimal quantities of intact protein are absorbed by the intestine, but in newborns the transfer of certain proteins, particularly immunoglobulins (IgA), from mother's milk is important for immune function. These antibodies are protected from digestion by the neonatal intestinal enzymes in part because pancreatic and intestinal secretions are less at this time. The mechanism of transfer involves a receptor-mediated endocytic process that yields phagosomes that coalesce with lysosomes to accomplish intracellular digestion. Some intact IgA leaves the basolateral membrane and enters the circulation.

Lipids

Lipids are hydrophobic molecules that in most cases contain **fatty acids**, straight-chain hydrocarbons having a carboxyl group at one end. A prevalent variety of lipid is **triglyceride** (or triacylglycerol), which is composed of a glycerol backbone, from which hang three fatty acid subunits. Other forms of fatty acid-containing lipids are glycolipids, phospholipids, and cholesterol esters. (A cholesterol ester is a cholesterol with one fatty acid attached, but unesterified cholesterol is also considered a lipid.) Fatty acids may also be present alone and as such are called *free fatty acids*.

Fatty acids are classified according to their size (short chain, medium chain, long chain) and according to the number of double bonds between carbons. If the fatty acid has no double bonds, it is said to be *saturated* (with hydrogens, since single bonds between carbon and hydrogen replace double bonds between carbons). If the fatty acid contains one or more double bonds, it is said to be *unsaturated*; if one double bond, then *monounsaturated*; if more, *polyunsaturated*. Sixteen- and 18-carbon fatty acids are the most common in the body, although shorter and longer fatty acids are also present.

Lipids, the major constituent of all cell membranes, are found in association with carbohydrates and proteins. Lipids are also stored in adipose tissue, where they act as an energy reserve for metabolism and as a thyroid-stimulated source of body heat. In the skin, fat stores insulate the body against heat loss. Therefore, lipids are particularly important for homeothermic animals, and such animals tend to store surplus calories as fat. Poikilotherms, which do not maintain a constant body temperature and whose metabolic rates are much more variable, do not require (and so do not have) as much body fat. The lipid **cholesterol** is an important constituent of steroid hormones and bile acids (and, like other lipids, is present in cell membranes). Dietary lipids are important for the absorption of the fat-soluble vitamins A, D, E, and K.

Lipids in the Diet About 98% of total dietary lipid is made up of triglycerides. The fatty acids in triglycerides are saturated or unsaturated to varying degrees. If triglycerides contain highly saturated fatty acids, they are called *saturated fats*. Saturated fats are primarily of animal origin and are generally solid at room temperature. These fats contribute to cardiovascular risk by raising serum low-density lipoprotein levels in both animals and humans. High levels of low-density lipoprotein are associated with atherosclerosis (fat deposition in arterial walls).

Triglycerides containing unsaturated fatty acids are called *unsaturated fats*. Unsaturated fats are generally liquid at room temperature and may be polyunsaturated or monounsaturated. There are two major categories of polyunsaturated fats: omega-3 and omega-6 fatty acids. Polyunsaturated fats provide the essential omega-6 fatty acid *linoleic acid*. Linoleic acid cannot be synthesized by the body and must be provided in the diet. It is required for the synthesis of arachidonic acid, the precursor of prostaglandins. Fish oils contain omega-3 fatty acids. Monounsaturated fats do not appear to raise levels of low-density lipoproteins. Canola oil and olive oil contain the highest percentage of monounsaturated fat. Oleic acid is the major fatty acid found in these oils.

Lipid Digestion The digestion of lipids is complicated by the fact that lipids are insoluble in water, while the enzymes necessary for lipid digestion are water-soluble. Therefore, lipids and their breakdown products are emulsified in the GI tract. **Emulsification** is a process whereby a water-insoluble oil is finely divided and mixed with water, sometimes with the help of an **amphipathic** substance, a substance that has both hydrophobic and hydrophilic properties—in other words, it possesses affinities for both oil and water. (Saponified fat, also known as soap, is an example of an amphipathic emulsifier.) In the GI tract, emulsification increases fat's contact area with water, thus increasing the size of the water–oil interface at which digestive enzymes act.

Lipid digestion begins with the secretion of *gastric lipase* in the stomach. (Lingual lipase has been found in animals but not in humans.) Here, the enzyme begins to hydrolyze and cleave lipid bonds. Because less than 10% of total dietary lipid is digested in the stomach, normal lipid digestion can occur in the absence of gastric lipase. The stomach does play an important role in emulsification, however, by mechanically agitating the food. This breaks fat into smaller globules, increasing the surface area for digestion.

Lipids then pass from the stomach into the small intestine. Emulsification continues as the emulsifier called **bile**, produced in the liver and stored in the gallbladder, is secreted into the duodenum. Bile is an emulsifier because it is composed of amphipathic substances—cholesterol-based **bile salts** and the phospholipid *lecithin*. The fat-soluble components of bile dissolve into the fat globules, while the hydrophilic components project outward into the surrounding water (FIGURE 27.11). This increases the solubility of the lipids and lowers the surface tension of the fat globule. With lower surface tension and increased solubility, fragmentation into smaller emulsion droplets is possible.

Once the lipids have been emulsified, they are subject to the action of the powerful pancreatic enzymes that have been secreted into the duodenum. *Glycerol ester hydrolase* is a pancreatic lipase that cleaves fatty acids from triglycerides to yield two free fatty acids and one 2-monoglyceride (glycerol with one fatty acid attached to the glycerol's second carbon). *Cholesterol esterase* cleaves cholesterol esters to produce one fatty acid and free cholesterol. *Phospholipase A2* cleaves a fatty acid from phospholipids (leaving behind lysophospholipid).

As the lipids in the emulsion droplet are cleaved, the products of cleavage drift away and fresh dietary lipids from within the hydrophobic core of the emulsion droplet rise to the surface, where they too are cleaved. The cleavage products are handled in a special way that enables fat absorption (see below), and once inside the enterocytes, the cytoplasmic enzyme *enteric lipase* makes a small contribution to lipid digestion. See FIGURE 27.12 for a summary of lipid digestion.

Lipid Absorption   As noted above, the process of lipid absorption begins when lipid cleavage products are released from the emulsion droplets. At this

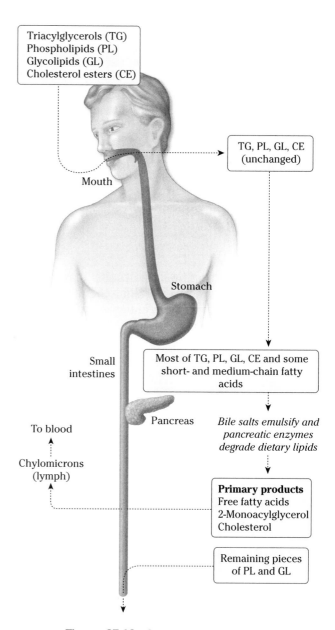

Figure 27.12   Summary of lipid digestion.

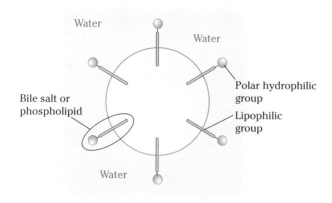

Figure 27.11   Emulsification of fats in the small intestine. Emulsion droplets form when lipids first mix with bile. Pancreatic digestion follows.

point, the cleavage products are organized into smaller emulsion droplets called **micelles** by the amphipathic bile salts (FIGURE 27.13). Micelles are 3 to 6 nm in diameter and contain approximately 20 to 40 molecules of bile salt. The cholesterol portions of the bile salt molecules aggregate in the center of the micelle along with the products of lipid digestion and fat-soluble vitamins, as in the emulsion droplet. The outer surface of the micelle is covered with the polar groups of the bile salts, making the micelle water-soluble so it can interact with the enterocytes' brush border. After contacting the brush border, the free fatty acids, 2-monoglycerides, and free cholesterol diffuse freely from the micelle through the enterocytes' luminal plasma membrane and into the interior of the cells. Meanwhile, the bile salts of the emptied

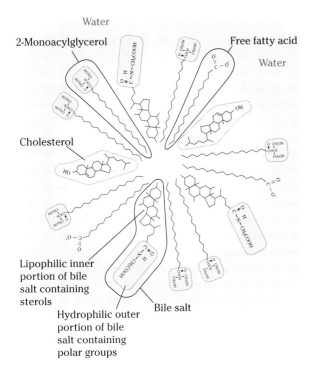

Figure 27.13 Role of micelles. Micelles emulsify the products of pancreatic digestion and deliver them to enterocytes for absorption.

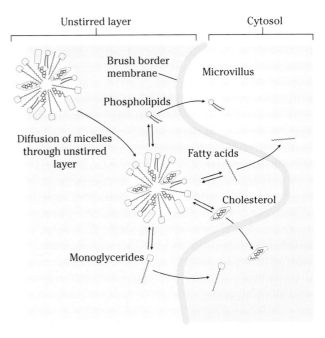

Figure 27.14 Absorption of lipid cleavage products by enterocytes.

micelle return to the intestinal lumen to form new micelles loaded with fresh cleavage products. A critical mass of bile salts is necessary for micelle formation. Impairments in the production, delivery, or activity of bile salts result in impaired fat absorption and the excretion of excess fat in the stool (steatorrhea).

The rate-limiting step in the absorption of lipids is the diffusion of micelles through the **unstirred layer**, the fluid immediately surrounding the brush border (FIGURE 27.14). This fluid does not mix readily with the rest of the lumen contents. However, a concentration gradient favors the passive diffusion of the lipid digestion products across the unstirred layer, toward the brush border, and into enterocytes. A pH gradient also exists across the unstirred layer: The side closest to the brush border has a lower pH. This favors the protonation of free fatty acids, which enhances their rate of diffusion into the intestinal cells.

Once inside the enterocyte, the products of lipid digestion are transported to the smooth endoplasmic reticulum (ER), where they are reconstituted into their original forms by a series of **re-esterification** reactions (FIGURE 27.15). These reactions reattach the fatty acids that were cleaved in the emulsion droplets. Free fatty acids and 2-monoglycerides are re-esterified to form new triglycerides. Lysophospholipid molecules and free fatty acids are re-esterified into new phospholipid molecules. Free cholesterol molecules and free fatty acids are re-esterified to form new cholesterol esters. In addition, after being

absorbed, some of the 2-monoglyceride molecules are digested into glycerol and free fatty acids by intracellular lipases. Inside the ER, these free fatty acid molecules are also reconstituted into new triglycerides.

After the process of re-esterification is complete, the new lipid particles aggregate in the Golgi apparatus and are processed to form lipoprotein spheres called **chylomicrons**. The chylomicron core contains cholesterol esters, triglycerides, and the hydropho-

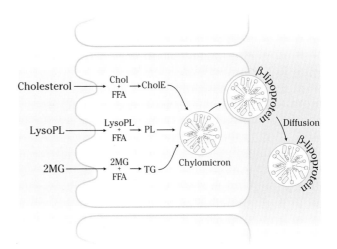

Figure 27.15 Formation and exocytosis of chylomicrons. (1) Products of lipid digestion are reconstituted by re-esterification, the reattachment of fatty acids. (2) The reconstituted fats are organized into chylomicrons. (3) Apoproteins are attached to the chylomicrons to allow exocytosis and entry into the lymphatic system.

bic fatty portions of the phospholipids. The chylomicron surface bears **apoproteins**, which serve as ligands that bind to specific receptors in other parts of the body and activate enzymes. In so doing, the chylomicron apoproteins mediate the transfer of fats from one location to another.

The apoprotein *apoB-48* mediates the egress of chylomicrons from the enterocyte. ApoB-48 attaches to sites on the basolateral enterocyte cell membrane, causing exocytosis of chylomicrons from the basolateral membrane. Chylomicrons are too large to enter capillaries. However, they can enter the lymphatics, whose endothelial cells are more widely spaced than those of capillaries. The chylomicrons then pass through the lymphatics to the thoracic duct and into the bloodstream via the left subclavian vein.

The vast majority of ingested lipid is absorbed in the form of chylomicrons. However, small- and medium-chain fatty acids are more water-soluble than longer-chain fatty acids. Consequently, they can diffuse through the enterocyte into the capillaries of the villi, which drain into the mesenteric portal venous system.

Lipid Transport in the Blood   There are two lipid transport systems in the blood (FIGURE 27.16). One system processes lipids absorbed in the diet (exogenous fat) and the other system shuttles fats and cholesterol back and forth between the liver and the peripheral tissues (endogenous fat). Lipoproteins are the shuttles for the transport of both exogenous and endogenous fat. Lipoproteins for shuttling endogenous fat include **low-density lipoprotein (LDL)** and **high-density lipoprotein (HDL)**, which are released into the bloodstream by the liver and intestinal tissues. The lipoprotein shuttle for exogenous fat is the chylomicron, whose delivery of fat to the tissues is guided by interactions with the capillary endothelium and with the lipoproteins of the endogenous system. The various lipoproteins are distinguished from one another by their lipid content (LDLs have a lower protein-to-lipid ratio) and by the particular apoproteins they bear.

The processing of exogenous fat begins with the action of **lipoprotein lipase** upon the chylomicron. Lipoprotein lipase is an enzyme found on the capillary walls of most tissues (but predominantly cardiac and skeletal muscle) and is activated by the apoprotein *apoCII* on the surface of the chylomicron. The capillary enzyme hydrolyzes triglycerides to monoglyceride, glycerol, and fatty acids. These digestion products are free to enter cells of the surrounding tissue. As the chylomicron circulates, more and more triglyceride is progressively removed, and thus the particle decreases in size and increases in density. The resulting *chylomicron remnant* is then removed from circulation by the liver (see Figure 27.16). Inside the liver, the apoproteins, cholesterol esters, and other components are degraded to amino acids, free cholesterol, and fatty acids.

Endogenous fat that is stored in the liver is transported from the liver by *very-low-density lipoprotein (VLDL)*. Like chylomicrons, VLDLs bear apoCII and activate lipoprotein lipase, hydrolyzing triglycerides in their core to glycerol and fatty acids, which can then enter nearby cells. VLDL, which grows denser and changes from VLDL to LDL as it unloads fat, is much richer in cholesterol esters than chylomicrons and receives added cholesterol esters from HDL. The delivery of cholesterol to the tissues is probably the most important function of VLDL and LDL. Peripheral tissues bind VLDL and LDL apoproteins and absorb

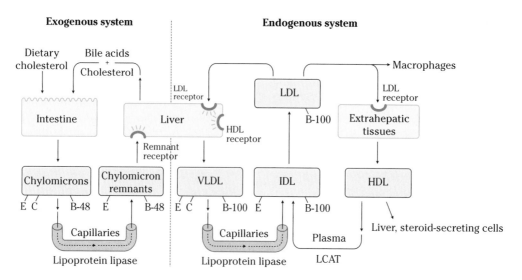

Figure 27.16   Transport of exogenous and endogenous lipids in the blood.

cholesterol from them. Macrophages also bear such apoprotein receptors and absorb cholesterol. In the context of injury to the arterial walls, cholesterol-bearing macrophages may inhibit the arterial walls and contribute to the formation of atherosclerotic plaques that constrict the arterial lumen. **Atherosclerosis** is the cause of *coronary artery disease (CAD)* and a major cause of *cerebrovascular accidents (CVAs)*, also known as strokes.

HDL particles shuttle cholesterol esters back to the liver, where they are degraded. The resulting cholesterol molecules are converted into bile acids, secreted into bile, or packaged into new lipoproteins. In addition, HDL plays an important role in the regulation of both endogenous and exogenous systems for lipid transport. It does so by delivering apoproteins to other lipoproteins and mediating the uptake and esterification of free cholesterol. Low levels of HDL and high levels of LDL both contribute to the risk of developing atherosclerosis.

Nucleic Acids

Nucleic acids—deoxyribonucleic acid (DNA) and ribonucleic acid (RNA)—are composed of polymers of nucleotides bound together through *phosphodiester linkages*. (Recall that nucleotides are molecules made of a pentose ring, a nitrogenous purine or pyrimidine base, and a group of phosphate esters.) Since all animals and plants have genomes and transcriptional capabilities based on DNA and RNA, these nucleic acids are present in all food. Accordingly, the digestive tract has evolved the ability to break down and absorb nucleic acids.

The digestion of nucleic acids begins in the small intestine, where **pancreatic ribonucleases** and **deoxyribonucleases** in pancreatic secretions hydrolyze phosphodiester bonds that link the nucleotides in a chain. The resulting oligonucleotides are further hydrolyzed by pancreatic phosphodiesterases to form a mixture of absorbable mononucleotides with a phosphate at either the 3′ or 5′ carbon of the pentose ring. These molecules can be further digested to free bases before absorption. Purine bases can also be converted to uric acid by enzymes found in the intestinal mucosa. The 3′ and 5′ mononucleotides and free bases are absorbed in the intestine through active transport. In addition, uric acid is absorbed by enterocytes and excreted from the body in urine. FIGURE 27.17 summarizes nucleic acid digestion and absorption.

Water and Electrolytes

Nearly 9 L of water passes through the digestive tract each day. Approximately 2 L of this fluid is ingested, and 7 L of water is contained in gastrointestinal secretions: 1,500 mL in saliva, 2,500 mL in gastric secretions, 500 mL in bile, 1,500 mL in pancreatic secretions, and 1,000 mL in intestinal secretions. The small intestine absorbs an amount roughly equal to that secreted (7 L), leaving 2 L to enter the large intestine (colon), which absorbs all but around 100 to 200 mL. *The large intestine is the site of net water intake by the GI tract.* Water absorption in the small intestine and colon is driven by solute absorption. The transport of electrolytes from the lumen into the blood results in an osmotic gradient, and water flows passively from the intestinal lumen into the bloodstream.

The reasons behind the body's need for a net absorption of 2 L of water per day lie in the governance of the osmolality (solute concentration) of the extracellular fluid volume (see Chapter 23). Losses of water in excess of solute occur every day in the human body. At least 1 L water is lost each day through evaporation from the skin and respiratory epithelium. About 500 L of water without salt is lost each day due to the excretion of nitrogenous wastes. This "free water" must be replaced by drinking. Otherwise, the plasma osmolality will rise, with adverse consequences for the brain and other body tissues.

Water Absorption Water can be absorbed through either the *cellular route*, through the plasma membrane, or the *paracellular route*, through tight junctions between intestinal epithelial cells. Water absorption across the intestinal cells involves the family of water channels called aquaporins. The permeability of tight junctions depends on the segment of the intestine in which they are located. In the small intestine, the junctions are more permeable than they are in the colon.

As suggested above, the principal mechanism for water absorption is via diffusion. The direction of the flow of water is determined by the concentration of solutes in the intestinal lumen versus that in the bloodstream. The chyme that is delivered into the duodenum from the stomach is hypertonic. Thus, the net direction of water flow in the duodenum is from the blood into the lumen (secretion). As solutes are absorbed, however, the tonicity of chyme decreases. This causes a reversal in the direction of water flow. Net water absorption occurs in the remainder of the small intestine. *In the colon, water follows the active absorption of sodium.*

Sodium Absorption Sodium is quantitatively the major cation present in the extracellular fluid. It creates the osmotic pressure that holds water inside the extracellular space consisting of interstitial and plasma volume. Humans have perhaps inherited a "salt hunger" from evolutionary experience with salt

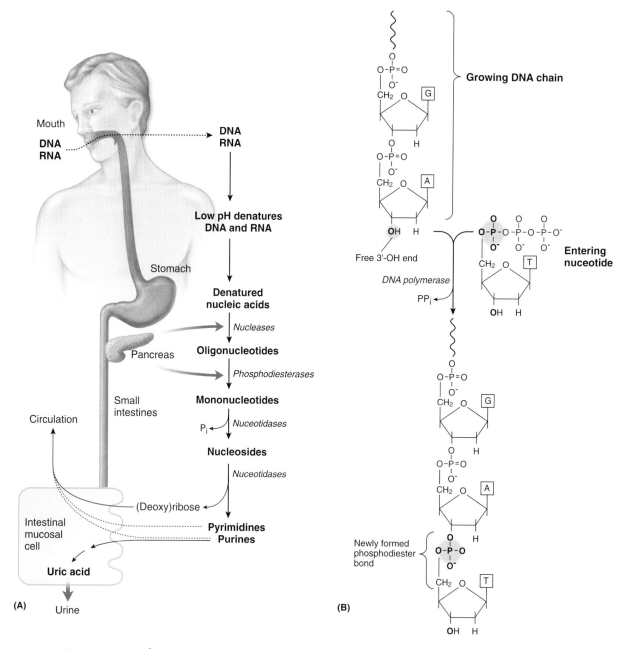

Figure 27.17 Summary of nucleic acid digestion. **A.** Nucleic acid digestion at each location in the GI tract. **B.** The structure of a nucleotide chain. The chain elongates when a phosphodiester forms between the free hydroxyl group of the nucleotide at the 3′ end of the chain and the phosphate at the 5′ end of the entering nucleotide. This bond is broken during digestion by various ribonucleases and deoxyribonucleases.

scarcity. We tend to eat foods high in salt; the hypothalamus and kidney then manage the intake and output of free water to normalize the osmolality of the extracellular fluid volume (see Chapter 23).

Sodium transport can occur by a variety of mechanisms. As mentioned earlier, the absorption of sodium in the small intestine occurs via active transport. The basolateral Na^+/K^+-ATPase in enterocytes pumps sodium across the basolateral membrane and into the interstitial fluid and the paracellular spaces. Na^+ then diffuses down its concentration gradient into the cell. It crosses the apical cell membrane through a variety of secondary active transporters, including SGLT1, Na^+-coupled amino acid transport, and Na^+/H^+ exchange (NHE). In addition, high luminal concentrations of glucose and peptides drive sodium absorption by creating a gradient favorable to the functioning of the sodium-solute symporters. (Thus, diffusion of glucose or amino acids into the enterocytes coupled to Na^+ can drive Na^+ absorption, in addition to the other way around.) In the ileum, the rate of sodium absorption decreases because the concen-

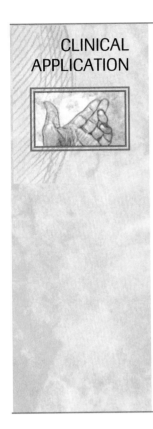

ORAL REHYDRATION THERAPY

Some intestinal infections and the toxins they produce interfere with the active transport of sodium from the intestinal lumen and promote the secretion of chloride. This not only lessens the gradient for water absorption in the GI tract but also can cause the passive secretion of water from the blood into the intestinal lumen. With salt trapped in the intestines, the lumen solute concentration can exceed that of plasma, causing water to diffuse into the lumen. *Diarrhea* results. Drinking more water does not help, because without salt absorption there is no way for the water to enter the plasma. The water remains in the intestinal lumen, and the diarrhea intensifies. The ingestion of salty water exacerbates the problem. Without the capacity to absorb salt, the gradient for the secretion of water into the intestinal lumen is even worse.

Oral rehydration therapy, an important treatment for diarrhea, employs a different strategy to restore water absorption in the intestine. It makes use of glucose/sodium coupling in the small intestine. With oral administration of a solution with a high glucose concentration and some salt content (e.g., 20 g glucose and 3.5 g sodium chloride in 1 L of water), glucose may diffuse across the glucose/sodium symporter, bringing sodium along with it from intestinal lumen to the blood. This movement of solutes is followed by the diffusion of water into the bloodstream.

The importance of oral rehydration cannot be overstated, given that diarrhea with dehydration is the second greatest cause of infant mortality in the world and given that access to intravenous hydration is limited in most afflicted areas.

---

trations of sugars and amino acids are lower than in more proximal portions of the small intestine. (See Clinical Application Box *Oral Rehydration Therapy*.)

In the colon, the action of the basolateral Na^+/K^+-ATPase and diffusion of Na^+ through apical channels become the most important means for sodium absorption. The apical membrane channel is known as the epithelial Na^+ channel (ENaC), also found in the renal cortical collecting duct. This process is increased by the presence of the adrenal hormone aldosterone, whose secretion is governed by the blood pressure-sensitive renin-angiotensin-aldosterone (RAA) axis. Compared to the small intestine, sodium absorption in the large intestine occurs against a larger luminal concentration gradient. Short-chain fatty acids, products of bacterial metabolism, and major anions in the stool have a stimulatory effect on colonic NaCl absorption. This has been the basis of the use of pectins and other carbohydrate fibers to treat diarrheal illnesses since the bacterial production of propionate and butyrate stimulates NaCl and water absorption in the colon. (See Integrated Physiology Box *Intestinal Flora*.)

Chloride and Bicarbonate Absorption and Secretion

The absorption of chloride is linked to that of Na^+. The absorption of sodium ions in the duodenum and jejunum creates a slightly electronegative potential in the intestinal lumen, driving Cl^- across the lumen and into plasma. Most of the absorption of Cl^- ions is by passive diffusion via a paracellular route in accordance with this electrical gradient. Another mechanism of Cl^- absorption is by Na^+/Cl^- cotransport. In the ileum and colon, the main means of Cl^- absorption is by Cl^-/HCO_3^- exchange.

Net Cl^- absorption also depends on how much Cl^- is secreted in pancreatic and other digestive fluids. The primary mechanism for Cl^- secretion in intestinal epithelia is the colonic apical membrane Cl^- conductance, mediated by the cystic fibrosis transmembrane conductance regulator (CFTR). The several ways in which Cl^- secretion may be regulated have great clinical significance and demonstrate the integration and complexity of intracellular signaling pathways. The basolateral membrane has the ubiquitous Na^+/K^+-ATPase, which serves to lower cell Na^+. A K^+ channel at the basolateral membrane returns the K^+ to the extracellular fluid, and in so doing maintains cell electronegativity. A basolateral $Na^+/K^+/2Cl^-$ (NKCC) transporter, similar to the cotransport mechanism in the renal thick ascending limb of Henle, is the mechanism that allows Cl^- to enter the cell from the extracellular fluid. The driving force is the inwardly directed Na^+ gradient provided by the Na^+/K^+-ATPase.

These steps provide the intracellular Cl^- and the intracellular negativity needed for a functioning CFTR to secrete Cl^- into the lumen. CFTR is stimulated by cyclic nucleotides, in particular cAMP and protein kinase A (basolateral adenyl cyclase receptor) and cGMP (apical guanylate cyclase receptor). The K^+ channel action is increased by rises in cell calcium,

Intestinal Flora

Symbiotic relationships are important to many species. They are the basis for aerobic respiration and photosynthesis in eukaryotic cells, whose mitochondria and chloroplasts are derived from ancient prokaryotic cell lines. Symbiotic relationships are also the means by which eukaryotic organisms obtain reactive nitrogen for making proteins. Finally, symbiotic bacteria inhabit our skin and other epithelia, conferring protection and performing metabolic functions for the benefit of our eukaryotic cells. In no place is this more important than in the intestines. These symbiotic microbes are called *intestinal microflora*.

Flow through the human upper GI tract is normally too fast to allow significant bacterial colonization, but the terminal ileum and large intestine are loaded with bacteria. Eukaryotic cells are, in fact, vastly outnumbered by the microbial inhabitants of the colon, which may lead us to ask if we host our bacteria or if our bacteria host us (a favorite irony of the physician-philosopher Lewis Thomas). Hundreds of bacterial species, most of them anaerobic, are represented in the intestinal flora, and the particular distribution of species varies from individual to individual.

Besides making up more than half of the mass of feces, colonic bacteria have several physiologic functions. First, the microbes metabolize indigestible proteins and carbohydrates, yielding absorbable short-chain fatty acids. Some of these fatty acids supply energy to the colonic enterocytes, and some are absorbed into the portal-mesenteric blood. The microbial supply of fatty acids is important enough to colon cells that without it, the colon epithelial cells do not grow normally. Microbes also manufacture menaquinone, a form of vitamin K that may be absorbed in the terminal ileum. (Microbial metabolism yields gas, which mixes with swallowed air to form flatus in the colon. Flatus comes from the Latin *flare*, to blow.)

Second, the intestinal flora serves as an important barrier to infection. The organisms monopolize the binding sites on the colon epithelium and eat the nutrients that might otherwise sustain an unruly bacterial invader. The microbes even appear to be important in training the host's immune system to recognize bacteria. This is consistent with Lewis Thomas's view that the immune system evolved as a means of negotiating and regulating symbiotic relationships, and not as a means of killing microbes.

---

the NKCC is regulated by a process of cell fusion and endocytosis, and the Na^+/K^+ pump is controlled by gene transcription and translation.

This pathway is important not only in cystic fibrosis, a disease characterized by abnormally low Cl^- secretions in various tissues, but also in many common diarrheal diseases. For example, a mechanism by which cholera causes severe diarrhea is activation of the alpha subunit of the G protein, G_s, resulting in increased cAMP. Many common toxins associated with *Escherichia coli* increase cGMP. *Clostridium difficile*, the cause of a common diarrheal disease in hospitalized patients, appears to increase intracellular Ca^{2+}.

The transport of bicarbonate ions (HCO_3^-) varies according to location in the GI tract. In the duodenum, HCO_3^- is secreted mainly through pancreatic and biliary fluids. In the jejunum, however, a large amount of luminal HCO_3^- is absorbed. This occurs mainly through the combination of luminal H^+ and HCO_3^- to form carbonic acid (H_2CO_3) (FIGURE 27.18). The carbonic acid dissociates to form H_2O and CO_2. The CO_2 then diffuses through the apical cell membrane and dissociates into HCO_3^-, which is then absorbed. This mechanism for HCO_3^- absorption is similar to the process of HCO_3^- absorption in the renal tubules. In the ileum and colon, HCO_3^- is secreted into the lumen via Cl^-/HCO_3^- exchange. The secreted HCO_3^- is important in the neutralization of acidic products of bacteria, especially as the luminal contents reach the large intestine.

Potassium Absorption and Secretion The absorption of potassium ions occurs by passive diffusion in the small intestine. As water is absorbed from the intestinal lumen, the concentration of luminal K^+ in-

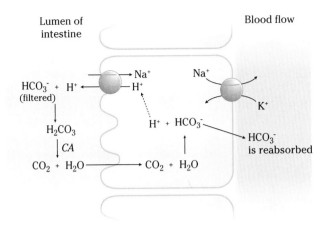

Figure 27.18 Bicarbonate absorption in the jejunum.

creases. This increase establishes a driving force favoring the absorption of K^+ through a paracellular route. In the large intestine, K^+ can be absorbed or secreted depending on the luminal concentration. When the luminal concentration is less than 25 mM, net secretion occurs; when luminal concentration is greater than 25 mM, net absorption occurs. A colonic H^+/K^+-ATPase, similar to the transporter in the renal collecting duct, is a mechanism that allows for K^+ absorption, and may be increased by potassium depletion. The secretion of K^+ is regulated by aldosterone, as it is in the distal nephron. Colonic K^+ secretion is particularly important in patients with kidney failure, adapting to the decreased ability of renal secretion to maintain K^+ balance. Apical membrane K^+ channels have been identified in colonic epithelial cells that are increased with increased plasma K^+ concentrations.

Vitamins and Minerals

Vitamins and minerals are *micronutrients*, constituents of the body tissues that make up a smaller percentage of the body weight than *macronutrients*—fats, proteins, and carbohydrates. **Vitamins** are organic compounds essential for many metabolic reactions in the body. Unlike macronutrients, they do not yield energy; instead, most vitamins serve as coenzymes. (Coenzymes are separate molecules integrated into the structure of enzymes and necessary for enzymatic function.) **Minerals** are inorganic elements, and like vitamins they do not furnish energy. With a few exceptions—vitamin D, vitamin K, and biotin—humans cannot synthesize vitamins and minerals; we acquire them in the diet. (Vitamin D is synthesized from its precursor in human skin. Vitamin K and biotin are produced by symbiotic microorganisms living in the intestines.) Vitamins are classified

as fat-soluble or water-soluble. TABLE 27.1 lists the essential vitamins and minerals.

The **fat-soluble vitamins**, A, D, E, and K, are present in micelles. They are absorbed into the lymph with the other products of lipid digestion. In general, the absorption of most **water-soluble vitamins** occurs by either facilitated diffusion or sodium-dependent active transport.

Vitamin B_{12} Absorption The absorption of vitamin B_{12} (cobalamin) is unique in that it occurs in two phases and requires the presence of a cofactor known as **intrinsic factor (IF)**. Without IF, only 1% to 2% of the ingested amount of vitamin B_{12} is absorbed. Most of the ingested B_{12} is bound to proteins. In the first phase of absorption, the *gastric phase*, the low pH of the stomach and the presence of pepsin cause the release of B_{12} from these proteins. At this point, vitamin B_{12} binds to glycoproteins from the saliva and gastric secretions known as R proteins. In the stomach, IF is secreted by parietal cells. IF binds to vitamin B_{12} with less affinity than the R proteins.

Table 27.1 **VITAMINS AND MINERALS**

VITAMINS	
Fat-Soluble Vitamins	*Water-Soluble Vitamins*
A (retinol, carotenes)	C (ascorbic acid)
D (cholecalciferol)	B_1 (thiamine)
E (tocopherols)	B_2 (riboflavin)
K (phylloquinone, menaquinone, menadione)	B_3 (niacin)
	B_5 (pantothenic acid)
	B_6 (pyridoxine)
	B_{12} (cobalamin)
	Folate (folic acid)
	Biotin

MINERALS	
Macrominerals (>0.005% body weight)	*Microminerals (<0.005% body weight)*
Sodium	Chromium
Chloride	Cobalt
Calcium	Copper
Phosphate	Fluoride
Potassium	Iodine
Magnesium	Iron
Sulfur	Manganese
	Molybdenum
	Selenium
	Zinc
	Arsenic[a]
	Boron[a]
	Cadmium[a]
	Lithium[a]
	Nickel[a]
	Silicone[a]
	Tin[a]
	Vanadium[a]

[a] Physiological role has not been established.

The second phase of absorption, the *intestinal phase*, occurs after the release of B_{12} complexes into the duodenum. There, pancreatic proteases digest R protein/B_{12} complexes. Vitamin B_{12} is then transferred to IF. These IF/B_{12} complexes are resistant to proteases. The absorption of vitamin B_{12} occurs in the terminal ileum, which contains receptors for IF/B_{12} complexes. After binding of the complexes to the receptors, the vitamin B_{12} is absorbed, exits the basolateral membrane, and enters the portal bloodstream. Within the portal system, vitamin B_{12} binds to *transcobalamin II*, a protein synthesized by the liver and intestinal epithelium. Transcobalamin II/B_{12} complexes are then taken into hepatocytes via receptor-mediated endocytosis. Stores of vitamin B_{12} are present in the liver.

Vitamin B_{12} is required for the normal development of red blood cells. Without B_{12}, *pernicious anemia* results. Apart from anemia, neurologic abnormalities and dementia are part of the clinical syndrome of B_{12} deficiency. Pernicious anemia can be caused by insufficient B_{12} (which occurs in gastrectomy, in gastric atrophy, and in the presence of antibodies to IF); the lack of pancreatic enzymes to digest R protein/B_{12} complexes (which occurs in pancreatic insufficiency); and the lack of a functioning terminal ileum (as might occur with surgical resection of the small intestine). Since IF is made by the parietal cells of the stomach, which also produce HCl, it is not uncommon for pernicious anemia to be associated with achlorhydria (absence of gastric acid). Congenital forms of pernicious anemia also exist, including specific transport defects due to deficient binding proteins.

The Schilling test is sometimes used to distinguish between a gastric IF deficiency and a disorder of the terminal ileum. A radioactive dose of cyanocobalamin is given orally, followed by an intramuscular dose of nonradioactive B_{12}, which saturates hepatic B_{12} uptake and prevents the liver from absorbing the radioactive cyanocobalamin. The radioactivity of the urine is tested; if low, it could represent either an IF deficiency or an ileal absorptive problem. However, if the urinary radioactivity remains low after the oral ingestion of combined IF and B_{12}, then an ileal disorder is suspected.

Serum levels of B_{12} can be measured directly but do not accurately reflect tissue B_{12}. Since B_{12} is important for the conversion of homocysteine to methionine, B_{12} deficiency is associated with elevated homocysteine levels. Conversion of propionic acid to succinic acid requires B_{12}, so patients with B_{12} deficiency accumulate and excrete the intermediate, methylmalonic acid.

Iron Absorption   The absorption of iron is critical to maintaining a steady level of iron at approximately 4 g in a healthy adult. Losses of approximately 1 to 2 mg/day occur through the sloughing of cells from skin and the GI tract; in women, losses secondary to menstrual bleeding occur. The recommended daily intake of iron is 20 mg/day. However, only 0.5 to 1.0 mg/day is absorbed by healthy men, and in women only 1.0 to 1.5 mg/d is absorbed. Iron ion absorption is limited by its formation of insoluble complexes with anions in intestinal secretions.

Iron can be absorbed in the form of *heme* (iron in the center of a porphyrin ring, as is present in the oxygen-carrying blood protein hemoglobin) or as free iron (mostly Fe^{2+}). Heme is absorbed by intestinal cells via endocytosis. Once inside cells, the iron (Fe^{2+}) is released from the heme molecule by the action of a cytosolic xanthine oxidase. The absorption of free iron is slightly more complicated. Enterocytes release **transferrin**, an iron-binding protein, into the intestinal lumen. Once in the lumen of the duodenum and jejunum, a single molecule of transferrin binds two iron molecules. Receptors on the brush border of the duodenum and jejunum bind the transferrin/iron complex. The complex is then absorbed by receptor-mediated endocytosis. Once inside the cell, iron is released from transferrin, and the transferrin is recycled by resecretion into the lumen.

Cytosolic iron has two fates. It can be bound irreversibly to the protein *ferritin* or transported across the basolateral membrane into the blood. In the bloodstream, it then binds plasma-borne transferrin and is transported to numerous sites in the body, including the bone marrow and liver, where it is used or stored.

The absorption of iron is a highly regulated process that is adjusted according to the body's needs. Excess iron absorption can lead to iron overload, which occurs in the condition of *hemochromatosis*. To prevent this, absorption is reduced by upregulating ferritin in the enterocyte cytoplasm. This leads to increased formation of iron/ferritin complexes, which are lost in feces when intestinal epithelial cells are sloughed off. In addition, the rate of iron absorption can be decreased by reducing the number of receptors for the transferrin/iron complexes. On the other hand, during periods when additional iron is required by the body (in pregnancy or after blood loss), the amount of ferritin is downregulated, and the receptors for transferrin/iron complexes are expressed in greater numbers.

The Function of the Exocrine Pancreas

The **exocrine pancreas** is essentially a factory and a warehouse for the production and storage of digestive enzymes. While its physiology is not as complex as that of the liver—a topic requiring its own chapter—a few details of pancreatic production, storage, and secretory processes are worth mentioning.

The pancreas possesses a well-developed endoplasmic reticulum and Golgi apparatus for the production of large amounts of protein: the zymogen precursors to digestive enzymes. Zymogen-loaded vesicles pinch off from the Golgi to form zymogen granules. The zymogen granules cluster near the apical side of the pancreatic acinar cells lining the pancreatic secretory ducts. Neurohormonal signals cause the zymogen granules to be exocytosed (see Chapter 28). (The pancreas stores digestive enzymes as inactive zymogens to protect itself from autodigestion.)

The pancreas must also secrete fluid to deliver its enzymes to the duodenum. Pancreatic secretions thus have an aqueous and an enzymatic component. The secretory rate of pancreatic cells varies; flow increases during the stimulation of a meal passing down the GI tract. The anions found in pancreatic secretions also vary. (The concentrations of cations, Na^+ and K^+, and the osmolality remain constant and similar to that of plasma.) When the secretory rate is low and no meal is present, chloride is the predominant anion in pancreatic fluid. The fluid secreted at high rates during the digestion of a meal, on the other hand, is rich with bicarbonate anions instead of chloride anions. This renders the fluid alkaline (pH 7.5 to 8.0). The alkalinity neutralizes the acidity of chyme coming from the stomach and creates the optimal pH for the functioning of the pancreatic enzymes. Bicarbonate (HCO_3^-) arises in the cell under the action of carbonic anhydrase, which catalyzes the transformation of H_2O and CO_2 to H^+ and HCO_3^-. The HCO_3^- is extruded across the apical membrane into the pancreatic ducts across a HCO_3^-/Cl^- antiporter. The H^+ left behind by the HCO_3^- is exchanged for Na^+ at the basolateral surface of the acinar cell.

The fate of the pancreatic enzymes (and all other digestive enzymes) subsequent to their digestive action has been a matter of controversy for nearly three decades. One theory says that the enzymes, which are made of protein, are themselves digested by proteases (in part by colonic bacteria) and absorbed. Another theory suggests that the pancreatic enzymes are absorbed by the intestines and recycled to the pancreas in what would be called an *enteropancreatic circulation*.

PATHOPHYSIOLOGY

Maldigestion occurs when there is a deficiency of digestive enzymes. A common cause of carbohydrate maldigestion is lactase deficiency in the brush border of the duodenum and jejunum. Under these circumstances, lactose remains in the lumen unabsorbed and is presented to the lower small intestine and colon. The luminal osmotic pressure is increased, which "pulls" water into the lumen. This results in an osmotic diarrhea. The undigested lactose is also metabolized by colonic bacteria to lactic acid and CO_2. The gas distends the colon and causes bloating and cramping. The condition is commonly referred to as **lactose intolerance**.

Maldigestion of lipids occurs in the context of a deficiency of pancreatic enzymes. This condition can be present in cases of pancreatic cancer, pancreatitis, and cystic fibrosis. **Acute pancreatitis** is most often caused by a gallstone obstructing the pancreatic duct and preventing the flow of pancreatic secretions into the duodenum.

Malabsorption arises in the context of abnormalities of the alimentary epithelium. Inflammation due to autoimmune disease or infection may decrease the absorptive surface area or render the absorptive surface dysfunctional. Surgery may also decrease the absorptive surface area. Malabsorption may be general to all nutrients, or it may affect specific classes of nutrients, depending on the pathogenesis. Autoimmune diseases, such as *Crohn's disease* and *ulcerative colitis*—the **inflammatory bowel diseases**—may lead to general malabsorption.

Following are examples of nutrient-specific malabsorptive syndromes.

Hartnup's disease is a rare autosomal recessive disorder in which the carrier system for neutral amino acids is absent. The patient cannot absorb neutral amino acids such as tryptophan from the lumen of the GI tract (or the renal tubule). However, dipeptides or tripeptides that contain tryptophan can sometimes be absorbed and can be transported to various tissues.

Lipid absorption can be disturbed by several processes. Reduced intestinal bile salt concentration can lead to impaired micelle formation. This condition can occur with liver disease because bile salts are produced in the liver. It can also occur in the context of conditions affecting the ileum. The process of bile salt secretion, modification, and return to the liver is known as **enterohepatic circulation** (FIGURE 27.19). Bile salts and primary/secondary bile acids, which are versions of bile salts that have been modified (deconjugated, dehydroxylated) by intestinal bacteria, are absorbed primarily in the ileum via active transport. They then move from the enterocyte into the portal blood and liver. Inside the liver, the primary and secondary bile acids are converted into bile salts, which are secreted into bile to further aid in the digestion of lipids. This process can be interrupted by ileal resection or inflammatory disease of the ileum, thereby leading to *lipid malabsorption*.

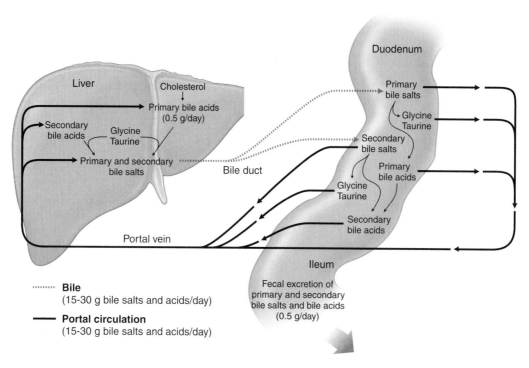

Figure 27.19   Enterohepatic circulation of bile salts. Bile acids are produced from cholesterol in the liver, where they undergo conjugation with glycine and taurine to form bile salts. Bile salts are secreted into the intestine, where they are modified/deconjugated to form primary and secondary bile acids. In the terminal ileum, the bile acids and bile salts are absorbed and return to the liver via the portal vein. In the liver, the bile acids undergo modification and are resecreted into the intestine.

The clinical presentation of salt and water malabsorption is **diarrhea**, which is defined as the excretion of 200 g or more of water in the stools of an adult over 24 hours. Diarrhea can be caused by a variety of mechanisms. Hypermotility of the gut leads to diarrhea due to the increased transit rate of chyme through the digestive tract. Water and salts are delivered to the colon faster than the intestinal epithelial cells can absorb them. An increased rate of transit through the intestines also decreases the absorption of nutrients, thereby raising the osmotic pressure of the intestinal lumen. Consequently, water is retained in the lumen. In *irritable bowel syndrome*, anxiety may lead to intestinal hypermotility. Various infectious pathogens may impair the enterocytes' capacity to absorb solutes, leading to high luminal osmotic pressure and retention of water in the lumen. In some cases of impaired sodium absorption and hyperosmolality in the intestinal lumen, secretion of water may take place.

Either maldigestion or malabsorption can lead to **malnutrition**. Inadequate caloric intake can result in muscle wasting and ketoacidosis. Deficient absorption of specific vitamins manifests clinically as particular diseases such as *scurvy* (vitamin C deficiency), *rickets* (vitamin D deficiency), and *beriberi* (thiamine deficiency).

Summary

- Anabolism is synthesis of macromolecules from building blocks, a process requiring energy. Catabolism is degradation of macromolecules into simpler substances, releasing energy. Metabolism is anabolism plus catabolism: the sum total of all chemical reactions in a living being.

- Both energy and building blocks for the construction and maintenance of body tissues come from the digestion (catabolism) and absorption of nutrients taken in by eating.

- The GI tract (alimentary canal) is a tube from the mouth to the anus that digests and absorbs dietary nutrients: carbohydrates, proteins, lipids, nucleic acids, water, vitamins, and minerals.

- Hydrolysis is employed in the digestion of all the macronutrients (carbohydrates, proteins, lipids, and nucleic acids). Its general formula is:

$$R''-R' + H_2O \rightarrow R''OH + R'H$$

- Much of digestion is accounted for by pancreatic enzymes that are released as inactive zymogens into the duodenum through the ampulla of Vater.

- Carbohydrates are digested by salivary α-amylase, pancreatic α-amylase, and intestinal disaccharidases, yielding the monosaccharides glucose, fructose, and galactose.

- Glucose and galactose are absorbed by secondary active transport involving an apical Na^+/monosaccharide symporter powered by a basolateral Na^+/K^+-ATPase. Fructose is absorbed by facilitated diffusion.

- Proteins are digested by gastric pepsin, pancreatic proteases, and intestinal peptidases. Pancreatic proteases are secreted as inactive zymogens and activated by intestinal enterokinase. This process yields amino acids, dipeptides, and tripeptides.

- Amino acids are absorbed by secondary active transport involving an apical Na^+/amino acid symporter powered by the basolateral Na^+/K^+-ATPase, as in carbohydrate absorption. Dipeptides and tripeptides are actively absorbed by cotransport with H^+ that is also coupled to the active Na^+ absorption.

- Lipids are digested in the following stages: first, cleavage by gastric lipases in the stomach plus mechanical emulsification in the stomach; second, emulsification into droplets by the amphipathic constituents of bile; third, digestion by pancreatic lipases and cholesterol esterase. This process yields free fatty acids, 2-monoglyceride, free cholesterol, and lysophospholipid.

- Lipids are absorbed by bile salt emulsification of the cleavage products into micelles, smaller amphipathic droplets that deliver the cleavage products to the intestinal brush border for diffusion into enterocytes, where fatty acids are reattached by re-esterification to the other cleavage products and bundled into chylomicrons, which are then exocytosed and taken up by lymphatics. Lipoprotein lipase in the capillaries again breaks down triglycerides into 2-monoglyceride and fatty acids so that cells can absorb the cleavage products by diffusion.

- Chylomicrons are the lipoprotein shuttles for transporting dietary (exogenous) fat in the bloodstream to the periphery. Low-density lipoprotein (LDL) transports endogenous cholesterol stores from the liver to the tissues. High-density lipoprotein (HDL) transports endogenous cholesterol from the tissues to the liver for disposal.

- Nucleic acids are digested by pancreatic ribonucleases and deoxyribonucleases into individual nucleotides and by pancreatic phosphodiesterases into free bases (purine, pyrimidine) and phosphorylated pentose rings. They are absorbed by active transport.

- A net water uptake of 2 L per day (equal to the amount taken in by drinking) occurs in the large intestine. The Na^+/K^+-ATPase drives Na^+ absorption, causing water to diffuse after it into the enterocytes and the bloodstream.

- Sodium is absorbed in the small intestine and large intestine by active transport. In the small intestine, this active transport is coupled to sugar and amino acid absorption.

- The volume of water and the concentration of Na^+ in the blood (salt and water balance) are not controlled at the level of the GI tract. Rather, the GI tract takes in salt and water in proportion to what is ingested, and the brain and kidney afterward modulate salt and water excretion to keep blood volume and salt concentration within normal limits.

- Chloride is absorbed with sodium because of electrical gradients established by the Na^+/K^+-ATPase pump.

- Bicarbonate (HCO_3^-) is secreted in pancreatic fluid and bile in the duodenum, neutralizing the gastric acidity of chyme. HCO_3^- is absorbed in the jejunum and again secreted in the ileum and colon, where it neutralizes acidic products of bacterial metabolism.

- The fat-soluble vitamins A, D, E, and K are in micelles and are absorbed into the lymph with the other products of lipid digestion. The absorption of most water-soluble vitamins occurs by either facilitated diffusion or sodium-dependent active transport.

- The absorption of vitamin B_{12} (cobalamin) depends on the gastric secretion of intrinsic factor (IF), which binds vitamin B_{12} and protects it from degradation by pancreatic proteases. Iron is absorbed bound to transferrin.

- Maldigestion results from a digestive enzyme deficiency. One cause is acute pancreatitis, in which pancreatic enzymes cannot flow down the pancreatic duct, usually due to blockage by a gallstone. The enzymes instead attack the pancreas.

- Malabsorption arises in the context of abnormalities of the alimentary epithelium. Inflammation due to autoimmune disease or infection may decrease the absorptive surface area or render the absorptive surface dysfunctional. Salt and water malabsorption results in diarrhea.

- Either maldigestion or malabsorption can lead to malnutrition.

Suggested Reading

Chan FK, Leung WK. Peptic-ulcer disease. Lancet. 2002; 360(9337):933–941.

Guarner F, Malagelada JR. Gut flora in health and disease. Lancet. 2003;361(9356):512–519.

Shiotani A, Graham DY. Pathogenesis and therapy of gastric and duodenal ulcer disease. Med Clin North Am. 2002;86(6):1447–1466.

Thielman NM, Guerrant RL. Clinical practice. Acute infectious diarrhea. N Engl J Med. 2004;350(1):38–47.

Thomas L. *The Lives of a Cell*. New York: Penguin, 1974.

Wallace JL, Tigley AW. Review article: new insights into prostaglandins and mucosal defence. Aliment Pharmacol Ther. 1995;9:227–235.

REVIEW QUESTIONS

Directions: Each of the numbered items or incomplete statements in this section is followed by answers or by completions of the statement. Select the ONE lettered answer or completion that is BEST in each case.

1. A 65-year-old woman is admitted to the hospital with severe nausea and vomiting and diffuse abdominal pain, including colicky pain in the right upper quadrant. Imaging studies suggest the presence of a gallstone that is occluding the common bile duct and the pancreatic duct. Which of the following would accurately describe the fluid in her duodenum after a meal?

   (A) Abnormally high pH
   (B) Abnormally low pH
   (C) Normal pH
   (D) Elevated volume
   (E) Infection with *Helicobacter Pylori*

2. A 10-year-old child is severely dehydrated after 1 week of copious watery diarrhea with high fever. Oral rehydration therapy could help by:

   (A) Slowing intestinal motility.
   (B) Increasing solute-coupled sodium transport.
   (C) Increasing the expression of aquaporins.
   (D) Decreasing the renal excretion of fluid.
   (E) Improving the digestion of sugars.
   (F) Healing dysfunctional absorptive cells.
   (G) Killing bacterial pathogens in the intestine.

3. An obese 50-year-old woman undergoes partial gastrectomy to control her appetite. Several months later she is found to be anemic, even though her incisions have healed nicely. The cause could be:

   (A) Inadequate vitamin B_{12} in her diet.
   (B) Inadequate production of intrinsic factor.
   (C) Poor transcobalamin II production.
   (D) Inadequate acid production.
   (E) Bone marrow failure.
   (F) Inadequate erythropoietin production.

ANSWERS TO REVIEW QUESTIONS

1. **The answer is B.** After a meal, pancreatic secretions are alkaline and hence raise the pH of the acidic chyme delivered to the duodenum from the stomach. Obstruction of the pancreatic duct would block these alkaline secretions from reaching the duodenum and would leave the chyme more acidic than usual. The pancreas accounts for 1,500 mL of fluid out of the 7 L secreted into the intestines each day. Obstruction of pancreatic secretion would *decrease* the fluid volume of the duodenum rather than increase it. *Helicobacter pylori* infection is associated with peptic ulcer disease, not acute pancreatitis.

2. **The answer is B.** Oral rehydration therapy acts on the glucose/sodium symporter. When intestinal infections compromise the capacity of the Na^+/K^+-ATPase in enterocytes, salt and therefore water absorption are impaired in the intestines. Oral rehydration therapy contains sugar and salt. The diffusion of glucose from the intestinal lumen into the enterocytes across the glucose/sodium symporter results in increased Na^+ and hence water absorption. Oral rehydration therapy does not treat the offending bacteria and does not repair damaged cells. In fact, it relies on the function of the remaining cells with an intact absorptive surface. It does not contain any drugs that distribute into the bloodstream.

3. **The answer is B.** The partial gastrectomy has resulted in decreased production of intrinsic factor owing to a decrease in the number of available parietal cells. Intrinsic factor protects vitamin B_{12} from degradation by pancreatic proteases; if production of intrinsic factor is inadequate, dietary vitamin B_{12} is digested instead of absorbed and cannot conduct its physiologic action of stimulating erythropoiesis (red blood cell production). Transcobalamin II is produced by the liver, which is unaffected by gastrectomy (it assists in the storage of vitamin B_{12} in the liver). The patient's gastric acid production might be below physiologic levels, but this would not affect vitamin B_{12} absorption per se. Bone marrow failure and decreased erythropoietin production (as occurs in renal failure) could also cause anemia in contexts other than the one presented here.

Control of Gastrointestinal Motility and Secretion

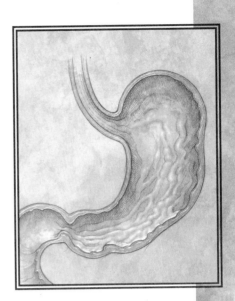

INTRODUCTION

In Chapter 27, we saw that the acquisition of energy and building blocks requires two gastrointestinal processes in tandem: digestion and absorption. We now focus on two other critical GI capabilities, without which digestion and absorption could not occur: motility and secretion. **Motility** is the muscular capacity for movement by which the digestive organs agitate food mechanically and propel it through the GI tract. **Secretion** is the process that delivers digestive enzymes, emulsifiers, and fluid at low or high pH into the intestinal lumen to enable digestion and absorption. Particular sequences of muscular contractions and secretions of specific digestive agents must be orchestrated perfectly in time for digestion and absorption to occur normally. Consequently, motility and secretion are controlled by an elaborate neurohormonal regulatory system.

There are three major components to this regulatory system:

1. The **central nervous system (CNS)**, which provides *extrinsic* innervation and control to the GI tract.

2. The **enteric nervous system (ENS)**, sometimes called the "minibrain" of the intestines, which provides *intrinsic* innervation and control to the GI tract.

3. **Enteroendocrine cells** distributed throughout the GI mucosa.

SYSTEM STRUCTURE

As described in the previous chapter, the entire length of the GI tract shares a similar structural foundation. Working from the inside wall out, the layers are the mucosa, submucosa, muscularis, and serosa (see Figure 27.1). Recall that the muscularis has an inner circular and an outer longitudinal sublayer of smooth muscle tissue. (The action of these two layers, which constrict the gut in diameter and in length, respectively, provides the basis for peristalsis.) Between the inner circular and outer longitudinal muscle layers of the muscularis lies the **myenteric plexus** (*Auerbach's plexus*), one major component of the ENS (FIGURE 28.1). The other major component of the ENS is the **submucosal plexus** (*Meissner's plexus*), found between the muscularis and the submucosa. Scattered widely throughout the GI tract epithelium are specialized enteroendocrine cells adapted for the detection of certain stimuli and for the release of various hormones.

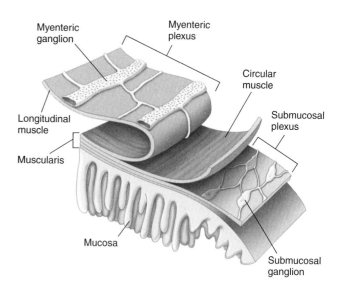

Figure 28.1 The enteric nervous system. The myenteric plexus, which controls motility, and the submucosal plexus, which controls secretion and blood flow, make up the ENS.

Muscles of the GI Tract

Many muscles are involved in chewing and swallowing food. The **masseter muscle** (a striated skeletal muscle) is particularly important to the closure of the mandible in the act of biting. The **tongue** (striated muscle), **pharyngeal muscles** (striated/smooth), and **upper esophageal sphincter (UES)** (striated/smooth) are particularly important in swallowing a bolus of chewed food and passing it into the esophagus. The UES is 1 to 3 cm long and demarcates the transition from the pharynx to the esophagus. The **esophagus** is composed of both skeletal and smooth muscle, with the proportion of smooth muscle increasing at the base; the last third of the esophagus is entirely smooth muscle. The **lower esophageal sphincter** is a tonically contracted zone in the terminal 2 to 4 cm of the esophagus that divides the esophagus from the stomach. The **pyloric sphincter** (or pyloric valve) separates the stomach from the duodenum, and the **ileocecal valve** separates the ileum from the large intestine. The **sphincter of Oddi** opens and closes the communication between the duodenum and the ampulla of Vater (which carries the bile and pancreatic secretions). The **stomach**, **small intestine**, and **large intestine** (also called the *colon*) are lined with smooth muscle and myenteric plexus. Gap junctions between adjacent smooth muscle cells allow for low-resistance electrical connections between the cells. This is important for coordinated contraction and relaxation of the GI tract. The large intestine also possesses three strips of longitudinal muscle called the **taenia coli**. Skeletal muscle does not reappear until the **rectum**.

Where the circular smooth muscle of the rectum thickens into the **internal anal sphincter**, the rectum is also sheathed in skeletal muscle. This voluntarily controlled striated muscle is the **external anal sphincter**, and it continues distally past the end of the internal anal sphincter.

Innervation of the GI Tract

As stated above, the regulatory system governing GI function includes three components: the CNS, ENS, and enteroendocrine cells. All three are interconnected by nerves, and neurons and enteroendocrine cells both serve as sensors and effectors for the combined CNS/ENS control center. The entire regulatory apparatus is referred to as the **brain-gut axis**. The transmission of information from the GI tract to the brain for processing is via afferent sensory axons whose cell bodies are located in the submucosal or myenteric plexus. Neural commands from the brain and spinal cord—the CNS—are sent in the opposite direction via efferent axons to the computational circuits in the enteric minibrain.

Intrinsic Innervation The ENS, composed of the submucosal and myenteric plexuses, provides intrinsic innervation of GI tract structures. Each plexus is composed of ganglia. The myenteric ganglia form a continuous network from the upper esophagus to the internal anal sphincter. The submucosal ganglia are concentrated in the small and large intestine. The ganglia within each layer are connected longitudinally and circumferentially via "highways" of internodal axons. The two plexuses are also connected via processes akin to bridges traversing the circular muscle layer. These internal highways and bridges are critical for the coordination of activity along the intestinal wall. The enteric neurons connect with the intestinal mucosa, secretory cells, blood vessels, smooth muscle cells, sympathetic neurons, parasympathetic neurons, and enteroendocrine cells.

The number of neurons that make up the ENS approximates that found in the spinal cord: 10 to 100 million. The types of motor neurons found in the ENS include excitatory and inhibitory motoneurons, secretomotor neurons, and vasodilator neurons. Enteric sensory neurons are responsive to mechanical and chemical stimuli. Interneurons participate in enteric reflexes and are regulated by the hormonal milieu created by surrounding enteroendocrine and neuroendocrine cells.

Extrinsic Innervation The GI tract is connected extrinsically to the CNS by nerves. Above the esophagus, this connection is partly through somatic nerves, which give the CNS partly voluntary control over chewing and swallowing. Muscles in the mouth and pharynx are innervated by cranial nerves V (trigeminal), IX (glossopharyngeal), X (vagus), and XII (hypoglossal). Taste in the oral cavity is mediated by cranial nerves VII and IX. Afferent and efferent neurons complete a reflex arc through the swallowing center in the brain stem. The external anal sphincter is also innervated with a somatic nerve (the pudendal), and therefore the CNS can consciously control either end of the GI tract. *Between the pharynx and the external anal sphincter, the GI tract is extrinsically innervated only by the autonomic nervous system.* The brain thus has little voluntary control over most of the GI tract; it is regulated involuntarily. The parasympathetic and sympathetic divisions of the autonomic nervous system (ANS) regulate the functions of the GI tract, as shown in Figure 28.2.

The **parasympathetic nervous system** connects the medulla to the myenteric and submucosal plexuses through the **vagus nerve** and the **pelvic nerve**. Both vagus and pelvic nerves contain efferent (motor) and afferent (sensory) fibers. The vagus innervates the GI tract from the upper esophageal sphincter to the transverse colon. Sensory-motor reflexes carried in the vagus nerve are called **vagovagal reflexes** (Figure 28.3). (The *vago*vagal reflex should not be confused with the *vaso*vagal reflex, which parasympathetically drops the heart rate in response to stress-related spikes in blood pressure.) The pelvic nerves, originating in the sacral spinal cord (S2–S4), innervate the GI tract from the splenic flexure of the colon to the internal anal sphincter. The parasympathetic nerves release acetylcholine (ACh).

The **sympathetic nervous system** innervates the entire GI tract with neurons that arise from the **sympathetic chain** (located alongside spinal cord levels T5–L2) and travel to the *prevertebral ganglia* (celiac, superior mesenteric, inferior mesenteric, and hypogastric). From the prevertebral ganglia, sympathetic neurons travel along blood vessels to penetrate the intestinal wall. Sympathetic fibers synapse with neurons in the enteric plexuses, as well as directly on smooth muscle cells, blood vessels, and the muscularis mucosa. The preganglionic neurons release ACh in the prevertebral ganglia, and the postganglionic neurons release norepinephrine (NE) at their targets in the gut.

Enteroendocrine Cells

Unlike the endocrine cells of the thyroid or pancreas, which are collected into discrete, isolated glands, GI endocrine cells are distributed over large

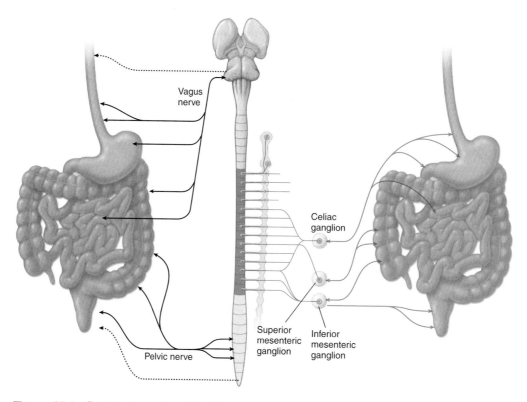

Figure 28.2   Extrinsic innervation of the GI tract. On the left side of the spinal cord, the parasympathetic nervous system is depicted. On the right, the sympathetic nervous system is depicted. C = celiac ganglion, SM = superior mesenteric ganglion, IM = inferior mesenteric ganglion.

mucosal areas and are more heterogeneous in nature. This distribution enables them to respond to a diversity of stimuli over the length of the GI tract with a wide variety of endocrine signals. GI endocrine cells are derived from the same crypt stem cells that differentiate into enterocytes, as well as

goblet cell and Paneth cell lineages. They are continuously differentiating from pluripotent intestinal stem cells into specialized cells that secrete one specific agent. Like other endocrine cells, they contain many secretory granules full of peptides. GI endocrine cells are stimulated at their apical (luminal)

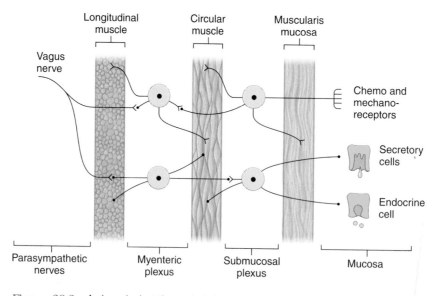

Figure 28.3   A closer look at the extrinsic innervation of the GI tract. The vagovagal reflex receives afferent signals from the mucosa and ENS and delivers efferent signals back to the ENS and mucosa.

surfaces by nutrients, by neural input, or by distention of the GI tract wall.

GI Hormones and Neurotransmitters

GI hormones and neurotransmitters are secreted by enteroendocrine cells and axon terminals; they are the final common pathway shared by the nervous and endocrine systems to control the GI system. In response to both luminal stimuli and nervous input, they govern enzymatic secretion from the stomach, pancreas, and intestines; bile secretion from the liver; the contraction and relaxation of GI smooth muscle; and blood flow to the digestive tract. GI regulatory substances communicate with other cells by endocrine, paracrine, or neurocrine routes (FIGURE 28.4).

Recall that **endocrine communication** occurs when a hormone is released from one tissue into the bloodstream to reach a distant target cell. The target tissues distinguish themselves by possessing receptors for that particular agent. Five of the GI peptides—secretin, gastrin, cholecystokinin (CCK), glucose-dependent insulinotropic peptide (GIP), and motilin—are considered endocrine hormones.

Paracrine communication occurs when an agent is released from endocrine cells into the interstitial fluid to affect neighboring cells. Target tissues must possess receptors for the agent and be located near the agent's source. The primary GI paracrine agents are somatostatin and histamine.

Neurocrine communication occurs when an agent is synthesized and released from neurons in response to an action potential and behaves as a neurotransmitter. The major neurotransmitters released into and by the ENS are ACh and NE. Other established neurotransmitters of the ENS include gastrin-releasing peptide (GRP), nitric oxide (NO), tachykinins (e.g., substance P), enkephalins, and vasoactive intestinal peptide (VIP).

Each regulatory agent exerts its action on the GI tract via binding to a specific receptor on the target cell membrane. Some hormones that share similar peptide structure can bind to the same receptor, albeit with different affinities (e.g., CCK and gastrin). Hormone receptors in the GI tract belong to a family of G-protein-linked receptors. Depending on the receptor, ligand binding activates one of two major intracellular pathways. The binding of gastrin, CCK, and ACh to their respective receptors activates *phospholipase C*, leading to increased intracellular calcium release. The binding of other substances, including secretin, VIP, and histamine, activates *adenylate cyclase*, which leads to an increased intracellular concentration of cAMP. Through the activation of these second messengers (Ca^{2+}, cAMP), hormones can elicit an immediate response, such as the activation of

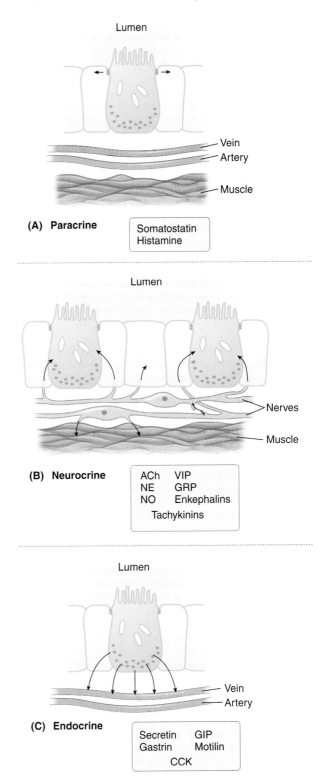

Figure 28.4 Classification of the neurohormonal substances of the GI tract. Endocrine substances are released into the bloodstream and circulate to their targets. Neurocrine substances are released directly onto their targets from neuronal axon terminals. Paracrine substances are released into the interstitium to affect neighboring cells. ACh = acetylcholine, NE = norepinephrine, NO = nitric oxide, VIP = vasoactive intestinal peptide, GRP = gastrin-releasing peptide, CCK = cholecystokinin, GIP = glucose-dependent insulinotropic polypeptide.

enzyme secretion or muscle contraction. Alternatively, hormone binding can elicit a delayed response, such as the activation of gene expression to exert a trophic effect on GI mucosa.

SYSTEM FUNCTION

As stated above, in order to digest and absorb nutrients, the GI tract must propel food through the tract and secrete digestive enzymes at the right moments in time. TABLE 28.1 shows the motile and secretory events in sequence, along with their neural and endocrine mediators. TABLE 28.2 describes the endocrine, paracrine, and neurocrine factors involved in digestion. While the regulation of each step of digestion is complex, it is useful to keep a few general principles in mind.

The parasympathetic nervous system and its end-product, ACh, tend to promote motility and secretion and relax GI tract sphincters. The sympathetic nervous system and its end-product, NE, tend to inhibit motility and secretion. The GI tract receives tonic sympathetic output (i.e., a constant, basal level of sympathetic output) so that the default setting of the GI tract is depressed motility, low secretion, and constricted sphincters. ACh tends to dilate blood vessels, promoting blood flow (and hence digestion), while NE tends to constrict vessels.

Peristalsis is the basic means of propulsion in all parts of the GI tract. In **peristalsis**, the GI tract wall contracts behind its luminal contents and relaxes in front of them (FIGURE 28.5). The contraction/relaxation pattern of the musculature then advances along the tract, pushing the luminal contents forward. The ENS achieves peristalsis without extrinsic help by sending nervous impulses forward and backward along the GI tract from a site of luminal distention. The backward impulses result in the release of signals to the smooth muscle to contract, such as ACh. The forward impulses result in the release of signals to relax, such as NO. Peristalsis is conducted by neurons in the myenteric plexus (as opposed to the submucosal plexus).

The smooth muscle of the GI tract manifests electrical pacemaker activity at all times, like the muscle tissue of the heart. Calcium ions are repeatedly flowing into the smooth muscle cells, depolarizing them, and potassium ions are repeatedly being released, repolarizing them. These actions lead to rhythmic increases and decreases in wall tension. Peristalsis is superimposed upon this underlying pattern of muscular activity. Likewise, the extrinsic influences of the parasympathetic and sympathetic nervous systems are superimposed on this basic pattern, with ACh tending to assist in depolarization (excitation) of the

Table 28.1   MOTILITY AND SECRETION: FROM HUNGER TO DEFECATION

Transit Time	Digestive Event	Regulatory Structure or Mediator Involved
N/A	Perception of hunger	Hypothalamus
	Procurement of food	Cerebral cortex
	Anticipation of eating (cephalic phase of digestion) and preparation of GI tract	Cerebral cortex, cranial nerves, brain stem (dorsal motor nuclei of vagus nerves, salivatory nuclei)
	Tasting of food (oral phase) and preparation of GI tract	Cranial nerves, brain stem (dorsal motor nuclei of vagus nerves, salivatory nuclei)
	Chewing (mastication)	Cerebral cortex, trigeminal nerve (cranial nerve V)
	Initiation of swallowing (deglutition)	Cerebral cortex
1–2 sec in pharynx, 5–8 sec in esophagus	Swallowing of food down esophagus into stomach	Vagovagal swallowing reflex, ENS peristalsis
30–45 min in stomach	Secretion of acid and pepsinogen (gastric phase)	Vagovagal reflex, gastrin from G cells, histamine from ECL cells
	Mixing and grinding of food in stomach, squirting of chyme into duodenum until stomach is empty	Vagovagal reflex, ENS peristalsis
2–4 hr in small intestine	Secretion of pancreatic fluid and bile into duodenum (intestinal phase)	Secretin from S cells, CCK from I cells, vagovagal reflex
	Propulsion through small intestine to colon	ENS peristalsis
12–30 hr in colon	Feces formation with water/salt absorption, propulsion toward rectum	ENS peristalsis, mass movement
Seconds to minutes	Defecation	ENS peristalsis, pelvic nerve spinal reflex, cerebral cortex

Table 28.2   ENDOCRINE, PARACRINE, AND NEUROCRINE FACTORS INVOLVED IN DIGESTION

Endocrine Factors

Factor	**Secretin**
Location	S cells of duodenum and jejunum
Stimulus	Low pH (<4.5) in duodenum → secretin release
Action	Neutralizes chyme by stimulating pancreatic water and bicarbonate secretion, causes exocytosis of pancreatic enzymes

Factor	**Gastrin**
Location	G cells of gastric antrum
Stimulus	Sight, smell, or taste of food → vagal output → gastrin release (cephalic phase) Gastric distention and presence of nutrients → gastrin secretion (gastric phase) Duodenal distention → gastrin secretion from duodenal G cells (intestinal phase)
Action	Stimulates acid secretion by parietal cells

Factor	**Cholecystokinin (CCK)**
Location	I cells and enteric neurons of duodenum and jejunum
Stimulus	Free fatty acids, triglycerides, peptides, amino acids, and gastric acid in small intestine → CCK release
Action	Causes gallbladder contraction and sphincter of Oddi relaxation, thus allowing bile to enter intestine; causes exocytosis of pancreatic enzymes

Factor	**Glucose-dependent insulinotropic polypeptide (GIP)[a]**
Location	Enteroendocrine cells in duodenum and jejunum
Stimulus	Glucose, triglycerides, or amino acids → GIP release
Action	Stimulates insulin release from endocrine pancreas

Factor	**Motilin**
Location	Upper portions of small intestine
Stimulus	Released in 90-min cycles during fasting state
Action	Initiates migrating myoelectrical complex (MMC)

Paracrine Factors

Factor	**Somatostatin**
Location	D cells in gastric antrum, near gastrin-secreting G cells
Stimulus	Low pH in stomach → somatostatin (inhibited by parasympathetic input, stimulated by sympathetic input)
Action	Inhibits acid secretion from parietal cells

Factor	**Histamine**
Location	Enteroendocrine cells and mast cells in gastric mucosa
Stimulus	Gastrin
Action	Stimulates gastric acid secretion via its activation of parietal cell H_2 type receptor

Factor	**Prostaglandin E_2 (PGE_2)**
Location	Stomach
Stimulus	
Action	Inhibits acid secretion, stimulates mucous production

(continued)

Table 28.2 *(Continued)*

Factor	**Acetylcholine (ACh)**	**Neurocrine Factors**
Location	Vagal axon terminals throughout GI tract	
Stimulus	Vagovagal reflexes	
Action	Enhances secretion and motility	
Factor	**Norepinephrine (NE)**	
Location	Sympathetic axon terminals throughout GI tract	
Stimulus	Tonically active	
Action	Inhibits secretion and motility	
Factor	**Gastrin-releasing peptide (GRP)**	
Location	Vagal axon terminals in stomach	
Stimulus	Vagovagal reflex	
Action	Gastrin release from G cells	
Factor	**Vasoactive intestinal peptide (VIP)**	
Location	Vagal axon terminals throughout GI tract	
Stimulus	Vagovagal reflex	
Action	Relaxes sphincters, circular muscle, and dilates blood vessels; stimulates intestinal and pancreatic secretion	
Factor	**Nitric oxide (NO)**	
Location	Vagal axon terminals throughout GI tract	
Stimulus	Vagovagal reflex	
Action	Relaxes sphincters, circular muscle, and dilates blood vessels	

[a] GIP is also called by its earlier name, gastric inhibitory peptide, but this name does not reflect its behavior at physiologic doses.

smooth muscle membranes and NE polarizing the membranes and inhibiting their excitability.

GI motility is controlled by the myenteric system, while the submucosal plexus is in perfect position to regulate blood flow and epithelial functions (secretion). Sensory receptors or chemoreceptors in the GI tract are sensitive to mechanical, thermal, osmotic, and chemical stimuli, while effector neurons result in motility, electrolyte and exocrine secretion, as well as neuroendocrine stimulation. A variety of reflexes within the GI system couple the functioning of two or more organs. For example, the intestine and stomach are linked by the enterogastric reflex, in which intestinal distention suppresses secretion and motility in the stomach.

Ingestion

Animals acquire nutrients by **ingestion** (eating), and mouths have been around since the pre-Cambrian beginnings of animal life more than 550 million years ago. Since that time, many organs have evolved in close alliance with the mouth: the sensory organs used to detect food, the muscles used for locomotion toward food sources, and the ganglia that coordinate the complex interaction between an animal and its prey. It is probably not an exaggeration to say that eating is responsible for the anatomic arrangement of our bodies into segments like those of ancient swimming tunicates and the placement of our organs of sight, audition, olfaction, and gustation in the head, near the mouth.

Anticipation of a Meal The human brain not only processes and regulates the interaction between our mouth and our food, but it also signals (via the hypothalamus) the need for food with the subjective sensation of hunger or **appetite**, plans for food procurement (via the cerebral cortex), and begins to prepare the digestive tract for action even before eating takes place. This anticipation of eating, sometimes called the *cephalic phase* of digestion, is the first

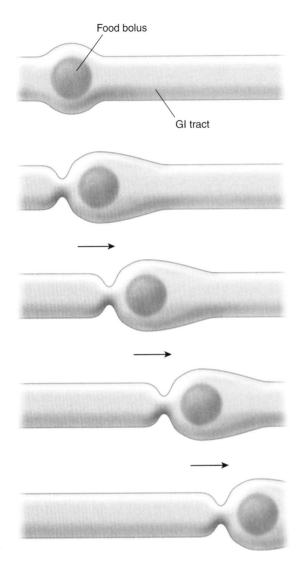

Food bolus

GI tract

Figure 28.5 Peristalsis. Distention of the GI lumen triggers a myenteric reflex that causes circular contraction proximal to the site of distention and dilatation distal to the site of distention. These contractions, termed peristalsis, move the bolus forward, triggering another myenteric reflex, and so on.

stage in the functioning of the GI tract. The cephalic phase includes thinking of food and registering the smells, sights, and sounds of food. The *oral phase* of digestion (taste) begins when food reaches the tongue. The stimuli of the cephalic and oral phases result in increased parasympathetic output from the *dorsal motor nuclei* of the vagus nerves and the *salivatory nuclei*. These signals, in turn, increase salivary, gastric, and exocrine pancreas secretion, enhance gallbladder contractility, and relax the smooth muscle of the body of the stomach and the sphincter of Oddi.

Ghrelin (ghre, a prefix for growth) is a peptide hormone secreted by epithelial cells of the gastric fundus that coordinates appetite and energy balance. Ghrelin's actions on receptors in the anterior

pituitary gland stimulate the release of growth hormone while hypothalamic receptor activation stimulates appetite. Ghrelin also appears to suppress fat utilization in adipose tissue. Levels of ghrelin are highest just prior to a meal, and in some obese individuals with extreme appetites, levels have been found to be elevated.

Mastication Mastication, commonly known as chewing, is both a voluntary and an involuntary process involving muscles innervated by cranial nerve V. Like the act of walking, chewing involves certain stereotyped patterns of movement that are partially automatic, though they can be controlled or interrupted with conscious attention. To be able to chew, one must have healthy teeth, gums, and mucous membranes. In edentulous persons (those without teeth), it is imperative that dentures fit well. The inability to chew properly can result in nutritional deficiencies due to the avoidance of certain foods (e.g., fruits and vegetables), as well as esophageal obstruction from swallowing overly large pieces of solid food. Chewing and grinding food enhance digestion by increasing the overall surface area of the food that will be exposed to digestive enzymes. Mastication also enhances future gastric emptying (the movement of food onward from the stomach to the duodenum) by decreasing the size of the material that must pass through the small-diameter pyloric sphincter.

Salivation Salivation, the production of saliva by the salivary glands, is important for many reasons, including lubrication, digestion, acid neutralization, and immunologic function. The salivary nuclei in the brain stem (which were already stimulated during anticipation of the meal) are further stimulated by the tactile and gustatory sensation of food in the mouth, transmitted to the brain by cranial nerves VII and IX. Efferent sympathetic and parasympathetic fibers in the same nerves also innervate the salivary glands of the mouth. Parasympathetic stimulation increases salivation. About 1,500 mL of saliva with a pH of 6.0 to 7.0 is secreted daily. This pH helps protect the mouth and esophagus from refluxed gastric acid. In addition to the digestive enzyme *salivary amylase*, the saliva contains *immunoglobulin IgA*, which protects against bacterial, fungal, and viral pathogens.

Deglutition Deglutition, the physiologic term for swallowing, is the process in which several muscles contract and relax under regulation by the *swallowing center* in the brain, located in the medulla and lower pons (FIGURE 28.6). Cranial nerves pass afferent information from the upper GI tract (mouth to esophagus) to the swallowing center. Efferent information from the swallowing center returns to the upper GI

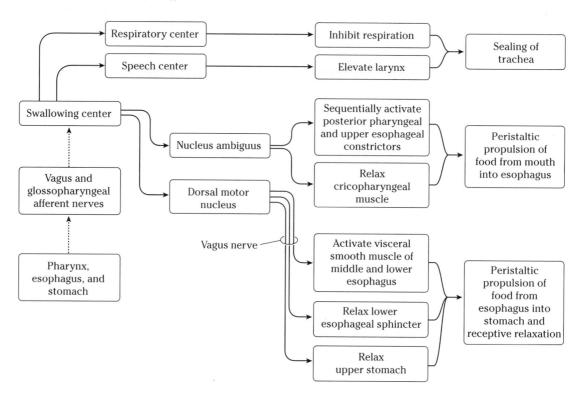

Figure 28.6 The swallowing reflex.

tract in multiple cranial nerves. Some of these fibers are somatic, arising in the *nucleus ambiguus* and terminating in striated muscle. Other efferent fibers arise in the dorsal motor nucleus of the vagus nerve and cast parasympathetic axons onto the upper GI smooth muscle.

Deglutition begins voluntarily, as the tongue pushes the food bolus into the posterior oropharynx. This initiates the involuntary **swallowing reflex**: the nasopharynx closes, the vocal cords and epiglottis close off the airway to the lungs, the pharynx contracts, and the upper esophageal sphincter (which is tonically constricted) relaxes. Pharyngeal peristalsis pushes the bolus into the esophagus in less than 2 s. The lower esophageal sphincter anticipates passage of the bolus by beginning to relax under parasympathetic influence 1 to 2.5 s after deglutition, and the peristaltic wave traveling down the esophagus pushes the bolus past the lower esophageal sphincter and into the stomach. If the entire food bolus does not make it through, a secondary peristaltic wave begins at the site of distention and clears the bolus.

The lower esophageal sphincter, like the upper one, is tonically constricted, which is important for preventing acid reflux from the stomach to the esophagus. The sphincter is reinforced by the diaphragm muscle surrounding it and by the positive intra-abdominal pressure (as opposed to the negative intrathoracic pressure). If the upper portion of the stomach slides up into the thorax (hiatal hernia),

the low pressure around the lower esophageal sphincter can cause acid reflux into the esophagus.

Finally, the swallowing reflex includes a vagally mediated reduction in the muscle tone of the stomach wall. This "receptive relaxation" allows the stomach to accommodate up to 2 L of fluid without an increase in intragastric pressure. Swallowing is the first of the vagovagal reflexes to occur in digestion. A second vagovagal reflex involving mechanoreceptors in the wall of the stomach contributes to receptive relaxation. (See Clinical Application Box *What Is Gastroesophageal Reflux Disease?*)

Gastric Motility and Secretion

During fasting, the stomach and small intestine are largely quiescent, aside from the small rhythmic contractions described above and what is known as the **migrating myoelectrical complex (MMC)**. The MMC is a pattern of motility that builds in intensity until it generates one large "housekeeper" contraction, a wave that sweeps from the stomach to the terminal ileum. The MMC, which arises every 75 to 90 min and lasts for 3 to 6 min, pushes any undigested, unabsorbed material from the stomach and small intestine into the large intestine for excretion. It also prevents stasis from occurring within the stomach and small intestine, thereby preventing overgrowth of the small number of bacteria normally present in these organs. The MMC is prompted by the neuroen-

WHAT IS GASTROESOPHAGEAL REFLUX DISEASE?

A 34-year-old man complains to his primary care physician of "burning pain" just below his sternum. The pain has bothered him for almost a year and is aggravated by spicy and fried foods, and especially by caffeine. He has experienced limited relief with over-the-counter treatments like Tums and Pepcid. The patient is instructed to avoid aggravating foods and is prescribed omeprazole (Prilosec). He is also referred to a gastroenterologist for an endoscopy, which shows normal esophageal mucosa. His pain resolves after a month of twice-daily omeprazole, and his dietary changes help in the months following, though he still has pain occasionally.

Reflux (gastroesophageal reflux), the medical term for *heartburn*, involves the backflow of acid and pepsin from the stomach across the lower esophageal sphincter and into the lower esophagus. Acid and pepsin injure the esophageal mucosa, causing pain because the esophageal mucosa does not share the protections of the gastric mucosa—mucus and bicarbonate production, for example. **Gastroesophageal reflux disease (GERD)** is chronic reflux; the reflux is present recurrently over a long period of time.

While gastric secretions do cause the pain, gastric secretion is *not* elevated in most cases of GERD. Rather, the problem is a failure of the lower esophageal sphincter. Aberrant swallowing may cause the lower esophageal sphincter to open without the appropriate lower esophageal peristalsis afterward. This results in failure to flush refluxed secretions back into the stomach. Postprandial overdistention or irritation of the stomach also increases the likelihood of reflux. Untreated GERD may eventually cause **Barrett's esophagus**, a metaplastic change wherein the esophageal mucosa begins to express features of the gastric mucosa to protect itself from acid. The development of Barrett's esophagus carries an increased risk of esophageal cancer.

Several medical treatments for GERD reduce the acidity of gastric secretions, but they do not address the underlying cause of the reflux. Tums ($CaCO_3$) acts as a base and neutralizes the stomach acid so that when it is refluxed, it is not harmful to the esophageal mucosa. H_2 blockers, such as ranitidine (Zantac), block the histamine receptor and hence interfere with gastrin's activation of parietal cell acid secretion. Proton pump inhibitors, such as omeprazole (Prilosec), inhibit the parietal cell H^+/K^+-ATPase. Dietary modification is more successful at eliminating the cause of GERD. The principal surgical treatment for GERD is fundoplication of the lower esophageal sphincter, in which part of the stomach is wrapped around the lower esophageal sphincter to reinforce it. This procedure can now be performed laparoscopically, which makes for an easier recovery than older approaches, but surgery is still reserved for patients in whom medical therapy and dietary modification have failed.

docrine mediator **motilin**. This 22-amino-acid peptide is secreted during fasting states by neuroendocrine cells in the proximal small intestine, possibly under the influence of an alkaline duodenal pH. (The antibiotic erythromycin is a non-peptide motilin receptor agonist that can be used clinically to stimulate GI motility, but when taken for usual reasons, it can also lead to abdominal discomfort.)

When food is delivered to the stomach, stretching the gastric walls, the pattern of motility changes. Gastric distention stimulates vagovagal pathways and the ENS, which initiate contractions in the stomach walls. Waves of contractions push food against a contracted pyloric sphincter three times a minute,

mixing and grinding the food and causing small amounts to squirt into the duodenum.

At the same time, gastric distention and the presence of food also stimulate gastric acid secretion from *parietal cells* through the action of ACh, gastrin, and histamine. The vagovagal response to distention deploys ACh to the muscarinic receptors on the parietal cells of the gastric mucosa, directly increasing acid secretion. Vagal stimulation of antral **G cells** and stimulation of the G cells by amino acids lead to **gastrin** release into the bloodstream. Gastrin reaches the parietal cells through the circulation and acts on the parietal cells directly, increasing H^+ secretion. Gastrin also affects the parietal cells

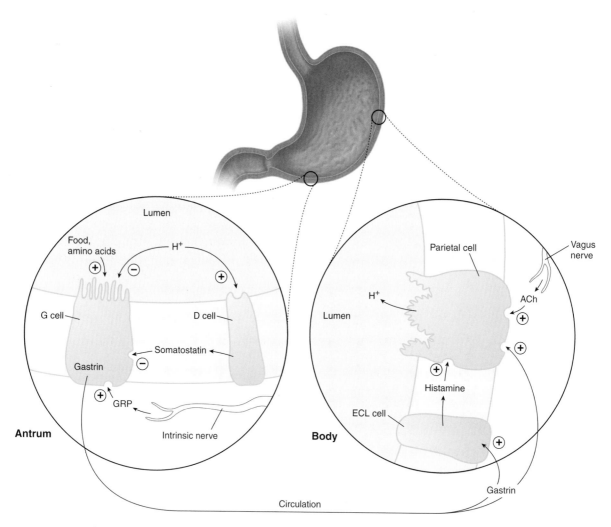

Figure 28.7   Controlled release of gastric acid from parietal cells. Gastrin, histamine, and ACh are the main triggers for acid secretion. Acid secretion involves the fusion of intracellular vesicles with the cell membrane. These vesicles carry H^+/K^+-ATPases. Their fusion also increases the surface area for acid secretion, as reflected in the more wrinkled morphology of the cell membrane. H^+ and somatostatin suppress acid secretion in a negative-feedback loop. GRP = gastrin-releasing peptide, ECL cell = enterochromaffin-like cell.

through the intermediary of histamine-containing enteroendocrine cells called *enterochromaffin-like (ECL) cells*. In response to gastrin, ECL cells secrete **histamine**, which binds the H_2 receptor on parietal cells and increases H^+ secretion. The common mechanism by which these various mediators increase H^+ secretion is translocation of H^+/K^+-ATPase from intracellular vesicles to the parietal cell membrane (with concomitant increase in the cell membrane surface area due to the addition of the vesicles). When the pH drops below 3.0, G cells stop secreting gastrin and *D cells* secrete the paracrine factor *somatostatin*. Somatostatin inhibits gastrin release. Thus, the acidification of the gastric contents is self-limiting (FIGURE 28.7). Finally, vagal input and gastrin (as well as other factors) stimulate the gastric *chief cells* to secrete *pepsinogen*. Pepsino-

gen is cleaved by acid pH to form pepsin, an important enzyme in the digestion of proteins.

Duodenal Regulation of Pancreatic and Hepatobiliary Secretion

The entry of food material (called chyme upon leaving the stomach) into the small intestine stimulates three different regulatory pathways that stimulate the pancreas and liver. Two of the signals are hormones secreted by intestinal enteroendocrine cells and one pathway involves the vagus nerve.

S cells in the mucosa respond to the low pH of chyme by releasing the hormone **secretin** into the bloodstream. Secretin circulates to acinar cells of the exocrine pancreas and binds basolateral receptors on those cells. This has two main effects: it causes the fusion of zymogen granules with the apical membrane, dumping zymogens (digestive enzyme precursors) into the pancreatic ducts; and it causes the translocation of H^+-ATPase to the basolateral membrane. This in turn results in increased clearance of H^+ from the cell, enabling the pancreatic cell to make and secrete HCO_3^-, which keeps the pancreatic secretions alkaline and enables neutralization of the acidic chyme.

I cells in the small intestine respond to luminal proteins, lipids, and their cleavage products by secreting the hormone **cholecystokinin (CCK)** into the bloodstream. CCK circulates to the pancreas and stimulates pancreatic secretion, as secretin does. CCK also circulates to the smooth muscle of the gallbladder and the sphincter of Oddi. It promotes gallbladder contraction and sphincter relaxation, resulting in the secretion of bile and pancreatic fluid into the duodenum. Pancreatic enzymes and bile acids in the duodenum may have an inhibitory effect on I cells, controlling CCK secretion (and thus pancreatic and hepatobiliary secretion) with negative feedback.

Vagovagal reflexes increase pancreatic and gallbladder secretion. Vagal afferents detect intestinal distention and high luminal osmolality, causing vagal efferents to stimulate the pancreas and gallbladder. CCK acts on the vagal neurons to potentiate these effects. Peristalsis moves the chyme onward through the small intestine until it arrives at the ileocecal valve. CCK has an additional role in signaling satiety to the hypothalamus of the brain.

Ileocecal Regulation of Motility

The terminal ileum regulates not only the passage of chyme into the colon, but also the motility in proximal parts of the small intestine. Lipids in the ileum suggest that chyme moved too fast through the small intestine for proper digestion and absorption to occur. Accordingly, the ileal mucosa reacts to lipids in the ileum by sending an inhibitory signal to the ENS of the upper small intestine. This phenomenon, sometimes called the **ileal brake**, constitutes a feedback system that slows GI motility to improve digestion and absorption. Distention of the ileum relaxes the ileocecal sphincter, enabling the chyme (at this point, mostly composed of indigestible matter and water) to flow into the colon.

Colonic Motility and Defecation

Because the large intestine retains waste material until almost all water can be absorbed, it is a slower-moving portion of the GI tract. The lower-flow conditions allow bacteria to thrive in the colon, unlike in the small intestine. While mammals have developed a symbiotic relationship with the **intestinal microflora** in the colon (see Chapter 27), even symbiotic bacteria

are unwanted in the small intestine. Here they would steal digestible nutrients from the host and obstruct the absorptive surface. However, because of the absence of a significant microflora population in the small intestine, this part of the GI tract is more susceptible to invasive pathogens than the large intestine. For all these reasons, the ileocecal sphincter is a one-way valve, and when the cecum is distended by incoming waste matter, a reflex closes the valve.

Wastes pass through the colon by a slower-wave peristalsis. In addition, segmental and nonpropulsive contractions occur randomly in the colon. These movements help release water from the waste material for absorption. Intermittently giant **mass movements** of fecal material also occur, often after the gastroduodenal distention of a meal. When a mass movement follows gastroduodenal stimulation, it is called the **gastrocolic reflex**. Its mechanism is not entirely understood.

Either the baseline slow peristalsis of the large intestine or a mass movement can push waste material (at this point termed *feces*) into the rectum. Distention of the rectum leads to the **defecation reflex** when the rectal pressure exceeds 18 mm Hg. The reflex includes ENS peristalsis and a spinal parasympathetic reflex (through the pelvic nerve) with relaxation of the internal anal sphincter. The internal anal sphincter is otherwise tonically constricted by sympathetic input.

When the involuntary defecation reflex has begun, several voluntary steps are necessary for **defecation**, the evacuation of feces from the rectum, to occur. First, the external anal sphincter must be consciously relaxed. Second, the *Valsalva maneuver* must usually be employed to some degree. This is the instinctual, but voluntary, event commonly called straining, in which the abdominal wall muscles are contracted against a closed epiglottis to increase intra-abdominal pressure, thereby helping propel the feces through the anal canal. The closure of the epiglottis is necessary to sustain the raised intra-abdominal pressure. With it open, the raised pressure would move the diaphragm up, forcing air out of the lungs and expanding the abdominal cavity volume at the expense of the thoracic volume. With a closed epiglottis, the diaphragm is fixed in place, and abdominal muscle contraction compresses the fixed volume of the abdominal cavity. (See Clinical Application Box *What Is Irritable Bowel Syndrome?*)

PATHOPHYSIOLOGY

Because disorders of motility or secretion lead to disordered digestion and absorption, some of the important derangements of motility and secretion were described in Chapter 27. To that material we will now add the three most common disorders of GI

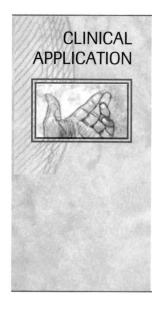

WHAT IS IRRITABLE BOWEL SYNDROME?

A 45-year-old woman complains of a long history of constipation, diarrhea, and abdominal cramps. She has three children, works hard at an exhausting and stressful job, and describes herself as "stressed out." She has been diagnosed repeatedly with irritable bowel syndrome and wants to know if there is anything else that can be done about her symptoms.

Irritable bowel syndrome (IBS) is a condition of chronic diarrhea, constipation, abdominal pain, or some combination of these three. It seems to be caused by stress and anxiety, which produce alterations in GI motility and in sensitivity to visceral stimuli, such as distention. Approximately 15% of American adults suffer symptoms consistent with a diagnosis of IBS, which is defined as 12 weeks of the above otherwise unexplained GI symptoms in a year. IBS is the most common diagnosis made by American gastroenterologists and may cost the U.S. economy more than $30 billion annually. Treatments are directed toward symptoms, with dietary changes and fiber playing an important role.

---

motility, and introduce several less common disorders of motility and secretion that were not touched upon previously.

Common Disorders

Vomiting, diarrhea, and constipation are frequent maladies of the digestive tract and often are brief and self-limiting. Although they account for a significant number of complaints heard by any general practitioner, treatments are less than perfect.

Vomiting   **Vomiting**, or *emesis*, serves the functional purpose of expelling potentially harmful luminal contents from the GI tract. The *vomiting center* in the medulla receives signals from both vagal and sympathetic afferents from the stomach and small intestine. The stimulus to vomit is often initiated through this pathway by mucosal irritation or overdistention in the GI tract. In addition, many metabolic and psychological stimuli are transduced into signals affecting the medullary vomiting center. The anticipation of vomiting is the subjective sensation of **nausea**. (Agents that inspire nausea are *nauseous* agents, and a sufferer of nausea is referred to as *nauseated*.)

Vomiting commences with **antiperistalsis**, or reverse peristalsis. It can bring contents from as far down the tract as the ileum all the way back to the duodenum. The retrograde accumulation of GI contents distends the duodenum until a threshold is reached. The upper GI sphincters relax, and strong contractions of the duodenum, stomach smooth muscle, and abdominal skeletal muscle force the GI contents up the esophagus and out of the mouth.

Diarrhea   **Diarrhea** is impaired GI water absorption. It results from derangements of the absorptive surface, from abnormalities in the osmotic gradient for small or large intestine water absorption, and from abnormally rapid transit of chyme and feces through the GI tract. (High transit rates do not expose the chyme to the absorptive surface long enough for adequate water absorption.) Infections of the GI tract may cause diarrhea by all three of the above mechanisms.

Inflammation around mucosal pathogens obstructs the absorptive surface and leaves solutes in the intestinal lumen that would normally be absorbed. Solutes in the lumen pose another obstacle for successful water absorption by creating osmotic pressure to retain water in the gut. The resulting distention of the intestine, in combination with inflammatory irritation of the intestinal wall, can provoke ENS and vagovagal reflexes that increase intestinal motility. Psychological factors (anxiety) may also increase parasympathetic input to the GI tract and increase motility.

Constipation   **Constipation** is impairment or infrequency of defecation, and it is generally caused by two factors, often seen together. One factor is decreased water content in the stool, which reduces the lubrication of the stool inside the colon, thereby impeding its forward movement. The other factor is depressed intestinal motility, which results in a failure to push the feces out toward the rectum and also causes dry stools. Depressed GI motility leads to dry stools because inadequate peristalsis or mass movements slows the transit time of the feces through the colon. With a longer transit time, the feces are exposed to the absorptive surface for a longer period of time, and more water is withdrawn from the stool.

Inadequate dietary intake of fiber and water is the most common cause of constipation. With too little water in the diet, too little water is left in the stool. Poor fiber content in the chyme delivered to the cecum leads to constipation in two different ways. First, less fiber in the diet means less waste matter in the chyme. Consequently, the waste matter delivered to the colon is less bulky. With a smaller mass of waste material, the colon does not experience as much distention, so the luminal contents inspire weaker peristaltic and parasympathetic reflexes. The diet may be low in fiber because of food choices or from decreased overall consumption (dieting or malnutrition). Second, less undigested fiber means a lower osmolality in the chyme entering the colon. This promotes water absorption, drying out the stool.

Behavioral factors may also contribute to constipation. A daily rhythm of gastrocolic reflexes and mass movements may be established by a regular eating schedule. Irregular meals may interfere with this rhythm and reduce mass movements. Similarly, irregular opportunities or uncomfortable circumstances for defecation can interfere with regular evacuation of the bowels. The longer the feces sit in one place, the more the GI tract's response to distention is attenuated. ENS peristalsis and spinal reflexes are suppressed, and GI motility declines in the distal colon, worsening the problem. Stoppage breeds more stoppage.

Certain populations are at increased risk for constipation. The combination of immobility (and hence decreased opportunities for defecation) and decreased fluid intake seen in the geriatric population makes constipation a frequent problem among the elderly or disabled. Pregnant women suffer depressed GI motility under the influence of such pregnancy hormones as *relaxin*. Anxiety-related irritable bowel syndrome (IBS) may also cause constipation. Patients in the hospital are susceptible to constipation owing to infrequent opportunities or uncomfortable circumstances for defecation. (Patients who must use a bedpan and require assistance from a nurse may have difficulty attending to this body function.)

Whatever the cause of the constipation, increased fluid and fiber intake can reverse it or prevent it. Stool softeners and laxatives may provide short-term help. Chronic constipation can decrease appetite and lead to **hemorrhoids**, which are congested and dilated anal and rectal veins due to high-pressure defecatory straining. Constipation can also compromise a person's sense of well-being. (See Clinical Application Box *What Is Small Bowel Obstruction?*)

CLINICAL APPLICATION

WHAT IS SMALL BOWEL OBSTRUCTION?

A 45-year-old man presents to the emergency department with 36 hours of nausea, vomiting, and unrelieved abdominal pain increasing in severity. His last stool was 24 hours ago, and since then he has not passed gas. On examination, his abdomen is distended and bowel sounds are high-pitched and hyperactive. An upright abdominal x-ray shows air-fluid levels; a supine view shows distended bowel proximal to a point in the right lower quadrant and no gas in the colon. Further questioning reveals a history of abdominal surgery, with an appendectomy performed 3 years previously. The patient is diagnosed with complete small bowel obstruction. He receives intravenous normal saline and precautionary antibiotics, a nasogastric (NG) tube is placed, and he is referred for immediate surgery. Laparotomy reveals an adhesion compressing the small bowel in the right lower quadrant. The adhesion is successfully lysed.

Small bowel obstruction (SBO) arises when the bowel is physically (mechanically) compressed. There are two major causes. One cause is **adhesions**, intra-abdominal scar tissue that binds together loops of intestine and can entangle or compress the bowel. Abdominal surgery can lead to adhesions. Another cause of SBO is the condition in which a loop of intestine herniates through the inguinal canal, cutting off luminal flow and blood flow to this portion of the bowel. This condition is called an **incarcerated hernia**. Whenever a segment of bowel is compressed in two places, as in an incarcerated hernia, the intestine between the compression sites becomes strangulated. **Bowel strangulation**, a loss of blood supply, can lead to necrosis of the intestine and **perforation**, or breakdown in the intestinal wall. Perforation introduces bacteria into the peritoneal cavity, where the bacteria can grow and lead to sepsis. **Sepsis** is infection of the blood associated with **shock**, which is widespread vasodilation and consequent hypotension (low blood pressure). Any obstructed intestine becomes inflamed, however, even if it is not strangulated and necrosed, because the obstruction of GI flow leads to bacterial overgrowth inside the GI tract.

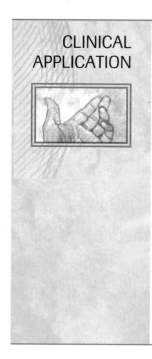

WHAT IS SMALL BOWEL OBSTRUCTION? (*Continued*)

Adynamic or **paralytic ileus** can mimic SBO. This condition arises in the context of gastroenteritis or after surgery. Gastroenteritis and abdominal surgery may acutely stun the myenteric plexus of the small intestine, temporarily abolishing peristalsis. Food fails to move through, causing backup, distention, and antiperistalsis in the upper GI tract. This is why patients are not allowed to eat after abdominal surgery until they recover their bowel motility, as evidenced by bowel sounds (detectable on auscultation of the abdomen).

Bowel sounds are gurgling sounds made by air and fluid passing through the GI tract. A gurgle is called a **borborygmus** (plural, borborygmi). SBO, by contrast, leads to high-pitched bowel sounds because the distention stretches the intestinal wall taut and raises the frequency of the sound waves it emits during borborygmi. In addition, distention triggers peristaltic and vagovagal reflexes, leading to hyperactive bowel sounds.

SBO is treated with normal saline to replace fluid lost to the intestinal wall, which is undergoing an inflammatory response. The NG tube decompresses the bowel proximal to the obstruction and relieves nausea and vomiting. Antibiotics guard against sepsis. Surgery relieves the causes of mechanical obstruction.

Less Common Disturbances of GI Regulation

Achalasia is a condition resulting from damage to the myenteric plexus in the lower esophagus. A patient with achalasia does not have normal esophageal peristalsis or normal lower esophageal sphincter opening and hence has an abnormal swallowing reflex. Difficulty swallowing is called **dysphagia**. **Carcinoid tumors** of the GI tract are tumors of enteroendocrine cells. A large proportion of tumors of the small intestine are carcinoid tumors; however, small bowel tumors are dwarfed in incidence compared to colon cancer. Well-differentiated carcinoid tumors may secrete hormones in an unregulated fashion. This leads to syndromes such as Zollinger-Ellison syndrome.

Zollinger-Ellison syndrome is a disorder caused by a gastrin-producing tumor (gastrinoma) in the pancreas or duodenum, which leads to gastric acid hypersecretion and severe peptic ulcer disease. Gastrinomas can be malignant or benign tumors, and they may be associated with other neoplasms in a *multiple endocrine neoplasia (MEN)* type of syndrome. There are three different types of MEN, all exceedingly rare.

Summary

- GI motility (motor activity) and secretion of enzymes and fluid enable digestion and absorption to take place.

- The GI tract's motility and secretion are controlled by the central nervous system (CNS), the enteric nervous system (ENS), and the enteroendocrine cells distributed throughout the GI mucosa.

- The ENS is composed of the myenteric plexus, which controls motility, and the submucosal plexus, which controls secretion and blood flow.

- The CNS and ENS communicate via the parasympathetic and sympathetic nervous systems. The parasympathetic nervous system carries afferent and efferent signals between the two in the vagus nerve (a cranial nerve) and the pelvic nerve (a sacral nerve).

- Motility, the propulsion of food, chyme, and feces through the GI tract, is achieved mainly through peristalsis and vagovagal reflexes. Peristalsis is a myenteric reflex in which luminal distention leads to contraction behind and dilatation in front of a bolus of food, driving the bolus forward. Vagovagal reflexes augment peristalsis and coordinate GI contractions with sphincter dilatations and secretions.

- A basal level of "sympathetic tone" inhibits motility and keeps sphincters closed.
- Cranial nerve reflexes lead to salivation even before food enters the mouth.
- Gastric acid secretion is controlled through enteroendocrine G cells. Vagal input and amino acids on the mucosa stimulate G cells to release the hormone gastrin, which triggers enterochromaffin-like (ECL) cells to secrete the paracrine factor histamine. Histamine and vagal input trigger the gastric parietal cells to secrete H^+.
- Enteroendocrine S cells in the duodenal mucosa respond to the low pH of chyme by releasing the hormone secretin into the bloodstream. Secretin stimulates pancreatic secretion.
- Enteroendocrine I cells in the duodenal mucosa respond to luminal proteins, lipids, and their cleavage products by secreting the hormone cholecystokinin (CCK) into the bloodstream. CCK stimulates pancreatic secretion and gallbladder contraction.
- When feces reach the rectum, an autonomic pelvic nerve reflex initiates defecation. Conscious, voluntary compliance with this reflex in the form of external anal sphincter relaxation (and often voluntary straining) is necessary for defecation to be completed.
- Vomiting occurs by antiperistalsis.
- Diarrhea is impaired GI water absorption. Hypermotility plays a role in diarrhea.
- Constipation is impairment or infrequency of defecation. A lack of bulk in the stool (i.e., lack of fiber) reduces colonic motility.

Suggested Reading

De Caestecker J. ABC of the upper gastrointestinal tract. Oesophagus: heartburn. Br Med J. 2001;323:736–739.

Diamant NE. Physiology of esophageal motor function. Gastroenterol Clin North Am. 1989;18:179–194.

Goyal RK, Hirano I. The enteric nervous system. N Engl J Med. 1996;334:1106–1115.

Hersey SJ, Sachs G. Gastric acid secretion. Physiol Rev. 1995;75:155–189.

Horwitz BJ, Fisher RS. The irritable bowel syndrome. N Engl J Med. 2001;344:1846–1850.

Owyang C. Neurohormonal control of the exocrine pancreas. Curr Opin Gastroenterol. 1994;10:491–495.

REVIEW QUESTIONS

Directions: Each of the numbered items or incomplete statements in this section is followed by answers or by completions of the statement. Select the ONE lettered answer or completion that is BEST in each case.

1. A woman with rectal bleeding is found on examination to have a thrombosed hemorrhoid. Which of the following conditions might predispose her to developing hemorrhoids?
   - (A) She has had repeated bouts of infectious gastroenteritis in the past year.
   - (B) She is a vegetarian with a high-fiber diet.
   - (C) She is in her third trimester of pregnancy.
   - (D) She has Zollinger-Ellison syndrome.
   - (E) She abuses laxatives.

2. H_2 blockers are sometimes used in the treatment of heartburn symptoms because:
   - (A) Overproduction of gastric acid is the most common cause of heartburn.
   - (B) H_2 blockers prevent reflux.
   - (C) H_2 blockers improve lower esophageal sphincter tone.
   - (D) H_2 blockers inhibit the H^+/K^+-ATPase.
   - (E) H_2 blockers can help control heartburn symptoms.

3. A 70-year-old man has suffered several small strokes in his medulla. Since then, he can initiate swallowing but has not been able to move food all the way from his esophagus to his stomach. The stroke has probably disabled:
   - (A) The salivatory nucleus.
   - (B) The nucleus ambiguous.
   - (C) The dorsal motor nucleus of the vagus nerve.
   - (D) ENS peristalsis.
   - (E) The myenteric plexus.

ANSWERS TO REVIEW QUESTIONS

1. **The answer is C.** Pregnancy slows GI motility, leading to constipation, which is the usual cause of hemorrhoids. Constipation causes hemorrhoids by requiring straining with high intra-abdominal pressures. Gastroenteritis, a high-fiber diet, and laxative abuse would cause diarrhea. Zollinger-Ellison syndrome would cause peptic ulcer.

2. **The answer is E.** H$_2$ blockers control heartburn symptoms by lowering the acidity of gastric secretions. They do not prevent reflux. They do not reinforce the lower esophageal sphincter as surgical fundoplication does. They do not inhibit the H$^+$/K$^+$-ATPase as omeprazole does. They block the histamine receptor and thereby prevent activation of the parietal cell. Overproduction of acid is not the cause of reflux; lower esophageal sphincter incompetence and gastric distention are.

3. **The answer is C.** The dorsal motor nucleus of the vagus nerve sends out signals that open the lower esophageal sphincter. The ENS is not affected by a CNS stroke.

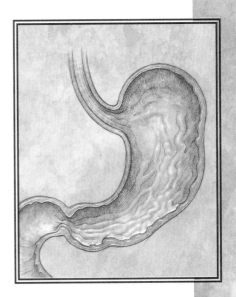

29

Hepatic Physiology

INTRODUCTION

The kidney modifies the contents of the plasma by filtering its components into the urine; the liver modifies the blood contents by metabolically transforming them. Liver cells, or **hepatocytes**, house a vast stable of enzymes for this purpose. The liver is where drugs, hormones, and toxic waste products such as ammonia are metabolized to inactive forms. Energy substrates are shifted from one form to another: Glucose is stored here (and in muscle) as glycogen; glucose is synthesized primarily in hepatic gluconeogenesis; in starved states, ketone bodies are produced in the liver from fatty acids. Nonessential amino acids are created in the liver. Fats are absorbed from the intestine with bile salts and phospholipids secreted by the liver, and cholesterol is shuttled to the tissues by hepatic lipoproteins and excreted from the body by the liver. The liver also synthesizes the major plasma proteins, including albumin and the clotting factors. Its roles in energy metabolism are regulated by pancreatic endocrine hormones, discussed in Chapter 30. The role of the liver in lipid digestion and transport is partly governed by enteroendocrine cells (see Chapter 27). This briefer chapter will focus on the liver's role in detoxification and the synthesis of blood proteins.

SYSTEM STRUCTURE

The **liver** is situated in the right upper quadrant of the abdomen. It has a dual blood supply from the hepatic artery and the portal vein. The **hepatic artery**, which branches off the celiac trunk, is oxygen-rich but nutrient-poor and provides the liver with 20% to 30% of its blood supply. The **portal vein**, which carries blood from the digestive tract, pancreas, and spleen, is oxygen-poor but nutrient-rich and provides the liver with 70% to 80% of its blood supply. Both of these vessels enter the liver at the **porta hepatis**, which is also the site at which the common hepatic bile duct leaves the liver. These three vessels—artery, portal vein, and bile duct—form the **portal triad**. The three vessels of the portal triad divide and subdivide together through the hepatic parenchyma, separating the liver into functional segments called lobules.

Lobules are hexagonal groups of hepatocytes bounded by portal triads at each corner. In the center of each hexagon is a **central vein**. The arterial and portal venous blood mix as they flow toward the center of the lobule in the spaces between hepatocytes called **sinusoids** (FIGURE 29.1). The sinusoids empty into the lobular central vein. The central veins come together in collecting veins, which come together in the hepatic veins and finally dump their blood into the vena cava. The plates of hepatocytes in the lobule

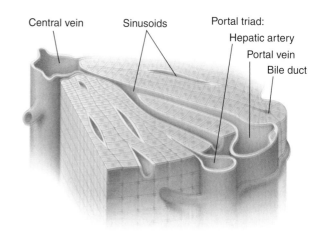

Figure 29.1   Hepatic microcirculation. The bile canaliculi arise between two cells, and the bile ducts arise within the lobule between two plates of hepatocytes apposed with one another.

are one or two cells thick, with sinusoids on either side. **Bile canaliculi**, into which bile is secreted, run between hepatocytes. The bile then collects between two layers of hepatocytes and flows away from the center of the lobule and out to the bile duct at the hexagon corners. The endothelium of hepatocytes lacks a basement membrane, which facilitates the exchange between hepatocytes and the blood.

The functions of the liver are performed by the various hepatocyte organelles. The mitochondria of hepatocytes have enzymes that take part in the urea cycle. The smooth **endoplasmic reticulum (ER)** is the site of glycogen synthesis, the conjugation of bilirubin, and the detoxification of foreign substances. The rough ER is the site of the synthesis of plasma proteins such as albumin, fibrinogen, and prothrombin. Lysosomes take part in the receptor-mediated endocytosis of lipoproteins such as LDL and HDL, as well as chylomicrons. Hepatocyte peroxisomes remove peroxide generated by oxidases, and they are the site of long-chain fatty acid oxidation. The Golgi apparatus is responsible for the glycosylation and secretion of plasma proteins, such as transferrin, and lipoproteins, such as VLDL.

SYSTEM FUNCTION

As stated above, this chapter will focus on just a few of the liver functions that have not been detailed in other chapters. Our interest here is also in laying the foundations for understanding the pathophysiology of liver failure. Particular aspects of liver physiology are helpful not only in predicting the consequences of disease, but also in understanding the clinical signs and symptoms by which liver disease is diagnosed.

Detoxifying Actions of the Liver

We will look at three significant detoxifying mechanisms in liver function: drug metabolism, ammonia metabolism, and the metabolism of bilirubin (a breakdown product of heme from red blood cells and the cause of jaundice). These processes are not hormonally controlled; they are governed by the kinetics of hepatic enzyme-substrate interactions. In other words, when more toxic substrate is present in the blood, the rate of enzymatic reactions in the liver increases. When the enzymes are saturated, which does not occur under physiologic circumstances, the toxic substrates accumulate in the blood and can have adverse effects.

Drug Metabolism   The liver plays a critical role in the transformation of drugs and xenobiotic compounds into inactive and hydrophilic (water-soluble) substances that are readily eliminated from the body through bile or urine. Two sets of enzymatic reactions take place in hepatocytes to serve these purposes (FIGURE 29.2). **Phase I reactions** are slow, energy-consuming reactions catalyzed by the heme-containing **cytochrome P-450 enzymes**. These reactions result in oxidation, reduction, or hydrolysis of the parent compound. Three gene superfamilies (I, II, III) encode different cytochrome P-450 enzymes, each with different substrate specificities. Sometimes a phase I reaction alone is adequate to inactivate a drug and prepare it for elimination. Often, however, the phase I product is a toxic intermediate such as a free radical that must be inactivated by a phase II conjugation reaction. **Phase II reactions**, which are much faster and less energy-dependent than phase I reactions, add bulky polar groups to the metabolites of the phase I reactions, inactivating them and rendering them even more water-soluble. Most of the enzymes involved in phase I and phase II reactions are located in the smooth ER of hepatocytes, so that toxic metabolites cannot interact with the rest of the cell.

Recall from renal physiology that the **clearance** of a compound from the blood by an organ is the volume of plasma rid of the substance by that organ per unit time. Drug clearance varies in different contexts. Newborns, whose cytochrome P-450 enzymes are poorly developed, clear drugs more slowly, as do older adults. Genetic cytochrome P-450 polymorphisms have been identified in members of different ethnic groups, which may contribute to altered metabolism of certain drugs. The presence of a second drug in the plasma may also affect the metabolism of the first drug (for example, by inducing the expression of cytochrome P-450 enzymes, thereby increasing clearance of the first drug). Other factors include gender and disease states. In chronic liver disease, phase I reactions are impaired in proportion to the loss of hepatocyte mass, while phase II reactions are relatively spared. This information needs to be considered when dosing drugs in patients with chronic liver disease.

The Elimination of Bilirubin   **Bilirubin** is a yellow pigment formed from the hemoglobin of old red blood cells by macrophages. Bilirubin gives the yellowish hue to a healing bruise, and the metabolites of bilirubin give the yellow color to urine and the brown color to feces. Before bilirubin gets into either urine or feces, however, it must be removed from the bloodstream and transformed by the liver.

Recall that hemoglobin contains *heme*—a porphyrin ring with iron at its center. Heme is metabolized inside macrophages to biliverdin (a green pigment, also seen in healing bruises), which is then metabolized to bilirubin (FIGURE 29.3). The bilirubin formed in this process is insoluble and is referred to as **unconjugated bilirubin**, or *indirect bilirubin*. Unconjugated bilirubin is carried in the blood tightly bound to the blood protein albumin and is taken up by hepatocytes.

In the hepatocytes, bilirubin is conjugated in the smooth ER to glucuronic acid by the enzyme glucuronyltransferase. After conjugation, it is known as **conjugated bilirubin** (also *bilirubin diglucuronide* or *direct bilirubin*), and it is water-soluble. It is finally secreted into the bile canaliculus and is expelled in bile from the gallbladder to the duodenum. Conjugated bilirubin is the only component of bile that does not take part in micelle formation (see Chapter 27), but it does give bile its yellow-brown color.

Conjugated bilirubin is deconjugated and reduced by intestinal bacteria to **urobilinogen**. Some of

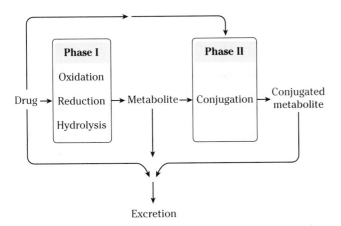

Figure 29.2 Drug inactivation. Some drugs are excreted without modification, some after phase I, some after phase II. Some drugs undergo phase II conjugation reactions without ever undergoing a phase I reaction by a cytochrome P-450 enzyme.

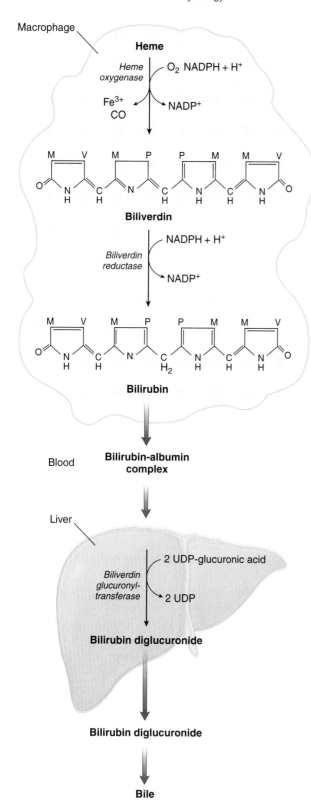

Figure 29.3 Metabolism of heme. The liver is the largest organ in the abdomen, while a macrophage is one cell. Drawing not to scale.

the urobilinogen is reabsorbed by the enterocytes. This urobilinogen circulates to the kidney where it is oxidized to **urobilin** and excreted in the urine (hence urine's yellow color). The urobilinogen remaining in the intestine is oxidized to **stercobilin**, which colors feces brown (Figure 29.4).

Jaundice, the yellow pigmenting of the skin, is due to **hyperbilirubinemia**, high levels of bilirubin in the blood. Hyperbilirubinemia may be caused by the increased breakdown of red blood cells (hemolysis) or the failed excretion of bilirubin in the bile. If the blood contains high levels of indirect (unconjugated) bilirubin, this is most consistent with a hemolytic cause of jaundice. If the blood contains high levels of direct (conjugated) bilirubin, it suggests a disorder of the liver. Severe hyperbilirubinemia in newborns can lead to **kernicterus**, where bilirubin accumulation in the basal ganglia, hippocampus, or brain stem causes neurologic impairment or death.

The Elimination of Ammonia Ammonia is formed during the metabolism of amino acids. If ammonia were not transformed into **urea** in the liver, it would bind α-ketoglutarate to form glutamate in the brain. Depletion of α-ketoglutarate saps the citric acid cycle of an important intermediary and leaves the neurons short on ATP. Additionally, glutamate can pick up another ammonia to form glutamine, decreasing glutamate and its metabolic product, gamma-amino butyric acid (GABA). Thus the major neurotransmitters are depleted (glutamate and GABA) while the excess glutamine within brain cells acts osmotically to increase cell water, leading to cerebral edema. These metabolic effects can lead to alterations in mental status and ultimately to coma and death. Hence, the hepatic **urea cycle** is critical for the organism's survival. (This cycle is described thoroughly in biochemistry texts.) When the liver fails to conduct the reactions of the urea cycle at an appropriate rate, **hyperammonemia** results. Hyperammonemia is likely to contribute to **hepatic encephalopathy**, the syndrome of altered mental status observed in liver failure.

Albumin

Hepatocytes are the site of the synthesis of clotting factors (see Chapter 10) and the synthesis of **albumin**, the most important blood protein. Albumin has three critical functions. One function is maintaining intravascular oncotic pressure. Albumin makes up half of the normal intravascular protein content and thus is essential for holding water inside the blood vessels. Albumin is also the main protein found in the interstitium or extravascular space (though it exists here in lower concentrations than in blood). Another

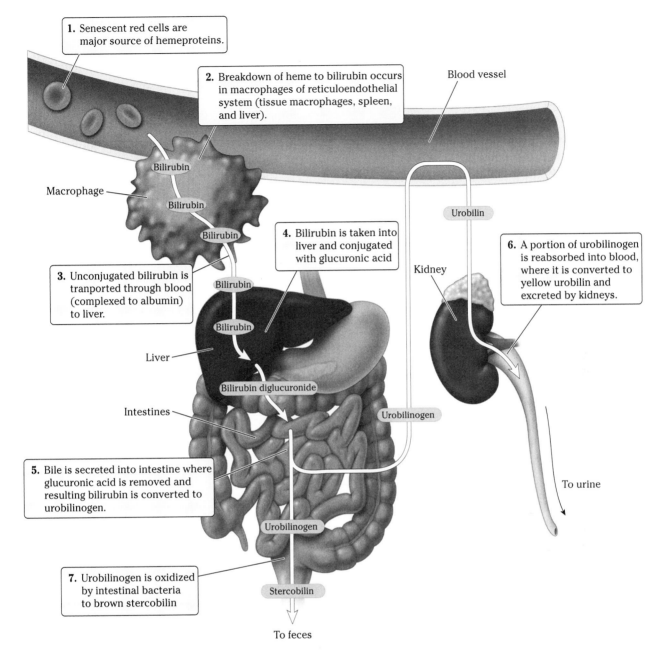

1. Senescent red cells are major source of hemeproteins.

2. Breakdown of heme to bilirubin occurs in macrophages of reticuloendothelial system (tissue macrophages, spleen, and liver).

Blood vessel

Bilirubin

Macrophage

Bilirubin

Bilirubin

3. Unconjugated bilirubin is tranported through blood (complexed to albumin) to liver.

Bilirubin

4. Bilirubin is taken into liver and conjugated with glucuronic acid

Kidney

Urobilin

6. A portion of urobilinogen is reabsorbed into blood, where it is converted to yellow urobilin and excreted by kidneys.

Bilirubin

Liver

Bilirubin diglucuronide

Intestines

Urobilinogen

5. Bile is secreted into intestine where glucuronic acid is removed and resulting bilirubin is converted to urobilinogen.

To urine

Urobilinogen

7. Urobilinogen is oxidized by intestinal bacteria to brown stercobilin

Stercobilin

To feces

Figure 29.4   Excretion of heme byproducts. While it is not shown, some of the reabsorbed urobilinogen is re-secreted in bile in addition to being excreted in urine.

primary function of albumin is the binding and transport of hormones, drugs, and other bloodborne factors. (The liver makes other important carrier proteins as well, such as sex hormone binding globulin.) Finally, albumin has the capacity to bind free radicals.

Hepatocytes synthesize and constitutively secrete albumin at a rate of 9 to 12 g per day. Because albumin is not stored, it cannot be released "on demand." At any time, 10% to 60% of hepatocytes are actively synthesizing albumin. The liver can only increase its albumin production by a factor of two to three, but albumin production is sensitive to changes in the intravascular oncotic pressure. When the intravascular oncotic pressure falls, the rate of albumin synthesis increases. Albumin production is also sensitive to nutritional status. A deficiency of amino acid precursors, such as leucine, arginine, isoleucine, valine, and tryptophan, can lead to a decrease in albumin synthesis. However, this is seen only in states of severe protein malnutrition. Albumin synthesis is also influenced by hormones, such as insulin, glucagon, thyroxine, and cortisol.

PATHOPHYSIOLOGY

A number of processes can lead to liver dysfunction. When the dysfunction is severe, it is called **liver failure**. Causes of liver failure include viral hepatitis (inflammation of the liver due to viral infection, such as infection with hepatitis B virus); drug toxicities (among them alcoholic hepatitis); autoimmune conditions like autoimmune hepatitis; and metabolic diseases such as Wilson's disease and hemochromatosis. In *Wilson's disease*, a hereditary disorder, the liver cannot excrete copper in bile, and the metal accumulates in liver (and other) tissues with injurious results. In *hemochromatosis*, an excess absorption of iron leads to an excess deposition of iron in the liver and elsewhere, with injury to the liver tissue. A common endpoint of all of these conditions, when present chronically, is scarring of the liver. Irreversible scarring is referred to as **cirrhosis**.

Inflammation and cirrhosis of the liver have predictable results. Because the liver is the principal site of energy metabolism, liver disease can interfere with these anabolic and catabolic functions. Altered carbohydrate metabolism in patients with cirrhosis can result in hyperglycemia or hypoglycemia. Altered lipid metabolism can result in hyperlipidemia, which can manifest as subcutaneous accumulations of cholesterol called xanthomas. Altered protein synthesis and degradation result in decreased levels of serum albumin and clotting factors, which contribute to the development of edema and coagulopathy (abnormal blood clotting), respectively. Reduced levels of albumin and other carrier proteins in the blood can also lead to increased levels of free (unbound) hormones or drugs, and hence increased hormone and drug activity. The metabolism of drugs, hormones, and toxic byproducts may be inadequate in liver failure. The consequences are longer drug and hormone half-lives and the accumulation of toxic agents like ammonia, as described above.

In addition to interfering with metabolic liver functions, cirrhosis also interferes with the function of the liver mechanically. Scar tissue prevents blood from flowing easily through the liver tissue. Consequently, low-pressure portal venous blood cannot easily get to the central veins of the liver lobules, and blood backs up in the portal system. As more portal blood is delivered than can be removed, portal blood pressure rises; this condition is called **portal hypertension**. Portal hypertension may cause fluid to weep from the liver capsule. This fluid is called **ascites**, and it accumulates in the peritoneal cavity, where it poses an infection risk (as low-flow conditions always do by providing bacteria purchase on cell membranes and extracellular proteins). In addition, the loss of fluid from the intravascular space decreases the systemic blood pressure, stimulating the kidneys to retain more salt and water. This worsens the portal hypertension, more ascites develops, and more water is retained in a vicious cycle. Low albumin may contribute to the formation of ascites. Patients with liver dysfunction may be observed to have distended abdomens from ascites.

Portal hypertension also forces portal blood into collateral paths from the portal system to the inferior vena cava. A portosystemic route of communication expands in the gastroesophageal area, leading to dilated veins known as **esophageal varices**. The development of untreated esophageal varices can be catastrophic because they are susceptible to bleeding into the upper gastrointestinal tract. Furthermore, portosystemic routes of venous return to the vena cava represent a shunt past the liver, which diminishes the liver's effect on the blood, thereby worsening the consequences of liver failure.

Finally, disease may also affect the biliary system. Inflammation of the gallbladder and bile ducts is called **cholecystitis**. A common cause of cholecystitis is gallstones (which in turn result from supersaturation of bile with cholesterol among other causes). When the biliary ducts (cystic duct, hepatic duct, or common bile duct) are blocked, the condition is described as **cholestasis**. Cholestasis prevents bile from reaching the intestine, where it normally emulsifies fats. This leads to maldigestion. When a gallstone blocks the pancreatic duct, it may lead to acute pancreatitis.

The Assessment of Liver Function

Liver dysfunction is reflected in various blood tests. The three best indicators of liver function are the prothrombin time, the serum bilirubin, and the serum albumin. *Prothrombin* is one of the blood clotting factors, and the **prothrombin time** is the rate at which prothrombin is converted to *thrombin* in the cascade of activation events that lead to blood clotting. The prothrombin time is hence an indicator of the time required for clot formation. When hepatic synthesis of clotting factors is impaired, the prothrombin time is increased. Clotting factors produced in the liver, with vitamin K as a cofactor, are factors II (prothrombin), VII, IX, and X. These factors have in common a post-translational protein modification of glutamic acid residues to **γ-carboxyglutamic acid (GLA),** which, as a dicarboxylic acid, allows for Ca^{2+} binding. These vitamin K-dependent and calcium-dependent reactions are blocked by the anticoagulant warfarin. As discussed in Chapter 28, vitamin K is a fat-soluble vitamin absorbed in the small intestine. Therefore, small intestinal disorders could lead to abnormal clotting by depletion of vitamin K; however, unlike in liver disease, the clotting abnormality can be overcome by the injection of vitamin K.

The depression of serum albumin in liver disease was discussed above. However, hypoalbuminemia takes weeks to develop because of the long half-life of albumin, and it is therefore not a reliable measure of hepatic synthetic function in acute liver disease. Serum bilirubin levels may be elevated in either hepatic or biliary disease, both of which impair the clearance of bilirubin from the blood. (As stated above, hemolysis also increases the serum bilirubin. Hemolysis should produce unconjugated hyperbilirubinemia, whereas hepatic elevations in bilirubin are expected to be in conjugated bilirubin.) The retention of bilirubin can lead to jaundice (discussed above), and the retention of bile salts can lead to pruritus (itching) due to the deposition of bile salts in the skin. Conjugated bilirubin is water-soluble and present in plasma water. Thus it is filtered by the renal glomeruli and appears as a pigment in the urine in the case of hepatic disease. In contrast, unconjugated bilirubin is heavily albumin-bound so it is not filtered, nor secreted into the urine when plasma levels are increased.

The presence of certain liver-specific enzymes in the blood also serves as an indicator of liver disease. **Aspartate aminotransferase (AST)** and **alanine aminotransferase (ALT)** are both found in the hepatocyte cytosol. AST is also found in hepatocyte mitochondria. The leakage of these enzymes into the circulation is a marker for ongoing hepatocellular inflammation. Whereas bilirubin levels may be elevated in cholestasis or intrinsic liver disease, AST and ALT are more specific for intrinsic liver disease. An AST/ALT ratio greater than 2:1 is found most often in alcoholic liver disease. ALT is more specific than AST for measuring hepatocellular injury, as AST is also found in muscle, kidney, brain, pancreas, and red blood cells.

Alkaline phosphatase (AP) is present in the hepatocyte canalicular plasma membrane and the luminal membrane of bile duct epithelium. In cholestatic states, the bile acid accumulation stimulates the synthesis and release of AP. Hence, elevated AP levels are indicative of cholestasis. AP is also found in a number of other tissues, including bone. The source of an elevated AP can be confirmed by measuring the levels of **5′-nucleotidase** and **γ-glutamyl transpeptidase (GGT)**. If 5′-nucleotidase and GGT levels are also increased, the elevated AP is likely from liver and not from bone. GGT is often elevated in people who consume three or more alcoholic drinks per day. It is a measure of immoderate intake and can be used to confirm sobriety in alcoholics. (See Clinical Application Box *What Is Alcoholic Hepatitis?*)

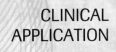

CLINICAL APPLICATION

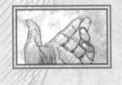

WHAT IS ALCOHOLIC HEPATITIS?

A 60-year-old woman presents with fatigue, nausea, vomiting, and abdominal distention. She noticed that her abdomen has been swelling slowly over the past few weeks. Her past medical history is significant for ovarian cancer, which was treated with chemotherapy without recurrence, and high blood pressure, for which she is taking a β-blocker called atenolol. She consumes, on average, two beers and mixed drinks each day with no concomitant illegal drug use. On physical examination, there is moderate ascites and an enlarged liver and spleen. Her laboratory findings include total bilirubin 1.4 mg/dL (normal 0.1–1.0 mg/dL), alkaline phosphatase 373 U/L (20–70 U/L), AST 79 U/L (8–20 U/L), ALT 34 U/L (8–20 U/L), albumin 2.9 g/dL (3.5–5.5 g/dL), and prothrombin time 16.9 s (11–15 s). CT scan reveals ascites and an enlarged liver with no masses. A liver biopsy shows hepatocyte injury and necrosis, fatty changes, inflammation, and fibrosis.

This is a classic example of **alcoholic hepatitis**. Alcohol abuse remains the leading cause of hepatitis and cirrhosis in the United States. The patient has a history of excessive alcohol consumption. She has an AST/ALT ratio of greater than 2:1. The pathologic changes evident on her liver biopsy are consistent with alcoholic hepatitis, which involves "fatty change," or steatosis. **Steatosis,** the deposition of excess fat in the liver, results from the activity of alcohol dehydrogenase, which yields excess NADPH. NADPH stimulates lipid production. The decreased serum albumin concentration and increased prothrombin time together reflect chronic liver disease, with the serum albumin contributing, along with portal hypertension, to the development of ascites. The increase in total bilirubin is consistent with impaired hepatic clearance due to injury and necrosis. The elevated alkaline phosphatase is reflective of the fatty liver changes and fibrosis, which interfere with biliary secretion.

Summary

- The liver modifies the blood contents by metabolically transforming them.
- The liver is a major site of the synthesis of glycogen, glucose, and ketone bodies, thereby playing a fundamental role in energy metabolism.
- The liver governs cholesterol metabolism, mediating its transport to the peripheral tissues and its excretion from the body. The liver also mediates fat absorption by secreting bile (an emulsifier) into the duodenum.
- The liver produces albumin and the clotting factors.
- The liver metabolizes drugs, hormones, and toxic byproducts.
- Hepatic cytochrome P-450 enzymes conduct phase I reactions to detoxify drugs, in which the drug is oxidized, reduced, or hydrolyzed. Phase II reactions are conjugation reactions that inactivate toxic metabolites from phase I. Both phase I and phase II render toxic agents more water-soluble to enhance their elimination in urine or bile.
- Bilirubin, a metabolite of heme from red blood cells, is conjugated in hepatocytes and excreted in bile. Bilirubin is reduced to urobilinogen in the intestine.
- Some urobilinogen is reabsorbed into the blood and oxidized and excreted by the kidney as urobilin. Some urobilinogen remains in the intestine and is oxidized to stercobilin.
- The hepatic urea cycle inactivates free ammonia, a product of protein metabolism.
- Albumin creates oncotic pressure in the blood, helping to hold water inside the blood vessels, and serves as a transport protein for hormones, drugs, electrolytes, and other agents.
- A common endpoint of various types of liver diseases is cirrhosis, the scarring and dysfunction of liver tissue.
- Liver failure reduces albumin production and clotting factor production with predictable results: edema and clotting abnormalities. Cirrhosis and hypoalbuminemia together contribute to the formation of ascites—cirrhosis by creating portal hypertension, hypoalbuminemia by lowering oncotic pressure.
- Cholestasis is obstruction of the biliary ducts.
- Hemolysis, intrinsic liver disease, and cholestasis lead to high levels of bilirubin in the blood and jaundice. Hepatic hyperbilirubinemia leads to high conjugated bilirubin levels; hemolytic hyperbilirubinemia leads to high unconjugated bilirubin levels.
- Levels of aspartate aminotransferase (AST) and alanine aminotransferase (ALT) are high in intrinsic liver disease. Levels of alkaline phosphatase (AP) are high in cholestasis.
- Alcoholism is the most common cause of cirrhosis.

Suggested Reading

Johnston DE. Special considerations in interpreting liver function tests. Am Family Phys. 1999;59:2223–2230.

Pratt DS, Kaplan MM. Evaluation of abnormal liver-enzyme results in asymptomatic patients. N Engl J Med. 2000;342:1266–1271.

Rothschild MA, Ortiz M, Schreiber SS. Serum albumin. Hepatology. 1988;8:385–401.

Spatzenegger M, Jaeger W. Clinical importance of hepatic cytochrome P450 in drug metabolism. Drug Met Rev. 1995;27:397–417.

REVIEW QUESTIONS

Directions: Each of the numbered items or incomplete statements in this section is followed by answers or by completions of the statement. Select the ONE lettered answer or completion that is BEST in each case.

1. A 48-year-old man with a long history of alcoholism suffers hematemesis and is treated with balloon tamponade. The source of his bleeding is likely to be:
   (A) The central veins of the hepatic lobules.
   (B) The hepatic sinusoids.
   (C) The left gastroepiploic artery.
   (D) Esophageal varices.
   (E) The splenic vein.

2. A 43-year-old woman is evaluated for jaundice. She has an elevated total bilirubin level and her direct (conjugated) bilirubin level is 1 mg/dL. AST is 35 U/L, ALT is 41 U/L, and alkaline phosphatase is 197 U/L. Her prothrombin time is 15 seconds and her albumin level is 3.4 g/dL. Sonography shows that her gallbladder diameter is more than 4 cm. The cause of her jaundice is probably:
   (A) Alcoholic steatohepatitis.
   (B) Autoimmune hepatitis.
   (C) Acute pancreatitis.
   (D) Hemolytic anemia.
   (E) Cholestasis.

3. Which of the following substances present in urine accounts for its yellow color?
   (A) Heme
   (B) Bilirubin
   (C) Urobilinogen
   (D) Urobilin
   (E) Stercobilin

ANSWER TO REVIEW QUESTIONS

1. **The answer is** D. Alcoholism is the most common cause of cirrhosis. Chronic cirrhosis leads to portal hypertension, which creates fragile venous collaterals called esophageal varices. Alcoholics with esophageal varices frequently bleed into the upper GI tract and vomit blood (hematemesis).

2. **The answer is** E. A distended gallbladder is suggestive of biliary obstruction and cholestasis.

The elevated direct bilirubin level rules out hemolysis as the cause of jaundice. Cholestasis can cause pancreatitis, but pancreatitis does not cause jaundice.

3. **The answer is** D. Bilirubin is secreted in bile and reduced to urobilinogen in the intestine. Urobilinogen is absorbed into the bloodstream. Before excreting it, the kidney oxidizes urobilinogen to urobilin, which gives urine its yellow color.

30

The Gastrointestinal Immune System

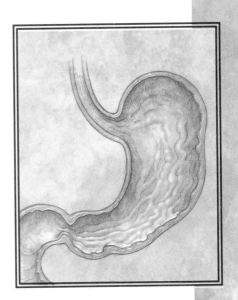

INTRODUCTION

As described in Chapter 11, the immune system is a complex cellular network that defends the body against danger. To carry out this function, the immune system must distinguish between the normal, healthy body ("self") and anything else ("nonself"), including invaders such as bacteria and dysfunctional body cells such as cancer, which might harm or impair the body. The cells of the immune system are prominent at those anatomic locations where the external environment borders the internal environment of the body: the skin, the respiratory tract, and the gastrointestinal (GI) tract. Although contact between nonself and self occurs in each of these places, the most dramatic example is in the GI tract.

Every time a person eats or drinks, he or she ingests an enormous number of nonself molecules. The small intestine must absorb nutrients, many of which are potential antigens (foreign substances that elicit an immune response; see Chapter 11). In addition, many benign or even helpful organisms, such as symbiotic bacteria of the large intestine that produce nutrients or aid digestion, reside in the GI tract. However, because of its great surface area, the GI tract is also a potential portal for dangerous invaders such as pathogenic bacteria, viruses, and parasites. The immune system of the GI tract must distinguish not only between self and nonself, but also between benign or helpful nonself and dangerous nonself. Harmless nutrients must be absorbed, self and benign nonself must be benevolently ignored, and potentially harmful nonself must be neutralized. A large amount of nonself material must be processed within the GI tract each day, but this processing must be done in such a way that neutralizing potentially harmful nonself does not cause a harmful and inappropriate inflammatory response on a regular basis, for if it did, the digestion and absorption of nutrients would not be possible.

The immune system of the GI tract, sometimes called the *enteric immune system*, is one of the largest immune organs in the body. It is estimated, for example, that 70% of the body's immune cells are found within the GI tract. This chapter describes the immunologic functions of the GI tract, emphasizing the clinical implications of the GI system as part of the immune system.

SYSTEM STRUCTURE

The immune system of the GI tract can be divided into "nonimmunologic" and "immunologic" defenses. Both operate throughout the GI tract, although in certain regions immunologic defense mechanisms predominate. The nonimmunologic defenses include mechanical barriers (such as epithelial cells and the mucous coating of the GI tract), mechanical actions (the peristaltic movement of the GI tract), components of GI secretions (such as gastric hydrochloric acid), and the nonpathogenic GI bacteria (which compete with potential pathogens for space and nutrients). The immunologic defenses include immune cells that either reside in or patrol the GI tract and the immune system molecules produced by such cells. The numbers and types of immune cells and the range of molecules can change dramatically from the healthy state to different disease states.

Gastrointestinal Immune System Tissues

Host defense tissues are found throughout the GI tract. The epithelial lining is arguably the most important nonimmune tissue component of the GI defenses. In the oral cavity, for example, where defenses are largely of the nonimmune type, there is a stratified, squamous epithelial lining that keeps bacteria from penetrating into deeper tissues. In the stomach, small intestine, and large intestine, epithelial cells held together by tight junctions provide a similar barrier through which antigens cannot pass (FIGURE 30.1; see Clinical Application Box *Antibiotic Prophylaxis When the GI Barrier Is Broken.*)

Among the immune tissues, the **gut-associated lymphoid tissue (GALT)** is a structure composed of innate and adaptive immune cells arranged in a pattern similar to those in lymph nodes and the spleen. These collections of lymphoid tissue are located throughout the GI tract in the lamina propria, just beneath the epithelial lining. While many small lymphoid collections are present in the floor of the oropharynx, those at the back, the *tonsils*, are the largest and can be seen on physical examination. Groups of subepithelial lymphoid follicles called **Peyer's patches** are found throughout the small intestine, although the majority of them are found in the ileum and jejunum. These circumscribed collections of lymphoid tissue contain anywhere from 200 to 400 lymphoid follicles. The large intestine does not have Peyer's patches but does have numerous GALT follicles. In the appendix, there are large aggregates of such lymphoid tissue.

Gastrointestinal Immune System Cells

Both innate and adaptive immune system cells are involved in defense of the GI tract. Some are resident cells stationed among epithelial cells or in the lamina propria. Others circulate through the body, exiting the blood at high endothelial venules to patrol tissues such as the GI mucosa in search of pathogens, and then entering the lymphatic system to return to the blood. An estimated one fourth of the cells

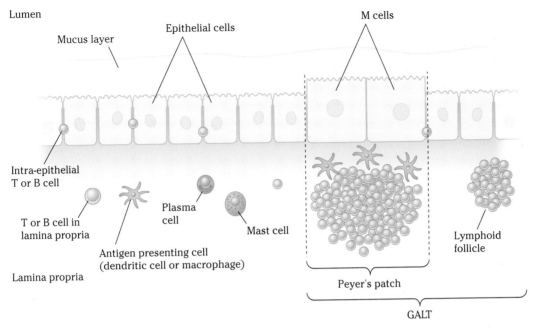

Figure 30.1 Tissue and cellular components of the GI immune system. Nonimmune defenses such as the mucus layer and epithelial layer are present throughout the GI tract. Innate immune cells such as antigen-presenting cells (macrophages and dendritic cells) and mast cells are present in the lamina propria. Adaptive immune system T cells, B cells, and plasma cells are found scattered among epithelial cells, in the lamina propria, or in the context of gut-associated lymphoid tissue (GALT), such as lymphoid follicles. Clusters of lymphoid follicles form Peyer's patches.

making up the intestinal mucosa are lymphoid cells, and approximately 70% of the body's antibody-secreting B cells are located in the intestine. In addition, nonpathogenic bacteria that normally reside in the large intestine and specialized macrophages in the liver make important contributions to the GI defense system.

Innate Immune Cells Among the innate immune cells are antigen-presenting cells (APCs) such as macrophages and dendritic cells, as well as mast cells. The top of each Peyer's patch is covered by a specific type of epithelial cell known as an **M cell**. M cells, also called "microfold cells," can sample luminal contents and shuttle these antigens into the lymphoid tissue of the Peyer's patches. Each M cell has a specialized membrane with numerous folds providing a large surface area for sampling antigen (FIGURE 30.2). They also contain vesicles believed to be important in the transport of antigen across the cell. M

CLINICAL APPLICATION

ANTIBIOTIC PROPHYLAXIS WHEN THE GI BARRIER IS BROKEN

The epithelial barrier of the GI tract keeps millions of bacteria from entering the bloodstream and causing serious infection. This epithelial layer, however, is broken on a daily basis during such routine activities as eating or brushing one's teeth. These relatively minor breaches usually only allow a small number of bacteria to enter the circulation, and they are usually neutralized quite easily. However, in some instances, such as during invasive dental procedures, a larger inoculum of bacteria can enter the blood, where it circulates until it can be cleared. In persons with damaged or artificial heart valves, however, these circulating bacteria can colonize the heart valves and lead to a condition called infective endocarditis. To prevent this life-threatening infection, persons at risk (e.g., those with mitral valve prolapse, artificial heart valves, rheumatic heart disease, or serious congenital heart diseases such as transposition of the great arteries) should receive prophylactic antibiotics for any procedure that breaches the GI epithelial barrier.

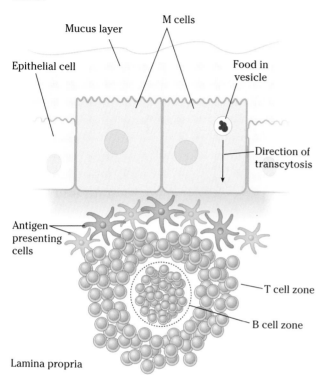

Lumen

Mucus layer

M cells

Epithelial cell

Food in vesicle

Direction of transcytosis

Antigen presenting cells

T cell zone

B cell zone

Lamina propria

Figure 30.2 Cellular structure of a Peyer's patch. The luminal "cap" of the patch is composed of M cells that transport luminal contents into the lamina propria via transcytosis. There, antigen-presenting cells such as dendritic cells and macrophages digest and present antigen to T cells. The germinal center of a Peyer's patch has a central area of B cells and a surrounding area of T cells.

cells do not contain specific receptors to bind antigens. Rather, they are located in pits where antigens are likely to deposit and are not covered with secretory immunoglobulins (see below) that prevent the binding of antigens. For these reasons, M cells can sample a large percentage of the antigens in the gut.

Adaptive Immune Cells   The lymphocytes of the adaptive immune system (T cells and B cells) are located in three anatomic areas: among epithelial cells, within the loose connective tissue of the lamina propria, and in the lymphoid follicles of the GALT and Peyer's patches. Each follicle is made up of a germinal center (containing mostly B cells) surrounded by collections of T cells and additional B cells as well as a number of APCs.

Nonpathogenic Bacteria   In the large intestine, billions of nonpathogenic bacteria are also important cells in preventing invasion by pathogenic microorganisms. These bacteria live in a mutually beneficial relationship with the human host, receiving a steady supply of nutrients while at the same time producing substances useful to the host (such as vitamin K) and preventing the colonization of the large intestine by other, more pathogenic bacteria. The importance of

the normal gut flora in protecting against infection can be seen in patients who are given antibiotics. In addition to killing the bacteria that are causing infection in the person, these antibiotics also kill the normal intestinal flora. This allows pathologic species of bacteria to colonize the gut. The classic example of this is colonic infection by *Clostridium difficile,* which may cause an inflammatory condition called pseudomembranous colitis.

Kupffer Cells   As described in Chapter 29, the liver is one of the organs responsible for removing damaging chemicals and potentially toxic compounds from the blood. Most of the intestinal venous blood flow enters the liver via the portal circulation, carrying the wide array of potentially infectious microbes and other antigenic materials that can bypass the GI tract defenses and enter the circulation. The liver is home to a population of fixed (i.e., noncirculating) macrophages called *Kupffer cells* located within the liver sinusoids. These cells encounter and engulf many soluble antigens from the portal circulation.

Gastrointestinal Immune System Molecules

Both nonimmune and immune molecules are important in the defense of the GI tract. In different segments of the GI tract, different defense molecules are present.

Nonimmune Molecules   In the oropharynx, saliva contains several nonimmune antibacterial molecules, including lactoferrin, lysozyme (also known as muramidase), and lactoperoxidase. Lactoferrin binds iron present in food or saliva, depriving bacteria of this needed element. Lysozyme hydrolyzes constituents of bacterial cell walls, compromising their integrity with consequences fatal to susceptible microbes. In the presence of hydrogen peroxide (H_2O_2), lactoperoxidase, like other peroxidase enzymes, catalyzes the oxidation of a number of target molecules, disrupting their functions in bacterial structure and/or metabolism.

One of the key ways in which the stomach prevents invasion by microorganisms is through the acid milieu. The pH in the stomach is usually less than 4 on the luminal side, and many bacteria (and other microorganisms) cannot survive in this acidic environment. (See Clinical Application Box *Helicobacter Pylori and Peptic Ulcer Disease.*)

The small intestine contains many digestive secretions, including bile salts and pancreatic enzymes such as trypsin, which are lethal to many bacteria.

Mucus, a complex mixture of glycoproteins and proteoglycans secreted by goblet cells interspersed among mucosal epithelial cells, is another important

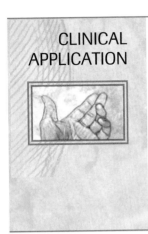

HELICOBACTER PYLORI AND PEPTIC ULCER DISEASE

Although the environment of the stomach is hostile to most microorganisms, some species of bacteria find it the optimal niche. One such bacterium is *Helicobacter pylori*. This organism is one of the major causes of peptic ulcer disease. It is found deep within the mucous layer covering gastric epithelial cells. It has an enzyme called urease that produces ammonia and buffers the acidic environment of the stomach, protecting the bacterium. Thus, it can overcome one of the GI tract's protective mechanisms and cause a substantial inflammatory disease. *H. pylori* infections can be treated with a combination of antibiotics, and the discovery of this pathogen and its association with peptic ulcer disease has changed the approach to and management of this common health problem.

nonimmune defense. In the stomach, the small intestine, and the large intestines, mucus forms a layer covering epithelial cells, prohibiting bacterial adherence and thus decreasing the probability that a pathogen will gain entry.

Immune Molecules Immunoglobulin A (IgA) is one of the most important immune molecules involved in the defense of the GI tract. IgA is secreted by plasma cells (mature, antibody-secreting B cells; see Chapter 11) located within the salivary ducts and within the mucosa of the stomach, the small intestine, and the large intestine. IgA coats bacteria and does not allow them to adhere to epithelial cells. Because bacteria must adhere to cells in order to invade, prevention of adherence by both nonimmune and immune molecules is a key immunoprotective mechanism in the GI tract.

In the gut, IgA is usually in a dimeric form with two individual IgA molecules joined by a joining protein called the *J chain*. Like all antibodies, IgA is a protein designed to bind antigens and allow these antigens to be handled by the immune system. Because each IgA molecule has two antigen binding sites (FIGURE 30.3), the dimeric structure of intestinal

IgA allows it to have four antigen-combining sites and to function as a molecule that causes agglutination. In addition to the J chain, IgA in the gut also has a component that allows it to be secreted into the lumen. This *secretory component (SC)* is a transmembrane protein located at the basolateral surface of intestinal epithelial cells. It binds to the dimeric IgA and causes the complex to be taken up by the epithelial cell and transported into the lumen. The entire complex of dimeric IgA, the J chain, and the SC is referred to as secretory IgA (sIgA).

SYSTEM FUNCTION

In addition to the fixed structural elements (e.g., the epithelium) of the GI tract that prevent infection, a number of dynamic processes at work in the gut participate in the handling of foreign materials. Some of these processes work on the macroscopic level, while others involve the interaction among cells and molecules. There are both nonimmune and immune mechanisms for GI tract defense, and they are integrated. After introducing the salient defense strategies, this section follows the course of ingested foreign matter as it traverses the GI tract.

Nonimmune Mechanisms

A major nonimmune, macroscopic defense process is **peristalsis**. The peristaltic motions of the esophagus, stomach, small intestine, and large intestine do not allow bacteria to remain in contact with one area for a prolonged period of time. This decreases the chances of bacterial adherence and translocation across epithelial cells. Peristalsis aids in the breakdown of ingested materials into smaller particles. In addition, by churning the contents of the GI tract, peristalsis increases the opportunity for contact between such small particles and the antigen-sampling cells of the gut.

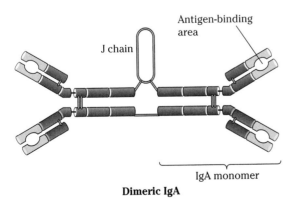

Figure 30.3   Structure of dimeric IgA. Dimeric IgA is composed of two IgA monomers linked by a joining or J chain. Since each IgA monomer has two antigen binding sites, dimeric IgA has a total of four such sites.

Immune Mechanisms

The immune system cells and molecules detailed earlier interact with one another and with ingested foreign material to elaborate a proper immune response. In many cases, this involves the neutralization of potential pathogens without creating a large inflammatory response. In other cases, such as contact between the GI immune system and beneficial proteins derived from foods, the best immune response is none at all, a situation called *tolerance*. To distinguish between beneficial nonself and potentially harmful nonself, the cells of the immune system must sample and analyze the contents of the GI tract, a procedure called antigen processing.

Antigen Sampling and Processing

Once antigens adhere to the apical surface of M cells, they are pinocytosed into the cell and packaged into vesicles for release on the opposite (basolateral) side where they are delivered to APCs such as dendritic cells and macrophages in the Peyer's patches. The APCs process the antigens by digesting them and present them to T cells by inserting antigenic peptides into the clefts of MHC II molecules and displaying them on the APC surface. T cells may recognize these antigenic peptides in MHC II clefts by means of their cell surface T-cell receptors.

A T cell that recognizes antigen may then respond in any of a number of ways, depending on the context in which the antigen is presented. If certain costimulatory signals are present, the T cell will generate signals to initiate inflammation. This may occur if antigens from a pathogenic bacterium or virus are detected and recognized. Another T cell response may instruct B cells in the gut to mature into IgA-secreting plasma cells. If the antigen is harmless, however, and costimulatory signals are absent, the T cell may ignore the information or even initiate a program to suppress inflammation in response to the antigen. This anti-inflammatory response is one type of tolerance mechanism.

Other cells in the small intestine also sample antigen from the lumen. Although their role is primarily in absorbing nutrients, the intestinal epithelial cells themselves may also take up antigen from the gut lumen. These antigens are then deposited on the basal side, where they are processed by APCs. Antigens may also pass between intestinal epithelial cells (called the paracellular route) and encounter immune cells in the lamina propria of the small intestine. This type of antigen movement is usually prevented by the tight junctions between epithelial cells. However, in situations where these junctions are disrupted (such as in infection, ischemia, or inflammation), antigen can pass from the intestinal lumen into the lamina propria.

The Kupffer cells of the liver can also engulf antigenic proteins and present them to T cells, thus triggering an immune response. In this way, many antigens and potentially infectious agents that are able to bypass the intestinal immune system are cleared by Kupffer cells in the liver.

IgA Production and Function

Once a B cell receives the appropriate signals from T cells, it can mature into a plasma cell that produces and secretes antigen-specific IgA. As described earlier, sIgA is composed of two IgA monomers joined by a J chain and a secretory component. Once released from the B cell, dimeric IgA binds to the basolateral surface of intestinal epithelial cells by means of a specific receptor and is transported to the apical side of the epithelial cell by the process of transcytosis. Since this carries IgA from the lamina propria into the lumen of the GI tract, it is essentially the reverse direction of the transcytosis by which M cells bring material from the lumen into the lamina propria. Once on the apical side, the epithelial cell receptor is enzymatically cleaved, releasing the sIgA. That portion of the epithelial cell receptor that remains bound to the dimeric IgA is the SC (FIGURE 30.4).

Once released into the lumen, sIgA binds to antigens and prevents them from adhering to the intestinal cells, entering the cells, and damaging the mucosa. In the case of viruses, bacteria, and parasites, this binding of sIgA in the GI lumen prevents infection. Secretory IgA can also bind to and neutralize potentially harmful products of pathogenic organisms, such as bacterial toxins.

Importantly, sIgA differs not only structurally but also functionally from other immunoglobulins in that it does not activate inflammatory and cytotoxic immune system responses. When one considers the immense antigen burden faced by the GI tract, it is clear that if classical immune responses (including inflammation and cell death) were induced by sIgA, the gut would be in a state of constant inflammation. If this were the case, the GI tract would no longer be able to carry out its degradative, secretory, and absorptive functions.

Encountering Pathogens

Consider the integrated functions of the GI immune system in the case of a person eating a poorly washed apple. The surface of the fruit may be heavily colonized with potentially pathogenic microorganisms, yet the person is protected from serious infection from the moment of the first bite and all the way through the processes of digestion, absorption, and elimination.

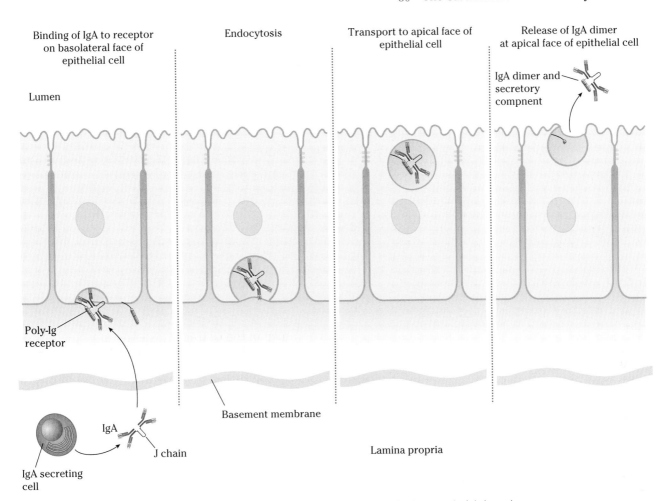

Binding of IgA to receptor on basolateral face of epithelial cell

Endocytosis

Transport to apical face of epithelial cell

Release of IgA dimer at apical face of epithelial cell

Lumen

IgA dimer and secretory compnent

Poly-Ig receptor

Basement membrane

IgA

J chain

Lamina propria

IgA secreting cell

Figure 30.4 Secretion of sIgA. Dimeric IgA is secreted from plasma cells in the lamina propria. It is bound by a receptor on the basolateral surface of GI epithelial cells and endocytosed. By the process of transcytosis, the vesicle carries the IgA to the basolateral surface, where it is released into the lumen. Enzymatic cleavage of the epithelial cell receptor frees the IgA, but part of the receptor remains attached and is called the secretory component.

In the oropharynx, salivary enzymes such as lactoferrin, lysozyme, and lactoperoxidase impair or damage the microorganisms. The epithelial barriers of the GI tract prevent access into the lamina propria and blood vessels beneath, and the mucous layer and sIgA even prevent adherence to the epithelium. After being swallowed, the food is pushed along by peristalsis, which also prevents adherence.

In the stomach, gastric acid may damage the microorganisms, and in the duodenum, bile and pancreatic digestive enzymes may do the same. In the jejunum and ileum, antigen is sampled by M cells processed by APCs. T cells and B cells in lymphoid tissues and Peyer's patches may respond by increasing the output of antigen-specific sIgA to neutralized microorganisms and their toxic products. In the large intestine, resident normal flora compete with pathogens for nutrients and space. If a pathogen should gain access despite the safeguards, the APCs, T cells, and B cells of the mucosa can respond by initiating an inflammatory reaction to destroy the invader. If a microorganism succeeds in entering the circulation, hepatic Kupffer cells may intercept it. Finally, the vast majority of ingested microorganisms are excreted in the stool.

The GI immune system does not work in isolation. Because T cells and B cells are mobile, they can encounter antigen in the GI tract and then move to other tissues. In the respiratory and genitourinary tracts, such cells may enter lymphoid tissues similar to GALT (called mucosa-associated lymphoid tissue, or MALT) where they may share information or carry out defensive functions. For example, after antigen processing occurs in the Peyer's patches and other lymphoid tissue in the gut, immature B cells are stimulated by T cells to begin producing IgA. Many of these B cells exit the small intestine through the lymphatic channels and enter the mesenteric lymph nodes. They are then transported into the systemic circulation. From here, the B cells not only return to the small intestine, but also travel to the salivary glands, the eye, the bronchial tissue, the genitourinary tract, and the mammary glands, where they may mature into plasma cells and produce large amounts of antigen-specific IgA. Thus, protection against antigen encountered in the gut can be conferred on the body as a whole, particularly on the other mucosal tissues, and in addition to providing local defense, the immune tissue in the small intestine also plays a role in systemic defense. Researchers have found higher rates of infection in critically ill patients who are fed via routes other than the alimentary tract, or "parenterally" (e.g., with total parenteral nutrition or TPN, a form of intravenous, liquid nutrition) than those who are fed via the gut. One hypothesis suggests that this is because decreased GI exposure to antigen results in poorer immune system education and thus weakened defenses at the skin and mucosal surfaces such as the respiratory, genitourinary, and GI tracts.

SYSTEM PATHOPHYSIOLOGY

As in the immune system as a whole, the GI immune system can malfunction in one or more of three ways that result in disease: by not defending the body from danger (immunodeficiency); by attacking normal, healthy body tissues or cells (autoimmunity); and by generating an inflammatory response against a benign nonself substance (hypersensitivity). While there are many examples of GI infections in immunodeficient patients and diseases such as pernicious anemia are examples of autoimmunity, this section focuses on hypersensitivity and inappropriate inflammatory reactions on the part of the GI immune system.

Food Allergy

When functioning properly, the immune tissues of the GI tract provide an impressive defense against a variety of microbial and other antigens. There are disease states, however, in which the GI immune system appears to be overly active. This hypersensitivity can cause multiple problems for the host. Take, for example, **food allergies**. An estimated 1% to 2% of the general population has some type of food allergy, a hypersensitivity reaction directed against one or more food antigens. Some more common foods that provoke allergies include eggs, cow's milk, peanuts, and shrimp. These reactions occur when antigen enters the lamina propria and binds to the surface of resident mast cell by means of membrane-bound antigen-specific IgE. The cross-linking of mast cell surface IgE by food antigens induces mast cell activation, with the release of many inflammatory mediators, such as histamine and leukotrienes. Once release, these chemical mediators cause vasodilation and leakage of fluid from the vascular space into the lamina propria. This causes edema, and if the permeabil-

ity barrier of the gut is breached, larger amounts of antigen may enter the systemic circulation. If this antigen load and mast cell mediators are carried throughout the body, mast cells at other sites and blood basophils may also be activated. This can lead to systemic responses such as hives, itching, and swelling of the mucous membranes, and in its most extreme form can be accompanied by low blood pressure from vasodilation and respiratory distress from bronchoconstriction. This general condition called "anaphylaxis" can be life-threatening.

Gluten–Sensitive Enteropathy

Gluten-sensitive enteropathy, also called celiac disease, celiac sprue, and nontropical sprue, is a disease of the small intestine that leads to intestinal malabsorption and consequent nutritional deficiencies. It is a hereditary disease and the prevalence varies by geographic location, ranging from 1 in 300 people in areas of Ireland to 1 in 5,000 people in North America. It can manifest at any age.

Gluten is a cereal protein found in wheat and rye. Gluten-sensitive enteropathy is linked to a specific component of gluten called the gliadin fraction. There are several theories as to the pathogenic nature of gliadin. Some investigators believe that gliadin (or some intermediary breakdown product of gliadin) is toxic to the intestinal epithelium. Other investigators point to an autoimmune mechanism in which an unchecked immune response is set up in the small intestine as the primary cause of intestinal epithelial damage. In essence, gluten-sensitive enteropathy is a disease in which the intestinal immune system responds inappropriately to gliadin by creating inflammation. Some research indicates that individuals with a specific type of immune genes called MHC DQ can process and present gliadin to T cells. These T cells then stimulate B cells to produce non-IgA antigliadin antibodies, which initiate an inflammatory response.

People with gluten-sensitive enteropathy make not only antigliadin antibodies but also antibody directed against various components of the intestinal basement membrane, including reticulin and endomysium (specifically, the molecule tissue transglutaminase). These are known as autoantibodies since they are directed against components of the body itself. It may be that the immune reaction to gliadin triggers this immune reaction to the intestinal basement membrane, leading to the inflammation and atrophy of the intestinal villi and hyperplasia of the crypts that characterize the disease. In support of this autoimmune mechanism, researchers have found that the basement membrane of the small intestine of people with gluten-sensitive enteropathy contains deposits of IgA. Furthermore, there is some evidence to suggest that antigliadin antibodies trigger an immune response that is in part mediated by IgG. This IgG leads to an inflammatory response not usually seen with IgA and may contribute to the villous atrophy seen in the disease. The specific mechanics of the disease still need to be established. However, it is clear that in gluten-sensitive enteropathy, the normal functioning of the intestinal immune system is disrupted, leading to a sloughing of intestinal epithelial cells and a decrease in the absorptive surface area of the small bowel.

The functional consequences of this loss of villi and decreased absorptive surface area are profound. Persons with the disease cannot absorb calories and needed nutrients. Furthermore, they sometimes lose enzymatic capacity within the brush border of the small bowel, including the loss of lactase. This can worsen malabsorption. In addition to loss of local enzymatic processes, there may be a decrease in the stimulation of other digestive organs, such as the pancreas and the gallbladder. Loss of their functions may lead to defects in fat absorption and further worsen the nutritional status of patients with gluten-sensitive enteropathy.

The clinical manifestations of the disease are varied and can range from mild diarrhea to severe malnutrition. Most patients have some degree of diarrhea and abdominal distention. Children may fail to grow properly or may lose a significant amount of weight. In addition to general signs of malabsorption, patients may manifest the signs and symptoms of more specific nutritional deficiencies, such as iron deficiency or folate deficiency resulting in anemia that may clinically appear as weakness, fatigue, and pallor. If the malabsorption is severe and patients develop hypoproteinemia, edema may be present. Oral ulcers may also be seen. Some patients present with metabolic bone disease and complain of bone pain and tenderness.

The disease is usually suspected on the basis of clinical history and physical examination. A family history of the disease may be present to guide the clinician as well. Three criteria must be met in order to make the diagnosis of gluten-sensitive enteropathy: evidence of malabsorption in the presence of a normal diet; an abnormal jejunal biopsy in which blunting of the villi is seen in conjunction with deepening of the crypts; and improvement after beginning a gluten-free diet (Table 30.1), which is the treatment.

Malabsorption can be assessed using a D-xylose absorption test. D-xylose is a pentose sugar that is well absorbed across normal intestinal mucosa but is not absorbed across abnormal mucosa. If the D-xylose is absorbed, it enters the bloodstream and is then excreted in the urine unchanged; if not, it is lost

Table 30.1	SOME GLUTEN-CONTAINING FOODS TO BE AVOIDED BY PATIENTS WITH GLUTEN-SENSITIVE ENTEROPATHY	
Baking soda	Graham flour	Rye
Beer	Gravy cubes	Scotch
Bran	Ground spices	Soy sauce
Bread flour	Malt	Starch
Bulgur	Malt vinegar	Vegetable starch
Caramel color	Mustard powder	Certain vitamins
Couscous	Nuts	Wheat
Dextrins	Pasta	White vinegar

in the stool. Thus, measuring urine D-xylose levels or serum D-xylose levels can be an indicator of D-xylose absorption and intestinal absorption in general. To perform the test, the patient fasts for 8 hours and is then given a 25 mg D-xylose load orally. The urine is then collected for 5 hours after the oral load and the total urinary D-xylose measured. If the urinary excretion is less than 15% of the given load, malabsorption is suggested. In patients with renal failure, serum D-xylose levels can be measured and any serum level less than 25 mg/dL is suggestive of malabsorption. Edema, severe diarrhea, intestinal bacterial overgrowth, or delayed gastric emptying time may interfere with the interpretation of the test results.

Endoscopy may show a characteristic scalloped appearance of the small intestine. Jejunal biopsy shows flat villi, deep crypts, and a cellular infiltrate in the lamina propria. Blood tests to assist in the diagnosis of gluten-sensitive enteropathy include antigliadin antibodies and antitissue transglutaminase antibodies.

Inflammatory Bowel Disease

The two major types of **inflammatory bowel disease**, *Crohn's disease* and *ulcerative colitis*, are disorders of GI immunity in which there is inappropriate and damaging inflammation that affects the GI tract. Both seem to have a genetic component, and if long-standing inflammation is left untreated, both diseases are associated with increased risks of GI cancer.

Crohn's disease is characterized by patchy inflammatory lesions that often start as aphthous ulcers but then progress to involve the full thickness of the gut wall (Figure 30.5A). Lesions may occur anywhere from the oropharynx to the anus. As the inflammation

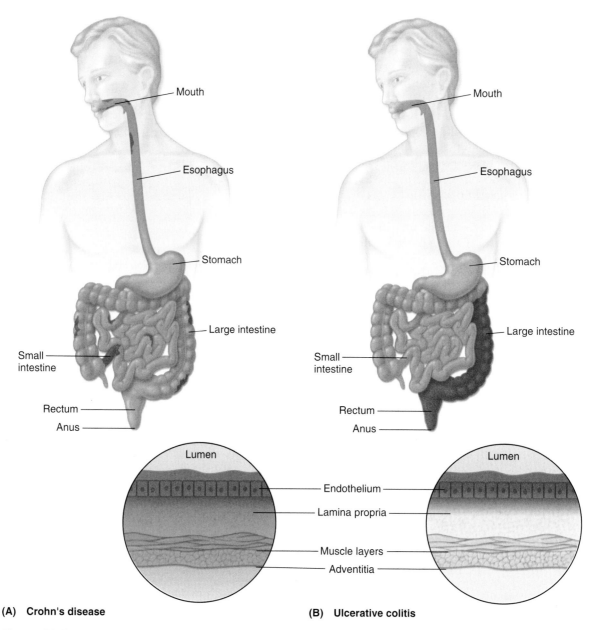

Mouth

Esophagus

Stomach

Large intestine

Small intestine

Rectum

Anus

Mouth

Esophagus

Stomach

Large intestine

Small intestine

Rectum

Anus

Lumen

Lumen

Endothelium

Lamina propria

Muscle layers

Adventitia

(A) Crohn's disease

(B) Ulcerative colitis

Figure 30.5   Inflammatory bowel diseases. **A.** In Crohn's disease, patchy inflammation affects the full thickness of the gut wall. Lesions may occur anywhere along the GI tract from oropharynx to anus. **B.** In ulcerative colitis, there is continuous inflammation affecting the more superficial GI mucosa. Lesions involve the distal large bowel at a minimum and may affect the entire large bowel.

worsens, ulcers and fissures may progress to cause perforation and fistulas. Scar formation may lead to obstruction by strictures. Symptoms include abdominal pain, diarrhea (often with visible blood in the stool), and weight loss partially due to malabsorption. Numerous other symptoms, including fever, skin rashes, joint disease, and anemia, may be present. The cause of the immune dysregulation is not known, but evidence suggests that there is an overly exuberant inflammatory response and/or a loss of tolerance to nonpathogenic gut bacteria. The diagnosis is made by a typical history and the gross and histologic pat-

terns of lesions as determined by abdominal radiographic imaging and endoscopy with biopsy. Medical treatments include anti-inflammatory and immunosuppressive drugs, and antibiotics are effective in some cases. Often, however, surgical resection of inflamed tissue is necessary, though disease often recurs after surgery.

Ulcerative colitis is also an inflammatory bowel disease, but it differs from Crohn's disease in that the inflammation is superficial instead of affecting the entire thickness of the gut wall and is continuous instead of patchy (see FIGURE 30.5B). While

Crohn's disease may affect any portion of the GI tract, ulcerative colitis by definition is limited to the colon, though the inflammation may involve as little as the rectum or as much as the entire large intestine. Typical symptoms of abdominal pain and bloody diarrhea may be accompanied by fever and extraintestinal symptoms that resemble Crohn's disease. Like Crohn's disease, the cause of the inflammation is unknown, but many hypotheses implicate abnormal reactivity of the GI immune system. The diagnosis of ulcerative colitis is made by a history of typical symptoms and visualization of the inflamed colonic epithelium by colonoscopy. Medical treatment includes anti-inflammatory and occasionally immunosuppressive drugs, but antibiotics do not seem to be efficacious. If severe disease called toxic megacolon or cancer arises, surgical resection of the entire large intestine (total proctocolectomy) is curative.

Summary

- The GI tract immune system not only protects the gut from the large antigenic and infectious burden it faces on a daily basis, but also contributes to mucosal immunity of the whole body. In defending the body, the GI immune system must distinguish not only between self and nonself, but also between benign/helpful nonself and potentially harmful nonself.

- Potentially dangerous nonself microorganisms and antigens are neutralized in a manner that does not cause frequent inflammation that would interfere with the digestive and absorptive functions of the GI tract.

- The GI tract integrates both nonimmune and immune strategies to protect the host. Although there are some regional differences along the gut, many of the *enteric immune system* defense mechanisms operate throughout the entire GI tract.

- Nonimmune mechanisms include the epithelial barrier, the mucous layer, and peristalsis. Immune mechanisms include the organized sampling of antigens by innate antigen-presenting cells (APCs) and the coordinated responses of adaptive T cells and B cells.

- The epithelial barrier is a critical nonimmune structure that prevents pathogens from entering the body via the GI tract.

- Innate immune cells such as APCs and mast cells and adaptive immune cells (T cells and B cells) are distributed throughout the gut

mucosa in three compartments: in the epithelial lining, in the loose connective tissue of the lamina propria, and in the more organized **gut-associated lymphoid tissues (GALT)**.

- GALT is present throughout the GI tract. In the small intestine, large collections of GALT follicles form the **Peyer's patches**.

- Nonpathogenic colonic bacteria (normal flora) benefit the host not only by aiding digestion and producing important metabolic factors such as vitamin K, but also by helping prevent infection by competing with potential pathogens for nutrients and space.

- **Mucus**, secreted by cells such as goblet cells, forms a layer in which potential pathogens are trapped.

- **IgA** is an important immune molecule secreted by plasma cells into the gut lumen by the process of transcytosis. sIgA binds to antigens and neutralizes them, preventing them from adhering to the epithelial lining and gaining access to the lamina propria, but without inducing inflammation.

- **M cells** overlying Peyer's patches are important in sampling luminal contents and transporting them into the lamina propria. There, APCs process antigens and present them to T cells.

- **Food allergies** occur when food antigens cross-link IgE on the surface of GI mast cells.

- **Gluten-sensitive enteropathy** is an inflammatory disease of the GI tract in which there is an inappropriate reaction to gliadin.

- **Inflammatory bowel diseases**, *Crohn's disease* and *ulcerative colitis*, are disorders in which chronic, inappropriate inflammation occurs in the gut.

Suggested Reading

Galperin C, Gershwin E. Immunopathogenesis of gastrointestinal and hepatobiliary diseases. JAMA. 1997;278(22):1946–1955.

Heel K, McCauley R Papadimitrou J, Hall J. Review: Peyer's patches. J Gastroenterol Hepatol. 1997;12:122–136.

James S. The gastrointestinal immune system. Digest Dis. 1993;11:146–156.

James SP. Immunologic, gastroenterologic, and hepatobiliary disorders. J Allergy Clin Immunol. 2003;111(2):S645–S658.

Toy L, Mayer L. Basic and clinical overview of the mucosal immune system. Semin Gastrointest Dis. 1996;79 (1):2–11.

REVIEW QUESTIONS

Directions: Each of the numbered items or incomplete statements in this section is followed by answers or by completions of the statement. Select the ONE lettered answer or completion that is BEST in each case.

1. In the small intestine, which of the following plays an important role in preventing bacterial adherence?

    (A) IgE
    (B) IgG
    (C) Mucus secreted by goblet cells
    (D) Nonpathogenic bacteria
    (E) Neutrophils

2. What properties of M cells allow them to sample antigen effectively from the small intestinal lumen?

    (A) They have a receptor-mediated active transport system for hundreds of antigens.
    (B) They are not covered by IgA.
    (C) They protrude above the epithelial cells and are thus able to capture antigen as it passes by.
    (D) They lack a nucleus, making them more efficient at antigen capture.

3. Gluten-sensitive enteropathy is characterized by which of the following histologic features?

    (A) Flattening of intestinal crypts and elongation of intestinal villi
    (B) Flattening of intestinal villi and elongation of intestinal crypts
    (C) Obstruction of intestinal crypts by mucus impaction and fibrosis
    (D) IgE antibodies against gliadin
    (E) Bleeding into the muscle layer of the gut wall

4. A 67-year-old man presents to the emergency department with a 1-week history of diarrhea. He had been taking antibiotics for pneumonia when

the diarrhea started. Which of the following elements would be the most appropriate part of his diagnostic and treatment plan?

(A) Evaluation of his PT and PTT
(B) Administration of vitamin K
(C) Assay of stool for *Clostridium difficile* toxins
(D) Abdominal CT
(E) Upper GI endoscopy

5. A 37-year-old, previously healthy patient has been in the intensive care unit for 2 weeks following a high-speed motor vehicle accident that has left him in a coma. He has been unresponsive since admission, and he has been losing weight. The ICU team discusses starting him on total parenteral nutrition (TPN). What concerns are germane when considering this strategy?

(A) He will be at higher risk of developing systemic infections if he is fed parenterally instead of via the GI tract.

(B) Feeding him with TPN will require placement of a central line and all the risks associated with placing that line.
(C) He will not be able to receive sufficient calories through TPN.
(D) The large volume of fluid of TPN will cause heart failure.

6. Inflammatory bowel disease such as Crohn's disease can be treated effectively by any or all of the following EXCEPT:

(A) Surgical resection of severely inflamed, fibrotic, or perforated tissues
(B) Antibiotics
(C) Anti-inflammatory agents
(D) Immunosuppressive agents
(E) Bone marrow transplant

ANSWERS TO REVIEW QUESTIONS

1. **The answer is** C. Both IgA and mucus secreted by goblet cells in the small intestine prevent bacteria from adhering to intestinal epithelial cells. Although IgE and IgG play smaller roles in small intestinal immunity, they are not major factors in preventing bacterial adherence. Nonpathogenic bacteria are normally found in the large intestine, not the small intestine. Neutrophils are normally rare in the lamina propria and do not prevent pathogen adherence.

2. **The answer is** B. M cells reside in pits between epithelial cells and antigen is likely to drop into these pits. M cells are not covered with mucus or IgA and thus are effective at sampling antigen. They do this through pinocytosis and not receptor-mediated active transport. Like most body cells except mature red blood cells, M cells have a nucleus.

3. **The answer is** B. Gluten-sensitive enteropathy is characterized both by a flattening of small intestinal villi and by elongation of intestinal crypts, but not by a flattening of crypts or elongation of villi. While patients may have IgA, IgG, or even IgE antibodies directed against the gliadin fraction of gluten, the presence of such antibodies is a serologic, not a histologic, feature of the disease. Bleeding generally does not occur in the deeper muscle layers of the gut wall in this disease.

4. **The answer is** C. The patient's history of antibiotic use raises the possibility of *C. difficile* infection. The patient's stool should be sent for *C.*

difficile toxin assay; if the result is positive, he should be treated with an antibiotic such as metronidazole. Neither abdominal CT nor upper GI endoscopy is indicated initially in this case. If the patient had a long history of antibiotic use coupled with malnutrition and the inability to eat, the possibility of vitamin K deficiency coagulopathy would exist and merit evaluation. In this case, however, it seems less likely.

5. **The answer is** A. TPN is used to provide nutritional support to patients who cannot maintain adequate oral intake. It is administered through a peripherally inserted central catheter (PICC line) or a central venous line, so this patient might not need the latter. TPN can provide sufficient calories to patients. However, these patients are often at increased risk of systemic infection owing in part to the fact that their GI tract is no longer seeing the amount of antigen it usually encounters and thus the immune system is stimulated less. In a previously healthy 37-year-old, heart failure from fluid overload is possible but is less likely.

6. **The answer is** E. Crohn's disease can be effectively treated with surgery when necessary, with antibiotics on occasion, with anti-inflammatory agents (such as sulfasalazine [Azulfidine]), with and immunosuppressive agents (such as corticosteroids). While removal of the colon is curative for patients with ulcerative colitis, Crohn's disease involves the entire GI tract from mouth to anus and thus surgery is a last resort for refractory disease. Bone marrow transplant, while it might theoretically be helpful, is not an accepted treatment for Crohn's disease.

Part VIII

ENDOCRINE PHYSIOLOGY

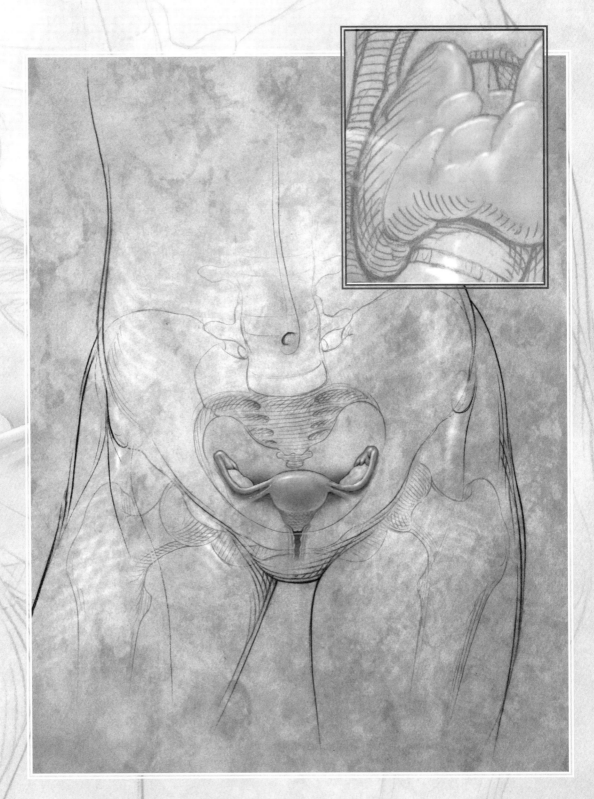

The Endocrine Pancreas: Fed and Fasted Metabolic States

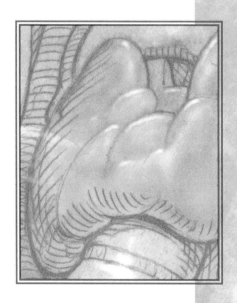

INTRODUCTION

The discovery of insulin was a dramatic moment in the history of medicine. When Canadians Frederick Banting and Charles Best isolated insulin and made possible the treatment and survival of millions of diabetics, they demonstrated the power of the scientific method in terms of spared suffering on an enormous scale. They helped initiate the era of modern medicine, in which the empiricism of the 18th century and its practice in the 19th came to fruition in the wondrous cures of the 20th.

The early research into pancreatic function that laid the groundwork for Banting and Best focused on the difference between the acini, the cells that secrete digestive enzymes, and those in the islets of Langerhans. At a time when scientists were beginning to appreciate the importance of hormones, researchers ascertained that the islets had an *endocrine function*, secreting hormones *into* the bloodstream, as opposed to the *exocrine function* of the acini, secreting enzymes *out of* the body and into the lumen of the intestines.

All endocrine organs deploy hormones into the bloodstream to act at distant target sites. The job of the major pancreatic hormones, insulin and glucagon, is to regulate the body's metabolism of carbohydrates, lipids, and proteins. By controlling the construction and breakdown of these energy-containing organic molecules, and their levels in the blood versus in tissue stores, the pancreatic hormones work to ensure a constant supply of energy to cells regardless of fluctuations in dietary intake. **Insulin** promotes storage of energy-laden molecules, while **glucagon** promotes the consumption of energy stores.

SYSTEM STRUCTURE: THE ISLETS OF LANGERHANS

The **pancreas** is an organ 80 to 100 g in volume that lies in the posterior abdomen. It extends from the curvature of the duodenum to the spleen (FIGURE 31.1). (For more detail on the vasculature and innervation of the pancreas, see Chapter 27.) The endocrine pancreas is organized histologically into **islets of Langerhans**, which are roughly spherical clusters of cells. These patches of endocrine tissue are buried amid the pancreatic **acinar cells** (**acini**), which make up the exocrine pancreas (FIGURE 31.2). This histology contrasts with the histology of many lower species, including some types of bony fish, where the islets constitute an anatomic structure entirely separate from the exocrine pancreas. In humans, the approximately 1 million islets make up 1% to 2% of the total weight of the pancreas.

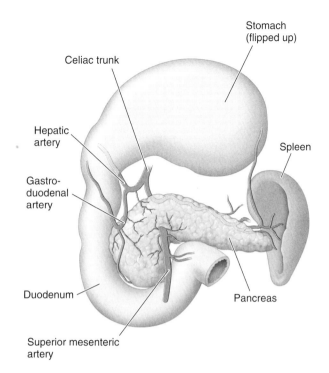

Figure 31.1 The pancreas. The pancreas is situated in the posterior abdomen. This drawing depicts its blood supply.

The islets of Langerhans consist primarily of beta cells and alpha cells, although other cell types are present in the islets too. **Beta cells** synthesize and secrete the peptide hormone insulin. **Alpha cells** make and secrete the peptide hormone glucagon. Less important cells are the delta cells, which synthesize

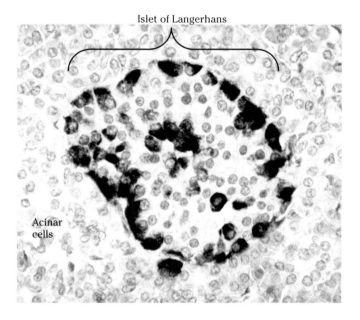

Figure 31.2 Histology of the pancreas. The islets of Langerhans (endocrine tissue) are surrounded by acinar cells. Within the islet, note the alpha cells at the periphery (large cells with a darker cytoplasm) and the central, lighter beta cells.

somatostatin; PP cells, which make pancreatic polypeptide; D1 cells, which secrete vasoactive intestinal peptide (VIP); and enterochromaffin cells, which secrete serotonin.

Hormonal Protein Structure

Because the major products of the endocrine pancreas—insulin and glucagon—are peptide hormones, the organelles involved in protein synthesis and secretion play important roles in the islet cells. The organelles involved are the cell nucleus, ribosomes, endoplasmic reticulum, Golgi apparatus, microtubules, and secretory vesicles. The intracellular production of an insulin molecule begins with a large peptide precursor called **proinsulin**, which is then cleaved to form insulin. The final product of this intracellular processing—the active hormone insulin—consists of two protein chains, known as A and B, which are 21 and 30 amino acids in length, respectively, bridged by a connecting C chain of 31 amino acids (FIGURE 31.3). Glucagon, meanwhile, is a 29-amino-acid, single-chain polypeptide created in the alpha cells. It is also synthesized in a precursor form called **preproglucagon**, which is then processed to glucagon.

The Insulin and Glucagon Receptors

Most tissues express the insulin receptor, but liver, muscle, and adipose tissue bear the receptor in especially high concentrations. The receptor is a transmembrane protein complex with four subunits. Insulin binds to the extracellular domain of the receptor and thereby activates the cytosolic domain, which is a *tyrosine kinase*. Glucagon binds to transmembrane receptors on hepatocytes, triggering the *adenylate cyclase/cAMP pathway*. (See Chapter 4 for a fuller explanation of tyrosine kinase and cAMP mechanisms.)

SYSTEM FUNCTION: THE REGULATION OF PLASMA GLUCOSE CONCENTRATION

As stated above, insulin and glucagon, the major products of the endocrine pancreas, regulate the availability of energy-storing organic molecules in the plasma. These energy molecules include carbohydrates, lipids, and proteins. While most body tissues can utilize any of these forms of fuel, and while the endocrine pancreas governs the metabolism, storage, and release of all of these forms, the pancreas's regulatory apparatus is tied most closely to the plasma glucose level. Plasma glucose control is critical because glucose is the primary fuel source for the brain (as well as for the retina and gonads). The brain contains no significant stores of **glycogen** (the polymerized storage form of glucose) and is inaccessible to other sources of energy, like fatty acids, because the blood-brain barrier limits neuronal absorption of fatty acids from the bloodstream. Hence, a drop in glucose availability in the plasma has severe consequences for neurologic function. Meanwhile, as we will discuss, excessive increases in plasma glucose concentration can have many different harmful effects—for the brain and for the entire organism.

After a meal, when the gut has digested carbohydrates and absorbed glucose into the bloodstream, the plasma glucose level is high. This is called the **fed state**, and in this state the pancreas secretes the hormone insulin. When plasma glucose is low—as in a so-called **fasted state** or starved state—the pancreas secretes the hormone glucagon. Insulin drives fed-state metabolic activities: the uptake and storage of glucose (**glycogenesis**), as well as the uptake and storage of amino acids and triglycerides (FIGURE 31.4). Glucagon drives the fasted-state metabolic activities: (1) **glycogenolysis**, the breakdown of glycogen, and **gluconeogenesis**, the synthesis of glucose, in the

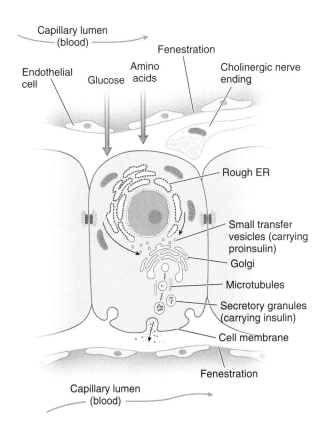

Figure 31.3 Insulin production in the beta cell. The nucleus transcribes mRNA that codes for proinsulin. Ribosomes on the rough endoplasmic reticulum (ER) translate the mRNA into the proinsulin peptide. Vesicles shuttle the proinsulin to the Golgi apparatus, which secretes granules loaded with proinsulin. Proinsulin is cleaved here, and the granules store the insulin, which is later exocytosed.

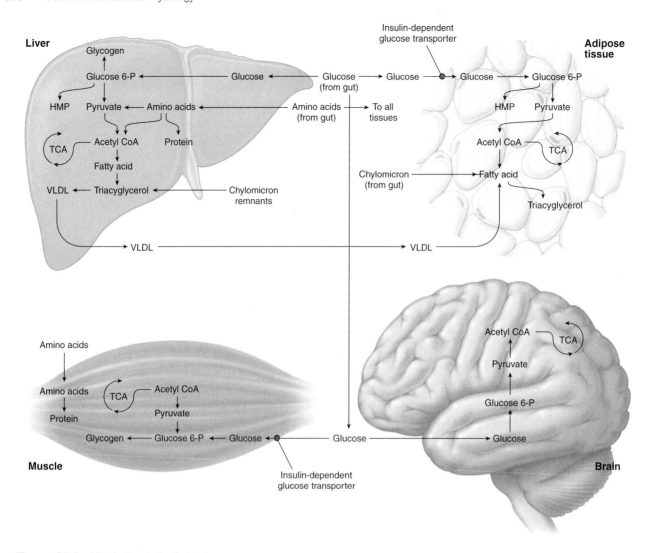

Figure 31.4   Metabolism in the fed state.

liver, which boosts the plasma glucose level to feed the glucose-requiring brain; and (2) the production of an alternate fuel substrate the rest of the body can use in the absence of glucose. The alternate fuel substrates are molecules known as **ketone bodies** (FIGURE 31.5).

Finally, glucagon is supported by several other hormones in the promotion of fasted-state metabolism: glucocorticoids, epinephrine, and growth hormone. Collectively, the four hormones of fasted-state metabolism are known as the **counterregulatory hormones**. (In pregnancy, human chorionic somatomammotropin also has counterregulatory effects.) While insulin decreases the plasma glucose level and drives fed metabolism, the counterregulatory hormones increase the plasma glucose level and drive fasted metabolism. We will delve more deeply into these subjects; meanwhile, let this overview and Figures 31.4 and 31.5 serve as a map to orient you as we proceed with the discussion.

Insulin Secretion

Insulin is secreted from the beta cells into the bloodstream principally in response to an elevated plasma glucose level. Beta cells detect the increased glucose level through the intracellular enzyme **glucokinase**. When the plasma glucose level rises (e.g., after absorption of glucose into the blood from the gut), glucose diffuses down its concentration gradient through the GLUT1 and GLUT2 transporters into the beta cells. Glucokinase, which is very sensitive to changes in the glucose concentration at physiologic levels, then phosphorylates the glucose so that it may undergo glycolysis. The consequent production of ATP inhibits ATP-sensitive K^+ channels, depolarizing the cell. This intracellular electropositivity triggers voltage-sensitive Ca^{2+} channels, Ca^{2+} flows into the cell and further depolarizes it, and the increased Ca^{2+} level promotes exocytosis of insulin granules (FIGURE 31.6). The set point at which glucokinase trig-

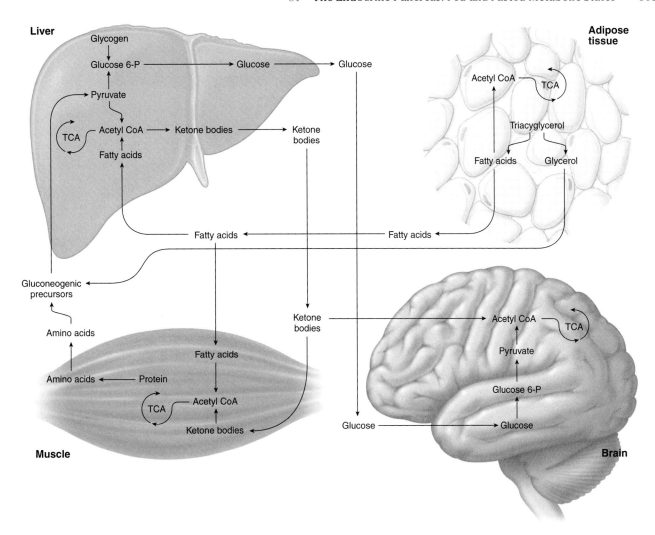

Figure 31.5 Metabolism in the fasted state.

gers insulin release is a plasma glucose concentration of 5 mmol/L (90 mg/dL).

By this sensing mechanism a postprandial (after-meal) increase in plasma glucose stimulates the beta cells of the pancreas and results in a biphasic increase

in plasma insulin levels (FIGURE 31.7). Within 3 to 5 min of beta-cell stimulation, the insulin concentration rapidly rises in the bloodstream to as much as 10 times the basal level; this represents the secretion of stored insulin from cytoplasmic granules. A second

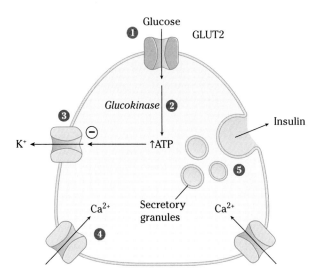

Figure 31.6 Glucose-sensing mechanism of the pancreatic beta cell. (1) Glucose binds the GLUT2 receptor of the beta cell. (2) In the presence of elevated glucose levels, glucokinase promotes glycolysis and hence oxidative phosphorylation, increasing the level of ATP. (3) ATP inhibits ATP-sensitive K^+ channels and decreases K^+ efflux. (4) Decreased K^+ efflux depolarizes the cell, which triggers voltage-gated Ca^{2+} channels and creates Ca^{2+} influx and further depolarization of the inside of the cell. (5) Ca^{2+} promotes exocytosis of insulin-laden granules.

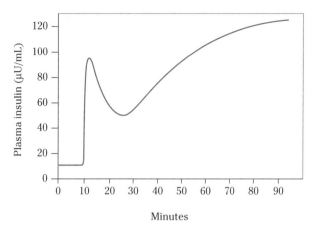

Figure 31.7 Insulin secretion. This graph charts a biphasic increase in plasma insulin concentration after the ingestion of a bolus of glucose (at time 0).

peak occurs gradually over the next 15 to 20 min, representing both further release of stored insulin and the release of newly synthesized insulin. The constitution of the meal will determine the amount of insulin secreted; thus, diabetic patients will inject amounts of insulin before a meal depending on the carbohydrate content (a process known to the diabetic as carbohydrate-counting). Other stimuli of insulin secretion include increased plasma levels of amino acids, increased plasma fatty acids, and acetylcholine (reflecting increased parasympathetic nervous activity). Endocrine signals from the gut called **incretins** (such as *GIP*, gastroinhibitory polypeptide, and *GLP-1*, glucagon-like polypeptide-1) are also known to promote insulin production and secretion in response to a meal. In contrast, insulin secretion is inhibited by conditions of low plasma glucose and by the sympathetic nervous system (norepinephrine and epinephrine). The autonomic nervous system may contain its own glucose-sensing capabilities, through which it controls insulin secretion in parallel with the direct effect of glucose on the beta cells. Glucose-sensing neurons in the hypothalamus detect low blood sugar levels and stimulate the sympathetic nervous system. In diabetic patients, this produces the warning signals of hypoglycemia, such as sweating, tachycardia, and restlessness. Fortunately, these warning signs occur before the glucose level is low enough to cause changes in consciousness. However, long-term diabetics with well-controlled blood sugar levels may lose their sensitivity to hypoglycemia, and the loss of warning signals may result in episodes of neurologic dysfunction as a first sign of hypoglycemia.

Insulin Action

Once again, insulin mediates fed-state metabolism. Accordingly, its functions are generally *anabolic* (i.e., promoting the synthesis and storage of

molecules rather than consumption). However, insulin also promotes the utilization of glucose by stimulating **glycolysis**, the breakdown of glucose into constituents that may enter into the citric acid cycle or undergo anaerobic energy extraction.

The Effects of Insulin on Carbohydrate Metabolism
Insulin responds to conditions of elevated plasma glucose by increasing the uptake of glucose into tissues, principally into liver, skeletal muscle, and adipose cells. It does so by upregulating the expression of GLUT glucose transporters on these tissues, and possibly also by increasing GLUT efficiency. Glucose is thus thought to be absorbed down its concentration gradient by facilitated diffusion. The resulting increased availability of glucose inside the cells drives glycogen synthesis and glycolysis by a mass effect. Insulin also directly enhances these metabolic pathways. It stimulates the storage of glucose as glycogen by activating *glycogen synthase*, an enzyme that links glucose molecules. It stimulates a glycolytic utilization of glucose by increasing the activity of several enzymes in the glycolytic pathway that convert glucose to pyruvate in the production of ATP (FIGURE 31.8).

Insulin also has inhibitory effects. It prevents the breakdown of glycogen by inhibiting *glycogen phosphorylase*, an enzyme that degrades glycogen. Insulin inhibits gluconeogenesis by decreasing the availability of key substrates for gluconeogenesis, such as free fatty acids. FIGURE 31.9 summarizes the effects of insulin on carbohydrate metabolism.

The Effects of Insulin on Lipid Metabolism
Insulin's main role in lipid metabolism is to promote fat storage in adipose tissue during the fed state. Insulin facilitates this action by inhibiting the enzyme *hormone-sensitive lipase*, found in the cytoplasm of adipose cells, where it works to release **free fatty acids (FFAs)**. FFAs are a freely diffusible constituent of **triglyceride** molecules (also known as triacylglycerol), which in turn are the storage form of fat (FIGURE 31.10). By inhibiting lipase, insulin decreases plasma levels of "traveling" fats (FFAs) and increases the level of the storage form of fat (triglycerides) in adipose tissue. This decrease in plasma FFA also has the indirect effect of stimulating glucose uptake by cells, since FFA normally inhibits glucose uptake by cells.

In addition to inhibiting the mobilization of fats, insulin increases the de novo synthesis of fat, particularly in liver and adipose cells. In the liver, as mentioned above, excess glucose is first converted to glycogen for storage; however, after the hepatocyte glycogen concentration exceeds a certain point, feedback inhibition prevents further glycogen synthesis. The excess glucose is then converted to fat. In adipose tissue, excess glucose is first converted to

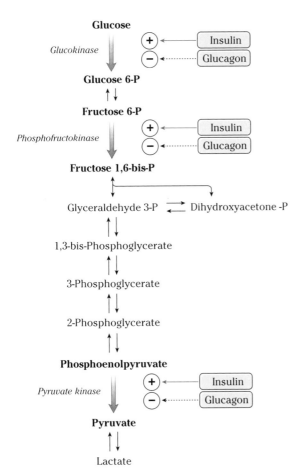

Figure 31.8 Insulin stimulation of glycolysis. Insulin activates enzymes at several stages along the glycolytic pathway, resulting in an increased utilization of glucose. Glucagon has an inhibitory effect on the same enzymes.

glycerol, which then forms triglyceride. Insulin's final contribution to fat storage is the hormone's stimulation of triglyceride uptake into adipose cells. It does so by stimulating the enzyme *lipoprotein lipase (LPL)*. LPL in tissue capillaries is activated by very-low-density lipoprotein (VLDL) and then hydrolyzes the

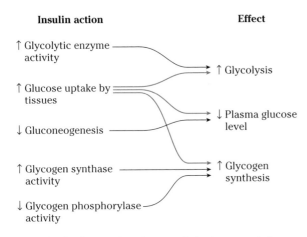

Figure 31.9 Effects of insulin on carbohydrate metabolism.

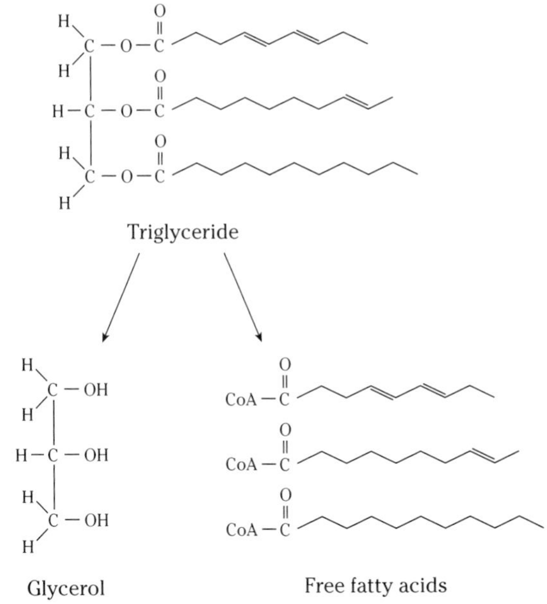

Triglyceride

Figure 31.10 Triglyceride (triacylglycerol), the storage form of fat, and its constituents: glycerol and FFAs. Insulin inhibits the breakdown of triglyceride into its components and keeps freely diffusible FFAs out of the bloodstream.

triglyceride of the VLDL to produce intermediate-density lipoprotein (IDL), fatty acids, and glycerol.

The Effects of Insulin on Protein Metabolism Insulin favors the storage of proteins in tissues in the fed state. The hormone stimulates the transport of free amino acids into liver and muscle cells, thus providing the building blocks for protein formation. At the same time, insulin inhibits the catabolism of proteins. (See Integrated Physiology Box *Insulin Effects on Plasma [K⁺].*)

Glucagon Secretion

A low plasma glucose level is the chief stimulus for glucagon secretion from the alpha cells of the islets of Langerhans. It is not completely clear how glucose sensing occurs in the alpha cells. Norepinephrine and epinephrine also stimulate the secretion of this most important counterregulatory hormone. Glucagon secretion is inhibited, conversely, by high plasma glucose levels, by insulin, and by fatty acids.

Glucagon Action

As the major counterregulatory hormone, glucagon functions to antagonize or counter insulin action. While insulin controls metabolism in the fed state, glucagon controls it in the fasted state. Hence, the important actions of glucagon are to raise the plasma glucose levels (via the stimulation of glycogenolysis and gluconeogenesis) and to increase the availability of fatty acids (via the activation of

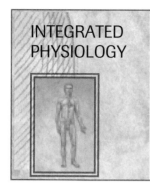

INTEGRATED PHYSIOLOGY

Insulin Effects on Plasma [K$^+$]

In addition to its many roles in the regulation of metabolism, insulin also has an effect on the plasma potassium level. When the insulin peptide binds its receptor, it alters the cell membrane's permeability to ions and hyperpolarizes the cell. The electronegativity created inside the cell by hyperpolarization creates an inward movement of K$^+$. Insulin thereby stimulates K$^+$ uptake by cells. This characteristic of insulin has therapeutic and physiologic importance, but it is unclear whether insulin helps govern the K$^+$ level as part of a feedback loop.

hormone-sensitive lipase in adipose cells). Like insulin, glucagon decreases plasma levels of amino acids by increasing uptake into liver cells. However, whereas amino acid uptake under insulin's influence leads to peptide synthesis, amino acid uptake under glucagon's influence provides additional carbon backbones to the gluconeogenesis pathway. (Because glucagon stimulates the gluconeogenesis pathway, it depletes gluconeogenesis precursors, so the increased amino acid levels owing to increased uptake are consumed by the gluconeogenesis pathway by a mass effect.)

When glucagon action predominates (and the body is therefore in an extreme or prolonged fasted-state metabolism), ketone bodies are produced. This occurs in the following manner. Under glucagon influence, lipid metabolism is shifted toward the breakdown of triglycerides. The activation of hormone-sensitive lipase increases the breakdown of adipose tissue triglyceride stores into FFAs. The FFAs are oxidized in the liver to *acetyl-CoA*. (The reverse occurs in fed-state, insulin-mediated metabolism.) Through glucagon's influence on protein metabolism, amino acids are catabolized to acetyl-CoA as well. It is this buildup of acetyl-CoA that drives the formation of ketone bodies—namely **acetoacetate** and **hydroxybutyrate**—by a mass effect (FIGURE 31.11). These ketone bodies serve as fuel substrates in the muscles and elsewhere to preserve any available glucose for use in the brain. The state called **ketosis**, meaning high levels of ketone bodies in the plasma, occurs in starvation and in pathologic conditions, such as diabetes.

Other Pancreatic Hormones

A third product of the endocrine pancreas is the peptide *somatostatin*. Somatostatin, which is also expressed in the central nervous system and the

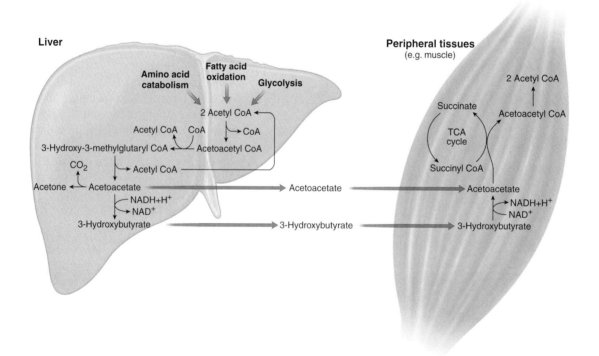

Figure 31.11   Ketone body production and utilization.

gastrointestinal tract, is produced in the islets by delta cells. Although its exact metabolic role is not completely clear, it likely acts in a paracrine fashion to inhibit insulin and glucagon secretion.

The fourth product of the endocrine pancreas is *pancreatic polypeptide*, which is synthesized in the PP cells of the islets. This peptide, secreted in response to protein-containing meals, stimulates the secretion of gastric and intestinal enzymes and inhibits intestinal motility. Other substances produced in the islets include VIP, made by D1 cells, which stimulates glycogenolysis, and serotonin, made by the enterochromaffin cells, whose pancreatic function is not yet elucidated.

In summary, the pancreas regulates metabolism, primarily through the secretion of insulin and glucagon. These hormones integrate activity in the liver, skeletal muscle, and adipose tissue during both fed and fasted states to maintain a constant level of plasma glucose.

PATHOPHYSIOLOGY: DYSREGULATION OF THE PLASMA GLUCOSE LEVEL

An abnormal glucose level may result from three sorts of conditions. First, pancreatic pathology may cause too much or too little production of pancreatic hormones. Second, the target sites of the pancreatic hormones may become insensitive to those hormones. Finally, an excess or deficiency of the extrapancreatic counterregulatory hormones (growth hormone, epinephrine, and glucocorticoids) may skew the plasma glucose level.

Low plasma glucose is called **hypoglycemia**. High plasma glucose is called **hyperglycemia**. Severe hypoglycemia may lead to confusion, stupor, loss of consciousness, and coma. Severe hyperglycemia raises the serum osmolality, which leads to **polydipsia** (excess thirst). If hyperglycemia is high enough to overwhelm the kidney's capacity for glucose reabsorption, an osmotic diuresis occurs and **polyuria** (excess urination) is observed. Hyperglycemia may also result in disturbances of mental status and coma. Chronic exposure to hyperglycemia injures the blood vessels and ultimately accelerates atherosclerosis.

Islet Cell Tumors

Islet cell tumors involve a proliferation, either benign or malignant, of any of the cell types that normally make up the islet. An increased number of any of the hormone-secreting cells elevates the plasma level of the hormone produced by those cells. The most common type is the beta-cell tumor, also called an **insulinoma**. As the name suggests, these tumors are associated with high levels of circulating insulin and hypoglycemia. Complicating the hypoglycemia is

the fact that glucagon, which normally functions to elevate blood sugar, cannot reverse the hypoglycemia because its secretion is inhibited by the high levels of circulating insulin. The other counterregulatory hormones then become more important in preserving the plasma glucose level, and high levels of epinephrine may result in adrenergic symptoms, such as tachycardia (high heart rate) and jitteriness. Tumors involving other cells of the islets, such as the alpha cells (glucagonomas) and the delta cells (somatostatinomas), have also been reported but are considerably rarer.

Diabetes Mellitus

Diabetes mellitus (DM) is a condition of impaired insulin action that leads to hyperglycemia. DM is the seventh leading cause of death in the United States today. The disorder has been classified into two different types, each with distinct clinical and pathologic features. Type I accounts for 10% to 20% of cases and type II for the rest. Type I was previously called insulin-dependent diabetes mellitus (IDDM) and juvenile-onset diabetes, though these names have fallen out of favor. Similarly, the alternate names for type II diabetes, non-insulin-dependent diabetes mellitus (NIDDM) and adult-onset diabetes, are no longer preferred.

The short-term signs and symptoms of DM include polydipsia, polyuria, polyphagia (excess hunger), and high plasma and urine glucose levels. The longer-term sequelae are usually categorized as *microvascular complications* and *macrovascular complications*. Microvascular complications include retinopathy, neuropathy, and nephropathy, frequently progressing to renal failure. The macrovascular complication is *atherosclerosis*, manifesting as coronary artery disease, cerebrovascular disease, or peripheral vascular disease. The combination of peripheral neuropathy, which can lead to foot injury owing to impaired sensation, and peripheral vascular disease, which compromises blood flow to the feet, can lead to nonhealing ulcers of the feet and ultimately to amputation.

One mechanism that has been considered important in causation of diabetic neuropathy involves the sorbitol pathway. Sorbitol is a 6-carbon polyalcohol that can be formed from glucose by aldose reductase. In the presence of hyperglycemia, glucose can enter the nerve, form sorbitol, and cause osmotic swelling due to the trapping of sorbitol within the cell. This mechanism has also been invoked in cataract formation, due to sorbitol accumulation within the lens.

Type I Diabetes   In **type I diabetes**, autoimmune attack on the islet beta cells destroys significant numbers of these cells. Consequently, the pancreas

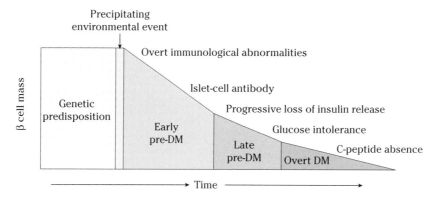

Figure 31.12 Progression of type I diabetes.

cannot make adequate amounts of insulin, and hyperglycemia follows. In type I diabetes, as in other autoimmune diseases, the immune system falsely recognizes a nonforeign protein as though it were foreign and mobilizes an inflammatory response against cells expressing that protein. Autoimmune responses are thought to be the product of genetic susceptibility (certain kinds of major histocompatibility complexes confer added risk) and environmental triggers, such as infectious pathogens or toxins whose chemistry is similar to endogenous proteins. Certain types of autoantibodies are associated with the autoimmune response to the beta cell. Consequently, there is interest in the possibility of early detection of type I diabetes and the prevention of further disease progression (FIGURE 31.12). Because of the very low levels of insulin manufactured by the pancreas in type I diabetes, these patients are often dependent on subcutaneous insulin administration.

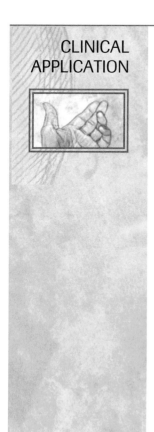

CLINICAL APPLICATION

TREATING DIABETES

Type I diabetes is treated with the administration of insulin. Human insulin is mass-produced for therapeutic purposes using recombinant bacteria. It is self-administered by patients daily, using subcutaneous injection. Because the half-life of insulin in the bloodstream is short, long-acting preparations are available (such as ultralente insulin) that distribute into the bloodstream slowly. These preparations thus maintain an insulin level in the blood over a longer period of time. Insulin pumps that feed insulin continuously into a subcutaneous port have made it possible to mimic normal pancreatic function quite closely. The pumps provide a steady flow of insulin to re-create the basal levels of insulin found physiologically, and the patient can dial in additional boluses of insulin to cover meals of varying caloric and carbohydrate content. Patient education is extremely important in the treatment of diabetes, because patients administer insulin to themselves and must learn to recognize the signs of hypo- and hyperglycemia in their bodies. Dietary modifications and assessments are a critical part of living with diabetes.

Type II diabetics may also progress to the point where they lack sufficient insulin production and may require insulin therapy. Before that point, obese type II diabetics are encouraged to lose weight, which can reduce insulin resistance and prevent progression of the disease. Oral hypoglycemic medication is also available to increase insulin secretion or potentiate its actions in the face of insulin resistance. The sulfonylureas are a class of oral hypoglycemics that promote insulin secretion by inhibiting the same K^+ channel involved in the glucokinase-mediated secretion of insulin from normal beta cells. Some examples of sulfonylureas are glyburide, glipizide, and chlorpropamide. Thiazolidinediones act at the insulin target tissues rather than at beta cells. Their mechanism of action is not well understood, but they are known to enhance the effects of insulin. Finally, injectable GLP-1 analogs have recently generated interest as a way of mimicking the gut's incretin effect on insulin secretion.

Type II Diabetes   **Type II diabetes** appears to begin with a syndrome of insulin resistance and progresses toward insulin deficiency. *Insulin resistance* means that the adipose, skeletal muscle, and hepatic tissues do not respond to insulin as they do under normal physiologic circumstances. Obesity is strongly correlated with insulin resistance, and it has been proposed that the increased intracellular levels of fatty acids in obese people interfere with insulin signaling. Other factors produced by adipose cells may interfere with insulin function and secretion. Because insulin does not have its intended effect in this context, plasma glucose levels remain high. Consequently, the pancreas produces higher-than-normal levels of insulin (*hyperinsulinemia*). The syndrome of insulin resistance is diagnosed by a high level of insulin for a given level of glucose. As the disease progresses, however, the capacity of beta cells to secrete insulin declines. Investigators have found that amyloid, which is normally secreted along with insulin, may deposit in beta cells and interfere with insulin secretion. Other researchers hypothesize that chronic exposure of beta cells to high glucose levels (and hence to increased glucose metabolism) creates increased levels of reactive oxygen species. These free radicals are thought to injure the genome and impair expression of the genes for proinsulin. (See Clinical Application Box *Treating Diabetes.*)

Summary

- The pancreas consists of exocrine tissue that secretes enzymes into the gut lumen and endocrine tissue that secretes hormones into the bloodstream. Exocrine structures called acinar cells surround smaller amounts of endocrine tissue, the islets of Langerhans.

- The islets of Langerhans are composed of alpha cells and beta cells. The peptide hormone glucagon is made in alpha cells, and the peptide hormone insulin is made in beta cells.

- Glucagon and insulin are synthesized as pre-proglucagon and proinsulin, respectively.

- Glucagon and insulin receptors occur in high concentrations on the cell membranes of adipose, skeletal muscle, and hepatic tissue. Glucagon's signal is transduced through a cAMP-mediated pathway. Insulin's signal is transduced through a tyrosine kinase-mediated pathway.

- Insulin and glucagon together regulate the plasma glucose level. Glucagon raises it to ensure an adequate supply of glucose to the brain; insulin lowers it to promote the storage and utilization of excess glucose. This decrease in plasma glucose also helps prevent the consequences of hyperglycemia: high plasma osmolality and, more chronically, damage to the blood vessels.

- High plasma glucose levels stimulate insulin secretion from beta cells through a glucokinase-mediated sensing mechanism. Glucokinase's effects on glycolysis and hence on intracellular ATP ultimately depolarize the cell and promote the exocytosis of granules of stored insulin. This occurs at plasma glucose values less than 5 mmol/L (90 mg/dL).

- Amino acids, fatty acids, acetylcholine, and incretins made in the gut also promote insulin secretion from beta cells.

- Inside liver, fat, and muscle tissue, insulin promotes the polymerization of glucose into glycogen, the storage form of glucose; promotes glycolysis; promotes the binding of free fatty acids to glycerol to form triglyceride, the storage form of fat; and promotes protein synthesis. Insulin also inhibits the degradation of these same macromolecules and inhibits glucagon secretion.

- Inside liver, fat, and muscle tissue, glucagon promotes glycogenolysis (the breakdown of glycogen into diffusible glucose that can be transported to the brain); promotes gluconeogenesis (the synthesis of glucose from carbon precursors such as fatty acids); promotes the degradation of triglycerides into fatty acids and glycerol to feed the gluconeogenesis pathway; and promotes the hepatic uptake of amino acids to feed the gluconeogenesis pathway.

- Counterregulatory hormones that share glucagon's plasma glucose-raising properties and counter insulin's actions are growth hormone, glucocorticoid, and epinephrine.

- Glucagon levels are chronically high when glucose levels are chronically low, as occurs in starvation. Glucagon levels may also be chronically high in uncontrolled type I diabetes due to insulin deficiency, because this deficiency reduces insulin's inhibition of glucagon secretion.

- When glucagon levels are chronically high, acetyl-CoA accumulates from the degradation of triglyceride and protein. Excess acetyl-CoA leads to the formation of ketone bodies, acetoacetate and hydroxybutyrate, which serve as alternate fuel sources for the body so that the brain can use any available glucose. Ketosis is an important feature of prolonged fasted metabolism and has special consequences for the blood's pH.

- Other hormones produced by the islet of Langerhans include somatostatin, pancreatic polypeptide, VIP, and serotonin.

- Low plasma glucose is called hypoglycemia. High plasma glucose is called hyperglycemia.

- Islet cell tumors lead to increased levels of pancreatic hormones. The most common type is the beta-cell tumor, also called an insulinoma, which leads to hypoglycemia.

- Diabetes mellitus is a condition of impaired insulin action that leads to hyperglycemia. The short-term signs and symptoms include polydipsia, polyuria, polyphagia (excess hunger), and high plasma and urine glucose levels. The longer-term sequelae are injuries to large and small blood vessels.

- In type I diabetes, autoantibodies against beta cells reduce beta-cell mass and hence reduce insulin secretion. Chronic lack of insulin-mediated glucagon inhibition can put the body into a fasted-state metabolism, worsening the hyperglycemia and leading to ketosis. The mainstay of therapy is subcutaneous injection of insulin.

- Type II diabetes begins with insulin resistance in fat, liver, and muscle tissue. Insulin resistance is correlated with obesity. As the disease progresses, insulin secretion also declines. Treatment options include weight loss, oral hypoglycemic medication, and administration of exogenous insulin.

Suggested Reading

Atkinson MA, Eisenbarth GS. Type 1 diabetes: new perspectives on disease pathogenesis and treatment. Lancet. 2001;358(9277):221–229.

Cryer PE. Glucose counterregulation: prevention and correction of hypoglycemia in humans. Am J Physiol. 1993;264(2 Pt 1):E149–155.

Drucker DJ. Enhancing incretin action for the treatment of type 2 diabetes. Diabetes Care. 2003;26(10):2929–2940.

Goldstein BJ. Insulin resistance as the core defect in type 2 diabetes mellitus. Am J Cardiol. 2002;90(5A):3G–10G.

Matschinsky FM, Glaser B, Magnuson MA. Pancreatic beta-cell glucokinase: closing the gap between theoretical concepts and experimental realities. Diabetes. 1998;47(3):307–315.

Porte D Jr, Kahn SE. Beta-cell dysfunction and failure in type 2 diabetes: potential mechanisms. Diabetes. 2001;50(Suppl 1):S160–163.

Zierler K. Whole body glucose metabolism. Am J Physiol. 1999;276(3 Pt):E409–426.

REVIEW QUESTIONS

Directions: Each of the numbered items or incomplete statements in this section is followed by answers or by completions of the statement. Select the ONE lettered answer or completion that is BEST in each case.

1. A 73-year-old woman comes to the emergency room with worsening disorientation and stupor. The workup reveals pronounced hypoglycemia, hyperinsulinemia, and a pancreatic mass. Which of the following explains the woman's failure to compensate for her hypoglycemia?

    (A) Glycogen deficiency
    (B) Excess free fatty acids
    (C) Decreased alpha-cell mass
    (D) Glucagon inhibition
    (E) Adrenal suppression

2. A 13-year-old girl is admitted to a psychiatric ward for treatment for an eating disorder. She is severely malnourished and underweight. It is likely that:

    (A) Her glucagon levels are low.
    (B) Her plasma glucose level is low.
    (C) Her tissues are insulin-resistant.
    (D) Her tissue glycogen stores are depleted.
    (E) Her gluconeogenesis enzymes are depleted.

3. An obese 50-year-old man notices a significant increase in his thirst and appetite over the past few months and complains of frequent urination. He has a long family history of type II diabetes but has never had any symptoms of it before now. The mechanism behind his hyperglycemia is likely to involve:

    (A) An impaired glucokinase-mediated signaling pathway.
    (B) An impaired tyrosine kinase-mediated signaling pathway.
    (C) Decreased beta-cell mass.
    (D) Impaired glucagon action.
    (E) Impaired insulin secretion.

ANSWERS TO REVIEW QUESTIONS

1. **The answer is D.** The woman has an insulinoma. The consequent high levels of insulin cause the hypoglycemia and also inhibit glucagon secretion, preventing counterregulatory compensation for the low plasma glucose level. Glycogen deficiency could interfere with the counterregulatory response to the low plasma glucose level since the counterregulatory hormones derive glucose from glycogenolysis; however, hyperinsulinemia *increases* glycogen stores rather than decreases them. Hyperinsulinemia *decreases* levels of free fatty acids, binding them into triglycerides by inhibition of hormone-sensitive lipase. Decreased alpha-cell mass would interfere with the compensation for hypoglycemia by limiting the amount of glucagon that can be produced. However, hyperinsulinemia does not reduce glucagon secretion by decreasing alpha-cell mass; rather, it inhibits secretion from alpha cells. Adrenal suppression would also interfere with the response to hypoglycemia because the adrenal glands produce glucocorticoid, a counterregulatory hormone. Hyperinsulinemia does not, however, suppress the secretion of any of the counterregulatory hormones besides glucagon.

2. **The answer is D.** The girl's metabolism is in a fasted state. Decreased consumption of carbohydrates initially lowers the plasma glucose level, and glucagon secretion increases. Glucagon levels would therefore be elevated, not low. Glucagon promotes glycogenolysis to increase the glucose level at the expense of glycogen stores, so glycogen stores would be depleted. The plasma glucose level may not be low because of successful counterregulatory compensation for the decreased dietary supply of glucose. Insulin resistance is associated with obesity, not malnourishment. While her liver would be conducting more gluconeogenesis to provide glucose to the bloodstream to feed the brain, increased metabolic activity is not associated with a decrease in enzyme levels.

3. **The answer is B.** The man has type II diabetes with insulin resistance. Because the insulin receptor in insulin's target tissues (liver, muscle, and fat) is a tyrosine kinase, peripheral insulin resistance is likely to involve this signaling pathway. The glucokinase signaling pathway mediates glucose sensing and insulin secretion in beta cells. Early in the progression of type II diabetes, insulin secretion and beta-cell mass are normal. There is no glucagon impairment in type II diabetes. Furthermore, impaired glucagon action would lead to hypoglycemia, not hyperglycemia.

32

The Pituitary Gland

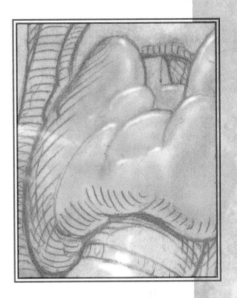

INTRODUCTION

The hypothalamus and pituitary gland constitute an elegant "command center" known as the **hypothalamic-pituitary (HP) axis**. Each hormone controlled by the pituitary is regulated separately along its own "axis." The HP axis integrates information from the body's internal and external environments with higher cortical input. It then orchestrates changes in the multiple physiologic systems controlled by the pituitary hormone axes. The centralization of the control of these axes makes possible the integration of sensory inputs from many stimuli in the formation of hormonal responses. Centralizing the sensory data and hormonal control also allows coordinated hormonal responses to stimuli. Efficient coordination is necessary for everyday activities, such as eating and sleeping, and essential for responding to illness or other stressful situations. In this chapter, there are many examples of how the individual systems that control each pituitary hormone interact to produce this coordination.

The **pituitary gland** (or *hypophysis*, meaning "undergrowth") is a small endocrine gland (0.5 to 0.9 g) located beneath the hypothalamus. It is divided into an anterior lobe, a posterior lobe, and an infundibulum, which connects the pituitary to the hypothalamus.

The **anterior pituitary** synthesizes and secretes six hormones (TABLE 32.1): adrenocorticotropic hormone (ACTH), thyroid-stimulating hormone (TSH), growth hormone (GH), follicle-stimulating hormone (FSH), luteinizing hormone (LH), and prolactin. The secretion of all these hormones except prolactin is regulated by stimulatory factors from the hypothalamus, and by hormonal feedback from the target organs they affect. Diverse influences further modulate their secretion. Prolactin is under tonic inhibition from the hypothalamus through dopaminergic pathways.

The **posterior pituitary** stores and releases two hormones synthesized in the hypothalamus: antidiuretic hormone (ADH) and oxytocin (see Table 32.1).

Pituitary hormones act on endocrine and nonendocrine sites, including the kidneys, adrenal glands, thyroid, ovaries, testes, breast, uterus, and vascular smooth muscle. These hormones are essential to metabolic and autonomic nervous system function and also support changes that occur throughout life.

SYSTEM STRUCTURE

The pituitary gland is located below the hypothalamus, attached to it by the pituitary **infundibulum**,

Table 32.1   PITUITARY HORMONES

Compound	Size	Structure	End Organ
Anterior pituitary			
ACTH	MW 4,500	39 aa[a]	Adrenal cortex
TSH	Glycoprotein MW 28,000	alpha subunit[b]: 89 aa beta subunit: 112 aa	Thyroid
GH	MW 21,500	191 aa polypeptide	IGF-1 production; growth and metabolic effects
FSH	glycoprotein MW 29,000	alpha subunit[b]: 89 aa beta subunit: 115 aa	Ovaries Testes
LH	glycoprotein MW 29,000	alpha subunit[b]: 89 aa beta subunit: 115 aa	Ovaries Testes
Prolactin	MW 22,000	198 aa polypeptide	Breast
Posterior pituitary			
ADH		Nonapeptide (9 aa)	Vascular smooth muscle; distal tubule of kidney
Oxytocin		Nonapeptide (9 aa)	Mammary gland smooth muscle; uterus

[a] aa, amino acid.
[b] The alpha subunits of TSH, FSH, and LH, as well as hCG (human chorionic gonadotropin, a compound released by the placenta), are identical; the beta subunits are distinct and give each its identity and function.

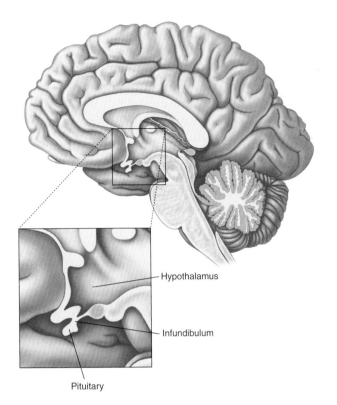

Figure 32.1 Midsagittal cross section of the hypothalamus. The infundibulum connects the pituitary with the hypothalamus.

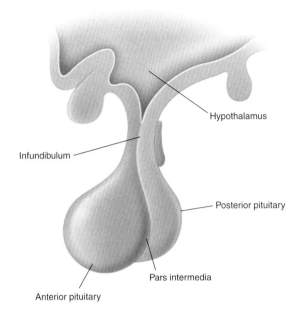

Figure 32.2 Anterior and posterior pituitary. The posterior pituitary comprises axonal projections from cell bodies in the hypothalamic nuclei. Both anterior and posterior pituitary cells secrete hormones into a capillary plexus supplied by the hypophyseal arteries and the pituitary portal circulation, bringing blood from the hypothalamus.

or neural stalk (FIGURE 32.1). The pituitary rests in the *sella turcica* (Latin for Turkish saddle) of the sphenoid bone and is separated from the brain and its surrounding arachnoid membranes and cerebrospinal fluid by a reflection of the dura mater called the *diaphragmatic sellae*.

The pituitary is inferior and slightly posterior to the optic chiasm. It lies posterior to the air-filled sphenoid sinus and adjacent to the venous cavernous sinuses through which travel cranial nerves III, IV, and VI and the internal carotid artery. Any of these anatomic structures may be compressed and disturbed by pituitary tumors. Surgeons often reach the pituitary via the sphenoid sinus.

Gross Anatomy

The important functional division of the pituitary is into the anterior and posterior lobes (FIGURE 32.2). These lobes are often referred to as the *adenohypophysis* (anterior lobe) and the *neurohypophysis* (posterior lobe), reflecting their respective ectodermal and neuroectodermal embryologic origins. The infundibulum makes up the rest of the pituitary and consists of the more proximal median eminence and the distal stalk. It contains vasculature carrying hypothalamic hormones to the anterior pituitary and

neural tracts that project from the hypothalamus to the posterior lobe.

Histology of the Anterior Lobe

The anterior lobe consists of cords of secretory cells, fibroblasts, and capillary endothelial cells. The secretory cells are named according to the staining properties of their granules as chromophils, divided into acidophils and basophils, and chromophobes. The chromophobes contain few or no secretory granules and may represent undifferentiated chromophils, or chromophils that have released their granules.

The acidophils and basophils are further classified on the basis of the hormones they produce (TABLE 32.2). There are two types of acidophils, **somatotrophs** and **lactotrophs**. The remaining four hormones are made by three basophilic cell types: **corticotrophs**, **thyrotrophs**, and **gonadotrophs**.

The anterior pituitary is dependent upon releasing factors from the parvocellular (small-diameter) neurons of the hypothalamus. These neurons originate in many clusters of neurons known as nuclei. Their axons release substances into the fenestrated capillaries of the median eminence. These capillaries coalesce into hypophyseal portal vessels that travel

Table 32.2 **ANTERIOR LOBE CELL TYPES**

Cell Type (% of anterior lobe cells)	Staining Properties	Secretory Granules (nm)	Hormone Product(s)
Somatotroph (50)	Acidophilic	300–400	GH (somatotropin)
Lactotroph (mammotroph) (10–25)	Acidophilic	200 (600 in pregnant or lactating women)	Prolactin
Corticotroph (15–20)	Basophilic	400–550	ACTH[a] (corticotropin)
Thyrotroph (<10)	Basophilic	120–200	TSH (thyrotropin)
Gonadotroph (10–15)	Basophilic	250–400	FSH, LH

[a] Corticotrophs synthesize and releases multiple peptides; see text.

down the infundibulum, form another capillary bed, and release substances to the anterior pituitary. This is the pituitary portal circulation. (See Integrated Physiology Box *Portal Circulations.*)

Histology of the Posterior Lobe

The posterior lobe contains the unmyelinated axons of hypothalamic neurosecretory cells, pituicytes (specialized glial cells), and capillary endothelial cells. No hormone synthesis occurs in the posterior lobe. Magnocellular (large-diameter) hypothalamic neurons originate in the paraventricular and supraoptic nuclei. Their axons carry hormones down the infundibulum into the posterior lobe, where they are stored. The axon terminals are adjacent to fenestrated capillaries and release hormones directly to the systemic circulation without making use of the pituitary portal circulation.

SYSTEM FUNCTION

Each pituitary hormone is controlled by an HP axis (FIGURE 32.3). Each axis has primary regulatory mechanisms, described below. This regulation is fine-tuned by other influences, particularly the regulatory agents of *other* HP axes. A hormone with a primary role in one system will play a secondary role in another system likely to be needed simultaneously. Thus, one axis easily adjusts the activity of other axes. This overlap may be of critical importance in marshaling the body's response to a particular challenge, from hypoglycemia to being chased by a bear! This overlap may also be maladaptive because pathologic changes and an imbalance along one pituitary axis can thereby disrupt others. Other influences on pituitary function include changes in body metabolism or electrolyte balance and higher central nervous system input.

The primary control mechanisms include positive and negative hypothalamic releasing factors and feedback loops (FIGURE 32.4). A positive **releasing factor** stimulates the release of a compound, and a negative factor inhibits its release. All the hypothalamic regulatory hormones are peptides, except dopamine, which is a biogenic amine. Most hypothalamic and pituitary hormones are secreted in a pulsatile fashion. Although the reason is not clear in all circumstances, pulsatility is required for the hormones to be effective.

In a **feedback loop**, the end-product of a chain of events feeds back to an earlier step and inhibits it (negative feedback) or stimulates it (positive feedback). Negative feedback is much more common. It

---

INTEGRATED PHYSIOLOGY

Portal Circulations

In the systemic circulation, the vascular sequence is arteries → capillaries → veins. In a portal circulation, such as in the pituitary or the liver, there is an additional set of veins and capillaries, yielding the sequence arteries → capillaries → veins → capillaries (or venules) → veins. A portal system is used to transport substances in a focused, undiluted fashion to a site for a specific purpose, such as detoxification (liver) or hormonal signaling (pituitary).

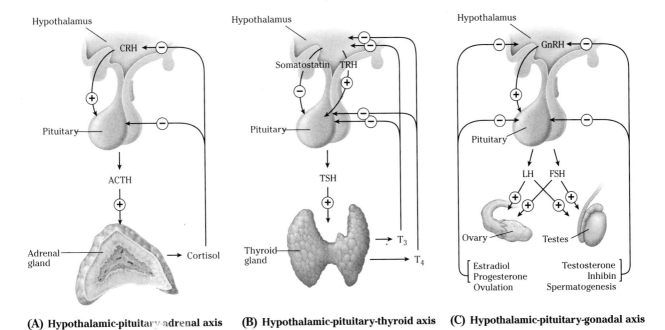

(A) Hypothalamic-pituitary-adrenal axis   **(B) Hypothalamic-pituitary-thyroid axis**   **(C) Hypothalamic-pituitary-gonadal axis**

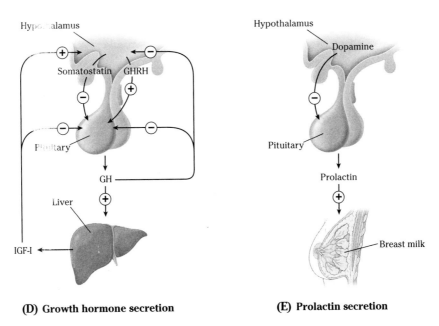

(D) Growth hormone secretion   **(E) Prolactin secretion**

Figure 32.3   Hypothalamic-pituitary axes. Plus signs represent stimulation; minus signs represent inhibition. Each axis diagram includes its feedback regulation.

prevents the overproduction of a compound; when a sufficient amount of a hormone has been produced, it shuts off its own releasing process. Feedback loops are not unique to the pituitary and are found throughout human physiology.

Consider the hypothalamic-pituitary-thyroid axis (HPT), an example of negative feedback. Hypothalamic TRH prompts TSH release by the pituitary, modified by hypothalamic somatostatin inhibition of TSH release. TSH causes thyroid hormone release by the thyroid. Thyroid hormone feedback in-

hibits the release of both TRH and TSH. These are long feedback loops because they involve the end-product. Short feedback loops involve intermediate products, as in the inhibition of TRH release by TSH.

The pituitary gland also provides the basis for adaptations at various life-cycle stages or during a chronic illness. In these settings, significant changes in pituitary hormones and the systems they regulate are made possible by changes in gland size. During pregnancy, for example, lactotroph hyperplasia occurs to provide a needed increase in prolactin.

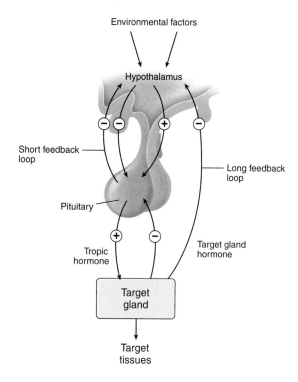

Figure 32.4 Feedback loops. The short and long feedback loops are depicted as having a negative (inhibitory) feedback effect, but they may also have a positive (stimulatory) feedback effect.

The Anterior Pituitary

The six hormones synthesized in the anterior pituitary (ACTH, TSH, GH, FSH, LH, and prolactin) individually affect the activity of one or more target organs (FIGURE 32.5).

The anterior lobe is under the influence of hypothalamic regulatory factors: corticotropin-releasing hormone (CRH), thyrotropin-releasing hormone (TRH), growth hormone-releasing hormone (GHRH), gonadotropin-releasing hormone (GnRH), and hypothalamic inhibitory factors, somatostatin and prolactin-inhibiting factor (PIF). Their roles are summarized in TABLE 32.3.

Corticotrophs **ACTH** is synthesized as pro-opiomelanocortin (POMC), a 28,000-molecular-weight prohormone whose primary breakdown product is ACTH. Other breakdown products include endorphin precursors. ACTH causes the release of glucocorticoids (and, to a lesser extent, mineralocorticoids and adrenal androgens) from the adrenal cortex. Over time, ACTH also promotes the growth of the adrenal cortex; in its absence, the gland atrophies. The role of ACTH in adrenal gland function and corticosteroid synthesis is described more fully in Chapter 34.

Pulsatile release of **CRH** from the hypothalamus stimulates a diurnal pattern of ACTH release, characterized by an early morning peak and an evening nadir. Cortisol feedback inhibits the release of CRH and ACTH. ACTH inhibits CRH release via a short feedback loop. A posterior pituitary hormone, ADH, is a less-potent stimulator of ACTH release and acts predominantly through the potentiation of CRH activity.

Both psychological and physical stressors, such as trauma and illness, increase ACTH levels by a variety of mechanisms. Fever, for example, is associated with cytokine-mediated release of CRH. Other compounds, including catecholamines and opioids, affect ACTH release, enabling the activation of this axis when its end-product, cortisol, is needed to respond to a stressor.

Thyrotrophs **TSH** regulates thyroid gland size and the synthesis and secretion of thyroid hormones (see Chapter 33). The hypothalamus creates a set point for the serum level of thyroid hormones and controls the level by secretion of **TRH** and *somatostatin*. Hypothalamic secretion of TRH causes TSH synthesis, post-translational glycosylation, and release. There is a pulsatile, circadian pattern of TSH release that peaks in the early morning and reaches its nadir in the late afternoon (a good time for a siesta). Somatostatin inhibits TSH release from the pituitary. The thyroid hormones thyroxine (T_4) and triiodothyronine (T_3)—primarily the more physiologically active T_3—inhibit TSH and TRH release via long feedback loops. TSH inhibits TRH release via a short negative-feedback loop.

Starvation, stress, exercise, and illness decrease TSH secretion. This occurs through many mechanisms, including increased cortisol, which is a stress response. Cortisol decreases TSH by decreasing the sensitivity of the pituitary to TRH. During starvation, the lowering of TSH decreases the overall basal metabolic rate and preserves scarce energy sources.

Somatotrophs Unlike other anterior pituitary hormones, **GH** does not prompt the release of another hormone from a specific endocrine gland. Instead, GH has direct effects at many sites in the body. GH also has indirect effects through the release and actions of **insulin-like growth factor-1 (IGF-1)**, also known as *somatomedin-C*. The liver secretes IGF-1 into the systemic circulation. Other tissues respond to GH by secreting IGF-1 locally, where it has a paracrine effect. IGF-1 circulates bound to IGF-binding protein-3, synthesized by the liver in response to GH.

GH is essential for the growth of long bones. Long-bone growth occurs at the epiphysis (growth plate) via a process known as endochondral ossification, in which chondrocytes (cartilage-producing cells) multiply, grow, and lay down cartilage that then undergoes calcification. The combined actions of GH and IGF-1 at the growth plate are explained by the *dual-effector hypothesis*. When GH binds to recep-

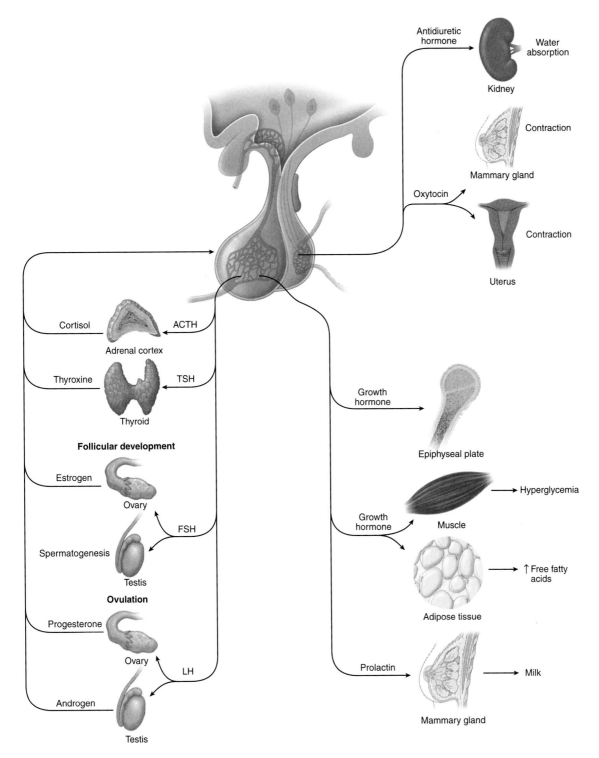

Figure 32.5 Actions of pituitary hormones on target tissues.

tors on epiphyseal prechondrocytes, they differentiate into chondrocytes and secrete IGF-1. IGF-1 then promotes chondrocyte proliferation and the subsequent long-bone growth.

The metabolic effects of GH make the body's energy supplies (in the form of stores of glucose and fat) available for building new proteins, which occurs

in growth. Therefore, GH has anabolic effects on protein metabolism and catabolic effects on glucose and lipid metabolism.

Much of the information about the actions of GH and IGF-1 comes from in vitro studies and studies of the administration of pharmacologic doses. GH and IGF-1 appear to be synergistic in their effects on

Table 32.3 HYPOTHALAMIC REGULATORY HORMONES

Hypothalamic Hormone	Structure	Function[a]
Thyrotropin-releasing hormone (TRH)	Tripeptide (3 aa[b])	Stimulates TSH release by thyrotroph; stimulates prolactin release by lactotroph
Corticotropin-releasing hormone (CRH)	41 aa polypeptide	Stimulates ACTH release by corticotroph
Gonadotropin-releasing hormone (GnRH)	Decapeptide (10 aa)	Stimulates FSH and LH release by gonadotroph
Growth hormone-releasing hormone (GHRH)	44 aa polypeptide	Stimulates GHRH release by somatotroph
Somatostatin	14 aa peptide	Inhibits GH release by somatotroph; inhibits TSH release by thyrotroph
Prolactin-inhibiting factor (PIF)	Dopamine[c]	Inhibits prolactin release from lactotroph

[a] Primary function. Almost all hypothalamic hormones have some effects on each of the anterior pituitary cell types.
[b] aa, amino acid.
[c] Evidence indicates that there may be additional PIFs. However, dopamine appears to be the primary PIF.

protein, but they generally have antagonistic effects on glucose and lipid metabolism.

GH and IGF-1 both have anabolic effects on protein metabolism. GH increases protein synthesis directly. IGF-1 appears to mediate the inhibition of protein breakdown.

GH's effects on carbohydrate metabolism are consistent with its role as one of the counterregulatory hormones that reverse hypoglycemia (along with glucagon, epinephrine, and cortisol). GH inhibits insulin action in the liver, thereby decreasing glucose uptake and utilization. However, unlike glucagon, GH preserves glycogen stores in the liver. This feature of both GH and cortisol is called a *glycostatic effect.*

IGF-1, as its name suggests, has structural similarity to insulin. Skeletal muscle cells, but not hepatocytes or adipocytes, have IGF-1 receptors that, when activated, result in insulin-like glucose uptake and utilization. GH's effects on glucose metabolism are antagonized by IGF-1.

The effects of GH on lipid metabolism are also consistent with its role as a counterregulatory hormone. GH has a lipolytic effect by increasing the activity of hormone-sensitive lipase. GH makes fat stores available as an energy source, just as it makes glucose available as an energy source. In contrast, short-term administration of IGF-1 appears to have an anti-lipolytic effect, which may occur via IGF-1 actions on adipocyte insulin receptors; recall that adipocytes do not have IGF-1 receptors. However, longer-term administration causes lipolytic effects via IGF-1-related decreases in insulin secretion.

There is a baseline pattern of GH release mediated by higher-order central nervous system centers, including the hippocampus and amygdala. GH release occurs mostly during sleep. Nocturnal release of GH accounts for approximately 70% of daily GH re-

lease (which may be why children need their sleep). It is not surprising to learn that GH levels peak during adolescence and decrease with age. By linking metabolic changes and growth induction through GH, the body ensures that it will have the metabolic substrate necessary for growth.

GH secretion is stimulated by **GHRH** from the hypothalamus and inhibited by somatostatin from the hypothalamus. GH leads to IGF-1 synthesis. IGF-2 provides feedback inhibition at the hypothalamus and pituitary. In addition, GH inhibits GHRH release via short-loop feedback inhibition.

GH secretion changes in response to virtually any stress or change in endocrine function or metabolism. Since GH is one of the counterregulatory hormones, it is appropriate that hypoglycemia is a potent stimulus to GH release. Strong evidence indicates that emotional deprivation can impair GH secretion and lead to growth failure in severely affected children. For example, institutional abuse and profound neglect have been found to produce dwarfism.

The GH axis interacts with almost every other pituitary axis. For example, cortisol increases GH release; the linking of these two counterregulatory hormones facilitates a more effective response to hypoglycemia. The thyroid hormone T_3 potentiates the pituitary response to GHRH, increasing GH levels. Consequently, in hypothyroidism, the GH response to GHRH is blunted, so hypothyroidism typically retards growth in children. Again, the pituitary coordinates events: when the body's thyroid function is low, as in illness, it is an inopportune time for growth.

Gonadotrophs   LH and FSH, the gonadotropins, act on the ovaries and testes. Their effects include both gametogenesis and the production of sex steroids. More detailed information may be found in Chapters 36 and 37.

Hypothalamic **GnRH** governs the secretion of pituitary gonadotropins LH and FSH. The secretion of GnRH, and consequently of LH and FSH, is pulsatile. The pacemaker for pulsatility is likely intrinsic to the hypothalamus, but the pulse rate is clearly altered by higher neural input, which may enable the changes in pulse frequency that occur with puberty. Pulsatility is necessary for gonadal activity. Continuously elevated GnRH leads to the suppression of LH and FSH, perhaps due to the downregulation of GnRH receptors. This phenomenon is used in the therapy of hyper-LH/FSH states, such as precocious puberty.

The regulation of LH and FSH by the sex steroids is complex. In women, traditional feedback loops exist: *estrogen* and *progesterone* inhibit GnRH secretion and may also have inhibitory effects at the pituitary via the modulation of GnRH effects. Gonadotropins also exert short-loop feedback inhibition at the hypothalamus.

Besides gonadal steroids, gonadal peptides also regulate gonadotropins. Inhibin is a polypeptide with alpha and beta subunits made in ovarian granulosa cells and testicular Sertoli cells. In women, in the late follicular phase of the menstrual cycle, inhibin acts synergistically with estrogen to inhibit FSH release. Inhibin does not affect LH release.

Under other circumstances, estrogen exerts positive feedback. During the follicular phase of the menstrual cycle, rising levels of estrogen and progesterone stimulate LH secretion and create a mid-cycle surge in LH. Although the mechanism for this positive feedback is controversial, it appears to involve hormonal sensitization of the pituitary to GnRH, including increased GnRH receptors.

In men, testosterone and dihydrotestosterone (DHT) from testicular Leydig cells suppress LH (but not FSH) via the suppression of GnRH. As in women, inhibin produced by the testes inhibits FSH secretion.

As with other hormonal systems, stress and other environmental changes modulate the activity of this system. In anorexia nervosa, for example, GnRH levels decline, with resultant decreases in the gonadotropins and the sex steroids, leading to amenorrhea and other clinical changes. Again, the pituitary effectively coordinates the hormonal response to its environment: in the setting of starvation, it averts the possibility of pregnancy.

Gonadotropin levels change over the course of development, again demonstrating the role of the hypothalamus and pituitary in adaptations during different life-cycle stages. In early childhood, there is central inhibition of GnRH secretion, and the pituitary is very sensitive to negative feedback by gonadal steroids. With the onset of puberty, central inhibition of GnRH release decreases, and heightened pituitary sensitivity to negative feedback declines. There is a transition to the adult pattern of pulsatile GnRH secretion. These pulses are initially primarily during sleep but soon change to the adult pattern of every 90 min. The pulsatile secretion of LH results in pubertal development. At menopause, with the lack of circulating sex steroids from the ovaries, levels of LH and FSH rise.

Lactotrophs **Prolactin** acts primarily at the mammary gland. Its two main roles are to promote breast development and lactation. Its effects on lactation are inhibited during pregnancy by high estrogen and progesterone levels. Like other anterior pituitary hormones, prolactin is secreted in a pulsatile fashion. Peak levels occur at the end of the night. Unlike other anterior pituitary hormones, prolactin regulation is predominantly through hypothalamic inhibition. The major inhibitory factor is **dopamine**. Through a short feedback loop, prolactin regulates hypothalamic dopamine release.

As with every pituitary hormone, there are secondary influences on prolactin regulation. Estrogen causes increased synthesis and release of prolactin; in fact, estrogen stimulation is responsible for intrapartum hyperplasia of the lactotrophs, resulting in the high prolactin levels characteristic of pregnancy, in preparation for postpartum lactation.

Prolactin release is triggered by a decrease in dopaminergic inhibition or by releasing factors. Many possible prolactin-releasing factors have been proposed. TRH and VIP (vasoactive intestinal peptide) are likely candidates, and probably act at the pituitary level, because lactotrophs have TRH and VIP receptors in their membranes. These substances may mediate the maternal prolactin release that occurs in response to suckling.

The Posterior Pituitary

The hypothalamic hormones released by the posterior lobe of the pituitary are two peptide hormones, ADH (also known as *vasopressin*) and oxytocin. Their structures are quite similar, differing by only two amino acids (see Table 32.1). Recall that these compounds are synthesized in neuronal cell bodies in the hypothalamus but stored in neuronal axons in the posterior pituitary.

ADH The primary role of **ADH** is to promote water retention at the level of the renal distal tubule. Via the V_2 receptor and a G-protein/cAMP/protein kinase cascade, ADH causes the fusion of water-channel (aquaporin)-containing vesicles with the luminal membrane of the distal tubules, increasing water permeability and thereby allowing water reabsorption.

Osmolarity is the most important regulator of ADH secretion. When plasma osmolarity rises from the normal 280 mOsm/kg H_2O, this is recognized by osmoreceptors in the anterior hypothalamus, which signal the supraoptic and paraventricular nuclei to release ADH. This system is very sensitive: a small increase in osmolarity causes rapid ADH release, water retention, and the restoration of normal osmolarity. The short plasma half-life of ADH, approximately 15 min, allows precise control and rapid adjustments. Once osmolarity is restored to normal, ADH secretion is turned off, and existing ADH breaks down. The ability to conserve water, of course, ultimately depends on the urine-concentrating ability of the kidney. ADH osmoreceptors also stimulate the body's thirst mechanism, providing another (external) source of water.

Decreased blood volume, sensed by low-pressure baroreceptors in the left atrium, and decreased blood pressure, sensed by high-pressure baroreceptors in the aortic arch and carotid arteries, result in signaling via the vagus and glossopharyngeal nerves to the brain stem and then to the hypothalamus for ADH release. This hemodynamic mechanism for ADH release is much less sensitive than the osmolarity system, and significant changes in blood pressure or volume are required to causes ADH release.

Oxytocin Oxytocin has two putative roles. It clearly plays a role in lactation by leading to the contraction of myoepithelial cells in the breasts, causing milk flow. Oxytocin may also play a role in maintaining labor. It causes uterine smooth muscle contraction, and myometrial cells express a large number of oxytocin receptors during pregnancy. Though its physiologic role is uncertain, oxytocin is frequently used at pharmacologic doses to induce labor by promoting uterine contraction, and it is also used to promote postpartum uterine contraction. Oxytocin's function in men is unclear. It may increase motility in seminiferous tubules and seminal vesicles.

Suckling induces the release of oxytocin. Interestingly, visual or psychological stimuli suggestive of suckling can also provoke this response. The suckling stimulus is carried by afferent sensory neurons that eventually transmit signals to the hypothalamus. Both beta-agonists and opioids appear to have an inhibitory effect on oxytocin secretion. During pregnancy, the increased endogenous opioids in response to stress have the effect of preserving oxytocin stores for parturition and uterine contraction.

PATHOPHYSIOLOGY

Pituitary pathology causes three types of problems: those due to insufficient pituitary hormone secretion, those due to excessive pituitary hormone secretion, and those due to mass effects of enlarging pituitary tumors. Typically, the disruption of one HP axis alters the others. This results from the normally adaptive interactions that exist among the pituitary axes. Additional disruption occurs when the overgrowth of one cell type leads to hypoplasia of the others. Pituitary pathology leads to a disruption of the endocrine and metabolic processes that the pituitary carefully regulates.

Anterior Pituitary Pathology

If the entire pituitary gland is damaged, as with infarction due to head trauma, all the pituitary hormones will be decreased or absent. This is known as **panhypopituitarism**. More commonly, through injury or developmental anomaly, a single cell type will be deficient or absent.

The effects of deficiencies of the various anterior pituitary hormones follow logically from their function. For example, GH deficiency in children leads to short stature. FSH/LH deficiency causes hypogonadism. ACTH deficiency leads to adrenal insufficiency, and TSH deficiency causes central hypothyroidism, much rarer than primary hypothyroidism, caused by disease of the thyroid gland itself.

In the anterior pituitary, the most common type of pathology is a **pituitary adenoma**, a tumor of one of the chromophil or chromophobe cells. Tumors may be either large (macroadenoma) or small (microadenoma), and functioning (hormone-secreting) or nonfunctioning. A functioning pituitary adenoma causes abnormal elevation of the hormone it produces and can cause hypofunction of other cell types by taking up necessary space and nutrients. The most common such tumor is a prolactin-secreting prolactinoma; also frequent are GH- and ACTH-secreting adenomas. Prolactinomas lead to hypogonadism. GH excess during childhood causes gigantism; during adulthood it leads to the clinical phenotype of acromegaly, characterized by soft tissue proliferation, bony changes at characteristic sites, generalized visceromegaly, and a spectrum of cardiovascular effects, endocrine abnormalities, and metabolic disturbances.

Posterior Pituitary Pathology

The most clinically significant disease involving the posterior lobe of the pituitary is a deficiency of ADH, a condition known as **diabetes insipidus (DI)**, which results in an inability to retain water. Patients excrete large amounts of dilute urine. ADH deficiency refers to central DI, not to be confused with nephrogenic DI, which occurs when ADH is present but the kidney cannot respond properly. Central DI can occur with any insult to the pituitary, and it is common after neurosurgical resection of tumors near the pituitary. It may be transient (secondary to postoperative swelling) or permanent. Because central DI is a deficiency of ADH, it can be treated with a synthetic form of ADH, DDAVP (desmopressin acetate).

Mass Effects from Pituitary Tumors

The classical presentation of a patient with an enlarging pituitary tumor is a *bitemporal hemianopsia* (bilateral loss of lateral vision fields) resulting from compression of the optic chiasm. Compression of the central optic nerve fibers that innervate the nasal retinae and supply the lateral visual fields causes a loss of peripheral vision. Tumors may also invade the nearby cavernous sinus, compromising the integrity of the internal carotid artery or of cranial nerves II, IV, or VI, which travel through it. Since the cranial nerves control extraocular movements, their compromise leads to diplopia or other vision changes.

Because pituitary adenomas often create pathology in two ways—by hormonal overproduction and by a mass effect on the optic nerves—vision changes with evidence of hormonal dysfunction should arouse clinical suspicion of a pituitary tumor. Acromegaly is an example of a condition that often combines hormonal and visual disturbances. The signs of hormonal disturbance in acromegaly are enlargement of soft tissue and bony structures, particularly the hands, feet, and facial bones, owing to an overproduction of growth hormone. (See Clinical Application Boxes *What Is a Prolactinoma?* and *How MRI Works.*)

Summary

- The pituitary is divided into anterior and posterior lobes. The anterior lobe, also known as the adenohypophysis, is an extension of the ectodermal tissue of the hypothalamus. The posterior lobe, also known as the neurohypophysis, is an extension of the neuroectodermal tissue of the hypothalamus.

- The anterior pituitary hormones are part of a hypothalamic-pituitary (HP) axis. The hypothalamus secretes a hormone that stimulates the pituitary to secrete a hormone, and the pituitary hormone in turn stimulates a target organ to secrete its hormone.

- The axes involve pulsatile release in circadian patterns, and hormones are released in response to stimulatory factors specific to each axis.

- The HP axes are also governed by negative (and in one case positive) feedback.

- In the hypothalamic-pituitary-adrenal (HPA) axis, corticotropin-releasing hormone (CRH) is secreted by the hypothalamus in a circadian rhythm in response to stress. The HPA

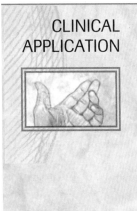

CLINICAL APPLICATION

WHAT IS A PROLACTINOMA?

A 51-year-old man is referred to the endocrinologist for decreased libido. He has also had episodes of impotence and worsening headaches for a period of several months. Recently, he was involved in a motor vehicle accident in which he did not see an oncoming car at a four-way stop sign. Neurologic examination reveals decreased peripheral vision and lab tests show low levels of serum testosterone, luteinizing hormone (LH), and follicle-stimulating hormone (FSH) and a high level of serum prolactin. MRI results suggest a pituitary macroadenoma encroaching on the inferior aspect of the optic chiasm.

Prolactinomas are the most common type of hormone-secreting pituitary tumors. They represent hyperplasia of the pituitary lactotrophs, which secrete prolactin. The high prolactin levels suppress LH and FSH, and low levels of those hormones lead to hypogonadal effects in men and women: suppression of testosterone secretion from the male gonads and irregular menses and infertility in females. The tumor may also compress structures adjacent to the pituitary. For example, compression of the optic chiasm, which sits on top of the pituitary, may lead to visual field deficits. Treatment may be medical—bromocriptine is a dopamine agonist that suppresses prolactin secretion—or surgical. Surgical resection is usually done through the sphenoid sinus.

CLINICAL APPLICATION

HOW MRI WORKS

Magnetic resonance imaging (MRI) works in a manner very different from that of an x-ray. X-rays are high-frequency electromagnetic waves that cast a shadow behind any object that absorbs their energy. By contrast, MRI—whose name was changed from *nuclear* magnetic resonance imaging (NMRI) in the 1970s for political reasons—relies on the spin properties of the protons in the nuclei of hydrogen atoms. The spin of individual protons lends them a magnetic polarity that makes them sensitive to magnetic fields. When exposed to a magnetic field, a proton may be aligned in agreement with the magnetic vector (a low-energy state) or in opposition to it (a high-energy state). A change in orientation of the proton from a high-energy state to a low-energy state gives off energy and a change from low to high absorbs energy. When energy is cast across hydrogen atoms by an NMR spectrometer in the form of radio waves, the exchange of energy (resonance) between the protons and the spectrometer creates a measurable signal. When the waves are cast across a plane of hydrogen atoms from all 360 degrees, a computer can track the signals and define the location of groups of atoms.

Because human tissues are mostly water, making hydrogen the most abundant element in the body, MRI is well suited to the visualization of soft tissues. Furthermore, the hydrogen composition of fat, bone, and other tissues differs from one to another, creating a distinct signal for each tissue type and enabling the imaging of distinct organic structures. MRI is also typically used to detect tumors such as pituitary adenomas. MRI does not pose a carcinogenic risk in the way that x-rays do, because radio waves are lower-energy waves than x-rays and do not break chemical bonds as x-rays do. However, radio waves can heat body tissues if the machinery malfunctions, and the powerful magnets of MRI machines can cause metal objects to fly through the air.

---

axis stimulates the pituitary corticotrophs to secrete adrenocorticotropic hormone (ACTH). ACTH acts on the adrenal glands to promote the secretion of cortisol.

- In the hypothalamic-pituitary-thyroid (HPT) axis, thyrotropin-releasing hormone (TRH) is secreted by the hypothalamus in a circadian rhythm to regulate the metabolic rate. TRH stimulates the pituitary thyrotrophs to promote the secretion of thyroid-stimulating hormone (TSH). TSH acts on the thyroid gland to promote the secretion of thyroxine, which acts peripherally on the tissues.

- In the growth hormone axis, growth hormone (GH) is secreted directly from the pituitary in response to growth hormone-releasing hormone (GHRH) from the hypothalamus.

- GH promotes the release of insulin-like growth factor-1 (IGF-1) into the bloodstream from the liver. It also promotes local (paracrine) secretion and the action of IGF-1 in other tissues.

- IGF-1 promotes the growth of long bones and mimics the action of insulin.

- GH promotes protein synthesis but is counterregulatory when it comes to carbohydrate and lipid metabolism. In other words, it promotes the breakdown of carbohydrate and lipid macromolecules.

- In the hypothalamic-pituitary-gonadal axis, gonadotropic-releasing hormone (GnRH) is secreted by the hypothalamus in accordance with complex long feedback loops. GnRH promotes the secretion of follicle-stimulating hormone (FSH) and luteinizing hormone (LH) from the gonadotrophs of the pituitary. FSH and LH promote the gonadal production of sex steroids.

- In the prolactin axis, the release of prolactin, unlike other pituitary hormones, from the pituitary is controlled by inhibitory rather than stimulatory signals from the hypothalamus. The hypothalamus inhibits the release of prolactin via dopamine.

- Prolactin is important in pregnancy; it promotes breast development and lactation.
- The posterior pituitary secretes antidiuretic hormone (ADH) and oxytocin. ADH is primarily important in the regulation of serum osmolality. Oxytocin promotes milk secretion and may promote the uterine contractions of labor.
- Pituitary pathology causes three types of problems: those due to insufficient pituitary hormone secretion, those due to excessive pituitary hormone secretion, and those due to mass effects of enlarging pituitary tumors.
- The most common form of pituitary pathology is the pituitary adenoma, and the most common functional pituitary adenoma is the prolactinoma.
- Mass effects of pituitary tumors may include visual field deficits, hemorrhage due to invasion of the cavernous sinus, and cranial nerve palsies.

Suggested Reading

Aron DC, Tyrell JB, Wilson CB. Pituitary tumors. Current concepts in diagnosis and management. West J Med. 1995;162(4):340–352.

Berneis K, Keller U. Metabolic actions of growth hormone: direct and indirect. Baillieres Clinical Endocrin Metab. 1996;10(3):337–352.

Butler AA, Le Roith D. Control of growth by the somatotropic axis: growth hormone and the insulin-like growth factors have related and independent roles. Annu Rev Physiol. 2001;63:141–164.

Ho KKY, O'Sullivan AJ, Hoffman DM. Metabolic actions of growth hormone in man. Endocrine J. 1996;43(Suppl):S57–63.

Spagnoli A, Rosenfeld RG. The mechanisms by which growth hormone brings about growth: the relative contributions of growth hormone and insulin-like growth factors. Endocrin Metab Clin North Am. 1996;25(3):615–631.

Wilson CB. Surgical management of pituitary tumors. J Clin Endocrinol Metab. 1997;82(8):2381–2385.

REVIEW QUESTIONS

Directions: Each of the numbered items or incomplete statements in this section is followed by answers or by completions of the statement. Select the ONE lettered answer or completion that is BEST in each case.

1. A 60-year-old man is diagnosed with a prolactin-secreting pituitary microadenoma after a thorough workup for impotence. He is given medication that suppresses prolactin secretion. This medication is likely to mimic the effects of which hypothalamic product?

   (A) GnRH
   (B) GHRH
   (C) CRH
   (D) TRH
   (E) Dopamine
   (F) Bromocriptine
   (G) ACTH
   (H) FSH
   (I) LH
   (J) Thyroxine

2. A 41-year-old man is diagnosed with acromegaly after a progressive enlargement of the hands and feet and prognathism. Which of the following lab abnormalities is likely to be observed?

   (A) Hypocalcemia
   (B) Hypoalbuminemia
   (C) Hypo-osmolality
   (D) Hyperglycemia
   (E) Hypernatremia

3. A 28-year-old woman presents with amenorrhea, galactorrhea, and bitemporal hemianopsia. The most likely cause is:

   (A) Gonadal failure.
   (B) Panhypopituitarism.
   (C) Pituitary adenoma.
   (D) Gigantism.
   (E) Acromegaly.

ANSWERS TO REVIEW QUESTIONS

1. **The answer is E.** Hypothalamic dopamine inhibits the secretion of prolactin from pituitary lactotrophs. GnRH, GHRH, CRH, and TRH are all hypothalamic hormones with stimulatory, not inhibitory, effects on pituitary tissues other than the lactotrophs. Bromocriptine is not a hypothalamic product; rather, bromocriptine is the medication that mimics dopamine action on the lactotrophs. ACTH, FSH, and LH are produced in the pituitary, not the hypothalamus. Thyroxine is produced in the thyroid gland.

2. **The answer is D.** GH, levels of which are elevated in acromegaly, is a counterregulatory hormone that mimics glucagon action in its effects on carbohydrate metabolism. It promotes gluconeogenesis and increases the plasma glucose level. High levels of GH also increase IGF-1 levels, which mimics the effect of insulin, not glucagon, thus driving down the serum glucose level. Clinically, it is more common to observe an increase in the counterregulatory effects and hyperglycemia.

3. **The answer is C.** The symptoms of hyperprolactinemia and cranial mass effects are indicative of a prolactin-secreting pituitary adenoma. Pituitary adenomas can lead to gigantism or acromegaly, but these produce a different clinical picture. Gonadal steroid production is suppressed in hyperprolactinemia, but gonadal failure alone would not explain galactorrhea (milk production) or cranial mass effects.

The Thyroid Gland

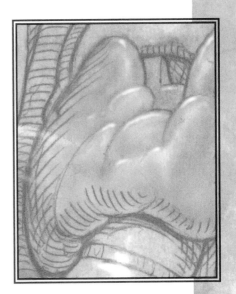

INTRODUCTION

The manifestations of thyroid disease have attracted attention for many millennia. The herbal medicine treatise, the *Pen-Tsao*, supposedly written by the Chinese emperor Shen-Nung around 2700 B.C., may contain the earliest known description of the swollen neck, or **goiter**, that we know today as pathologic thyroid enlargement. Galen wrote of the thyroid in the first centuries A.D. and the Roman satirist Juvenal observed "swollen necks" around the same time in the Alps. Ancient treatments for goiter included the administration of animal thyroid and iodine-containing Sargasso weed (pelagic seaweed). Various medieval practitioners also found the ashes of burnt sea sponge useful in the treatment of goiter, probably because sea sponges harbor iodine-containing scleroproteins. In the latter half of the 19th century, the Swiss surgeon Theodor Kocher performed thousands of thyroidectomies on goiter patients; after observing the disastrous results in his postoperative patients, he became the first to describe the symptoms of hypothyroidism (thyroid hormone deficiency) and received the Nobel Prize in 1909.

The etymology of the word thyroid—from the Greek *thureoeides*, meaning "shield-shaped"—reflects the fact that the gland's anatomy was understood long in advance of its possible function. Today we know that the iodine-containing thyroid hormone binds to a nuclear receptor to influence gene expression, just as the cholesterol-based steroids do. Thyroid hormone appears to have evolved earlier than the steroids, however, probably originating in the pre-Cambrian era over 500 million years ago, before the evolutionary divergence of arthropods and vertebrates. It is thought that the ancient thyroid hormone acquired a new role with the evolution of warm-blooded animals (homeotherms). In these animals, it maintains a metabolic rate necessary for homeothermic heat generation. Put another way, *thyroid hormone stokes the biochemical furnaces of all cells to maintain body heat.* Its other crucial role is in promoting normal growth and development from fetal life through childhood.

Roughly 5% of the U.S. population has a diagnosed thyroid disorder, and perhaps another 5% has undiagnosed thyroid disease, according to the American Association of Clinical Endocrinologists. In developing countries where dietary iodine is lacking, thyroid disease is even more widespread. Because of the prevalence of thyroid disease and its accessibility to treatment, an understanding of thyroid physiology is of great clinical importance.

SYSTEM STRUCTURE

The **thyroid gland** is located in the neck anterior to the trachea and inferior to the larynx and cricoid cartilage (FIGURE 33.1). It consists of right and left lobes connected by an isthmus and weighs around 15 to 20 g. When neuroendocrine signals demand more thyroid hormone for a sustained period of time, the gland may hypertrophy to many times its normal size and protrude visibly. This accounts for the development of goiter described by Shen-Nung, Juvenal, and other ancient observers.

The **follicles** are the functional units of the thyroid gland (FIGURE 33.2). They are spherical structures less than 0.5 mm in diameter and are filled with **thyroglobulin (Tg)**, the glycoprotein precursor to thyroid hormone. The pool of thyroglobulin molecules is referred to collectively as a substance called **colloid**. Each colloid-filled follicle is encapsulated by a capillary-laden basement membrane and lined on the inside by a one-cell-thick cuboidal epithelium. The epithelial cells, sometimes called *thyrocytes*, have different surface proteins on their **apical surface,** the luminal or colloid-facing side, than they do on their **basal surface**, the capillary-facing side. Accordingly, the apical and basal membranes perform different functions in the biosynthesis and transport of thyroid hormones. (Recall a similar segregation of surface proteins and similar terminology, from renal physiology, where the inner membranes of the renal tubular cells are called apical and the outer membranes called basolateral.)

The follicles are bundled into lobules by connective tissue, and along the planes of connective tissue

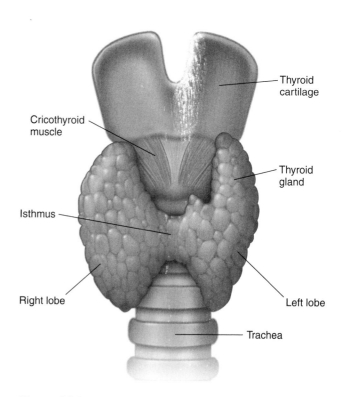

Figure 33.1 Anatomy of the thyroid gland. A normal variant of thyroid anatomy includes a pyramidal lobe extending upward from the isthmus.

(Figure labels: Thyroid cartilage; Cricothyroid muscle; Thyroid gland; Isthmus; Right lobe; Left lobe; Trachea)

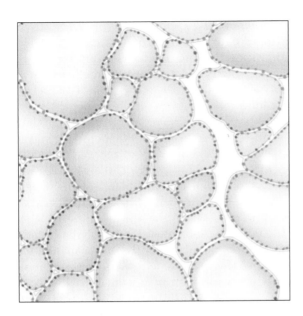

Figure 33.2 Thyroid follicles. The follicles are filled with colloid (thyroglobulin). Thyroglobulin is iodinated, and iodotyrosyls are coupled in the follicle lumina.

travel nerves (parasympathetic and sympathetic), blood vessels, and lymphatics. **Parafollicular cells** are scattered among the follicles. They produce *calcitonin*, a hormone that aids in the regulation of plasma calcium concentration (see Chapter 35).

The Biosynthesis of Thyroid Hormones

There are two primary types of thyroid hormone (FIGURE 33.3). The two varieties are identical, except that thyroxine (T_4) possesses four iodine moieties and triiodothyronine (T_3) possesses three. Thyroid hormone, like epinephrine and norepinephrine, is a modified molecule of the amino acid **tyrosine**. Whereas tyrosine has one benzene ring (a hydroxyl-bearing phenol group), thyroid hormone is equivalent to a tyrosine with a second benzene ring in its side chain. Thyroid hormone also has iodine moieties on both of its benzene rings; in T_4, there are two atoms of iodine on each ring, while in T_3, there are two atoms of iodine on one ring and one atom of iodine on the other. When T_3 is synthesized, either the phenol ring or the inner ring may receive two atoms of iodine. If the outer phenol ring bears two atoms of iodine, the molecule is inactive and is called **reverse T_3 (rT_3)**.

Ingredients: Thyroglobulin, I^-, and H_2O_2 Tyrosine is combined with iodine to form T_4 and T_3 in the follicle lumen under enzymatic control (FIGURE 33.4). First, a glycosylated protein scaffold (thyroglobulin) is constructed in the endoplasmic reticulum with multiple tyrosine groups (tyrosyls) along its length. The thyroglobulin molecules are then exocytosed into the follicle lumen. Meanwhile, dietary iodine dif-

fuses from the follicular capillaries across the basal **Na^+/I^- symporter (NIS)** and into the thyrocyte cytoplasm. The energy driving this I^- uptake comes from the **Na^+/K^+-ATPase**, which has suppressed the intracellular Na^+ concentration. Extracellular Na^+ flows down its concentration gradient across the NIS and into the cell, and because the NIS couples Na^+ movement to I^- movement, the influx of Na^+ drives an influx of I^-. This is an example of *secondary active transport*. The I^- accumulates inside the cell until

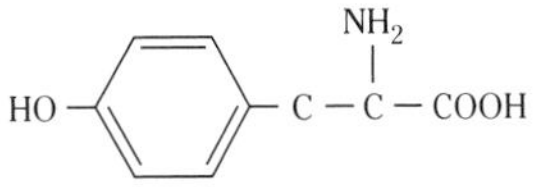

Tyrosine

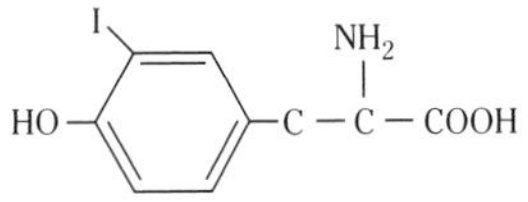

MIT (3-monoiodotyrosine)

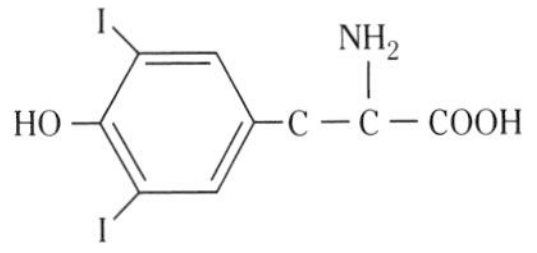

DIT (3,5-diiodotyrosine)

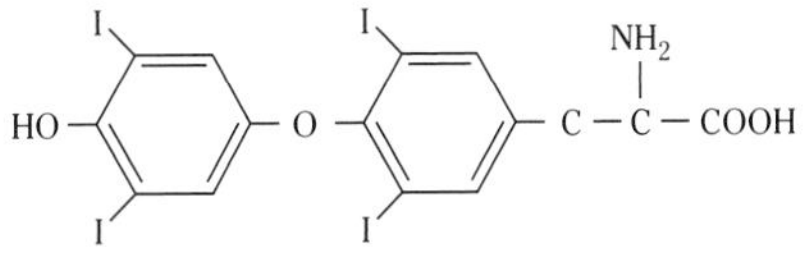

Thyroxine, T_4 (3,5,3',5'-tetraiodothyronine)

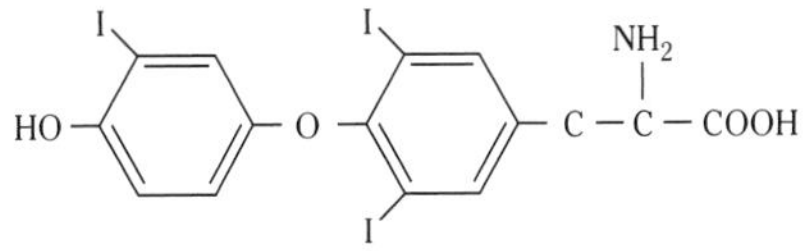

T_3 (3,5,3'-triiodothyronine)

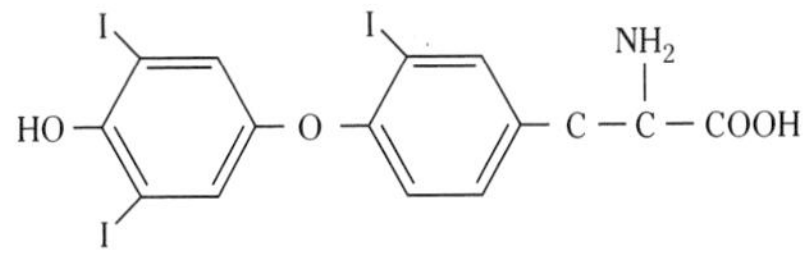

reverse T_3 (3,3',5'-triiodothyronine)

Figure 33.3 Structure of tyrosine, MIT, DIT, T_4, T_3, and rT_3. The iodinated carbons on the inner benzene ring are labeled 3 and 5. The carbons on the outer benzene ring are labeled 3' and 5'. T_3 has no iodine moiety at the 5' carbon. Thus, it is a 5' deiodinase that converts T_4 to T_3. Reverse T_3 has no iodine moiety at the 5 carbon. Thus, it is a 5 deiodinase that converts T_4 to rT_3, thereby inactivating it.

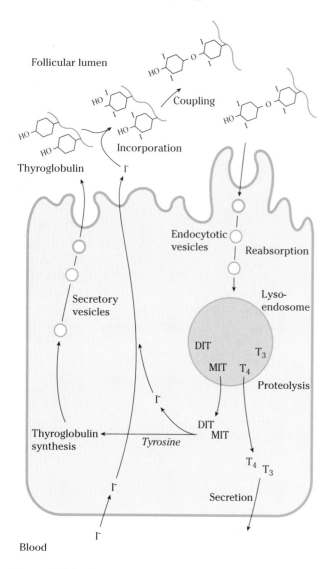

Figure 33.4 Biosynthesis of thyroid hormone.

there is a concentration gradient across the apical membrane. Then it flows through the I^-/Cl^- transporter (called pendrin) and into the follicular lumen. Finally, **hydrogen peroxide (H_2O_2)** is produced in the lumen by NADPH oxidase associated with the apical membrane.

Iodination   Once thyroglobulin, I^-, and H_2O_2 have been congregated in the follicle lumen near the apical membrane, **thyroid peroxidase (TPO)** catalyzes the oxidation of I^- to an intermediate species, possibly a free radical, using H_2O_2 as an electron acceptor. The oxidized iodine intermediate then binds the benzene rings of the tyrosyl groups, which are sitting on the thyroglobulin backbone. This is termed **iodination** of thyroglobulin (or *organification of iodine*). If the tyrosyl binds one iodine atom, the group is called **monoiodotyrosine (MIT)**. If the tyrosyl binds two iodine atoms, the group is called **diiodotyrosine (DIT)**.

The Formation of T_4 and T_3   At this stage, thyroid peroxidase catalyzes a second oxidation-reduction reaction. One tyrosine hydroxyl group loses its hydrogen and binds an adjacent tyrosine benzene ring, linking two iodinated rings together. Two DIT moieties join to form T_4, without the T_4 detaching from the thyroglobulin scaffold. Alternatively, a DIT and an MIT bind together to make T_3. Some DIT and MIT moieties remain uncoupled. An average molecule of thyroglobulin contains two or three residues of T_4, 0.7 of T_3, four or five of DIT, and five of MIT. The mature thyroglobulin, loaded with T_4, T_3, DIT, and MIT, is finally released from the apical epithelial surface into the large pool of mature thyroglobulin called the colloid. When signals from the brain mandate the secretion of thyroid hormone, mature thyroglobulin is endocytosed and transported into lysosomes. Here, T_4, T_3, DIT, and MIT are cleaved from the thyroglobulin backbone and the backbone is digested. The biologically inactive DIT and MIT are metabolized, and their iodine is recovered for another round of iodination. T_4 and T_3 are conducted by an unknown mechanism to the basal membrane and transported into the capillary blood. *Almost all the thyroid hormone released by the thyroid is in the form of T_4.* Roughly 80 to 100 μg of T_4 is secreted per day, versus a daily output of around 4 μg of T_3 and 2 μg of rT_3.

SYSTEM FUNCTION

The thyroid gland is one of the endocrine glands under the control of a neuroendocrine axis, a cascade of signals originating in the brain that controls the secretion of hormone from the thyroid gland. The hypothalamus first secretes thyrotropin-releasing hormone (TRH), which causes the pituitary to release thyroid-stimulating hormone (TSH)—also called thyrotropin. TSH triggers the production of thyroid hormone and also promotes its secretion from the thyroid gland. This axis is therefore called the **hypothalamic-pituitary-thyroid (HPT) axis** (FIGURE 33.5). The HPT axis features classic negative feedback control: the axis end-product, thyroid hormone, circulates back to the hypothalamus and the pituitary in the bloodstream and inhibits the release of its own control signals, TRH and TSH. Thyroid hormone thereby delimits its own production and secretion.

The Regulation of Thyroid Hormone Production and Secretion

We will begin our discussion of thyroid function at the top of the HPT axis, with the hypothalamus. Then we will proceed in sequence through the release of thyroid hormone, its transport, peripheral activation, and cellular recognition. We will conclude

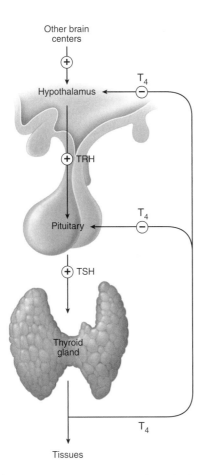

Figure 33.5 The hypothalamic-pituitary-thyroid axis. Plus signs represent stimulation; minus signs represent inhibition.

with the mechanisms by which the thyroid boosts metabolism and thermogenesis and influences growth and development.

TRH **Thyrotropin-releasing hormone (TRH)** was discovered in 1969, the first of the hypothalamic releasing factors to be specifically characterized. It consists of just three modified amino acids—pyroglutamine, histidine, and prolinamide. TRH is cleaved from a prohormone by *prohormone convertases* in the paraventricular nucleus of the hypothalamus. It is then shuttled along neuronal axons into the hypothalamic median eminence and secreted into the portal blood vessels that connect the hypothalamus to the anterior pituitary. When it reaches the pituitary in the portal blood, it acts on the **thyrotroph cells** (TSH-secreting cells) of the anterior pituitary.

TRH production and secretion is fairly constant, leading to a relatively constant plasma level of thyroid hormones. This is in keeping with thyroid hormone's task of ensuring a constant supply of body heat under any circumstances. Negative-feedback control by thyroid hormone appears to be the chief regulator of TRH output. Brain centers for the

perception of temperature may also have some influence on TRH production, with cold leading to TRH release. Neurons in the medulla, pons, and other areas of the brain synapse with the TRH-producing cells of the hypothalamus, but the physiologic role of these connections is not entirely clear.

TRH acts at the TRH receptor on the cell membranes of pituitary thyrotrophs (FIGURE 33.6). The TRH receptor is a G-protein-linked seven-transmembrane receptor that stimulates TSH gene expression through a Ca^{2+}-mediated signaling pathway. Increased TRH stimulation of the receptor leads to increased production of TSH. In addition, TRH controls the bioactivity of the TSH produced; that is, it exerts qualitative control as well as quantitative control over TSH. Specifically, TRH increases the bioactivity of TSH by promoting post-translational modification of oligosaccharide chains on TSH. These changes increase TSH bioactivity directly and by indirect contributions; by facilitating TSH secretion and by prolonging its half-life (delaying its degradation), the TRH-mediated changes support TSH's ability to act on the thyroid.

TSH **Thyroid-stimulating hormone (TSH)** is a glycoprotein hormone like the gonadotropic hormones of the pituitary, follicle-stimulating hormone (FSH) and luteinizing hormone (LH), and like one of the major

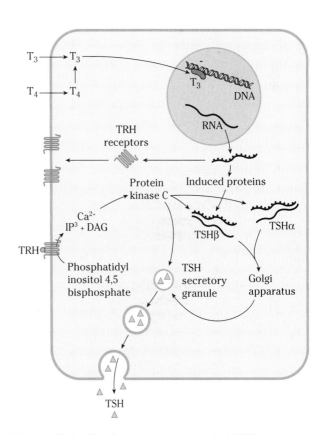

Figure 33.6 Signaling mechanisms by which TRH acts on pituitary thyrotroph cells.

placental hormones found in women's bloodstreams during pregnancy, human chorionic gonadotropin (hCG). TSH shares an alpha subunit in common with FSH, LH, and hCG, but the beta subunits of these hormones are unique and account for their differing physiologic actions. The related hormones may sometimes mimic one another's actions, however. For example, by virtue of its structural homology with TSH, hCG may in pregnancy stimulate the thyroid to make more thyroid hormone, thus recruiting thyroid hormone for the fetus until the fetus can make its own.

Like TRH, TSH also binds to a G-protein-linked receptor (FIGURE 33.7). The TSH receptor is located on the basal membrane of the thyroid follicle cells and triggers an increase in intracellular cAMP. The cAMP-mediated signaling cascade promotes increased thyroid hormone biosynthesis and secretion. A phospholipase C-mediated signaling pathway also participates. Specifically, the signaling effects include increased gene expression of proteins involved in thyroid hormone biosynthesis and secretion; phosphorylation and activation of proteins involved in thyroid hormone biosynthesis and secretion; and, with prolonged TSH exposure, growth and cell division of the thyrocytes (which accounts for goiter). Increased thyroidal blood flow to the follicles is also observed in the presence of TSH. This increases iodide and oxygen delivery to the thyroid and sweeps away secreted thyroid hormone at an increased rate, thereby creating an improved gradient for the secretion of hormone into the bloodstream.

TSH secretion is controlled by TRH, as described above, and it is also subject to the same negative-feedback effects that act upon the TRH-secreting cells. Increased levels of T_4 and T_3 dampen the pituitary response to TRH and hence suppress TSH production and secretion. Conversely, decreased levels of thyroid hormone disinhibit TSH secretion, and the plasma TSH level goes up, driving the thyroid gland to replenish the blood levels of thyroid hormone.

Clinically, the TSH level is the single most important indicator of thyroid function. If the thyroid is making a normal amount of thyroxine, the TSH level will be in the normal range. If the thyroid is underperforming (e.g., owing to the destruction of thyroid tissue), the TSH will be high. If the thyroid is overperforming (e.g., owing to unregulated hormone production), the TSH will be low.

Other Controls: Thyroglobulin and Iodine Levels   In addition to TRH/TSH-mediated control of thyroid hormone and negative feedback effects, at least two lesser factors affect the regulation of thyroid hormone production and secretion. First, thyroglobulin is thought to have its own negative feedback effect by autocrine action on the follicle that contains it. Accumulation of thyroglobulin in the follicle is thought to suppress the gene expression of proteins involved in thyroid hormone biosynthesis. Second, the availability of iodine limits the amount of thyroid hormone that can be produced. Without enough iodine substrate, thyroid hormone cannot be produced in adequate amounts, which is why dietary iodine deficiency can lead to hypothyroidism. Conversely, too much iodine in the blood can also inhibit the production of thyroid hormone. Excess iodine may monopolize the binding sites on follicular thyroid peroxidase, leading to inefficient iodination of thyroglobulin.

Finally, the body may regulate the proportions of T_3 versus rT_3 available to its tissues. Plasma levels of T_3 are known to drop and levels of rT_3 known to rise during prolonged fasting or in nonthyroidal illnesses. The mechanism is not completely understood, but the effect is probably to slow metabolism and conserve energy when food is scarce or when energy is needed for healing.

Thyroid Hormone Transport

As stated above, the thyroid makes roughly 20 to 25 times more T_4 than T_3 each day. While the liver converts some of the T_4 to T_3, T_3 is also absorbed by tissues and metabolized more quickly than T_4. The end result is that total T_4 concentrations in the plasma average somewhere around 100 nmol/L, while the total T_3 concentrations are somewhere around 2 nmol/L. Thus, *T_4 is the major circulating form of thyroid hormone.*

Like many other hormones, thyroid hormone binds to carrier proteins found in the blood. In fact,

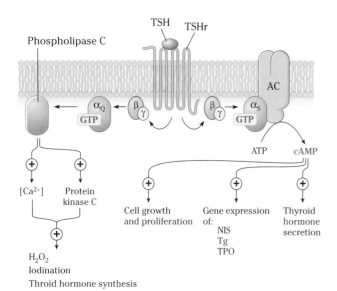

Figure 33.7   Signaling mechanisms by which TSH acts on thyroid cells. TSHr, TSH receptor.

once T_4 and T_3 enter the bloodstream, nearly all of these hormones are taken up by the plasma proteins that transport them (FIGURE 33.8). Whatever T_4 and T_3 remains unbound in the plasma is referred to as **free T_4** and **free T_3**. The association reaction of thyroid hormone and carrier protein is reversible and is governed by an equilibrium constant. For T_4, we would write:

$$\text{Free } T_4 + \text{carrier protein} \leftrightarrow \text{Bound } T_4$$

For T_3 we would write:

$$\text{Free } T_3 + \text{carrier protein} \leftrightarrow \text{Bound } T_3$$

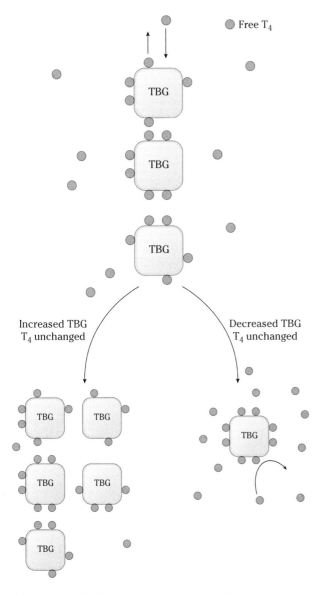

Figure 33.8 T_4 binding to TBG. If the amount of thyroxine-binding globulin (TBG) is increased without a change in T_4, more T_4 is bound. In normal physiology, this situation is transient, as the decreased free T_4 will result in increased TSH. This, in turn, will increase the free T_4 level until the TBG is loaded with T_4 and the free T_4 is back in the normal range, and it is how increased TBG levels yield increased total T_4 levels, as in pregnancy.

As in any reversible reaction, the reactants (free T_4/T_3 and carrier protein) combine more frequently when their concentrations are increased. When either of their concentrations is decreased, the reaction shifts leftward. *It is free T_4 and free T_3, not bound thyroid hormone, that enters cells to alter their functioning.*

When the transport proteins pass by the cells in the periphery, they unload the T_4 and T_3. Unloading occurs because of the cellular uptake of T_4 and T_3 from the extracellular fluid (by simple diffusion or by a specific transporter that has not been clearly identified). This action drops the plasma concentration of free T_4 and T_3, which in turn shifts the equilibrium between protein and thyroid hormone toward dissociation. (In addition, factors associated with the microvasculature may promote enhanced dissociation of thyroid hormone from plasma proteins.) Hormone unloading is analogous to the unloading of oxygen from hemoglobin in the periphery; free, dissolved hormone and free, dissolved oxygen enter the cells by diffusion while the carrier protein remains in the bloodstream.

Three proteins bind T_4 in the blood: albumin, transthyretin (TTR), and **thyroxine-binding globulin (TBG)**. TBG, not to be confused with thyroglobulin (the thyroid hormone precursor), carries the vast majority of T_4 in plasma. It thus serves as an extrathyroidal reservoir of T_4, protecting the T_4 supply from fluctuations in thyroidal output. If T_4 production falls in the thyroid (e.g., due to low dietary iodine intake), the TBG reservoir of T_4 can buffer the peripheral tissues against T_4 shortage until adequate T_4 production is resumed. However, if T_4 underproduction is sustained—as in chronic autoimmune thyroiditis, for instance—the TBG buffer supply will eventually be exhausted and the level of free T_4 will fall. Under physiologic conditions, the plasma protein reservoir also prevents losses of T_4 and T_3 to the urine since the large carrier proteins are not filtered at the glomerulus.

In pregnancy, placental estrogen increases hepatic production and decreases hepatic clearance of TBG, thus increasing the size of the TBG reservoir. This increases the **total T_4** (bound T_4 + unbound T_4) in the mother without increasing the free T_4 concentration. The sequence likely works as follows:

1. Estrogen increases plasma levels of TBG.

2. Increased levels of TBG shift the TBG-free T_4 equilibrium toward binding. The excess TBG soaks up some of the free T_4.

3. The free T_4 level transiently drops.

4. The pituitary thyrotrophs experience less T_4 inhibition of TSH secretion. TSH secretion rises.

5. Under the influence of increased TSH levels, the thyroid cells secrete more T_4.

6. New T_4 binds TBG, shifting the equilibrium between bound and unbound T_4 toward unbound T_4. The old concentration of free T_4 is again achieved. The transient dip in T_4 is erased, while the total T_4 level is now increased.

The increase in total T_4 enables the mother to supply the fetus with thyroid hormone without compromising her own supply. As T_4 diffuses across the placenta (from the intervillous maternal blood to the villous fetal capillaries), T_4 is progressively unloaded from TBG, maintaining the level of free T_4 so that T_4 can continue to diffuse across the placenta and into maternal tissues. (See Clinical Application Box *The Free Thyroxine Index*.)

The Actions of Thyroid Hormone

While T_4 is the major circulating form of thyroid hormone, T_3 is the active form of thyroid hormone inside cells. Because the majority of the thyroid hormone supply is in the form of T_4, the majority of thyroid hormone in the plasma must be converted to T_3 if it is to act upon the cells. The **deiodinases** are the enzymes responsible for converting T_4 to active T_3, and they are present throughout the body.

Activation and Inactivation by Deiodinases   Deiodinases in the liver create T_3 that circulates to sites of action in the tissues, and deiodinases in the peripheral tissues also create T_3 that acts locally. The type I 5′ deiodinase in the liver is chiefly responsible for manufacturing circulating T_3. Circulating T_3, which is less well bound to the plasma proteins, diffuses quickly into the cells and stimulates the intracellular T_3 receptor. Type I and type II 5′ deiodinases inside many different body tissues convert T_4 to locally acting T_3. An example of local T_3 activation is found in the pituitary. For thyroid hormone to have its negative-feedback effect on TSH secretion, T_4 must enter the thyrotroph and be deiodinated to T_3. The T_3 then acts inside the thyrotroph to suppress TSH production and secretion. The 5 deiodinase (as opposed to 5′ deiodinase) in the tissues *inactivates* both T_4 and T_3. It inactivates T_4 by converting it to rT_3 and inactivates T_3 by converting it to T_2 (diiodothyronine). Peripheral activation and inactivation may constitute a form of regulation of thyroid function, but more remains to be learned about such regulation.

The Thyroid Hormone Receptor   Thyroid hormone binds intracellular **thyroid hormone receptors (TRs)** that complex with **thyroid hormone response elements (TREs)** and bind nuclear DNA, thereby influencing gene expression. TRs have a much higher affinity for T_3 than they do for T_4, which accounts for the importance of T_3 as the active form of thyroid hormone. TRs are present in most body tissues, but particular TR subtypes or isoforms ($TR\alpha_1$, $TR\alpha_2$, $TR\beta_1$, $TR\beta_2$, $TR\beta_3$) may predominate in one tissue or another. Different isoforms may complex differently with TREs, producing different thyroid hormone effects in different tissues. TR-TRE complexes may also interact with other signaling pathways (a phenomenon known as *cross talk*), and the variation in TR isoforms may also vary the pattern of cross talk.

In addition to actions mediated by the well-known TR, research has begun to illuminate other pathways of thyroid hormone action. First, investigators have identified faster, *nongenomic actions* of thyroid hormone that are not mediated by intracellular TRs. Receptors for T_4 and T_3 at the cell surface may mediate these actions instead of the slower mechanism of altered gene expression. Such nongenomic signaling mechanisms include the activation of various protein kinases and alterations in solute transport. Finally, thyroid hormone appears to act

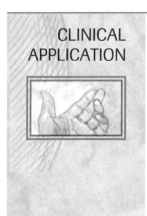

CLINICAL APPLICATION

THE FREE THYROXINE INDEX

Various methods are available for evaluating the serum free T_4 level, although the reliability and clinical utility of these methods are controversial. Calculation of the *free thyroxine index (FTI)* is one way to estimate the level of free T_4. The FTI may be calculated following a *resin T_3 uptake test*. In the test, TBG is exposed to a special form of T_3 bearing a radioisotope of iodine. The radio-T_3 binds any available binding sites on the TBG and the remaining radio-T_3 is taken up by a resin. Less resin uptake of radio-T_3 means there were more available TBG binding sites to be filled by radio-T_3. Hence, TBG was initially less saturated with T_4, a situation that corresponds with low T_4. The FTI is calculated by multiplying the total T_4 by the percentage of radio-T_3 taken up by the resin.

PHARMACEUTICAL IMPLICATIONS OF TR ISOFORMS

The physiologic significance of the various TR isoforms is not completely understood. However, researchers may be able to capitalize on the knowledge of isoform distribution alone. Because the heart contains a higher proportion of TRα versus TRβ, investigators have become interested in developing a chemical ligand that preferentially binds TRβ. Such a drug could stimulate thyroid activity in the liver (increasing cholesterol clearance) without stimulating thyroid activity in the heart (leading to tachycardia).

directly on transcription factors associated with the *mitochondrial genome*. Nongenomic and mitochondrial mechanisms may contribute to many of the physiologic and developmental end results of stimulation by thyroid hormone. (See Clinical Application Box *Pharmaceutical Implications of TR Isoforms.*)

Metabolic and Thermogenic Actions   How, after all, does thyroid hormone influence metabolism and thermogenesis? The most important answer is probably this: T_3 *stimulates increased mitochondrial* O_2 *consumption.* This is the definitive metabolic process by which aerobic cells extract energy from foodstuffs. The T_3 stimulation increases the rate of ATP synthesis and consumption. The increased churning of the oxidative phosphorylation machine results in more molecular motion, and hence more dissipation of energy as heat. T_3 increases mitochondrial O_2 consumption and the heat dissipation associated with it by a number of different direct mechanisms:

- T_3 increases the expression of mitochondrial proteins that enhance oxidative phosphorylation. It causes such expression by binding the nuclear receptor, TR, and perhaps by direct effects on mitochondrial DNA.

- Over a period of days, T_3 promotes mitochondriogenesis.

- T_3 may also render the mitochondrial membrane more permeable to protons. Recall that during oxidative phosphorylation, the electron transport chain concentrates protons in the intermembrane space of the mitochondrion. The proton gradient then causes protons to flow through the ATP synthetase, making ATP from ADP (FIGURE 33.9). By increasing the membrane's proton permeability, the process of making ATP becomes more inefficient. More molecular motion of protons (and more NADH) is needed to generate each molecule of ATP, and more energy is hence wasted as heat.

In addition, T_3 increases mitochondrial O_2 consumption through actions at a slightly farther remove from the mitochondrion itself:

- T_3 promotes an increased expression of the ubiquitous Na^+/K^+-ATPase. This is perhaps another form of fuel-burning to promote energy consumption and heat dissipation.

- T_3 promotes an early increase in lipogenesis, followed by lipolysis, which it promotes by inducing the expression of lipolytic enzymes. This provides fatty acids as substrate to the citric acid cycle and thus stimulates more energy release. (T_3 also increases LDL receptors in the liver, thus promoting decreases in plasma cholesterol, but this is thought to occur separately from T_3 stimulation of metabolism.)

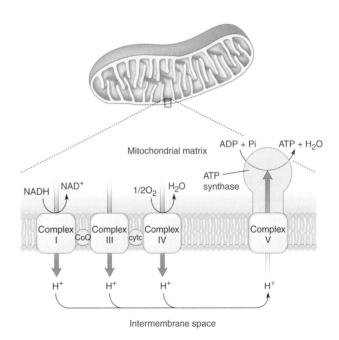

Figure 33.9   ATP synthesis in oxidative phosphorylation. A proton gradient from the intermembrane space to the mitochondrial matrix drives ATP synthesis.

• Finally, T_3 increases cardiac contractility and heart rate, which increases oxygen delivery to the tissues and burns large amounts of fuel in cardiac muscle cells. T_3 increases contractility and heart rate via several mechanisms. First, T_3 increases the expression of a myosin isoform with greater ATPase activity in the cardiac muscle cells, which increases the force and speed of contraction of the muscle fibers; and second, T_3 increases the expression and activity of the sarcoplasmic Ca^{2+} ATPase, which does the same. T_3 increases venous return to the heart by venoconstriction, which increases contractility by increasing preload (see Chapter 13). Finally, T_3 may potentiate sympathetic effects on the heart by increasing the expression of adrenergic beta receptors.

Influences on Growth and Development   While the mechanisms behind thyroidal involvement in growth and development are not completely understood, it is clear that thyroid hormone plays a major role. Deficiencies in thyroid hormone in fetal life or in infancy can retard neurologic development. Since T_3 does not appear to increase O_2 consumption in the brain, it is not known exactly how thyroid's effects are mediated in nervous tissue. Thyroid hormone promotes growth hormone synthesis in the pituitary, and data suggest that increased mitochondrial activity in general also contributes to development and cell differentiation. Normal levels of thyroid hormone are important for both male and female fertility.

PATHOPHYSIOLOGY: THYROID HORMONE EXCESS AND DEFICIENCY

The implications of **hyperthyroidism** (thyroid hormone excess) and **hypothyroidism** (thyroid hormone deficiency) follow logically from a knowledge of thyroid function. By promoting energy consumption in all tissues, thyroid hormone indirectly promotes all energy-requiring processes—which is to say that it adds impetus to all life processes. (Indeed, energy-requiring processes are definitive of life.) Thus, hyperthyroidism presents with signs and symptoms of hyperfunctioning in many organ systems, especially those tissues directly involved in energy metabolism. These findings may include weight loss, increased appetite, palpitations or racing heart, heat intolerance and sweating, nervousness, hyperdefecation, and muscle weakness. Symptomatic hyperthyroidism is called *thyrotoxicosis.* Infrequently, severe thyrotoxicosis leads to the sudden onset of *thyroid storm,* a life-threatening condition marked by very high fever. Hypothyroidism, by contrast, may present with

weight gain, low appetite, constipation, intolerance to cold, fatigue, depression, dry skin and hair, and heavy menstrual periods. In severe hypothyroidism, proteins and sugars may accumulate in the skin owing to sluggish metabolism, and they in turn may promote a form of superficial edema called *myxedema.*

Hyperthyroidism is most commonly caused by an autoimmune condition called **Graves' disease,** or a thyroxine-secreting tumor of the thyroid gland. In Graves' disease, antibodies to the TSH receptor stimulate the receptor in the same way that TSH itself does. This leads to an unregulated and constant overactivity of the thyroid gland. Under the influence of TSH-like stimulation, the thyroid gland hypertrophies, forming a protruding goiter. Because proteins in the extraocular muscles resemble the TSH receptor, the anti-TSH receptor antibodies also cause inflammation in the eye sockets, causing the eyes to protrude—a condition called *exophthalmos.* When the thyroid escapes pituitary control and secretes too much T_4, the pituitary thyrotrophs are suppressed and secrete less TSH. Hyperthyroidism is associated with a low TSH except in the circumstance of a TSH-secreting pituitary tumor. In that case, hyperthyroidism is accompanied by a high TSH level, and treatment would involve resection of the pituitary tumor.

Antithyroid drugs propylthiouracil (PTU) and methylmercaptoimidazole (MMI), also called methimazole, inhibit thyroid peroxidase. PTU also inhibits peripheral activation of T_4. Other treatments include administration of radioactive iodine to ablate the malfunctioning thyroid tissue, or surgery to remove the thyroid gland. Beta-adrenergic receptor blockers, such as propranolol, can help control symptoms, especially palpitations and tachycardia.

Hypothyroidism is most commonly caused by an autoimmune condition called **autoimmune thyroiditis**, also known as *Hashimoto's thyroiditis.* In this condition, antibodies to thyroglobulin or thyroid peroxidase interfere with thyroid hormone synthesis. Antibodies that attack the TSH receptor but do not stimulate it, as in Graves' disease, can also cause autoimmune thyroiditis. In this condition, thyroid hormone levels in the blood are low and the TSH level is high. Chronic stimulation of the thyroid tissue by TSH may lead to goiter. However, inflammation may fibrose the thyroid, keeping it small. (Technically, Hashimoto's refers to autoimmune thyroiditis with a goiter present.) Iodine deficiency, other forms of thyroiditis (e.g., viral), and drug side effects (lithium, amiodarone) may also cause hypothyroidism.

Hypothyroidism is treated with exogenous thyroxine, administered in the form of a daily pill. Dosages increase for hypothyroid mothers during pregnancy by 25% to 50%. However, whether the patient is pregnant or not, dosage is always titrated to normalize the plasma TSH level. The TSH is the most important lab test in the diagnosis and treatment of thyroid disease.

Summary

- Thyroid hormone stokes the biochemical furnaces of all cells to maintain body heat. Its other crucial role is in promoting normal growth and development from fetal life through childhood.

- Thyroxine (T_4) is the major circulating form of thyroid hormone, and triiodothyronine (T_3) is the active form.

- T_4 is made in thyroid follicles from tyrosine-containing thyroglobulin, I^-, H_2O_2, and thyroid peroxidase.

- T_4 is produced and secreted by the thyroid gland under the control of hypothalamic thyroid-releasing hormone (TRH) and pituitary thyroid-stimulating hormone (TSH) as part of the hypothalamic-pituitary-thyroid (HPT) axis. The HPT axis is governed by negative-feedback effects of T_4 on TRH and TSH-secreting cells.

- Thyroglobulin accumulation and iodine availability also limit T_4 production.

- T_4 is transported in the blood bound to thyroxine-binding globulin (TBG). It is converted to T_3 (activated) by deiodinases in the liver and in the tissues themselves, where thyroid hormone acts.

- T_3 binds an intracellular thyroid receptor (TR) that binds thyroid response elements (TREs). The TR-TRE complex binds nuclear DNA and alters its transcription. Complexes may also bind to mitochondrial DNA and surface receptors may mediate nongenomic effects of thyroid hormone.

- The primary action of T_3 is to stimulate increased mitochondrial O_2 consumption, which concomitantly increases heat dissipation.

- This metabolic/thermogenic effect is mediated by six mechanisms: increased expression of mitochondrial proteins, increased mitochondriogenesis, increased proton permeability in the inner mitochondrial membrane, increased expression of the Na^+/K^+-ATPase, increased lipogenesis and lipolysis, and increased cardiac contractility and heart rate.

- In fetal life, infancy, and childhood, thyroid hormone contributes to cell differentiation and neurologic development and facilitates the action of growth hormone.

- Hyperthyroidism is thyroid hormone excess. Hypothyroidism is thyroid hormone deficiency. Graves' disease and autoimmune thyroiditis are two common autoimmune conditions that cause hyperthyroidism and hypothyroidism, respectively.

- Hyperthyroidism is treated with medical and surgical methods of reducing thyroid activity. Hypothyroidism is treated with exogenous thyroxine.

- Measurement of the serum TSH level is the critical instrument of diagnosis and treatment of thyroid disorders.

Suggested Reading

Dillmann WH. Cellular action of thyroid hormone on the heart. Thyroid. 2002;12(6):447–452.

Dunn JT, Dunn AD. Update on intrathyroidal iodine metabolism. Thyroid. 2001;11(5):407–414.

Harvey CB, Williams GR. Mechanism of thyroid hormone action. Thyroid. 2002;12(6):441–446.

Köhrle J. Local activation and inactivation of thyroid hormones: the deiodinase family. Mol Cell Endocrinol. 1999;151(1-2):103–119.

Ladenson PW, et al. American Thyroid Association guidelines for detection of thyroid dysfunction. Arch Intern Med. 2000;160(11):1573–1575.

Silva JE. The thermogenic effect of thyroid hormone and its clinical implications. Ann Intern Med. 2003;139(3):205–213.

REVIEW QUESTIONS

Directions: Each of the numbered items or incomplete statements in this section is followed by answers or by completions of the statement. Select the ONE lettered answer or completion that is BEST in each case.

1. A woman has been taking 100 µg qd of levothyroxine for autoimmune thyroiditis for the past 4 years. During that time, her TSH has remained below 2.0 mU/L. She is now pregnant, and in the 11th week of pregnancy, she has an elevated TSH level of 7.5 mU/L (normal, 0.4 to 5.0 mU/L). A possible cause of her elevated TSH is the fact that:

   (A) Antibodies are stimulating her TSH receptors.
   (B) Her levothyroxine dose is too high.
   (C) Her thyroxine-binding globulin (TBG) levels are increased.

(D) High human chorionic gonadotropin (hCG) levels are mimicking TSH action.

(E) The placenta is producing TSH.

(F) The fetus's pituitary gland is producing TSH.

(G) The fetus's thyroid gland is producing T_4.

(H) She has a toxic thyroid adenoma.

2. A 10-year-old child with congenital hypothyroidism might be expected to exhibit which of the following signs?

(A) Tall stature, cachexia, and low IQ

(B) Short stature, a potbelly, and low IQ

(C) Tall stature, cachexia, and high IQ

(D) Tall stature, a potbelly, and low IQ
(E) Short stature, cachexia, and low IQ

3. Propylthiouracil interferes with more than one process essential to normal thyroid function, but methimazole interferes with just one. Which is it?

(A) Thyroid hormone synthesis
(B) Thyroid hormone transport
(C) Conversion of T_4 to T_3
(D) Binding of T_3 to thyroid receptor
(E) T_3 stimulation of mitochondrial O_2 consumption

ANSWERS TO REVIEW QUESTIONS

1. **The answer is C.** TBG levels increase in pregnancy because placental estrogen stimulates hepatic TBG production and decreased hepatic clearance of TBG. TBG soaks up T_4, transiently decreasing the level of free T_4, lifting negative feedback on the pituitary, and yielding increased TSH secretion. Because the woman cannot increase her endogenous T_4 production in response to the high TSH level, her TSH level remains elevated. All the other possible causes listed, aside from (E) and (F), are states of high T_4 and hence low TSH. TSH receptor-stimulating antibodies are found in autoimmune thyroid disease, but they are present in Graves' disease, not autoimmune thyroiditis, and Graves' antibodies cause high T_4 and low TSH levels. Serum hCG is thought to mimic TSH action during pregnancy, but again this would increase T_4 and depress TSH. (E) and (F) are not true causes of high maternal TSH.

2. **The answer is B.** Sustained thyroid deficiency from birth impairs growth hormone secretion (short stature), lipolysis in adipose tissues (leading to fat accumulation and potbelly), and neurologic development (low IQ).

3. **The answer is A.** Both propylthiouracil and methimazole inhibit thyroid peroxidase inside thyroid follicles, preventing normal iodination and coupling of thyroid hormone precursors. Propylthiouracil also interferes with deiodination of T_4 to T_3.

34

The Adrenal Gland

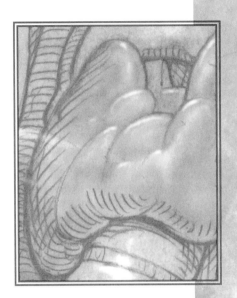

INTRODUCTION

The **adrenal gland** plays a pivotal role in human endocrine physiology. Although considered one gland anatomically, the adrenal gland functions as two distinct entities: the cortex and the medulla. These two portions of the adrenal originate from different embryonic tissues and have distinctly different physiologic roles.

The outermost shell of the adrenal gland, the **adrenal cortex**, produces three kinds of steroid hormones: aldosterone, cortisol, and androgens. **Aldosterone**, a mineralocorticoid, modulates electrolyte and fluid balance by stimulating sodium retention in the kidney's collecting ducts. **Cortisol**, a glucocorticoid, plays a crucial role in the body's stress response, in the regulation of protein, glucose, and fat metabolism, in the maintenance of vascular tone, and in the modulation of inflammation. The adrenal **androgens** are most important during fetal life as a substrate for placental estrogen production, but they play a minor role during adult life. The **adrenal medulla** is the inner core of the adrenal gland; it produces the catecholamines **epinephrine** and **norepinephrine**, which are also important components of the stress response.

Adrenal function is essential to human life. Adrenalectomy will lead to cardiovascular collapse and death within a few days from a lack of cortisol, which maintains blood vessel tone and blood pressure.

SYSTEM STRUCTURE: ADRENAL ANATOMY AND EMBRYOLOGY

The adrenals are triangular retroperitoneal organs located at the superior poles of the kidneys, lateral to the 11th thoracic and 1st lumbar vertebrae. These glands receive blood from the superior adrenal artery, a branch of the inferior phrenic; the middle adrenal artery, a branch of the aorta; and the inferior adrenal artery, a branch of the renal artery (FIGURE 34.1). This rich blood supply from three distinct locations explains why the adrenals are a frequent site of metastases from distant primary cancers. More importantly, the rich blood supply ensures the adrenals access to the bloodstream to facilitate hormonal secretion. The adrenal arteries anastomose (network) into a subcapsular plexus, which in turn branches into arteries that flow inward. Some of these arteries form capillary networks in the cortex and some form capillary networks in the medulla (FIGURE 34.2). The left adrenal vein drains into the left renal vein, while the right adrenal vein drains directly into the inferior vena cava (IVC). This drainage is analogous to the

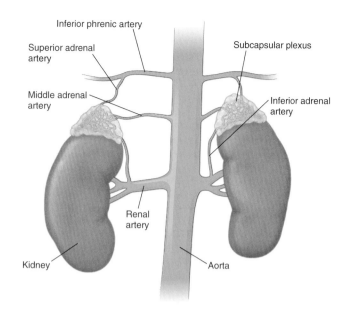

Figure 34.1   Arterial supply to the adrenal glands. The adrenal arteries are not drawn to scale, nor drawn in their exact anatomic locations.

testicular and ovarian veins. The left testicular/ovarian vein drains into the left renal vein, while the right testicular/ovarian drains right into the IVC.

The medulla and cortex of the adrenal glands are separate in structure, function, and embryologic origin. The cortex arises from the mesoderm, while the medulla derives from the ectoderm. The mesodermal gonadal ridge gives rise to the steroidogenic cells of the ovaries and testes as well as the adrenal cortex precursor cells, which migrate to the retroperitoneum. These mesodermal cortical cells are invaded by migrating ectodermal neural crest cells, which will become the medulla. Encapsulation of the adrenal gland around week 8 of fetal life creates a unified organ out of these two originally separate entities.

SYSTEM FUNCTION: THE ADRENAL CORTEX

The adrenal cortex makes up 80% to 90% of the adrenal gland by volume and comprises three histologically and functionally distinct zones, each of which makes a different steroid (FIGURE 34.3). Starting from the outermost, these layers are the **zona glomerulosa,** which produces aldosterone; the **zona fasciculata,** which produces cortisol; and the **zona reticularis,** which produces adrenal androgens, primarily DHEA (dehydroepiandrosterone) and androstenedione. (Some cortisol is produced in the zona reticularis.)

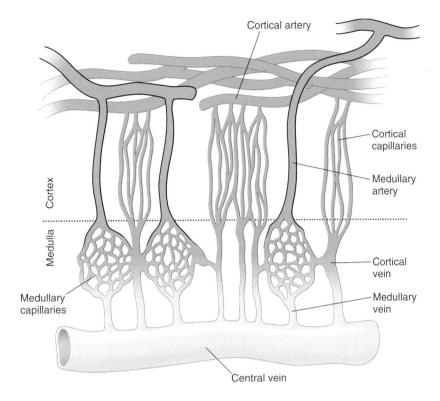

Figure 34.2   Vasculature inside the adrenal glands. The subcapsular plexus gives rise to arteries that form medullary capillary beds and to arteries that form cortical capillary beds.

CRH and ACTH

Production of the steroids in the adrenal cortex is regulated by the **hypothalamic-pituitary-adrenal (HPA) axis** (FIGURE 34.4). At the top of the HPA axis, the hypothalamus releases **corticotropin-releasing hormone (CRH)**, which stimulates the anterior pituitary to release *pro-opiomelanocortin*, a precursor molecule that is cleaved into four main products: *melanocyte-stimulating hormone, beta-lipotropins, beta-endorphins*, and **adrenocorticotropic hormone (ACTH)**. ACTH, also known as corticotropin, is released into the bloodstream and acts in the cortex, stimulating the synthesis and release of over 50

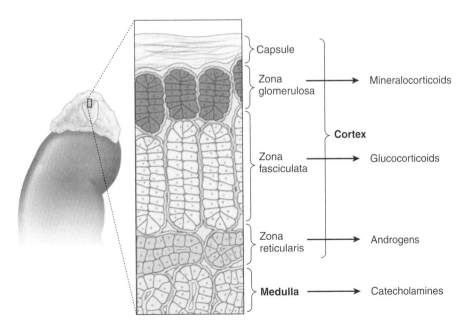

Figure 34.3   Adrenal zonation.

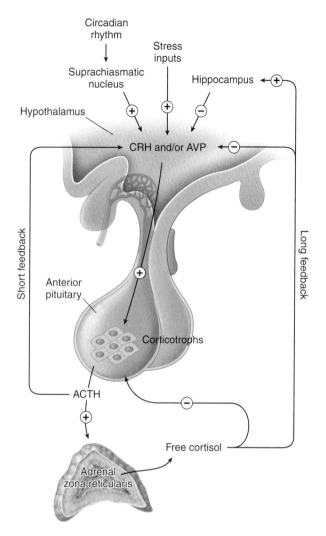

Figure 34.4 Hypothalamic-pituitary-adrenal axis. Stress, circadian rhythms, and negative feedback from cortisol all influence the paraventricular nucleus of the hypothalamus and modulate CRH output. Stressors may be organic in nature (such as hypoglycemia or infection) or psychological.

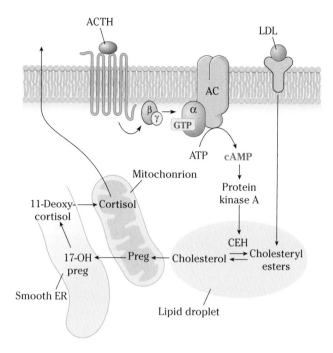

Figure 34.5 Action of ACTH on the adrenal cortex. AC, adenylyl cyclase; CEH, cholesteryl ester hydrolase; G, G protein (linking the receptor to the adenylyl cyclase); LDL, low-density lipoprotein; Preg, pregnenolone (cortisol precursor); R, ACTH receptor; Smooth ER, smooth endoplasmic reticulum.

steroid products, the most important of which are cortisol, the adrenal androgens, and aldosterone, although aldosterone is largely regulated in direct response to serum potassium levels and by *angiotensin II*, a hormone that helps to regulate blood pressure. In a classic endocrine feedback loop, cortisol directly inhibits both CRH production at the hypothalamic level and ACTH at the pituitary level, thereby acting as the main control mechanism for all adrenal cortical hormone production, with the exception of aldosterone.

The cortex responds dramatically to stimulation from ACTH, which elevates steroid production within minutes. It does so by activating a receptor on the cortical cell membranes that is linked to a G protein (FIGURE 34.5). The G protein, in turn, activates adenylyl cyclase and raises the cAMP level, activating a protein kinase. The kinase phosphorylates and hence

activates the enzyme **cholesteryl ester hydrolase (CEH)**, which promotes the conversion of cholesteryl esters into free cholesterol. The free cholesterol then supplies the steroid synthesis pathways, as described below. Chronic stimulation with excessive ACTH causes bilateral adrenal hypertrophy, while removal or destruction of the pituitary, which is responsible for producing ACTH, conversely leads to adrenal atrophy.

Cortical Hormones: Their Actions and Regulation

As steroids, the cortical hormones all share certain functional features. They are all secreted into the adrenal blood vessels and circulate from the adrenal veins to target tissues all over the body. At the target tissues, they dissolve into the lipid membranes of the tissues and pass into the intracellular cytosol. There, the steroids bind cytosolic receptor proteins, which in turn bind to particular DNA sequences, thereby initiating the transcription of mRNA, resulting in the synthesis of new proteins.

As mentioned above and described in more detail below, the secretion of steroid hormones from the cortex is regulated by various kinds of negative-feedback loops. TABLE 34.1 summarizes the actions of the cortical steroids.

Table 34.1 ACTIONS OF THE CORTICAL STEROIDS

Adrenal Hormone	Main Actions
Aldosterone	• Increases salt and water reabsorption from kidney tubules • Increases K^+ secretion in kidneys
Cortisol	• Counterregulatory effects: increases blood sugar, increases catabolism of triglyceride and protein • Anti-inflammatory/immunosuppressant effects • Maintains blood vessel tone and hence blood pressure
Androgens	• Help determine male sex characteristics during fetal development and puberty

Aldosterone Action Aldosterone plays a key role in the regulation of fluid balance by enhancing the ability of kidney tubules to absorb salt and water in two ways. First, aldosterone directly stimulates the production and activity of Na^+/K^+-ATPase pumps located in the basolateral side of the cortical collecting ducts. These pumps exchange sodium for potassium, and aldosterone stimulation of these pumps leads to increased sodium reabsorption in exchange for potassium excretion. Remember that increased reabsorption of sodium leads to passive water reabsorption and increased extracellular fluid volume (see Chapter 22).

Second, aldosterone increases salt and water reabsorption in the kidney by creating more apical Na^+ channels, directly increasing sodium permeability on the luminal side of the cortical collecting ducts. Aldosterone also drives K^+ secretion through its effects on the translocation of Na^+. Increased Na^+ reabsorption creates tubular electronegativity and drives paracellular K^+ secretion (see Chapter 24).

Finally, aldosterone acts on the H^+-ATPase in the renal tubule and has other effects on acid-base balance (see Chapter 25). Because it acts on the levels of these inorganic (mineral) electrolytes, it is termed a **mineralocorticoid.**

Aldosterone Regulation Aldosterone regulation is unique in that it is the only adrenal cortical hormone that is secreted largely independently of ACTH. A small amount of ACTH from the pituitary is required for aldosterone release, but aldosterone is regulated mainly by two other control mechanisms: the serum potassium level and the renin-angiotensin-aldosterone (RAA) system. Elevated potassium levels trigger aldosterone secretion, which in turn stimulates renal potassium excretion via the Na^+/K^+ exchange pump to rectify the hyperkalemia. Low blood pressure stimulates the adrenal to secrete aldosterone through the RAA system. This increases salt reabsorption and raises the extracellular fluid volume and blood pressure.

Cortisol Action Cortisol has a multitude of actions, and derivatives of this hormone are used frequently in medical therapy. Cortisol is consequently one of the most challenging adrenal hormones to understand and at the same time one of the most clinically relevant. Cortisol is produced mostly by the fasciculata, with some production in the reticularis. Although mainly exerting glucocorticoid activity (explained below), cortisol also functions as a weak mineralocorticoid, with effects similar to those of aldosterone. Cortisol's precursor, **corticosterone,** also exhibits some glucocorticoid activity. About 20 to 30 mg of cortisol is secreted per day by the adrenals, with 90% to 95% of circulating cortisol bound in the plasma to *cortisol-binding globulin.*

Glucocorticoid action can be thought of mainly in two broad categories: metabolic and anti-inflammatory. Although the myriad metabolic actions of cortisol can be daunting, it is useful to remember that cortisol acts to prepare the body for stress. Teleologically speaking, in times of stress the body does not have the energy surplus to build protein or add to triglyceride and glycogen stores; instead it requires rapidly usable energy for the brain in the form of glucose. Therefore, the body under stress will mobilize amino acids and fatty acids as substrates for gluconeogenesis (see Chapter 31). Under glucocorticoid influence, an increase in all gluconeogenic enzymes raises hepatic gluconeogenesis sixfold. Blood sugar levels climb, while peripheral uptake and utilization of glucose are decreased. To fuel this upregulated gluconeogenic activity, cortisol increases the production of amino acids from muscle breakdown. Synthesis of protein and fat is halted, as the main focus is on survival and the mobilization of stores (catabolism) rather than on growth and repair (anabolism).

This bolus of glucose is liberated from tissue energy stores instead of from the diet. Thus, glucocorticoids are *counterregulatory hormones,* alongside glucagon, epinephrine, and growth hormone. Glucocorticoids reproduce glucagon action and oppose insulin action. However, glucocorticoids do not

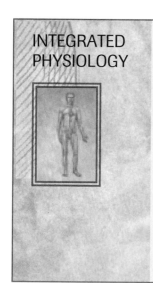

The Insulin/Counterregulatory Balance

The stress response induced by cortisol is intended to be only temporary. If exposure to cortisol is prolonged, as in long-term treatment with *prednisone* (a glucocorticoid administered as medicine), the body suffers deleterious effects. A constant elevation of cortisol levels disrupts the normal balance between insulin and cortisol, leaving the body in a prolonged state of catabolism, which can be very destructive.

In *Cushing's disease*, excess ACTH production leads to an abnormal elevation of cortisol and disruption of the metabolic balance. Skin striae, skin thinning, and muscle weakness ensue from excessive protein and collagen breakdown due to cortisol action. In *diabetes mellitus*, low insulin production disrupts the balance between cortisol and insulin. When diabetics experience physical stress such as illness or infection, cortisol levels increase and blood sugar levels increase, and therefore their insulin requirement goes up.

---

promote glycogen breakdown as does glucagon. This phenomenon is known as glucocorticoid's *glycostatic effect*. (See Integrated Physiology Box *The Insulin/Counterregulatory Balance.*)

Cortisol also has powerful effects on the immune system, which accounts for the widespread use of glucocorticoids as anti-inflammatories and as immunosuppressants. Cortisol reduces the inflammatory response by both blocking the early stages of inflammation and speeding up the resolution of inflammation. Inflammation is decreased in a number of specific ways:

- Stabilization of white cell granules, which release proteolytic enzymes during inflammation

- Decreased capillary permeability (which decreases edema)

- Decreased production of prostaglandins and leukotrienes, both of which are powerful stimuli of inflammation

- Decreased leukocyte migration

- Decreased interleukin-1 (IL-1) and IL-6 release

- Direct suppression of T cells

- Decreased production of lymphocytes and antibodies

Because of the powerful immunosuppressant effects of cortisol, patients taking glucocorticoids for prolonged periods should be considered immunocompromised and at an increased risk for infections.

Cortisol is also a powerful modulator of the allergic response, acting to decrease eosinophil production, increase eosinophil apoptosis, and limit the inflammation that can be deadly in anaphylaxis. Interestingly, cortisol increases red blood cell production in an unknown manner. Finally, cortisol acts to maintain blood pressure by potentiating catecholamines and by directly supporting blood vessel tone.

Cortisol Regulation   Cortisol is regulated by the HPA axis, as mentioned above. The median eminence of the hypothalamus is responsible for the production of CRH, which is produced in response to a host of stressful stimuli: trauma, infection, catecholamines, surgery, and so on. How the hypothalamus detects these stimuli has not been completely worked out. CRH is also released in a circadian manner, leading to a diurnal variation with cortisol levels peaking in the early morning. CRH triggers ACTH release from the anterior pituitary. ACTH is also modulated by **antidiuretic hormone (ADH)**, which acts synergistically with CRH to stimulate ACTH release. Cortisol is almost exclusively regulated by ACTH, which activates cholesteryl ester hydrolase (CEH) and ultimately increases the production of *pregnenolone*, a cortisol precursor. Cortisol inhibits CRH and ACTH in a classic negative-feedback loop.

The Androgens   The adrenal androgens, like the gonadal androgens, are male sex hormones—that is, they help determine and maintain male sex characteristics. The principal adrenal androgens are **androstenedione, dehydroepiandrosterone (DHEA)**, and **DHEA-S**. These hormones have a negligible effect on adult physiology compared to the gonadally produced hormones (such as *testosterone*), which account for the majority of sex hormone effects. They are about one fifth as potent as testosterone. Androstenedione can be converted to testosterone, which is in turn converted to *dihydrotestosterone (DHT)* and *estradiol* in extra-adrenal tissues. These androgens are most important during fetal development and puberty.

In the fetus, the adrenal glands are much larger proportionally than in the adult, and a layer known as the provisional or fetal cortex exists, which is analogous to the adult reticularis. This layer produces DHEA-S, which is converted by the placenta into androgens and estrogens. Overproduction of DHEA-S, as in congenital adrenal hyperplasia (discussed below), can lead to fetal virilization in female infants.

Adrenal androgens are also important during adolescence, when they stimulate the development of pubic and axillary hair in women, which is know as *adrenarche*. Adrenarche and puberty normally coincide, but they are actually two physiologically separate events. Androgen production continues into adulthood and declines with age. Androgens continue to cause groin and axillary hair growth in adult women. Many claims have been made about DHEA as a "youth hormone," but at this point, there is little scientific evidence for the efficacy of DHEA replacement as a fountain of youth.

Steroid Biosynthesis

All the products of the adrenal cortex are steroid hormones, which have a standard four-ring structure and are produced by a similar biosynthetic pathway. Enzymes specific to each layer of the cortex influence the structural differences of the hormones produced. Cholesterol provides the basic four-ring steroid framework. Although the adrenals can synthesize cholesterol de novo from acetyl CoA, 80% of the cholesterol used in adrenal hormone synthesis comes from dietary cholesterol packaged as cholesteryl ester in circulating low-density lipoprotein (LDL) particles. CEH converts the esters to free cholesterol in response to ACTH. The rate-limiting step in hormone biosynthesis is the transfer of cholesterol to the inner mitochondrial membrane of adrenal cells via the *steroidogenic acute regulatory protein (StAR)*, followed by the conversion of cholesterol to pregnenolone. This reaction is catalyzed by the enzyme *desmolase*.

Once pregnenolone is made from cholesterol, the pregnenolone flows downhill through each zone of the cortex, undergoing successive modifications to the basic steroid ring. These modifications result in a distribution of various steroid products throughout the adrenal cortex (FIGURE 34.6). The steroids are released immediately after synthesis; very little of the cortical hormones are stored. This is in direct contrast to the medulla, which packages and stores its products for release under stimulus at a later time.

Some enzymes in the steroid biosynthetic pathways are common to all three zones, while others are unique to a specific adrenal zone. Pregnenolone flows across zones and also undergoes progressive transformation along each zone's unique enzymatic

pathway unless an enzyme deficiency in one pathway acts as a roadblock. Such a condition prevents further modification of the steroid product, leading to an excess of premodification substrate that will spill over into the remaining open routes. An example of this hormonal roadblock is found in the pathologic condition **congenital adrenal hyperplasia (CAH)**. (See Clinical Application Box *What Is Congenital Adrenal Hyperplasia?*)

PATHOPHYSIOLOGY: DISEASES OF CORTICAL OVER- AND UNDERPRODUCTION

Levels of cortisol and aldosterone normally vary in response to changing conditions in the body. During stress, cortisol levels rise. When blood pressure is low, aldosterone levels rise. Pathologic conditions, however, may interfere with the adrenal cortex's normal response to stimuli. These conditions are classified as those that cause the overproduction of a hormone and those that cause underproduction. In cases of overproduction, the hormone is secreted at levels out of proportion to adrenal stimuli. In cases of underproduction, the adrenal cortex cannot mount the normal response to stimuli.

Diseases of Overproduction

Diseases of overproduction may be primary to the adrenal gland, or they may originate outside the adrenal (in which case hyperproduction is called secondary). For example, ACTH overproduction in the pituitary can stimulate a perfectly normal adrenal gland to overproduce cortisol. Chronic stimulation of the RAA system due to renal disease can cause a normal adrenal to overproduce aldosterone. Isolated overproduction of androgens is much less common and usually arises from CAH and less commonly from adrenal carcinomas or adenomas.

Hypercortisolism Excess glucocorticoid exposure, called **hypercortisolism**, can lead to a variety of disease manifestations and is one of the most serious adrenal derangements. Excess glucocorticoids may be the result of endogenous overproduction or exogenous administration of glucocorticoid drugs in higher-than-normal amounts. Endogenous cortisol overproduction can be classified into two categories: ACTH-dependent and ACTH-independent. *ACTH-dependent* causes account for 85% of endogenous hypercortisolism and include Cushing's disease (also known as pituitary adenoma), ectopic ACTH production (as occurs with some lung cancers), and ectopic CRH production, which is rare. *ACTH-independent* causes are primary to the adrenal gland. They include adrenal adenoma and adrenocortical carcinoma. Exogenous glucocorti-

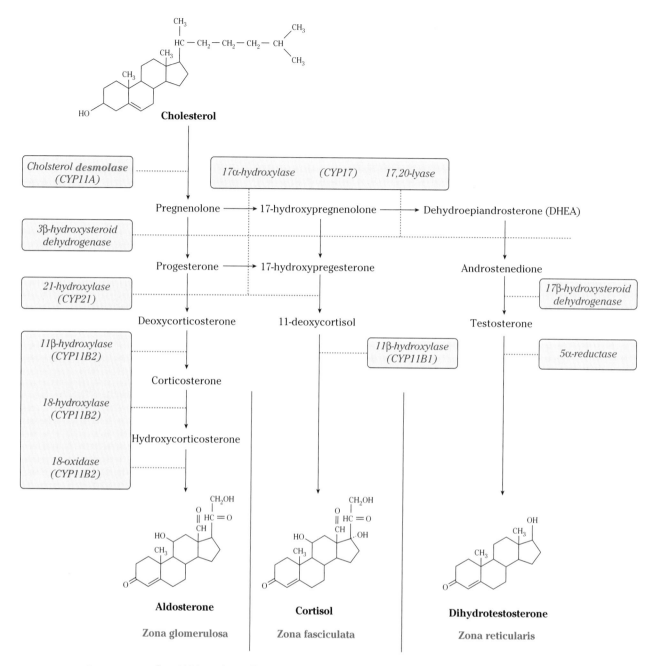

Figure 34.6 Steroid biosynthesis. The line next to 21-hydroxylase is highlighted to indicate the barrier to aldosterone and cortisol synthesis posed by 21-hydroxylase deficiency. Such a barrier causes progesterone and 17-hydroxyprogesterone to build up, which decreases the rate of conversion of pregnenolone to progesterone and of 17-hydroxypregnenolone to 17-hydroxyprogesterone. In turn, pregnenolone and 17-hydroxypregnenolone build up and drive increased DHEA formation.

coids—drug preparations like prednisone or large quantities of steroid inhalers—can also lead to hypercortisolism. Rarely, hypercortisolism is caused by excess secretion of CRH from the hypothalamus.

Hypercortisolism due to any cause yields a constellation of clinical findings known as **Cushing syndrome** (as opposed to Cushing's disease, which is one of many causes of Cushing syndrome). The signs and symptoms of cortisol excess, first described by

Harvey Cushing in 1932, include truncal obesity, a round and full face ("moon facies"), a "buffalo hump" of fat on the posterior neck, pigmented skin striae, thinned skin and easy bruising, muscle weakness, osteoporosis, hypertension, and hyperglycemia. The catabolic effects of cortisol cause muscle weakness, osteoporosis, striae, bruising, and hyperglycemia. The abnormal fat distribution is believed to be due to increased lipolysis, which affects the extremities more than the trunk, but a clear explanation for the moon facies and buffalo hump has yet to be found. Virilizing symptoms of hirsutism and acne can accompany ACTH-dependent hypercortisolism as a result of androgen overproduction from excessive ACTH. Hyperpigmentation is also seen with elevated ACTH levels and is believed to be caused by ACTH cross-reacting with melanocyte-stimulating hormone (MSH) receptors on melanin-producing cells. (See Clinical Application Box *Diagnosing Cushing Syndrome with Lab Tests.*)

Hyperaldosteronism   As with hypercortisolism, **hyperaldosteronism** can be classified into two categories: primary (arising from the adrenal) and secondary (extra-adrenal). *Primary hyperaldosteronism*, known as *Conn's syndrome*, arises most often from an aldosterone-producing adrenal adenoma. Hypokalemia, hypernatremia, diastolic hypertension, polyuria, and muscle weakness (secondary to low potassium levels) are characteristics of hyperaldosteronism. Plasma renin levels are low owing to the negative feedback from elevated aldosterone levels.

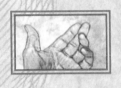

CLINICAL APPLICATION

WHAT IS CONGENITAL ADRENAL HYPERPLASIA?

A newborn girl in the hospital nursery is discovered to have abnormal findings on examination of her genitals. She has an enlarged clitoris and a single urogenital sinus instead of separate openings for the vagina and urethra. She also has low blood pressure and a high plasma K^+ level. With a putative diagnosis of congenital adrenal hyperplasia, the infant receives hydrocortisone and fludrocortisone (a medicinal mineralocorticoid) and is placed on daily salt supplements. The family is referred to a surgeon and a psychiatrist for consultation.

Patients with **congenital adrenal hyperplasia (CAH)** have a genetic deficiency of *21-hydroxylase*, an enzyme that transforms progesterone to corticosterone in the glomerulosa and transforms *17-hydroxyprogesterone* to cortisol in the fasciculata. When this enzyme is absent, the aldosterone and cortisol precursors encounter a "block" and accumulate. Encountering this backup, progesterone and 17-hydroxy progesterone can overflow into the androgen biosynthetic pathway, where they are converted by *17, 20-lyase* into DHEA and androstenedione, creating a surplus of androgenizing hormones (and a deficiency of aldosterone and cortisol, which cannot be made without 21-hydroxylase). Because of the lack of cortisol, which normally provides negative feedback to the brain, the hypothalamus and pituitary continue to churn out CRH and ACTH to make up for the cortisol deficit, leading to adrenal hypertrophy and even more pregnenolone production.

Excess pregnenolone in the context of 21-hydroxylase deficiency results in more DHEA production. Normally, DHEA has only a minor effect on females, as a stimulus for pubic and axillary hair growth and as a substrate for testosterone production. However, in female fetuses undergoing sexual differentiation, large amounts of DHEA result in clinically significant levels of testosterone, which in turn can lead to virilized external genitalia. At birth, female infants with CAH may be mistaken for male or may have what is known as *ambiguous genitalia*. Male infants with CAH initially may go undiagnosed as they do not have ambiguous genitalia. (They are exposed to virilizing testosterone in utero as part of normal genital development.)

A lack of cortisol and aldosterone can be disastrous for both male and female infants. Aldosterone deficiency in many cases leads to a *salt-wasting crisis* with profound hyponatremia, hyperkalemia, hypotension, and acidosis. Lack of cortisol impairs carbohydrate metabolism and can lead to death from loss of blood vessel tone and blood pressure normally maintained by cortisol.

Glucocorticoid administration makes up for cortisol deficiency and suppresses ACTH, thereby decreasing excess pregnenolone and hence androgen production. Mineralocorticoid and salt administration counteract the salt wasting due to aldosterone deficiency, which is present in the majority of cases. Now that the genetic basis of CAH has been clearly elucidated, prenatal diagnosis and even treatment are possible.

CLINICAL APPLICATION

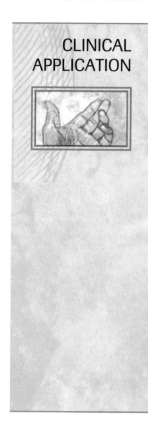

DIAGNOSING CUSHING SYNDROME WITH LAB TESTS

Several tests are available to help diagnose **Cushing syndrome**, each with varying degrees of sensitivity and specificity. The first and most direct test is measurement of the plasma cortisol level, which is done at night. Normally, circadian rhythms dictate a drop in cortisol secretion during the night. However, because night-time depression in cortisol levels does not occur to the same extent in patients with Cushing syndrome, their late-night plasma cortisol levels may be elevated. A salivary cortisol test has also been recently introduced to assess night-time cortisol secretion. In addition, because increased plasma cortisol leads to increased renal cortisol filtration and excretion, Cushing syndrome can be detected with a 24-hour collection of urine-free cortisol.

The *dexamethasone-suppression test* is used to detect ACTH-dependent causes of Cushing syndrome. The test entails the administration of dexamethasone, followed by measurement of ACTH levels. Dexamethasone is a glucocorticoid and normally suppresses ACTH secretion just as cortisol does. However, ACTH-secreting pituitary adenomas or ectopic sources of ACTH do not respond to negative feedback normally but continue to secrete ACTH even in the presence of increased cortisol levels. (This, indeed, is the pathologic reason for the hypercortisolism in the first place.) Therefore, a failure to suppress the ACTH level upon dexamethasone-suppression testing is indicative of an ACTH-dependent cause of hypercortisolism. Imaging studies can then help locate the tumor that might be secreting ACTH. The sensitivity and specificity of this test, however, are not ideal.

Diagnosis is made by demonstrating a failure to suppress aldosterone production after intravenous saline loading.

The hypertension seen in primary hyperaldosteronism is typically mild, due in part to the phenomenon of *aldosterone escape* (also called mineralocorticoid escape). Because primary hyperaldosteronism affects only one of several renal modes of control over the extracellular fluid volume, the kidney can compensate through its other modes of volume control. The unregulated aldosterone secretion increases salt reabsorption in the distal tubule, leading to increased water reabsorption and increased fluid volume; however, other renal mechanisms respond to the increase in circulatory volume and pressure by reducing salt reabsorption and promoting diuresis. Decreased expression of distal NaCl cotransporters may also contribute to aldosterone escape.

Secondary hyperaldosteronism results from activation of the RAA system via a primary overproduction of renin or a primary kidney disorder involving decreased renal perfusion, such as renal artery stenosis.

Diseases of Underproduction

In 1849, Thomas Addison described the classic features of *adrenal insufficiency*. Six years later he summarized those features: "The leading and characteristic features of the morbid state to which I would direct attention, are, anaemia, general languor and debility, remarkable feebleness of the heart's action, irritability of the stomach, and a peculiar change of colour in the skin, occurring in connexion with a diseased condition of the supra-renal capsules (*On the constitutional and local effects of disease of the suprarenal capsules*, 1855).

Like hyperaldosteronism, adrenal insufficiency can be categorized as primary (disease originating in the adrenal gland) and secondary (disease originating outside the adrenal). **Primary adrenal insufficiency**, or *Addison's disease*, is characterized typically by both aldosterone and cortisol deficiency. It is caused by adrenal cortex destruction, most often owing to *autoimmune adrenalitis* mediated by lymphocytic attack, but also arising from a host of other causes. Adrenal hemorrhage, tuberculosis, cytomegalovirus (CMV) infection, certain medications, metastases, HIV infection, and rare familial disorders such as adrenal leukodystrophy may all cause destruction of the adrenal cortex. (The medulla is generally spared.)

One case of primary adrenal insufficiency *not* caused by cortical destruction is a genetic deficiency of synthetic enzymes—most commonly deficiency of 21 hydroxylase, as seen in CAH. CAH can lead to an underproduction of cortisol and aldosterone, with concurrent overproduction of adrenal androgens.

Because primary adrenal insufficiency is most commonly caused by destruction of the entire adrenal cortex, glucocorticoid, mineralocorticoid, and androgen production can all be affected at once. Cortisol deficiency leads to fatigue, weakness, anorexia, weight loss, hypotension, and hypoglycemia. If aldosterone is deficient, hyperkalemia and salt craving may be present as well. Because androgens have little effect on adults, symptoms of androgen deficiency are limited to decreased hair growth in women. The lack of cortisol feedback on the pituitary leads to increased ACTH production, which can be detected serologically or upon dermatologic examination, which reveals ACTH-related hyperpigmentation. *Cortrosyn*, an ACTH analog, can also be used to challenge the adrenals and test for primary adrenal insufficiency.

Primary adrenal insufficiency may present initially as an acute *Addisonian crisis*. This occurs when a patient with underlying undiagnosed adrenal disease encounters a stressor such as surgery or infection and cannot mount an appropriate cortisol response. The crisis is characterized by anorexia, nausea, vomiting, abdominal pain, hyponatremia, and hyperkalemia. Addisonian crises can be fatal if not rapidly treated with cortisol replacement, fluids, and glucose.

Secondary adrenal insufficiency arises from pituitary ACTH deficiency and usually results in a lack of cortisol only, as aldosterone production does not rely on ACTH. There are two main causes of ACTH deficiency. The less common cause is pituitary damage resulting from necrosis, nonfunctioning adenoma, or head trauma. The more common cause is the suppression of a pituitary production of ACTH owing to long-term use of exogenous glucocorticoids, which exert negative feedback on the pituitary. When a patient is treated with steroids, it can take some time for the pituitary to recover fully after the steroids have been stopped. Patients on high-dose or chronic steroids should always be tapered off the drugs to allow for adequate recovery of pituitary function. Similarly, patients taking glucocorticoids chronically, which causes suppression of their HPA axes, may often require "stress-dose steroids"—an increased amount of exogenous corticosteroids when undergoing surgery, trauma, or major illness—to mimic the physiologic response to stress. Such patients require stress-dose steroids because the normal pituitary response has been suppressed and they cannot provide themselves with the physiologic boost in steroid secretion.

SYSTEM FUNCTION: THE ADRENAL MEDULLA

At the core of the adrenal glands are the adrenal medullae, which are part of the sympathetic nervous system and are responsible for the production of catecholamines, epinephrine and norepinephrine. Catecholamines are essential modulators of the rapid response to stress, triggering a variety of fight-or-flight responses, including increased heart rate, elevated cardiac output, and increased blood glucose levels. The parenchymal cells of the medulla, known as **chromaffin cells**, are derived from neural crest cells, as are postganglionic sympathetic neurons, which share a similar structure and function. Like postganglionic sympathetic neurons, the medulla is innervated by cholinergic preganglionic sympathetic neurons. Chromaffin cells are widely distributed throughout the body during fetal life, but the majority degenerate after birth, leaving the adrenal medulla as the main locus of chromaffin cells. However, extra-adrenal chromaffin cells may persist in adult life, especially adjacent to the abdominal aorta, in clusters know as *paraganglia*.

In contrast to adrenal cortical cells, which do not store their products, medullary cells are full of secretory granules, which are storehouses for catecholamines, ATP, opiate-like enkephalins, and proteins called *chromogranins*, which bind to catecholamines. It is believed that two separate types of medullary cells exist, epinephrine-producing and norepinephrine-producing cells. About 80% of the medulla's output is epinephrine.

The Synthesis, Storage, and Release of Catecholamines

Catecholamines are amines with a phenyl ring; they include *dopamine*, *norepinephrine*, and *epinephrine* (FIGURE 34.7). Just as cholesterol is the common precursor of adrenal cortical hormones, tyrosine is the precursor for catechol synthesis. Tyrosine comes from the diet, or it can be synthesized from phenylalanine. Catecholamines are produced in both peripheral and central neural tissues.

Tyrosine hydroxylase is the rate-limiting enzyme and catalyzes the production of dihydroxyphenylalanine (DOPA) from tyrosine. Acetylcholine (ACh), the preganglionic sympathetic neurotransmitter, stimulates both tyrosine hydroxylase activity and synthesis. DOPA is converted to dopamine and then to norepinephrine (NE). At this point, catechol synthesis is cytosolic. NE is then taken up into granules by an ATP-driven monoamine transport or is converted to epinephrine in the cytosol by phenylethanolamine-*N*-methyltransferase (PNMT) and packaged into secretory granules. Both NE and epinephrine are stored in granules until release is triggered. The adrenal medulla is the main producer of epinephrine in the body, while adrenergic axons make mostly NE. The CNS makes dopamine, norepinephrine, and small amounts of epinephrine.

The release of secretory granules occurs by exocytosis of the entire granule contents directly into the extracellular space and circulatory system. ACh

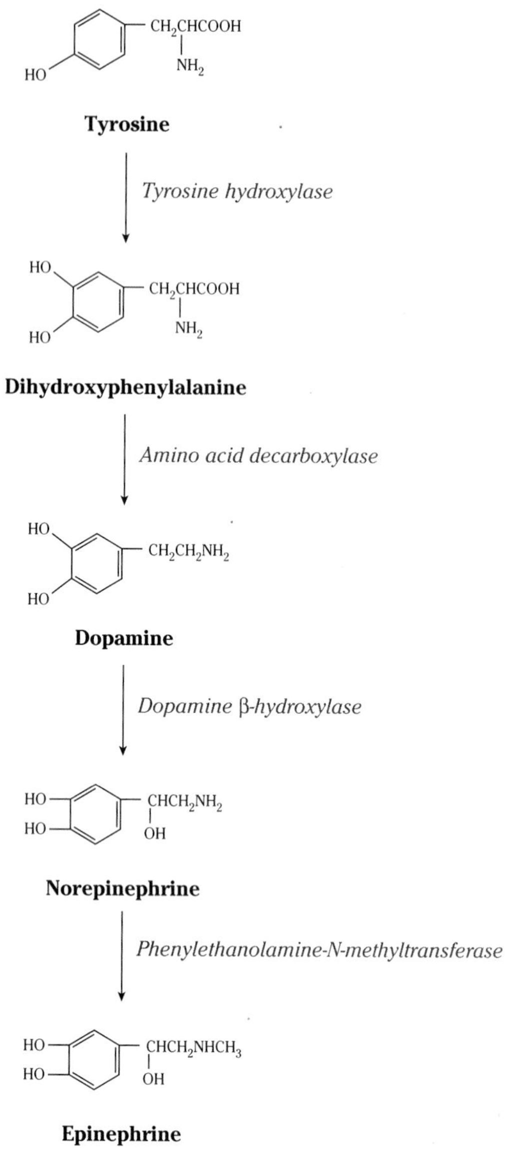

Tyrosine

$\downarrow$ *Tyrosine hydroxylase*

Dihydroxyphenylalanine

$\downarrow$ *Amino acid decarboxylase*

Dopamine

$\downarrow$ *Dopamine β-hydroxylase*

Norepinephrine

$\downarrow$ *Phenylethanolamine-N-methyltransferase*

Epinephrine

Figure 34.7 Catecholamine biosynthesis. Catecholamines are produced from a tyrosine precursor in the adrenal medulla. This pathway is stimulated by input from the sympathetic nerves.

stimulates voltage-gated calcium channels to open, causing an influx of calcium, which triggers the union of the granule and external plasma membrane. Blood flow to the medulla increases significantly during the secretion of catecholamines, likely as a means of expediting the distribution of the catecholamines to the rest of the body. Vasodilation is controlled neurally and by local vasoactive factors. Once in the bloodstream, NE and epinephrine are active for 10 to 30 s, then exert weaker activity for up to several minutes. Catecholamines are metabolized by two systems, monoamine oxides (MAO), found in nerve endings, and catechol-*O*-methyltransferase (COMT), which is present in many tissues throughout the body. The

main product of epinephrine degradation is vanillyl-mandelic acid (VMA).

Catecholamine Actions and Regulation

Like cortisol, the catecholamines have a wide variety of effects in a great many tissues. They are not steroids, however, and do not bind to cytosolic receptors; they bind to receptors on the surface of target tissues. They are regulated centrally by the nervous system.

Catecholamine Actions Catecholamines have two main types of effect: hemodynamic and metabolic. Hemodynamically, they increase heart rate, cardiac output, blood vessel tone, and extracellular fluid volume (all of which raise the blood pressure). NE and epinephrine both act at adrenergic receptors, of which there are two types, **alpha receptors** and **beta receptors**. NE has greater alpha activity, while epinephrine has an equal effect on alpha and beta receptors. Acting on alpha receptors, NE causes the constriction of blood vessels, which elevates total peripheral resistance and arterial blood pressure. It also stimulates the kidneys to secrete renin, initiating the RAA cascade and leading to tubular salt reabsorption and extracellular fluid volume expansion. Stimulation of β_1 receptors by NE leads to increased cardiac activity; stimulation of β_2 receptors leads to bronchodilation and decreased gastrointestinal motility. Epinephrine has a greater effect on myocardial contractility and heart rate via the β_1 receptors.

Metabolically, NE and epinephrine are counterregulatory hormones like cortisol, opposing insulin action and mimicking glucagon action. Epinephrine is up to 10 times more metabolically active than NE and acts to increase the metabolic rate and stimulate glycogenolysis. Both NE and epinephrine elevate plasma glucose levels by suppressing glucose utilization, increasing glucagon levels, and decreasing insulin production.

Regulation of the Adrenal Medulla Both the postganglionic sympathetic nerve endings and the adrenal medulla release catecholamines in response to signals from the nervous system. The brain registers stress or hypotension (detected by the body's baroreceptors; see Chapter 22) and discharges impulses along the sympathetic nerves. When the sympathetic nerves that innervate the adrenal gland are stimulated, the adrenal medulla releases NE and epinephrine, a sympathetic stimulus that affects the body globally by traveling in the bloodstream. Recall that NE and epinephrine have a short half-life. They do not regulate their own medullary release by negative feedback as cortisol does. Instead, they are regulated by the central nervous system.

PATHOPHYSIOLOGY: MEDULLARY DYSFUNCTION

As in the adrenal cortex, medullary pathology can be classified as diseases of overproduction and those of underproduction. Once again, these conditions arise because of a dissociation between hormone secretion and the usual stimuli for hormone secretion. In the case of overproduction, unregulated secretion occurs. In the case of underproduction, the adrenal medulla cannot respond to stimuli in the normal manner.

Catecholamine Overproduction

Pheochromocytomas are catecholamine-producing tumors of chromaffin cells, either within the adrenal (90% of cases) or in extra-adrenal chromaffin islands that persist after fetal life. They are rare and are perhaps most remarkable for their overrepresentation as a favorite "zebra" on medical boards. Pheochromocytomas usually produce both NE and epinephrine and are characterized by headache, pallor, palpitations, diaphoresis (sweating), and hypertension. Classically, these symptoms are paroxysmal, but pheochromocytomas may also cause persistent symptoms. Diagnosis is made by collecting a 24-hour urine sample and testing for catecholamines, metanephrines, and VMA.

Catecholamine Underproduction

Isolated adrenal underproduction of catecholamines usually does not lead to any sequelae, as the rest of the sympathetic nervous system can adequately perform the same functions. However, autonomic dysfunction that involves the sympathetic nerves can occur. Autonomic dysfunction may be idiopathic or secondary to diabetes, autoimmune disorders, or central nervous system infections. This dysfunction typically leads to postural hypotension.

Summary

- The two portions of the adrenal gland are the medulla, which secretes catecholamine hormones, epinephrine and norepinephrine, and the cortex, which surrounds the medulla.
- The three layers of the cortex from outermost to innermost are the zona glomerulosa, which secretes the mineralocorticoid aldosterone; the zona fasciculata, which secretes the glucocorticoid cortisol; and the zona reticularis, which secretes adrenal androgens, DHEA, and androstenedione.
- The adrenal glands are very well perfused. The adrenal arteries arise from three separate larger vessels, and when the medulla is stimulated, adrenal blood flow increases far in excess of that needed to meet adrenal oxygen demands. The vascular anatomy and vasodilatory capacity facilitate hormonal secretion.
- The HPA axis regulates adrenal secretion from the cortex. The hypothalamus releases CRH, which stimulates the anterior pituitary to release ACTH.
- ACTH triggers increased CEH conversion of cholesteryl ester to cholesterol, thereby increasing intracellular cholesterol levels. Steroid production from cholesterol, in particular cortisol, increases. Cortisol inhibits the secretion of CRH and ACTH in a classic negative-feedback loop.
- Steroids bind to intracellular receptors and modify DNA transcription.
- Aldosterone increases salt and water reabsorption in the kidney and K^+ secretion in the kidney. Its secretion is regulated primarily by the RAA system (which responds to blood pressure) and the plasma K^+ level.
- Cortisol's major effects are anti-inflammatory, metabolic (as a counterregulatory hormone that mimics glucagon action), and cardiovascular, by potentiating the response to catecholamines and supporting blood vessel tone, thereby helping maintain the blood pressure. Its secretion is regulated by CRH and ACTH. CRH is released in response to physiologic stress and in accordance with circadian rhythms and is suppressed by negative feedback from cortisol.
- The adrenal androgens are physiologically important during fetal development and puberty but are less important and less potent than the gonadal androgens (such as testosterone) during the other periods of life. Adrenal androgen secretion is governed by CRH and ACTH levels.
- All steroids are derived from cholesterol and pregnenolone, a modified form of cholesterol. Cholesteryl esters are delivered to the adrenal by LDLs in the blood and converted to cholesterol by CEH. They are translocated to the inner mitochondrial membrane by the StAR protein and converted to pregnenolone by the enzyme desmolase.

- Enzyme deficiencies can cause roadblocks in the biochemical pathways that lead from pregnenolone to the final end-products cortisol, aldosterone, and the androgens. Such conditions may cut off the production of some end-products and may result in excessive levels of steroid precursors. The precursors may then overflow into parallel biochemical pathways and cause an excess production of other end-products of steroid biosynthesis.

- In the disease congenital adrenal hyperplasia, 21-hydroxylase deficiency causes decreased production of cortisol and aldosterone, an overflow of precursors into the androgen pathways, and excess production of adrenal androgens.

- Hypercortisolism, an overproduction of cortisol, leads to Cushing syndrome. Hypercortisolism may have ACTH-dependent causes, such as pituitary adenoma and ectopic ACTH-secreting tumors, or ACTH-independent causes, such as adrenal tumors or exogenous glucocorticoid administration.

- Hyperaldosteronism may arise from adrenal tumors or kidney disease.

- Destruction of the adrenal glands owing to various causes leads to primary adrenal insufficiency (Addison's disease). Secondary adrenal insufficiency results from decreased ACTH production, whether due to pituitary pathology or the suppression of ACTH by the administration of exogenous glucocorticoids.

- The catecholamines epinephrine and norepinephrine mediate the fight-or-flight response, which includes increased heart rate, elevated cardiac output, and increased blood glucose levels.

- Catecholamines are made from the common amino acid precursor tyrosine.

- Many CNS-processed signals, including stress and hypotension, cause increased sympathetic nervous output, thereby driving the release of adrenal catecholamines.

- Pheochromocytomas are extremely rare catecholamine-secreting tumors of the adrenal medulla. Destruction of the adrenal medulla does not have significant sequelae, since the sympathetic nervous system can compensate for the effects of circulating catecholamines.

Suggested Reading

Christenson LK, Strauss JF III. Steroidogenic acute regulatory protein: an update on its regulation and mechanism of action. Arch Med Res. 2001;32(6):576–586.

Hasinski S. Assessment of adrenal glucocorticoid function. Postgrad Med. 1998;104(1):61–70.

Raff H, Findling JW. A physiologic approach to diagnosis of the Cushing syndrome. Ann Intern Med. 2003;138(12):980–991.

Speiser PW, White PC. Congenital adrenal hyperplasia. N Engl J Med. 2003;349(8):776–788.

Ten S, New M, Maclaren N. Clinical review 130: Addison's disease. J Clin Endocrinol Metab. 2001;86(7):2909–2922.

Vinson GP. Adrenocortical zonation and ACTH. Microsc Res Tech. 2003;61(3):227–239.

REVIEW QUESTIONS

Directions: Each of the numbered items or incomplete statements in this section is followed by answers or by completions of the statement. Select the ONE lettered answer or completion that is BEST in each case.

1. A newborn girl is observed to have ambiguous genitalia, low blood pressure, and hyperkalemia and is diagnosed with congenital adrenal hyperplasia. Her 21-hydroxylase deficiency has caused which of the following patterns of adrenal hormone derangement?

   (A) Decreased cortisol, decreased aldosterone, increased adrenal androgens
   (B) Decreased cortisol, increased aldosterone, increased adrenal androgens
   (C) Increased cortisol, decreased aldosterone, decreased adrenal androgens
   (D) Increased cortisol, increased aldosterone, decreased adrenal androgens
   (E) Increased cortisol, decreased aldosterone, increased adrenal androgens

2. A 27-year-old man is treated with oral prednisone (a glucocorticoid) to control a severe asthma exacerbation. After 2 weeks on the medication, his wheezing resolves and he decides to stop taking the prednisone without tapering his doses as prescribed. Two days later, he comes to the emergency room with symptoms of fatigue, weakness, and anorexia. He is hypotensive and hypoglycemic. He probably has adrenal insufficiency because:

   (A) His adrenal cortex is unresponsive to ACTH.
   (B) His ACTH secretion is low due to pituitary dysfunction.
   (C) His ACTH secretion has been suppressed by exogenous glucocorticoids.
   (D) His adrenal glands have been destroyed by lymphocytic infiltration.
   (E) He has an ACTH-secreting pituitary adenoma.
   (F) He has an adrenal adenoma.
   (G) He has an adrenal pheochromocytoma.
   (H) Exogenous glucocorticoids have injured his adrenal glands.

3. A 25-year-old woman with type I diabetes is hospitalized with a severe case of double pneumonia. During her hospital stay, she requires higher-than-usual doses of insulin. This is because:

   (A) Elevated glucagon secretion has increased her plasma glucose level.
   (B) Alveolar inflammation has liberated glucose into the blood.
   (C) Her intake of carbohydrates has increased dramatically.
   (D) Elevated cortisol secretion has increased her plasma glucose level.
   (E) Her adrenal function has been suppressed.

ANSWERS TO REVIEW QUESTIONS

1. **The answer is A.** The 21-hydroxylase deficiency in CAH results in a failure to convert progesterone into deoxycorticosterone in the aldosterone pathway and a failure to convert 17-hydroxyprogesterone into 11-deoxycortisol in the cortisol pathway. Pregnenolone levels consequently rise and drive conversion to 17-hydroxypregnenolone and then DHEA, an androgen. CAH therefore decreases cortisol and aldosterone output, while it increases the secretion of androgens, leading to the development of ambiguous genitalia in female infants.

2. **The answer is C.** Administration of an exogenous glucocorticoid (prednisone) has suppressed ACTH production from his pituitary. When the prednisone is abruptly withdrawn, his pituitary cannot immediately generate enough ACTH to stimulate the adrenals to make normal amounts of cortisol. The patient has a form of secondary adrenal insufficiency. Exogenous glucocorticoids are always prescribed on a taper (i.e., with progressively decreasing doses of the glucocorticoid) to relieve ACTH suppression gradually. Destruction of the adrenals causes primary adrenal insufficiency, which also leads to low cortisol levels, but there is no indication of primary adrenal pathology in this case. A functioning pituitary or adrenal adenoma causes hypercortisolism, not adrenal insufficiency. A pheochromocytoma is a rare tumor of the adrenal medulla that does not cause adrenal insufficiency, but rather increased catecholamine secretion.

3. **The answer is D.** The stress of infection has driven the patient's hypothalamus to increase CRH secretion, which in turn elevates the level of ACTH and then cortisol in the bloodstream. Cortisol's insulin-opposing, counterregulatory effect elevates the plasma glucose level. The insulin dose must therefore be increased to cover the higher level of glucose. Other causes of hyperglycemia would also require an increased insulin dose, but we know that infection has engaged her CRH response to stress. Her adrenal function is fine, as it is mounting an effective response to stress.

35

Hormonal Regulation of Calcium and Phosphate Metabolism

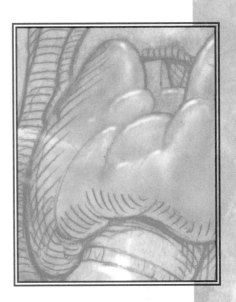

INTRODUCTION

Calcium plays fundamental roles in the physiology of all living organisms. At the macroscopic level, calcium is essential to maintaining the structural integrity of the skeleton; at the molecular level, calcium is central to the excitation of muscle and nervous tissue and to the control of enzymes. Calcium is integrally involved in many physiologic processes, including neurotransmitter release, signal transduction, and blood coagulation. Over the course of the evolution of living things from a seawater environment abundant in calcium to a terrestrial one relatively scarce in calcium, organisms have evolved mechanisms for closely regulating and conserving calcium. Parathyroid hormone (PTH), the main product of the parathyroid glands, and vitamin D together regulate the serum calcium level.

SYSTEM STRUCTURE: THE PARATHYROID GLANDS AND THE DISTRIBUTION OF CALCIUM AND PHOSPHORUS

The **parathyroid gland** synthesizes and secretes parathyroid hormone. There are usually four parathyroid glands, with pairs located at the superior and inferior margins of the thyroid capsule (FIGURE 35.1).

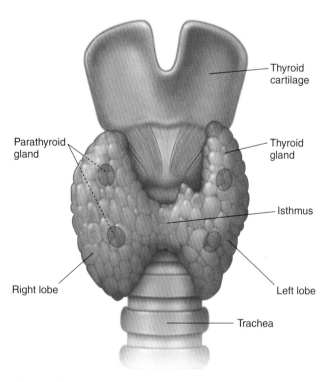

Figure 35.1 Anatomy of the parathyroid glands. The four small parathyroid glands are found in the capsule of the posterior thyroid or embedded in the thyroid tissue. They share the thyroid's blood supply.

The parathyroid gland is small, averaging $6 \times 4 \times 2$ mm in size and weighing 40 mg. The parathyroid develops at 5 to 14 weeks of gestation from the third and fourth branchial pouches. There are two types of cells in the parathyroid: chief cells and oxyphil cells. The *chief cells*, the principal cells of the parathyroid, are crucial to the synthesis and secretion of PTH. The function of the *oxyphil cells* is unknown.

Extracellular and Intracellular Pools of Calcium

The extracellular pool of calcium (the concentration of calcium in the plasma) is tightly regulated and remains remarkably constant, varying from 8.8 to 10.4 mg/dL (2.2 to 2.6 mM). This extracellular pool consists of three fractions: free, ionized calcium (50%); protein-bound calcium (40%); and calcium complexes with anions such as citrate and phosphate (10%). *The free, ionized calcium fraction is physiologically active and under close regulation by PTH.*

The equilibrium between free, protein-bound, and complexed fractions may change under certain conditions. Acidosis increases the proportion of free, ionized calcium, while alkalosis decreases it. Thus, hyperventilation can decrease ionized calcium levels to the point where the patient becomes symptomatic. Increases in citrate and phosphate concentration can also decrease ionized calcium levels. For example, hypocalcemia by these mechanisms may occur during blood transfusions, in which citrate is used as an anticoagulant, and in crush injuries to muscle, where there is an acute release of phosphate into the circulation.

On an intracellular level, the concentration of free calcium is only 0.1 μM, 1/10,000th of the extracellular concentration. The magnitude of this gradient allows for rapid flow of calcium into the cell when calcium channels are opened, transiently increasing the intracellular concentration 10-fold to 100-fold. Calcium pumps and exchangers actively restore and maintain this large gradient. The endoplasmic reticulum, microsome, and mitochondria store calcium in bound form where it is available for rapid intracellular release when signaled.

Inputs and Outputs of Calcium

For calcium levels to remain stable, the daily amount of calcium absorption must equal the amount of excretion. The dietary intake of calcium of an American adult averages 0.4 to 1.5 g of calcium per day (FIGURE 35.2). For reference, a quart of milk contains about 1.0 g of calcium. Only half of the dietary intake is absorbed by the gastrointestinal tract, and this amount is regulated by the actions of vitamin D

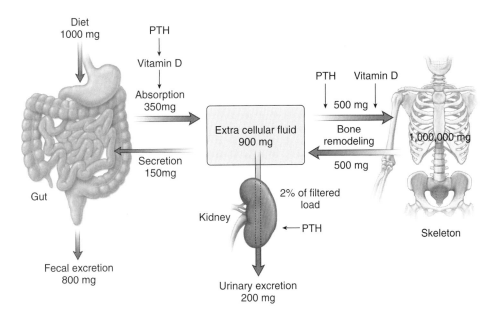

Figure 35.2 Daily calcium flux. Average Ca^{2+} flux values are shown. However, the amount of flux varies in accordance with changes in the serum Ca^{2+} and accompanying changes in PTH and vitamin D levels. The kinds of Ca^{2+} flux affected by PTH and by vitamin D are indicated.

(discussed later). During periods of growth, pregnancy, and lactation, vitamin D increases the absorption of calcium. In addition, the body secretes calcium into the lumen of the gastrointestinal tract in digestive juices. Incomplete absorption of dietary and secreted calcium results in an average of 0.35 to 1.0 g of calcium lost in the stool every day. This balances out to a net gut absorption of 0.15 to 0.4 g of calcium per day. Net inputs from the gut are matched by losses from the urinary tract. The kidney filters 10.0 g of calcium per day. It reabsorbs 98% of the calcium, excreting only 0.15 to 0.3 g in the urine.

The last component in the equation between inputs and outputs is the role of the skeleton. About 98% of the body's 1- to 2-kg total store of calcium is found in the skeleton as *calcium hydroxyapatite* $[Ca_{10}(PO_4)_6(OH)_2]$. The extracellular fluid (ECF) described earlier contains a small fraction—only 0.9 g. There is a dynamic balance between the pool of calcium in the skeleton and in the ECF. During the course of normal day-to-day bone remodeling, 0.25 to 0.5 g of calcium enters and leaves the ECF from the skeleton, for a net skeletal balance of zero. However, when necessary, the skeleton can rapidly mobilize its pool of calcium and replenish the calcium in the critical ECF pool in a matter of hours. This skeletal reservoir is sufficient to prevent hypocalcemia for months to years. Maintenance of appropriate levels of calcium in the ECF takes precedence over the strength of the skeleton.

The size of this skeletal reservoir of calcium changes with aging. Strictly speaking, the net skeletal balance of zero described above exists only between the ages of 20 and 30. During the period of growth and development of childhood, a gradual positive skeletal balance occurs, and more calcium enters than leaves the skeleton. After about age 30, there is a progressive negative skeletal balance; in its more extreme forms, the deficit may lead to osteoporosis. While aging changes the flux of calcium in and out of the skeleton, however, the calcium concentrations in the ECF remain stable.

In light of the effects of aging on bone mass, the U.S. Recommended Daily Allowance (RDA) for calcium changes with age:

- 1,200 to 1,600 mg calcium per day for ages 11 to 24.
- 1,000 mg per day for women ages 24 to 49, women on estrogen replacement therapy, and men ages 25 to 64.
- 1,500 mg per day for postmenopausal women not on estrogen replacement therapy and for men over age 65.

By increasing dietary calcium levels, the body relies less on the skeletal calcium reservoir for maintaining appropriate levels of calcium in the body. The skeletal reservoir is thus protected.

Phosphorus

The hormones that regulate calcium homeostasis also regulate phosphorus or phosphate homeostasis. In addition to being a component of the calcium hydroxyapatite that forms bone, phosphorus, in the form of phosphate ions, covalently modifies enzymes and substrates during signal transduction. It also participates in energy transactions (e.g., ATP, creatine phosphate).

The distribution of phosphorus is similar to calcium. The adult human body contains roughly 600 g of phosphorus, and most of it (85%) is stored in crystalline form in the skeleton. About 100 g is found in the soft tissues as phosphate esters. The extracellular pool contains approximately 550 mg of phosphate. This pool is in equilibrium with soft tissues and bone. The gastrointestinal tract absorbs phosphorus considerably more efficiently than calcium, and inputs from the gastrointestinal tract are more than ample for daily requirements. Phosphorus, generally in the form of inorganic phosphate (HPO_4^{2-} and $H_2PO_4^{-}$), circulates at concentrations of 2.8 to 4 mg/dL (0.9 to 1.3 mM). Calcium and phosphate circulate at concentrations close to their saturation point. This fact underscores the importance of coordinating the regulation of calcium and phosphate.

The regulation of phosphate levels takes place primarily at the level of the kidney by PTH, where increasing levels of PTH lower plasma phosphate levels by enhancing urinary phosphate excretion. Vitamin D defends against hypophosphatemia by inhibiting the production of PTH. However, overall, the regulation of calcium balance is much tighter than the regulation of phosphate.

SYSTEM FUNCTION: PTH AND VITAMIN D

PTH and vitamin D are the two principal hormones that regulate plasma levels of calcium in response to rapid, daily fluxes of calcium inputs and outputs. 1,25-dihydroxyvitamin D ($1,25(OH)_2D$) is the active metabolite of vitamin D; in this chapter, we will use the two interchangeably. PTH and vitamin D work in concert to raise calcium levels. PTH regulates calcium minute to minute. Vitamin D, on the other hand, acts on a longer time frame and facilitates the effects of PTH.

Parathyroid hormone (PTH) increases calcium levels by three mechanisms: increasing bone resorption, increasing the renal reabsorption of calcium at the proximal tubule, and increasing the synthesis of active vitamin D by the kidney. **Vitamin D** increases calcium levels by two mechanisms: increasing the intestinal absorption of calcium and increasing bone resorption. FIGURE 35.3 summarizes the actions of and interactions between PTH and vitamin D in response to a hypocalcemic challenge. These interactions will be presented in greater detail below.

Calcitonin, a peptide hormone secreted by C cells in the thyroid, also plays a role in calcium

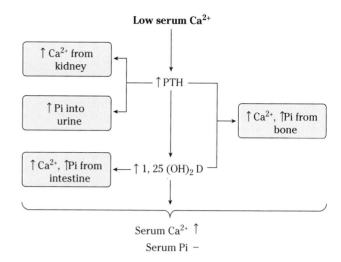

Figure 35.3 Response to hypocalcemia. Low serum calcium levels lead to an increased release of PTH and increased synthesis of $1,25(OH)_2D$, the active metabolite of vitamin D. The increase in PTH stimulates bone resorption (thereby increasing the flux of calcium from the skeleton to the ECF), the renal reabsorption of calcium, and the synthesis of vitamin D by the kidney. The increase in vitamin D in turn increases the intestinal absorption of calcium and increases bone resorption. PTH promotes the wasting of phosphate (P_i) in the kidney, while vitamin D increases its absorption in the intestine.

homeostasis by lowering plasma calcium levels. However, the participation of calcitonin in calcium regulation is much smaller than PTH and vitamin D and will be discussed below.

Parathyroid Hormone

As the most significant mediator of calcium homeostasis, PTH requires a detailed discussion. We will explore which stimuli promote and inhibit PTH secretion and what effects PTH produces and by what mechanisms of action. We will also touch upon the subject of parathyroid hormone-related protein, which interacts with the PTH receptor in the context of some malignancies.

PTH Secretion and Calcium Levels   The secretion of PTH is exquisitely sensitive to circulating free, ionized calcium levels. (Recall that it is the free, ionized calcium in the circulation that is physiologically active.) Decreases in calcium levels increase PTH secretion. FIGURE 35.4 illustrates the steep, inverse sigmoidal relationship between calcium and PTH secretion. The steep portion of the curve corresponds to the normal range of calcium, reflecting the sensitivity of the parathyroid to minor changes in calcium levels. Thus, small decreases in calcium concentrations dramatically increase PTH secretion.

The parathyroid detects calcium levels through the calcium-sensing receptor, an extracellular, 120-kD G protein-linked receptor. This receptor is a member of the seven-transmembrane domain family of

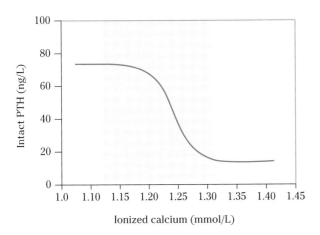

Figure 35.4 The inverse sigmoidal relationship between serum ionized calcium levels and PTH. Parathyroid sensitivity is maximal within the normal range, indicated by the shaded area.

receptors (another example of which is the beta-adrenergic receptor). Calcium ions are the ligand for this receptor. Stimulation of this receptor depresses PTH secretion through the activation of G_q, which is coupled to phospholipase C. This initiates the inositol trisphosphate and diacylglycerol signaling pathway common to many other cell types. The same calcium-sensing receptor is also present in renal tubule cells and in the thyroid C cells, which secrete calcitonin.

Mutations that inactivate the calcium-sensing receptor affect calcium homeostasis. One example is *familial hypocalciuric hypercalcemia (FHH)*, an autosomal dominant, benign condition. FHH is remarkable, as the name states, for the finding of hypocalciuria in the presence of PTH-mediated hypercalcemia. In FHH, the mutation alters the set point for calcium in the parathyroid, leading to inappropriate PTH release and in turn hypercalcemia. Simultaneously, the same abnormal receptor in the kidney inhibits the renal excretion of calcium, exacerbating the hypercalcemia. Signs and symptoms of hypercalcemia will be discussed below.

Other Modulators of the PTH Level   Other factors that influence PTH secretion include magnesium, lithium, and aluminum. Magnesium influences PTH secretion in a manner similar to calcium. Low serum levels of magnesium stimulate PTH secretion, and high levels suppress it. However, paradoxically, chronic, severe hypomagnesemia (<1.0 mg/dL, 0.4 mM) suppresses PTH secretion. In this setting, prolonged magnesium deficiency depletes *intracellular* magnesium levels, thereby interfering with the secretion and response to PTH. Lithium stimulates PTH secretion by changing the set point for PTH secretion. This becomes clinically important because hypercalcemia may be seen in patients who receive lithium for manic

depression. Aluminum, on the other hand, inhibits PTH secretion. High levels of aluminum, for example, may be seen in patients with renal failure who are dialyzed against solutions containing aluminum, or who are being treated with aluminum-containing phosphate binders for the hyperphosphatemia observed in renal failure. Catecholamines, phosphodiesterase inhibitors, histamine, and glucocorticoids have also been found to stimulate PTH secretion, but the physiologic significance of these effects is not clear.

So far we have discussed PTH secretion. The regulation of PTH synthesis through negative feedback loops is also important to calcium homeostasis. Vitamin D and high levels of calcium suppress transcription of the PTH gene. (Later, we will see that PTH increases the production of the active vitamin D metabolite; so vitamin D suppresses PTH as a form of negative feedback.) Conversely, hypocalcemia stimulates the synthesis of PTH. TABLE 35.1 summarizes the regulation of PTH secretion and synthesis.

PTH Structure   PTH is a small protein composed of 84 amino acids with a molecular weight of 9,300. As with many secreted proteins, the PTH gene encodes a precursor of PTH, prepro-PTH, which has a 23-amino-acid signal sequence and a 6-amino-acid prohormone sequence located at its amino terminus. Once PTH is processed and secreted, the circulating intact PTH is rapidly metabolized by the liver and kidney and has a half-life of only 2 to 4 min. The rapid breakdown of PTH thus allows the body to respond quickly to changing calcium levels.

The metabolism of PTH becomes clinically relevant when determining the levels of PTH. Newer assays for PTH quantify *intact PTH* and avoid the pitfalls of earlier approaches, which tended to detect only the carboxyl terminal fragments produced during the breakdown of intact PTH. These carboxyl terminal fragments are cleared by the kidney and accumulate in renal failure, and thus may potentially skew the measurements of earlier assays toward higher PTH values.

The Actions of PTH   PTH has direct effects on two organ systems where calcium flux occurs: bone and kidney. Before discussing the effects of PTH on the skeletal system, a short overview of skeletal physiology may be helpful. The skeletal system is not a static

Table 35.1   THE REGULATION OF PTH SECRETION

↑ Secretion	↓ Secretion
↓ [Ca^{2+}]	↑ [Ca^{2+}] (negative feedback)
↓ [Mg^{2+}]	↑ [Mg^{2+}] Vitamin D (negative feedback via synthesis inhibition)

system but a dynamic one. Bone is continuously resorbed and reformed; 5% to 10% of the skeleton turns over annually. There are three types of cells in bone: osteoblasts, osteocytes, and osteoclasts. **Osteoblasts** develop from the mesenchymal stem cells of the bone marrow and synthesize the collagen matrix, or osteoid, where mineralization takes place. As long as calcium and phosphate are present in the appropriate concentrations, mineralization occurs spontaneously on the collagen scaffolding laid down by osteoblasts. Mineralization is complete within 2 to 3 weeks. **Osteocytes** are osteoblasts that are embedded in cortical bone during remodeling. Their physiologic role is not as clear.

Osteoclasts are multinucleated giant cells that resorb bone and in the process release calcium and phosphate. In contrast to osteoblasts, osteoclasts emerge from hematopoietic granulocyte-macrophage stem cells (these cells also give rise to monocytes and macrophages). As will be clearer later, osteoblasts and osteoclasts coordinate their activities, with osteoblasts generally issuing most of the orders to osteoclasts through cytokines.

In bone, PTH acts via osteoblasts to increase the activity and number of osteoclasts. PTH increases the magnitude of bone resorption and therefore the efflux of calcium from bone into the circulation. Phosphate is also liberated concurrently. *Osteoclasts do not express any PTH receptors; PTH receptors are found on osteoblasts.* Osteoblasts mediate the signal from PTH by releasing cytokines, which increase osteoclast activity (FIGURE 35.5). PTH also recruits more osteoclasts by accelerating the maturation of osteoclast precursors. Chronic elevations in PTH inhibit osteoblast activity, and unless the calcium is replaced, the increased osteoclast-mediated bone resorption will be at the expense of skeletal mass and integrity. Because osteoblasts possess PTH receptors, *intermittent* PTH administration paradoxically leads to clinically significant osteoblast activity and enhanced bone formation. This phenomenon has shown some therapeutic promise.

In the kidney, PTH performs two functions for calcium homeostasis: stimulation of calcium reabsorption and increased synthesis of the active metabolite of vitamin D, 1,25(OH)₂D. Because of its direct actions on the kidney, PTH raises calcium levels faster and in greater magnitude through the kidney than through bone resorption. As mentioned earlier, the kidney filters 10 g of calcium per day, returning 98% of it to the body. About 90% of this calcium reabsorption takes place in the *proximal* convoluted tubule, and this process is not regulated by PTH. *The fate of the remaining 10% is modulated by PTH at the distal tubule; the presence of PTH increases calcium reabsorption at the distal tubule.* (Its mechanism is controversial.) Furthermore, PTH

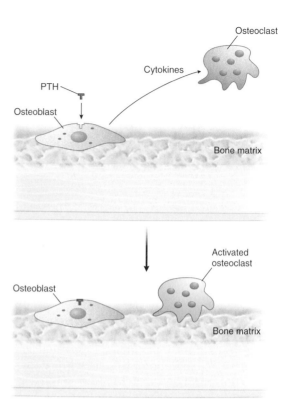

Figure 35.5 PTH's activation of osteoclasts via osteoblasts. Osteoblasts, but not osteoclasts, possess receptors for PTH. When activated by PTH, osteoblasts release cytokines that directly and indirectly stimulate osteoclasts, leading to increased bone resorption and increased release of calcium into the circulation.

activates 25-hydroxyvitamin D-1α-hydroxylase, the enzyme responsible for converting vitamin D to its most active metabolite, 1,25(OH)₂D. This enzyme is found in the mitochondria of the proximal tubule. TABLE 35.2 summarizes the actions of PTH.

Phosphate balance is also regulated by PTH in the kidney. The kidney is the principal site for phosphate regulation, and PTH determines the set point for serum phosphate levels. *PTH inhibits phosphate reabsorption at the proximal and distal tubule.* The phosphaturia produced by PTH compensates for and indeed outweighs the release of phosphate from bone due to PTH. Hence, PTH overall decreases

Table 35.2 THE ACTIONS OF PTH

↑ Osteoclast activity and number (via osteoblasts)

↑ Calcium reabsorption at distal tubule

↑ Synthesis of 1,25(OH)₂D

↓ Activity of vitamin D-24-hydroxylase (deactivator of vitamin D metabolites)

↑ Urinary phosphate excretion

serum phosphate levels. Through these coordinated effects, the body can increase the levels of calcium without excessively increasing phosphate levels. This avoids the risk of precipitating calcium phosphate crystals in the bloodstream.

FIGURE 35.6 summarizes the actions of PTH on its target organs to raise serum calcium levels and decrease serum phosphate levels. FIGURE 35.7 illustrates the changes in calcium and phosphate levels when PTH is administered pharmacologically.

The PTH Receptor The **PTH receptor** is found in bone and the kidney. It has a molecular weight of 80,000 and is a member of the G-protein receptor superfamily with a seven- transmembrane domain, similar to the calcium-sensing receptor in the parathyroid. This receptor is coupled to two receptor-associated G proteins, G_s and G_q. The G_s receptor is linked to adenylyl cyclase, which in turn increases cAMP. The G_q receptor is coupled to phospholipase C and the inositol trisphosphate and diacylglycerol signaling pathway. In the kidney, the increase in intracellular cAMP from PTH activation is large enough that cAMP spills over into the urine. Measurements of urinary cAMP can be used clinically to determine responsiveness to PTH.

PTHrP **Parathyroid hormone-related protein (PTHrP)** is a protein secreted in certain malignancies that mimics the calcium-raising effects of PTH. Binding of the PTH receptor requires only the first 34 residues of PTH (intact PTH has 84 residues), and activation of the receptor requires only the first 6 residues. It turns out that PTHrP is homologous with PTH only at the amino terminus, where they share 8 of the first 13 amino acid residues. This homology becomes clinically important because the secretion of PTHrP by certain malignancies can activate the PTH receptor and cause hypercalcemia. Examples of malignancies that secrete PTHrP are renal cell carcinoma, squamous cell carcinoma, and breast cancer.

In addition to its relationship to malignancy, PTHrP also has a physiologic role that is currently being determined. It is found in multiple tissues such as the breast, the central nervous system, and smooth muscle, where it is believed to be active locally. PTHrP may play a role in breast differentiation, and it has also been found to relax smooth muscle, particularly uterine and gastric smooth muscle.

Vitamin D

As mentioned earlier, vitamin D is another key player in calcium homeostasis. Vitamin D increases calcium levels by two principal mechanisms: increasing the intestinal absorption of dietary calcium and stimulating the maturation of bone-resorbing osteoclasts. Vitamin D is not a vitamin in the strictest sense because the body can synthesize it in sufficient quantity with appropriate exposure to sunlight. Vitamin D

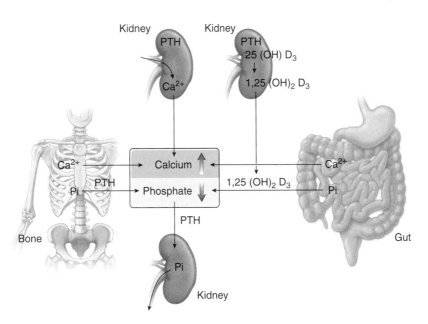

Figure 35.6 Actions of PTH. PTH increases serum calcium levels by increasing bone resorption, increasing calcium reabsorption in the kidney, and stimulating the synthesis of 1,25(OH)$_2$D, the active metabolite of vitamin D, which in turn leads to increased intestinal absorption of calcium. Phosphate levels are reduced by PTH through decreased renal reabsorption of phosphate, which outweighs the increase in phosphate flux from bone and the intestine.

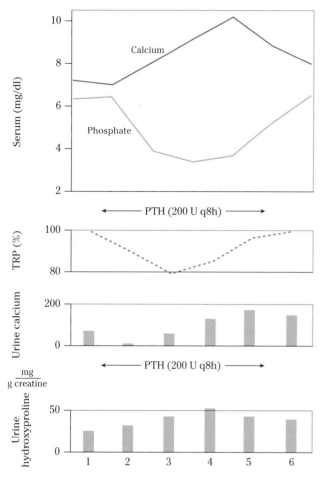

Figure 35.7 Effect of PTH on a PTH-deficient patient with low plasma calcium and high plasma phosphate levels. PTH increases serum levels of calcium and decreases serum levels of phosphate. Tubular resorption of phosphate (TRP) decreases with PTH administration, and hence the urinary excretion of phosphate increases. Urinary calcium levels initially decrease owing to increased calcium reabsorption mediated by PTH. However, urinary calcium levels eventually increase because the filtered load of calcium increases with rising serum calcium concentrations. Rising urinary hydroxyproline levels reflect PTH-mediated bone resorption.

is a sterol prohormone that needs to be converted (through a sequence of reactions) to its active metabolite, $1,25(OH)_2D$, before it can participate in calcium regulation. These conversions take place in the skin, liver, and kidney.

There are two forms of vitamin D: vitamin D_3 (cholecalciferol), which is found in animal sources (such as cod liver oil), and vitamin D_2 (ergocalciferol), which is found in plant sources. Both are metabolically equivalent, with the same actions and potency in the body.

Vitamin D Synthesis The skin synthesizes vitamin D (Figure 35.8). The starting substrate is 7-dehydrocholesterol (7-DHC) or *provitamin D*, the immediate precursor of cholesterol. In the epidermis, ultraviolet

light from 290 to 310 nm transforms 7-DHC to *previtamin D*. (UVB is from 290 to 320 nm, sun-burning range.) Thermal energy then converts previtamin D to vitamin D over the course of several days. This allows for a steady supply of vitamin D after brief UV radiation exposure.

Several factors modulate the production of vitamin D. Melanin pigmentation and exogenous factors such as sunscreen compete for the UV energy available for making vitamin D. Age is a significant factor. With advancing age, the amount of 7-DHC in the epidermis decreases; for example, a 70-year-old person produces only 30% of the amount of vitamin D a young adult produces when exposed to similar amounts of UV light. Additional UV radiation converts previtamin D and vitamin D to inert compounds.

Once vitamin D is synthesized, circulating vitamin D-binding protein draws vitamin D from the skin into the bloodstream; vitamin D-binding protein has a 1,000-fold higher affinity for vitamin D compared to previtamin D. Once in the circulation, vitamin D is brought to the liver, where it is hydroxylated by a mitochondrial cytochrome P_{450} vitamin D-25-hydroxylase to create $25(OH)D$, the major circulating form of vitamin D. It is also its major storage form in adipose and muscle. Vitamin D-25-hydroxylase in the liver is loosely regulated by a negative-feedback mechanism by $25(OH)D$. Since this is not a tight regulation, measurements of $25(OH)D$ are used clinically for assessing vitamin D deficiency or intoxication.

However, $25(OH)D$ is not biologically active at its physiologic levels. It is transported to the kidney, where another hydroxylation takes place by a mitochondrial cytochrome P_{450} $25(OH)D$-1α-hydroxylase to **$1,25(OH)_2D$**. *The $1,25(OH)_2D$ is the most biologically potent form of vitamin D.* It is 100 to 1,000 times more potent than its precursor. Specifically, this hydroxylation occurs in the proximal convoluted tubule, where $25(OH)D$ is filtered, reabsorbed, then transformed into $1,25(OH)_2D$. This is the rate-limiting step in the metabolism of vitamin D and is the enzymatic step that is under the tightest regulation.

The Regulation of $1,25(OH)_2D$ Production There are several regulators of $1,25(OH)_2D$ synthesis. PTH is the principal determinant; increases in PTH increase the conversion of $25(OH)D$ to $1,25(OH)_2D$ by increasing the synthesis of $25(OH)D$-1α-hydroxylase. Hypocalcemia (both independently and through increased PTH) and hypophosphatemia increase $1,25(OH)_2D$ production, and conversely hypercalcemia and hyperphosphatemia inhibit it. Hormonal influences such as estrogen, prolactin, and growth hormone also stimulate $25(OH)D$-1α-hydroxylase activity, thereby increasing levels of calcium during

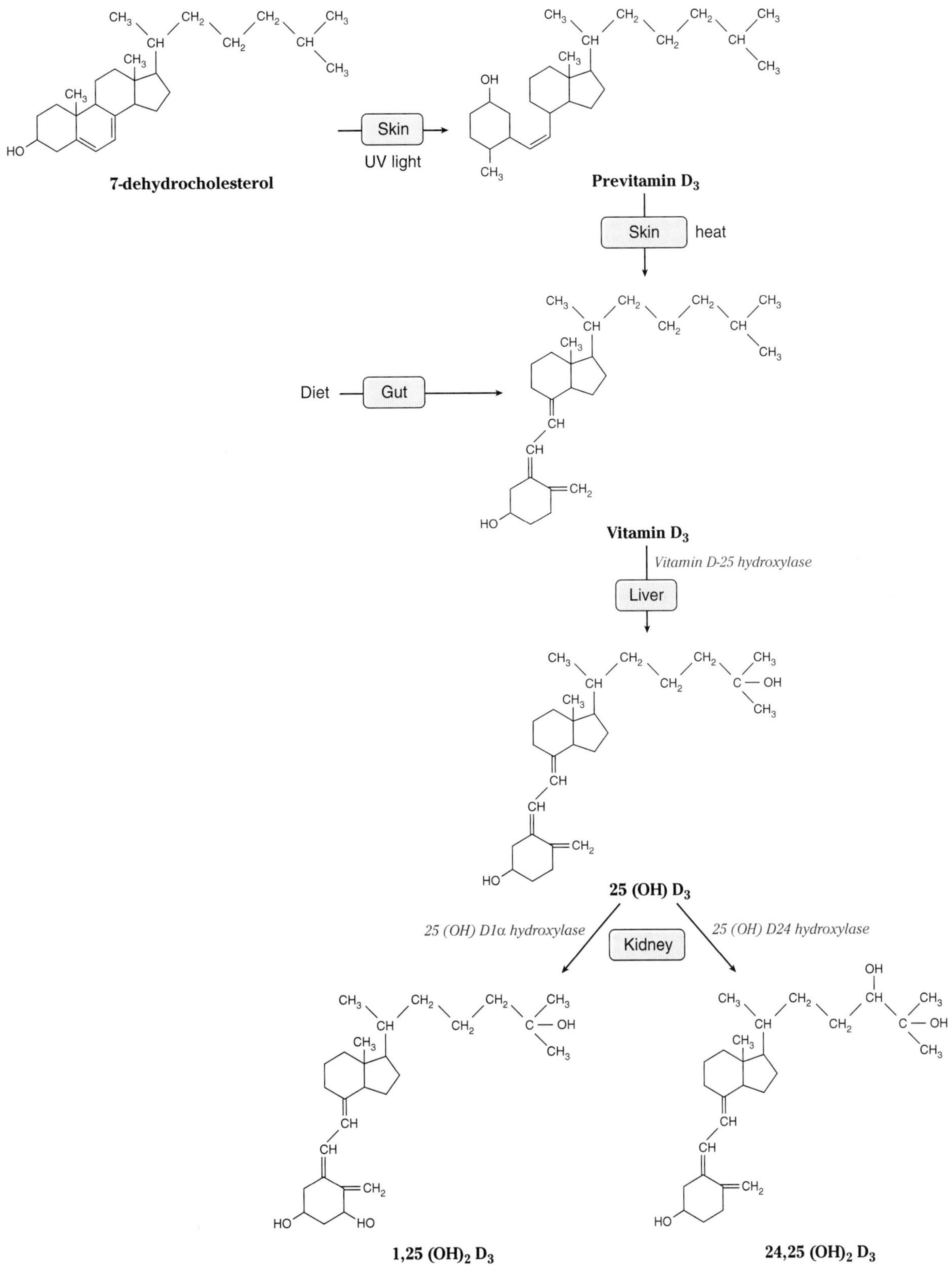

Figure 35.8 Photochemical, thermal, and metabolic pathways for the synthesis of vitamin D. Vitamin D is synthesized in the skin through the actions of ultraviolet and thermal energy. Vitamin D then undergoes a series of hydroxylations in the liver and in the kidney to become its most active form, 1,25(OH)$_2$D. Vitamin D$_3$ (cholecalciferol) is found in animal sources, while vitamin D$_2$ (ergocalciferol) is found in plant sources. Vitamin D$_2$ closely resembles vitamin D$_3$, except that it bears an extra methyl group at carbon 24. Cholecalciferol and ergocalciferol are both ingested as part of the diet.

pregnancy, lactation, and growth. In addition, 1,25(OH)$_2$D itself participates in negative-feedback regulation by inhibiting the transcription of the 25(OH)D-1α-hydroxylase gene. TABLE 35.3 summarizes the regulation of 25(OH)D-1α-hydroxylase.

The Mechanism of Vitamin D Action The mechanism of action of vitamin D is similar to other steroid hormones, such as estrogen and glucocorticoids (FIGURE 35.9). Vitamin D diffuses across cell membranes of its target tissues and forms complexes with specific intracellular receptors. The 1,25(OH)$_2$D first binds to the vitamin D receptor (VDR), a member of the nuclear hormone receptor superfamily. This receptor has an affinity for 1,25(OH)$_2$D that is 1,000-fold greater than for 25(OH)D. This 1,25(OH)$_2$D-VDR complex in turn interacts with the retinoic acid X receptor (RXR) to form a heterodimeric complex, which acts as a transcription factor on specific DNA sequences. These DNA sequences are known as vitamin D response elements (VDREs). The interactions between the VDR complex and DNA's VDREs enhances or inhibits the transcription of various genes.

Actions of Vitamin D In the intestinal tract, vitamin D plays a crucial role by increasing the absorption of calcium (FIGURE 35.10). Most of the active absorption of calcium takes place in the duodenum, while passive transport occurs throughout the rest of the small intestine. The efficiency of calcium absorption increases from 10% to 70% in the presence of vitamin D. Vitamin D stimulates the transcription of multiple proteins, including calbindin and calcium pumps. *Calbindin*, a calcium-binding protein, is thought to be one of the principal proteins that mediates the increased flux of calcium from the lumen into the mucosa. Vitamin D also increases calcium absorption by directly opening calcium channels in the cell membrane, an effect that is independent of transcription. This phenomenon, known as *transcaltachia*, occurs over a period of seconds to minutes, whereas the effects on transcription take hours.

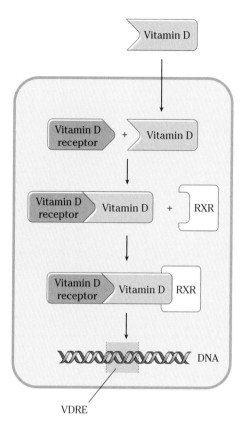

Figure 35.9 A proposed general mechanism of action of vitamin D (1,25(OH)$_2$D). Free vitamin D enters the cell and binds to the vitamin D receptor (VDR). The vitamin D-VDR complex then interacts with the retinoic acid X receptor (RXR) to form a heterodimer, which in turn binds to vitamin D response elements (VDREs). This binding enhances or inhibits the transcription of the target genes of vitamin D.

Vitamin D also increases the absorption of phosphate in the gastrointestinal tract. This absorption occurs primarily in the jejunum. However, the effect of the kidney on phosphate balance is more significant than the effect of the gastrointestinal tract.

In bone, vitamin D enhances mobilization of skeletal calcium stores through its effects on osteoblasts and ultimately osteoclasts. The osteoblast is the principal target of 1,25(OH)$_2$D. Vitamin D stimulates osteoblasts to produce cytokines that accelerate maturation of osteoclasts from their precursor; cytokines also stimulate osteoclast activity. (Mature osteoclasts, in the same way they lack PTH receptors, also do not directly respond to vitamin D.)

In addition to increasing serum calcium levels, the increase in osteoclast activity through vitamin D may facilitate the bone remodeling process. Furthermore, in osteoblasts, 1,25(OH)$_2$D upregulates the synthesis of a variety of proteins involved in matrix formation, including alkaline phosphatase, osteocalcin, and osteopontin. *Despite its array of effects on osteoblasts, the primary role of vitamin D in skeletal*

Table 35.3 THE REGULATION OF 25(OH)D-1α-HYDROXYLASE

↑ Activity	↓ Activity
PTH	1,25(OH)$_2$D (negative feedback)
↓ [Ca^{2+}]	↑ [Ca^{2+}]
↓ [P$_i$]	↑ [P$_i$]
Estrogen	
Prolactin	
Growth hormone	

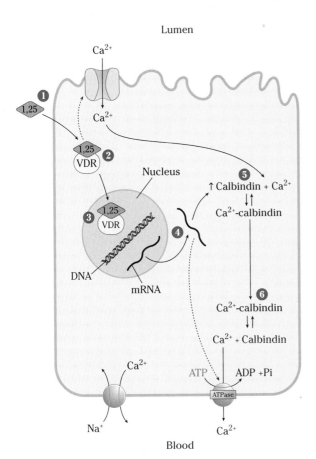

Lumen

Blood

Figure 35.10 A proposed mechanism of action of vitamin D (1,25(OH)$_2$D) on the intestine. Vitamin D, through a series of interactions with the VDR, drives the transcription of a variety of genes, including calbindin. Calbindin is a calcium-binding protein believed to transport calcium through the cell. Circled numbers indicate the sequence of the steps depicted.

physiology is to maintain appropriate concentrations of calcium and phosphate through its effects on intestinal absorption.

In the parathyroid gland, vitamin D inhibits the transcription of PTH, completing the feedback loop between PTH and vitamin D. This effect is mediated through a vitamin D response element in the parathyroid chief cells. TABLE 35.4 summarizes the actions of vitamin D.

The Biodegradation of Vitamin D When calcium levels are sufficient, there is no longer a need for 1,25(OH)$_2$D. In response, 25(OH)D may be diverted away from 1,25(OH)$_2$D production in the kidney and instead deactivated to 24,25(OH)$_2$D through a 24-hydroxylation in the kidney by 25(OH)D-24-hydroxylase. This represents the first step in the biodegradation of vitamin D, ultimately resulting in the water-soluble calcitroic acid. This enzyme is regulated by 1,25(OH)$_2$D and PTH. As may be predicted, 1,25(OH)$_2$D stimulates this enzyme as part of a

negative feedback loop. PTH inhibits 25(OH)D-24-hydroxylase, as ultimately the role of PTH is to increase the production of 1,25(OH)$_2$D. 24,25(OH)$_2$D is also a substrate for 25(OH)D-1α-hydroxylase, though the metabolite, 1,24,25(OH)$_3$D, is inactive.

Other Actions of Vitamin D Vitamin D also has functions unrelated to its role in calcium homeostasis. Receptors for vitamin D are found in many tissues not classically considered to be target organs, including skin, breast, pituitary, brain, and skeletal muscle. For example, as a steroid hormone, vitamin D inhibits the proliferation of keratinocytes and fibroblasts and inhibits the differentiation of keratinocytes. It also inhibits the production of IL-2 by activated T lymphocytes. Clinically, the antiproliferative effects of vitamin D can be used to treat psoriasis, a disorder where there is hyperproliferation of keratinocytes. Calcipotriene, an analog of vitamin D, is used for this purpose.

Nutritional Requirements for Vitamin D Nutritionally, the RDA for vitamin D for adults is 200 IU (international units). For infants, children, and pregnant and lactating women, it is 400 IU. In general, these demands are met by endogenous synthesis from casual exposure to UV radiation. For example, a whole-body dose of sunlight that produces minimal erythema in Caucasians generates an equivalent oral dose of 10,000 to 25,000 IU. However, the generation of vitamin D depends on a range of factors that affect the intensity of UV radiation, including altitude, geographic location, and time of day, along with factors such as amount of skin exposed, skin pigmentation, and age, as mentioned earlier. In higher latitudes, such as Boston (42°N), there is insufficient UV radiation to synthesize vitamin D between the months of November and February. During the spring, summer, and fall months in Boston, 5 to 15 min of sunlight exposure is all that is necessary to meet daily requirements.

Dietary fortification of vitamin D also helps prevent against vitamin D deficiency; a quart of milk contains roughly 400 IU of the vitamin. In the United

Table 35.4 ACTIONS OF 1,25(OH)$_2$D (ACTIVE VITAMIN D)

↑ Intestinal absorption of calcium

↑ Intestinal absorption of phosphate

↑ Osteoclast maturation (via osteoblasts)

↓ PTH synthesis (feedback inhibition)

↑ Synthesis of vitamin D-24-hydroxylase (deactivator of vitamin D metabolites) (feedback inhibition)

States, milk has been fortified with vitamin D since the 1930s. However, despite these measures, a significant proportion of the population is deficient in vitamin D. A recent study of medical inpatients found that 60% of them did not have adequate amounts of vitamin D. Given the importance of vitamin D for calcium homeostasis, vitamin D deficiency has ramifications for skeletal strength, and chronic deficiencies in vitamin D may result in osteoporosis and osteomalacia (discussed below).

Calcitonin

Calcitonin is a 32-amino-acid peptide that modestly lowers serum calcium concentrations by inhibiting bone resorption by osteoclasts. Calcitonin is secreted by the parafollicular C cells of the thyroid, which make up 0.1% of the mass of the thyroid. Embryologically, these cells originate from the neural crest and fill the ultimobranchial body during development. The C cell shares the same calcium-sensing receptor as the parathyroid. However, in the C cell, increasing calcium levels stimulate secretion of calcitonin (by contrast, increasing calcium levels suppress PTH secretion in the parathyroid). The calcitonin gene encodes two different proteins, depending on how the mRNA is spliced. This splicing varies from tissue to tissue. In the C cell, it produces calcitonin. However, in tissues such as the central nervous system, splicing at alternative sites creates calcitonin gene-related peptide (CGRP), a potent vasodilator.

Calcitonin decreases levels of calcium and phosphate. These effects are mediated by osteoclasts and by proximal renal tubule cells, both of which express receptors for calcitonin. Calcitonin inhibits osteoclasts, causing them to shrink and withdraw their bone-resorbing processes. In the kidney, calcitonin promotes the excretion of calcium, phosphate, sodium, potassium, and magnesium. Elevations in serum calcium are the main stimuli for calcitonin secretion. In addition, food ingestion, through a variety of gastrointestinal hormones, also leads to calcitonin secretion. Gastrin is the most potent of these hormones, and this phenomenon is used clinically for diagnosing medullary thyroid cancer (see below).

However, the physiologic role of calcitonin in humans is not clear given the following observations. Calcitonin deficiency secondary to thyroidectomy (and hence removal of the C cells) has no effect on calcium or bone metabolism. In addition, excess levels of calcitonin, as in medullary thyroid carcinoma, have little if any effect on calcium homeostasis.

Clinically, calcitonin is important as a marker for medullary thyroid cancer and as a therapeutic agent. Increased calcitonin secretion in medullary thyroid cancer can be provoked with calcium or pentagastrin infusions. Calcitonin is useful for treating metabolic bone conditions such as Paget's disease and osteoporosis, and also for treating hypercalcemia secondary to malignancy. Salmon calcitonin is generally used because it is 10-fold to 100-fold more potent than mammalian calcitonin.

PATHOPHYSIOLOGY: DERANGEMENTS OF THE SERUM CALCIUM LEVEL

In the absence of pathophysiology, PTH and vitamin D maintain serum calcium levels within normal limits. However, derangements in these regulatory systems can lead to hypercalcemic or hypocalcemic states.

Hypercalcemia

The vast majority of cases of **hypercalcemia** are due to hyperparathyroidism or malignancy. The possible mechanisms of hypercalcemia reflect the body's inputs and outputs of calcium: increased bone resorption, increased gastrointestinal absorption, and decreased renal excretion. Of these three, increased bone resorption is the most common mechanism.

Symptoms Signs and symptoms of hypercalcemia occur when calcium levels exceed around 10.0 mg/dL. Normally, calcium and phosphate circulate at concentrations close to their saturation point. When calcium levels rise above 13 mg/dL, calcifications begin to develop at multiple sites. Calcium levels exceeding 15 mg/dL are a medical emergency, as coma and cardiac arrest may occur.

In the heart, hypercalcemia has two major effects: a positive inotropic effect (more forceful pumping) and altered conduction. Acute rises in calcium increase contractility but shorten systolic ejection time, slowing the heart rate. On the ECG, a shortened QT interval and widened T waves are seen. Hypertension is also common due to systemic vasoconstriction (smooth muscle contraction). Hypercalcemia worsens digitalis toxicity, as both calcium and digitalis increase intracellular calcium levels.

Calcium always has a steep gradient from out to in (extracellular concentrations are in millimolar quantities, intracellular in nanomolar), so that it has a significant depolarizing potential when it enters. On the basis of only the calcium gradient, one might think that hypercalcemia, with its greater gradient, would depolarize the cell and lead to greater excitability. In fact, the opposite occurs because high extracellular calcium actually diminishes calcium entry across the cell membrane through inhibition or closing of voltage-gated calcium channels (VGCCs). The result is depression of neural reflexes, mental depression, and muscle weakness. In other words, when there is a greater calcium gradient and cell depolarization, intracellular calcium actually decreases owing to the effects on these calcium channels (T-type).

Hypercalcemia produces a variety of symptoms, including fatigue, depression, mental confusion, anorexia, nausea, vomiting, constipation, and increased urination. The nausea, vomiting, and constipation observed result from the inhibitory effects of hypercalcemia on gastrointestinal smooth muscle contraction.

Hypercalcemia also affects the concentrating ability of the renal system. Hypercalcemia interferes with the actions of antidiuretic hormone on the distal convoluted tubule, leading to polyuria. The mnemonic "stones, bones, groans, and moans" reviews the symptoms of hypercalcemia. "Stones" refers to kidney stones, "bones" to signs and symptoms of bone resorption seen in hyperparathyroidism, "groans" to a wide variety of gastrointestinal complaints and maladies, and "moans" to an array of mental symptoms, from lethargy to behavioral changes. The following is a brief discussion of some of the etiologies of hypercalcemia.

Primary Hyperparathyroidism **Primary hyperparathyroidism (PHP)** occurs when there is excessive secretion of PTH. This condition has an estimated prevalence of more than 1%, with a higher prevalence in the elderly. In 80% of cases, primary hyperparathyroidism is caused by a single parathyroid adenoma, or focal expansion from a single abnormal cell. Primary hyperplasia of the whole parathyroid accounts for another 15% of cases; in many instances, it is a manifestation of one of the multiple endocrine neoplasia syndromes. Parathyroid carcinoma is rare and accounts for only 1% to 2% of cases.

Symptoms of primary hyperparathyroidism reflect those of hypercalcemia, hypercalciuria, and the effects of long-standing PTH-mediated bone resorption. However, with the advent of routine determinations of serum calcium levels, 85% of patients who are diagnosed with primary hyperparathyroidism are asymptomatic or minimally symptomatic. One of the manifestations of chronically elevated PTH levels is osteitis fibrosa cystica. This skeletal manifestation stems from the increased number and activity of osteoclasts, resulting in classic subperiosteal resorption of cortical bone, bone cysts, and a "salt-and-pepper" appearance of the skull, for example. Treatment for primary hyperparathyroidism is surgical, involving resection of the tumor or some of the enlarged parathyroid glands. (See Clinical Application Box *What Is Primary Hyperparathyroidism?*)

Malignancy Malignancy is the most common cause of hypercalcemia in hospitalized patients, with an incidence of 15 in 100,000 per year. Lung cancer, breast cancer, and multiple myeloma account for 50% of these cases. In many instances, the secretion of PTHrP, as discussed earlier, is responsible for the hypercalcemia. However, direct bone resorption by lytic metastases and the release of other mediators by tumors can also lead to hypercalcemia.

Sarcoidosis The kidney is not the only place where there is 25(OH)D-1α-hydroxylase activity. Interestingly, in certain pathologic states, activity of this enzyme may occur at extrarenal sites. For example, in *sarcoidosis*, a chronic multisystem granulomatous disorder of unknown etiology, hypercalcemia is seen in 10% of cases. This is due to the presence of 25(OH)D-1α-hydroxylase activity in macrophages from sarcoid tissue. The same mechanism can give rise to hypercalcemia in other granulomatous disorders, including tuberculosis, berylliosis, coccidioidomycosis, histoplasmosis, and leprosy.

Hypocalcemia

Hypocalcemia generally occurs when the decrease in calcium levels overwhelms the body's homeostatic mechanisms. Under such circumstances, PTH and/or 1,25(OH)$_2$D fail to boost the calcium level adequately in the face of low plasma calcium. This can happen when PTH or vitamin D production fails, in conditions where the body becomes resistant to the action of these hormones, or when the plasma calcium level drops too dramatically to be compensated. Calcium levels can drop precipitously if phosphate levels rise (e.g., in a crush injury), causing precipitation of calcium phosphate.

Symptoms Most of the signs and symptoms of hypocalcemia revolve around increased neuromuscular excitability or irritability. Low extracellular calcium levels (hypocalcemia) might be expected to create a smaller gradient of calcium concentration from out to in, and thus to create a hyperpolarizing effect on cell membranes with decreased excitability. However, in the nervous system particularly, hypocalcemia is a hyperexcitable state characterized by hyperreflexia and, if severe, seizures. Muscle cramps, tingling, and twitching are common in the hypocalcemic state known as *tetany*. The reason for the hyperexcitable state is that low extracellular calcium leads to greater opening of membrane calcium channels. Any hyperpolarizing effect, including low ECF calcium, actually disinhibits these channels and allows greater calcium uptake, which ultimately depolarizes the cells and activates them.

CLINICAL APPLICATION

WHAT IS PRIMARY HYPERPARATHYROIDISM?

Mary Murphy, age 68, has felt fatigued and has had trouble remembering things for quite some time. She has been diagnosed with depression; suffered constant constipation, nausea, thirst, and urinary frequency; and was treated for a kidney stone a month ago. Her physical exam is completely benign. Her total calcium level is 11.8 mg/dL (normal 8.8–10.4 mg/dL), and her phosphorus level is 3.2 mg/dL (3–4.5 mg/dL). Having noted her hypercalcemia, her doctors are concerned about primary hyperparathyroidism or malignancy since these two illnesses account for 90% of cases of hypercalcemia. Further lab tests reveal a PTH level of 90 pg/mL (10–60 pg/mL) and a 24-hour urine Ca^{2+} level of 500 mg (50–250 mg/day). Mrs. Murphy is diagnosed with primary hyperparathyroidism and referred to a surgeon for treatment.

Primary hyperparathyroidism (PHP) is a condition of parathyroid overgrowth and concomitant overproduction of PTH. A diagnosis of PHP begins with the detection of hypercalcemia. All of the symptoms of hypercalcemia are common complaints; however, the constellation of all these complaints in one patient leads one to entertain the diagnosis of hypercalcemia. Once hypercalcemia is established, PHP and malignancy rise to the top of the differential diagnosis, because they account for the majority of cases of hypercalcemia. The availability of new diagnostic tools to measure intact PTH levels facilitates the diagnosis of PHP, and further workup is generally unnecessary. The differential for hypercalcemia associated with elevated PTH, in addition to PHP, includes familial hypocalciuric hypercalcemia and lithium use. (To confound matters, lithium also produces hypocalciuria.) By comparison, in hypercalcemia of malignancy, the PTH level is low or undetectable.

PHP is most often diagnosed in asymptomatic patients on the basis of abnormally high calcium levels during routine laboratory tests; only 20% of patients with PHP present with symptoms. Renal stones are the most common complication of PHP, but they occur in only 15% to 20% of patients, down from 40% in the past. (Only 5% of patients with renal stones have PHP.) The classic skeletal manifestation of PHP, *osteitis fibrosa cystica* with subperiosteal bone resorption, bone cysts, and so on, is present in fewer than 10% of patients.

The treatment for PHP is surgical. In experienced hands, parathyroidectomy is curative in more than 90% of cases. The indications for surgery include severe calcium elevation (>11.4 to 12 mg/dL); a previous episode of life-threatening hypercalcemia; evidence of overt bone disease or where bone mass is less than 2 SD below normal; reduced renal function, stone disease, or significant hypercalciuria (>400 mg per day); or patients who are young, under age 50 years.

These neuronal changes first lead to numbness and tingling around the fingertips, toes, and circumoral regions. Eventually tetany results, classically seen as the carpopedal spasm, also known as the *main d'accoucheur* posture, where there is flexion of the wrist and metacarpophalangeal joints, extension of the interphalangeal joints, and adduction of the thumb (FIGURE 35.11). Spasms from tetany may be life-threatening, particularly if they involve the laryngeal muscles and block the airway.

Chvostek's and Trousseau's signs are additional classic indicators of hypocalcemia that reflect the increased neuromuscular excitability. *Chvostek's sign* can be elicited by tapping the facial nerve just

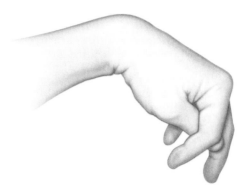

Figure 35.11 The main d'accoucheur posture of the hand. This posture is seen in the carpal spasm caused by hypocalcemia.

anterior to the ear and looking for facial muscle contractions. About 10% of people have a positive Chvostek's sign but are otherwise normocalcemic. *Trousseau's sign* is positive when there is carpopedal spasm following the inflation of a blood pressure cuff to 20 mm Hg above systolic pressure for 3 min. Ischemia unmasks the heightened excitability of the nerves. Trousseau's sign is more specific than Chvostek's sign, with only 1% to 4% of normal subjects having a positive Trousseau's sign. On the ECG, the QT interval is prolonged due to delayed repolarization.

Hypoparathyroidism   In general, a diagnosis of **hypoparathyroidism** should be considered when the findings of hypocalcemia and hyperphosphatemia occur in the setting of normal renal function and a normal magnesium level. (Recall that severe hypomagnesemia from gastrointestinal or renal losses, alcoholism, and so forth temporarily paralyzes the parathyroid.)

The most common cause of hypoparathyroidism is surgery. Because of the anatomy in this region, the parathyroid glands may be inadvertently removed during neck surgery. Hypoparathyroidism may also be idiopathically caused by autoimmune disease in cases where there are circulating antiparathyroid antibodies in the setting of type I polyglandular autoimmune syndrome. Another cause of hypoparathyroidism is *DiGeorge syndrome,* a rare congenital disorder characterized by an absence of thymus and parathyroid gland development, giving rise to neonatal hypoparathyroidism.

Pseudohypoparathyroidism   **Pseudohypoparathyroidism** is a genetic condition characterized by a defect in responsiveness to PTH. There are two types of pseudohypoparathyroidism. *Type 1B* is a disorder only of resistance to PTH, giving rise to symptoms of hypocalcemia, hyperphosphatemia, and secondary hyperparathyroidism (increased PTH secondary to PTH resistance). In addition to the symptoms of 1B, *type 1A* has a distinct phenotype known as *Albright's hereditary osteodystrophy.* This syndrome is characterized by short stature, a round face, a short neck, brachydactyly (particularly of the fourth and fifth metacarpal bones), subcutaneous ossifications, and reproductive abnormalities secondary to hypothyroidism. Patients with type 1A, but not type 1B, pseudohypoparathyroidism have a nonfunctional copy of the $G_s\alpha$ subunit that transmits the signal from the PTH receptor to adenylyl cyclase.

Osteomalacia and Rickets   Vitamin D deficiency results in two well-known conditions, osteomalacia and rickets. **Osteomalacia** is a defect in mineralization of the bone matrix or osteoid deposited during normal bone remodeling. In addition to the poor bone mineralization of osteomalacia, **rickets** is characterized by inadequate mineralization of the epiphyseal cartilage or growth plate in growing skeleton. Therefore, rickets by definition occurs only in children. (By contrast, in osteoporosis, there is a loss of bone mass overall with a *normal* mineral-to-collagen ratio, while in osteomalacia, there is a *decreased* mineral-to-collagen ratio from poor bone mineralization.)

Vitamin D deficiency has a variety of etiologies. They include nutritional deficiency (rare in the United States because of dietary fortification), inadequate endogenous production of vitamin D, increased catabolism of vitamin D (as may occur with stimulation of hepatic enzymes by anticonvulsants), malabsorption of vitamin D from gastrointestinal disorders, defective activation of vitamin D, and resistance to vitamin D owing to genetic disorders.

In both osteomalacia and rickets, insufficient vitamin D levels result in decreased intestinal absorption of calcium and phosphate. Although severe hypocalcemia develops only late in the course of vitamin D deficiency, a suboptimal supply of calcium and phosphate hinders proper bone mineralization. Indeed, increases in PTH compensate for deficient calcium absorption by increasing bone resorption with consequent phosphaturia and phosphate losses. It is not clear whether the effects of vitamin D on osteoblasts per se are of immediate importance in the pathology of rickets or osteomalacia, as experimental models of osteomalacia can be remedied solely with calcium replacement.

Rickets produces multiple characteristic skeletal findings, reflecting its effects on an active growth plate. These findings include growth failure, pigeon-breast deformity of the sternum, and bowing of the long bones. Children with rickets have an increased frequency of fractures and diffuse bone pain. Osteomalacia, on the other hand, does not result in prominent skeletal findings; rather, osteomalacia may present as diffuse skeletal pain, bone tenderness, proximal muscle weakness, and fractures from minimal trauma.

Summary

- The skeleton is a major reservoir of calcium for maintaining calcium plasma levels.
- Parathyroid hormone (PTH) and vitamin D are the two main hormones involved in calcium regulation.
- PTH raises calcium levels by increasing bone resorption, increasing renal reabsorption of calcium, and increasing the production of activated vitamin D.

- Vitamin D raises calcium levels by increasing the intestinal absorption of calcium and increasing the production of osteoclasts.

- Phosphate levels are regulated primarily at the kidney by PTH; increasing PTH decreases plasma phosphate concentrations.

- The physiology of calcium and phosphate metabolism can be summarized by looking at the response to a hypocalcemic challenge, a decrease in calcium intake. A decrease in serum calcium levels is rapidly met with an increase in PTH secretion. This leads to an efflux of calcium and phosphate from bone through the stimulation of osteoclast bone resorption via osteoblasts.

- At the same time, PTH increases renal reabsorption of calcium at the distal tubule and promotes wasting of phosphate in the urine to compensate for the increased phosphate load from bone. The net effect is to restore calcium levels without excessively increasing phosphate levels.

- On a long-term basis, the increase in PTH leads to increased renal conversion of $25(OH)D$ to its active metabolite, $1,25(OH)_2D$. It increases the intestinal absorption of dietary calcium and phosphate, further

boosting the levels of calcium and phosphate in the ECF. Elevated levels of $1,25(OH)_2D$ increase the pool of osteoclasts available for resorption and hence the quantity of calcium available for the body's use.

- In response to hypophosphatemia, vitamin D plays a central role. Hypophosphatemia stimulates renal production of $1,25(OH)_2D$, which in turn increases intestinal absorption of phosphate (as well as calcium). Moreover, $1,25(OH)_2D$ inhibits the synthesis of PTH, thereby reducing the renal phosphate excretion mediated by PTH. The net effect restores phosphate levels in the ECF.

Suggested Reading

Bushinsky DA, Monk RD. Electrolyte quintet: calcium. Lancet. 1998;352(9124):306–311.

Clark OH. How should patients with primary hyperparathyroidism be treated? J Clin Endocrinol Metab. 2003;88(7):3011–3014.

Martin TJ. Actions of parathyroid hormone-related peptide and its receptors. N Engl J Med. 1996;335:736–737.

Marx SJ. Medical progress: hyperparathyroid and hypoparathyroid disorders. N Engl J Med. 2000;343: 1863–1875.

Strewler GJ. The physiology of parathyroid hormone-related protein. N Engl J Med. 2000;342(3):177–185.

Zahrani AA, Levine MA. Primary hyperparathyroidism. Lancet. 1997;349:1233–1238.

REVIEW QUESTIONS

Directions: Each of the numbered items or incomplete statements in this section is followed by answers or by completions of the statement. Select the ONE lettered answer or completion that is BEST in each case.

1. An 11-year-old boy with a history of epilepsy, short stature, and bone deformities is discovered to have low levels of vitamin D as a chronic side effect of his seizure medication. Which of the following responses to hypocalcemia is most significantly impaired in this child?

   (A) Increased bone resorption
   (B) Increased hydroxylation of inactive vitamin D by the kidney
   (C) Increased reabsorption of Ca^{2+} by the proximal tubule in the kidney
   (D) Increased secretion of PTH
   (E) Increased intestinal absorption of dietary Ca^{2+}

2. A 55-year-old man is diagnosed with sarcoidosis and hypercalcemia. If macrophages are secreting vitamin D-25-hydroxylase, thereby increasing the conversion of vitamin D to its major circulating (and still inactive) form, the macrophages are mimicking a physiologic function of which other tissue?

   (A) Skin
   (B) Liver
   (C) Kidney
   (D) Bone
   (E) Parathyroid
   (F) Intestine

3. After suffering from a kidney stone, a man is diagnosed with hypercalcemia due to primary hyperparathyroidism, which has increased the levels of PTH in his plasma. The PTH is creating hypercalcemia by acting at receptors on which cells?

   (A) Chief cells in the parathyroid gland
   (B) Osteoclasts in bone
   (C) Osteoblasts in bone
   (D) Duodenal cells in the gut
   (E) Parafollicular C cells in the thyroid gland

ANSWERS TO REVIEW QUESTIONS

1. **The answer is E.** Vitamin D alone promotes increased intestinal absorption of Ca^{2+}, so a deficiency in vitamin D is likely to impair intestinal absorption. While vitamin D does also promote bone resorption to liberate Ca^{2+} from bone, PTH is the more significant mediator of bone resorption, so bone resorption would not be affected to the same extent as intestinal absorption. The ability of the parathyroids to secrete PTH is normal in this child and so are PTH actions, including bone resorption, increased renal hydroxylation (and activation) of inactive vitamin D, and increased renal Ca^{2+} reabsorption.

2. **The answer is B.** Inactive vitamin D is newly synthesized in the skin or absorbed in the intestine, converted to its major circulating form by vitamin D-25-hydroxylase in the liver, and converted to its active form in the kidney.

3. **The answer is C.** PTH promotes the liberation of Ca^{2+} from bone by acting on the PTH receptor in osteoblasts, which in turn augment the activity of osteoclasts through cytokines. The osteoclasts promote bone resorption and the release of Ca^{2+}. The chief cells of the parathyroid produce PTH. While negative feedback loops do affect the chief cells, the negative feedback is mediated through vitamin D influence on the cells and not PTH directly. Vitamin D, not PTH, acts on the duodenal cells of the intestine to promote Ca^{2+} absorption. The parafollicular C cells in the thyroid produce calcitonin in response to high levels of serum Ca^{2+}.

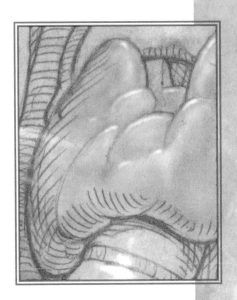

36

The Female Reproductive System

INTRODUCTION

The menstrual cycle defines the reproductive years of a woman's life. This era begins with menarche (the onset of menstruation) at about age 8 to 13 and ends with menopause, which begins at about age 50. Teleologically, the purpose of each menstrual cycle is to create the opportunity for pregnancy. Preparation for potential pregnancy is achieved through two concurrent cycles: the ovarian cycle and its dependent uterine cycle, which together make up the menstrual cycle. Once a month, the ovarian cycle produces one egg or oocyte (the female haploid gamete cell) and expels it into the fallopian tubes, where it may encounter a sperm or spermatozoon (the male haploid gamete cell) and become fertilized, thus creating a diploid zygote. The uterine cycle concomitantly produces a favorable environment within the uterus in which an embryo can implant and grow. If the egg is not fertilized, this nutritive uterine lining is shed, menstruation occurs, and the cycle begins anew. If a pregnancy does occur, a transient organ called the placenta creates a new and unique hormonal milieu to support the growth of a fetus. When the baby is delivered and the placenta passed from the body, the menstrual cycle resumes.

SYSTEM STRUCTURE

Unlike animals that lay eggs that are fertilized and develop outside the mother's body, human eggs are produced, are fertilized, and develop within a human female's body in a specialized environment. This section describes the anatomic, histologic, and hormonal elements of the female reproductive system.

Gross Anatomy

First we will consider the reproductive tract—that is, the reproductive organs located in the abdominal cavity. Then we will mention the cranial structures that secrete important reproductive hormones and help regulate reproductive function and development.

The Reproductive Tract   The **ovaries** are the gonads of the human female. They are located in the pelvis, one on either side of the uterus within the broad ligaments (FIGURE 36.1). They are almond-shaped organs, each about 2 to 3 cm long. The ovarian ligaments contain the ovarian artery and vein, which enter and leave the ovary at its hilum. Ovarian steroid hormones control the menstrual cycle with their monthly fluctuations.

The **fallopian tubes**, or *oviducts*, are hollow structures on either side of the uterus. The space inside each tube is continuous at the distal end with the peritoneal cavity and at the proximal end with the

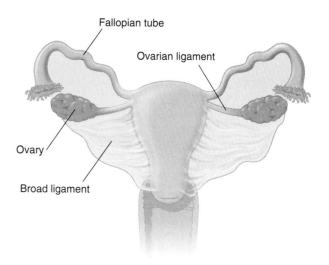

Figure 36.1   Anatomy of the ovaries.

cavity of the uterus. Each tube is subdivided into a distal infundibulum with tentacle-like projections called *fimbriae*, an ampulla, and a proximal isthmus (FIGURE 36.2). Fertilization of the ovum by the sperm occurs in the fallopian tube. The fallopian tube conducts the egg from the ovary into the tube and the fertilized egg from the tube into the uterus.

The **uterus**, or *womb*, is the chamber in which the fetus grows. It is a muscular organ located in the pelvis posterior to the bladder, anterior to the rectum, and superior to the vagina. The most superior portion is called the *fundus*; the upper, pear-shaped portion of the uterus is called the *corpus* (body); and the lower, cylindrical portion is called the **cervix**. The ends of the cervix are the *internal* and the *external cervical os*. (*Os* is Latin for mouth or opening.)

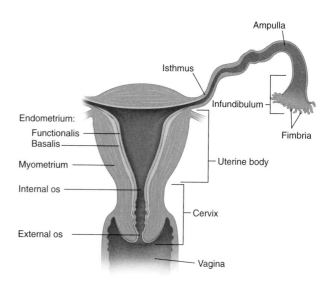

Figure 36.2   Anatomy of the uterus and fallopian tubes.

The **vagina**, or birth canal, is the passageway leading from the internal female reproductive tract to the external genitalia. The mons pubis, the labia majora, the labia minora, the clitoris, the hymen, and the greater vestibular (or Bartholin's) glands make up the female external genitalia.

The Brain   The generation of an egg, the establishment and maintenance of an appropriate environment for fertilization and development, the process of birth, and the nourishment of an infant all require precise functioning of a number of hormone-producing organs in the brain. The **hypothalamus** is located in the diencephalon, the part of the brain that lies above the brain stem and between the two cerebral hemispheres. The **pituitary gland** is a bilobed structure in the sella turcica, in the midline of the brain, just inferior to the hypothalamus. As described in Chapter 32, the pituitary gland consists of the *anterior pituitary* (adenohypophysis) and the *posterior pituitary* (neurohypophysis). The axons of hypothalamic neurons project directly into the posterior pituitary through the infundibular stalk. The anterior pituitary is not connected to the hypothalamus by neuronal tissue, but the pituitary blood supply makes the adenohypophysis the recipient of venous blood draining directly from the hypothalamus (the hypothalamic-pituitary portal system).

Histology

Each ovary has an inner *medulla* that contains the ovarian blood vessels and an outer *cortex* that contains the **follicles**, the functional components of the ovary (Figure 36.3). A follicle is composed of three different cell types: oocytes, granulosa cells, and theca cells. Each follicle contains one **oocyte**, or central egg. Depending on the stage of development of the follicle, the oocyte is surrounded by a number of other cells and associated structures. A clear area called the *zona pellucida* insulates the oocyte with a

layer of mucopolysaccharides. The cells closest to the oocyte are **granulosa cells**, which are surrounded by a basal lamina or basement membrane. Outside this basal lamina are the **theca cells**. When an oocyte leaves the follicle in the process of ovulation, the remaining parts of the follicular tissue—granulosa cells, theca cells, and ovarian fibroblasts—change organization and function and are called the **corpus luteum** (Latin for "yellow body"). When the corpus luteum degenerates, it turns into a scar-like structure called the *corpus albicans* (literally, the "body being white").

The wall of the fallopian tubes contains smooth muscle, while the cells of their luminal surfaces are lined with long cilia. These project into the fallopian tube lumen to help propel an egg down the tube from ovary to uterus.

The walls of the uterus are composed of an outer serosa (mesothelium), a thick smooth muscle layer called the **myometrium**, and an inner mucosal layer called the **endometrium** (see Figure 36.2). The superficial layer of the endometrium, the *stratum functionalis*, is composed of porous connective tissue (called the stroma) invested with secretory glands. The functionalis grows up to a centimeter thick and then is sloughed during menstruation. A deeper layer, the *stratum basalis*, proliferates to create a new functionalis. Arcuate arteries run through the myometrium parallel to the mucosal surface. Two sets of vessels branch off of the arcuates perpendicularly to supply the endometrium: the straight arteries, which supply the basalis, and the coiled or *spiral arteries*, which supply the functionalis. (See Clinical Application Box *What Are Uterine Fibroids?*)

The hypothalamus has numerous collections of nerve cells called nuclei. The **hypothalamic nuclei** relevant to the female reproductive system are the arcuate nucleus in the medial basal hypothalamus, and the paraventricular and supraoptic nuclei, which contain the magnocellular cells. Some cells important for female reproduction are also distributed diffusely throughout the hypothalamus and are not localized in nuclei. At least five different cell types inhabit the anterior lobe of the pituitary, but the ones most important for the female reproductive system are the **gonadotrophs** and the **lactotrophs** (also called mammotrophs).

Molecules: The Reproductive Hormones

Many of the hormones required for the proper functioning of the female reproductive system are members of the steroid family. Steroids are derivatives of cholesterol; other hormones involved in reproductive function are protein hormones. Before

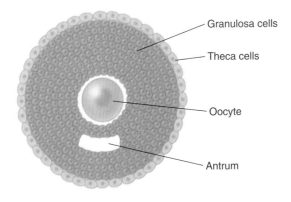

Figure 36.3   An antral ovarian follicle.

Granulosa cells

Theca cells

Oocyte

Antrum

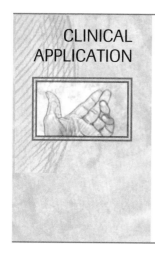

CLINICAL APPLICATION

WHAT ARE UTERINE FIBROIDS?

A 30-year-old woman complains of extreme cramping with menstruation, irregular periods, and pain during intercourse. An abdominal examination reveals a firm mass in the hypogastric region. An ultrasound scan shows a large pelvic mass, compressing her uterus.

A fibroid, or *leiomyoma*, is a benign tumor of the uterine myometrium. Leiomyomata occur in 20% to 40% of women of reproductive age and are a cause of pelvic pain. Estrogen and progesterone both contribute to the growth of fibroid tumors. In postmenopausal women or in women who do not require continued fertility, hysterectomy (removal of the uterus) is the most definitive treatment. Myomectomy (removal of the fibroid) is also possible, but fibroids often recur. Laparoscopic myomectomy and uterine artery embolization are newer treatment options.

---

detailing the function and interaction of these hormones, it may be useful to get briefly acquainted with the hormones' names, molecular structures, and sites of action. You may want to refer back to this list when you are considering system function.

The members of the steroid family germane to female reproduction are pregnenolone, **progesterone**, dehydroepiandrosterone (DHEA), androstenedione, testosterone, and the **estrogens**. The estrogens constitute a steroid subfamily. The three members of this subfamily are estrone, estradiol, and estriol. The name of each molecule indicates the subtle structural differences. *Estrone* has one OH group, *estradiol* has two such groups, and *estriol* has three. **Estradiol**, with two OH groups, is the most abundant and physiologically important of the three. All steroid hormones bind to intracellular receptors to exert their influences. The distribution of the receptors determines the distribution of the effects of the steroid hormones: the fact that a particular cell possesses the receptor for a steroid hormone makes that cell a target for that hormone. Progesterone and estrogen receptors are located throughout the body, but most importantly in the uterus, breast, hypothalamus, and pituitary.

Sex steroids are produced by the cells of the ovaries, the maternal and fetal adrenal glands, and the placenta, but many other tissues (e.g., the liver and fat tissues) are also involved in the synthesis, metabolism, and catabolism of these molecules (FIGURE 36.4). Estrogen and progesterone are transported in the blood bound to proteins called *sex hormone-binding globulins*.

Gonadotropin-releasing hormone (GnRH) is a protein hormone produced by the arcuate nucleus of the hypothalamus. The gonadotrophs of the anterior pituitary possess GnRH receptors. The pituitary produces two protein hormones critical for the proper functioning of the female reproductive system. These

hormones are called *gonadotropins* because they are intimately involved in the function of, and have an affinity (or tropism) for, the gonads. The pituitary gonadotropins are **luteinizing hormone (LH)** and **follicle-stimulating hormone (FSH)**. LH and FSH are produced and secreted by the gonadotroph cells of the anterior pituitary. They are both glycoproteins composed of alpha and beta subunits. The alpha subunit is common to both and is the same as that of thyroid-stimulating hormone (TSH) and human chorionic gonadotropin (hCG). The beta subunit is unique to each hormone and determines the specific action at the target organ or tissue. Ovarian granulosa cells possess LH and FSH receptors, and theca cells have LH receptors but no FSH receptors.

Activin, follistatin, and inhibin are glycoprotein hormones and members of the transforming growth factor beta (TGF-β) superfamily. All three appear to be produced in the ovary as well as in other body tissues. Activin acts in a paracrine fashion on sites near to its release. (Its role is not yet well understood. In the ovary, it has been shown to promote and to suppress follicular development, a subject covered below.) Follistatin binds to and inhibits activin. Inhibin circulates in the blood from the ovarian follicles to the pituitary, where it acts at receptors on the FSH-secreting gonadotrophs to attenuate FSH secretion. These hormones are an area of active research.

FIGURE 36.5 illustrates the structure of the hormonal system and its feedback mechanism, collectively known as the **hypothalamic-pituitary-gonadal (HPG) axis**. Generally speaking, GnRH promotes the secretion of FSH and LH; FSH and LH stimulate ovarian responses, including the secretion of estrogen and progesterone; estrogen and progesterone promote reversible (and at puberty some irreversible) developments of the reproductive tract and feed back negatively on FSH and LH secretion; and ovarian inhibin inhibits FSH secretion. While this abbreviated

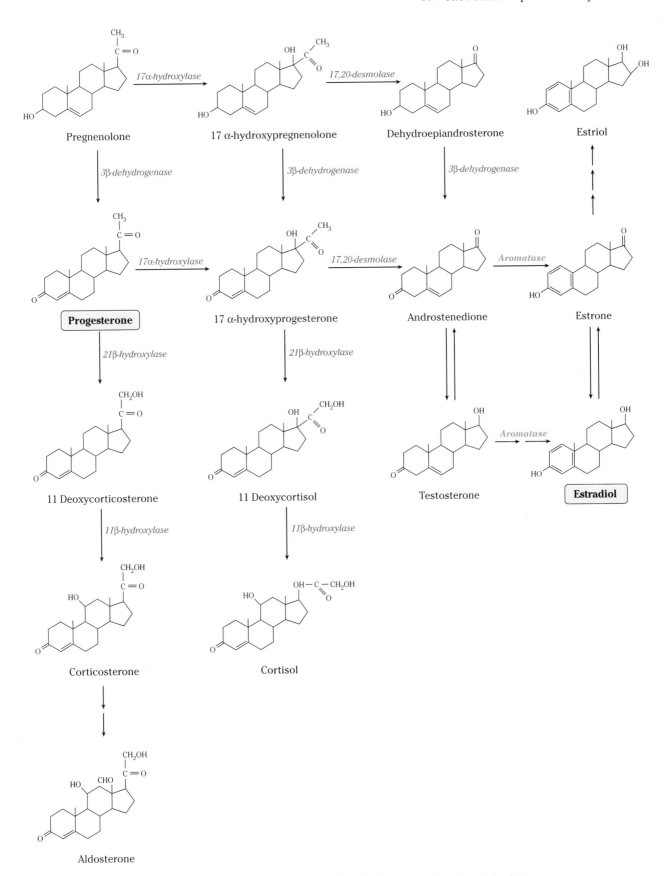

Figure 36.4   Biosynthesis of the sex steroids. Androgens are made in the theca cells of ovarian follicles, but only the granulosa cells contain aromatase. Therefore, androgens must pass from theca to granulosa to be converted to estrogens.

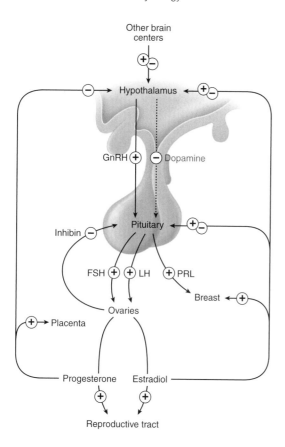

Figure 36.5 Hypothalamic-pituitary-gonadal axis: an overview. PRL, prolactin. Plus signs represent stimulation; minus signs represent inhibition.

account and Figure 36.5 may suggest that the HPG axis operates much like the other neuroendocrine axes, with hypothalamic control and negative feedback from target organ products, the reproductive axis is more complex than the other axes. The function of this system will be explored in detail below.

SYSTEM FUNCTION

Like all other organ systems, the female reproductive system starts developing before birth. Unlike the cardiovascular, pulmonary, renal, and other systems, however, the reproductive system does not need to be operational at birth. It continues to develop throughout childhood and becomes fully functional later. In fact, the achievement of total reproductive system function is the definition of both female and male biological maturity, distinguishing childhood from adulthood. Reproductive function therefore changes over the lifespan of an individual—and these changes over time are even more pronounced in the female than in the male. One function in particular—**oogenesis,** the production of eggs—begins in the first weeks of fetal life and is not completed for many years. Because of the reproductive system's evolving character, we will survey the development of female repro-

ductive function, from fetal life to middle age, when reproductive function ceases in women.

Fetal Life

A genetically distinct individual comes into being the moment that a sperm and egg fuse—the moment of **fertilization**, or *conception*. Each sperm and egg cell contains 23 unpaired chromosomes and is called **haploid** (having *half* a set of chromosomes). When the cells merge at fertilization, they form a **zygote** with 23 pairs of chromosomes for a full **diploid** set of 46. Twenty-two of these pairs are called *autosomes*; the single remaining pair are the *sex chromosomes*. There are two types of sex chromosomes: an X and a Y. When a fertilized egg has two X chromosomes, all the cells derived from the division of this fertilized egg will also have a pair of X chromosomes, and the resulting fetus is genetically female. If the zygote has one X and one Y chromosome, it is genetically male. Thus, by the time conception has occurred, sexual differentiation and sexual functioning have already begun; in the first moments of life, the organism is already preparing for the next generation.

The genetic sex of the fetus is not immediately translated into the phenotypic features of that gender, however. Initially, the developmental paths of the male and female gonads and genital systems are identical. The reproductive structures begin to take shape in the fifth week of gestation, when **germ cells** migrate from the yolk sac into the *coelom* (body cavity) inside the tiny embryo (FIGURE 36.6). They undergo mitotic division during their journey and settle into the inner surface of the embryo's dorsal

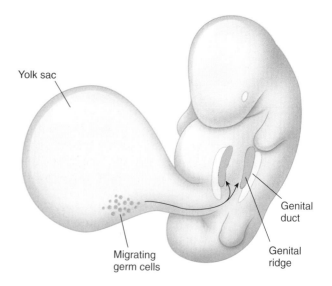

Figure 36.6 Primordial genitals around the fifth week of life. At this early stage of development, male and female genital structures are undifferentiated.

body wall. The germ cells signal the coelomic epithelium to grow and differentiate into two *genital ridges* lateral to the developing vertebral column. The genital ridges are the primordial gonads, and at this time they are still gender-indifferent (neither male nor female). They possess a medulla and cortex. By the sixth week, two pairs of genital ducts also have developed in every fetus lateral to the genital ridge: the **Wolffian ducts**, male genital precursors, also called the mesonephric ducts; and the **Müllerian ducts**, or paramesonephric ducts, the female genital precursors. (These pairs of ducts are named after 18th- and 19th-century German anatomists, but they sound as if they were named for their gender affiliations, making them easier to remember: *Müllerian* like the Latin word *mulier*, meaning woman, and *Wolffian* like *wolf*, an animal that connotes the hairiness and aggression associated with testosterone.) The rudiments of the external genitalia are also indifferent at this stage.

If a normal Y chromosome is present (i.e., if the fetus is genetically male), a gene on the Y yields a zinc finger DNA-binding protein called *testis-determining factor (TDF)*. TDF will set the gonads and genitals on the path of development into a male, preserving the Wolffian ducts and causing regression of the Müllerian ducts. If, however, the fetus has two X chromosomes, it will develop into a female without any particular single factor to tell it to do so. The "default program" of the human fetus is to form the female reproductive tract.

The first step in this default path of development is regression of the gonadal medulla and growth of the cortex (the inverse of what happens in the male), so that the indifferent gonads develop into ovaries. This begins after the sixth week of gestation. The multiplying germ cells bundled into the immature ovary differentiate into **oogonia**, egg-producing cells. The coelomic epithelial tissue surrounding the oogonia in the ovaries develops into granulosa cells, while the mesenchymal stromal cells become theca cells. By the 12th week there are millions of oogonia, and some of them begin to undergo meiosis. Signals from the granulosa will stop them, however, from completing meiosis and hence delay complete egg development until puberty many years later. It is widely believed that all the oogonia have entered meiosis by the third trimester (though some researchers have recently challenged this notion).

Meanwhile, without any TDF around to dictate otherwise, the Müllerian duct remains and the male sex precursor, the Wolffian duct, regresses. By the 9th or 10th week of gestation, the upper Müllerian ducts form the fallopian tubes, while the lower Müllerian ducts fuse to produce the uterus, cervix, and upper vagina. The genital tubercle transforms into the clitoris, the urethral folds transform into the labia minora, the genital swellings transform into the labia majora, and the urogenital sinus transforms into the lower vagina.

In all fetal body cells outside the ovarian germ cells, one or the other of the two X chromosomes is selected at random to be inactivated and thereafter condenses to form the Barr body. This is called *X inactivation*. In some body cells, the paternal X chromosome has been inactivated, in others the maternal. Once a given cell has selected either the paternally derived or the maternally derived X chromosome for inactivation, all of its subsequent daughter cells will have the same X chromosome inactivated. In a normal female, about 50% of the somatic cells have paternal X inactivation and 50% have maternal X inactivation.

During gestation of a normal female, the hypothalamus produces GnRH, the pituitary synthesizes LH and FSH, and the fetal adrenal glands and the placenta are active endocrine organs. Although the ovaries can synthesize and secrete some estrogens, these hormones are not necessary for female reproductive tract development in utero.

Oogenesis

We mentioned above that by the third trimester of fetal life, all or most oogonia have entered meiotic division. This is the beginning of oogenesis—the production of eggs or ova. Because the meiotic phases of oogenesis are spread out over years and are intimately linked with adult reproductive function, a detailed acquaintance with meiosis is helpful to understand adult reproductive physiology in the female. For this reason, we will briefly review the process and the purpose of meiosis and then examine its special time course in the human female.

Let's say that a man and a woman want to have a baby. To do so, each one must produce a gamete carrying genetic information, and the fusion of these gametes (conception) will create a new individual. Like all normal humans, both the man and woman have 46 chromosomes (23 pairs) each in their somatic cells. Because the fusion of sperm and ovum at conception adds paternal and maternal chromosomes up into the new individual's genetic repertoire, each gamete has to have half the number of chromosomes of a normal somatic cell if the chromosome number of a species is going to stay the same from one generation to the next. Instead of having 23 *pairs* of chromosomes, each normal sperm and ovum has 23 *single* chromosomes, so that at conception, the 23 chromosomes in the man's sperm combine with the 23 chromosomes in the woman's ovum to produce a new set of 46 (23 pairs) chromosomes. Otherwise, if the man's sperm and the woman's ovum each had 46 chromosomes, the new zygote would have 92 chromosomes and (presuming their child made 92-chromosome gametes and had a baby with a similarly endowed 92-chromosome person), the man and woman would have grandchildren with 184 chromosomes! Like all cells, however, the man's sperm are descendants of the single cell (zygote) that he was, and the woman's ova are descendants of the zygote that she was, and each of those zygotes had 46 chromosomes. While "simple" **mitosis** produces two daughter cells, each with the same 46 chromosomes as the parent cell, a

different process is needed to produce cells with only 23 chromosomes; this process is called **meiosis**.

Recall from cell biology that mitosis is divided into six phases (FIGURE 36.7):

1. **Interphase**: This is the nondividing phase in which human cells spend most of their time. At the end of interphase, internal and external signals prompt DNA replication to occur. Interphase is sometimes divided into G_1

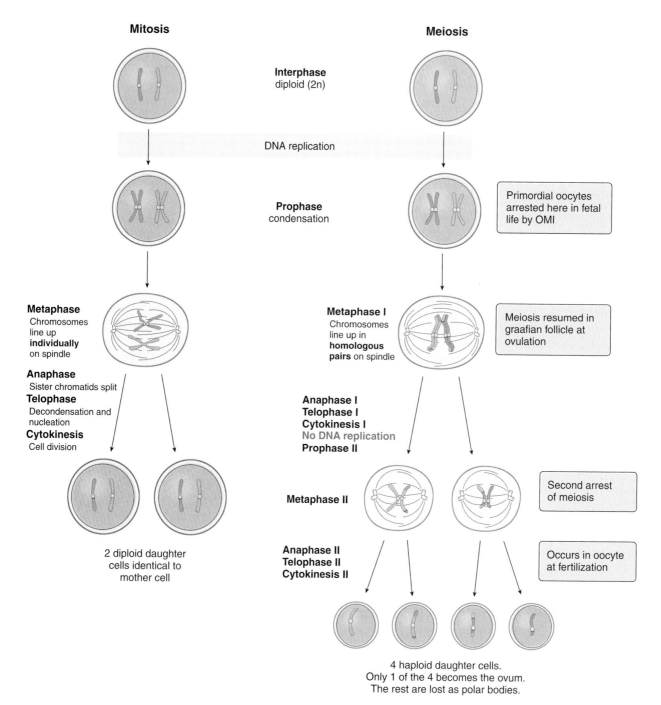

Figure 36.7   Mitosis and meiosis. Mitosis is the process of cell division. Meiosis produces gametes. In the development of the female gamete, meiosis is arrested in prophase I during fetal life, resumes at ovulation once menarche has occurred, is arrested in metaphase II, and resumes at fertilization.

phase (quiescent), *S phase* (DNA replication), and G_2 *phase* (pre-cell division).

2. **Prophase**: Chromosomes condense. Owing to replication, every one of the 46 chromosomes has an identical sister called a *chromatid*. The cell has gone from the usual amount of genetic material, called 2n (diploid), to 4n.

3. **Metaphase**: Chromosomes attach to a spindle of microtubules and line up in the midline of the cell, an area designated the *metaphase plate*.

4. **Anaphase**: Identical sister chromatids are pulled away from each other along the microtubule spindle with the help of ATP-requiring dynein motor proteins.

5. **Telophase**: Two sets of 46 chromosomes decondense and nucleate on each side of the mother cell.

6. **Cytokinesis**: The mother cell's cytoplasm splits, and two diploid daughter cells are formed.

Meiosis is divided into two subphases, meiosis I and meiosis II, each with five steps. **Meiosis I** consists of prophase I, metaphase I, anaphase I, telophase I, and cytokinesis I. **Meiosis II** consists of prophase II, metaphase II, anaphase II, telophase II, and cytokinesis II.

The quintessential differences between mitosis and meiosis are the following. In mitosis, each of the somatic cell's 46 chromosomes is replicated and lines up *individually* on the metaphase plate. This means that when the cell separates, each of the two daughter cells is identical to the mother cell, with a full set of 46 chromosomes. In meiosis, all the chromosomes replicate as in mitosis, but during metaphase I, **homologous chromosomes** pair up and these 23 *pairs* line up on the metaphase I plate. Consequently, with the first division each of the two intermediate cells receives a single double-stranded chromosome from each homologous pair. The two daughter cells are *not* identical to each other or to the mother cell. In meiosis II, *there is no further DNA replication*, and these 23 double-stranded chromosomes line up *individually* on the metaphase II plate. The double strands separate from each other. When meiosis is complete, four gametes (two pairs) have been produced from one somatic cell, each with only 23 chromosomes.

Meiosis and gametogenesis (the process by which gametes are formed and mature) differ significantly between the male and female reproductive systems. In the male, spermatogenesis occurs continuously throughout life, and a single germ cell normally produces four viable sperm. In the female, however,

meiosis is not a continuous process, and meiosis does not produce four fully functional gametes.

As we stated above, most oogonia begin the process of meiosis between the 12th and 20th week of fetal life. The first meiotic division (meiosis I) has only just begun, however, when the process is suspended in prophase I, with DNA replicated and chromosomes condensed but unattached to the spindle. Consequently, at birth, the ovarian cortex houses **primordial follicles**, which consist of 4n *oocytes* that are suspended in division, and a surrounding layer of ovarian granulosa cells. It is thought that the granulosa cells suspend the meiotic division of the primordial oocytes by synthesizing and secreting a substance called **oocyte maturation inhibitor (OMI)**. Although the primordial oocytes are "frozen" in prophase I, most do not survive to resume meiosis. While approximately 7 million primordial germ cells migrate to the ovaries during embryogenesis, by the time of birth, there has been such atrophy that only about 2 million follicles remain. This atrophy continues in postnatal life. By menarche (the onset of menstruation in adolescence), 400,000 follicles are distributed throughout the ovarian stroma. Only 300 to 400 will be released from the ovary (ovulated) before menopause; the rest will degenerate.

Surviving oocytes resume their meiotic division many years after birth, as individual follicles are recruited for meiotic completion each month in the menstrual cycle, at the time of ovulation. When meiosis does continue for the few selected oocytes, the first and second cytokinesis stages are characterized by a great disparity in the allocation of cytoplasm. With cytokinesis I, one daughter cell receives the majority of the cytoplasm and has the metabolic capacity to function, while the other daughter cell forms the first **polar body**, a sort of cellular "runt." Ovulation then occurs, with meiosis arrested again in metaphase II. At the time of fertilization, meiosis resumes again, and the secondary oocyte divides, again unequally. The final ovum takes almost all the cytoplasm, while another polar body is formed, which carries away an identical but superfluous set of chromatids and degenerates.

Adolescence and Puberty

From infancy until adolescence, the reproductive system is largely quiescent. Development of the reproductive organs begins between ages 8 and 13 in girls, a phase of life known as **puberty**. It is possible that metabolic factors contribute to the onset of puberty, perhaps with a signal related to body mass or nutritional status. However, it is not precisely known how puberty begins; it is only known that GnRH levels increase at this time. Increased GnRH levels, in turn, stimulate the pituitary to increase its output of LH and FSH. LH stimulates the theca cells of the ovarian follicles to synthesize androgens, and FSH stimulates the granulosa cells to proliferate and make more of the enzyme **aromatase**, which converts androgens to estrogens (FIGURE 36.8). (LH and FSH's effects are mediated by a cAMP-dependent mechanism.) The estrogen level rises in the blood, exposing the entire body to its effects, and inside the ovary, estrogen acts in a paracrine fashion to potentiate the influence of LH and FSH. As we will see shortly, the LH/FSH-mediated development of the follicle and of estrogen secretion

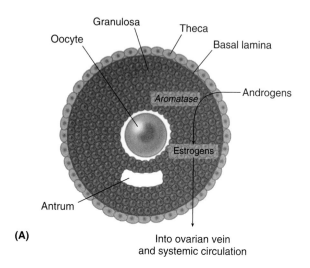

(A)

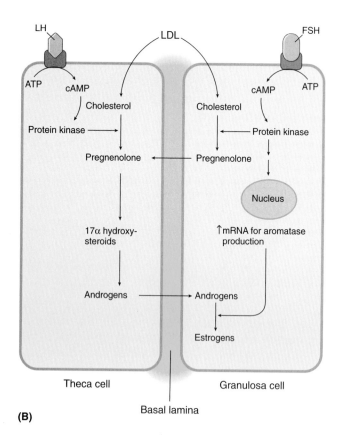

(B)

Figure 36.8   Estrogen production by the ovarian follicle. **A.** histologic view. **B.** A biochemical view.

occurs in a cyclical fashion once it is well underway, but for now it is enough to know that the adolescent body is exposed overall to higher levels of estrogen.

The increased exposure to estrogen has two primary developmental effects: the first is usually **thelarche**, the beginning of breast development. **Menarche**, the onset of menstruation, follows. (The suffix *-arche* is Greek for beginning.) Menarche begins because the gonadotropins have initiated development of the ovarian follicles, and ovulation has begun. Once follicular development has begun, the reproductive system enters into a self-sustaining monthly cycle of ovarian and uterine changes, including the vaginal bleeding of menses. (Consistent with the hypothesis of a metabolic signal to begin puberty is the observation that the average age of menarche has dropped over the past 200 years in accordance with improved nutrition in the general population. It was recorded at age 17 years in Norway in 1840 and over the past several decades has stabilized at around age 12 or 13.) Around the time of menarche or before adrenal androgens also promote the growth of pubic and axillary hair, which is known as **adrenarche**, growth hormone levels rise to promote the growth of the long bones.

Reproductive Maturity: Follicular Development and the Menstrual Cycle

It is customary to think of the neuroendocrine axes as controlled "from the top down." In other words, in most endocrine systems the hypothalamus stimulates target tissues and modulates their hormone production in accordance with feedback data, data on physiologic parameters, and circadian central nervous system rhythms. The situation is different, however, in the HPG axis. While hypothalamic GnRH does initiate puberty, it does not control postpubertal ovarian hormone secretion in the same way that it controls, for example, thyroxine production. Rather, once puberty has begun, the hypothalamic-pituitary-ovarian axis is largely controlled "from the bottom up"; that is, events initiated in the ovary dictate further ovarian developments and even dictate responses from the hypothalamus. The ovarian follicles, on a predestined course much like that of embryologic development, set the pace of monthly ovulation, uterine buildup, and uterine shedding: the **menstrual cycle**.

The Follicular Phase   As mentioned above, hundreds of thousands of follicles are embedded in the ovary with oocytes inside them arrested during meiosis prophase I. In fact, while the oocytes are all suspended at this meiotic stage, the primordial follicles have continued to develop throughout childhood (FIGURE 36.9). The granulosa cells have multiplied, a thecal cell layer has developed around the granulosa, and the oocytes

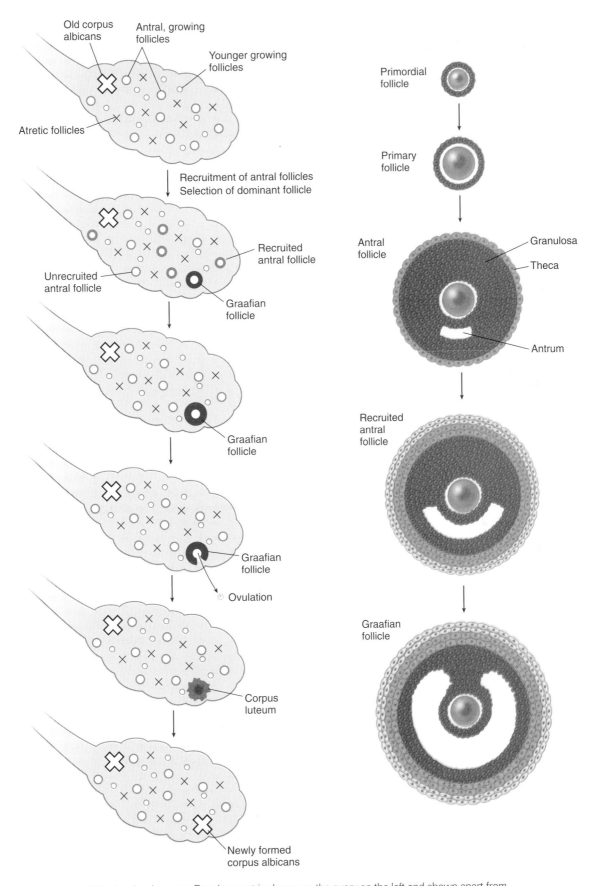

Figure 36.9 Follicular development. Development is shown on the ovary on the left and shown apart from the ovary on the right. The arrows represent the passage of time. Although the drawings are not to scale, they correlate roughly with the actual size of the structures involved. The corpus luteum in particular takes up a substantial portion of the ovarian cortex before it regresses. Only the ovarian cortex is shown; the ovarian medulla, containing the ovarian blood vessels, is not depicted.

have increased in size. Eventually, the granulosa cells secrete a fluid into the middle of the follicle containing mucopolysaccharides, electrolytes, proteins, and numerous steroid and peptide hormones (including OMI). The resultant lake of follicular fluid is called the **antrum**. The formation of **antral follicles** takes place continuously over the entire reproductive lifespan, but before puberty their destiny is **atresia**—follicular *apoptosis*, programmed cell death.

At puberty, pulsatile GnRH secretion increases in amplitude and frequency (one pulse every 60 to 200 min), in turn increasing the size and frequency of LH and FSH pulses. This exposes the ovary to increased long-term blood concentrations of LH and FSH. Under the increased pubertal influence of LH and FSH, **recruitment** begins from among those follicles at the antral stage. In each cycle, a group of around 10 follicles is recruited to develop further. They grow large, while the antral follicles not recruited take the default path of atresia. The granulosa cells of the large recruited follicles make estrogen, which stimulates the uterine endometrium to grow (FIGURE 36.10).

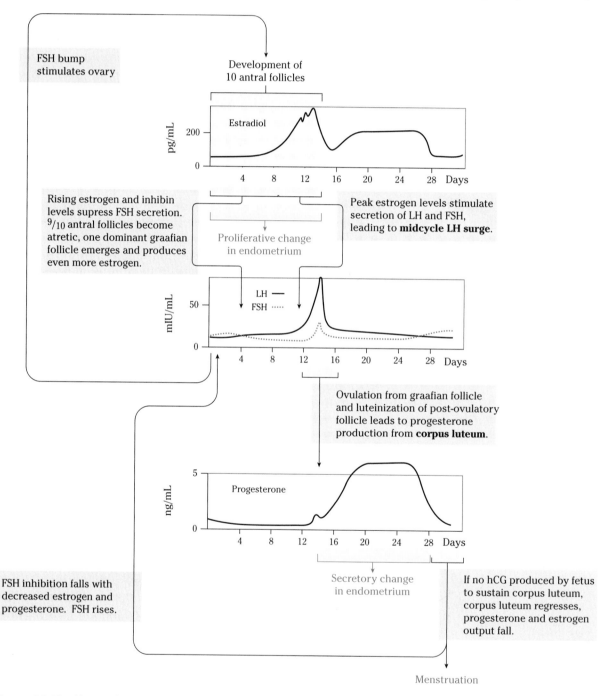

Figure 36.10   Hormonal signaling in the menstrual cycle, under the control of follicular development. The text in red refers to the uterine cycle. The text in black refers to the ovarian cycle.

Finally, for reasons not completely understood, 1 of the 10 follicles achieves a metabolic advantage and grows larger than the others. The process is sometimes referred to as **selection**. This single fully grown follicle is called the **Graafian follicle** (after the 17th-century Dutch physician Regnier de Graaf). Perhaps due to increased expression of the FSH receptor, the Graafian follicle is especially sensitive to FSH from the pituitary, which enhances its advantage over the other follicles. As all the follicles pour estrogen and inhibin into the bloodstream, these ovarian hormones begin to inhibit FSH secretion from the pituitary gonadotrophs. Lacking the Graafian follicle's enhanced FSH sensitivity, and hence lacking the growth stimulus received by the Graafian follicle, the other follicles become atretic and die. This 2-week cultivation of a Graafian follicle is called the **follicular phase** of the **ovarian cycle**. Follicular estrogen production yields endometrial growth during these 2 weeks, so that the follicular phase of the ovarian cycle coincides with the **proliferative phase** of the uterine cycle.

Ovulation   By mechanisms that are also not precisely clear, the climbing estrogen level of the follicular phase has a remarkable effect on the hypothalamus and pituitary: once it reaches a concentration of more than 100 pg/mL in the blood for more than 36 hours, it no longer inhibits LH and FSH secretion, but rather stimulates it. *The high estrogen level results in a shift from negative feedback to positive feedback.* This results in the 48-hour **midcycle surge** of LH and FSH. (LH levels increase in excess of FSH levels.) LH stimulates a burst of activity in the follicle, antagonizing the effects of OMI, and meiosis resumes. LH promotes follicular inflammation, activates proteolytic enzymes,

and initiates ovarian contractions. The contractions, the pressure accumulated in the antrum by continued fluid secretion, and the weakening of the follicular wall together lead to follicular rupture. The oocyte inside the follicle is ejected into the peritoneal cavity and clings to the ovarian capsule until it is removed by the fallopian fimbria. It then begins its journey to the uterus via the fallopian tube. This is the process known as **ovulation**. (See Clinical Application Box *How Oral Contraceptive Pills Work.*)

The Luteal Phase   FSH in the follicular phase has increased the expression of LH receptors on the granulosa of the follicle. This, in combination with the LH surge, puts the follicle under the heavy influence of LH. Under this influence, the ruptured Graafian follicle transforms into a new tissue called the **corpus luteum** (Latin for yellow body). This transformation is called **luteinization** and accounts for LH's name, luteinizing hormone.

The two major luteinizing effects of LH are a shift in enzyme expression and an alteration in the proliferative characteristics of the follicular cells. The shift in enzyme expression diverts the cells' steroidogenic pathway away from estrogen production and toward progesterone production. (The corpus luteum does produce estrogen as well, however.) Meanwhile, the follicular cells begin proliferating at an enormous rate and become heavily vascularized. They receive a copious blood supply into which they pour progesterone, which ceases the estrogen-mediated buildup of the uterus and over the next 2 weeks of the luteal phase renders the uterine lining secretory and supportive of a potential embryo. Thus, the **luteal phase** of the ovarian cycle corresponds with the **secretory phase** of the uterine cycle.

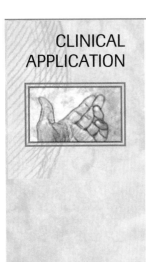

CLINICAL APPLICATION

HOW ORAL CONTRACEPTIVE PILLS WORK

Oral contraceptive pills (OCPs) capitalize on estrogen and progesterone's negative feedback effect on the hypothalamus and pituitary. By delivering daily doses of an estrogen and a progestin (which acts at the progesterone receptor), the pills inhibit the pituitary LH surge that is responsible for ovulation. (By the same mechanism, the placenta inhibits follicular development during pregnancy.) The estrogen and progesterone combination also interferes with the normal changes of the uterine cycle so that the endometrium cannot mature to its full extent. An estrogen/progestin pill is typically taken daily for 3 weeks, when a sugar pill is substituted for 1 week. This withdrawal of steroidal support from the endometrium allows menstruation in mimicry of a normal menstrual cycle.

Because of concerns about thrombotic and breast cancer risks, the estrogen content of OCPs is lower today than it was when the contraceptive pill was introduced in 1960. Today most OCPs contain 20 to 35 micrograms of ethinyl estradiol. For nonsmoking women under the age of 35, these risks are considered low enough for the benefits to outweigh the risks.

The corpus luteum is a transitory structure, fated for degeneration in 2 weeks' time unless rescued by the influence of a hormone called **human chorionic gonadotropin (hCG)**. This hormone is produced only in the context of pregnancy. It is structurally similar to, but distinct from, LH and stimulates the LH receptors of the corpus luteum, thereby enabling the survival of the corpus luteum. The corpus luteum continues to produce progesterone, maintaining the endometrial lining of the uterus in a condition supportive of a developing embryo. hCG is produced by a part of the embryo itself called the **trophoblast cells**, which will later develop into the placenta—the structure that will establish a vascular connection between mother and fetus in the womb. Home pregnancy tests measure the presence of hCG in the urine with impressive accuracy and can be confirmed in the doctor's office with a blood test for the exact hCG level.

If pregnancy does not occur, no hCG is produced and the corpus luteum degenerates. The granulosa and theca cells become necrotic, and the corpus luteum is invaded by macrophages and leukocytes, a process called **luteolysis**. Luteolysis ends with the transformation of the corpus luteum into the *corpus albicans*, a scar-like structure in the ovary. As the corpus luteum degenerates, progesterone production falls and the endometrium degenerates, having lost its supporting hormone. It is sloughed off in the bleeding of menses.

Meanwhile, the decreased progesterone and estrogen production that follows luteolysis removes inhibition from the hypothalamus and pituitary. Estrogen and progesterone have been feeding back negatively on the brain during the luteal phase, suppressing LH and FSH. The removal of this negative feedback results in a bump in FSH secretion, which initiates recruitment of another 10 antral follicles for growth. A new follicular-proliferative phase has begun. This cycle repeats for all the reproductive years of a woman's life until the supply of antral follicles is exhausted.

The Uterine Cycle   The **uterine cycle** begins with the **proliferative phase**, in which endometrial growth occurs (FIGURE 36.11). The proliferative phase coincides with the follicular phase of the ovarian cycle and takes place under the influence of estrogen from the growing follicles. As basal endometrial cells proliferate, the stratum functionalis grows and its glands and arteries elongate. The endometrium increases in thickness from 1 to 2 mm to 8 to 10 mm by day 14 (ovulation), when the proliferative phase ends. Estrogen also promotes the expression of progesterone receptors in the endometrium, preparing the endometrium for the transition into the progesterone-dominated luteal-secretory phase.

After ovulation, progesterone from the corpus luteum initiates the **secretory phase** of the uterine cycle, lasting from day 15 to day 28. The secretory phase thus coincides with the luteal phase of the ovarian cycle. During the secretory phase, endometrial maturation takes place. Estrogen levels fall, and progesterone downregulates the expression of estrogen receptors. Consequently, the high mitotic rate of the stratum basalis decreases, stopping endometrial growth. The endometrial mucus gland cells accumulate glycogen, glycoprotein, and glycolipid, and the glands and arteries become more coiled. Overall, the functionalis layer becomes a highly vascularized and nutrient-rich layer ready to support an embryo if one should arrive from a fallopian tube.

If conception does not occur, the uterine lining must be refreshed in anticipation of another ovarian cycle and possible conception. In the absence of pregnancy, the corpus luteum reaches the end of its allotted lifespan and degenerates into the corpus albicans. The functionalis, meanwhile, degenerates in parallel to the demise of its endocrine patron. The two main mechanisms of endometrial remodeling are vasoconstriction and inflammation. Vasoconstriction of the spiral arteries may occur in response to increased levels of **prostaglandins**. The **ischemia**, or lack of blood flow, results in death of the spiral arteries' endothelium, with artery rupture, bleeding, and functionalis cell necrosis. Infiltration of the lining by inflammatory cells leads to enzymatic breakdown of the endometrium. Fibrinolytic factors maintain bleeding to create a flow out of the uterus, and the entire functionalis is sloughed off over several days. The blood and shed endometrium exit the uterus by passing out of the cervix and then the vagina, resulting in menstruation—a woman's monthly period. (See Integrated Physiology Box *The Regulation of Receptor Expression and Distribution.*)

Systemic Effects of Estrogen and Progesterone in Maturity   The breasts, vagina, cervix, hypothalamic thermoregulating center, and other parts of the body are also affected by the changing hormonal milieu during the menstrual cycle. Estrogens are **mitogenic**; that is, they cause tissue to proliferate. Therefore, during the relatively estrogen-rich follicular phase, there is growth not only at the follicles of the ovary and the functionalis of the uterus, but also at the breasts, cervix, and vagina. Estrogen causes breast swelling in the first half of the menstrual cycle and breast engorgement during pregnancy. A lack of estrogen leads to flattened breasts and decreased tissue turgor at menopause.

Estrogen leads to the production of thin, clear, watery, and elastic mucus by the endocervical glands. *Spinnbarkeit* refers to the elasticity of cervical

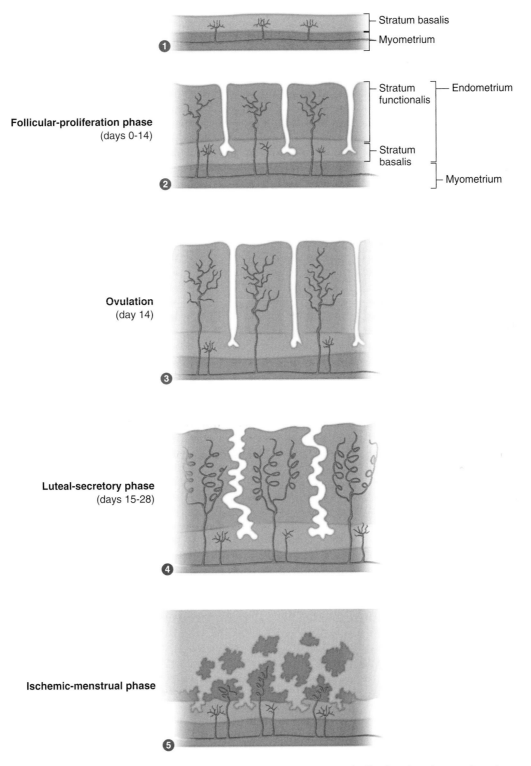

Follicular-proliferation phase
(days 0-14)

Ovulation
(day 14)

Luteal-secretory phase
(days 15-28)

Ischemic-menstrual phase

Figure 36.11 The endometrium through the phases of the uterine cycle. The first three images show the progressive growth of the endometrium under the influence of follicular estrogen. The fourth image shows the increased tortuosity of the spiral arteries and endometrial glands under the influence of progesterone from the corpus luteum. The fifth image shows the breakdown of the endometrium and bleeding from ruptured spiral arteries under the influence of ischemia.

The Regulation of Receptor Expression and Distribution

Many hormones promote changes in gene expression, and this signaling mechanism is put to a very particular use in some organ systems. In the female reproductive system, for example, hormones signal a tissue to manufacture and express a new class of *receptors*. One hormone can alter a tissue's receptivity to the signal of another hormone. When the second signal arrives in the bloodstream, the tissue has been primed to respond to it in a different way than previously. By this mechanism, hormones can reversibly alter the function of certain tissues in a highly controlled manner.

Here are two important examples of such regulation of receptor distribution and reversible tissue transformation in the female reproductive system. (1) FSH stimulates the expression of LH receptors in the Graafian follicle, thereby preparing the follicular tissue for differentiation into another tissue (the corpus luteum) capable of executing LH-mediated commands. (2) Estrogen stimulates the uterine endometrium to express progesterone receptors, enabling transformation of the endometrium into a secretory, nutrient-rich layer under the influence of progesterone. It is as if one hormone were "teaching" a tissue the "message-language" of another hormone, thereby translating the tissue from one class of functions to another. Progesterone also "teaches" the endometrium to *stop* listening to the message-language of estrogen.

Although there are many other examples of the regulation of receptor expression in biology, the mechanism seems to be particularly important in the female reproductive system. (FSH stimulates the expression of the androgen receptor in Sertoli cells in the testis of the male. Thyroid hormone may increase the expression of cardiac beta-adrenergic receptors.) One reason this form of signaling may be rare in other systems is that the female reproductive system relies on the genesis and degeneration of transient organs like the corpus luteum, the stratum functionalis, the placenta, and the lactating breast lobule. The female reproductive system thus relies on the temporary genetic differentiation of tissues, and it accomplishes this by switching the receptor classes expressed in those tissues.

mucus, and it is measured by physical stretching. Because this sort of mucus is associated with high estrogen levels, it is most prominent during the follicular phase and immediately before the midcycle surge. An increased spinnbarkeit (with stretching of mucus >10 cm) has been interpreted clinically as a sign of midcycle ovulation. The vaginal mucosa also responds to estrogen levels, subtly thickening and thinning over the menstrual cycle and noticeably undergoing atrophy at menopause. Estrogen has also been shown to maintain bone density, which is one reason postmenopausal women suffer a decline in bone mass (osteoporosis).

Progesterone also has systemic effects, many of which share the function of tissue differentiation into secretory units. Whereas estrogen stimulates the ductal elements of the breast to grow, progesterone stimulates the secretory acinar glands to develop. (This will be discussed below under the topic of pregnancy.) Similarly, estrogen stimulates the functionalis to grow during the proliferative phase, and progesterone then induces it to produce mucus during the secretory phase. Progesterone converts the endocervical mucus from a thin, watery type to thick, opaque, viscous mucus. During pregnancy, this mucus becomes so thick that it forms a plug in the cervix.

Progesterone causes an increase in the basal body temperature of about 0.6°F. This increased temperature is apparent within 24 hours of ovulation and remains elevated for 11 or 12 days (or more, if a pregnancy occurs and maintains the corpus luteum). Finally, progesterone causes many symptoms commonly referred to as *premenstrual syndrome*, which occur just before menses, in concurrence with peak progesterone levels. These symptoms include breast tenderness, bloating, swelling of the extremities, and mood changes. Women who have no progesterone, such as anovulatory women, prepubescent girls, and postmenopausal women, do not have these symptoms.

Menopause

As we saw above, the vast majority of antral follicles are not recruited for further growth and undergo atresia. Over many years, atresia of unrecruited follicles results in exhaustion of the oocyte store. As a woman approaches age 50 years, the groups of follicles recruited begin to dwindle in number. Fewer maturing follicles each month leads to decreased estrogen and inhibin production, because there is less follicular tissue available to make these hormones. The decline in estrogen and inhibin output lessens the inhibition of FSH secretion from the pituitary, and FSH levels rise. Increased FSH levels may hasten the development of the follicle and shorten the cycle, leading to lighter or irregular menstrual periods. Small follicle cohorts and abnormal patterns of follicular stimulation may also mean that some cycles do not lead to ovulation. The period may in this case be skipped entirely, and prolonged uterine proliferation can result in a heavy period at the next menstruation.

This time of waning follicular recruitment and irregular periods is a transitional phase known as **menopause**. As the transition progresses toward total exhaustion of the stored oocyte pool and cessation of the menstrual cycle, women often experience a few characteristic symptoms in addition to irregular menses. The most common one is *hot flashes*—an intermittent and uncomfortable (but harmless) disturbance in temperature regulation related to decreasing estrogen levels. Hot flashes and other symptoms may be treated with short-term *hormone replacement therapy (HRT)*—exogenous estrogen—as is administered in oral contraceptives.

After the menopause transition is complete and the final menstrual period has occurred, estrogen levels decline in women. The putative risks of low estrogen levels, such as fractures due to osteoporosis, are a subject of ongoing research and controversy, as is the risk-benefit analysis of long-term HRT. However, the medical community is generally moving away from long-term HRT as a preventative of chronic disease in postmenopausal women. Studies have shown associated risks (e.g., breast cancer, blood clotting, and coronary artery disease). HRT is the best current treatment for symptoms of menopause, however. Balancing these concerns can be complicated for women at this life stage.

SYSTEM STRUCTURE: PREGNANCY

As mentioned, the functions of the female reproductive system depend on the ongoing development of new tissues and structures. Pregnancy involves not only the structures discussed in the previous section, but also several others. Like the corpus luteum or stratum functionalis, these other structures are transient and last only as long as they are needed to support pregnancy or breast feeding.

The Organs of Pregnancy

The **placenta** serves as the point of exchange between the circulatory systems of the mother and fetus; it is also a hormone-producing organ. The fully developed placenta is a round oval organ 15 to 20 cm in diameter and 2 to 3 cm thick, embedded in the uterine wall. It connects to the developing fetus via the **umbilical cord** (FIGURE 36.12A). Along with the baby, it is expelled from the uterus during birth.

The placenta is composed of segments called *cotyledons*. Fingers of placental tissue (**chorionic villi**) extend into a pool of arterial maternal blood in the uterine wall, the **intervillous space** (see FIGURE 36.12B). The intervillous space is supplied by uterine spiral arteries, which have developed under the influence of progesterone; its location in the uterine wall is designated the *decidua basalis*. The villi contain fetal capillary plexuses. Bathed in the maternal blood of the intervillous space, the fetal capillaries of the villi passively absorb oxygen and nutrients and pass carbon dioxide and waste products into the maternal blood. The intervillous blood then drains back into the maternal circulation through the uterine veins in the decidua basalis.

The outer sheath of the villi is a layer called the **chorion**, which is composed of trophoblast cells. The chorionic barrier between the fetal villous blood and the maternal intervillous blood blocks the passage of most cells and large proteins, including peptide hormones. It allows the passage of steroid hormones. The chorion not only covers the villi but also extends beyond the placenta to envelop the entire **amnion**, the sac that contains the developing fetus in its **amniotic fluid**.

After a baby is born, the mother's body can continue to provide nourishment via the paired milk-producing **mammary glands**, or breasts (FIGURE 36.13). Breasts can be thought of as a collection of sweat glands that have through evolution acquired the ability to produce milk. They lie beneath the skin and subcutaneous fat but above the deep fascia of the thorax (with the exception of the axillary tail of the breast, which lies beneath the fascia). The breasts are composed mainly of fat and connective tissue.

The mammary glandular tissue is divided into 15 to 20 *lobules* arranged in a radial pattern around the areola of the nipple. Each lobule connects to the outside world through a network of *lactiferous ducts*. The lactiferous ducts merge with each other as they approach the nipple, and there are about 5 to 10 duct openings on the nipple surface. The lobules are composed of individual **mammary alveoli**. Each

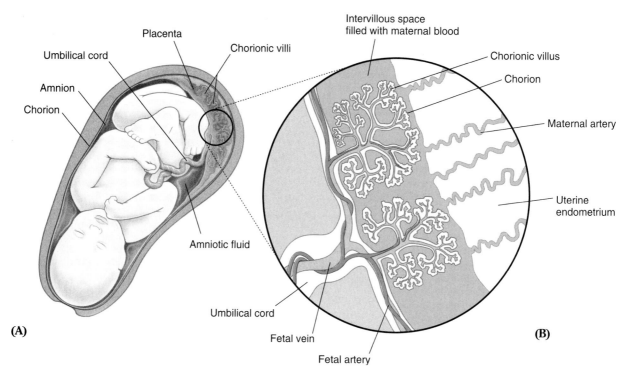

Figure 36.12 The placenta, chorionic villi, and intervillous space. **A.** The position of the fetus and placenta within the uterus. **B.** A closer view of the villi and intervillous space.

alveolus is lined with epithelial cells and a sublayer of myoepithelial cells. Fat is scattered generously between the lobules and the ducts. Ligaments of connective tissue network from the deep fascia of the thorax to the skin overlying the breasts. These are called the *suspensory ligaments of Cooper.* Lymphatic drainage from the breast is mainly to the axillary lymph nodes.

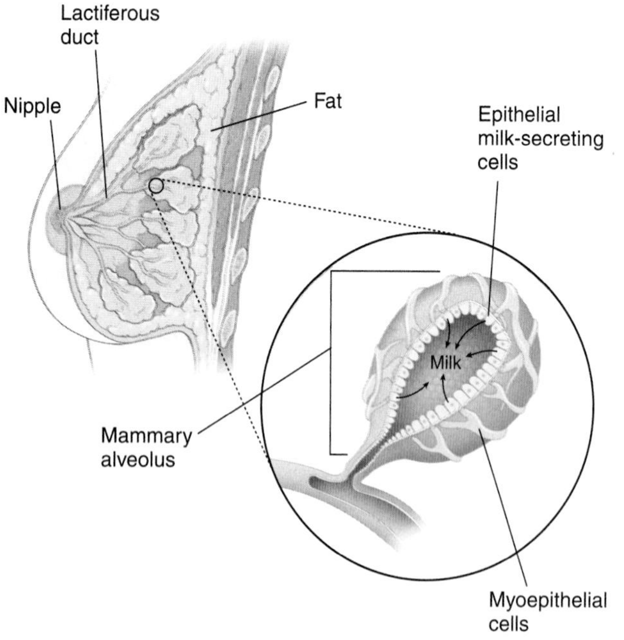

Molecules: The Hormones of Pregnancy

Because of the complexity of hormonal interactions during pregnancy, we will once again begin with a list of the names of the hormones involved, their structures, and sites of production and action. You may want to refer back to this list when you are considering system function in later sections of the chapter. We have already mentioned hCG and described a little of its function in maintaining the corpus luteum and progesterone production. **hCG** is a heterodimeric glycoprotein synthesized and secreted by trophoblast cells of the placenta. Like LH, FSH, and TSH, hCG has an alpha and a beta subunit. The alpha subunit has the same amino acid sequence as that of LH, FSH, and TSH. The beta subunit is almost identical to that of LH but differs by having 31 extra amino acids at the carboxy terminus. hCG differs from the other three hormones in the number and type of carbohydrate side chains on the polypeptide subunits. Because hCG is more heavily glycosylated than LH, FSH, and TSH, it has a much longer half-life. The ovarian corpus luteum has hCG receptors.

Relaxin, a polypeptide hormone secreted by the ovaries and other tissues, is active in many of the

Figure 36.13 The mammary gland and mammary alveoli. The mammary alveoli are not drawn to scale; in reality, they are much smaller and more numerous.

structures of pregnancy. One of its functions is to relax the birth canal by proliferative effects on the surrounding tissues, which facilitates the delivery of a baby. The G-protein-linked relaxin receptor (LGR7) is expressed in the connective tissue of the uterine endometrium and the connective tissue of the breast. Relaxin likely also acts in the small intestine through a nitric oxide-mediated mechanism to depress intestinal motility (which may be the reason for many of the gastrointestinal symptoms of pregnancy), and decreases blood vessel tone through nitric oxide.

Prolactin is a polypeptide hormone synthesized and secreted by lactotroph cells in the anterior pituitary. It is structurally similar to growth hormone, as is its receptor. Breast tissue alveolar epithelial cells have prolactin receptors.

Oxytocin is a peptide product of hypothalamic magnocellular neurons and is released from the posterior pituitary. The cell bodies of the magnocellular neurons are located in the hypothalamic supraoptic and paraventricular nuclei. After production in these cell bodies, the oxytocin is packaged into secretory granules, transported down the axons within the infundibular stalk, and secreted at the axon terminals within the posterior pituitary. Oxytocin receptors are found on uterine myometrial cells and breast tissue myoepithelial cells.

Human chorionic somatomammotropin (hCS), also called human placental lactogen (hPL), is another protein hormone synthesized and secreted by the placenta. It strongly resembles prolactin and growth hormone and mimics their effects in the mother's body.

The **prostaglandins** are a family of related molecules derived from arachidonic acid. Among the many members of this family, prostaglandins E_2 (PGE$_2$) and $F_{2\alpha}$ (PGF$_{2\alpha}$) are important in labor.

SYSTEM FUNCTION: PREGNANCY

With the achievement of a pregnancy, the female reproductive system changes function. The ovaries and uterus abandon their monthly cycles and instead promote the growth of the fetus, the changes in the pelvis necessary to facilitate delivery, and the development of the breasts necessary for **lactation**, or milk production, during the *postpartum period*, the period of time after birth.

Sexual Response in the Female

Fertilization may result from **sexual intercourse** between a male and female. The sexual response cycle consists of four phases: *excitement, plateau, orgasm,* and *resolution*. In males and females, sexual intercourse is preceded by the condition of libido or desire, which leads to arousal or excitement in a sexual encounter. In the female, the excitement and plateau phases involve secretory lubrication of the vagina and elevation of the uterus in the pelvis. Orgasm is associated with spasm of the vaginal walls. Females can usually achieve arousal again shortly after orgasm, unlike males, who have a refractory period that increases with age.

Chronic disease states of all varieties may alter an individual's self-image with respect to sexuality or sexual performance, or that of his or her partner. Consequently, chronic disease may interfere with desire and excitement, thereby disrupting the normal cycle of human sexual response. In addition, psychological problems often include or manifest as disturbances in the capacity for desire or excitement.

Fertilization

Once ejaculated into the vagina, sperm must undergo *capacitation*—cytologic changes that prepare the sperm for fusion with an egg. Capacitation occurs inside the female reproductive tract and involves the loss of sperm surface glycoproteins and lipids as well as an increase in sperm motility. The process takes more than 1 hour. Capacitated sperm can last up to 2 days in the female reproductive tract, but for fertilization to occur, sperm must reach the oocyte within 24 hours of ovulation. Therefore, for fertilization to occur, intercourse must usually take place from 1 to 2 days before ovulation to 1 day after.

Pregnancy begins with a spermatozoon's fertilization of a secondary oocyte—an ovulated oocyte arrested in metaphase II of meiosis. The sperm swim from the vagina, through the cervix and uterus, and into the fallopian tube, where they encounter or wait for the oocyte in the ampulla. Estrogen-dependent proliferative-phase changes in the female reproductive tract encourage the sperm's progress: vaginal glycogen production acidifies the vagina and enhances sperm motility, and watery cervical fluid promotes the sperm's passage, as does the enhanced contractility of the myometrium. Still, only one sperm in about a million reaches the ampulla. Shortly before or after the sperm's arrival, the oocyte is waved into the ampulla by the cilia lining the fallopian tube. The oocyte has endured countless waves of atresia in the ovary to become one of several hundred ovulatory oocytes out of the 7 million initial candidates.

Each sperm cell in the ampulla penetrates the outer shell of the secondary oocyte, the *corona radiata*, by driving forward with flagellar movements. When one reaches the zona pellucida, a glycoprotein in the zona triggers the release of proteolytic enzymes from the **acrosome**, or head of the sperm (FIGURE 36.14). The enzymes break down the zona and the sperm drives into the oocyte. Although hundreds of tiny sperm may encounter the gigantic oocyte at nearly the same time, once a single sperm makes it through the zona pellucida, cortical granules in the oocyte release proteases in what is called the *zona reaction* and render the zona impenetrable to other sperm, thus preventing multiple fertilization. Once inside the zona pellucida, the cell membranes of the sperm and egg fuse, making their cytoplasm continuous. This stimulates the nucleus of the secondary oocyte to complete meiosis II and form the mature haploid ovum while casting off a second polar body. The nuclei of the mature ovum and the spermatozoon then fuse, forming a zygote with 46 chromosomes.

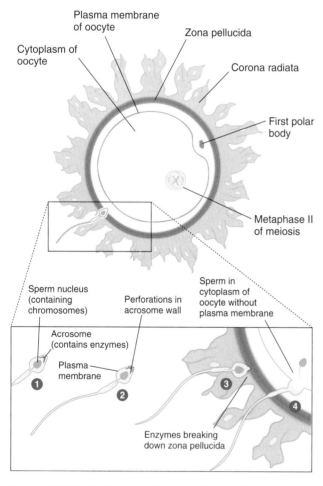

Figure 36.14 Fertilization. After capacitation, the acrosome of the sperm can release its digestive enzymes. The enzymes digest part of the zona pellucida around the oocyte and ultimately merge the cytoplasm of the two gametes. The oocyte, arrested in metaphase II of meiosis, now resumes meiosis and generates a second polar body.

Development From Zygote to Embryo

When the zygote begins to divide, it is called an embryo. The embryo slowly drifts down the fallopian tube, dividing as it travels, and enters the uterus approximately 3 days after fertilization. It increases in cell number along the way, but not in size, which prevents it from getting stuck in the fallopian tube; once in the uterus, the embryo consists of about 12 cells clustered into a ball and is called a **morula** (FIGURE 36.15). The morula develops into a **blastocyst**, an asymmetric ball of cells with a cavity of fluid inside, before it implants into the wall of the uterus. Blastocyst formation takes roughly another 3 days. Thus, the time from fertilization to implantation in the uterus is about 6 days. Some of the cells of the blastocyst differentiate and grow into the maternal endometrial tissue. This insinuation of fetal tissue into the endometrium is called **implantation,** and the embryonic cells that invade the endometrium are known as **trophoblasts**. It appears that the trophoblasts lack the *major histocompatibility complexes* by which a maternal immune response could be mounted against the foreign embryonic tissue. Other mechanisms also appear to defend the embryo against the mother's immune system (but some maternal autoimmune conditions, such as autoimmune thyroiditis, are associated with increased rates of spontaneous abortion, ostensibly due to attack by the maternal immune system). Soon after implantation, the trophoblasts begin to produce hCG.

The Placenta and the Hormones of Pregnancy

The placenta is a transient organ derived from embryonic tissue. As stated above, it not only serves as a site of exchange between maternal and fetal circulations, but also secretes hormones that maintain pregnancy. Its hormones are derived from two sources: de novo synthesis of polypeptide hormones and conversion of hormonal precursors. Hormones synthesized from scratch include hCG and hCS. The high levels of steroid hormones (progesterone and estrogen) characteristic of pregnancy are due to placental conversion of precursors: maternal cholesterol into progesterone and fetal adrenal androgens into estrogens.

hCG and hCS   hCG from placental trophoblasts mimics the effects of LH and preserves the corpus luteum, and hence the endometrial functionalis, as described above. The trophoblastic hormone is the basis of all pregnancy tests because it is a hormone unique to the pregnant state, and because its serum level doubles approximately every 1.7 to 2 days during the early weeks of pregnancy. It is thus easily

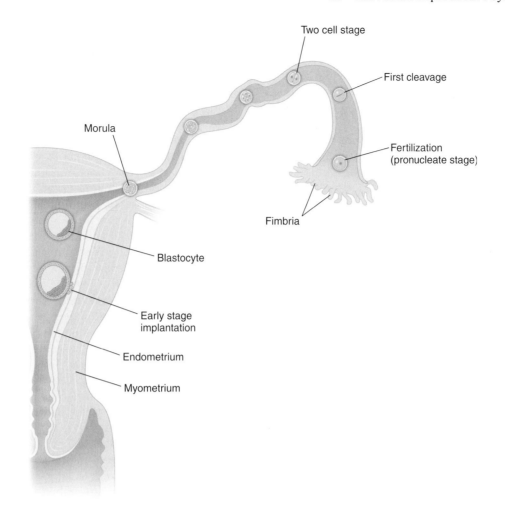

Figure 36.15 Implantation.

detected and quantified in maternal peripheral blood. Trophoblastic production of hCG peaks at around the 10th week of gestation, then drops off and plateaus at a lower level.

Progesterone secreted under the aegis of hCG prolongs pregnancy not only by maintaining the endometrium but also by keeping the myometrium silent. If there is an early fetal demise and the production of hCG stops, the myometrium begins to contract and the endometrium begins to shed. This is known as **spontaneous abortion**, or *miscarriage*. Progesterone secreted during pregnancy also thickens the cervical mucus and closes the cervical os to seal the uterus.

hCS is produced by the placenta beginning in the fourth or fifth week of gestation. In accordance with its structural similarity to growth hormone, hCS functions as a counterregulatory hormone, just as growth hormone does. The counterregulatory hormones (glucagon, cortisol, epinephrine, and growth hormone) oppose the effects of insulin and raise the blood glucose. By mimicking growth hormone in this

respect, hCS makes more circulating glucose available for fetal consumption. For this reason, it may contribute to gestational diabetes—high blood sugar levels associated with pregnancy. While production of hCS begins early in pregnancy, it plays a larger role later in pregnancy. The placenta also produces many other hormones with a vast array of effects on other organ systems, some of which will be explored below.

Progesterone and Estrogen During Pregnancy Also at around 10 weeks, the developing placenta acquires the ability to convert maternal cholesterol into progesterone, thereby eliminating the dependence on the corpus luteum for progesterone to maintain the pregnancy. Meanwhile, placental signals such as hCG also lead to high estrogen levels in the maternal circulation. They do so by stimulating the fetal adrenal glands to produce large amounts of androgens (mainly DHEA), which circulate to the aromatase-rich placenta and are converted to estrogens. *The placenta thus keeps the maternal circulation high in progesterone and estrogen.*

High levels of progesterone and estrogen feed back negatively on the hypothalamus and pituitary, suppressing LH and FSH secretion and thereby inhibiting follicular development and ovulation until the pregnancy ends. Progesterone continues to maintain the quiescence of the myometrium and opposes the softening of the cervix seen at birth; it thereby helps to prevent premature birth. Estrogen causes the breasts to develop in anticipation of lactation and stimulates prolactin production in the pituitary lactotrophs. During pregnancy, prolactin also stimulates the development of breast tissue. (See Clinical Application Box *The "Abortion Pill."*)

The Effects of Pregnancy Outside the Reproductive System

A woman's body undergoes significant physiologic changes during pregnancy, and these changes are of two general types. First, the altered hormonal milieu established by the placenta drives changes in the functioning of many organ systems. Second, the fetus puts new metabolic and mechanical stresses on normal organ systems. Whether by hormonal alterations in function or by physiologic adaptations to new stresses, the organ systems must meet the added demand for energy, oxygen, and nutrients posed by the developing fetus. The etiology of the many physiologic changes of pregnancy is complex and incompletely understood, but their outcomes are known. These changes explain many of the symptoms experienced by pregnant women and account for the fact that many reference values for lab tests are different in pregnancy than in nongravid (nonpregnant) physiology.

Changes in Metabolism *Early pregnancy is characterized by anabolism, later pregnancy by catabolism.* Early pregnancy features the maternal storing of energy and the building of macromolecules, while later pregnancy involves the consumption of maternal energy stores to feed the anabolic growth of the fetus. From one point of view, pregnancy constitutes a transfer of potential energy from mother to child. In the earlier phase of pregnancy, the synthesis of lipids, glycogen, and protein increases under the influence of insulin. In the later phase, high levels of hCS promote the degradation of maternal lipids, glycogen, and proteins to supply fatty acids, glucose, and amino acids to the growing fetus. Maternal cortisol production is also increased during pregnancy, partly under the influence of placental corticotrophin-releasing hormone (CRH). As a counterregulatory hormone, cortisol may contribute to the catabolic phase of pregnancy.

In the case of bone, the transfer of building blocks from maternal stores to the fetus would compromise the integrity of the maternal skeleton. Consequently, the placenta tries to recruit the calcium needed for fetal ossification not from maternal bones, but directly from the outside world. It does so by activating more vitamin D, which increases calcium absorption from the maternal intestines. Finally, placental estrogen increases the hepatic synthesis of thyroid-binding globulin (TBG) and decreases the hepatic clearance of TBG. Increased levels of TBG

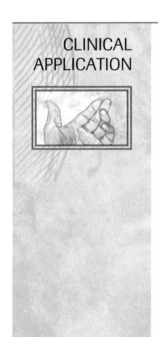

CLINICAL APPLICATION

THE "ABORTION PILL"

Mifepristone (trade name RU-486 from Roussel-Uclaf) is the controversial drug sometimes referred to as the "abortion pill." Its mechanism of action is competitive inhibition of progesterone at the progesterone receptor. Its antiprogesterone effect enables it to interfere with both fertility and pregnancy. Because progesterone acts during pregnancy to oppose myometrial contractions and to stabilize the cervix, mifepristone's antagonism of progesterone can cause cervical softening and uterine contraction, and it thereby acts as an effective abortifacient in the first 9 weeks of pregnancy. It is sometimes used in combination with an orally or vaginally administered prostaglandin analog, **misoprostol**, which activates collagenases and softens the cervical connective tissue, just as endogenous prostaglandins do during labor.

Despite the strong links between mifepristone and abortion in the minds of the public, the drug has other potential uses. If administered within 3 days of unprotected sex, it can prevent implantation of an embryo by opposing progesterone's supportive actions on the endometrium. It could thus act similarly to the "morning-after pill," also called emergency contraception, which is a high-dose ethinyl estradiol pill. Mifepristone can also promote fetal expulsion after miscarriage and may have other applications, such as the induction of labor.

result in increased total maternal thyroxine levels, as more thyroid hormone is produced in order to fill the TBG reservoir. Maternal thyroxine demand also increases independently of changes in TBG, which may reflect first-trimester losses of thyroxine to the fetus. Untreated hypothyroidism in pregnant mothers is known to retard the neurologic development of the fetus.

Renal, Cardiovascular, and Hematologic Changes

During pregnancy, systemic vascular resistance (SVR) drops. This is in part a result of systemic vasodilation, which may be due to the elaboration of prostaglandins that decrease blood vessel sensitivity to angiotensin II, a vasoconstrictor. SVR also drops because the decidua basalis represents an addition to the systemic vasculature of a new path of blood flow. The spiral arteries, intervillous space, and uterine veins are a circuit added in parallel. Recall that with more parallel pathways, the cross-sectional area of the circulatory system increases, thereby dropping resistance.

Decreased SVR is compensated for by increased cardiac output and by increased activity of the renin-angiotensin-aldosterone (RAA) system, which together maintain blood pressure. Since angiotensin II's vasoconstrictive effects appear to be partly blocked during pregnancy, the RAA system probably maintains blood pressure more through extracellular fluid volume expansion than through vasoconstriction. RAA activity increases plasma volume by as much as 45% by the third trimester, and increased fluid volume can account for 6 to 8 kg of the weight gained during pregnancy.

Erythrocyte volume also increases (by 20% to 40%, depending on the availability of iron stores) under the influence of elevated erythropoietin levels. Because the plasma volume generally increases in excess of the increase in blood cell mass, the hematocrit is expected to drop by 4% to 7%. (Recall that the hematocrit is the percentage of the blood volume accounted for by red blood cells.)

Increased systemic blood flow translates into an increased renal blood flow and an increased glomerular filtration rate (GFR). The GFR increases by nearly half again (then plateaus) by week 10. The increased GFR results in lower serum creatinine and urea nitrogen levels and increased urine volume. Later in pregnancy, the uterus compresses the bladder, limiting bladder volume and increasing the frequency and urgency of urination. When the uterus attains this size, it can also compress the inferior vena cava, especially when the pregnant mother lies in the supine position (on her back). This compression results in impaired venous return to the heart and may lead to lightheadedness. Finally, osmoregulation

is somewhat different in pregnancy because the hypothalamic threshold for the secretion of antidiuretic hormone (ADH) is lower, meaning that the plasma-diluting effect of ADH is invoked more quickly. This may be another means of supporting the blood volume to adequately perfuse the blood vessels under circumstances of enlarged SVR.

Pulmonary Changes

Pulmonary function during pregnancy is influenced by two factors: decreased lung volumes owing to pressure from the enlarging uterus and progesterone's stimulatory effect on the respiratory drive. As the uterus grows, it pushes up on the diaphragm, thus decreasing the space available in the thorax. Functional residual capacity (FRC)—the lung volume just before inhalation with breathing muscles at rest—thus declines. However, the diaphragm can still contract normally and airway function is normal. Tidal volume, the size of each normal inhalation, increases during pregnancy because of progesterone's stimulation of increased central respiratory drive. Increased tidal volumes raise the PO_2 and lead to respiratory alkalosis, which is compensated by increased renal excretion of bicarbonate. Increased PO_2 in maternal blood helps drive the diffusion of oxygen from the intervillous blood into the chorionic capillaries. The high oxygen affinity of fetal hemoglobin compared with adult hemoglobin further supports this oxygen transfer. TABLE 36.1 summarizes the maternal changes during pregnancy.

Parturition

Parturition is the medical term for birth, which takes place after roughly 40 weeks of gestation in humans. (Obstetricians count weeks of gestation from the date of the last menstrual period rather than from conception, since the exact time of conception can be difficult to define with certainty.) Uncoordinated uterine contractions (called Braxton-Hicks contractions) and cervical softening begin around 1 month before the end of gestation, and parturition commences with the accelerated cervical dilation and coordinated uterine contractions known as **labor**. The contractions of labor, unlike Braxton-Hicks contractions, get increasingly stronger, longer, and closer together. A decrease in fetal movement can also signal the onset of labor. Close to or during labor, the chorionic and amniotic membranes rupture under pressure (commonly referred to as "water breaking"). The contractions ultimately drive the fetus out of the uterus and through the dilated cervix and vagina.

The proliferative effects of relaxin have helped prepare the perineum for its role as birth canal. The placenta is expelled soon afterward, and intense uterine contractions, possibly driven by oxytocin, help

Table 36.1   MATERNAL CHANGES DURING PREGNANCY

Maternal Organ or Parameter Affected During Pregnancy	Change During Pregnancy	Cause of Change
Myometrium	Contractions are suppressed	Progesterone At first produced in corpus luteum under influence of trophoblastic hCG, then produced directly by placenta
Cervix	Cervical os is closed, cervical connective tissue stabilized	Progesterone From corpus luteum and then placenta

Pituitary	LH and FSH secretion suppressed
	
	Prolactin production increased
		Progesterone and estrogen
		    From corpus luteum, then placenta
		Estrogen
		    From placenta

Ovary	Follicular development and ovulation suppressed	Low LH and FSH
Breast	Development of secretory apparatus, increase in size	Estrogen (from placenta) and prolactin (from pituitary)
Energy stores	Increased early in pregnancy Depleted to release fatty acids, glucose, and amino acids to fetus later in pregnancy	Insulin and other factors? hCS, cortisol?
Serum calcium	Maternal ionized calcium remains stable, but gut absorption increases	Vitamin D (activated by placenta)
Thyroxine-binding globulin (TBG) and thyroxine level	Hepatic synthesis of TBG increased, hepatic clearance of TBG decreased; total thyroxine level thus increased	Estrogen From placenta
Systemic vascular resistance (SVR)	Decreased	Prostaglandins (which decrease vessel sensitivity to angiotensin II) Addition of decidua basalis circuit
Cardiac output	Increased	?
ECF volume	Increased	RAA system
Red blood cell mass	Increased	Erythropoietin
Hematocrit	Decreased	ECF volume increased out of proportion to increases in RBC mass
Pedal edema	May appear in late pregnancy	Increased ECF volume
Venous return to the heart	May be decreased late in pregnancy in supine position	Uterine compression of inferior vena cava
GFR	Increased	Increased cardiac output Increased ECF volume
Bladder	Increased urinary frequency	Increased GFR Later in pregnancy, uterine compression of bladder
Osmoreceptor complex	ADH set point decreased; ADH more easily released	?
Functional residual capacity	Decreased	Uterine compression of diaphragm at rest
Tidal volumes and P_aO_2	Increased	Progesterone From placenta

staunch uterine bleeding. When the placenta vacates the uterus, its hormonal influence goes with it. Placental hormones remain in the maternal blood for a duration dictated by their respective half-lives, then disappear. Placental progesterone and estrogen levels fall, releasing the hypothalamus and pituitary from their inhibition. LH and FSH are once again secreted and follicular development resumes.

The initiation of parturition in humans is not well understood. Oxytocin and locally acting prostaglandins promote uterine contractions, but they do not seem to be the initial or crucial elements in the signaling pathway. Some investigators have suggested that at labor, the myometrium expresses increased numbers of oxytocin receptors. It has also been theorized that a change in the uterine ratio of progesterone and estrogen allows the myometrium to escape the inhibitory influence of progesterone, but no significant change in the levels of these hormones has been observed in humans prior to birth. A critical fetal mass may also stretch the uterus to the point where reflex contractions begin. Finally, fetal or maternal stress may trigger a rise in placental CRH levels, which in turn may somehow trigger the cascade of events leading to birth; or alternatively, increased placental CRH and fetal cortisol levels may gird the fetus for the stresses of birth. In this sense birth is, as Sigmund Freud once speculated, the inaugural stress in a life that is loaded with it.

Lactation and Mammary Physiology

The American Academy of Pediatrics advocates breast feeding as "the ideal method of feeding and nurturing infants." Indeed, evolution has refined the breast's principal function—*lactation*—so that it serves the newborn child in every way possible. The reflex arc that governs milk production ensures that the supply of milk will always meet but not exceed the demands of the baby, thereby conserving maternal energy stores. In addition, a baby's suckling suppresses further menstrual cycles in its mother. This helps prevent another pregnancy too close to the first, so that maternal resources are conserved for the newborn exclusively. Breast milk is readily available to the infant, it is easily ingested by a naïve nervous and digestive system, and it fortifies the naïve immune system. Feeding from the breast is one of the first instances of satisfaction and relief for the baby.

Breast Development The breasts are organs found only in women because their growth and development depends on estrogen and progesterone. If these hormones are artificially or pathologically present in a male, he, too, can develop breasts. Breast tissue first begins to grow during puberty in response to increased levels of estrogen and progesterone. Initial changes include a darkening of the areola (the area around the nipple) and the development of a mound of breast tissue directly underneath the areola. The breasts will continue to increase in size, mostly owing to fat deposition, for roughly 5 more years. They also grow slightly and transiently during each menstrual cycle. During pregnancy, the breasts undergo a second phase of growth and development under the influence of estrogen, progesterone, prolactin, and hCS. In this state, the breasts differentiate into functional lactational units. The inactive terminal alveolar cells in the mammary gland lobules are converted into active milk-secreting units. After the birth of the baby, prolactin will be the main stimulus to the breast to produce milk. During pregnancy, however, the high levels of progesterone block this effect by inhibiting the action of prolactin at its receptors.

Postpartum Breast Function While progesterone helps the secretory apparatus to develop, it also inhibits the activation of that apparatus—unlike prolactin, which promotes development *and* milk production. Under the high progesterone exposure of pregnancy, the breast cannot produce milk but instead produces colostrum. **Colostrum** is a thin fluid rich in nutrients and antibodies. The breasts secrete it for the first 3 to 4 days of breast feeding postpartum. Then, as maternal levels of estrogen and progesterone drop in the wake of placental expulsion, prolactin acts on the breasts unimpeded. (Prolactin is cleared more slowly, taking at least 7 days to reach prepregnancy levels.) This brief period of high prolactin levels without the inhibitory progesterone leads to the production of milk within the lobules of the mammary gland. After this initial milk production, the newborn must suckle the nipples to maintain milk production and to elicit milk secretion. This is the **reflex arc of lactation** (FIGURE 36.16). Milk secretion, or milk letdown, and milk production are both mediated by the hypothalamus.

Milk letdown is activated by oxytocin. When the infant suckles at the breast, tactile sensors in the areola are activated, stimulating the hypothalamus and triggering the release of oxytocin from the posterior pituitary. Oxytocin travels through the bloodstream to the breast ductal systems, where it causes the myoepithelial cells that line the lactiferous ducts to contract, secreting preformed milk from the ducts.

The production of new milk is governed in a similar fashion but is activated by prolactin. Suckling at the breast not only promotes oxytocin secretion from the neurohypophysis, but also inhibits the hypothalamic production of the neurotransmitter dopamine. Because dopamine inhibits prolactin release from the anterior pituitary, decreased dopamine output leads

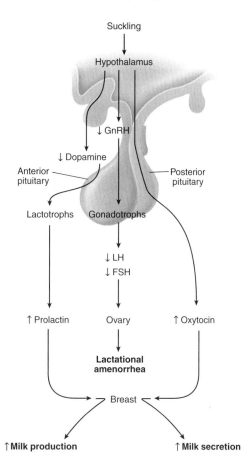

Suckling

Hypothalamus

↓ GnRH

↓ Dopamine

Anterior pituitary — — Posterior pituitary

Lactotrophs   Gonadotrophs

↓ LH
↓ FSH

↑ Prolactin   Ovary   ↑ Oxytocin

Lactational amenorrhea

Breast

↑ **Milk production**   ↑ **Milk secretion**

Figure 36.16   The reflex arc of lactation.

to increased prolactin output. Prolactin then travels to the terminal ducts and causes milk production there. The longer the infant suckles, the more prolactin is secreted and the more milk is produced. In this way, the infant regulates its own food supply. If the infant is not satisfied by the amount of milk in the breast at a given meal, it will suckle longer, the prolactin released during this feeding episode will be greater, and a larger supply of milk will be produced for the next meal. If a given meal is too large, the infant will stop suckling when full and the next meal will consequently be smaller. When suckling is discontinued for a prolonged period, milk production ceases and the breasts gradually return to their prepregnancy state.

Breast feeding also suppresses ovarian function and fertility. This delay in return to normal menstrual cycles in a breast-feeding mother is called *lactational amenorrhea.* Though the exact signal is unclear, suckling disrupts the pulsatile pattern of GnRH release from the hypothalamus and LH and FSH release from the pituitary. Follicular development, ovulation, and endometrial development are suppressed. As mentioned above, the contraceptive function of breast feeding may serve to protect the infant and, from an evolutionary perspective, may be advantageous to

mammalian societies by controlling population. In addition, breast feeding provides other forms of protection. Breast milk transmits to the infant physiologic gut flora (the symbiotic bacteria that inhabit the intestinal tract and protect against harmful pathogens) and may pass on antibodies and factors that activate and modulate the naïve infantile immune system.

PATHOPHYSIOLOGY

Just as the life cycle of the female reproductive system guided our discussion of physiology, the life cycle will set the course of our much briefer discussion of pathophysiology. When broken down this way, disorders of female reproduction fall into the following categories: disorders of sexual development, disorders of fertility, disorders of pregnancy, and disorders of parturition.

Disorders of Sexual Development

When the reproductive system does not develop in accordance with the XX or XY genotype, or when the sex chromosomes are abnormal or not intact, the result may be **ambiguous genitalia** at birth. The genitals are malformed or simultaneously possess both male and female phenotypes. Enzyme deficiencies in the fetus, the placenta, or the mother can create excess androgens and virilize a genotypically female fetus. Likewise, androgen insufficiencies or insensitivities can divert a genotypic male's reproductive development toward the default female phenotype. Flaws in, or an absence of, the *SRY* gene that codes for testis-determining factor (TDF) can have a similar result. Finally, abnormal sex genotypes can be caused by errors in chromosomal division during gametogenesis or during embryologic cell division. Some abnormal genotypes may result in phenotypically normal males or females with infertility or other forms of pathology. Other abnormal genotypes lead to ambiguous phenotypes. Individuals who possess both male and female sex characteristics are described as *hermaphroditic* or *hermaphrodites* (from Hermaphroditos, the double-sexed child of the Greek gods Hermes and Aphrodite).

Disorders of Fertility

Once a couple has decided to have a child, the time to conception varies from one couple to another. The first ovulatory cycle may result in fertilization, or a number of cycles may pass before conception occurs. The diagnosis of **infertility** is made once a couple has tried to conceive without success for 1 year. Defects in sperm production or delivery lead to male infertility, while a broader array of defects leads to female infertility.

Ovulatory defects account for a substantial portion of the cases of female infertility. The uncommon disorders of sexual development, mentioned above, may lead to an inability to ovulate (and in males, an inability to make sperm). In such cases, patients often have never ovulated. In *premature ovarian failure*, ovulation ceases long before normal menopause from injury to the ovaries—whether ischemic, toxic, traumatic, infectious, neoplastic, or autoimmune. The single largest cause of ovulatory infertility is *polycystic ovary syndrome*, in which excess ovarian androgens are thought to impair normal development of the Graafian follicle. Malnutrition, as seen in anorexic patients, and strenuous exercise, as seen in some female athletes, can suppress pituitary LH and FSH production, leading to a failure to ovulate; this is called *hypogonadotropic hypogonadism*. Finally, *hyperprolactinemia* from a prolactin-secreting pituitary tumor can also suppress the pituitary gonadotrophs, leading to failed follicular development and anovulation.

Tubal defects may arise from insults to the peritoneum such as *pelvic inflammatory disease*, which may accompany sexually transmitted infections. Scarring or closure of the fallopian tubes for any reason, however, obstructs oocytes from traveling into the tube where they may be fertilized, and obstructs the passage of sperm.

Endometriosis is a common condition in which endometrial cells grow in the peritoneum outside the uterus. While this is a form of uncontrolled cell growth, endometriosis is not cancerous and does not threaten the patient, except with pelvic pain and possible infertility. It does not always cause infertility, however, and when endometriosis does accompany infertility, the precise causal connection between the two is not always clear. It appears that endometriotic tissue can sometimes lead to the development of peritoneal adhesions that distort the anatomy of the fallopian tubes and ovaries; this may mechanically interfere with the meeting of egg and sperm in the fallopian tube. Endometriomas on the ovary itself may also interfere with ovulation. (See Clinical Application Box *In Vitro Fertilization*.)

Disorders of Pregnancy

Once a pregnancy has been established, a number of pathophysiologic events can endanger the mother and the fetus. An **ectopic pregnancy**, also known as a *tubal pregnancy*, is a pregnancy in which the embryo never passed from the fallopian tube to the uterus. The embryo grows, some of its cells differentiate into trophoblasts, and the trophoblasts ultimately begin to invade the fallopian tube as they would the endometrium. This can lead to severe hemorrhage. While hCG is still produced by the ectopic trophoblasts, hCG levels are usually lower than in intrauterine pregnancies.

A **spontaneous abortion** (miscarriage), mentioned above, is a fairly common complication of pregnancy. While it usually represents a psychological more than a physical threat to the mother, retained products of conception can lead to bleeding or infection. Consequently, the contents of the uterus must be passed. Miscarriages are most often managed surgically (by vacuum aspiration), but in pregnancies of less than 8 weeks' gestation, expectant management is possible and the body may expel the pregnancy on its own.

Certain medical conditions are specifically associated with pregnancy. As described above, the placenta dictates that in late pregnancy, maternal metabolism is shifted toward catabolism in order to make nutrients available to the fetus. Different mothers have different capacities for dampening the catabolic state with insulin. If there is a low insulin reserve, the blood sugar level rises inordinately—a condition known as **gestational diabetes mellitus**.

Another disorder seen in pregnant women is **pre-eclampsia**, in which reduced placental perfusion and maternal constitutional factors likely combine to release vasoconstrictive factors into the maternal bloodstream. This results in multiple organ dysfunction, and the diagnosis is made upon observing hypertension and protein in the urine during the third trimester. (*Eclampsia* means lightning in Greek and refers to the seizures seen in this condition.) Magnesium sulfate is used in pre-eclampsia and eclampsia to prevent seizures by a largely unknown mechanism.

Disorders of Parturition

Parturition is pathological for mother and fetus if it comes too soon and leads to preterm birth, or if it results in injury to mother or child at term. A **preterm birth** is one that occurs before 37 weeks of gestation. It may occur spontaneously, or it may be induced by a doctor to protect the well-being of the mother or fetus. Preterm birth threatens the premature infant because its lungs and other organs are not fully developed and are not ready to negotiate extrauterine life. Inadequate surfactant production in the infant's lungs is a major complication of preterm birth because it compromises the infant's ability to breathe and oxygenate. Causes of preterm labor include infection of the reproductive tract or placental tissues, infection of the urinary tract, premature rupture of membranes (PROM), pre-eclampsia (for which labor is artificially induced), cervical incompetence, placental abruption (premature detachment of the placenta from the uterus), multiple gestation, and fetal distress (which may arise from many causes,

IN VITRO FERTILIZATION

The Centers for Disease Control and Prevention reported that in the year 2000, over 25,000 babies were born with the help of assisted reproductive technology. The best-known example of such technology is **in vitro fertilization (IVF)**, which involves several phases: superovulation, egg collection, sperm preparation, in vitro insemination, and embryo transfer.

Superovulation is achieved by pharmacologic stimulation of the ovary with recombinant FSH, resulting in the production of several Graafian follicles, which are then aspirated from the ovary through a needle. (The needle is inserted through the wall of the vagina under sonographic guidance while the patient is under IV sedation; it is an outpatient procedure.) Semen is meanwhile washed and centrifuged to select healthy sperm and to promote the capacitation process that sperm normally undergo en route to the egg in vivo. (*In vitro* is from Latin, meaning "in glass," while *in vivo* means "in that which is *vivus* [alive].") Several oocytes are then placed in a test tube or Petri dish with tens of thousands of sperm, and in vitro insemination occurs. If sperm quality is poor, this phase of IVF may be achieved through *intracytoplasmic sperm injection (ICSI)*, in which one sperm is injected into one oocyte.

Several days later, a number of viable embryos suspended in medium are deposited into the uterus through a catheter. (Other viable embryos may be frozen in a glycerin-treated solution that prevents the formation of ice crystals.) Supplemental progesterone is given to the mother to ensure that the endometrium is hospitable to implantation, because ovulation by needle aspiration does not leave behind a normally functioning corpus luteum.

Although IVF is an effective solution for many types of infertility, it is not the first line of defense. Diagnosing any underlying cause of the infertility in both partners is the first step, although in one third of cases, the cause is idiopathic (unknown). Any underlying causes are medically or surgically treated. In ovulation defects, ovulation may be induced by recombinant FSH or by clomiphene citrate, an estrogen antagonist that promotes FSH and LH release.

Intrauterine insemination (IUI) may also be tried before IVF. In IUI, prepared sperm are placed in the uterus shortly before ovulation—either natural ovulation or by superovulation and needle aspiration. All forms of assisted reproductive technology run the risk of multiple pregnancy, though IVF would not if one embryo at a time could be transferred with an acceptable success rate.

---

including placental insufficiency). **Fetal distress** is assessed by monitoring the fetal heart rate (FHR), and **fetal bradycardia** (FHR <120 beats per minute) is suggestive of fetal distress.

If labor begins too soon, its underlying cause may sometimes be treated; for example, antibiotics may be administered for an infection of the membranes. Medicines called *tocolytics* may also be used to forestall labor. Terbutaline and magnesium sulfate are tocolytics; terbutaline relaxes smooth muscle by sympathomimetic beta-2 agonism, while magnesium sulfate's mechanism of tocolysis, like its antiseizure mechanism, is still not understood. Conditions such as pre-eclampsia, PROM, or fetal distress, on the other hand, may necessitate **induced labor** with intravenous oxytocin and transvaginal prostaglandins to avert further risk to mother and fetus. Placenta previa (a placenta covering the cervix and positioned between the cervix and fetus—"placenta first"), unusual fetal positioning within the mother's pelvis, unsuccessful labor, hemorrhage, fetal distress, or other factors complicating vaginal delivery may necessitate a **cesarean section**—abdominal surgery to deliver the fetus. A cesarean section may be performed in response to labor complications, or it may be planned. A complicated labor process may lead to hypoxic injury to the infant and consequent brain damage.

Parturition is a time when fetal and maternal blood may mix in the uterus, and this event also carries certain risks. If the fetus has inherited from its father a different blood type than the mother's, the mother's immune system may develop antibodies against that fetal red blood cell antigen. Then, if the mother carries a second child with the same fetal blood antigens, the maternal antibodies may cross the placenta and attack the fetal red blood cells. This results in hemolytic anemia in the fetus, which may continue into infancy, when it is called *hemolytic disease of the newborn (HDN)*. HDN can occur in response to foreign A or B blood types (ABO incompatibility), but it more commonly occurs in response to **Rh factor** on the fetal red blood cells. If the fetus is Rh positive and the mother is Rh negative, blood mixing will provoke a maternal immune reaction. For this reason, Rh-negative mothers are administered intravenous RhoGAM before parturition. *RhoGAM* is a preparation of antibody to Rh factor. If any fetal red blood cells bearing the Rh factor mix with maternal blood, the RhoGAM antibodies bind to them. Once bound to RhoGAM antibody, the Rh antigen does not elicit a maternal immune response. The maternal immune response to Rh factor is called **Rh disease**, or erythroblastosis fetalis.

Summary

- The female reproductive system is composed of the reproductive tract, the GnRH-producing center in the hypothalamus, and the pituitary gonadotrophs. The reproductive tract includes the vagina, cervix, uterus, fallopian tubes, and ovaries.

- The neuroendocrine system by which reproductive function is regulated is called the hypothalamic-pituitary-gonadal (HPG) axis. Hypothalamic GnRH promotes the secretion of FSH and LH; FSH and LH stimulate ovarian responses, including the secretion of estrogen and progesterone.

- Estrogen and progesterone promote reversible (and at puberty irreversible) developments of the reproductive tract and feed back negatively on FSH and LH secretion. Ovarian inhibin inhibits FSH secretion.

- Ovarian follicles are the functional endocrine units of the ovary. A follicle is composed of one oocyte, theca, and granulosa cells.

- Mitosis is divided into six phases: interphase (quiescence, then DNA replication); prophase (chromosomal condensation); metaphase (chromosomes line up individually on spindle); anaphase (sister chromatids separate); telophase (chromosomes decondense and nucleate); and cytokinesis (cell division). Mitosis produces diploid replicas of the mother cell.

- Meiosis follows the same interphase with DNA replication as above, but then is divided into two subphases, meiosis I and meiosis II, each with five steps. Meiosis produces haploid gametes.

- The key differences between mitosis and meiosis are that in metaphase I of meiosis, chromosomes line up in homologous pairs, not individually, and before prophase II, there is no interphase with DNA replication.

- The default pathway of fetal gonadal and genital development is into the female. By week 5 of gestation, germ cells form oogonia in the primordial gonads. By week 12, they begin meiosis, initiating the process of oogenesis, and are now called primordial follicles. Meiosis is immediately arrested in prophase I by oocyte maturation inhibitor (OMI) produced in the granulosa cells of the primordial follicles.

- Meiosis remains arrested until puberty, when it is resumed in one egg per month at the time of ovulation. Then it is arrested again in metaphase II. Meiosis resumes the second time and is completed only when the sperm penetrates the egg at fertilization.

- GnRH levels increase at puberty in response to an unidentified signal, possibly related to body mass. Increased GnRH leads to increased plasma estrogen levels.

- Increased estrogen levels lead to thelarche, the onset of breast development, and menarche, follicular development and the onset of menstruation. At the same time, increased adrenal androgen levels lead to adrenarche, the growth of pubic and axillary hair, and increased growth hormone levels lead to the "growth spurt."

- The ovarian follicles are the pelvic clock that controls the HPG axis from the bottom up.

- Throughout childhood, the primordial follicles (with oocytes arrested in prophase I) grow into antral follicles. The milieu of higher FSH levels of puberty results in monthly recruitment of roughly 10 antral follicles for further growth and development. Unrecruited antral follicles undergo atresia (degeneration).

- From among the recruited antral follicles, one follicle is selected for dominance and grows larger over a 2-week period. The dominant or Graafian follicle will be the only one of the antral follicles to undergo ovulation.

- This 2-week cultivation of a Graafian follicle is called the follicular phase of the ovarian cycle. Follicular estrogen production stimulates endometrial growth in these 2 weeks, so that the follicular phase of the ovarian cycle coincides with the proliferative phase of the uterine cycle.

- When the estrogen level exceeds 100 pg/mL for more than a day, its influence on the pituitary shifts from negative feedback to positive. It prompts the midcycle LH surge. LH inhibits OMI (causing meiosis to resume) and causes the Graafian follicle's wall to break down and rupture, leading to ovulation.

- LH also transforms the ruptured Graafian follicle into the corpus luteum, whose predominant steroidogenic pathway is shifted from estrogen production to progesterone production.

- Over the next 2 weeks of the luteal phase, progesterone renders the uterine lining secretory and supportive of a potential embryo. Thus, the luteal phase of the ovarian cycle corresponds with the secretory phase of the uterine cycle.

- If fertilization and pregnancy occur, hCG from embryonic trophoblast cells mimics LH action and preserves the corpus luteum. Progesterone continues to be secreted and the endometrium is maintained. If no pregnancy occurs, luteolysis, the degeneration of the corpus luteum, results, according to its own 2-week time clock.

- Decreased progesterone and estrogen production withdraws support for the endometrium, which undergoes ischemia and is sloughed off in the menses. Decreased progesterone and estrogen levels also relieve the pituitary from inhibition, resulting in a rise in LH and FSH, which recruits a new crop of antral follicles, and the menstrual cycle begins again.

- Endometrial breakdown occurs via two main mechanisms: vasoconstriction and inflammation. Vasoconstriction of the spiral arteries may occur in response to increased levels of prostaglandins.

- Estrogen has mitogenic (proliferative) effects on the endometrium, breast, vagina, and bones. Progesterone has secretory effects on the endometrium, breast, cervix, and vagina.

- Over many years, atresia of unrecruited follicles results in exhaustion of the oocyte store. This leads to menopause—the cessation of monthly menstruation and fertility—beginning at around age 50.

- After the male ejaculates during intercourse, capacitated sperm swim to the fallopian ampulla, where they can remain fertile for 2 days. An egg must be fertilized within a day of ovulation. Fertility, therefore, lasts from around 2 days before ovulation to 1 day after.

- Fertilization stimulates the nucleus of the secondary oocyte to complete meiosis II and sperm and egg nuclei fuse, leading to the formation of a diploid zygote. Implantation takes place in the uterus 6 days later when embryonic trophoblasts invade the endometrium and start making hCG.

- The placenta develops from embryonic tissue, including trophoblasts, which make up the chorion. The placenta serves as the point of exchange between the circulatory systems of the mother and fetus and is also a hormone-producing organ. Bathed in the maternal blood of the intervillous space, the fetal capillaries of the villi passively absorb oxygen and nutrients and pass carbon dioxide and waste products into the maternal blood.

- The placenta produces hCG and hCS. Late in pregnancy, hCS acts like a counterregulatory hormone to raise the maternal plasma glucose level. Early pregnancy is characterized by anabolism, later pregnancy by catabolism.

- The placenta converts fetal androgens into estrogens and converts maternal cholesterol into progesterone. The placental sex steroids inhibit the pituitary gonadotrophs and suppress the ovarian cycle during pregnancy. They also prevent premature parturition. They do not contribute significantly to the development of the fetal sex organs.

- Systemic vascular resistance (SVR) drops during pregnancy. Cardiac output and glomerular filtration rate (GFR) increase. Functional residual capacity (FRC) decreases, but tidal volume and P_aO_2 increase.

- Labor is the acceleration of uterine contractions and cervical softening and dilation that together lead to parturition (birth). Oxytocin, prostaglandins, and placental CRH all likely play a role in the initiation of parturition.

- During pregnancy, the breasts differentiate into functional lactational units under the influence of estrogen, progesterone, prolactin, and hCS. Progesterone inhibits prolactin's stimulus to milk production until parturition, when the progesterone-producing placenta is expelled from the mother's body.

- Suckling stimulates prolactin secretion, which results in continued milk production. Suckling also stimulates oxytocin secretion from the posterior pituitary, which in turn results in milk secretion.

- Disorders of reproductive development may lead to ambiguous genitalia at birth.

- Infertility in women may be caused by ovulatory defects, tubal defects, or endometriosis. Male infertility is caused by a low sperm count.

- Disorders of pregnancy include ectopic pregnancy, spontaneous abortion, gestational diabetes, and pre-eclampsia.

- The major disorder of parturition is preterm birth. Preterm labor may be forestalled with tocolytics. Labor may also be induced with oxytocin and prostaglandins. A cesarean section may be performed to avert harm to mother or fetus, as in a case of fetal distress.

Suggested Reading

Apter D, Hermanson E. Update on female pubertal development. Curr Opin Obstet Gynecol. 2002;14(5):475–481.

McGee EA, Hsueh AJ. Initial and cyclic recruitment of ovarian follicles. Endocrinol Rev. 2000;21(2):200–214.

Niswender GD, et al. Mechanisms controlling the function and life span of the corpus luteum. Physiol Rev. 2000; 80(1):1–29.

Park SJ, Goldsmith LT, Weiss G. Age-related changes in the regulation of luteinizing hormone secretion by estrogen in women. Exp Biol Med (Maywood). 2002;227(7):455–464.

Rowell P, Braude P. Assisted conception. I: General principles. Br Med J. 2003;327(7418):799–801.

Welt C, Sidis Y, Keutmann H, Schneyer A. Activins, inhibins, and follistatins: from endocrinology to signaling. A paradigm for the new millennium. Exp Biol Med (Maywood). 2002;227(9):724–752.

REVIEW QUESTIONS

Directions: Each of the numbered items or incomplete statements in this section is followed by answers or by completions of the statement. Select the ONE lettered answer or completion that is BEST in each case.

1. A 26-year-old woman and her 28-year-old husband have been trying to conceive without success for more than a year. The man's sperm count and sperm quality are normal. Blood chemistries show a normal LH surge in the woman. If the woman has a history of pelvic inflammatory disease, the most likely cause of this couple's infertility is:

   (A) Endometriosis.
   (B) An ovulatory defect.
   (C) Abnormal female reproductive tract anatomy.
   (D) Retrograde ejaculation.
   (E) Contraception.

2. A 65-year-old postmenopausal woman who has been taking hormone replacement therapy (HRT) for 10 years is diagnosed with breast cancer. If the HRT contributed to the development of the carcinoma, it most likely did so through which mechanism?

   (A) The mitogenic effect of estrogen
   (B) The secretory effect of progesterone
   (C) Progesterone's inhibition of prolactin
   (D) Increased prolactin secretion
   (E) Excess human chorionic somatomammotropin

3. A 29-year-old woman, 7 weeks pregnant, comes to the emergency room with a complaint of spotty vaginal bleeding and pelvic cramping. A transvaginal ultrasound shows no fetal heartbeat. A decrease in the plasma level of which of the following hormones may have caused her vaginal bleeding?

   (A) Relaxin
   (B) Human chorionic somatomammotropin
   (C) Estrogen
   (D) Oxytocin
   (E) Progesterone

ANSWERS TO REVIEW QUESTIONS

1. **The answer is** C. Scarring due to pelvic inflammatory disease can alter the anatomy of the female reproductive tract and prevent the egg from reaching the fallopian tube or prevent capacitated sperm from meeting the egg. The normal LH surge in the woman argues against an ovulatory defect, and the normal sperm count in the man argues against retrograde ejaculation as the cause of infertility.

2. **The answer is** A. Estrogen has a mitogenic (proliferative) effect on breast tissue, so estrogen-containing HRT can increase the risk of breast cancer in postmenopausal women. Progesterone, prolactin, and hCS all act on the breast, but they are not the principal ingredients of HRT and are not primarily mitogens.

3. **The answer is** E. The woman has likely had a spontaneous abortion. Fetal demise has led to trophoblast cell death and decreased hCG production. This in turn has led to luteolysis and decreased progesterone production. Decreased progesterone production has allowed the endometrium to begin to be sloughed off. Human chorionic somatomammotropin (hCS), different from hCG, affects maternal metabolism but does not support the corpus luteum.

37

The Male Reproductive System

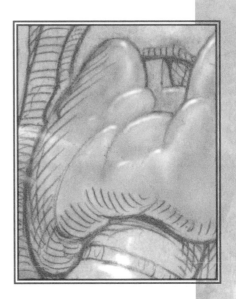

INTRODUCTION

The male reproductive system has three principal functions:

1. The differentiation and maintenance of the primary and secondary sex characteristics under the influence of the hormone testosterone, made in the testes.

2. Spermatogenesis—the creation of the male gametes inside the testes.

3. The penile delivery of sperm from the testes into the female's vagina in the act of procreation. This includes penile erection and ejaculation.

SYSTEM STRUCTURE

The male reproductive system comprises not only the male genitals, but also the cranial structures that help regulate the performance of the male reproductive system—namely, the hypothalamus and pituitary. At the hypothalamic and pituitary level, however, male and female anatomy and histology are more or less the same. For more details on the hypothalamic and pituitary structures involved in human reproduction, see Chapter 36. In the section that follows, we will focus on the anatomy and histology of the testes, the penis, and the ductal connections between the testes and penis.

The Testes

The male gonads, or **testes**, are suspended from the perineum in an external contractile sac called the **scrotum** (FIGURE 37.1A). Each testis is about 4 cm long, and the testes are perfused by the spermatic arteries. The spermatic arteries are closely apposed with the spermatic venous plexus, and this close contact allows countercurrent heat exchange between artery and vein, cooling the blood that flows to the testes. Countercurrent heat exchange helps keep the testicular temperature cool enough for optimal spermatogenesis (1°C to 2°C cooler than body temperature). The external location of the testes in the scrotum serves as a second important cooling mechanism. Because the testes develop within the abdomen, they descend into the scrotum during fetal life, reaching the deep inguinal rings around week 28 of gestation and inhabiting the scrotum by birth. In some instances (3% of the time in full-term male infants), the testes do not descend—a condition called *cryptorchidism*. Cryptorchidism must be corrected if the male is to have properly functioning, fertile gonads.

The testes are composed of coiled seminiferous tubules embedded in connective tissue (see Figure

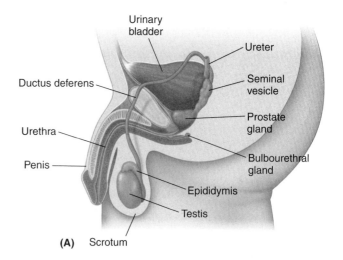

(A)   Scrotum

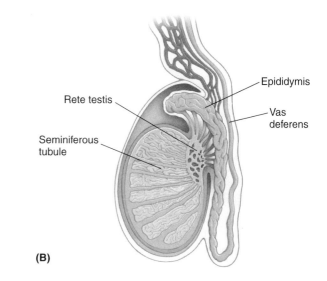

(B)

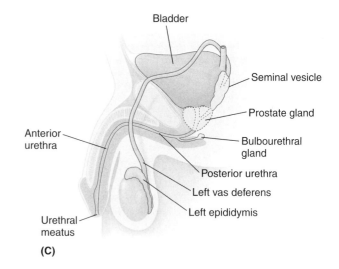

(C)

Figure 37.1 Anatomy of the male reproductive system. **A.** Overview. **B.** A closer look at the testis. **C.** The ducts of the reproductive system shown in isolation. The ducts arising from both testes are depicted, converging on the posterior urethra inside the prostate gland.

37.1B). The connective tissue, which makes up about 20% of the testicular mass, contains **Leydig cells**, which make testosterone. The **seminiferous tubules**, constituting 80% of the testicular mass, generate the sperm. The tubules contain two main cell types: spermatogonia and Sertoli cells. **Spermatogonia** are the germ cells that undergo meiosis to give rise to *spermatids*, the immediate precursors to spermatozoa. The copious cytoplasm of the **Sertoli cells** completely envelops and protects the spermatids, sealing them off from any contact with the tubules' outer basement membrane or blood supply. This Sertoli sheath hence forms a **blood-testis barrier** to protect the male gametes from any harmful bloodborne agents, and to prevent the immune system from attacking the unique sperm-specific proteins as though they were foreign antigens. By virtue of their position between the blood and the spermatids, the Sertoli cells also transport nutrients, oxygen, and hormones, such as testosterone, to the spermatids.

The spermatogonia sit outside the blood-testis barrier near the basement membrane. Here, they continuously conduct mitosis. The products of mitosis are pushed toward the tubule lumen and undergo meiosis and differentiation into sperm cells. The Sertoli barrier is fluid and accommodates the passage of cells developing into spermatids. The testes make around 120 million sperm a day. As they differentiate, the sperm migrate into the tubule lumen for transport distally to the *rete testis*, a plexus of ducts that collects sperm from each of roughly 900 seminiferous tubules. The rete testis empties into the **epididymis**, a single coiled tubule running from the top of the testis down its posterior aspect. In the epididymis, sperm are stored and undergo maturation before continuing their voyage outside the testis.

The Ducts and Penis

Each epididymis leads to a long, straight tube called the **vas deferens** (see Figure 37.1C). The vas deferens from the epididymis of each testis rises in the scrotum, ranges laterally through the inguinal canals, runs along the pelvic wall toward the posterior, and descends along the posterior aspect of the bladder. Here the two vas deferens tubes widen into ampullae, which are attached to glands called the **seminal vesicles**. (There are two seminal vesicles, one for each vas deferens.) The seminal vesicles secrete more than half the volume of the semen. The two ampullae each send an ejaculatory duct through the prostate gland, and the ejaculatory ducts join the urethra inside the tissue of the prostate gland. From this point onward, the male urethra serves as part of both the reproductive and urinary tracts, unlike female anatomy, in which the reproductive and urinary tracts are completely separate. Male physiology ensures that micturition and ejaculation do not occur simultaneously.

The urethra next passes through the muscle tissue of the **urogenital diaphragm**, a consciously controllable sphincter. Sitting just under the urogenital diaphragm are the **bulbourethral glands** (also called *Cowper's glands*), which lubricate the urethra with mucus. Finally, the urethra enters the penis. The cylindrical **penis** houses the urethra in erectile tissue, which helps effect the transition between the excretory and reproductive functions of the urethra (FIGURE 37.2). This erectile tissue contains **cavernous sinuses** that fill with blood under circumstances of increased penile blood flow, leading to erection of the penis. When erect, the penis may be inserted into the vagina so that sperm may be delivered to the fallopian tubes.

The erectile tissue is present in three cylinders inside the penis, each called a **corpus cavernosum** and together called the *corpora cavernosa*. Two of the corpora lie dorsally and are sheathed by the *ischiocavernosus muscles*. One lies ventrally and is sheathed by the *bulbospongiosus muscle*. The ventral corpus cavernosum is also called the **corpus spongiosum**, and it is special in that it contains the urethra and forms the *glans penis*, the spongy head of the penis. The corpora are each supplied by a **cavernous artery** that gives out helicine arteries. The penis averages 8.8 cm (3.5 in) in length when flaccid and 12.9 cm (5.1 in) when erect, indicating no correlation between flaccid and erect size.

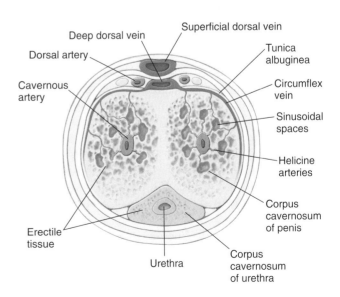

Figure 37.2 Cross section of the penis.

SYSTEM FUNCTION

Just as the female reproductive system is coordinated by the hypothalamus and pituitary, the activities of the male reproductive system are coordinated by the HPG axis, in this case the **hypothalamic-pituitary-testicular (HPT) axis** (FIGURE 37.3). (The gonadal HPT axis is not to be confused with the hypothalamic-pituitary-thyroid axis, also labeled HPT.) The male axis shares with the female the exact same hypothalamic hormone, **gonadotropin-releasing hormone (GnRH)**, and the same pituitary gonadotropins, **follicle-stimulating hormone (FSH)** and **luteinizing hormone (LH)**. (The gonadotropins are named for their female reproductive functions, but they act in the male nonetheless.) The same array of gonadal steroid hormones that is produced by the ovary is also synthesized by the male reproductive system, but in different proportions. Because of differential expression of enzymes in the steroid synthesis pathway, the female gonad makes predominantly progesterone and estrogen, while the male gonad predominantly makes the androgen steroid hormone **testosterone**. Testosterone inhibits the secretion of GnRH, LH, and FSH in a classic negative-feedback loop.

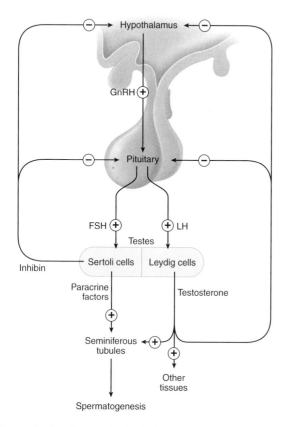

Figure 37.3 Hypothalamic-pituitary-testicular axis. Plus signs represent stimulation; minus signs represent inhibition.

The HPT Axis

GnRH is the initial driver of testicular function. It is secreted in a pulsatile fashion (one pulse every 1 to 3 hours) and distributes to the pituitary gonadotrophs through the hypothalamic-pituitary portal circulation. There, the releasing hormone stimulates the LH- and FSH-secreting cells. Each GnRH pulse directly prompts an LH pulse from the gonadotrophs. More frequent or larger-amplitude GnRH pulses result in more frequent or larger-amplitude LH pulses. GnRH also increases FSH release, but the correlation between GnRH and FSH release is not as exact.

LH acts on the Leydig cells. The LH signal is transduced by a seven- transmembrane receptor linked through a G protein to adenylyl cyclase, which produces cAMP. LH-dependent elevations in cAMP promote testosterone synthesis from cholesterol and promote the growth of Leydig cells. Testosterone synthesis is increased by the activation and increased expression of key proteins involved in steroidogenesis, such as the *steroidogenic acute regulatory protein (StAR)*. StAR shuttles cholesterol into steroid-manufacturing cells. The Leydig cells of the testis are unique in their ability to make testosterone in large amounts (FIGURE 37.4). While the zona reticulata cells of the adrenal gland also make androgens, the adrenal pathway stops at androstenedione, the immediate precursor to testosterone. (Some peripheral tissues can make testosterone from androstenedione in small amounts.)

FSH, meanwhile, binds to receptors on the Sertoli cells, activating the production of proteins involved in spermatogenesis. FSH also stimulates glucose metabolism, thereby providing energy to the sperm precursors. (Spermatogenesis will be discussed in more detail below.) Finally, FSH upregulates the expression of the androgen receptor in Sertoli cells, thereby potentiating the influence of testosterone upon spermatogenesis.

Like all steroids, testosterone binds an intracellular receptor, which binds DNA transcription factors and influences gene expression. The distribution of testosterone receptors in the body tissues determines the targets of testosterone action. In addition, target tissues express an enzyme that converts testosterone to its more active form, **dihydrotestosterone (DHT)**. This enzyme is *5α-reductase*. DHT binds more avidly to the androgen receptor than does testosterone itself. Testosterone from the Leydig cells passes through the Sertoli cells and into the seminiferous tubules, where, alongside FSH, it promotes spermatogenesis. The Sertoli cells make **androgen-binding protein (ABP)**, which helps them to retain testosterone. Testosterone also acts systemically, promoting growth and sustaining gene expression in many peripheral tissues. Testosterone is transported

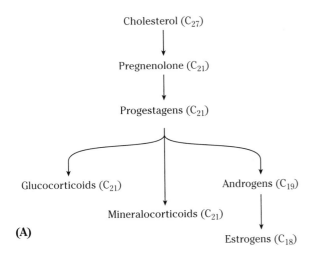

(A)

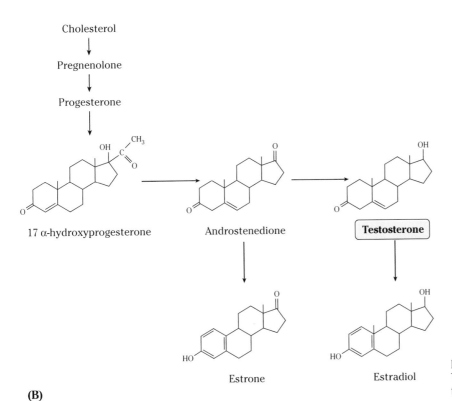

(B)

Figure 37.4 Biosynthesis of androgens. **A.** The steroidal family tree. **B.** A closer look at testosterone and its androgen precursors.

in the blood by **sex hormone-binding protein (SHBP)**, also called *sex hormone-binding globulin*, a liver-produced carrier protein that is structurally similar to ABP. It is thought that testosterone and SHBP itself may act at cell membrane receptors, in addition to testosterone's genomic effects. This is parallel to the genomic and nongenomic modes of signal transduction employed by thyroid hormone.

Finally, testosterone inhibits GnRH and gonadotropin secretion. Thus, testosterone limits its own production and action. **Inhibin** from the Sertoli cells also inhibits the pituitary and hypothalamus. Inhibin is a TGF-β glycoprotein hormone. Investigations suggest that additional feedback mechanisms link Sertoli cell behavior with Leydig cell behavior. Table 37.1 summarizes the actions of testosterone.

Table 37.1   **TESTOSTERONE ACTIONS**

Causes and sustains expression of the male sex characteristics:
    Embryologic development of male genitals and ducts
    Growth of penis, testes, and prostate at puberty
    Growth of hair, larynx
    Promotion of positive nitrogen balance in muscles, bones,
        and skin (promotion of increased protein anabolism,
        requiring retention of more nitrogen-containing amino acids)
    Increased libido and aggression

Causes spermatogenesis

Inhibits HPT axis (negative feedback)

The Expression of Male Sex Characteristics

The male reproductive system begins to function during embryonic life. As soon as the testes form and are capable of secreting testosterone, the androgen begins to act on the body tissues. At this stage, the hormone differentiates the fetus into a male with the appropriate *primary sex characteristics*—the male genitals. At puberty, testosterone causes sustained expression of the *secondary sex characteristics*, which are gender-based phenotypes other than the genitals, such as hair growth, muscle development, and a low voice.

Fetal Life and Infancy (Primary Sex Characteristics)

While the testes do act in utero, they cannot act before they have formed, and they do not form right away. In fact, before 6 weeks of gestation, the gonads of genotypically male or female embryos have not begun to differentiate into either ovaries or testes. The so-called "indifferent gonad" has an inner medullary (male) and an outer cortical (female) layer. In addition, the anatomic precursors of both males (the Wolffian ducts) and females (the Müllerian ducts) are present. Only at 6 to 8 weeks of gestation is male sexual development initiated by the *SRY* gene, a gene on the short arm of the Y chromosome. *SRY* encodes a zinc finger DNA-binding protein called *testis determining factor (TDF)*. Under the influence of TDF, the medullae of the indifferent gonads develop while the cortices regress. The previously indifferent gonads differentiate into testes: embryonic germ cells form spermatogonia, coelomic epithelial cells form Sertoli cells (6 to 7 weeks of gestation), and mesenchymal stromal cells form Leydig cells (8 to 9 weeks of gestation).

Now the testes can begin to act. The Sertoli cells secrete a *Müllerian-inhibiting factor (MIF)*, which causes regression of the Müllerian ducts. Human chorionic gonadotropin (hCG)—which is structurally related to LH—stimulates the Leydig cells to proliferate and secrete testosterone. The testosterone is reduced to DHT in target tissues by 5α-reductase. As long as target tissues contain the androgen receptor and 5α-reductase, DHT induces those tissues to form the primary male sex characteristics, the male reproductive organs. Under the influence of DHT, the Wolffian ducts differentiate into the epididymis, vas deferens, and seminal vesicles. The genital tubercle transforms into the glans penis, the urethral folds grow into the penile shaft, and the urogenital sinus becomes the prostate gland. Finally, DHT causes the genital swellings to fuse, forming the scrotum.

At its peak, the fetal testosterone level reaches 400 ng/dL, but by birth it falls below 50 ng/dL. There is a brief spike in the male infant's testosterone level between 4 and 8 weeks after birth, but its function is not well understood. Otherwise, the testosterone level remains low throughout childhood, until puberty.

Puberty and Beyond (Secondary Sex Characteristics)

Puberty is the process by which males and females achieve reproductive capacity, and it begins in both sexes with an increase in hypothalamic GnRH secretion. It is possible that this increase is in response to decreasing hypothalamic sensitivity to testosterone's negative-feedback effects. As the child approaches adolescence, the hypothalamus gradually escapes inhibition and GnRH secretion rises. LH and FSH secretion in turn rise, and testosterone secretion from the testes increases. Gradual maturation of hypothalamic neurons probably plays a role in this pubertal change in GnRH secretion.

Increased testicular production of testosterone and other androgens at puberty has a host of effects. The earliest one is enlargement of the penis and testes. From the beginning to the end of puberty, the testicular volume more than quadruples. Spermatogenesis commences (with testosterone effects perhaps being most important on the spermatids), and the prostate gland is stimulated to grow. Growth occurs in many tissues outside the reproductive system as well.

Androgens are **anabolic steroids**; they promote the storage of energy in complex molecules. While androgens promote protein synthesis, an anabolic hormone like insulin has a greater effect on the formation of complex carbohydrates and fats. Increased protein synthesis is associated with the growth of skeletal muscle, bones, skin, and hair (pubic, axillary, facial, chest, arms, and legs) and the growth of the larynx (which deepens the voice and causes the thyroid cartilage, or Adam's apple, to protrude). Men on average have around 50% more muscle mass than women; they have stronger, denser bone matrices and thicker skin. Muscle does not contain 5α-reductase, so it appears that testosterone, not DHT, promotes muscular protein anabolism. However, testosterone or DHT may promote muscular anabolism via extramuscular effects, such as the stimulation of growth hormone and insulin-like growth factor (IGF-1) production.

Collectively, the development of the secondary sex characteristics is called **virilization** (after the Latin *vir* for man). It appears that while testosterone promotes all of these effects—genital growth and spermatogenesis, hair growth, behavioral changes, and anabolism in peripheral tissues—certain androgen precursors, metabolic byproducts, and pharmaceutical androgen analogs preferentially serve peripheral anabolism. Many of these metabolites and drugs are abused by bodybuilders and athletes. (See Clinical Application Box *The Use and Abuse of Anabolic Steroids.*)

Testosterone, combined with a genetic predisposition, also influences hair growth on the head. Male-pattern baldness typically begins with a decrease in hair growth on the top of the head and progresses to a complete lack of hair growth extending from the top of the head down. Both factors, the androgens and the genes, are necessary for baldness to occur; a man without the genetic predisposition will not become bald regardless of his testosterone level. A woman with the genetic predisposition will usually not become bald unless she suffers from excess androgen production. Similarly, a castrated male with low testosterone levels will not become bald even if he has a genetic predisposition.

Once testosterone levels rise during puberty, they reach a plateau and remain elevated until a man reaches his seventies, when they begin to decline. This event, called the male *climacteric*, may create some symptoms resembling those of female menopause. However, hormone replacement therapy (HRT) is not commonly used to treat these symptoms. One reason is that men in this age group are at increased risk for prostate cancer. Because testosterone has proliferative effects on the prostate, HRT might further increase the risk of prostate cancer. While testosterone does promote spermatogenesis, this testicular function is remarkably well preserved in men even after the climacteric.

The Haploid Life Cycle in the Male

As mentioned above, spermatogenesis begins with puberty and continues into the eighth decade of life. Spermatogenesis has three phases: **spermatocytogenesis**, during which the primordial spermatogonia divide by mitosis and differentiate into *spermatocytes*; **meiosis**, resulting in four haploid gametes called spermatids, each with a quarter of the cytoplasm of the original spermatogonium (see Chapter 36); and **spermiogenesis**, during which the

---

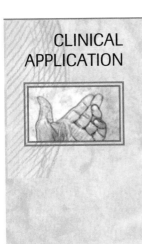

CLINICAL APPLICATION

THE USE AND ABUSE OF ANABOLIC STEROIDS

Some athletes at amateur and professional levels use regimens of anabolic steroids as a strength and muscle-building strategy despite the fact that such a practice is illegal. The risks of anabolic steroid use include:

- Suppression of the HPT axis by negative feedback on the hypothalamus and pituitary, leading to decreased FSH, LH, and testosterone levels. This leads to gonadal atrophy and impaired spermatogenesis.

- Increased peripheral metabolism of those androgens to estrogens, with feminizing effects such as gynecomastia (breast development in males).

- High cholesterol, high blood pressure, abnormal blood clotting, and other hematologic and cardiovascular risks.

- Irreversible virilization in women.

The effectiveness of anabolic steroids in building muscle has been controversial. However, recent literature has begun to support the notion that anabolic steroids do increase muscle mass in athletes. Older studies generally failed to reproduce the context, duration, and dosage used by competitive athletes.

Anabolic steroids are obtained illegally via the black market. However, "dietary supplements" provide a legal way to obtain some varieties of anabolic steroids. The baseball player Mark McGwire is known to have used an androstenedione-containing dietary supplement during his record-breaking season. While the effects of the supplement on athletic performance are a subject of controversy, data suggest that androstenedione does indeed have harmful cardiovascular effects.

spermatids are nourished and physically reshaped by the surrounding Sertoli cells. The product of spermiogenesis is spermatozoa, or sperm (FIGURE 37.5). After spermiogenesis, the epididymis and reproductive tract glands help prepare the sperm for fertilization.

Spermatocytogenesis and Meiosis   The evolving group of cells spanning from spermatogonia to spermatozoa is sometimes called the **spermatogenic series**. Not all spermatogonia enter into the spermatogenic series. If they did, they would be consumed—as happens to the oogonia in the ovary, eventually leading to menopause. Instead, the testis continually replenishes its own supply of spermatogonia. As they undergo mitosis, some of the new ones are committed to the spermatogenic series, while some remain undifferentiated. The undifferentiated stem cells are called **type A spermatogonia**, and the differentiated spermatogonia committed to becoming spermatocytes are called **type B spermatogonia**.

Once this allocation of mitotic products into one group or another occurs, spermatocytogenesis continues as follows. Type A spermatogonia remain on the outside of the blood-testis barrier, while type B spermatogonia cross it, becoming enveloped by the cytoplasmic processes of the Sertoli cells. These type B spermatogonia differentiate further and enlarge to become *primary spermatocytes*. The primary spermatocytes then enter meiosis, a process that takes around 3.5 weeks to complete, almost all of which is spent in prophase (when the newly replicated chromosomes condense). Each primary spermatocyte divides into two *secondary spermatocytes*, which in turn divide again into a total of four haploid spermatids. Each spermatid contains either an X chromosome or a Y chromosome. The male's gamete thus decides the sex of his offspring.

Spermiogenesis   Spermiogenesis begins once the spermatids are created and delivered into the embrace of the amoeboid Sertoli cells (FIGURE 37.6). The spermatid elongates and reorganizes its nuclear and cytoplasmic contents into a spermatozoon with a distinct head and tail. The head consists of a condensed nucleus surrounded by a thin layer of cytoplasm. The rest of the retained cytoplasm and cell membrane is shifted toward the opposite end of the sperm, the tail. A large amount of the spermatid's cytoplasm is shed into the surrounding Sertoli cell during spermiogenesis. As the transformed sperm is extruded into the seminiferous tubule lumen, the discarded cytoplasm

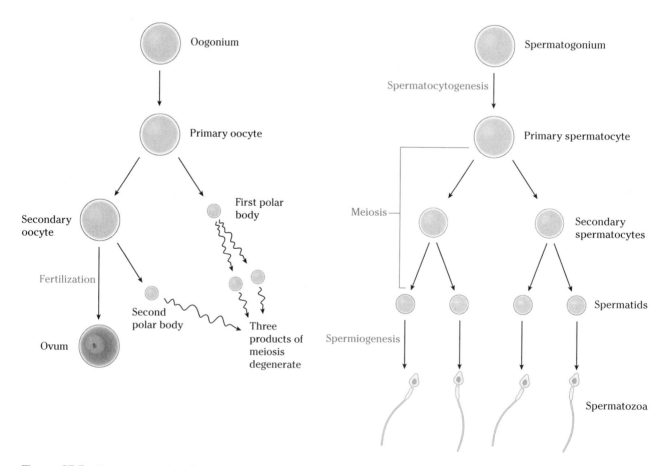

Figure 37.5 Spermatogenesis and oogenesis compared.

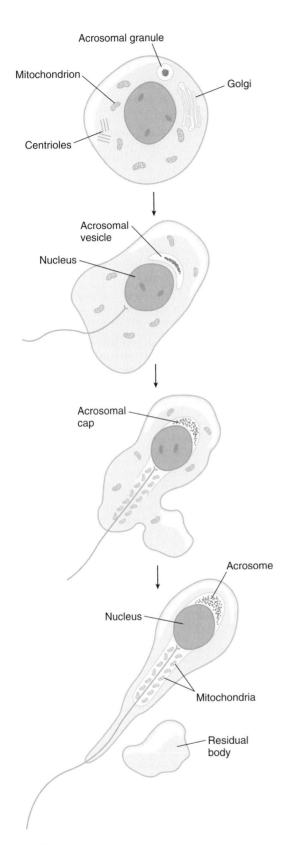

Figure 37.6 Spermiogenesis.

remains embedded in the cytoplasm of the Sertoli cell, where it is ultimately phagocytized.

The structure of sperm cells enables them to swim up the female reproductive tract and fertilize oocytes. The tail of a sperm contains a *flagellum* for motility. Originating from one of the centrioles of the sperm cells, the flagellum consists of a central skeleton of microtubules called the *axoneme*. The axoneme is arranged in the ancient 9 + 2 pattern characteristic of eukaryotic cilia and flagella across all kingdoms and phyla of life: 9 pairs of microtubules surrounding 2 central tubules, linked via a complex array of protein bridges. The sperm cell's mitochondria aggregate along the proximal end of the flagellum and supply energy for movement to the flagellum. The flagellum enables the sperm to swim.

The anterior two thirds of the head of the sperm cell is surrounded by a thick capsule known as the **acrosome**, formed from the Golgi apparatus. The Golgi apparatus contains numerous hydrolytic and proteolytic enzymes, similar to those found in lysosomes, and ultimately facilitates the sperm's penetration of the egg for fertilization. There is also evidence to suggest a role for the acrosomal enzymes in penetrating the mucus of the female cervix.

Epididymal Sperm Maturation and Storage   After spermiogenesis is complete, the sperm pass out of the testis (through the rete testis) and into the epididymis, where growth and differentiation continue. After the first 24 hours in the epididymis, the sperm acquire the potential for motility. However, the epithelial cells of the epididymis secrete inhibitory proteins that suppress this potential. Thus, the 120 million sperm produced each day in the seminiferous tubules are stored in the epididymis, as well as in the vas deferens and ampulla. The sperm can remain in these excretory genital ducts in a deeply suppressed and inactive state for over a month without losing their potential fertility.

The epididymis also secretes a special nutrient fluid that is ultimately ejaculated with the sperm and is thought to mature the sperm. This fluid contains hormones, enzymes (such as glycosyltransferases and glycosidases), and nutrients that are essential to achieving fertilization. The precise function of many of these factors is not known, but enzymes like gamma-glutamyl transpeptidase are thought to serve as antioxidants defending against mutations in the sperm.

Potentiation in the Ejaculate   The accessory genital glands—the seminal vesicles, prostate gland, and bulbourethral glands—also contribute to potentiation. During ejaculation, their secretions dilute the epididymal inhibitory proteins, allowing the sperm's motile potential to be realized. In addition, the glands make individual contributions to sperm preparation and support. The seminal vesicles secrete **semen**, a mucoid yellowish material containing nutrients and sperm-activating substances such as fructose, citrate, inositol, prostaglandins, and fibrinogen. Carbohydrates such as fructose provide a source of energy for the sperm mitochondria as they power the sperm's flagellar movements. The prostaglandins are believed to aid the sperm by affecting the female genital tract—making the cervical mucus more receptive to the sperm, and dampening the peristaltic contractions of the uterus and fallopian tubes to prevent them from expelling the sperm.

The prostate gland secretes a thin, milky, and alkaline fluid during ejaculation that mixes with the contents of the vas deferens. The prostatic secretion contains calcium, zinc, and phosphate ions, citrate, acid phosphatase, and various clotting enzymes. The clotting enzymes react with the fibrinogen of the seminal fluid, forming a weak coagulum that glues the semen inside the vagina and facilitates the passage of sperm through the cervix in larger numbers. The alkalinity imparted to semen by the prostate counteracts vaginal acidity, which is a natural defense against microbial pathogens and which can kill sperm or impair sperm motility. By titrating the acidity, the prostate ensures that the sperm can elude this antimicrobial defense.

Capacitation in the Female Reproductive Tract
Ejaculated sperm is not immediately capable of fertilizing the female oocyte. In the first few hours after ejaculation, the spermatozoa must undergo **capacitation** inside the female reproductive tract. This is the final step in preparation for fertilization. First, the fluids of the female reproductive tract wash away more of the inhibitory factors of the male genital fluid. The flagella of the sperm hence act more readily, producing the whiplash motion that is needed for the sperm to swim to the oocyte in the fallopian tube. Second, the cell membrane of the head of the sperm is modified in preparation for the ultimate acrosomal reaction and penetration of the oocyte. Capacitation is an incompletely understood phenomenon.

Fertilization
Once capacitated, the spermatozoa travel to the oocyte. There is an enormous rate of attrition among the hundreds of millions of ejaculated sperm, and at most a few hundred reach the oocyte. However, the female reproductive tract is simultaneously increasing receptivity to the male gametes (see Chapter 36).

When the few hundred sperm reach the egg, they begin to try to penetrate the granulosa cells surrounding the secondary oocyte. The sperm's acrosome contains hyaluronidase and proteolytic enzymes, which open this path. As the anterior membrane of the acrosome reaches the zona pellucida (the glycoprotein coat surrounding the oocyte), it rapidly dissolves and releases the acrosomal enzymes. Within minutes, these enzymes open a pathway through the zona pellucida for the sperm cytoplasm to merge with the oocyte cytoplasm. From beginning to end, the process of fertilization takes about half an hour.

Penile Erection and Ejaculation

The practice of internal fertilization, in which the male deposits gametes directly into the reproductive tract of the female, is at least 300 million years old. Early cartilaginous fishes probably were its innovators. These elasmobranchs retained their concepti internally until the eggs could be waterproofed and thus protected from the osmotic stress of seawater. Eventually, almost all the higher vertebrates would practice internal fertilization for the sake of defending the next generation.

For this reason, the male vertebrate possesses a special apparatus for penetrating the body of the female and delivering semen to an internal location. There are two physiologic events crucial to this internal delivery of semen: penile **erection**, which makes it possible for the penis to penetrate the vagina, bringing the urethral opening, or meatus, into close contact with the female cervix; and **ejaculation**, in which the semen is secreted into the male reproductive ductal system, mixed with sperm, and then mechanically squirted out of the penis. Both of these events are initiated and controlled by the nervous system in connection with the subjective state of sexual arousal.

Sexual Response in the Male
William H. Masters and Virginia E. Johnson in 1966 described four phases of sexual response in males and females: *excitement, plateau, orgasm,* and *resolution* (FIGURE 37.7). Desire or libido precedes excitement, and testosterone is known to increase libido. Excitement that leads to erection derives from a combination of psychological factors and genital stimulation. Erotic feelings can initiate an erection without physical stimulation, and physical stimulation can initiate erection in the absence of psychological stimuli. The *pudendal nerve* transmits sensory information from the penis to the spinal cord and brain.

Erection
As excitement builds in the central nervous system, efferent parasympathetic fibers in the *pelvic nerve* discharge more and more impulses

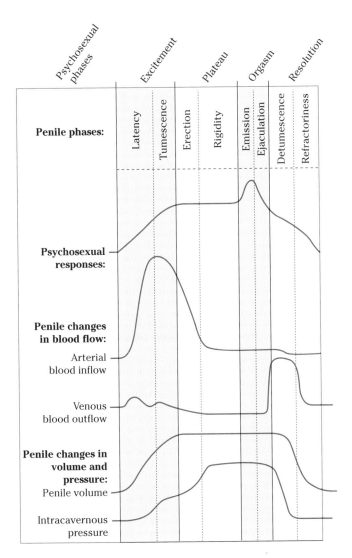

Figure 37.7 Sexual response and changes in the penis.

Ejaculation As sexual excitement continues to build, bulbourethral and urethral secretions lubricate the urethra. These secretions are small in volume compared with the ejaculate, but they do contain sperm and can by themselves lead to fertilization. As genital stimulation excites the pudendal nerve more and more, a subjective sensation of **orgasm** ensues, followed immediately by the **ejaculatory spinal cord reflex**. (While the ejaculatory reflex is involuntary, it can be suppressed and delayed by input from the cerebral cortex; it is possible that at orgasm, the central nervous system releases the spinal reflex from its inhibition.) Once the reflex is initiated, sympathetic nerves stimulate the closure of the bladder neck and contraction of the ampulla of the vas deferens, the seminal vesicles, and the prostate. The contractions cause the seminal vesicles and prostate to secrete their semen into the ejaculatory duct just as the sperm are propelled from the ampulla into the ejaculatory duct. The semen briefly pools in the **posterior urethra**. This first stage of ejaculation is called **emission**.

Emission is directly followed by the rhythmic contraction of muscles surrounding the urethra: the bulbospongiosus muscle that surrounds the corpus spongiosum, the urethral smooth muscle, and other pelvic floor muscles. These contractions expel the semen from the posterior urethra and out the penile meatus in spurts.

Resolution The total ejaculate contains about 400 million sperm in about 3 to 4 mL of secretions. The normal sperm concentration ranges anywhere from 35 million to 200 million sperm per milliliter of fluid. If the sperm have been delivered into an ovulatory female reproductive tract, they now begin their journey toward the egg. Meanwhile, the resolution phase occurs a few minutes after ejaculation with *detumescence* (drainage of blood from the penis) and a *refractory period* of varying lengths, in which erection and ejaculation cannot be repeated. The cavernous arteries constrict, preventing arterial inflow, and venous outflow lowers the intracavernous pressure. As the pressure falls, the veins decompress and venous outflow increases further. This shift from net inflow to net outflow rapidly returns the penis to its flaccid state. Elastic tissues in the corpora cavernosa also assist in this shrinkage.

PATHOPHYSIOLOGY

Common problems associated with the male reproductive tract include prostatitis, erectile dysfunction, infertility, and benign and malignant growth of the prostate.

Prostatitis is inflammation of the prostate, usually due to the ascent of a urinary tract infection.

through the pelvic plexus to the smooth muscle of the penile cavernous artery, which runs down the center of each of the corpora cavernosa. These parasympathetic impulses lead to the secretion of nitric oxide (directly from the parasympathetic nerve terminals and also from the endothelial cells in the arterial vasculature). The nitric oxide (NO) diffuses into the smooth muscle in the wall of the cavernous artery and relaxes it. (New data suggest that testosterone is also involved in the regulation of NO secretion.) NO-mediated arterial dilation leads to up to a 60-fold increase in penile blood flow. The penis swells with blood. When the spongy tissues are stretched to their full extent, intracavernous pressure then begins to rise. The penis becomes rigid and elevates. The increasing pressure eventually compresses the cavernous veins and reduces venous outflow, building the pressure even higher.

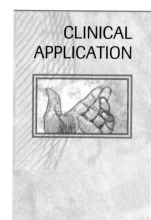

CLINICAL APPLICATION

TREATING ERECTILE DYSFUNCTION

The popular drug Viagra (generic name, sildenafil citrate), introduced in 1998, is used to treat **erectile dysfunction (ED)**. An internet search on the name at the time this chapter was written produced 17.4 million hits—an indication of the number of men seeking help for ED.

Viagra works by inhibiting the action of cGMP-specific phosphodiesterase type 5 (PDE5). PDE5 is specific to the penis. When this enzyme is inhibited, the cGMP levels in smooth muscle rise, mimicking the effect of nitric oxide on the smooth muscle of the penile cavernous arteries. The smooth muscle relaxes, and penile blood flow increases. Cross-reactivity with other PDEs can cause vasodilation elsewhere in the body, however, leading to hypotension (low blood pressure).

Some 10 to 20 million men suffer from **erectile dysfunction (ED)**, also known as *impotence*. Any cause of vascular insufficiency, including atherosclerosis, diabetes mellitus, and antihypertensive medication can lead to ED, as can psychological factors. (See Clinical Application Box *Treating Erectile Dysfunction.*)

An estimated 10% to 15% of couples cannot conceive after 1 year of trying; they are considered to have infertility. In 20% of infertile couples, the cause is never discovered. In the remaining 80%, around half of the cases of infertility are due to a problem in the male reproductive system.

Prostate cancer is by far the most common cancer in men and the second most frequent cause of male cancer deaths. Benign prostatic hyperplasia affects nearly all men as they age.

Male Infertility

Some of the causes of male **infertility** have been discussed previously. Cryptorchidism results in sterility, as the spermatogonia cannot survive at the increased temperatures of the body cavity. Other abnormalities of the testes and genital tract may also impair fertility, including varicoceles, trauma, and scarring. A careful history may reveal environmental exposures (chemical, radiation [e.g., due to cancer treatment], heat [due to tight underwear, fever, etc.]); sexually transmitted infections; mumps orchitis (which can destroy the seminiferous tubular epithelium); trauma; or previous surgery around the urogenital tract. (See Clinical Application Box *What Is a Varicocele?*)

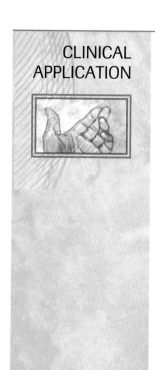

CLINICAL APPLICATION

WHAT IS A VARICOCELE?

A 20-year-old man presents to his university health service with testicular pain. On palpation, he has a mass in the region of his left spermatic cord, and his left testicle is slightly smaller than his right. After referral to the urologist, Doppler ultrasonography confirms a backflow of blood in the pampiniform plexus of the left spermatic vein. The patient is scheduled for varicocelectomy.

A **varicocele** is a dilatation in the plexus of veins leading away from the testis along the spermatic cord. This plexus, called the *pampiniform plexus*, has no physiologic function in humans. It is an ancient and vestigial remnant from the days when our ancestors were fish. These early fish employed a disorganized venous plexus in the peritubular reabsorption and secretion of solutes from the primitive renal tubule. Later, the reproductive system came to appropriate part of the embryologic duct that had given rise to the urinary system. The reproductive system took with it this venous plexus (now useless), and through evolution, the renal tubules received a glomerular blood supply for their peritubular capillaries.

Perhaps because it is vestigial, the pampiniform plexus is vulnerable to valvular defects and a backflow of venous blood. This backflow leads to venous pooling, which in turn can lead to painful venous enlargement (varicosity) and can impair cooling of the scrotum. The heat from the pooled blood can interfere with the temperature-sensitive process of spermatogenesis. It is a very common cause of male infertility.

The workup includes a *semen analysis*, which assesses ejaculate volume, sperm count, sperm morphology and motility, semen pH, and white blood cell count. Sperm counts of less than 20 million sperm per milliliter render a male infertile. Abnormal morphology of the sperm, including multiple heads or tails and abnormally shaped heads or tails, will impair fertility. Abnormal functioning of the sperm heads (acrosomes) or tails (flagella), despite seemingly normal morphology, can also impair fertility.

A postcoital test may also be performed to evaluate the interaction between the sperm in the semen and the female cervical mucus. The inability of the sperm to penetrate the cervical mucosa may suggest an abnormality of the fluid contents of the semen or an abnormality of the acrosomal head of the sperm itself.

Analysis of serum FSH and testosterone levels may also be helpful in diagnosing testicular disease. If the testes are damaged and failing to make testosterone, the testosterone level will be low and the FSH level will be high, resulting from hypothalamic disinhibition. Thyroid function tests are also indicated (most importantly a TSH level), since abnormal thyroid function interferes with spermatogenesis.

Benign Prostatic Hyperplasia and Prostate Cancer

The development and growth of the prostate gland are stimulated by testosterone. This mitogenic (proliferative) effect on the prostate continues throughout life, often resulting in the development of **benign prostatic hyperplasia (BPH)**. As many as 20% of men are affected by BPH before the age of 40, and the number increases with age: about 70% of men at age 60 and 90% of men in their seventies show evidence of some BPH. The main symptoms of BPH result from the enlarged prostate impinging on or obstructing the urethra, and include urinary frequency, urgency, nocturia (waking at night to urinate), urinary retention, and even urinary obstruction. As its name implies, BPH is otherwise benign and is not considered to be a premalignant lesion.

Prostate cancer is a slow-growing cancer. Its incidence increases with age, and it often has an insidious onset; that is, it may grow for a long time asymptomatically before coming to the attention of the patient or his doctor. Therefore, the cancer is frequently metastatic by the time of presentation. Because prostate cancer is so common and because it has an insidious onset, the medical community encourages screening by digital rectal exam (DRE) or the prostate-specific antigen (PSA) test for men above a certain age. (There is no consensus, however, on whether such screening would reduce mortality rates.) Questionable results from a rectal exam are usually followed with transrectal ultrasound and/or an ultrasound-guided transrectal biopsy. Testosterone is a growth stimulant for prostate cancer, just as it is for BPH. Certain therapies, especially those used in cases of known metastases, therefore aim at inhibiting testosterone production or preventing testosterone from stimulating the prostatic tissue, thereby slowing the growth and spread of the cancer. Men with both BPH and prostate cancer are candidates for transurethral prostate resection (TURP).

Heart Disease Male gender is a risk factor for atherosclerosis. In 1999 in the United States, 49% more men than women died of heart disease. Many of the phenotypic differences between men and women may account for this statistic. One particular explanation may be that testosterone increases the plasma level of low-density lipoproteins (LDL, or "bad" cholesterol) and decreases the level of high-density lipoproteins (HDL, or "good" cholesterol). High LDL levels and low HDL levels are both cardiac risk factors.

Summary

- There are three principal functions of the male reproductive system: the expression of male sex characteristics, spermatogenesis (the creation of sperm), and the delivery of sperm into the female for procreation.

- Male reproduction is coordinated by the hypothalamic-pituitary-testicular (HPT) axis, which is characterized by classic negative feedback. The hypothalamus secretes GnRH, which releases FSH and LH from the pituitary.

- FSH acts on the Sertoli cells in the seminiferous tubules of the testis and stimulates spermatogenesis.

- LH acts on the Leydig cells in the testicular parenchyma and stimulates secretion of the androgen steroid, testosterone. Testosterone inhibits GnRH and FSH/LH release.

- Testosterone is converted to its active form, dihydrotestosterone (DHT), at its sites of action.

- Testosterone causes development of the male genital system in utero and at puberty. It causes growth of the genitals; hair growth; the start of spermatogenesis; deepening of the voice; protein anabolism in muscle, bone, and skin; and increased libido and aggression.

- Spermatogenesis takes place in the seminiferous tubules of the testis and has three phases: spermatocytogenesis (mitosis and differentiation of some spermatogonia into spermatocytes), meiosis (resulting in four haploid spermatids), and spermiogenesis (the production of spermatozoa from spermatids). Testosterone and FSH promote this process.

- Newly created sperm pass from each of 900 seminiferous tubules into the epididymis of each testis. Here, sperm acquire potential motility, are bathed in inhibitory proteins, and are stored. Stored, suppressed sperm fill the vas deferens, the tube connecting the epididymis to the urethra, where they await ejaculation (expulsion from the penis) in the fluid called semen.

- Ejaculation is preceded by sexual excitement and penile erection.

- Excitement develops via psychological stimuli and tactile stimulation of the genitals. The pudendal nerve transmits afferent sensory information from the genitals to the brain.

- During excitement, the pelvic nerve transmits efferent parasympathetic impulses to the smooth muscle of the cavernous arteries in the erectile tissues of the penis, cylindrical bodies called the corpora cavernosa. These impulses dilate the penile arteries through a nitric oxide-mediated mechanism. Blood flow increases into the two dorsal corpora cavernosa and into the special ventral one, which houses the urethra; it is called the corpus spongiosum.

- When the three corpora cavernosa fill with blood, they eventually increase intracavernous pressure and reduce venous outflow, further increasing penile pressure. The penis becomes fully erect (that is, rigid and elevated).

- Increasing tactile stimulation of the pudendal nerve builds excitement until orgasm is reached, accompanied by release of the ejaculatory spinal cord reflex. The efferent limb of the reflex sends out impulses along sympathetic nerves that close the bladder neck and contract the seminal vesicles, prostate, and ampulla of the vas deferens. Contractions of urethral and pelvic muscles expel semen through the ejaculatory ducts and into the posterior urethra, an event called emission.

- If sperm are deposited into the vagina, they are capacitated, or rendered more motile and ready to fertilize, by the female reproductive tract. The acrosome, the head of the sperm cell, releases enzymes that digest a path into the oocyte, and fertilization occurs.

- Common problems associated with the male reproductive tract include prostatitis, erectile dysfunction, infertility, and benign and malignant growth of the prostate gland. Male gender is itself a cardiac risk factor.

Suggested Reading

Andersson KE, Wagner G. Physiology of penile erection. Physiol Rev. 1995;75(1):191–236.

Barry MJ, Roehrborn CG. Benign prostatic hyperplasia. Br Med J. 2001;323(7320):1042–1046.

Hiort O. Androgens and puberty. Best Pract Res Clin Endocrinol Metab. 2002;16(1):31–41.

Kandeel FR, Koussa VKT, Swerdloff RS. Male sexual function and its disorders: physiology, pathophysiology, clinical investigation, and treatment. Endocrinol Rev. 2001;22(3):342–388.

Kuhn CM. Anabolic steroids. Recent Prog Horm Res. 2002; 57:411–434.

REVIEW QUESTIONS

Directions: Each of the numbered items or incomplete statements in this section is followed by answers or by completions of the statement. Select the ONE lettered answer or completion that is BEST in each case.

1. The hypogastric nerve supplies sympathetic tone to the bladder and genitals. Its most important role in male reproductive function is probably that of stimulating:

   (A) Spermatogenesis.
   (B) Testosterone production.
   (C) Urethral lubrication.
   (D) Erection.
   (E) Detumescence.
   (F) Capacitation of sperm.
   (G) Spermiogenesis.
   (H) Ejaculation.

2. A 35-year-old man who is an avid bodybuilder complains of having developed what look like female breasts. A history reveals several years of drug abuse with a form of testosterone. Physical exam reveals acne, gynecomastia, and small testes. The mechanism behind his gynecomastia is:

   (A) Negative feedback on the hypothalamus.
   (B) Suppression of gonadal function.
   (C) Positive nitrogen balance.
   (D) Increased testosterone metabolism.
   (E) Increased testosterone action.

3. A 31-year-old man undergoes semen analysis after 1 year of trying unsuccessfully to impregnate his wife. If some of his sperm have abnormal flagella, this most likely reflects an error during which phase of sperm development?

   (A) Spermatocytogenesis
   (B) Epididymal maturation
   (C) Mixing with seminal and prostatic fluid in the posterior urethra
   (D) Spermiogenesis
   (E) Meiosis

ANSWERS TO REVIEW QUESTIONS

1. **The answer is** H. Ejaculation is mediated by sympathetic impulses from the spinal cord. Remember "point and shoot": "p" for parasympathetic mediation of erection and "s" for sympathetic mediation of ejaculation. The pudendal nerve carries afferent information to the central nervous system, and the pelvic nerve carries efferent parasympathetic impulses.

2. **The answer is** D. The drug has increased the testosterone level, thereby increasing the peripheral metabolism of testosterone to estrogen, which has proliferative effects on the breast tissue of males and females. While increased testosterone action at the androgen receptor, hypothalamic inhibition, and gonadal suppression all occur in this context, they do not cause gynecomastia.

3. **The answer is** D. Spermatids acquire their tails and become spermatozoa at the spermiogenesis phase of spermatogenesis. Thus, it is here that abnormalities in tail morphology are likely to arise. Abnormalities at other stages of sperm development are more likely to lower the sperm count or reduce sperm motility or penetrative ability.

CASE STUDY: INTRODUCTION TO DIAGNOSIS

The philosopher Carl G. Hempel wrote in 1948, "To explain the phenomena in the world of our experience, to answer the question 'why?' rather than only the question 'what?,' is one of the foremost objectives of empirical science." **Diagnosis** is the medical term for scientific explanation or hypothesis. An explanation takes a set of facts and seeks a general law of the universe from which those facts might be logically deduced. The explanation of *why* the apple falls downward from the limb of the tree is: The apple has mass, the earth has mass, and two bodies with mass attract each other—the law of gravity.

A patient's fever, runny nose, and cough could be explained on the basis of three laws: (1) people commonly get bacterial and viral infections in the upper respiratory tract—a law of microbiology; (2) infections activate macrophages—a law of immune response; and (3) macrophages secrete interleukins that alter the hypothalamic set point for temperature regulation, causing fever, and inflammatory cells at membranes cause mucus production—a law of immune system behavior. The term "upper respiratory infection" represents all these medical-biological laws. In addition, since the clinical phenomenon of fever, runny nose, and cough all at once could be deduced from the laws called "upper respiratory infection," those general laws could be the explanation for these specific clinical observations. However, we could also consider a rival explanation. For example, we could ask if the fever, runny nose, and cough could be caused by allergies.

A list of more than one possible explanation for clinical observations is called a **differential diagnosis**. The only way to distinguish between two equally plausible explanations is to gather more data and to reconsider the two explanations in light of the new data. For example, we could ask the patient about his exposures to other sick people and to possible allergens, such as dust, pets, or pollen. We could draw the patient's blood and measure the numbers of various kinds of immune cells. If the patient denies any contact with allergens and any history of allergies, if he suddenly remembers that his cousin who came to dinner had a terrible cold, if the complete blood count (CBC) shows high numbers of neutrophils (which are elevated in the response to some infections but not in response to allergies), and if all those things are revealed by our inquiries and tests, then one explanation now looks better than the other. The "upper respiratory infection" better explains all the data than the "allergy" explanation.

Thus, we test clinical hypotheses to select one diagnosis from a pool of differential diagnoses. Our hypothesis testing falls into two broad categories: (1) asking questions about the history of the present illness and other medical history and (2) obtaining objective information from the physical exam, from blood tests, imaging studies, etc. Subjective complaints that can be predicted by (deduced from) the presence of an underlying illness are termed **symptoms** of an illness. Objective findings that can be predicted by (deduced from) the presence of an underlying illness are called **signs**. A report of frequent coughing is a symptom, while a temperature of 102°F is a sign.

After gathering subjective and objective data, we try to narrow down the number of explanations from among many possibilities and plan a course of action. The plan may include more tests and inquiries to acquire more data, which would be used to narrow down the list of possible explanations even further. (We aim for the fewest possible explanations or diagnoses, in keeping with Isaac Newton's first rule of philosophical reasoning: "We are to admit no more causes of natural things than such as are both true and sufficient to explain their appearances.") The plan may also include treatments to reduce or control symptoms. Once a likely explanation is found, the plan will include a treatment aimed at relieving the underlying illness(es). The mnemonic SOAP summarizes the format of clinical thinking used in most medical presentations and in notes in the medical chart: S, subjective; O, objective; A, assessment; and P, plan. You may see the actual letters "S," "O," and "A/P" used as headings in doctors' or nurses' notes.

Knowledge of physiology is particularly important to making diagnoses. Illnesses may begin at the cellular level and their treatments may act at the cellular level, but illnesses are generally known to their sufferers by dysfunction or reaction at the organ level. To trace a path from an illness to its manifestations, we must know what the organ systems do, how one system affects the others, and the consequences when an organ system under- or over-performs.

As you go through the case studies, try not to concern yourself too much with mastering the details of the featured illnesses and their treatment protocols. Rather, take the opportunity to familiarize yourself with the process of diagnosis, by which physiologic principles are used to infer an explanation from among several possibilities. Follow the course of the illness and try to appreciate how its progression can be predicted (and hence better treated) from a knowledge of the physiologic laws of the body.

At the end of each study, we've provided questions as food for thought. Take these questions as an opportunity to discuss, review, do further research, and to learn to think physiologically about clinical medicine.

Part I CASE STUDY FOR **GENERAL PRINCIPLES**

J.K. is an 8-year-old girl who presented to the emergency room with severe pain and swelling in her right wrist after tripping on the sidewalk outside school.

PRESENTATION

J.K. and her mother were confused by the injury because its severity was out of proportion to the severity of the fall, which had been a minor tumble on the sidewalk due to an untied shoelace. The emergency room doctor suspected a routine Colles fracture (radial fracture), but unusual findings from an x-ray raised larger concerns. Medicine was called to consult.

On further questioning, it turned out that J.K. had had other troubles besides the injury to her arm. Over the last year, J.K.'s mother noticed that J.K. had developed a slight limp and that her left hip seemed to protrude. J.K. had been an attentive, engaged student in the first grade, but this year, her teachers had observed her to be a little "spacey," not infrequently failing to respond when called or questioned. J.K. complained of occasional pain in her left hip which was worse with activity. Her appetite and food intake were excellent. There was no known family history of bone disease or inherited disorders. Her mother reported that J.K. had been born by normal vaginal delivery after an uneventful pregnancy and that she had met all developmental milestones normally to her knowledge.

On physical exam, J.K. had a slightly elevated pulse of 83 beats per minute and was afebrile with otherwise normal vital signs. She appeared uncomfortable owing to the pain in her arm, but she was bright and attentive. Her height and weight were in the 75th percentile for her age, and she appeared well-nourished. Her temples were noted to be slightly asymmetrical, with a bumpy contour to the right temporal bone. On exam of her ears, tympanic membranes were normal, but hearing was decreased in the right ear on whispered speech test and on Weber and Rinne tests. The rest of the cranial nerve exam was normal. Her thyroid gland was slightly enlarged and nodular on palpation. Abdominal inspection revealed a 7-cm café-au-lait spot with irregular borders on the upper left quadrant of the abdomen close to the midline. J.K.'s spine was observed to be normally aligned. Breasts and genitals suggested Tanner stage 2 of pubertal development, with palpable breast buds and some pigmented pubic hair. Exam of the extremities revealed strong and equal radial and tibial pulses, capillary refill <2 s in the nail beds, and a slight varus deformity of the left hip (coxa vara) plus mild hip pain with abduction of the left femur. The left leg was noted to be 3 cm shorter than the right. The right wrist was swollen, red, hot, and tender.

Lab values were significant for a low thyroid-stimulating hormone (TSH) of 0.42 μIU/mL, an elevated alkaline phosphatase of 211 IU/L, a normal serum calcium level of 9.1 mg/dL, and a normal erythrocyte sedimentation rate of 17 mm/h. X-rays showed thickened bone with a "ground glass" appearance in the distal right radius and left proximal femur and a displaced, comminuted fracture of the distal right radius. Computed tomography (CT) scan also showed thickening in the right temporal bone of the skull.

Discussion

J.K. has abnormal bone anatomy in three skeletal locations, impaired hearing, and a low TSH, suggestive of hyperthyroidism. However, by Newton's first rule of philosophical reasoning (a principle also called Occam's Razor), we should pursue the smallest possible number of explanations for all these findings. Could disease in so many organ systems be traced to one or two causes? Any pathogenic agent that is distributed throughout the body by the bloodstream can theoretically affect multiple organ systems, so we might consider in a broad differential metastatic cancer, an autoimmune disease, a hormonal disorder, septicemia, or toxicity. Idiopathic bone disease like Paget's disease could be entertained, as could malnourishment, or a genetic illness affecting all or many cells.

By reviewing the evidence, we can begin to eliminate some of the possibilities from the differential diagnosis. The imaging studies do not show the lytic bone lesions we would expect in a metastatic cancer affecting the bones, and J.K.'s normal calcium level and normal growth and nutrition are not consistent with lytic malignancies of the bones. There are no signs of infection or of the widespread inflammation that would be seen in an autoimmune disease (fever and an elevated erythrocyte sedimentation rate are two nonspecific indicators of inflammation). Paget's lesions in bone do not have a "ground glass" radiographic appearance, and Paget's disease is more common in adults. Rickets due to vitamin D deficiency in the diet could cause weak bones, making them susceptible to pathologic fractures, but J.K.'s normal growth and nutrition point away from malnourishment. The normal calcium level argues against hyperparathyroidism and against the multiple endocrine neoplasia syndromes, in which we would also expect to see a wider variety of endocrine abnormalities.

The café-au-lait spot, present from birth, might support a genetic etiology. Such spots are sometimes found in disease-free individuals, but they can be markers for a genetic condition, especially neurofibromatosis or McCune-Albright syndrome. McCune-Albright syndrome usually involves a large, irregular café-au-lait spot close to the midline, as seen here in J.K.

McCune-Albright syndrome is a nonheritable genetic disease caused by a sporadic mutation in the somatic cell line early in embryonic development. Patients with McCune-Albright are thus mosaics of cells affected by the mutation and cells unaffected by it. The mutation results in an alteration of the G protein associated with adenylyl cyclase, causing overproduction of cAMP, altered signal transduction, and widespread hyperfunctioning of tissues. It is not known precisely why McCune-Albright affects particular tissues more than others, but McCune-Albright patients often suffer polyostotic fibrous dysplasia (bone lesions at multiple sites in the skeleton), hyperthyroidism and, in females, precocious puberty. J.K. has all of these signs of McCune-Albright. (At age 8 and Tanner stage 2, her pubertal development borders on precocious.) Enlargement of the temporal bone with impingement on the right vestibulocochlear nerve probably accounts for J.K.'s decreased hearing in the right ear. That, in turn, might explain her purported inattention in school.

TREATMENT AND SUBSEQUENT COURSE

With a putative diagnosis of McCune-Albright syndrome, J.K. was sent for orthopedic surgery on her right arm and left leg. Her radius underwent open reduction with osteotomy and internal fixation (open reduction means alignment of fragments through surgical intervention; osteotomy, removal of pieces of bone; internal fixation, placement of hardware to hold fragments in place), and her left leg underwent osteotomy, bone graft, and internal fixation, which successfully relieved the discrepancy in the length of her legs. She was discharged from the hospital a week later with pain medication and a prescription for 25 mg qd (once a day) propylthiouracil for hyperthyroidism. During follow-up, ultrasonography revealed an ovarian cyst, for which J.K. was followed by a gynecologist.

Case Study Questions

1. Why is the TSH low in McCune-Albright syndrome? How might increased cAMP lead to increased levels of thyroxine, and how does a high thyroxine level affect TSH secretion?

2. How might increased cAMP affect signal transduction in the ovary? Why might this lead to precocious puberty?

3. Would you expect the luteinizing hormone (LH) and follicle-stimulating hormone (FSH) levels to be elevated or normal? Why?

4. Could a somatic mutation inherited from the parents in the germ line affect the offspring in a mosaic fashion? What about an X-linked mutation?

Part II CASE STUDY FOR **MUSCULOSKELETAL PHYSIOLOGY**

S.O. is a 6-year-old boy who presented to his pediatrician with a waddling gait on tip-toe and a several-year-long history of falls and fatigue when engaged in play with other children.

PRESENTATION

S.O.'s parents had been concerned for some time about their son's energy level. He had walked late (at 20 months) and always appeared to them to be weak or fatigued. When engaged in play with other children, he could barely jump off the floor. In the last few months, S.O. at times seemed to have added difficulty getting up from a sitting to a standing position. This difficulty was unrelieved by rest and had slowly gotten worse. S.O.'s heels had also begun to lift off the ground when he walked.

On inspection, S.O. displayed some mild proximal muscle wasting and slight hypertrophy of the calves. There was scoliosis of the spine. He had a toe-walking gait with a slightly lordotic posture (abdomen pushed forward, versus hunched or kyphotic posture) and symmetrical proximal muscle weakness in the arms and legs. Neck muscles displayed symmetrical weakness, and deep tendon reflexes were diminished bilaterally. Muscle tone was floppy. No fasciculations (small, visible jerks in the muscle) were noted.

Lab tests were normal except for a creatine kinase of 2500 U/L, far above normal. S.O. was referred to a pediatric neurologist, who took a muscle tissue biopsy and performed a blood test looking for a mutation to the X-linked dystrophin gene. The biopsy revealed nearly undetectable levels of dystrophin, and the genetic blood test was positive, confirming the diagnosis of Duchenne muscular dystrophy.

Discussion

One of S.O.'s main presenting problems was weakness. Diseases can create weakness by acting at the muscles themselves, but also by acting anywhere along the chain of neural command that terminates at the muscles—anywhere from the neuromuscular junction up to the cerebral cortex. Neurologists can localize the cause of weakness with a number of inquiries: Is the weakness symmetrical or focal? Was its onset slow or sudden? Genetic or metabolic derangements are often symmetrical (nonfocal) and more gradual in onset, whereas a cerebrovascular accident (stroke) affecting the motor cortex or descending motor pathways is often focal and acute. Are the muscle tone and reflexes decreased or increased? Damage to lower motor neurons hampers reflexes, decreases muscle tone, and causes muscle fasciculations. Damage to upper motor neurons also creates weakness, decreasing the patient's ability to control the affected muscle, but such damage does not abolish reflexes or muscle tone. Instead, upper motor neuron disease cuts off inhibitory spinal input to peripheral neurons, causing increased muscle tone and hyperreflexia. Is the weakness proximal or distal? Disease of the peripheral nerves (peripheral neuropathy) preferentially affects the long nerves and thus it commonly presents with distal sensory and motor deficits. Muscle diseases, on the other hand, often present with proximal weakness. Is the weakness constant or can it be relieved? Disease of the neuromuscular junction, such as myasthenia gravis, is characterized by weakness that comes and goes.

The depressed reflexes and decreased muscle tone in S.O.'s case suggest a problem distal to the upper motor neurons, and the absence of fasciculations points away from a lower motor neuron disease. The steady, unfluctuating nature of the weakness argues against a disease of the neuromuscular junction. The proximal weakness points away from a neuropathy and toward a muscle disease. Finally, the high creatine kinase and absence of dystrophin on biopsy are strongly associated with Duchenne muscular dystrophy. Becker muscular dystrophy, which is clinically similar but less severe, is associated with higher levels of dystrophin on biopsy.

It is not known exactly how the dystrophin deficiency injures the muscle cells, but the result is progressive muscle cell death with atrophy, scarring, and contractures. The contractures pull up on the heel cords and account for the toe-walking. The apparent hypertrophy of the calves may at first be due to muscular compensation for the failing proximal muscles and later due to the replacement of wasted muscle with fat.

TREATMENT AND SUBSEQUENT COURSE

S.O. began a course of steroids—10 mg qd of prednisone—which limited his muscle pain and slowed the progress of the muscular cell death a little. He discontinued the steroids at age 9 because of the uncomfortable weight gain. A physical therapist worked with him to help him stretch and prevent painful contractures. By age 10, he was wheelchair-bound, and family members, visiting nurses, and other caregivers kept him on a turning schedule in bed to prevent pressure sores (decubitus ulcers). They also monitored his skin for signs of breakdown, since pressure sores are a constant threat for immobile patients. In his late teens, the scoliosis and atrophy of his diaphragm began to impair S.O.'s ability to breathe. By age 20, he required mechanical ventilation, and after a few weeks on the machine, he contracted pneumonia and died.

Case Study Questions

1. Why would impaired ventilation lead to a susceptibility to respiratory infection?

2. Why does the mutation found in Becker muscular dystrophy allow more dystrophin to be produced?

3. Why does lower motor neuron disease cause fasciculations? Why does disease of the neuromuscular junction create muscle fatigue that resolves in time?

4. How should a doctor deliver the news of a tragic diagnosis like Duchenne muscular dystrophy?

Part III CASE STUDY FOR BLOOD AND LYMPH

M.R. is a 25-year-old woman with no previous history of illness who was admitted to the neurology service overnight after what family members described as a dizzy spell.

INITIAL PRESENTATION

When M.R. arrived at the hospital, she was drowsy but alert and oriented. Her family members said she had been talking to her brother at a family barbecue when she began to stare and became unresponsive. She did not fall, but she did smack her lips repeatedly in a manner the family described as "strange." The staring, unresponsiveness, and lip-smacking lasted for 2–3 min.

M.R. remembered only a feeling of falling backward, followed by a gap in her memory. The family sat her down, gave her lemonade to drink, and called an ambulance. M.R. was taking no medications and had had no alcohol or drugs that day, and she reported no cardiac history or history of seizures.

At the time of admission, she had a fever of 99.5°F, a blood pressure of 110/76 mmHg, a heart rate of 88 beats per minute, and a respiratory rate of 20 breaths per minute. Her neurologic exam was nonfocal, carotid pulses were strong with no bruits, and her cardiac exam showed normal heart sounds, regular rate and rhythm, with no rubs or murmurs detected. Testing for orthostatic hypotension was negative. Blood tests were significant for a normal serum glucose of 97 mg/dL, normal creatine kinase of 154 U/L, a slightly elevated creatinine of 1.3 mg/dL, a low hematocrit of 30%, a low white blood cell count of 2,800/μL, and a low platelet count of 80,000/μL. Hemeoccult was negative, and electrocardiogram (ECG) showed sinus rhythm with no ischemic changes. Cerebrospinal fluid (CSF) from lumbar puncture was normal with no indicators of meningitis. A head computed tomography (CT) scan was also normal with no evidence of infarcts. It was determined that M.R. probably had a complex partial seizure, and she was kept overnight for observation and further testing.

Discussion

Whenever a patient has experienced a loss or alteration of consciousness, it is important to eliminate life-threatening causes from the list of differential diagnoses (or as clinicians say, to "rule them out"). Causes of decreased consciousness may be divided broadly into several categories: derangements of blood composition, derangements of blood flow to the brain, and intrinsic neurologic conditions. Intrinsic neurologic conditions generally affect consciousness in either of two ways: pathology involving both cerebral hemispheres or pathology in the brain stem, where the ascending reticular activating system (ARAS) is located. (One functional hemisphere and an intact ARAS are sufficient to sustain consciousness; either the ARAS or both hemispheres must be disordered to lose consciousness.) See TABLE CS3.1 for a categorized list of these causes of altered consciousness. Some of the conditions listed, such as brain herniation, are not consistent with partial or transient losses of consciousness; an experienced clinician hence would not need to consider everything on the table in this case. They are included here in order to demonstrate a part of the thought process that is second nature to experienced practitioners.

Table CS3.1   CAUSES OF DECREASED OR ALTERED CONSCIOUSNESS

Derangements of Blood Composition	Derangements of Blood Flow to the Brain		Intrinsic Neurologic Conditions	
	Impaired Blood Flow	Excess Blood Flow	Bilateral Cerebral Conditions	Brainstem Pathology
• **Hypoxia** • **Intoxication** (alcohol, illicit drugs, poisons, medications) • **Metabolic abnormalities** (hypoglycemia; hyperammonemia— i.e., hepatic coma; others) • **Electrolyte abnormalities**	• **Cardiac pathology** (MI; heart failure; valvular disease; arrhythmia; vasovagal response) • **Decreased ECF volume** (GI bleed; dehydration; 3rd spacing—i.e., loss of intravascular fluids to interstitial edema) • **Vascular disease** (vertebrobasilar ischemia; subclavian steal)	• **Hypertensive encephalopathy**	• **Inflammation** (meningitis/ encephalitis due to infection; vasculitis) • **Head trauma** (concussion; intracranial bleeding; depressed skull fracture) • **Intracranial bleeding** (non-traumatic, as from massive stroke or subarachnoid hemorrhage) • **Bilateral strokes** • **Generalized or complex partial seizures** (75% of generalized seizures are idiopathic; generalized seizures may also arise from focal lesions and from other generalized insults to the brain)	• **Increased intracranial pressure** (mass lesion or bleeding, leading to herniation) • **Inflammation** (meningitis) • **Infarction** (i.e., brainstem stroke)

Many pertinent negative findings (normal findings) emerged from M.R.'s initial workup that helped to rule out possible causes of her spell. The normal creatine phosphokinase (CK) level, normal ECG, normal cardiac exam, normal blood pressure, as well as her young age all suggest that she had no myocardial infarction and no pathologic drop in cardiac output. The negative hemeoccult (analysis of stool for blood content) suggests M.R. was not suffering gastrointestinal bleeding. She had no other signs of depleted intravascular volume. (Orthostatic hypotension reflects volume depletion and is measured by taking the pulse in a lying and then in a standing position—a significant increase in pulse is a positive test.) She was not intoxicated and had no obvious electrolyte or metabolic derangements of the blood. We can infer from the transient nature of the spell that brainstem pathology (herniation, infarction) or other catastrophic event is unlikely; and the normal neurologic exam and normal CT scan rule out mass lesions, bleeding, and infarction. While M.R. did have a low fever, her white count was not elevated, and her lumbar puncture showed no signs of infection or inflammation. She had no headache or nuchal (neck) rigidity—symptoms of meningitis. An infectious cause seems unlikely.

Some of the positive findings point to a complex partial seizure. The duration of minutes, the stare, the lip-smacking (a typical "automatism") are expected findings for a complex partial seizure. The underlying cause at this point remains unclear. Could it have something to do with the mild fever, elevated creatinine, and abnormal blood counts, which showed anemia (low red blood cell count), leukopenia (low white cell count), and thrombocytopenia (low platelet count)?

THE NEXT DAY

In the morning, M.R. was able to give a more complete medical history. Over the last two weeks, it turned out she had been suffering from fatigue and from pain in the wrists and knuckles of both hands, as well as in her knees and along her neck. The pain was worse in the morning. She had a very physical job as a nanny of three small children and attributed the pain to being overworked. She had had three other episodes of similar joint pain and fatigue over the last 5 years, each lasting about 2 weeks. On one of those occasions she also remembered suffering a sore throat and a red swollen rash on the back of her neck and on the extensor surfaces of her arms. At the time of this admission, she had no rash, and her knuckles and fingers appeared normal without any deformities.

Her fever remained slightly high at 99.7°F. More tests were performed. A T_2-weighted magnetic resonance imaging (MRI) of the head showed two small foci of increased signal intensity in the subcortical white matter of the temporal lobe. Urine dipstick revealed 2+ proteinuria and hematuria. The levels of several autoantibodies were measured. Anticardiolipin antibody was negative. The following were positive: ANA (antinuclear antibody), anti-dsDNA antibody (dsDNA is double-stranded DNA), anti-Sm antibody (Sm stands for Smith antigen, a ribonuclear protein). C3 complement was low at 59 mg/dL, while other complement levels were within normal limits. Bilirubin levels were normal. Blood cultures were negative. A renal biopsy revealed mild focal proliferative nephritis.

Discussion

After the second day, M.R.'s problem list has grown, but the explanation of her symptoms—and hence the treatment plan—has come into much clearer focus. She has fever, which might be expected in the context of widespread inflammation, and she has arthritis (inflammation of the joints), possible cerebritis (inflammation of the brain, as indicated by foci of subcortical edema picked up on MRI and by history of complex partial seizure), and nephritis (inflammation of the kidney as indicated by the renal biopsy, increased creatinine, proteinuria, and hematuria). The episode of inflammation appears to be part of a recurrent pattern, with previous flares having possibly included dermatitis (rash), and pharyngitis.

Various infections, autoimmune diseases, allergic drug reactions, even malignancies, can create widespread inflammation of this kind, but our suspicions are focused on an autoimmune disease by the autoantibodies detected by serology. The particular antibodies detected—ANA, anti-dsDNA, and anti-Sm—are all directed against elements of cell nuclei, and antibodies against cell nuclei are a cardinal sign of **systemic lupus erythematosus**. The exact pathogenesis of lupus is still being elucidated but, in general, it is thought that a wide variety of cells become subject to autoimmune attack (possibly due to a nonspecific polyclonal stimulation of B cells by heat-shock proteins or T cell superantigens or due to B cell activation by specific endogenous or exogenous antigens). This attack has several consequences: it leads to so much immune complex formation in the blood that the liver and spleen cannot remove it all and the inflammatory immune complexes end up deposited in vascular beds all over the body; lupus also appears to inflame the peripheral tissues by direct autoimmune attack; and it causes the liver and spleen to remove normal hematologic cells from the blood, especially thrombocytes (platelets). The anemia seen frequently in lupus is usually not due to attack on red blood cells (RBCs), though this can occur. (Destruction of red cells is called hemolytic anemia, and in hemolytic anemia, indirect bilirubin spills from lysed red cells—note that M.R.'s anemia is not likely hemolytic given her normal bilirubin level.) The leukopenia seen in lupus may be related to increased white blood cell (WBC) clearance or impaired hematopoiesis. Hypocomplementemia, as indicated by M.R.'s low C3, reflects complement activation by immune complexes and is seen especially often in lupus nephritis.

TREATMENT AND SUBSEQUENT COURSE

M.R. was treated with oral predisone, starting at 50 mg qd for three weeks, at which point a repeat MRI was normal with no high-intensity foci, her proteinuria and hematuria had resolved, her creatinine level had dropped to normal range, and her joint aches had gone. She was then tapered off the prednisone. She remained free of lupus signs or symptoms for 3 years, when a screening exam of the urine revealed mild proteinuria, despite the absence of any other signs or complaints. She was trying to conceive a child at the time, and was advised that pregnancy was possible but should be postponed until the lupus flare was controlled. Another short steroid taper was prescribed, during which she contracted pneumonia and required hospitalization to receive intravenous (IV) antibiotics. At the end of the steroid taper, the proteinuria again resolved.

Case Study Questions

1. Why would volume depletion cause an increase in heart rate when a patient moves from lying to standing?

2. What blood tests are used to assess blood clotting? Which one is specific for platelet function?

3. What might be the cause of the nonhemolytic anemia often seen in lupus?

4. How can a massive stroke in the left hemisphere impair consciousness?

5. How do immune complexes activate the complement system?

6. Name two reasons M.R. might have been predisposed to contract pneumonia during treatment with glucocorticoids.

7. What kind of acute renal failure might M.R. have had?

Part IV CASE STUDY FOR CARDIAC PHYSIOLOGY

L.B. is a 50-year-old male cellist who cannot complete the second movement of Elgar's cello concerto without shortness of breath.

PRESENTATION

He was well until 6 months ago, when he began to notice extreme fatigue. Since then, he has had light-headedness when moving from a sitting or lying to a standing position. After long orchestra practices, L.B. noted swelling in his feet and reported difficulty sleeping at night. He was troubled by shortness of breath in bed, relieved by propping himself up on two pillows, and had to make frequent trips to the bathroom to urinate during the night. He could no longer climb a flight of stairs without stopping to rest and found himself thirsty all the time. There was no known history of rheumatic fever or heart murmur and a remote history of smoking less than a pack a week. L.B. was not a current smoker and drank socially. He had no history of hypertension, diabetes, high cholesterol, or heart disease.

On exam, L.B. appeared pale. His blood pressure was 100/75 mmHg, heart rate 102 beats per minute, respirations 22 per minute, and he was afebrile. There was jugular venous distension to 10 cm. Lung exam revealed inspiratory rales. Cardiac exam was significant for an S3 gallop and a 2/6 holosystolic murmur of mitral regurgitation, which increased with handgrip. The liver was palpable below the right costal margin. He had 2+ pitting edema in the pretibial and ankle regions, and his nail beds appeared cyanotic. His hands were cool and clammy. Mental status was normal.

Laboratory tests revealed a low serum sodium of 130 mEq/L and a low normal serum potassium of 3.6 mEq/L. Chloride was 94 mEq/L, and bicarbonate was low at 15 mEq/L. Creatinine was slightly elevated at 1.6 mg/dL (nl < 1.3 mg/dL). Blood urea nitrogen (BUN) was high at 45 mg/dL (nl 10–20 mg/dL). Twenty-four-hour urine collection revealed urine output of 500 mL/day (low), urine sodium concentration of 2 mEq/L (low), and urine osmolality of 800 mOsm/kg (toward the concentrated end of the spectrum). Electrocardiogram (ECG) showed sinus tachycardia, and chest x-ray (CXR) showed bilateral pulmonary edema in the lower lung fields and an enlarged heart.

Discussion

It is useful in taking a history to ask a patient what, if anything, among his accustomed activities he can no longer do or can do only with difficulty; L.B.'s chief complaint is that he has experienced fall-off in tolerance for his usual level of activity. This complaint is part of a larger picture of shortness of breath (dyspnea) during various kinds of exertion. Dyspnea on exertion is in turn a symptom of pulmonary edema, signs of which were also heard on lung exam and observed on chest x-ray. Pulmonary edema can be caused by primary lung pathology, or more commonly, by left-sided **congestive heart failure (CHF)**. When the left ventricle fails to pump enough blood to the aorta, the pulmonary veins become congested with unpumped blood. Fluid weeps from the pulmonary vessels into the alveolar spaces, covering part of the gas exchanging surface and impairing oxygenation. Such patients do not easily tolerate exercise, which requires increased oxygenation. Subjectively, this congestion is perceived as shortness of breath.

If L.B.'s pulmonary edema is caused by left-sided heart failure, he ought to have other signs of decreased cardiac output (CO), and indeed he does. The fatigue and light-headedness are symptomatic of low cardiac output, as is "two-pillow" orthopnea (meaning he has shortness of breath when lying supine, relieved when propping himself up in bed to a height of two pillows). When lying flat, sufferers of CHF exacerbate their pulmonary edema because this position increases the venous return of blood volume to the heart. The heart fails to pump out this added volume, and the pulmonary vessels become congested and weep fluid into the air spaces. Poor cardiac output also causes congestion upstream of the lungs in the systemic venous circulation. This is evident in distension of the external jugular veins, which is observed in L.B. Such venous "backup" also leads to engorgement of the liver (L.B. has a large liver by abdominal palpation) and peripheral edema, especially in the lower extremities where gravity pools the venous blood, causing extravasation of fluid into the interstitium. Such patients may have increased urine volumes at night (nocturia) when their feet are elevated, as L.B. does. The lesser opposition of gravity to venous return from the feet mobilizes the pooled fluid and relieves the pressure in the pedal vessels. The interstitial fluid flows back into circulation and raises the intravascular perfusion pressure—hence the nighttime urinary output.

During the day, however, the combination of third-spacing (loss of intravascular volume to interstitial edema) and decreased pumping action of the heart drops the perfusion pressures in the arterial system. Decreases in perfusion of the kidney may cause a decline in the glomerular filtration rate (GFR). The GFR may be decreased enough to manifest as an elevated creatinine, which L.B. has.

The decreased perfusion pressures in CHF also lead to a number of compensatory changes that are observable in L.B.'s exam and lab values. The baroreceptor reflex activates the sympathetic nervous system, the renin-angiotensin-aldosterone hormonal axis, and when hypoperfusion is severe, the secretion of antidiuretic hormone (ADH). Increased sympathetic tone and increased levels of angiotensin II vasoconstrict the arteries to increase the systemic blood pressure (SBP) by increasing the systemic vascular resistance (SVR). (Recall that in analogy to Ohm's Law, SBP = CO × SVR. If CO drops, but SVR increases, SBP can be preserved.) Peripheral vasoconstriction explains L.B.'s pale appearance and cool, clammy palms.

The baroreceptor reflex also works to increase CO by increasing extracellular fluid (ECF) volume. The sympathetic nervous system and angiotensin II achieve this by increasing proximal tubular salt reabsorption in the kidney. Water (and urea) follow the salt. A low urine output is observed. Increased urea reabsorption under these circumstances is evident in an increased BUN relative to the creatinine level (BUN/Cr > 20:1, as seen in L.B.). Finally, increased sympathetic tone raises the heart rate (L.B.'s is high at 102 beats per minute) to boost the cardiac output (CO) (CO = stroke volume × HR), and angiotensin II leads to secretion of aldosterone, which increases distal tubular salt reabsorption and potassium secretion in the kidney. Note that L.B.'s serum potassium is slightly low, which probably reflects increased aldosterone action.

Antidiuretic hormone (ADH; also known as vasopressin) is also secreted in order to maintain blood pressure, and thirst is also activated to promote ingestion of free water. The normal function of ADH, however, is to reabsorb water without salt; and drinking water also adds water without salt to the ECF. Consequently, baroreceptor-induced secretion of ADH creates an incidental dilution of the plasma (worsened by drinking) and incidental concentration of the urine. Thus L.B.'s low serum sodium concentration and hyperosmolar urine are to be expected.

One might expect atrial natriuretic peptide (ANP) and brain natriuretic peptide (BNP) to be low under these circumstances since these hormones vasodilate and oppose salt and water reabsorption, leading to diuresis. However, these hormones are also present in high levels because the congestion of the heart chambers leads to high atrial pressures. ANP and BNP may contribute to L.B.'s nocturia, but in general, their blood pressure-lowering effect is overridden by the effects of the other hormones.

The blood pressure–preserving baroreceptor effects might explain some of L.B.'s normal findings as well. Probably by compensatory effects, his blood pressure is maintained in the normal range. The extent of his renal failure is also limited by angiotensin II, which vasoconstricts the efferent arteriole to maintain the GFR under these circumstances and avoid or mitigate prerenal failure.

It is not clear at this point what has caused L.B.'s CHF because the history was not very indicative and because his clinical picture describes the common endpoint of many forms of heart disease—**dilated cardiomyopathy**: CHF with an enlarged heart (which was observed on chest x-ray). Rheumatic heart disease can lead to mitral regurgitation of the sort heard over the precordium, and chronic regurgitation could dilate and injure the myocardium. However, there is no prior history of murmur. Enlargement of the heart owing to other causes could, on the other hand, create mitral regurgitation by enlarging the mitral valve and rendering it incompetent. The most common cause of dilated cardiomyopathy is ischemic heart disease, though L.B.'s history does not indicate many risk factors for ischemic disease, besides his gender and his age. Viruses can cause cardiomyopathy, as can toxicity, including chronic exposure to alcohol.

TREATMENT AND SUBSEQUENT COURSE

L.B. was treated with furosemide, a diuretic, to relieve his pulmonary and peripheral edema and with KCl to preserve his potassium level. Several days after beginning this treatment, however, he lost consciousness while practicing the cello. He was taken to the hospital by ambulance and admitted to the intensive care unit (ICU). In the ICU, a Swan-Ganz catheter was inserted, and more data were obtained. L.B.'s radial artery pressure was 100/70 mmHg. His cardiac index was 2.4 L/min/m^2 (the cardiac index is a measure of the CO per minute, heart rate $\times$ stroke volume, corrected for body surface area, and the normal range is around 2.5–4.2). The calculated SVR was high, and L.B. was tachycardic. The pulmonary capillary wedge pressure (which is equal to the left ventricular end-diastolic pressure) was elevated at 30 mmHg. The right atrial pressure was high. Oxygenation was 88% by pulse oximeter and improved with administration of oxygen by face mask.

The diuretic was maintained and in addition dobutamine was administered. The shortness of breath and light-headedness improved. The creatinine dropped to 1.3 mg/dL, his BUN fell to 25 mg/dL, and his serum sodium rose to 136 mEq/L. The pulmonary capillary wedge pressure dropped, his cardiac output improved, and his urine output rose. L.B. went home on an ACE inhibitor. The cardiomyopathy was later attributed to viral myocarditis.

Discussion

Prior to treatment, L.B.'s baroreceptor reflex resulted in a number of compensations for low CO and blood pressure, which we reviewed above. The sympathetic and angiotensin II–mediated vasoconstriction elevated the SBP by increasing SVR. The salt and water retention brought more fluid into circulation, which would distend the vessels and thereby raise the intravascular pressure. However, these compensations made affairs worse for the heart and lungs.

Volume expansion increases the preload (the end-diastolic volume) for the heart and, in a healthy heart, increases the force of contraction and the stroke volume by the Frank-Starling mechanism. However, in dilated cardiomyopathy with CHF, increased preload worsens the pulmonary edema. Thus, the diuretic was employed to reduce some of this preload.

The systemic vasoconstriction made things harder on the heart by increasing the afterload that the left ventricle was working against. This reduced the stroke volume and worsened the mitral regurgitation, further reducing the CO. (The relation of afterload to mitral regurgitation was evident when the murmur worsened while L.B. squeezed his hands closed, increasing peripheral resistance.) Therefore, dobutamine, a peripheral vasodilator, was used to relieve the afterload on the heart, reducing the mitral regurgitation and improving the CO. (Dobutamine is also a positive inotrope, meaning it increases cardiac contractility, which helps to improve stroke volume.) With improved CO and improved perfusion of the kidney, the GFR rose (and the creatinine hence fell), and the urine output rose. The excretion of water partially corrected the hyponatremia. The high pulmonary vascular pressure was relieved which alongside the diuretic lessened the pulmonary edema.

Case Study Questions

1. Why was the bicarbonate low on L.B.'s initial presentation?

2. This case featured systolic dysfunction. Should a preload-lowering diuretic be given in the context of diastolic dysfunction? Why or why not?

3. Explain the low urine sodium concentration.

4. This case demonstrates that it is preferable to maintain SBP by increasing the CO rather than by increasing the SVR. Do you agree or disagree? Why?

Part V CASE STUDY FOR **PULMONARY PHYSIOLOGY**

V.G. is a 69-year-old female former smoker with a history of chronic obstructive pulmonary disease and morbid obesity, who initially presented to the emergency room with shortness of breath, fever, and chills. We will follow V.G. from her initial presentation through her hospital discharge.

PRESENTATION: HISTORY

V.G. was in her usual state of health until several weeks ago, when she developed a cough, and became less active than usual. Three days ago, her cough worsened, and she began to experience back pain with breathing as well as increasing fatigue and shortness of breath. V.G. normally uses 3 L of oxygen by nasal cannula when sleeping; however, with the increase in symptoms, she began to use supplemental oxygen when awake. She also uses daily β_2-agonist inhalers for treatment of her chronic obstructive pulmonary disease (COPD), and with her worsening symptoms, her frequency of β_2-agonist treatment increased. On the day of admission, her symptoms intensified, and she reported the onset of a fever, myalgias, chills, and periods of sweating. Her cough was productive of greenish-gray sputum. At the time of admission, she had no chest pain and no gastrointestinal symptoms. She also reported no leg swelling and no change in the number of pillows upon which she slept at night.

Discussion

As clinicians, we should review V.G.'s symptoms: cough productive of greenish-gray sputum, dyspnea (shortness of breath), fever, myalgias (muscle aches), chills, sweating, and back pain with breathing.

What do these symptoms lead us to include in the differential diagnosis? A productive cough accompanied by fever and chills might be indicative of an infection, more likely bacterial than viral. Pleurisy (chest or back pain with breathing) can be a sign of pneumonia. Worsening dyspnea could be the result of a respiratory infection, but also might result from an exacerbation of V.G.'s underlying COPD, perhaps triggered by an infection. (COPD is a combination of emphysema and chronic bronchitis due to smoking. Both forms reduce outflow from the lung; emphysema because of increased lung compliance, and chronic bronchitis through increased airway resistance. COPD can result in hypercarbia and hypoxemia.) The absence of edema (swelling) in V.G.'s legs and the absence of orthopnea (dyspnea exacerbated by lying flat) are significant. The presence of either might have suggested pulmonary edema, perhaps secondary to congestive heart failure, but their absence in V.G.'s case makes such a diagnosis less likely.

PRESENTATION: PHYSICAL EXAM AND LAB VALUES

On initial examination, V.G.'s temperature was elevated at 102.7°F, and her blood pressure was 145/85. V.G. was alert and cooperative, but looked uncomfortable, with labored breathing. Pulmonary examination revealed tachypnea (rapid breathing) at 26 breaths per minute, crackles at the bases of her left lower lobe, and decreased breath sounds in all lobes by auscultation. An occasional wheeze was audible. Her oxygen saturation was 89% while breathing room air and 95% on 2 L of supplemental oxygen by nasal cannula. Her cardiovascular examination was unremarkable except for her mild tachycardia (rapid heart rate) at 103 beats per minute. V.G.'s abdominal and neurological examinations were unremarkable. She had no lower extremity edema.

V.G.'s laboratory tests were notable for an elevated white blood cell count of 15,770/mm^3, with 88% polymorphonuclear cells and 6% lymphocytes. Her arterial blood gas on room air demonstrated a pH of 7.46, a P_aO_2 of 56 mm Hg, a P_aCO_2 of 33 mm Hg, and a bicarbonate of 23 mEq/L. Her chest radiograph revealed an infiltrate in the left lower lobe.

Discussion

The examination confirms suspicions that V.G. has a pulmonary infection. Fever will increase the minute ventilation requirement and therefore produce tachypnea. Additionally, activation of J receptors by bacterial toxins in the pulmonary circulation can trigger tachypnea. Decreased breath sounds are consistent with V.G.'s history of COPD, but when localized to a particular lobe can indicate the consolidation of pneumonia. Wheezing results from the difficulties with expiration in COPD. The crackles at the base of her left lower lobe indicate that a process such as consolidation or fluid retention might be present there. If the crackles were equal at the bases of both lungs, this would be more consistent with pulmonary edema. However, the appearance of crackles in only one lung is more consistent with consolidation from pneumonia or perhaps atelectasis.

V.G.'s blood work also indicates the presence of an infectious process. Her elevated white blood cell count, with a predominance of polymorphonuclear cells, is consistent with bacterial infection. Her arterial blood gas demonstrates an A-a gradient of 46 mm Hg, which suggests the presence of low $\dot{V}_A/\dot{Q}$. Pneumonia can cause low $\dot{V}_A/\dot{Q}$ when infection in the alveoli leads to inflammation and exudate. Pneumonia would also explain her alkalotic blood pH. As stated above, fever and activation of J receptors by bacterial toxins in the pulmonary circulation can trigger tachypnea (hyperventilation). Second, with a P_aO_2, below 60 mmHg, her peripheral chemoreceptors would begin to drive hyperventilation to increase the P_aO_2. Hyperventilation secondary to fever, to J receptor stimulation, and to hypoxemia would create a respiratory alkalosis. The left lower lobe infiltrate found on chest radiograph confirms the diagnosis of pneumonia.

TREATMENT AND SUBSEQUENT COURSE

V.G. responded favorably to intravenous antibiotics to treat her pneumonia and β_2-agonist inhalers for her COPD, along with continued use of supplemental oxygen. Over the next several days, her fever and chills resolved. After five days of intravenous antibiotics, she was switched to oral antibiotics, and plans were made for discharge. The night prior to discharge, however, V.G. began to experience dyspnea once more and demonstrated wheezes audible to the ear without a stethoscope. Physical examination demonstrated tachypnea at 30 breaths per minute and wheezes in all lobes on lung auscultation. Her chest radiograph was unchanged from admission.

V.G. was placed on the anticholinergic agent ipratropium bromide, increased frequency of β_2-agonist nebulizers, corticosteroids, and maintained on supplemental oxygen. Her dyspnea and wheezing resolved to her baseline (preillness level) after a day of treatment. She had no further complications during her hospital stay. Once arrangements were ready for transfer, she was discharged to a pulmonary rehabilitation facility on β_2-agonist therapy, a short course of corticosteroids and supplemental oxygen for her COPD, and oral antibiotics for the remaining days of her treatment for pneumonia.

Discussion

V.G.'s new dyspnea and wheezing are most consistent with an exacerbation of her known COPD. Both are classic signs of obstructive pulmonary disease, especially in the absence of focal findings on examination (i.e., in the absence of findings localized to one area of the lung fields). β_2-agonists relax the smooth muscle of the airways, alleviating the obstructive symptoms of COPD. Anticholinergic agents such as ipratropium bromide also act as bronchodilators.

Case Study Questions

1. What would be the typical profile for a patient with COPD on pulmonary function tests?

2. If a ventilation-perfusion scan had been obtained during V.G.'s initial presentation with pneumonia, what would have been the results for her left lower lobe?

3. COPD can result in hypercarbia and hypoxemia. Pneumonia can cause hypoxemia.

   a. What effect does CO_2 retention have on hemoglobin's transport of oxygen?

   b. What effect does hypoxemia have on hemoglobin's interaction with CO_2?

4. Tachypnea can result from activation of a variety of receptors. Which receptors might be involved in each of the following situations?

   a. COPD exacerbation

   b. Pneumonia

   c. Pulmonary embolism

Part VI CASE STUDY FOR **RENAL PHYSIOLOGY**

G.G. came to medical attention several times over the course of his childhood. We will follow G.G. from infancy onward, stopping along the way to discuss his presentation, diagnosis, and treatment.

PRESENTATION IN INFANCY: HISTORY

G.G. was the first child born in his family. During the first six months of life, he grew slowly despite the fact that he nursed extremely well. At 7 months of age, his interest in food seemed to decrease, and he became more cranky, and sometimes sleepless. He had always been an avid bottle drinker, so much so that Mr. and Mrs. G. remembered there seemed to be the never-ending task of changing wet diapers. By 1 year of age, he had not yet begun to stand on his own; he sometimes seemed too weak to sit up.

When G.G. was 13 months old, his mother rushed him to the emergency room of the nearby municipal hospital. He had become increasingly sleepy to the point that Mrs. G. was unable to arouse him long enough to feed him. Two days earlier, he had developed vomiting and diarrhea after playing with his cousin, who was recovering uneventfully from a bout of gastroenteritis. Mrs. G. also noted that during the last 2 days, G.G. had continued to make large quantities of urine despite his poor fluid intake. The ER physician treated G.G. with an IV and promptly admitted him to the hospital.

Discussion

What should we as clinicians be thinking about at this point? First, we should take stock of the list of symptoms: lethargy, polyuria (increased urinary volume), and a history of poor growth.

How do we explain these symptoms? Is there one underlying explanation or several? He may be dehydrated from gastroenteritis-related vomiting and diarrhea and lethargic from the dehydration; however, his history raises concerns about a more chronic problem. Polyuria in a state of dehydration is not explained by gastroenteritis and was even recognized as unexpected by G.G.'s mother. The history of never-ending diaper changing may indicate that the polyuria has been of long-term duration. G.G.'s poor recovery from gastroenteritis compared to that of his cousin suggests that he may have been dehydrated to begin with. Finally, a history of slow growth despite good appetite suggests abnormal development. Our suspicions are pointed toward a chronic disorder.

So how do we explain chronic polyuria and slow growth? Diabetes can cause polyuria, but this would be early for a presentation of that disease. There are other types of polyuria, including diabetes insipidus (decreased antidiuretic hormone [ADH] action) and other renal tubular disorders. By interfering with the normal reabsorption of solute, tubular disorders can cause an excess loss of solutes in the urine, leading to osmotic diuresis. Some of these kidney disorders can also retard growth.

PRESENTATION IN INFANCY: PHYSICAL EXAM AND LAB VALUES

The admitting pediatrician observed that G.G. was only in the third percentile in height and weight. The physical exam revealed signs of dehydration, including tachycardia (high heart rate) and a low blood pressure. Ophthalmologic changes included corneal opacities. The muscles were diffusely weak, and the child was listless. There was poor muscular development and bilateral varus deformities of the knees (knees pointing away from the midline). There was enlargement of the wrists, ankles, and the costochondral junctions of the ribs (the cartilaginous joints where the ribs insert into the sternum), all findings consistent with rickets. The heart and lungs were normal, and the abdominal exam revealed hepatomegaly (enlarged liver). The lab values showed significant abnormalities in blood chemistries (Table CS6.1). X-rays included films of the extremities, which revealed metaphyseal widening and a loss of bone density suggestive of rickets.

Discussion

The exam confirmed some of the suspicions raised by G.G.'s history and brought up others. The tachycardia, hypotension, and listlessness observed on exam confirmed the suspicion of dehydration. The exam also revealed growth retardation, corneal opacities, evidence of rickets (impaired mineralization of growing bone owing to vitamin D deficiency), and hepatomegaly. The labs showed hypokalemia, hypocalcemia, hypophosphatemia, low serum bicarbonate, acidosis, and glycosuria.

Table CS6.1   G.G.'S LAB VALUES, AGE 1

	At Age 1	
Blood	**G.G.'s Values**	**Normal Child's Values**
Potassium (K^+)	3.0 mmol/L	3.5–4.5 mmol/L
Sodium (Na^+)	148 mmol/L	135–148 mmol/L
Chloride (Cl^-)	120 mmol/L	95–110 mmol/L
Bicarbonate (HCO_3^-)	15 mmol/L	24–29 mmol/L
pH	7.30	7.38–7.42
PCO_2	30 mm Hg	35–45 mm Hg
Glucose (fasting)	70 mg/100 mL	60–100 mg/100 mL
Phosphate (PO_4^{3-})	1.9 mg/100 mL	4–6 mg/100 mL
Calcium (Ca^{2+})	8.0 mg/100 mL	9–11 mg/100 mL
BUN	30 mg/100 mL	10–20 mg/100 mL
Creatinine	0.7 mg/100 mL	0.2–0.5 mg/100 mL
Hematocrit	45%	35–42%
Urine	**G.G.'s Values**	**Normal Child's Values**
Osmolality	300 mosm/kg water	[a]
pH	5.0	[a]
Glucose	4+	Negative

[a] There are no "normal" values for urine osmolality and urine pH because these values vary widely as a part of the kidney's normal efforts to regulate the osmolality and pH of the blood. In this setting of acidosis, the urine pH is expected to be acid, and it is. BUN, blood urea nitrogen.

How do we explain the other signs? Earlier, we wondered if a disorder of the renal proximal tubule could be causing G.G.'s polyuria and dehydration. A proximal tubular disorder could also account for many of the findings on physical and laboratory examination.

Such disorders can cause rickets and derangements in serum calcium and phoshate. Because the active form of vitamin D is synthesized by hydroxylation in the mitochondria of the renal proximal tubule, many kidney diseases result in vitamin D deficiency and consequent decreases in intestinal calcium and phosphate absorption. Proximal tubular disorders can also result in decreased reabsorption of calcium and phosphate and hence wastage of those electrolytes in the urine. The net result of wastage coupled with poor intestinal absorption may be severe degrees of hypocalcemia and hypophosphatemia. In children, this can lead to rickets.

Bicarbonate may also be poorly reabsorbed in renal tubular disorders, which in turn affects both acid-base and K^+ balance. Excess loss of bicarbonate in the urine decreases serum bicarbonate and creates a nonanion gap metabolic acidosis. That would explain G.G.'s low serum pH and bicarbonate. Also, whenever bicarbonate losses in the urine are excessive, K^+ excretion increases for two reasons. First, the excreted anionic bicarbonate must be accompanied by balancing cations—the negatively charged bicarbonate draws cations into the urine with it for excretion—and K^+ is excreted in this way. Second, K^+ losses occur because increased K^+ secretion is occurring in exchange for Na^+ at the distal nephron in response to high aldosterone. The osmotic diuresis caused by the loss of excess solute depletes extracellular fluid volume, the low extracellular fluid volume stimulates the RAA system, and the high aldosterone pumps Na^+ in and K^+ out. These pathologic mechanisms could explain G.G.'s hypokalemia.

In the lab values, also notice that there is glycosuria (glucose in the urine) but not hyperglycemia; this again reflects the presence of a renal tubular disorder. In diabetes mellitus, urine glucose and serum glucose are high. Normal blood sugar means diabetes mellitus is not present, and the defect lies in the proximal tubular reabsorption of glucose.

Since nearly all of G.G.'s findings are consistent with a disorder of the proximal tubule, our suspicions are now high for that diagnosis. See TABLE CS6.2 for further discussion of the lab values.

TREATMENT IN INFANCY

G.G. responded favorably to treatment with IV fluids and was discharged 15 days later on oral Na^+ and K^+ bicarbonate, phosphate, calcium, and vitamin D. The discharge diagnosis was dehydration associated with Fanconi's syndrome.

Because of the clinical presentation and the laboratory abnormalities, a number of special tests were performed. The results of these tests were known only after G.G.'s discharge. Twenty-four-hour urinary excretion of amino acids revealed increases—as much as ten times normal. The creatinine clearance was 90 mL/min/1.73 m^2 of body surface area (normal). The percent phosphate reabsorbed was 50% (usually about 90%). A sample of white blood cells showed a cystine content of 8 nmol/mg protein (normal less than 0.2).

When G.G. was seen as an outpatient over the next few years, his clinical situation was improved dramatically. He maintained a good state of hydration and continued to grow, although he maintained a short stature. He made large volumes of urine, at times 2 L per day, and continued to have glycosuria. His acid-base balance returned to normal, as did his serum levels of K^+, Na^+, Ca^{2+}, and phosphate. He was maintained on 1,25 hydroxy vitamin D and large supplements of K^+ bicarbonate.

Discussion

Because of the dehydration, G.G. received isotonic saline (154 mM NaCl, which dilutes in plasma water to 140 mM NaCl) to expand his extracellular volume. The metabolic acidosis was treated with bicarbonate. The other electrolyte disorders, including hypokalemia, hypocalcemia, and hypophosphatemia, were treated with replacement therapy; in addition, vitamin D was administered to increase G.G.'s serum phosphate and calcium levels.

Table CS6.2   A COMPARISON OF G.G.'S FLUID AND ELECTROLYTE HOMEOSTASIS

Test	13 Months: Interpretation		10 Years: Interpretation	
Hematocrit (%)	45	**High**: Fluid losses lead to hemoconcentration.	25	**Low**: Chronic renal failure causes anemia owing to decreased production of erythropoeitin.
BUN (mg %)	30	**High**: Urea is filtered and reabsorbed. In dehydration, tubular urea reabsorption is increased.	50	**High**: Decreased urea clearance owing to fall in GFR and decreased filtration of urea.
Creatinine (mg %)	0.7	**Slightly high**: Since creatinine is filtered, only a fall in GFR will cause creatinine to rise. GFR was only slightly reduced by dehydration.	6.0	**High**: Decreased creatinine clearance owing to fall in GFR, which was profoundly reduced due to renal disease.
Na$^+$ (mmol/L)	148	**High normal**: Results from urinary water losses owing to glycosuria. Note high Na$^+$ concentration despite decreased extracellular volume (clinical dehydration).	134	**Low normal**: Results from inability of kidney to excrete ingested water because of low GFR. Note low Na$^+$ concentration despite increased extracellular volume on exam (1+ edema).
HCO$_3^-$ (mmol/L)	15	**Low**: Since pH is also low, this is metabolic acidosis. PCO$_2$ falls in respiratory compensation.	15	**Low**: Acid blood pH indicates metabolic acidosis.
Anion gap	13	**Normal**: Na$^+$ - (Cl$^-$ + HCO$_3^-$) = anion gap, owing to unmeasured anions (e.g., albumin). Fall in HCO$_3^-$ is matched by rise in Cl$^-$. HCO$_3^-$ losses are due to defect in proximal tubule bicarbonate reabsorption/proximal renal tubule acidosis.	20	**High**: Low GFR results in retention in plasma of anions such as phosphate, sulfate. Fall in HCO$_3^-$ is matched by these increased inorganic anions, not Cl$^-$. Acidosis of renal failure is primarily due to decreased ammonia synthesis rather than bicarbonate wasting.
Urine pH	5.0	**Acid**: In proximal renal tubular acidosis, HCO$_3^-$ is lost until serum HCO$_3^-$ concentration falls. At that point, decreased filtered load of HCO$_3^-$ can be reabsorbed by proximal and distal nephron so urine pH falls to acid levels. However, when NaHCO$_3$ given, proximal tubule cannot accommodate increased filtered load and urine becomes alkaline.	5.0	**Acid**: Even though diseased kidneys cannot eliminate a normal amount of net acid, pH falls in urine because of decreased amount of urinary buffer (i.e., NH$_3$).
K+ (mol/L)	3.0	**Low**: Owing to urinary K$^+$ loss. Increased urinary flow rate and distal Na$^+$ delivery coupled with increased aldosterone owing to dehydration causes increased K$^+$ secretion by distal tubule. Note that with treatment, increased distal NaHCO$_3$ delivery increased urinary K$^+$ loss and serum K$^+$ fell further.	5.0	**High**: Diseased kidney is less responsive to aldosterone and has limited capacity to increase K$^+$ secretion. Dietary K$^+$ is underexcreted, leading to hyperkalemia.
Phosphate (mg/100 mL)	1.9	**Very low**: Phosphate reabsorption in proximal tubule is abnormal, resulting in phosphaturia and hypophosphatemia, causing renal rickets.	7.0	**High**: Owing to decreased phosphate filtration as GFR falls in renal failure.
Ca (mg/100 mL)	8.0	**Slightly low**: Decreased proximal tubule calcium reabsorbtion.	7.0	**Low**: Owing to decreased 1,25 vitamin D synthesis by diseased kidney.
Urine glucose test strip	4+	**High**: Not due to diabetes because blood glucose was normal. Therefore, it is due to abnormal proximal reabsorption.	0	**Normal**: Even though proximal tubule is abnormal, so little glucose is filtered by the diseased kidney with low GFR that this small amount can be reclaimed.
Urine osmolality or specific gravity	300	**Isosmotic**: Increased solute load resulting from impaired proximal reabsorption obliges water excretion. Result is polyuria due to osmotic diuresis.	1.010	**Isosmotic**: A normal solute load now excreted by fewer nephron units obligates isosmotic water excretion.
Urine protein	1+	**Abnormal**: Tubular proteins (e.g., β_2 microglobulin) appear in urine in this tubular disorder.	4+	**Abnormal**: Albuminuria indicates glomerular disease with leak of plasma proteins.

BUN, blood urea nitrogen; GFR, glomerular filtration rate.

Fanconi's syndrome is a form of proximal tubule dysfunction defined by amino-aciduria, glycosuria (without hyperglycemia), phosphaturia, bicarbonaturia, and rickets. The syndrome is the common endpoint for several underlying types of pathology; in children, the most common cause is a congenital *metabolic disorder* in which normal metabolic reaction pathways are blocked. This leads to the excessive accumulation of one or more compounds in cells throughout the body and multiorgan dysfunction. It is thought that in the kidney, this accumulation results in a depletion of the ATP necessary to drive the reabsorption of amino acids, glucose, phosphate, and bicarbonate across the wall of the proximal tubule.

G.G.'s aminoaciduria and glycosuria without hyperglycemia support the diagnosis of Fanconi's syndrome. A clue as to the cause of the syndrome was the finding of a high cystine content in the white blood cells, diagnostic of a metabolic disorder called cystinosis. *Cystinosis* is a disorder of cystine metabolism that results in the intracellular accumulation of free, nonprotein cystine crystals in lysosomes of cells in a variety of body organs. In retrospect, someone with experience with cystinosis may have recognized that G.G.'s corneal opacities were due to cystine accumulation.

TREATMENT AFTER THE DIAGNOSIS OF CYSTINOSIS

At age 3, after the diagnosis of cystinosis was established, G.G. was referred to a specialist in this area, who placed him on cysteamine. The specialist kept an eye on G.G.'s kidney function. The serum creatinine was measured repeatedly, and while his serum creatinine continued to rise, the cysteamine slowed its rate of increase.

Discussion

During infancy, while G.G. suffered many symptoms of defective proximal tubular reabsorption, he had a nearly normal serum creatinine, the index of glomerular filtration rate (GFR). His GFR was therefore nearly normal, and his glomeruli were functioning well. Over the course of years, however, G.G.'s GFR declined along with his tubular function. Cysteamine is a sulfhydryl-containing compound that can form a disulfide with cysteine, decreasing the production of the disulfide cystine which is responsible for the disease. This treatment slowed but did not stop the progression of renal failure.

PRESENTATION AT AGE 10

By age 10, G.G.'s renal failure had worsened to the point where he was a candidate for hemodialysis, in which a machine performs the work of clearance normally performed by the kidney. The nephrologist learned from Mrs. G. that G.G. was an average student in the public schools. He had frequently missed class, because of both physical and emotional problems. Kids teased him because he was short; in fact, at 8 years of age he looked more the size of a 4-year-old. As his renal function declined, he became progressively anemic. His creatinine had risen to 3 mg/100 mL. He had not been taking any medication; his electrolyte supplements were discontinued more than a year previously.

The nephrologist examined G.G., a blond-haired child with a fair complexion and noticed that he was markedly photophobic. As expected, he was short of stature. There was mild hepatosplenomegaly (enlargement of liver and spleen), some muscle weakness, 1+ peripheral edema, and a normal neurologic exam. G.G.'s lab results are listed in TABLE CS6.3.

Discussion

Mrs. G. revealed that G.G. has suffered physical and emotional problems because of his short stature, which is characteristic of his disease and of chronic metabolic acidosis and rickets. His anemia was likely due to erythropoetin deficiency associated with chronic renal disease. The very high creatinine indicates advanced renal failure. Fortunately, he had stopped taking the supplemental minerals, since at this stage of low renal function (i.e.,

Table CS6.3 **G.G.'S LAB VALUES, AGE 10**

Blood	At Age 10	
	G.G.'s Values	Normal Child's Values
Potassium (K^+)	5.0 mmol/L	3.5–4.5 mmol/L
Sodium (Na^+)	135 mmol/L	135–148 mmol/L
Chloride (Cl^-)	100 mmol/L	95–110 mmol/L
Bicarbonate (HCO_3^-)	15 mmol/L	24–29 mmol/L
pH	7.30	7.38–7.42
Phosphate (PO_4^{3-})	7.0 mg/100 mL	4–6 mg/100 mL
Calcium (Ca^{2+})	7.0 mg/100 mL	9–11 mg/100 mL
BUN	30 mg/100 mL	10–20 mg/100 mL
Creatinine	3.0 mg/100 mL	0.2–0.5 mg/100 mL
Hematocrit	25%	35–42%
Urine	**G.G.'s Values**	**Normal Child's Values**
Albumin	Positive (2+)	Negative
Glucose	Negative	Negative
pH	5.0	[a]
Osmolality	300 mosm/kg water	[a]

[a] There are no "normal" values for urine osmolality and urine pH, because these values vary widely as a part of the kidney's normal efforts to regulate the osmolality and pH of the blood. In this setting of acidosis the urine pH is expected to be acid, and it is. BUN, blood urea nitrogen.

low GFR) he would have had difficulty excreting potassium, phosphate, and even bicarbonate, which might have resulted in very high serum levels of these compounds. The advancement of glomerular disease has impaired electrolyte clearance—the opposite of the tubular disease, which promotes excessive clearance. The physical exam was typical for cystinosis: blond hair, photophobia, short stature, large liver, weak muscles, and corneal opacities. His edema is characteristic of renal failure, in which the extracellular fluid volume expands, hydrostatically causing fluid leakage into the tissues. (The albuminuria is not of sufficient magnitude to constitute the nephrotic syndrome.) The electrolytes are to be contrasted to his earlier admission; for further discussion, see Table CS6.2. Most notably, he was hyperkalemic, mildly hyponatremic (which occurred despite edema), acidotic, hyperphosphatemic, and hypocalcemic. There was now evidence of albuminuria, consistent with glomerular disease. This finding, along with the high serum creatinine, indicates that any chronic renal disease eventually affects the glomeruli, even if it starts as a tubular disorder.

TREATMENT AT AGE 10 AND AFTERWARD

G.G.'s parents were anxious to find out whether they could donate a kidney to their son. Over the next 6 months, G.G., his physicians, and his family made preparations for dialysis, which eventually was started.

Soon after starting dialysis, arrangements were made for G.G. to receive a kidney transplant from his father. Within a year he received the transplant, which functioned well, and he is currently feeling better than ever and is back in school.

Discussion

Because cystinosis is an inherited defect in metabolism, it is produced by the affected cells themselves. G.G.'s father does not have cystinosis, and his kidney cells do not accumulate cysteine. Therefore, there will not be recurrent cystinosis in the transplanted kidney. However, it is likely that the extrarenal organs will continue to deposit the amino acid, and therefore therapy may be continued.

Case Study Questions

1. Distinguish between glomerular and tubular functions of the normal kidney. How were these affected by G.G.'s disease? Distinguish between proximal and distal tubular functions. What evidence exists in this case to pinpoint the tubular site of injury?

2. What is rickets, and what role does the kidney play in vitamin metabolism? Why is G.G. anemic?

3. What is (are) the mechanism(s) underlying metabolic acidosis in this case?

4. Why did G.G.'s Fanconi syndrome disappear in the latter stage of the disease?

Part VII CASE STUDY FOR GASTROINTESTINAL PHYSIOLOGY

B.C. is a 42-year-old accountant who was seen by his primary care physician with a loss of appetite and a 10-lb weight loss occurring over several months.

PRESENTATION

B.C. noted that he was particularly weak in the morning, finding it hard to start the day, and would fatigue easily with little exertion. He began to notice easy bruising on his extremities and flank with minimal or no trauma. His parents came for a visit recently, and commented on the color of his eyes, which had a yellowish tint.

At first, he was reluctant to discuss his habits with his physician but acknowledged that he had had a "drinking problem" since college. He had at times consumed 3–4 drinks of whiskey in an evening after work; after social occasions on which he drank heavily, he had trouble remembering the events of the previous night.

In reviewing his recent history, B.C. also noted that he had been losing the muscle mass in his upper extremities, and yet his waist size had increased. He had also developed hemorrhoids, with some rectal bleeding. His breasts had enlarged, causing him some embarrassment. He had been hospitalized once, having hit his head in a period of heavy drinking at a party, and had had a single seizure at that time, years ago. On another occasion, he had tried to stop drinking, but experienced nausea and vomiting, as well as extreme restlessness and shakes; none of these symptoms has recurred. He does not smoke. The only medication that he takes is an occasional acetaminophen for headache.

On physical examination, B.C. had a blood pressure of 102/58 mmHg, a pulse of 92 beats per minute, respiration of 16 breaths per minute, and he was afebrile. He had wasting of his deltoids and chest muscles. There was normal jugular venous pressure, a normal cardiac exam, ascites with superficial dilated veins in the abdomen. The liver and spleen were not palpable. There was gynecomastia and testicular atrophy. Peripheral edema was noted. Other findings included clubbing of the fingers, palmar erythema, spider angiomata, and scleral icterus.

Laboratory tests included a hematocrit of 33%, with an elevated mean corpuscular volume; the urine tested positive for bilirubin; the serum aspartate aminotransferase and alkaline phosphatase were mildly elevated; and the serum prothrombin time was prolonged. An ammonia level was mildly increased, and the blood sugar was 52 mg/dL in a fasting sample. The serum albumin was 2.8 g/dL. Hepatitis B and C serologies were negative. An ultrasound of the abdomen did not reveal signs of biliary obstruction, and there were no masses in the small liver.

Discussion

B.C. has many of the signs of **alcoholic cirrhosis,** the most common form of liver failure in the United States. Alcoholic cirrhosis follows a long history of alcohol abuse and can be seen in high-functioning individuals. It may follow other complications of alcohol abuse, such as seen in this case: a history of loss of consciousness, withdrawal seizures and other withdrawal symptoms, head trauma, and alcohol hepatitis.

While this patient presents with a vague complaint (weight loss and low appetite) and suffers a dizzying array of signs and symptoms, a thorough knowledge of hepatic physiology makes the diagnosis clear because many of the signs and symptoms can be traced back to the failure of normal liver function and to the consequences of alcoholism. That said, it is important in such a case to exclude other causes of liver disease, such as gallstones causing obstruction of the biliary tract, and liver cancers, which can occur in the setting of cirrhotic liver. The abdominal ultrasound helps to rule out those conditions.

Now let's try to identify those findings in B.C.'s case that are typical of cirrhosis, with special attention to those signs and symptoms that could be predicted by a consideration of hepatic physiology. The liver is responsible for synthesizing important blood proteins, including the vitamin K–dependent clotting factors and albumin. Scarring of the liver reduces its synthetic capacities, leading to decreased levels of clotting factors and albumin. The lack of clotting factors often manifests in a prolonged prothrombin time, as it has in this case, and can predispose toward bruising and even bleeding. Low albumin in the blood reduces the oncotic pressure of the blood and may lead to the peripheral edema seen in B.C. The edema is worsened by direct sodium-retaining effects of the liver disease on the kidney (the poorly understood hepatorenal syndrome). In the extreme, patients with advanced liver disease may develop kidney failure owing to the hepatic factors influencing the renal circulation, rather than to damage to the kidney per se.

Patients with cirrhosis develop portal hypertension, owing to the scarring within the liver and decreased flow from the portal circulation through the liver into the systemic circulation. This can result in ascites, which is an accumulation of fluid within the abdominal space. The increased abdominal girth often is associated with hyperventilation (due to irritation of the diaphragm) and consequent respiratory alkalosis. When patients are severely ill with portal hypertension, they may present with gastrointestinal hemorrhage owing to dilated veins or varices, which typically occur in the esophagus or stomach. These dilated vessels represent collateral blood flow around the scarred liver.

Endocrine abnormalities such as increased peripheral formation of estrogen are seen in cirrhosis and may be associated with findings noted in B.C., including gynecomastia (breast enlargement) and softening of the testes. The increased estrogen may be responsible for spider angiomata, the small vessel vasodilation seen in the skin.

Because the liver normally clears many metabolites from the bloodstream, liver disease can result in symptomatic accumulation of those metabolites. The failure of urea cycle enzymes in the liver leads to increased ammonia in the blood. B.C.'s ammonia levels were just above normal, but in extreme cases, ammonia can rise to very high levels. In the central nervous system, this leads to increased formation of glutamate and glutamine in brain cells and disrupted neurotransmission—a condition known as portosystemic encephalopathy or hepatic encephalopathy. The jaundice in B.C., evident in the yellow eyes, is due to accumulation of conjugated bilirubin in the circulation. This is the form of bilirubin that is not bound to albumin and can be filtered by the kidneys and excreted in the urine, usually as a dark pigment. Drugs are also cleared more slowly and some medicines metabolized in the liver to toxic intermediates may worsen liver damage. B.C.'s use of acetaminophen to treat his hangovers actually poses an added danger to his liver function owing to the toxic effect of that drug when combined with alcohol.

Finally, the diet of patients with alcoholic cirrhosis is often poor and leads to characteristic signs and symptoms. B.C.'s anemia may be caused by folate deficiency, and the weight loss may be due to a general decline in caloric intake. Poor diet is compounded by the liver's decreased capacity to conduct gluconeogenesis, which may be reflected in B.C.'s low blood sugar.

TREATMENT AND SUBSEQUENT COURSE

B.C. received I.V. fluid with dextrose and vitamins, and 0.5 L of ascites fluid was drained by paracentesis and sent to the lab. A course of norfloxacin was prescribed. B.C. was prescribed folate pills and referred to an alcohol addiction treatment program. During the first week of treatment at the program, he awoke at night with severe nausea and shakes and he vomited repeatedly. The emesis had a "coffee ground appearance." He suffered variceal hemorrhaging in the ambulance, which was controlled in the emergency room (ER) with balloon tamponade. B.C. was transfused and rehydrated. The varices were surgically sclerosed, and a transhepatic intrajugular portosystemic shunt (TIPS) was placed. He was treated for delirium tremens with I.V. benzodiazepines.

B.C. was able to return to the treatment program, which he completed with a renewed commitment. After 6 months of alcohol-free treatment, he became eligible for liver transplant but was rehospitalized with symptoms of worsening hepatic encephalopathy.

Case Study Questions

1. Why would peripheral estrogen production increase in the context of chronic liver failure? Why would clubbing of the fingers appear in chronic liver failure?

2. Why might the antibiotic norfloxacin have been prescribed? What is spontaneous bacterial peritonitis?

3. What is the significance of "coffee ground emesis"?

4. Why are benzodiazepines useful in the treatment of alcohol withdrawal?

5. How does the TIPS placement relieve pressure on esophageal varices?

Part VIII CASE STUDY FOR ENDOCRINE PHYSIOLOGY

A.D. is a 30-year-old woman who presented with a complaint of infertility.

PRESENTATION: HISTORY AND PHYSICAL EXAM

A.D. was in good health until the birth of her only daughter 5 years ago, when immediately postpartum she developed severe uterine bleeding, followed by a loss of consciousness and a long intensive care unit (ICU) stay. She had developed severe hypoglycemia and hypotension. During the stay in the ICU, she also began to produce large urine volumes, as much as 1 L per hour. Fortunately, she was stabilized and discharged on only a small amount of medication that included desmopressin and hydrocortisone, which she required only briefly.

Over the last several years, she noted menstrual irregularities, notably oligoamenorrhea, and she has been unable to conceive. Her body hair had become scant, and she felt sluggish. Other problems included constipation, a feeling of being cold all the time, and a gain in weight that seemed not to correlate with increased appetite.

On physical exam, A.D. was obese, had a blood pressure of 150/90 mmHg, a regular pulse of 52 beats per minute, and a temperature of 96.8°F. Her skin was coarse, as was her hair, and she had lost the lateral third of her eyebrows. There was no axillary sweat and no axillary or pubic hair. There was no thyroid palpable on her neck exam. The lungs were normal, but the heart sounds were distant. There was no peripheral edema. Her mental status was normal, but her deep tendon reflexes showed a slow relaxation phase. The skin did not show hyperpigmentation.

Discussion

Even before obtaining any labs, it is possible to draw some conclusions about this patient. A.D. has many symptoms of hypothyroidism: sluggishness, cold intolerance, constipation, and weight gain. A small thyroid gland on exam and coarse skin could also be consistent with hypothyroidism and loss of the lateral third of the eyebrows and other body hair is sometimes seen in this condition. Her oligoamenorrhea and difficulty conceiving a child may suggest estrogen deficiency. The regression of secondary sex characteristics (such as pubic hair) could be due to either hypothyroidism or low estrogen or both.

In addition, she has a history of what sounds like diabetes insipidus (lack of antidiuretic hormone [ADH] action) and hypocortisolism. The production of large urine volumes, resolved with administration of desmopressin (exogenous ADH), suggests she has central diabetes insipidus. The hypotension and hypoglycemia, resolved with administration of hydrocortisone, suggest hypocortisolism. (Recall that two critical functions of cortisol are to sustain blood pressure and blood sugar.) Thus, it appears that she has suffered from deficiencies in the products of 3 hypothalamic-pituitary axes and a deficiency in one product of the posterior pituitary—ADH. This implies some pathology in her pituitary gland.

Is it possible that the high intracranial pressures of labor and delivery ruptured a saccular aneurysm or arteriovenous malformation, leading to subarachnoid hemorrhage? And could such bleeding and inflammation—or trans-sphenoidal surgery to control the hemorrhaging—have damaged her pituitary gland? There is also a known pituitary injury associated with childbirth called Sheehan's syndrome. It has become rare in developed countries but remains common in the developing world.

Sheehan's arises because at the time of parturition the pituitary is enlarged owing to hyperplasia of prolactin-secreting lactotrophs—the preparation for suckling. This enlargement renders it vulnerable to insult by low blood flow. If there is massive blood loss due to uterine hemorrhage, the resultant hypotension can actually cut off blood flow to the pituitary and infarct it. Pituitary infarction, also called pituitary apoplexy, can lead to decreased pituitary function, or **hypopituitarism**. In Sheehan's syndrome, the signs of hypopituitarism can present gradually over a period of years, which fits with the time course of presentation seen here. If A.D. has hypopituitarism, lab tests should be able to demonstrate that her thyroid hormone, estrogen, and cortisol deficiencies are due to a lack of pituitary hormones and not to failure of the thyroid gland, ovary, or adrenal.

PRESENTATION: LABORATORY TESTS

Laboratory tests included a urine specific gravity of 1.005, a serum sodium of 143 mEq/L, a serum potassium of 4.2 mEq/L, a random serum glucose of 78 mg/dL, and a low prolactin level. The free thyroxine was low, and thyroid stimulating hormone (TSH) level normal. There was a low estrogen and basal luteinizing hormone (LH) and follicle-stimulating hormone (FSH) levels. In response to a small dose of insulin, the blood sugar fell to 40 mg/dL without increase in growth hormone or cortisol levels. Thyrotropin-releasing hormone was given without an increase in TSH and corticotropin-releasing hormone (CRH) administration was without significant elevation in adrenocorticotropic hormone (ACTH) levels.

Discussion

The labs confirm a low thyroxine and estrogen level and also offer proof that the problem is in the pituitary. If A.D.'s pituitary were functioning normally, a low thyroxine level would disinhibit the pituitary thyrotrophs and would be associated with a high TSH as the pituitary demands more thyroxine from the thyroid gland. Similarly, a low estrogen level disinhibits a normal pituitary, increasing the production of LH and FSH. Basal levels of LH and FSH in the context of low estrogen indicate pituitary failure. Failure of the hypothalamo-pituitary axis counterregulatory hormones (cortisol and growth hormone) to respond to a hypoglycemic challenge suggests dysfunction in these axes. Finally, the pituitary's failure to secrete TSH and ACTH in response to hypothalamic hormones TRH and CRH confirms panhypopituitarism.

In addition to the direct measurements of hormone levels, there are further indirect proofs that the problem is in the pituitary. Recall that the skin showed no hyperpigmentation on physical exam. If the defect were in the adrenal, ACTH secretion would be elevated, and this often manifests as skin hyperpigmentation since pro-opiomelanocortin (POMC), the precursor cleaved to release ACTH, also releases melanocyte-stimulating hormones (MSHs) when it is cleaved. If the defect were in the adrenal, we might also expect aldosterone deficiency, manifested by a high serum potassium. (We would not expect aldosterone deficiency with pituitary pathology because aldosterone is controlled by the renin-angiotensin-aldosterone axis and not by the hypothalamic-pituitary-adrenal axis.) The potassium is within normal limits in this case, indicating intact mineralocorticoid function.

The decreased prolactin level is interesting because hypopituitarism is often seen with an *increased* prolactin level. Prolactinomas are the most common tumor of the pituitary and can lead to hypopituitarism by compression of the pituitary or bleeding; in such a case, prolactin secretion alone might be preserved. Prolactin secretion can also be increased in injuries to the pituitary stalk and hypothalamus because the infundibular dopaminergic neurons normally suppress prolactin secretion. A low prolactin level is more consistent with Sheehan's syndrome than with some of the other etiologies of pituitary dysfunction.

The low-normal urine specific gravity (dilute urine) and high-normal serum sodium concentration (hyperosmolar plasma) suggest A.D. may still have mild ADH deficiency as well, which impairs A.D.'s ability to concentrate the urine and to dilute the plasma. Dilution of the plasma is especially important given that she is likely retaining salt at the kidneys as a compensation for hypoadrenal hypotension.

TREATMENT

A.D. was treated with desmopressin, prednisone, L-thyroxine, and conjugated estrogen/progesterone. Her symptoms began to resolve, and her endocrinologists followed her closely in order to titrate her complex and long-term drug regimen to her particular needs.

Case Study Questions

1. Hormone replacement therapy cannot mimic physiologic perfectly. What adjustments to her usual dosing might be necessary in the context of an infection?

2. Why might A.D.'s temperature be low?

3. Given A.D.'s hypocortisolism, we might expect her to have hypotension. Why might her blood pressure be high?

4. What is the reason for A.D.'s bradycardia (pulse of 52 beats per minute)?

Credits

FIGURE CREDITS

1.2   Based on Vander A, Sherman J, Luciano D. Human Physiology: The Mechanisms of Body Function, 2nd ed. Philadelphia: WB Saunders, 1975.

B1.1   Based on Lilly LS. Pathophysiology of Heart Disease, 2nd ed. Baltimore: Williams & Wilkins, 1998. Figure 9.9

2.2   Based on Alberts B, Johnson A, Lewis J, et al. Molecular Biology of the Cell, 4th ed. New York: Garland Science, 2002. Figure 10-10

2.4   Based on Alberts B, Johnson A, Lewis J, et al. Molecular Biology of the Cell, 4th ed. New York: Garland Science, 2002. Figure 10-17

2.10   Based on Alberts B, Johnson A, Lewis J, et al. Molecular Biology of the Cell, 4th ed. New York: Garland Science, 2002. Figure 11-13

2.11   Based on Alberts B, Johnson A, Lewis J, et al. Molecular Biology of the Cell, 4th ed. New York: Garland Science, 2002. Figure 11-9

4.7   Based on Alberts B, Johnson A, Lewis J, et al. Molecular Biology of the Cell, 4th ed. New York: Garland Science, 2002. Figure 15-36

5.4   Based on Kandel, ER, Schwartz, JH, Jessell, TM. Principles of Neural Science, 4th ed. New York: McGraw-Hill, 2000. Figure 8-6

5.5   Based on Kandel, ER, Schwartz, JH, Jessell, TM. Principles of Neural Science, 4th ed. New York: McGraw-Hill, 2000. Figure 9-9

5.6   Based on Kandel, ER, Schwartz, JH, Jessell, TM. Principles of Neural Science, 4th ed. New York: McGraw-Hill, 2000. Figure 9-10

5.7   Based on Kandel, ER, Schwartz, JH, Jessell, TM. Principles of Neural Science, 4th ed. New York: McGraw-Hill, 2000. Figure 8-8

5.10   Based on Rhoades RA, Tanner GA. Medical Physiology. Boston: Little, Brown, 1995. Figure 6-1

6.8   Based on Junqueira JL, Carneiro J, Kelley, RO. Basic Histology, 7th ed. Norwalk, CT: Appleton and Lange, 1992. Figure 10-6

6.11B   Photo from Ross MH, Kay GI, Pawlina W. Histology: A Text and Atlas, 4th ed. Baltimore: Lippincott Williams & Wilkins, 2003. Original slide specimen courtesy of Scott Ballinger.

6.12   Based on Berne RM, Levy MN. Physiology, 3rd ed. St. Louis: Mosby-Year Book, 1993. Figure 18-6

6.13   Based on Berne RM, Levy MN. Physiology, 3rd ed. St. Louis: Mosby-Year Book, 1993. Figure 17-8

7.1A   Based on Junqueira, JL, Carneiro, J, Kelley, RO. Basic Histology, 7th ed. Norwalk, CT: Appleton and Lange, 1992. Figure 11-1

7.1B   Based on Junqueira, JL, Carneiro, J, Kelley, RO. Basic Histology, 7th ed. Norwalk, CT: Appleton and Lange, 1992. Figure 11-12

7.2   Based on Junqueira, JL, Carneiro, J, Kelley, RO. Basic Histology, 7th ed. Norwalk, CT: Appleton and Lange, 1992. Figure 17-7

7.3   Based on Junqueira, JL, Carneiro, J, Kelley, RO. Basic Histology, 7th ed. Norwalk, CT: Appleton and Lange, 1992. Figure 15-1

7.4A   Based on Junqueira, JL, Carneiro, J, Kelley, RO. Basic Histology, 7th ed. Norwalk, CT: Appleton and Lange, 1992. Figure 10-21

7.4B   Photo from Ross MH, Kay GI, Pawlina W. Histology: A Text and Atlas, 4th ed. Baltimore: Lippincott Williams & Wilkins, 2003.

7.4C   Photo from Ross MH, Kay GI, Pawlina W. Histology: A Text and Atlas, 4th ed. Baltimore: Lippincott Williams & Wilkins, 2003.

7.14A-C Based on Rhoades RA, Tanner, GA. Medical Physiology. Boston: Little, Brown, 1995. Figure 9-20A-C

7.14D   Based on Rhoades RA, Tanner, GA. Medical Physiology. Boston: Little, Brown, 1995. Figure 9-21

7.14E   Based on Johnson, LR. Essential Medical Physiology. New York: Raven Press, 1992. Figure 9-11

7.15A-C   Based on Cotran, RS, Kumar, V, Robbins, SL. Robbins Pathologic Basis of Disease, 5th ed. Philadelphia: WB Saunders, 1994. Figure 11-11A,D, and E

8.1   Based on Netter FH (ed). The CIBA Collection of Medical Illustrations. Vol. 8: Musculoskeletal System, Part I. Anatomy, Physiology and Metabolic Disorders. Summit: New Jersey: CIBA-Geigy Corp., 1987. Plate 20

8.2   Based on Netter FH (ed). The CIBA Collection of Medical Illustrations. Vol. 8: Musculoskeletal System, Part I. Anatomy, Physiology and Metabolic Disorders. Summit: New Jersey: CIBA-Geigy Corp., 1987. Plate 24

8.5   Based on Netter FH (ed). The CIBA Collection of Medical Illustrations. Vol. 8: Musculoskeletal System, Part I. Anatomy, Physiology and Metabolic Disorders. Summit: New Jersey: CIBA-Geigy Corp., 1987. Plate 36

9.2   Photo from Gartner LP, Hiatt JL. Color Atlas of Histology, 4th ed. Baltimore: Lippincott Williams & Wilkins, 2006.

9.3   Photo from Ross MH, Kay GI, Pawlina W. Histology: A Text and Atlas, 4th ed. Baltimore: Lippincott Williams & Wilkins, 2003.

9.4   Photos from Gartner LP, Hiatt JL. Color Atlas of Histology, 4th ed. Baltimore: Lippincott Williams & Wilkins, 2006.

9.8   Photo from McClatchey KD. Clinical Laboratory Medicine, 2nd ed. Philadelphia: Lippincott Williams & Wilkins, 2002.

10.2   Photo from Ross MH, Kay GI, Pawlina W. Histology: A Text and Atlas, 4th ed. Baltimore: Lippincott Williams & Wilkins, 2003.

10.3   Photo from Ross MH, Kay GI, Pawlina W. Histology: A Text and Atlas, 4th ed. Baltimore: Lippincott Williams & Wilkins, 2003.

10.4   Based on Cotran, RS, Kumar, V, Robbins, SL. Robbins Pathologic Basis of Disease, 5th ed. W.B. Philadelphia: WB Saunders, 1994. Figure 4-12

10.8   Photo from Berne RM, Levy MN, Koeppen BM, et al. Physiology, 5th ed. St Louis: Mosby, 2004.

10.9   Based on Gartner LP, Hiatt JL. Color Atlas of Histology, 3rd ed. Baltimore: Lippincott Williams & Wilkins, 2000.

11.3   Photo from Ross MH, Kay GI, Pawlina W. Histology: A Text and Atlas, 4th ed. Baltimore: Lippincott Williams & Wilkins, 2003.

11.5   Based on Berne RM, Levy MN. Physiology, 3rd ed. St. Louis: Mosby-Year Book, 1993. Figure 28-7

11.6   Based on Olszewski WL, Engeset, A. Immune proteins, enzymes and electrolytes in human peripheral lymph. Lymphology. 1978 11:156–164.

14.4   Based on Schnapp B. "Cardiac Electrophysiology" lecture, Harvard Medical School, November 29, 1994.

14.8   Based on Lilly, LS. Pathophysiology of Heart Disease, 2nd ed. Baltimore: Williams & Wilkins, 1998. Figure 4-27

15.1   Based on Vander A, Sherman J, Luciano D. Human Physiology: The Mechanisms of Body Function, 7th ed. Boston: WCB-McGraw Hill, 1998. Figure 14-67

15.2   Based on Guyton AC, Hall JE. Textbook of Medical Physiology, 9th ed. Philadelphia: Harcourt Health Sciences, 1996. Figure 84-10

15.3   Based on Vander A, Sherman J, Luciano D. Human Physiology: The Mechanisms of Body Function, 7th ed. Boston: WCB-McGraw Hill, 1998. Figure 15-37

15.4   Based on Vander A, Sherman J, Luciano D. Human Physiology: The Mechanisms of Body Function, 7th ed. Boston: WCB-McGraw Hill, 1998. Figure 15-35

17.1   Photo from Ross MH, Kay GI, Pawlina W. Histology: A Text and Atlas, 4th ed. Baltimore: Lippincott Williams & Wilkins, 2003.

17.2   Photo from Ross MH, Kay GI, Pawlina W. Histology: A Text and Atlas, 4th ed. Baltimore: Lippincott Williams & Wilkins, 2003.

19.6   Based on Bullock J, Boyle J, Wang MB. Physiology, 2nd ed. Baltimore: Williams & Wilkins, 1991

19.9   Based on West JB (ed). Best and Taylor's Physiologic Basis of Medical Practice, 12th ed. Baltimore: Williams & Wilkins, 1990. Figure 5.83

20.14   Based on West JB (ed). Best and Taylor's Physiologic Basis of Medical Practice, 12th ed. Baltimore: Williams & Wilkins, 1990. Figure 4.14

27.16   Ganong, WF. Review of Medical Physiology, 20th ed. New York: McGraw Hill, 2001. Figure 17-29

27.19   Based on Champe PC, Harvey RA. Biochemistry, 2nd ed. Philadelphia: Lippincott, 1994. Figure 20.9

28.1   Based on Wood JD. Physiology of the enteric nervous system. In LR Johnson (ed). Physiology of the Gastrointestinal Tract. New York: Raven, 1971.

28.3   Based on Wood JD. Physiology of the enteric nervous system. In LR Johnson (ed). Physiology of the Gastrointestinal Tract. New York: Raven, 1971.

28.6   Based on Jacobson ED, Levine JS. Clinical GI Physiology for the Exam Taker. Philadelphia: WB Saunders, 1994.

29.2   Based on Grant DM. Detoxification pathways in the liver. J Inherit Metab Dis. 1991;14:421–430.

29.3   Based on Champe PC, Harvey RA. Biochemistry, 2nd ed. Philadelphia: Lippincott, 1994. Figure 23.6

29.4   Based on Champe PC, Harvey RA. Biochemistry, 2nd ed. Philadelphia: Lippincott, 1994. Figure 23.7

31.4   Based on Champe PC, Harvey RA. Biochemistry, 2nd ed. Philadelphia: Lippincott, 1994. Figure 25.7

31.5   Based on Champe PC, Harvey RA. Biochemistry, 2nd ed. Philadelphia: Lippincott, 1994. Figure 26.8

31.8   Based on Champe PC, Harvey RA. Biochemistry, 2nd ed. Philadelphia: Lippincott, 1994. Figure 7.3

31.11   Based on Champe PC, Harvey RA. Biochemistry, 2nd ed. Philadelphia: Lippincott, 1994. Figure 17.23

31.12   Based on Atkinson MA, Eisenbarth GS. Type I diabetes: new perspectives on disease pathogenesis and treatment. Lancet. 2001 Jul 21;358(9277):255.

32.3   Based on Vance ML. Hypopituitarism. N Engl J Med. 1994;330:1651–1662. Figure 1

32.4   Based on Goodman MH. Basic Medical Endocrinology, 2nd ed. New York: Raven, 1994.

33.2   Based on Burkitt HG, Young B, Heath JW. Wheater's Functional Histology: A Text and Color Atlas, 3rd ed. New York: Churchill Livingstone, 1993. Figure 17.7a

34.3   Based on Breslow MJ. Regulation of adrenal medullary and cortical blood flow. Am J Phys. 1992;262:H1317–H1330. Figure 1

35.3   Based on Favus MJ (ed). Primer on the Metabolic Bone Diseases and Disorders of Mineral Metabolism. Philadelphia: Lippincott-Raven, 1996.

35.4   Based on Conlin PR, Fajtova VT, Mortensen RM, et al. Hysteresis in the relationship between serum ionized calcium and intact parathyroid hormone during recovery from induced hyper and hypocalcemia in normal humans. J Clin Endocrinol Metab. 1989;69:593.

35.7   Based on Berne RM, Levy MN. Physiology, 3rd ed. St. Louis: Mosby-Year Book, 1993.

36.4   Based on Berne RM, Levy MN. Physiology, 3rd ed. St. Louis: St. Louis: Mosby-Year Book, 1993.

TABLE CREDITS

5.1   From Hardman JG, Limbird LE, Gilman AG. Goodman & Gilman's The Pharmacological Basis of Therapeutics, 10th ed. New York: McGraw-Hill, 2001.

20.1   Adapted and reprinted with permission from Pitts RF. *Physiology* of the Kidney and Body Fluids, 3rd ed. Chicago: Year Book Medical Publishers, 1974.

21.1   Adapted and reprinted with permission from Brenner BM, Mackenzie HS. Disturbances of Renal Function. In: Fauci AS, et al., eds. Harrison's Principles of Internal Medicine, 14th ed. New York: McGraw-Hill, 1998. Esson ML, Schrier RW. Diagnosis and treatment of acute tubular necrosis. Ann Intern Med. 2002;137:744–752.

23.1   Adapted from Rose BD, Post TW. Clinical Physiology of Acid-Base and Electrolyte Disorders, 5th ed. New York: McGraw-Hill, 2001, Table 9-1, and Smith HW. From Fish to Philosopher. Garden City: Doubleday, 1961.

25.1   Adapted and reprinted with permission from Rose, BD, Rennke HG. Renal Pathophysiology—The Essentials. Baltimore: Williams and Wilkins, 1994.

30.1   From the celiac disease web site. 2005. Available at: http://www.celiac.com. Accessed July 14, 2005.

Note: Page numbers followed by *b* indicate boxed material
Page numbers followed by *f* indicate a figure
Page numbers followed by *t* indicate a table